Tropical Viral Diseases Of Large Domestic Animals- Part 1.

Advances in Medical & Veterinary Virology,
Immunology, and Epidemiology- Vol. 7.

Series Editor: Thankam Mathew

Tropical Viral Diseases of Large Domestic Animals- Part 1.

Editor:
Thankam Mathew

Series Editor: Thankam Mathew
31. Glenview Dr.
West Orange
NJ 07052 USA

E mail:thajema@aol.com
Tel:973-731-6209
Fax:973-731-6209

Library of Congress Control Number: 2009909777
ISBN: Hardcover   978-1-4415-8160-0
               Softcover   978-1-4415-8159-4

Notice to the Reader

Publisher: Thajema Publishers
Executive Editor: Dr. Thankam Mathew
Developmental Editor: Dr. Taji Susan Abraham
Project Editor: Dr. Tripthi Mary Mathew
© 2010 Thajema Publishers
Total Pages 785
For information, contact

Thajema Publishers
31 Glenview Drive,
West Orange, NJ 07052-1010, USA
Tel/Fax: 973-731-6209
E-mail: *Thajema@aol.com*

Printed in the United States of America at Xlibris Corporation, 1663 Liberty Drive, Suite 200, Bloomington, IN 47403: Tel: 888-795-4274, Ext. 7420; Fax: 610-915-0294.

The book includes bibliographical references and index.

Cover illustration is provided by Dr. Thankam Mathew; one of her passions is embroidery. Shown here are the large animals susceptible for the tropical viruses drawn by her and stitched by Dr. Thankam Mathew herself.

To order additional copies of this book, contact:
Xlibris Corporation
1-888-795-4274
www.Xlibris.com
Orders@Xlibris.com
E-mail: *Thajema@aol.com*
58163

DEDICATIONS

To My Teachers

My teachers who always encouraged me, especially Dr. S. S. Rao, who was my PhD guide; Dr. K. P. C. Nair, professor of pathology; late Dr. U. K. Menon, professor of microbiology; late Dr. V. S. Alwar, professor of parasitology; late Dr. M. N. Menon, professor of surgery; and Dean of Kerala, Veterinary College and Animal Husbandry commissioner, government of India.

To My Late Parents and Late Brothers

My father, Mr. P. P. Devassy, Puzhaken master; my mother, Mrs. Mary K. Kattikaren; my brothers Prof. Francis Thekkinyath and Mr. Paul John Thekkinyath; and my loving sister-in-law, late Mrs. Thresiamma Francis (Mini), who all helped me and encouraged me to advance in my professional carrier.

To My Late In-laws

My late in-laws, Mr. C. J. Zachariah and Mrs. Susan Zachariah, who encouraged me to pursue in my research and teaching career after my marriage.

To My Late Aunts and Uncles

Late Mrs. Thelma Domnic and my late uncle Mr. Domnic, who all encouraged me in my studies while I was studying for my masters MVSc. in Madras; and Mr. Thariath Kattikaren to get admission in Maharajas College; Ernakulam and Aunt, Mrs. Thankamma Thariath, with them I stayed and studied for my BSc.

To My Family

My dear husband, Dr. Zachariah Mathew; my son-in-law, Mr. Bijou Thomas Abraham; and my three daughters, Dr. Taji Susan Abraham, Dr. Tripthi M. Mathew, and Dr. Trini Ann Mathew, who all encouraged me to establish my Thajema Publishing Co. to come up and publish this seventh series of the book.

Acknowledgment

I, Dr. Thankam Mathew, editor of the book, is thankful to all the authors of the book *Tropical Viral Diseases of Large Domestic Animals Part 1*. I am also thankful to my husband, Dr. Zachariah Mathew, for his encouragement and support and also contribution on some disease topics. Heartfelt thanks to my daughter, namely, Dr. Taji Susan Abraham, for all the support. Thanks are also due to Xlibris press for printing and publishing the book after proofreading, indexing, book review, marketing, and also printing on demand. Last but not the least, I want to thank God the Almighty, who provided me the talent to edit, make the cover page by embroidery, publish the book, and who gave me good health to complete the book.

Preface

After releasing the book *Modern Concepts of Immunology in Veterinary Science, Poultry Immunology* in 2002, I was planning to write the *Tropical Viral Diseases of Large Domestic Animals* as part 1 and *Tropical Viral Diseases of Aves* as part 2. Meanwhile, I could publish three books more. As I have pointed out earlier, there is a time for any or all planned events, God's time. God's time has come only now, and I got various authors from tropical countries to write the various tropical viral diseases of large animals, namely, equines as section 1, bovines and ovines as section 2, swines as section 3, and camels as section 4. I thank God for answering my prayers and helping me to materialize the long-planned task of publishing this book.

Dr. Thankam Mathew
Managing Director
Thajema Publishers
31 Glenview Dr.
West Orange, NJ 07052, USA
December 27, 2008

About the Editor

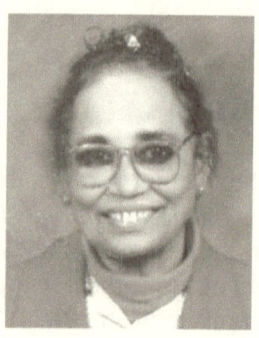

Dr. Thankam Mathew BSc, BVSc, MVSc, PhD, FISCD
Consultant Technomark and Managing Director
Thajema Publishers
31 Glenview Dr.
West Orange, NJ 07052, USA.
Tel./Fax: 973-731-6209
E-mail: <Thajema@aol.com>

Dr. Thankam Mathew was born in Ernakulam, state of Kerala, India. She passed the SSLC from St. Antony's High School, Pudukad, and graduated her bachelor of science, BSc, in botany (because of that, she is interested in herbs and spices) from Maharajas College, Ernakulam. Her love and affection for the dumb and suffering animals attracted her to study veterinary science and took her bachelor's degree (BVSc) from Madras Veterinary College in 1958, with high credits and awards. She later became a lecturer at Kerala Veterinary College in Mannuthy, Trichur, as the first lady veterinarian to work in the state of Kerala. She took her postgraduate degree in microbiology and immunology from Madras Veterinary College in 1962. ICAR awarded her a senior research fellowship in the subject of virology, leading to her PhD degree in 1967. She was the recipient of the Diamond Jubilee Postdoctoral Fellowship of Haffkine Institute in Bombay, where she received her PhD, and also worked as a CSIR pool officer (scientist). She had the assignment till 1971, working on antilymphocyte serum as an immune suppressor and also on some immune enhancers. Since then, she had worked as a senior research officer of the Indian Council of Medical Research (ICMR) virus unit, at Stanley Medical College, Madras, and the National Institute of Communicable Disease, Delhi, until 1979. Later, she worked as the principal scientific officer and head of the Veterinary Public Health Laboratory, Federal Livestock Department, Kaduna, Nigeria, until 1983. After her return from Nigeria, she took up the senior research associate fellowship of the ICMR and worked on "Basic Research on the Pathogenic Mechanism of Diarrhea by Different Bacterial Agents and Genetic Studies on Enterogenic Plasmids, Etc." at Maulana Azad Medical College, New Delhi, until October 31, 1984.

Later, she established a diagnostic laboratory, Thankam Laboratories, for diseases diagnosis of human, animal, and poultry, and she worked as director of the laboratory until 1993 when she migrated to the USA. While working in the laboratory, she also worked as managing director of Thajema Publishers and published two books and the *Bulletin of Indian Association of Lady Veterinarians*. After coming to the USA as a permanent resident, she worked as manager of the Quality Control Laboratory at IGI Inc., Vineland, for poultry vaccine production.

Later, she concentrated on book-publishing work, established Thajema Publishing, and continued the series publication of the book *Advances in Medical and Veterinary Virology, Immunology, and Epidemiology*. She already published six series of the books, and the seventh series, *Tropical Viral Diseases of Large Domestic Animals*, is publishing now.

She has ninety-three scientific papers and a few scientific booklets to her credit in addition to the six books published in 1987, 1993, 2002, 2004, 2005, and 2006. Dr. T. Mathew had various awards from universities and from different associations for her credits in various subjects and activities. She has also presented scientific papers and posters during the various national and international conferences in India, Nigeria, Germany, USA, Australia, France, Canada, and Brazil. She is the founder secretary and was president of the Indian Association of Lady Veterinarians and a member of World Women Veterinarians. She is also a member of various international organizations. With her talent in cross-stitching and embroidery work, she has designed the cover pages of the books, including this book.

TROPICAL VIRAL DISEASES OF LARGE DOMESTIC ANIMALS-PART 1.

AUTHORS' NAMES AND DESIGNATIONS

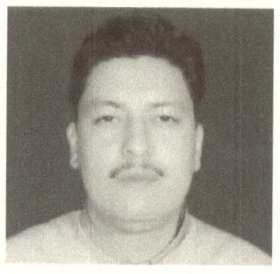

Dr. P. Bhatt, BVSc, MVSc
Assistant Professor
Dept. of Veterinary Clinics
College of Veterinary Sciences
GB Pant University of Agriculture
and Technology
Pantnagar 263145
Uttaranchal, India

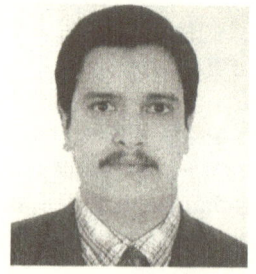

Dr. P. K. Dash, BVSc and AH, MVSc,
PhD Scientist, C.
Division of Virology
Defence R & D Establishment,
Indian Veterinary Research Institute (IVRI)
Jhansi Road, Gwalior 474002 (MP)
India

No Photo
Provided

Dr. R. S. Chauhan, BVSc and AH,
MVSc, PhD
FNAVS, FSIIP, FIAVP
Joint Director
Center for Animal Disease Research
and Diagnosis
Indian Veterinary Research Institute (IVRI)
Izatnagar, Bareilly (UP) 243122, India

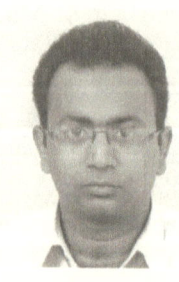

Dr. D. K. Gupta, MVSc
Assistant Scientist
Dept. of Clinical Veterinary Medicine
Ethics and Jurisprudence
GADVASU, Ludhiana, Punjab, India

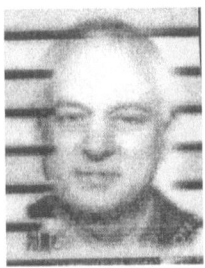

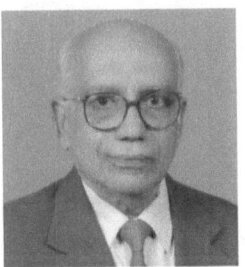

**No Photo
Provided**

**Dr. Prof. E. Gruys, DVM, PhD, Reg.Vet.
Pathol., RNVA, and ECVP
Em. Prof. Vet. Pathol.** (Utrecht 1981–2006)
Dept of Pathobiology
Faculty of Veterinary Medicine
Utrecht University, Utrecht, the Netherlands
Present Affiliation: Veterinary
Extension Services
3971HJ-9, Driebergen
The Netherlands

**Dr. H. Kothalawala, BVSc
(Sri Lanka)
Dip Path. (Osaka), MVSc Utrecht**
Veterinary Research Officer
Veterinary Research Institute
Peradeniya, Sri Lanka

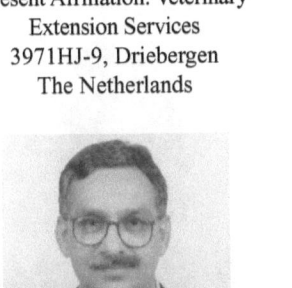

**Dr. S. Kapoor, BVSc, MVSc,
PhD Professor**
Dept. of Veterinary Microbiology
College of Veterinary Science
Chaudhary Charan Singh-Haryana
Agricultural University
CCS-HAU, Hisar 125004, India

**Dr. Prof. M. Krishnan Nair, BVSc,
MVSc, PhD
FRVCS, FNAVSc
Former Dean and Director, Prof. and
Head Dept of Pathology**
College of Veterinary and Animal Sciences
Kerala Agricultural University
Mannuthy, Thrissur, Kerala, India 680651

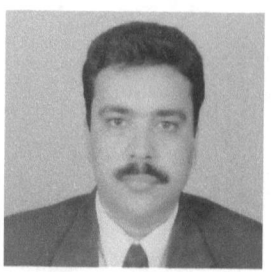

Dr. Kuldeep Dhama, BVSc, MVSc, PhD
Senior Scientist
Division of Pathology
Indian Veterinary Research Institute (IVRI)
Izatnagar, Bareilly (UP) 243122, India

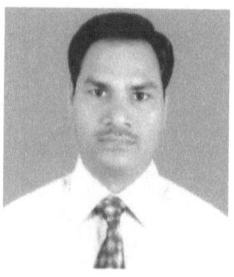

Dr. R. V. S. Pawaiya, BVSc and AH,
MVSc, PhD
Senior Scientist
Division of Pathology
Indian Veterinary Research Institute (IVRI)
Izatnagar, Bareilly (UP) 243122, India

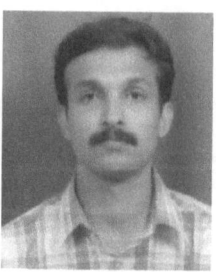

Dr. M. Mahendran, BVSc and AH,
MVSc, PhD
Veterinary Officer
Animal Husbandry Dept.
Gov't of Kerala,
Manjadi, Thiruvalla
Kerala State, India

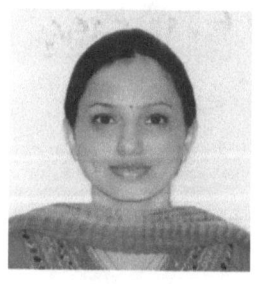

Dr. Rinku Sharma, BVSc and AH, MVSc,
PhD Scientist
Referral Veterinary Polyclinic
Indian Veterinary Research Institute (IVRI)
Izatnagar, Bareilly (UP) 243122, India

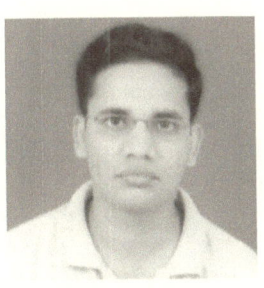

Dr. D. Nandi, BVSc and AH, MVSc, PhD
Doctoral Research Fellow
CSM Laboratory
Division of Medicine
Indian Veterinary Research Institute (IVRI)
Izatnagar, Bareilly (UP) 243122, India

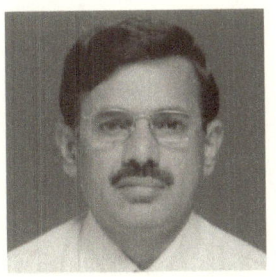

Dr. Prof. M. R. Saseendranath, BVSc and
AH, MVSc, PhD, FNASc
Professor and Head
Dept of Veterinary Epidemiology and
Preventive Medicine
College of Veterinary and Animal Sciences
Mannuthy
Thrissur, Kerala, India, 680651

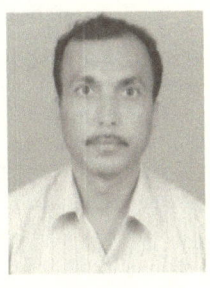

Dr. S. Nandi, BV Sc and AH, MVSc, PhD
Senior Scientist
Molecular Virology Laboratory
Center for Animal Disease Research and
Diagnosis
Indian Veterinary Research Institute (IVRI)
Izatnagar, Bareilly (UP) 243122, India

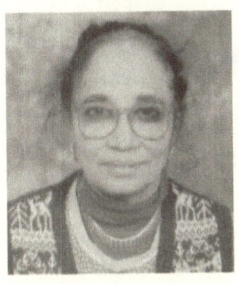

Dr. Thankam Mathew, BSc, BVSc, MVSc,
PhD, FISCD
Consultant, Technomark
Managing Director
Thajema Publishers
31 Glenview Dr.
West Orange, NJ 07052, USA

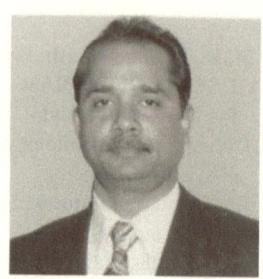

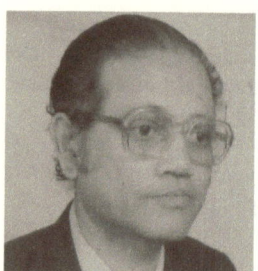

Dr. G. Saikumar, BVSc and AH, MVSc, PhD
Senior Scientist
I/C Swine Disease Laboratory
Division of Pathology
Indian Veterinary Research Institute (IVRI)
Izatnagar, Bareilly (UP) 243122, India

Dr. Z. Mathew, BVSc, MVSc, PhD,
MAMS
Ret. Scientist
Consultant, Technomark
31 Glen View Dr.,
West Orange, NJ 07052, USA

TROPICAL VIRAL DISEASES OF LARGE DOMESTIC ANIMALS- PART I.

TABLE OF CONTENTS

SECTION A

LIST OF EQUINE TROPICAL VIRAL DISEASES

SECTION B

List of Bovine and Ovine Tropical Viral Diseases

SECTION C

LIST OF SWINE TROPICAL VIRAL DISEASES

SECTION D

LIST OF TROPICAL VIRAL DISEASES OF CAMELS
R. S. Chawan, K. Dhama, and M. Mahendran

INTRODUCTION

OTHER VIRAL DISEASES OF CAMEL

SECTION A

LIST OF EQUINE TROPICAL VIRAL DISEASES

1. African Horse Sickness
(Perdesiekte, Pestis Equorum, La Peste Equina)

K. Dhama, R. V. S. Pawaiya, P. Bhatt, and S. Kapoor

Introduction

African horse sickness (AHS) is a highly fatal and infectious disease of horses and mules and generally a subclinical disease in other Equidae like donkeys and zebra. It is an insect-borne disease caused by African horse sickness virus (AHSV). Various forms of the disease—viz, acute, subacute, and mild forms—have been reported (Radostits et al., 2000), and 90% of the immunologically naive animals die of the disease (Guthrie, 2007). It presents a potential threat to the horse industry, especially in countries of the Western world. The effects of the disease, particularly in susceptible populations of horses, can be devastating, and mortality rates for this species may exceed 90% (Mellor and Hamblin, 2004). AHS has been allocated by the OIE (Office International des Epizooties) a list A status as a consequence of its severity and ability to expand rapidly without apparent warning in endemic areas. AHSV is reported to be enzootic in most of Africa and occasionally spread to other areas with devastating effects on the susceptible equine population. The disease is capable of persisting anywhere in the world when the climatic conditions favor the multiplication of the vector and its survival during the winter months. Epidemics have been reported in the Middle East, Asia, and the Mediterranean countries, including Spain, Portugal, and Morocco (Higgins and Snyder, 2006). Global warming could increase the risk for spread of arthropod-borne diseases such as AHS. AHS does not affect human although it has a significant impact of international trade in live Equidae and their products.

In horses, AHS is characterized by clinical signs, which develop as a result of damage to the circulatory and respiratory systems giving rise to serous effusion and hemorrhage in various organs and tissues. On the basis of extent and severity of the clinicopathological findings, the disease has been classified into four forms. In ascending order of severity, these are horse sickness fever (which usually affects only mules, donkeys, and partially immune horses), the subacute or cardiac form, the cardiopulmonary or mixed form, and the peracute or pulmonary form. All the forms of disease can be observed in any one outbreak, but in susceptible populations of horses, the mixed and pulmonary forms predominate, leading to a very high mortality. The clinical signs and lesions of the disease are the result of selective increase in vascular permeability, leading to impairment of the respiratory and circulatory systems. Clinical signs of the disease in natural infection and experimental study have been reported by many workers (Theiler, 1921;

Maurer and Mc Cully, 1963; Awad et al., 1981a; Newsholme et al., 1983; Lubroth, 1988; Crafford et al., 2003; Guthrie, 2007).

HISTORICAL ASPECT OF THE DISEASE

Moule (1896) reported the first epidemic of AHS in the Yemen in 1327, suggesting ancient history of the disease. It was believed that the virus originated in Africa and was first recognized there when horses were first introduced during the exploration of Central and East Africa (Theal, 1899). Father Monclaro's report of travels of Francisco Boro in East Africa in 1569 also reported AHS in horses imported from India (Henning, 1956, and Theiler, 1921). In South Africa, the virus was recognized after the first introduction of horses in 1657, the first major outbreak of the disease occurring in 1719 when over 1,700 animals died (Henning, 1956). Subsequently at least ten major and several lesser outbreaks of AHS have been recorded in Southern Africa, the largest being in South Africa in 1854–1855 when over seventy thousand horses died (Barnard, 1998; Coetzer and Erasmus, 1994a). Several losses due to AHS have been reported in 1780, 1801, 1839, 1855, 1862, 1891, 1914, 1918, 1923, 1940, 1946, and 1956 (Henning, 1956). The most recent outbreaks outside of the endemic area were in Spain, Morocco, and Portugal between 1987 and 1990 (House, 1993). The disease was earlier confused with anthrax and piroplasmosis, but in early 1900s, viral etiology of the disease was confirmed by many workers, including M'Fadyean (M'Fadyean, 1900, and Guthrie, 2007). Later in 1908, Sir Theiler Arnold revealed the plurality of immunologically distinct strains of AHSV, which did not always afford protection against infection by heterologous strains (Theiler, 1905, 1907, 1908a, b, 1921). It was demonstrated that viscerotropic isolates of AHSV became neurotropic without losing their immunogenecity after several intracerebral passages in mice (Alexander, 1933 and 1935). As a result of this finding, the first polyvalent vaccine against AHS was developed in the 1930s (Alexander and Du Toit, 1934; Alexander, 1936). In 1903, Pitchford and Theiler proposed the transmission of disease by biting insects, which was later confirmed by Du Toit in 1944, who suggested *Culicoides* species to be the vector of both AHS and bluetongue. As a result of decrease in the horse and zebra populations and the introduction of AHS vaccines, the frequency, extent, and severity of the disease has declined significantly over the last century in South Africa (Mellor and Hamblin, 2004). AHS is an important disease to be considered with international movement of equids, but appropriate quarantine and testing procedures can safely accomplish the movement (EC, 1997; OIE, 2000).

ETIOLOGY

The etiological agent of AHS is a typical *Orbivirus* of Reoviridae family. The virion is composed of a double-layered protein shell and is morphologically similar to bluetongue virus (BTV) of ruminants and equine encephalosis virus (EEV) (Verwoerd et al., 1979; Stanley, 1981; Sellers and Mellor, 1993; Radostits et al., 2000). The virus is present in the blood and certain organs—such as spleen, lung, and lymph nodes—in reasonably high concentration, whereas only traces are found in serum, tissue fluids, excretions, and secretions (Erasmus, 1972). At present, nine antigenic strains of the virus are known to exist and up to forty-two are suspected. The viruses can be grown in tissue culture, chick embryo, and the brains of mice (Radostits et al., 2000). The virion is an unenveloped particle composed of double-stranded RNA about 68–70 nm in diameter and is made up of a two-layered icosahedral capsid composed of thirty-two capsomers (Coetzer and Erasmus, 1994a) and ten double-stranded RNA segments in the genome (Grubman and Lewis, 1992), which encode seven structural proteins (VP1-7), most of which have been completely sequenced for AHSV serotypes 4, 6, and 9 and four nonstructural proteins (NS1, NS2, NS3, NS3A). The genome comprises of two major proteins, VP3 and 7, and three minor proteins, VP 1, 4, and 6 (Bremer et al., 1990; Roy et al., 1991; Patakakis, 2003). Together they make up the group specific epitopes (Hewat et al., 1992; Prasad et al., 1992; Grimes et al., 1995). The core particle is surrounded by the outer capsid composed of two proteins, VP2 and 5. VP2 protein is mostly responsible for antigenic variation (Burrage et al., 1993; Vreede and Huismans, 1994; Martinez Torrecuadrada and Casal, 1995). It was demonstrated that AHSV VP2 alone is sufficient to induce a protective immune response in horses and indicate the usefulness of ELISA-reactive antibodies for differentiation of vaccinated and naturally exposed horses (*Stone-Marschat* et al., 1996).

Nine antigenically distinct serotypes have been identified (Howell, 1962) with relatedness between the serotypes, especially AHSV types 1 and 2, 3 and 7, 5 and 8, and 6 and 9, although there is no evidence from the field that there is any intratypic variation (Coetzer and Erasmus, 1994a). Of the nine serotypes, types 1 to 8 are typically found only in restricted areas of sub-Saharan Africa while type 9 is more widespread (Mellor and Hamblin, 2004). The AHS virus is relatively heat stable and can be stored for at least six months at 4°C in saline containing 10% serum. Blood in OCG as preservative can remain infective for more than twenty years, and lyophilization may preserve infectivity for as long as forty years. The virus is readily inactivated at pH values lower than 6.3, but it is relatively stable between values ranging from 6.5–8.5. The viruses can be grown in tissue culture, chick embryo, and the brains of mice (Radostits et al., 1995). Viremia generally lasts for about four to eight days and roughly parallels the febrile reaction. In exceptional cases, viremia may last as long as seventeen days in the horse and twenty-eight days in zebra and donkeys (Erasmus, 1972).

Animals that recover from the disease develop a solid lifelong immunity against the infecting virus and a partial immunity against heterologous serotypes. Horses which recover from AHS exhibit solid humoral immunity against homologous challenge. Protective antibodies appear to be directed toward neutralizing epitopes on AHS virus VP2 (Burrage and Laegreid, 1994). Foals from immune dams have a passive immunity that may protect them for up to six months.

HOST SUSCEPTIBILITY

Zebras for long have been considered the natural vertebrate host and reservoir of AHSV, rarely exhibiting the clinical signs of infection. All other equid species and crossbreeds are also susceptible to infection, but the high mortality rates are frequently recorded in horses and occasionally in mules (Mellor and Hamblin, 2004). The horse is extremely susceptible with a mortality of more than 95% in epizootic and a morbidity of 85% (Rafyi, 1961). The mule is less susceptible with 50% morbidity during epizotics. The South African donkey (*Equus asinus somalicus*) is resistant (Theiler, 1921). The zebra (*E. burchelli*) may show a clinically evident disease (Howell, 1964). Dogs are susceptible to experimental infection with AHSV (Theller, 1906) and may die from the effects of the virus. Infection also occurs readily following ingestion of infected horse meat (Theiler, 1910; Bevan, 1911 and Van Rensburg et al., 1981). It is believed that dogs do not play a role in the spread or maintenance of AHSV due to low-level and transient viremia and as vector insects are rarely attracted to them (McIntosh, 1955). Camels can ostensibly become inapparently infected with AHS virus, but few details are available as to the level and duration of viremia in this species and its role, if any, in the epizootiology of the disease. It is likely that, like dog, this species has no significant role in the epidemiology of AHS (Awad et al., 1981b). Horses, mules, and donkeys have historically been known as hosts for AHS virus as reflected in the name of the disease. In view of the high mortality rate suffered by horses and mules, these species should be regarded as accidental or indicator hosts (Mellor and Hamblin, 2004). A high percentage of African elephant serum samples reacted positively against AHS virus in complement fixation tests (Davies and Otieano, 1977), but no neutralizing antibodies could be demonstrated in such samples. No evidence of virus replication could be found in elephants artificially infected with AHS virus (Erasmus et al., 1976). Therefore, it was suggested that the African elephant is not susceptible to infection and that the putative serological evidence resulted from abnormal reactions of elephant sera in a complement fixation test. Barnard et al. (1995) reported that the elephants seroconvert when exposed to infection but are not important reservoirs. The Angora goat, not susceptible under natural condition, produces febrile response to virus inoculation (Theiler and Stockman, 1905).

EPIDEMIOLOGY

AHS is an infectious but not contagious disease of equids spread by the bite of blood-feeding insects. The disease is enzootic in sub-Saharan Africa causing clinical disease in various species of animals (Radostits et al., 2000). The disease has a seasonal occurrence, and its prevalence is influenced by climatic and other conditions that favor breeding of *Culicoides* species (Guthrie, 2007). Other insects have been suggested as possible vector of AHSV, but none have been shown to play role in natural conditions.

GEOGRAPHIC DISTRIBUTION

The cradle of the disease lies in Africa, especially countries on either side of equator with dry tropical climate between the isohyets from 250–1000 mm (Bourdin, 1972). AHSV is endemic in tropical and subtropical areas of Africa south of the Sahara occupying a broad band, stretching from Senegal in the west to Ethiopia and Somalia in the east, and extending as far south as northern South Africa (Howell, 1963; Mellor and Boorman, 1995). The Sahara desert, however, seems to provide an effective geographical barrier, which has prevented the virus from establishing itself permanently in Northern Africa or beyond. The virus may also be endemic in one place outside Africa, in Yemen in the Arabian Peninsula (Sailleau et al., 2000), although its long-term status in this area is so far uncertain.

In the recent historic times, AHSV has been endemic across the whole of South Africa, and outbreaks of AHS in horses have been recorded on countrywide basis throughout the whole of the nineteenth century and into the first few decades of the twentieth century (Anwar and Qureshi, 1972). However, with the elimination of the large free-ranging populations of zebra (considered to be the reservoir), there was decline in the annual number of AHS outbreaks, particularly in the southern areas of South Africa. Restricting the populations of zebra to game parks in twentieth century in the northeastern parts of South Africa made AHSV endemic (Anwar and Qureshi, 1972). Outbreaks of AHS occurred in the surveillance zone of the Western Cape in 1999 and 2004 with the policy of maintaining a large population of unvaccinated horses in the surveillance zone (Venter et al., 2006).

Of late, AHSV was believed to be confined to sub-Saharan Africa except for occasional excursions into North Africa or the Arabian Peninsula (Rafyi, 1961; Mirchamsy and Hazrati, 1973). However, in the period 1959 to 1961 AHSV-9 spread in a broad swathe across Saudi Arabia, Syria, Lebanon, Jordan, Iraq, Turkey, Cyprus, Iran, Afghanistan, Pakistan, and India (Howell, 1960, 1963; Rafyi, 1961; Gohre et al., 1964; Mirchamsy and Hazrati, 1973). Nevertheless, by the end of 1961 in the face of a massive vaccination campaign and the death of over three hundred thousand equids, the disease in Asia ended (Anwar and Qureshi, 1972). The inability of the virus to persist in these regions was probably due to a combination of factors, including vaccination, vector-control campaigns, and adverse climatic conditions, that reduced or prevented adult vector activity during the winter periods (Mellor, 1994). During 1965, AHSV-9 again spread beyond its sub-Saharan endemic zones and appeared first in Morocco then spreading into Algeria and Tunisia before crossing the Strait of Gibraltar into Cadiz Province, Spain, in October 1966 (Diaz Montilla and Panos Marti, 1967 and 1968; Mornet et al., 1967; Laaberki, 1969). The virus was eliminated from Spain within three weeks, following the application of a vigorous vaccination and slaughter policy, but overall it persisted in North Africa for almost two years (Diaz Montilla and Panos Marti, 1967). The appearance of AHSV in North Africa was thought to be due to the movement of nomads and their animals, particularly donkeys, across the Sahara from West Africa where AHSV-9 is endemic (Maurice and Provost, 1967; Pilo-Moron et al., 1969). In July 1987, an outbreak of AHS due to serotype 4 of the virus was reported in central Spain, in the provinces of Madrid, Toledo, and Avila (Lubroth, 1988). The outbreak was apparently caused by the importation of a number of subclinically infected zebra from Namibia into a safari park at Aldea del Fresno (Lubroth, 1988).

Hyera and Baipoledi (2008) conducted a retrospective serological survey of AHS in Botswana covering a ten-year period (1995–2004). The survey involved horses showing clinical symptoms of the disease; and the horses had not been vaccinated against AHS. Serological evidence suggestive of infection with AHS virus was found in ninety-nine clinical cases out of which 41.4% (41/99) cases were found during the first half (1995–1999) and 58.6% (58/99) cases were found in the second half of the survey period (2000–2004).

CLIMATE AND TOPOGRAPHY

The incidence of AHS is seasonal because of seasonal variation in the number vector species present (Radostits et al., 2000). A high level of humidity following abundant rains and heat favors the spread of disease whereas cold and drought are unfavorable factors (Bourdin, 1972). Topographically the zones favoring the spread of AHS are the low swampy regions, the humid valleys with abundant flora (Hening, 1956), water courses, wells, puddles, mud holes, and boreholes (Laaberki, 1969; Reid, 1961; Sers, 1965). In mountainous region, AHS is restricted to the lower zones.

TRANSMISSION AND SPREAD

The ecology of African horse sickness is not properly understood. There is no doubt that the disease is spread by insects, but much of the evidences are circumstantial. AHS is a noncontagious disease, and the virus was the first shown to be transmitted by midges (*Culicoides* spp.) (Du Toit, 1994). The disease is spread by the passive transfer of very small quantities of blood by biting insects, and spread does not occur between animals in direct contact unless the requisite insect vectors are present. The tick *Hyalomma dromedarii* has been shown to transmit the virus between horses (Awad et al., 1981a). Biting midges or gnats, *Culicoides* species, are the most probable other vectors, and climatic conditions, which govern the breeding status and movement of these insects, also govern the spread and morbidity rate of horse sickness. These insects have almost worldwide distribution so that spread of the disease could be universal. Many other biting insects have been named as vectors, but there is a lack of satisfactory evidence in many reports. The mosquitoes *Aedes aegypti*, *Anopheles stephensi*, and *Culex pipiens* have been shown to be true biological carriers (Radostits et al., 2000).

The most significant vector seems to be *Culicoides imicola*, but other species, such as *C. variipennis*, which is common in many parts of the United States, should also be considered as potential vectors (Boorman et al., 1975). The virus is transmitted biologically by midges, and these insects are most active just after sunset and at about sunrise. Although other insects, such as mosquitoes, have been implicated as biological vectors, and large biting flies (e.g., *Stomoxys*, *Tabanus*) may transmit AHS virus mechanically, the role of these insects in the epizootiology of the disease is regarded as absolutely minimal compared with that played by the *Culicoides* species. Generally, midges disperse only a few kilometers from their breeding sites, but it has been postulated that they can be borne for longer distances on air currents (Seller et al., 1977). Analysis of field observations on the progression of outbreaks indicates that wind-borne spread of midges may assist the short-distance spread of the disease, but that long-distance jumps of the infection are invariably the result of movement of infected Equidae.

AHSV has long been thought to be transmitted between its equid hosts by biting arthropods, and during the last century, suspicion fell, at one time or another, on a wide variety of species and genera. However, in more recent times, it has become apparent that certain species of *Culicoides* are by far the most important vectors of AHSV. Du Toit (1944) first showed that wild-caught *Culicoides* species (mixed pools) were infected with AHSV and later in 1945 (Wetzel et al., 1970) demonstrated the transmission of the virus by *Culicoides* bite from an infected to a susceptible horse twelve days after the insects' infecting blood meal. It was demonstrated for the first time that AHSV is able to replicate in a species of *Culicoides* subsequent to ingestion by a factor of up to ten-thousand-fold and that transmission was also possible after seven to ten days incubation at 26°C (Mellor and Hamblin, 2004).

Wilson et al. (2009) reviewed the ways in which AHSV may have adapted to the mode of transmission involving insect vector. The virus particle can be modified by the pH or proteolytic enzymes of its immediate environment, altering its ability to infect different cell types.

AHSV infection rates of vector *Culicoides* and rates of virogenesis within them are temperature dependent (Wellby et al., 1996). Infection rates increase as temperature increases, virogenesis becomes faster, and transmission occurs sooner. Furthermore, replication of AHSV does not seem to occur below 15°C, and at temperatures below this level the apparent infection rate rapidly falls to zero. In related studies, other workers have shown that adults of *C. imicola*, the major vector of AHSV, are active at temperatures as much as 3°C lower than the minimum required for AHSV replication (Sellers et al., 1993). This finding suggests that AHSV transmission may be possible only over the warmer parts of a vector's range while in the cooler areas, even if the virus were to be introduced, transmission would be impossible or only possible at certain times of the year (e.g., summer) or in climatically sheltered localities.

Major epidemics of AHS occur every ten to fifteen years in South Africa with uncertain cause. However, a link between the timing of these epidemics and the warm (El Niño) phase of the El Niño–Southern Oscillation (ENSO) has been suggested (Baylis et al., 1999; Mellor and Hamblin 2004). A combination of heavy rain and drought due to ENSO and the *C. imicola*, the vector of AHSV, have been linked. It is due to breeding of *C. imicola* in wet soil, and its populations increase by over two-hundred-fold (Meiswinke, 1998). Baylis et al. (1999) have also shown that since 1803, thirteen of the fourteen major epidemics of AHS in South Africa have coincided with a warm-phase ENSO.

Mellor and Hamblin (2004) postulated the following over wintering mechanism for African horse sickness virus:

1. AHSV seems to require temperatures ≥15°C to replicate in and be transmitted by vector *Culicoides*.
2. Adults of the vector *C. imicola* are active at temperatures as low as 12°C and can survive even lower temperatures in an inactive state.
3. Since AHSV requires a higher minimum temperature than the vector, this suggests that transmission may be possible over only part of the range of the vector.
4. However, during cold periods, virus can survive at very low levels in adult vectors, whose life span is extended significantly at these temperatures.

5. When temperature rises to permissive levels (≥15°C), e.g., in spring, replication of this surviving virus commences, and transmission becomes possible.
6. This sequence of events could constitute an AHSV over wintering mechanism in the absence of vertebrate involvement.

PATHOGENESIS

African horse sickness is a disease of vascular endothelium, with virus serotypes affecting endothelium in different organs, resulting in a variety of "forms" of the disease. On entry into the vertebrate host, initial multiplication of AHSV occurs in the regional lymph nodes followed by dissemination throughout the body via the blood (primary viremia) and subsequent infection of target organs and cells, namely the lungs, spleen, and other lymphoid tissues, and certain endothelial cells (Coetzer et al., 1994a). The virus is present in the bloodstream from the first day of clinical illness and persists for about thirty days and up to ninety days. It can be recovered from defibrinated blood by intracerebral inoculation into infant mice (Radostits et al., 2000).

Virus multiplication in these tissues and organs gives rise to a secondary viremia, which is of variable duration and titer dependent upon a number of factors, including host species. Under natural conditions, the incubation period to the commencement of secondary viremia is less than nine days although experimentally it has been shown to vary between two and twenty-one days (Mellor, 1994). In horses, a titer of up to $10^{5.0}$ $TCID_{50}$ of virus/ml may be recorded but viremia usually lasts for only four to eight days and has not been detected beyond twenty-one days (Coetzer and Erasmus, 1994a). In donkeys and zebra the levels of viremia are lower ($<10^{3.0}$ $TCID_{50}$/ml) but may extend for up to four weeks (Coetzer and Erasmus, 1994a; Hamblin et al., 1998). In experimentally infected horses, high concentrations of AHSV rapidly accumulate in the spleen, lungs, cecum, pharynx, choroid plexus, and most lymph nodes. Subsequently, virus is found in most organs, probably due to their blood content. In the blood, virus is associated with the cellular fraction both red blood cells (Henning, 1956, and Theiler, 1921) and the buffy coat, while very little is present in the plasma (Laegreid, 1996). In AHS, the onset of viremia usually corresponds with the appearance of fever and persists until it disappears (Laegreid et al., 1993). Wohlsein et al. (1998) have shown that in experimentally infected horses with the peracute form of disease antigen is found primarily in the cardiovascular and lymphatic systems and, to lesser extent, throughout the body. In animals with horse sickness, fever antigen is concentrated in the spleen, with lesser amounts elsewhere. The main locations of antigen were endothelial cells, suggesting them to be a primary target of the virus and large cells of the red pulp of the spleen. The presence of antigen in large mononuclear cells, resembling phagocytic cells and surrounding lymphoid follicles, suggests that these cells might also be involved in virus replication and in the transport of viral protein to the lymphoid follicles (Zientara et al., 1993). The development of the various forms of the disease depends on the envelope chemistry of the individual strain of virus concerned the chemistry dictating the tissue to which the serotype will be directed (Bremer et al., 1990).

CLINICAL FINDINGS

The incubation period is about five to seven days in natural infections and two to twenty-one days in artificially produced infections. AHSV can cause four forms of disease: horse sickness fever, cardiac form, mixed form, and the pulmonary form (Erasmus, 1973). An intermittent fever of 40–41°C (105–106°F) is characteristic of all forms (Radostits et al., 2000).

1. *Horse sickness fever.* It is usually invariably mild, involving only mild to moderate fever and edema of the supraorbital fossa; there is no mortality. It frequently occurs following infection with less virulent strains of virus or when some degree of immunity exists and is the only form of disease exhibited by the African donkey and zebra (Howell, 1963). This is the mildest form and is frequently overlooked in natural outbreaks. The febrile reaction is usually of the remittent type, with morning remissions and afternoon exacerbations, and lasts for three to eight days but rarely exceeds 104°F (40°C). Apart from the febrile reaction, other clinical signs are rare and inconspicuous. The conjunctivae may be slightly congested, the pulse rate may be increased, and a certain degree of anorexia and depression may be present. This form of the disease is usually observed in donkeys and zebra or in immune horses infected with a heterologous serotype of AHS virus.

2. *The subacute edematous or cardiac or dikkop form.* This is most common in horses in enzootic areas. The incubation period may be longer, up to three weeks, and the fever develops more slowly and persists far longer than in the acute disease. The most obvious sign is edema in the head region, particularly in the temporal fossa, the eyelids and the lips, and this may spread to the chest. This may not develop until the horse has been febrile for a week. The oral mucosa is bluish in color, and petechiae may develop under the tongue. Restlessness and mild abdominal pain are often evident. Auscultation of the heart and lungs reveals evidence of hydropericardium, endocarditis, and pulmonary edema. Paralysis of the esophagus, with inability to swallow and regurgitation of food and water through the nose, is not uncommon. The mortality rate is not as

high as in the acute disease, but recovery is prolonged. A fetal course may be as long as two weeks (Radostits et al., 2000). Colic is often a feature, and mortality rates may exceed 50% (Coetzer and Erasmus, 1994a).

3. *The mixed form.* This is often the most common form of AHS, which is rarely diagnosed clinically and seen at necropsy in majority of fatal cases (Guthrie, 2007). It is a combination of the cardiac and pulmonary forms of disease. Initially, pulmonary signs are mild and not progressive followed by edematous swelling and effusions. A primary pulmonary syndrome may subside, but cardiac involvement causes death. In most cases, the subclinical cardiac form is suddenly followed by marked dyspnea and other signs typical of pulmonary form. The mortality rate is approximately 70%, and death usually occurs within three to six days after onset of fever (Coetzer and Erasmus, 1994a).

4. *The peracute pulmonary or dunkop form.* It is peracute form and may develop so rapidly that an animal can die without previous indication of illness. This form is characterized by very marked and rapidly progressive respiratory involvement. An acute febrile reaction may be the only clinical sign for a day or two, reaching a maximum of about 104–106°F (40–41°C). This is followed by various degrees of respiratory distress. The breathing may increase to sixty or even seventy-five respirations per minute, and the animal tends to stand with its forelegs spread apart, its head extended, and the nostrils fully dilated. Expiration is frequently forced with the abdomen showing heave lines. Profuse sweating is common, and spasmodic coughing may be observed terminally with frothy, serofibrinous fluid exuding from the nostrils. The onset of dyspnea is usually very sudden, and death often occurs within thirty minutes to a few hours after its appearance. The prognosis for horses suffering from this form of AHS is extremely grave, and mortality rates commonly exceed 95% (Coetzer and Erasmus, 1994a; Mellor, 1994). The pulmonary form of AHS is also the form most usually seen in dogs (Coetzer and Erasmus, 1994a). If animal recovers, the fever subsides gradually, but breathing remains labored for several days (Guthrie, 2007).

NECROPSY FINDINGS
The lesions observed at necropsy examination depend largely on the clinical form of disease manifested by the animal before death (Erasmus, 1972).

In *pulmonary form*, the most characteristic lesions are hydrothorax and edema of the lungs. The subpleural and interlobular tissues are infiltrated with a yellowish gelatinous exudate, and the entire bronchial tree may be filled with frothlike substance (Mellor and Hamblin, 2004). Ascites can occur also occur, and the mucosa of the stomach may appear hyperemic and edematous. Occasionally, the lungs may appear reasonably normal, but the thoracic cavity may contain as much as 8 L of fluid. Other less commonly observed lesions are periaortic and peritracheal edematous infiltration, diffuse or patchy hyperemia of the glandular fundus of the stomach, hyperemia and petechial hemorrhages in the mucosa and serosa of the small and large intestines subcapsular hemorrhages in the spleen, and congestion of the renal cortex. Most of the lymph nodes are enlarged and edematous, especially those in the thoracic and abdominal cavities. Cardiac lesions are usually not conspicuous, but epicardial and endocardial petechial hemorrhages are sometimes evident.

In *cardiac form*, the most prominent lesions are the presence of gelatinous yellow infiltration in the subcutaneous and intermuscular fascia primarily of the head, neck, and shoulders. Occasionally the lesion may also involve the brisket, ventral abdomen, and rump. Hydropericardium is observed with hemorrhages on the epicardial and/or endocardial surfaces. Petechial hemorrhages and/or cyanosis may also be observed on the serosal surfaces of the cecum and colon. The lungs are usually normal or only slightly engorged, and the thoracic cavity rarely contains excess fluid. A clear demarcation may sometimes be seen between affected and unaffected parts due to a selective involvement of endothelial cells. Ascites may occur as in the pulmonary form of the disease with absence or slight edema of the lungs (Mellor and Hamblin, 2004). The lesions in the gastrointestinal tract are generally similar to those found in the pulmonary form, except that submucosal edema of the cecum, large colon, and rectum tends to be far more pronounced.

In *mixed form of AHS*, lesions common to both the pulmonary and cardiac forms of the disease occur. In general, gross findings in acute cases include severe hydrothorax and pulmonary edema and a moderate ascites. The liver is acutely congested, and there is edema of the bowel wall. The pharynx, trachea, and bronchi are filled with yellow serous fluid and froth. In cases of cardiac horse sickness, there is marked hydropericardium, endocardial hemorrhage, myocardial degeneration, and anasarca, especially of the supraorbital fossa (Radostits et al., 2000).

MICROSCOPIC LESIONS

The histopathological changes are observed due to increased permeability of the capillary walls and circulatory impairment. The interlobular tissues of lungs show serous infiltration with distension of the alveoli and capillary congestion (Mallor and Hamblin, 2004). The central hepatic veins are also distended, and interstitial tissue contains erythrocytes and blood pigments while the parenchymous cells show fatty degeneration. Cellular infiltration can be observed in the renal cortex, and the spleen appears heavily congested. Congestion may also be seen in the gastrointestinal mucosae with cloudy swelling in the myocardial and skeletal muscles (Maurer and McCully 1963; Mirchamsy and Hazrati, 1973; Hess, 1988).

Diagnosis

The epizootic nature of the disease makes rapid and accurate diagnosis of AHS absolutely essential. Currently, diagnosis of AHS is based on typical clinical signs and lesions, a history consistent with vector transmission, and confirmation by laboratory detection of virus and/or anti-AHS virus antibodies (Laegreid, 1994). A battery of tests is available for viral identification, including the rapid capture (indirect sandwich) enzyme-linked immunosorbent assay (ELISA), using either polyclonal antibodies (PAbs) or monoclonal antibodies (MAbs), to the polymerase chain reaction (PCR) test, including a new reverse-transcription (RT) PCR for discrimination of the nine AHSV serotypes, or cell culture and inoculation of newborn mice. The better way is to perform more than one test to diagnose an outbreak of AHS, especially the index case, starting with a quick test such as ELISA or PCR, followed by virus isolation in tissue culture. Virus neutralization (VN) for serotype identification should be performed as early in the outbreak as possible so that the correct vaccine can be selected. Subsequently, the ELISA may be very useful in laboratory diagnosis (OIE, 2008).

Clinical signs and lesions in association with previous epidemiological information may be sufficient for clinical diagnosis; however, because most of the clinical signs and macroscopic lesions are not pathognomic, AHS must be confirmed by virus isolation. Virus isolation is particularly important when outbreaks are seen outside endemic areas. The diagnosis of AHS traditionally depends on the isolation of the infectious virus from whole blood collected in anticoagulant (preferably EDTA) during the febrile stage of infection (Hazrati et al., 1973). Because susceptible horses usually die following an acute infection, virus may also be readily recovered and identified after death directly from tissues such as spleen, lung, lymph nodes, and salivary glands (Erasmus 1973, Hamblin et al., 1992). Whole blood should be washed and lysed as soon as possible after collection to remove the anticoagulant and any antibody that might be present in the serum component. AHSV can be isolated in embryonated eggs, by intracerebral inoculation of newborn mice, or in cell cultures. Several mammalian-derived cell lines—including baby hamster kidney (BHK), African green monkey (Vero), and monkey kidney (MS)—cells are available for AHSV isolation, all of which usually show CPE within seven days (Erasmus, 1963 and 1964; Mirchamsy and Hazrati, 1973). Virus isolation in mice is the preferred technique for primary isolation.

There are no international standards for viruses or diagnostic reagents, and there is no standard methodology for the determination of AHSV. However, a viral panel has been evaluated, and comparative studies between different ELISAs for AHSV antigen determination have been carried out in different laboratories. The results have demonstrated a high level of correlation for antigen detection (Rubio et al., 1998) using the indirect sandwich ELISAs for antigen studies. Group-specific antibody against AHSV can be detected using a several diagnostic assays that are directed primarily toward the VP7, including complement fixation (Blackburn and Swanepoel, 1988), agar gel immunodiffusion (Anonymous, 1991), immunofluorescence (Davies and Lund, 1974), and ELISA (Hamblin et al., 1991; Hamblin et al., 1992; Laviada et al., 1992a, b). An indirect ELISA based on the detection of antibody against segment 10 (NS3) has also been described for AHSV serotype 4 (Laviada et al., 1995). This assay can be used to distinguish between naturally infected animals and those vaccinated with purified, inactivated vaccine. Serotype-specific antibody can be detected using serum neutralization tests (SNT) (Blackburn and Swanepoel, 1988; House et al., 1990). The SNT is not often used for primary diagnosis but may have value in epidemiological surveillance and transmission. In endemic regions where multiple AHSV serotypes are likely to be present, it is essential that paired sera collected at a minimum of two-week intervals be assayed serologically to confirm a diagnosis. The binding of antibodies to viral proteins separated by electrophoresis and transferred to nitrocellulose paper known as immunoblotting has been used for the determination of anti-AHSV antibodies (Laviada et al., 1992a).

AHSV can be identified directly in whole blood and other tissues using molecular probes (Venter et al., 1992; Moulay et al., 1995) and RT-PCR using group-specific primers for segment 3 (Sakamoto et al., 1994) and VP7 (Zientara et al., 1993). The indirect sandwich ELISA is also extremely useful for the rapid identification of AHSV antigen in solid tissues taken from animals that have died following an acute infection (Du Plessis 1990; Hamblin et al., 1991; Laviada et al., 1992a, b). In addition, isolated viruses can be identified by group-specific tests such as complement fixation (McIntosh, 1956) and direct and indirect fluorescence (Davies and Lund, 1974). Sailleau et al. (2000) reported the identification and differentiation of the nine AHSV serotypes by RT-PCR amplification of the serotype-specific genome segment 2, which have provided a method of confirming the identity of AHSV in tissue samples within twenty-four hours. A significant advantage of this method is that it can be used to type very low levels of AHSV antigen in samples that do not contain live virus, and the results are available within a few hours.

Fernandez-Pinero et al. (2009) have developed and standardized a highly sensitive and specific TaqMan-MGB real-time RT-PCR assay for the detection of AHSV. Currently, only conventional (gel-based) RT-PCR protocols are available for its detection; however, these methods are cumbersome and difficult to apply when large numbers of samples are to be tested as in the case of epizootics. To overcome this problem, a real-time RT-PCR method has been developed, based on a 5'-Taq nuclease-3'-minor groove binder-DNA probe (TaqMan MGB) for detection of a wide range of AHSV serotypes and strains designed to the highly conserved region of the VP7 gene (segment 7). The method was able to detect all prototype strains from the nine known serotypes of the virus, with a high analytical sensitivity; no cross-reactions were observed with other *Orbiviruses* or with other viruses affecting horses (Agüero et al., 2008). A coupled RT-PCR for the detection of AHSV dsRNA has been developed using genome segment 7 as the target template for primers (Zientara et al., 1998). Novel gel-based and real-time PCR assays for the improved detection of AHSV with high sensitivity and specificity have been developed (Rodriguez-Sanchez et al., 2008).

DIFFERENTIAL DIAGNOSIS

The clinical signs of AHS, particularly when not fully developed, may be confused with other infections like equine viral arteritis, equine infectious anemia, Hendra virus infection, purpura hemorrhagica, and equine piroplasmosis. Many aspects of the epidemiology of the diseases caused by the two viruses notably equine encephalosis and equine viral arteritis (EVA) are also similar in having a similar geographical distribution and vertebrate host range and the same vector species of *Culicoides* (Coetzer and Erasmus, 1994a, b; Venter et al., 2002). As a result, both can occur simultaneously in the same locations and even in the same animal. Fortunately, rapid, sensitive, and specific ELISAs are available to enable the detection of the antigen and antibody of both AHSV and EEV (Hamblin et al., 1991, 1992; Williams et al., 1993; Crafford et al., 2003), and if used in conjunction with each other can provide a rapid and efficient differential diagnosis. The hemorrhages and edema reported in cases of purpura hemorrhagica and EVA may be similar to those seen in the pulmonary form of AHS, although with AHS, the edema tends to be less extensive, and the hemorrhages are less numerous and widespread (Coetzer and Erasmus, 1994a). In purpura hemorrhagica, the hemorrhages and edema usually involve the limbs and lower abdomen. The highly sporadic occurrence of purpura also aids in differentiation. Horses suffering from equine encephalosis usually do not have characteristic lung edema or subcutaneous edema, and the mortality rate is considerably lower than in AHS.

Several other diseases may also be confused with one or other of the forms of AHS. Toxins, anthrax, and other causes of sudden death, as well as diseases that result in severe respiratory distress, should also be considered. The early stages of babesiosis (*Babesia equi* and *B. caballi*) can be confused with AHS, particularly when the parasites are difficult to demonstrate in blood smears (Coetzer and Erasmus, 1994a). In countries where piroplasmosis occurs, the early stage of this disease, before blood parasites can be demonstrated and anemia develops, may be confused with AHS. Pulmonary horse sickness resembles equine infectious pneumonia, but the latter is rare nowadays and is restricted in its occurrence almost entirely to large groups of horses in confined quarters and under poor hygienic and management conditions. Cardiac horse sickness has much in common with equine infectious anemia, babesiosis, and purpura hemorrhagica. Equine viral arteritis also has a passing resemblance to this form of the disease. Severe cases of EVA may readily be confused with AHS. The presence of ventral edema (in EVA), particularly of the lower limbs, and the much lower mortality rate should allow differentiation. The paucity of diagnostic signs in horse sickness fever would make it difficult to differentiate from many mild, sporadic diseases were it not for the rare occurrence of the disease separate from obvious clinical cases of the other forms of horse sickness (Radostits et al., 2000).

THERAPY

There is no specific treatment for AHS (House, 1993; Radostits et al., 2000). The affected animals should be provided with supportive therapy, adequate nursing, and rest as the slightest exertion may result in death. Animals that survive should be rested for at least four weeks after recovery before returning to light work. A careful monitoring for complications like piroplasmosis should be undertaken (Guthrie, 2007).

PREVENTION AND CONTROL

AHSV is noncontagious and can only be spread via the bites of infected vector species of *Culicoides*. Control may therefore be affected by restricting animal movement to prevent initiating new foci of infection, slaughter of viremic animals, in certain circumstances to prevent them acting as a source of virus for vector insects, husbandry modification, vector control, and vaccination (Mellor and Hamblin, 2004). A control program is essential to verify that the virus has been eradicated from the affected area. The main objective of such a program includes regular clinical examination of the sentinel horses, the investigation of deaths among Equidae, and the monitoring of the *Culicoides* population (Higgins and Snyder, 2006). Complicating and secondary infections should be treated appropriately during the recovery period. The following may be undertaken for effective prevention of the disease:

1. *Husbandry modification and the vector control.* It is aimed at denying or reducing vector access to susceptible animals, especially during times of maximum vector activity (i.e., the crepuscular periods and during the night). Vector belonging to *Culicoides* species, including *C. imicola*, are exophilic (Meiswinkel et al., 2000). Stabling the susceptible equids during the period of maximum vector activity will significantly reduce biting rates and the likelihood of infection. Windows, doors, and others suspected routes of vector entry to the stables are screened with fine mesh or with coarser material impregnated with insecticide like a synthetic pyrethroid. This will further reduce biting rates (Braverman, 1989). Recently, Carpenter et al. (2008) reviewed some prevailing methods of controlling *Culicoides* spp. (*Diptera: Ceratopogonidae*), namely (a) application of insecticides and pathogens to habitats where larvae develop; (b) environmental interventions to remove larval breeding sites; (c) controlling adult midges by treating either resting sites, such as animal housing, or host animals with insecticides; (d) housing livestock in screened buildings; and (e) using repellents or host kairomones to lure and kill adult midges. The data extrapolated from the results of vector-control operations indicated that the treatment of livestock and animal housing with pyrethroids, the use of midge-proofed stabling for viremic or high-value animals and the promotion of good farm practice to at least partially eliminate local breeding sites are the best options currently available.

It is rarely possible to completely eliminate populations of vector *Culicoides*. The main aim is to reduce the number of potentially infecting bites that susceptible animals receive to levels where maintenance of an epidemic becomes unsustainable. *C. imicola* usually breeds in organically enriched moist but not waterlogged soils. Such areas may be bare or covered with short grass (e.g., irrigated pastures) and need to remain moist for sufficient time to complete the developmental part of the vector's life cycle (i.e., at least seven to ten days). Targeted application of insecticides of known low mammalian toxicity (e.g., the synthetic pyrethroids) in and around stables and directly to equids themselves can be efficacious against *Culicoides* species and are more likely to be environmentally acceptable (Braverman, 1989, Braverman et al., 1995). Application of systemic insecticides such as ivermectin may also be effective at killing biting *Culicoides* (Standfast et al., 1985). An additional advantage with this system, and with such insecticidal food additives as tetrachlorvinphos, is that these drugs are eliminated in the feces that, should they be deposited on breeding sites, are toxic to the immature stages of *Culicoides* (Jackson, 1989; Standfast et al., 1985). Application of a larvicide to *Culicoides* breeding sites provides a slow but sustained release of the insecticide and may be effective for periods as long as thirty days

(Holbrook, 1985). Such preparations are effective even when used on breeding sites that are rich in organic matter, which makes them particularly suitable in *Culicoides* control (Braverman, 1989). Biological control of larval *Culicoides* by agents such as *Bacillus thuringensis* has apparently not proved successful (Lacey and Kline, 1983). Several repellents have been tested on *Culicoides*; however, none are completely effective, and the deterrent effect rarely persists for more than a few hours except for diethyl toluamide (DEET), which have a significant deterrent effect against *Culicoides* for periods of up to four hours (Braverman and Chizov-Ginsburg, 1997). Since *C. imicola* attacks apparently peak during the first four hours of the night, DEET may have a significant but temporary effect in reducing the biting rate of this species if applied nightly to susceptible animals (Mellor and Hamblin, 2004).

2. *Preventive measures.* The most important means of introducing AHS into disease-free country is by the introduction of equid animals incubating the disease. Zebra and African donkeys that do not develop any clinical sign of disease are particularly dangerous. Equid animals imported from infected countries should be quarantined in insect-proof facilities at the point of entry. It is possible that infected horses may introduce the disease, again especially if they are shipped by air. This eventuality can be prevented by restricting the importation of horses from countries known to have the disease, by vaccination and quarantining horses at the point of embarkation, by quarantining them in insect-proof enclosures at the point of entry, and by vaccination all horses within a 16-km (10-mile) radius of where horses are permitted to enter from abroad. At present, there is a minimum sixty-day quarantine period for horses brought into the United States from Asia, Africa, and the Mediterranean countries (Mellor and Hamblin 2004).

AHS should be reported immediately to state or federal authorities upon diagnosis or suspicion of the disease. If AHS is detected in a country where it is not endemic, a strict quarantine zone and movement controls should be established. Euthanasia of infected and exposed animals may be considered. After the disease has entered a region, numerous preventive measures should be employed to prevent further spread and eventually to exterminate the scourge in the shortest-possible time. Although the isolation and identification of causal virus is essential, it is imperative that control measures be implemented even before the final diagnosis has been made. The area of control should be delineated, taking into consideration geographical borders such as mountains and rivers. The movement of all equid animals within, into, and out of the control zone should be banned, and this restriction strictly enforced. Furthermore, all equid animals should be restricted within stable, at least from dusk to dawn, and sprayed with insect repellents to mitigate the probability of insects feeding on the animals. In case of insufficient stabling facilities, barns could be used, which will provide protection from insects to a good deal. In addition, regular (preferably twice daily) recording of the rectal temperatures of all equid animals in the zone should be taken to detect infected animals as early as possible because overt disease is generally preceded by viremia for about three days. Pyrexic animals should be killed or housed in insect-free stables until the etiology of the pyrexia has been established. Immediate vaccination of all equid animals and proper identification of vaccinated animals must be undertaken to control an outbreak of AHS. It is imperative to use a polyvalent vaccine before the viral serotype is identified, but once the virus type has been established, a monovalent vaccine can be employed (Higgins and Snyder, 2006).

The guidelines provided by International Animal Health Code (OIE, 2000) for the importation of domestic horses from AHS-infected countries or zones should be strictly followed. These include the housing of the animals in vector-protected quarantine facilities for at least forty days and testing for absence of AHSV or demonstration of a stable or declining AHS antibody titer.

3. *Vaccination.* Attenuated (monovalent and polyvalent) live vaccines for use in horses, mules, and donkeys are currently commercially available. The early vaccines were based on virus strains, attenuated by multiple suckling mouse brain passage (Alexander et al., 1936). They gave solid immunity but occasionally resulted in serious side effects, including fatal cases of encephalitis in horses and donkeys, particularly after primary vaccination (Nobel and Neumann, 1961; Parvi and Anderson, 1963). These problems were minimized by further attenuation of the vaccine virus strains through passage in cell culture (Mirchamsy and Taslimi, 1964). These cell-culture-adapted viruses still form the basis of the currently available vaccines. The AHS vaccines currently used in Southern Africa are supplied in two polyvalent vials containing AHSV types 1, 3 and 4, and 2, 6, 7 and 8, respectively. AHSV-5 is currently not included having been withdrawn in October 1993 because of reports of severe reactions and deaths in some vaccinated animals (Erasmus, 1994). AHSV-9 is also not included because type 6 is strongly cross protective and because type 9 is rarely present in Southern Africa and is considered to be of low virulence. In South Africa, most susceptible animals in areas considered to be at risk to AHS are vaccinated, routinely, twice in the first and second years of life, annually thereafter. The polyvalent AHS attenuated live vaccine (ALV) produced by Onderstepoort Biological Products (OBP) Ltd., South Africa, has been associated with some safety concerns and alleged cases of vaccine failure or vaccine-induced disease due of reassortment and reversion to virulence. However, study conducted by von Teichman and Smit (2008) showed no indications that vaccine

reassortants were pathogenic or lethal after inoculation in susceptible horses. No clinical symptoms typical of AHS were observed in inoculated horses, and all showed a good immune response. Attenuated vaccines are routinely used for control in endemic regions, but may not be licensed in other areas. These vaccines result in viremia, and the viruses could theoretically reassort with an outbreak virus. Attenuated vaccines may not be safe in AHS-free countries. They are also teratogenic.

Inactivated vaccines have the advantage that they do not contain a live and potentially dangerous agent. However, they may be expensive to produce, and multiple inoculations may be required to elicit and maintain high levels of protective immunity. It may also be difficult to ensure complete vaccine inactivation (Laegreid, 1996). There are no inactivated AHS vaccines available on the market though such vaccines have previously been developed (Mirchamsy and Taslimi, 1968; House et al., 1992). During the 1987–1991 AHSV epidemics in Spain, Portugal, and Morocco, one of these, a formalin inactivated vaccine Equipest was developed commercially (Dudourget et al., 1992). The initial clinical trials were carried out in France and were followed by two field trials in Spain and Morocco. Although this vaccine proved to be reasonably efficacious, it was withdrawn shortly after the eradication of AHSV from Europe and is no longer available.

A considerable amount of research has been undertaken on development of subunit vaccines against AHS. The development of baculovirus expression system for the preparation of the synthetic, outer capsid proteins, VP2 and VP5, of AHSV-4 have been described (Roy and Sutton, 1998). These were used together or VP2 was used alone to form the basis of experimental AHS vaccines for use in horses. With both the vaccines, animals developed neutralizing antibodies that apparently conferred protection against challenge with virulent homologous virus six months after vaccination. AHSV serotype 4 outer capsid protein VP2 and VP5 plus inner capsid protein VP7, derived from single and dual recombinant baculovirus expression vectors, have also been used in different combination to immunize horses (Martinez et al., 1996). Viremia was not detectable in vaccinated horses. However, these vaccines are not commercially available. The full protection of horses immunized with a soluble recombinant VP2 protein (AHSV serotype 5) administered with saponin to a lethal AHSV challenge has been reported (Scanlen et al., 2002).

PUBLIC HEALTH CONSIDERATIONS
Humans are not natural hosts for the African horse sickness virus, and no cases have been seen after contact with field strains. However, nonfatal

encephalitis and chorioretinitis resulting in partial or complete loss of vision have been reported in workers packing mouse brain attenuated strains of AHSV (House, 1993). These neurotropic strains have since been removed from AHS vaccine (Guthrie, 2007).

CONCLUSION

African horse sickness (AHS) is a severe, noncontagious, and one of the most fatal disease of horses and other solipeds caused by an arthropod-borne *Obivirus* of the family Reoviridae. Host susceptibility for the disease in decreasing order is horses, mules, donkeys, and zebras. AHS can cause mortality up to 95% and is classically divided into four clinical forms: the pulmonary, cardiac, mixed, and horse fever forms. The most prominent pathologic changes in affected animals are subcutaneous and intermuscular edema and lung edema. The most consistent clinical signs include fever, nonpurulent conjunctivitis, and increased respiratory rate. Although AHS is currently restricted to sub-Saharan Africa, it has expanded beyond this core region on several occasions, demonstrating a capacity to persist in these regions for several years. This suggests that the geographical area potentially suitable for AHSV transmission is considerably greater than that in which it is currently found. The distribution of the disease is controlled largely by the abundance, prevalence, and seasonal incidence of its insect vectors, which are certain species of *Culicoides* biting midge. Climate change has resulted in the major vector species *C. imicola*, expanding northward into many areas of Europe previously considered to AHS risk free. The related bluetongue virus, which is transmitted by the same vector species of *Culicoides*, has already entered many of these locations and is causing unprecedented outbreaks of disease in ruminants. This strongly suggests that at some stage in the future, AHSV could do the same. Developments have taken place in virus detection, and a real-time RT-PCR method has been developed with high sensitivity and specificity. There is no specific treatment for AHS apart from rest and good nursing. At present, *Culicoides* vector-control measures are poorly developed, and the only vaccines available are live, attenuated preparations that are not registered for use in Europe and whose deployment would be viewed with concern by some veterinary authorities. There is need to further improve our understanding of how variations in the virus can alter its capacity to infect and cause clinical signs in different host species, as well as influencing its transmission between *Culicoides* vectors and equid hosts in different ecosystems and under different environmental conditions. There is, therefore, an urgent need to enhance our predictive ability, improve vector-control measures and develop efficacious, inherently safe, inactivated vaccines for AHS.

REFERENCES

1. Agüero, M., Gómez-Tejedor, C., Angeles Cubillo, M., Rubio, C., Romero, E. and Jiménez-Clavero, A. 2008. Real-time fluorogenic reverse transcription polymerase chain reaction assay for detection of African horse sickness virus. *J. Vet. Diagn. Invest.* 20:325–328.

2. Anderson, R. M. and May, R. M. 1991. *Infectious diseases of humans: Dynamics and control.* Oxford: Oxford University Press.

3. Anonymous. 1991. African horse sickness. In *Manual of recommended diagnostic techniques and requirements for biological products for lists A & B diseases*, vol. 3. Paris, France: OIE.

4. Anwar, M. and Qureshi, A. A. A. 1972. Control and eradication of African horse sickness in Pakistan. In *Control and eradication viral diseases in the CENTO region*, ed. M. M. Lawrence, 110–112. Ankara: Central Treaty Organisation.

5. Awad, F. I., Amin, M. M., Salama, S. A. and Khide, S. 1981a. The role played by *Hyalomma dromedarii* in the transmission of African horse sickness in Egypt. *Bull. Anim. Health Prod. Afr.* 29:337–340.

6. Awad, F. I., Amin, M. M., Salama, S. A. and Aly, M. M. 1981b. The incidence of African horse sickness in animals of various species in Egypt. *Bull. Anim. Health Prod. Afr.* 29:285–287.

7. Alexander, R. A. 1933. Preliminary note on the infection of white mice and guinea pigs with the virus of horse sickness. *J. S. African Vet. Med. Assoc.* 4:1–9.

8. Alexander, R. A. 1935. Studies on the neurotropic virus of horse sickness. I. Neurotropic fixation. *Onderstepoort J. Vet. Sci. Anim. Ind.* 4:291–322.

9. Alexander, R. A. 1936. Studies on the neurotropic virus of horse sickness. V. The antigenic response of horses to simultaneous trivalent immunization. *Onderstepoort J. Vet. Sci. Anim. Ind.* 7:11–16.

10. Alexander, R. A. and Du Toit, P. J. 1934. The immunization of horses and mules against horse sickness by means of the neurotropic virus of mice and guinea pigs. *Onderstepoort J. Vet. Sci. Anim. Ind.* 2:375–391.

11. Alexander, R. A., Neitz, W. O. and Du Toit, P. J. 1936. Horse sickness: Immunization of horses and mules in the field during the season 1934–1935 with a description of the technique of preparation of polyvalent mouse neurotropic vaccine. *Onderstepoort J. Vet. Sci. Anim. Ind.* 7:17–30.

12. Barnard, J. H. 1998. Epidemiology of African horse sickness and the role of the zebra in South Africa. *Arch. Virol. Suppl.* 14:13–19.

13. Barnard, B. J., Bengis, R. G., Keet, D. F. and Dekker, E. H. 1995. Epidemiology of African horse sickness: Antibodies in free-living elephants (Loxodonta africans) and their response to experimental infection. *Onderstepoort J. Vet. Res.* 62:271–275.

14. Baylis, M. and Rawlings, P. 1998. Modelling the distribution and abundance of *Culicoides imicola* in Morocco and Iberia using climate data and satellite imagery. *Arch. Virol. Suppl.* 14:137–153.

15. Baylis, M., Mellor, P. S. and Meiswinkel, R. 1999. Horse sickness and ENSO in South Africa. *Nature* 397:574.

16. Bevan, L. E. W. 1911. The transmission of African horse sickness to the dog by feeding. *Vet. J.* 67:402–408.

17. Blackburn, N. K. and Swanepoel, R. 1988. African horse sickness in Zimbabwe 1972 to 1981. *Trop. Anim. Health Prod.* 20:169–176.

18. Boorman, J., Mellor, P. S., Penn, M. and Jennings, M. 1975. The growth of African horse sickness virus in embryonated hen eggs and the transmission of virus by *Culicoides variipennis* Coquillett (Diptera: Ceratopogonidae). *Arch. Virol.* 47:343–349.

19. Bourdin, P. 1972. Ecology of African horse sickness. Proc. 3rd Int. Conf. Equine Infectious Diseases, Paris, 12–30.

20. Braverman, Y. 1989. Control of biting midges *Culicoides* (Diptera: Ceratopogonidae), vectors of bluetongue and inducers of sweet itch: A review. *Isr. J. Vet. Med.* 45:124–129.

21. Braverman, Y. and Chizov-Ginsburg, A. 1997. Repellency of synthetic and plant derived preparations for *Culicoides imicola*. *Med. Vet. Entomol.* 11:355–360.

22. Braverman, Y., Wilamowsky, A. and Chizov Ginsburg, A. 1995. Susceptibility of *Culicoides imicola* to cyhalothrin. *Med. Vet. Entomol.* 9:443–444.

23. Bremer, C. W., Huismans, H. and Van Dijk, A. A. 1990. Characterisation and cloning of the African horse sickness genome. *J. Gen. Virol.* 72:793–799.

24. Burrage, T. G., Trevejo, R., Stone Marschat, M. and Laegreid, W. W. 1993. Neutralising epitopes of African horse sickness virus serotype 4 are located on VP2. *Virology* 196:799–803.

25. Burrage, T. G. and Laegreid, W. W. 1994. African horse sickness: pathogenesis and immunity. *Comp. Immunol. Microbiol. Infect. Dis.* 17:275–85.

26. Carpenter, S., Mellor, P. S. and Torr, S. J. 2008. Control techniques for Culicoides biting midges and their application in the U.K. and northwestern Palaerctic. *Med Vet Entomol.* 22: 175–87.

27. Coetzer, J. A. W. and Erasmus, B. J. 1994a. African horse sickness. In *Infectious diseases of livestock with special reference to southern Africa*, vol. 1., ed. J. A. W. Coetzer, G. R. Thomson, and R. C. Tustin, 460–475. Cape Town: Oxford University Press.

28. Coetzer, J. A. W. and Erasmus, B. J. 1994b. Equine encephalosis. In *Infectious diseases of livestock with special reference to southern Africa*, vol. 1, ed. J. A. W. Coetzer, G. R. Thomson, and R. C. Tustin, 476–479. Cape Town: Oxford University Press.

29. Crafford, J. E., Guthrie, A. J., van Vuuren, M., Mertens, P. P. C., Burroughs, J. N., Howell, P. G. and Hamblin, C. 2003. A group specific, indirect sandwich ELISA for the detection of equine encephalosis virus antigen. *J. Virol. Methods* 112:129–135.

30. Davies, F. G. and Lund, L. J. 1974. The application of fluorescent antibody techniques to the virus of African horse sickness. *Res. Vet. Sci.* 17:128–130.

31. Davies, F. G. and Otieno, S. 1977. Elephants and zebras as possible reservoir host for African horse sickness virus. *Vet. Rec.* 100:291–292.

32. Diaz Montilla, R. and Panos Marti, P. 1967. Epizootologiadela peste equina en Espana. *Bull. Off. Int. Epizoot.* 86:705–714.

33. Diaz Montilla, R. and Panos Marti, P. 1968. La peste Equina. *Bull. Off. Int. Epizoot.* 70:647–662.

34. Diaz Yubero, M. A. 1987. Situacion de la Peste Equina. *Epizootiological Inf.* No. ESP. 87(6): 145.

35. Du Plessis, D. H., van Wyngaardt, W. and Bremer, C. W. 1990. An indirect sandwich ELISA utilizing F(ab')2 fragments for the detection of African horse sickness virus. *J. Virol. Methods* 29:279–289.

36. Du Toit, R. M. 1944. The transmission of blue tongue and horse sickness by *Culicoides*. *Onderstepoort J. Vet. Sci. Anim. Ind.* 19:7–16.

37. Dudourget, P., Preaud, J. M., Detraz, F., Lacoste, A. C., Erasmus, B. J., and Lombard, M. 1992. Development, production and quality control of an industrial inactivated vaccine against African horse sickness virus serotype 4. In *Bluetongue, African horse sickness and related orbiviruses*, ed. T. W. Walton and B. I. Osburn, 874–886. Boca Raton: CRC Press.

38. EC. 1997. 97/10/EC: Commission decision of 12 December 1996 amending council decision 79/542/EEC and commission decisions 92/160/EEC, 92/260/EEC, and 93/197/EEC in relation to the temporary admission and imports into the community of registered horses from South Africa. *Official Journal* L003:9–24.

39. Erasmus, B. J. 1963. Cultivation of horse sickness virus in tissue culture. *Nature* 200:716–719.

40. Erasmus, B. J. 1964. Some observations on the propagation of horse sickness virus in tissue culture. *Bull. Off. Int. Epizoot.* 62:923–928.

41. Erasmus, B. J. 1972. The pathogenesis of African horse sickness. In *Proc. of the Third International Conference on Equine Infectious Diseases*, 1–11. Paris, Basel: Karger.

42. Erasmus, B. J. 1973. The pathogenesis of African horse sickness. In *Equine infectious diseases III, Proc. 3rd Int. Conf. Equine Inf. Dis.*, ed. J. T. Bryans and H. Gerber, 1–11. Paris, France (1972), Basel: Karger.

43. Erasmus, B. J., Young, E., Pieterse, L. M., and Boshoff, S. T. 1976. The susceptibility of zebra and elephants to African horse sickness virus. Proc. of the Fourth International Conference on Equine Infectious Diseases, Lyon. Princeton, NJ: Veterinary Publications Inc.

44. Erasmus, B. J. 1994. African horse sickness vaccine information. Circular to veterinary surgeons in practice in South Africa, Onderstepoort Biological Products, Department of Agriculture, Republic of South Africa.

45. Fernández-Pinero, J., Fernández-Pacheco, P., Rodríguez, B., Sotelo, E., Robles, A., Arias, M. and Sánchez-Vizcaíno, J. M. 2009. Rapid and sensitive detection of African horse sickness virus by real-time PCR. *Res. Vet. Sci.* 86:353–358.

46. Gohre, D. S., Khot, J. B., Paranjpe, V. L. and Manjrekar, S. L. 1965. Observations on the outbreak of South African horse sickness in India during 1960–1961. *Bombay Vet. Coll. Mag.* 1964–65:15.

47. Grimes, J., Basak, A. K., Roy, P. and Stuart, D. I. 1995. The crystal structure of blue tongue virus VP7. *Nature* 373:167–170.

48. Grubman, M. J. and Lewis, S. A. 1992. Identification and characterization of the structural and nonstructural proteins of African horse sickness virus and determination of the genome coding assignments. *Virology* 186:444–451.

49. Guthrie, A. J. 2007. African horse sickness. In *Equine infectious diseases*, ed. D. C. Sellon and M. T. Long, chapter 15, 164–170. Philadelphia, USA: Saunders, Elsevier Inc.

50. Hamblin, C., Mertens, P. P. C., Mellor, P. S., Burroughs, J. N. and Crowther, J. R. 1991. A serogroup specific enzyme linked immunosorbent assay for the detection and identification of African horse sickness viruses. *J. Virol. Methods* 31:285–292.

51. Hamblin, C., Anderson, E. C., Mellor, P. S., Graham, S. D., Mertens, P. P. C. and Burroughs, J. N. 1992. The detection of African horse sickness virus antigens and antibodies in young Equidae. *Epidemiol. Infect.* 108:193–201.

52. Hamblin, C., Salt, J. S., Mellor, P. S., Graham, S. D., Smith, P. R. and Wohlsein, P. 1998. Donkeys as reservoirs of African horse sickness. *Arch. Virol. Suppl.* 14:37–47.

53. Hazrati, A., Mirchamsy, H. and Bahrami, S. 1973. Comparative studies on the serological responses of horses to African horse sickness virus. In *Equine infectious diseases III, Proc. 3rd Int. Conf. Equine. Inf. Dis.*, ed. J. T. Bryans and H. Gerber, 69–80. Paris, France (1972), Basel: Karger.

54. Henning, M. W. 1956. African horse sickness, perdesiekte, Pestis equorum. In *Animal diseases in South Africa*, 3rd ed, Central News Agency, 785–808. South Africa: Ondertepoort.

55. Hess, W. R. 1988. African horse sickness. In *The arboviruses: Epidemiology and ecology*, vol. 2, ed. T. P. Monath, 1–18. Boca Raton: CRC Press.

56. Hewat, E. A., Booth, T. F., Loudon, P. T. and Roy, P. 1992. Three dimensional reconstruction of baculo virus expressed bluetongue virus core-like particles by cryo electron microscopy. *Virology* 189:10–20.

57. Higgins, A. J. and Synder, J. R. 2006. African horse sickness and equine encephalosis. In *The equine manual*, 2nd ed., 25–29. Elsevier Saunders.

58. Holbrook, F. R. 1985. Research on the control of bluetongue in livestock by vector suppression. In *Blue tongue and related orbiviruses*, ed. T. L. Barber and M. M. Jochim, 617–620. New York: A. R. Liss Inc.

59. House, J. A. 1993. African horse sickness. *Vet. Clin. North Am. Equine Pract.* 9:355–364.

60. House, C., Mikiciuk, P. E. and Berringer, M. L. 1990. Laboratory diagnosis of African horse sickness. Comparison of serological techniques and evaluation of storage methods of samples for virus isolation. *J. Vet. Diagn. Invest.* 2:44–50.

61. House, J. A., Lombard, M., House, C., Dubourget, P. and Mebus, C. A. 1992. Efficacy of an inactivated vaccine for African horse sickness serotype 4. In *Bluetongue, African horse sickness and related orbiviruses*, ed. T. W. Walton and B. I. Osburn, 891–895. Boca Raton: CRC Press.

62. Howell, P. G. 1960. The 1960 epizootic in the Middle East and SW Asia. *J. S. Afr. Vet. Med. Assoc.* 31:329–334.

63. Howell, P. G. 1962. The isolation and identification of further antigenic types of African horse sickness virus. *Onderstepoort J. Vet. Res.* 29:139–149.

64. Howell, P. G. 1963. African horse sickness. In *Emerging diseases of animals*, FAO, Rome. *FAO Agricultural Studies* 61:71–108.

65. Howell, P. G. 1964. La peste equine africaine. *Maladies nouvelles des animaux*, 75–116.

66. Hyera, J. M. and Baipoledi, E. K. 2008. A serological survey of African horse sickness in Botswana. *J. S. Afr. Vet. Assoc.* 79: 44–45.

67. Jackson, H. C. 1989. Ivermectin as a systemic insecticide. *Parasitol. Today* 5:146–156.

68. Laaberki, A. 1969. Evolution d'une dpizootic de P.E.A. au Maroc. *Bull. OIE* 71:921–936.

69. Lacey, L. A. and Kline, D. L. 1983. Laboratory assay of *Bacillus thuringensis* (H-14) against *Culicoides* spp. and *Leptoconops* spp. (Ceratopogonidae). *Mosq. News* 43:502–503.

70. Laegreid, W. W. 1994. Diagnosis of African horse sickness. *Comp. Immunol. Microbiol. Infect. Dis.* 17:297–303.

71. Laegreid, W. W. 1996. African horse sickness. In *Virus infections of vertebrates*. Vol. 6 *Virus infections of equines*, ed. M. J. Studdert, 101–123. Amsterdam: Elsevier Press.

72. Laegreid, W. W., Skowronek, A., Stone-Marschat, M. and Burrage, T. 1993. Characterisation of virulence variants of African horse sickness virus. *Virology* 195:836–839.

73. Laviada, M., Roy, P. and Sanchez-Vizcaino, J. M. 1992a. Adaptation and evaluation of an indirect ELISA and immunoblotting test for African horse sickness antibody detection. In *Bluetongue, African horse sickness and related orbiviruses*, ed. T. W. Walton and B. I. Osburn, 646–650. Boca Raton: CRC Press.

74. Laviada, M. D., Babin, M., Dominguez, J. and Sanchez-Vizcaino, J. M. 1992b. Detection of African horse sickness virus in infected spleen by sandwich ELISA using two monoclonal anti-bodies specific for VP7. *J. Virol. Methods* 38:229–242.

75. Laviada, M. D., Roy, P., Sanchez-Vizcaino, J. M. and Casal, J. I. 1995. The use of African horse sickness NS3 protein expressed in bacteria, as a marker to differentiate infected from vaccinated horses. *Virus Res.* 38:205–218.

76. Lubroth, J. 1988. African horse sickness and the epizootic in Spain 1987. *Equine Pract.* 10:26–33.

77. Martinez-Torrecuadrada, J. L. and Casal, J. I. 1995. Identification of a linear neutralisation domain in the protein VP2 of African horse sickness virus. *Virology* 210:391–399.

78. Martinez, J., Diaz-Laviada, M., Roy, P., Sanchez, C., Vela, C., Sanchez-Vizcaino, J. M. and Casal, I. 1996. Full protection against African horse sickness (AHSV) in horses induced by baculovirus-derived AHS virus serotype 4 VP2, VP5 and VP7. *J. Gen. Virol.* 77:1211–1221.

79. Maurer, F. D. and McCully, R. M. 1963. African horse sickness with emphasis on pathology. *Am. J. Vet. Res.* 26:235–266.

80. Maurice, Y. and Provost, A. 1967. La peste équine a type 9en Afrique Centrale enquête sérologique. *Rev. Elev. Med. Vet. Pays Trop.* 20:21–25.

81. McIntosh, B. M. 1955. Horse sickness antibodies in the sera of dogs in enzootic areas. *J. South African Vet. Med. Assoc.* 26:269–272.

82. McIntosh, B. M. 1956. Complement fixation with African horse sickness. *Onderstepoort J. Vet. Res.* 27:165–169.

83. Meiswinkel, R. 1998. The 1996 outbreak of African horse sickness in South Africa: The entomological perspective. *Arch. Virol. Suppl.* 14:69–83.

84. Meiswinkel, R., Baylis, M. and Labuschagne, K. 2000. Stabling and the protection of horses from *Culicoides bolitinos* (Diptera: Ceratopogonidae), a recently identified vector of African horse sickness. *Bull. Entomol. Res.* 90:509–515.

85. Mellor, P. S. 1993. African horse sickness: transmission and epidemiology. *Vet. Res.* 24:199–212.

86. Mellor, P. S. 1994. Epizootiology and vectors of African horse sickness virus. *Comp. Immunol. Microbiol. Infect. Dis.* 17:287–296.

87. Mellor, P. S. and Boorman, J. 1995. The transmission and geographical spread of African horse sickness and bluetongue viruses. *Ann. Trop. Med. Parasitol.* 89:1–15.

88. Mellor, P. S. and Hamblin, C. 2004. African horse sickness. *Vet. Res.* 35:445–446.

89. Mellor, P. S., Capela, R., Hamblin, C., Hooghuis, H., Mertens, P. P. C., Plateau, E. and Vizcaino, J. M. 1994. African horse sickness in Europe, epidemiology. In *Conf. equine inf. dis.*, ed. N. Nakajima and W. Plowright, 61–64. Proc. 7th Int. Tokyo, Japan, 8–11 June 1994, R&W Publications, Newmarket.

90. M'Fadyean, J. 1900. African horse sickness. *J. Comp. Pathol. Ther.* 13:1–20.

91. Mirchamsy, H. and Taslimi, H. 1964. Immunisation against African horse sickness with tissue culture adapted neurotropic viruses. *Brit. Vet. J.* 120:481–486.

92. Mirchamsy, H. and Taslimi, H. 1968. Inactivated African horse sickness virus cell culture vaccine. *Immunology* 14:81–88.

93. Mirchamsy, H. and Hazrati, A. 1973. A review of the aetiology and pathology of African horse sickness. *Arch. Inst. Razi.* 25:23–46.

94. Mornet, P., Toma, B. and Sers, J. L. 1967. Une nouvellemaladie réputée légalement contagieuse: lapeste equine. *Rec. Med. Vet.* 143:119–139.

95. Moulay, S., Zientara, S., Sailleau, C. and Cruciere, C. 1995. Detection of African horse sickness viruses by dot blot hybridisation using a digoxigenin labelled probe. *Mol. Cell Probes* 9:233–237.

96. Moule, L. 1896. Histoire de la Médecine Vétéri-naire, Maulde, Paris, 38.

97. Newsholme, O., Bedford, G. A. H. and Du Toit, R. M. 1983. A morphological study of the lesions of African horse sickness. *Onderstepoort J. Vet. Res.* 50:7–24.

98. Nobel, T. A. and Neumann, F. 1961. Vaccination against African horse sickness and post vaccination reactions in Israel. *Refu. Vet.* 18:168–173.

99. OIE. 2000. African horse sickness. In *International Animal Health Code*, Paris.

100. OIE. 2008. African horse sickness. In *OIE Terrestrial Manual*, 823–838.

101. Pavri, K. M. and Anderson, C. R. 1963. Isolation of vaccine strains of African horse sickness virus from brains of two horses given polyvalent vaccine. *Indian J. Vet. Sci. Anim. Husb.* 33:215–219.

102. Patakakis, J. M. 2003. *Culicoides imicola* in Greece. Proc. 3rd OIE Bluetongue International Symposium, 26–29th October, Taormina, Sicily, http://www.bluetonguesymposium.it/index.htm.

103. Pilo-Moron E., Vincent J., Ait-Mesbah O. and Forthomme G. 1969. Origine de la peste équine en Afrique du Nord; résultats d'une enquête surles ânes du Sahara Algérien. *Arch. Inst. Pasteur Alger.* 47:105–118.

104. Pitchford, N. and Theiler, A. 1903. Investigations into the nature and causes of horse sickness. *Agric. J. Cape Good Hope* 23:153–156.

105. Prasad, B. V. V., Yamaguchi, S. and Roy, P. 1992. Three dimensional structure of single shelled bluetongue virus. *J. Virol.* 66:2135–2142.

106. Radostits, O. M., Blood, D. C. and Gay, C. C. 1995. African horse sickness. In *Veterinary Medicine* 8th ed. W. B. Saunders Co. 946–949.

107. Radostits, O. M., Gay, C. C., Blood D. C. and Hinchcliff, K. W. 2000. African horse sickness. In *Veterinary Medicine*, 9th ed., 1038–1040. W. B. Saunders Co.

108. Rafyi, A. 1961. Horse sickness. *Bull. Off. Int. Epizoot.* 56:216–250.

109. Rodriguez-Sanchez, B., Fernandez-Pinero, J., Sailleau, C., Zientara, S., Belak, S., Arias, M. and Sanchez-Vizcaino, J. M. 2008. Novel gel-based and real-time PCR assays for the improved detection of African horse sickness virus. *J. Virol. Methods* 151:87–94.

110. Roy, P. and Sutton, G. 1998. New generation of African horse sickness virus vaccines based on structural and molecular studies of the virus particles. *Arch. Virol. Suppl.* 14:177–202.

111. Roy, P., Hirasawa, T., Fernandez, M., Blionov, V. M. and Sanchez-Vizcaino J. M. 1991. The complete sequence of the group-specific antigen, VP7, of African horse sickness virus serotype 4 reveals a close relationship to bluetongue virus. *J. Gen. Virol.* 72:1237–1241.

112. Reid, N. R. 1961. African horse sickness. The 1959–1969 epizootic of African horse sickness in the Near East region and India and a note on technical assistance provided by the FAO of the United Nations. *Brit. Vet. J.* 117:137–142.

113. Rubio, C., Cubillo, M. A., Hooghuis, H., Sanchez-Vizcaino, J. M., Diaz-Laviada, M., Plateau, E., Zientara, S., Cruciere, C. and Hamblin, C. 1998. Validation of ELISA for the detection of African horse sickness virus antigens and antibodies. *Arch. Virol. Suppl.* 14:311–315.

114. Sailleau, C., Hamblin, C., Paweska, J. Y. and Zientara, S. 2000. Identification and differentiation of the nine African horse sickness virus serotypes by RT-PCR amplification of the serotype-specific genome segment 2. *J. Gen. Virol.* 81:831–837.

115. Sakamoto, K., Punyahotra, R., Mizukoshi, N., Ueda, S., Imagawa, H., Sugiura, T., Kamada, M. and Fukusho, A. 1994. Rapid detection of African horse sickness by the reverse transcriptase polymerase chain reaction (RT-PCR) using the amplimer for segment 3 (VP3 gene). *Arch. Virol.* 136:87–97.

116. Scanlen, M., Paweska, J., Verschoor, J. and Dijk, A. 2002. The protective efficacy of a recombinant VP2-based African horse sickness subunit vaccine candidate is determined by adjuvant. *Vaccine* 20:1079–1088.

117. Sellers, R. F. and Mellor, P. S. 1993. Temperature and the persistence of viruses in *Culicoides* spp. during adverse conditions. *Rev. Sci. Tech. Off. Int. Epizoot.* 12:733–755.

118. Sellers, R. F., Pedgley, D. E. and Tucker, M. R. 1977. Possible spread of African horse sickness on the wind. *J. Hyg.* (Camb.) 79:279–298.

119. Sers, J. L. 1965. La peste equine en Algeric; Etude surl epizootied' automne 1965; these doct. vet., Alfort.

120. Standfast, H. A., Muller, M. J. and Wilson, D. D. 1985. Mortality of Culicoides brevitarsis fed on cattle treated with Ivermectin. In *Bluetongue and related orbiviruses*, ed. T. L. Barber and M. M. Jochim, 611–616. New York: A. R. Liss.

121. Stanley, N. F. 1981. Reoviridae: Orbivirus and reo-virus infections of mammals and birds. In *Comparative diagnosis of viral diseases*, vol. 4b, ed. E. Kurstak and C. Kurstak, 67–104. New York: Academic Press.

122. Stone-Marschat, M. A., Moss, S. R., Burrage, T. G., Barber, M. L., Roy, P. and Laegreid, W. W. 1996. *Virology* 220:219–222.

123. Theal, G. M. 1899. Records of South-Eastern Africa collected in various libraries and archive departments in Europe. *Gov. Cape Colony* 3:224.

124. Theiler, A. 1905. Horse sickness: Introduction. *Rep. Govern Vet. Bacteriol.* 131–162.

125. Theiler, A. and Stockman, S. 1905. On the correlation of viral diseases in stock in South Africa. *J. Comp. Pathol.* 18:155–160.

126. Theiler, A. 1906. Transmission of horse sickness into dogs. *Rep. Govern. Vet. Bacteriol.* 160–162.

127. Theiler, A. 1907. On the co-relation of various disease of stock in South Africa. *Rep. Govern. Vet. Bacteriol.* 67–80.

128. Theiler, A. 1908. Further notes on immunity in horse sickness, *Rep. Govern. Vet. Bacteriol.* 89–161.

129. Theiler, A. 1908. The immunization of mules with polyvalent serum and virus. *Rep. Govern. Vet. Bacteriol.* 192–213.

130. Theiler, A. 1910. The susceptibility of dog to African horse sickness. *J. Comp. Pathol.* 23:315–373.

131. Theiler, A. 1921. African horse sickness *(Pestis equorum). South Afr. Dept. Ag. Sci. Bull.* 19:30.

132. Van Ransburg, L. B. J., De Clerk, J., Groenewald, H. B. and Botha, W. S. 1981. An outbreak of African horse sickness in dogs. *J. South. Afr. Vet. Assoc.* 52:323–325.

133. Venter, E. H., Van Dijk, A. A., Huismans, H. and Van der Lugt, J. J. 1992. The detection of blue tongue and African horse sickness using dot-spot and conventional in situ hybridization. In *Blue tongue, African horse sickness and related orbiviruses*, ed. T. E. Walton and B. I. Osburn, 671–678. Boca Raton: CRC Press.

134. Venter, G. J., Groenewald, D., Venter, E., Hermanides, K. G. and Howell, P. G. 2002. A comparison of the vector competence of the biting midges, *Culicoides* (*Avaritia*) *bolitinos* and *C.* (*A.*) *imicola*, for the Bryanston serotype of equine encephalosis virus. *Med. Vet. Entomol.* 16:372–377.

135. Venter, G. J., Koekemoer, J. J. and Paweska, J. T. 2006. Investigations on outbreaks of African horse sickness in the surveillance zone in South Africa. *Rev. Sci. Tech.* 25:1097–109.

136. Verwoerd, D. W., Huismans, H. and Erasmus, B. J. 1979. Orbiviruses. In *Comprehensive virology*, vol. 14, ed. H. Fraenkel Conrat and R. R. Wagner, 285–345. London: Plenum Press.

137. von Teichman, B. F. and Smit, T. K. 2008. Evaluation of the pathogenicity of African horse sickness (AHS) isolates in vaccinated animals. *Vaccine* 26:5014–5021.

138. Vreede, F. T. and Huismans, H. 1994. Cloning, characterisation and expression of the gene that encodes the major neutralisation-specific antigen of African horse sickness virus sero-type 3. *J. Gen. Virol.* 75:3629–3633.

139. Wellby, M. P., Baylis, M., Rawlings, P. and Mellor, P. S. 1996. Effects of temperature on the rate of virogenesis of African horse sickness virus in *Culicoides* (Diptera: Ceratopogonidae) and its significance in relation to the epidemiology of the disease. *Med. Vet. Entomol.* 86:715–720.

140. Wetzel, H., Nevill, E. M. and Erasmus, B. J. 1970. Studies on the transmission of African horse sickness. *Onderstepoort J. Vet. Res.* 37:165–168.

141. Williams, R., Du Plessis, D. H. and van Wyngaardt, D. 1993. Group-reactive ELISAs for detecting antibodies to African horse sickness and equine encephalosis viruses in horse, donkey and zebra sera. *J. Vet. Diagn. Invest.* 5:3–7.

142. Wilson, A., Mellor, P. S., Szmaragd, C., Mertens, P. P. 2009. Adaptive strategies of African Horse Sickness virus to facilitate vector transmission. *Vet Res.* 40:16.

143. Wohlsein, P., Pohlenz, J. F., Salt, J. S. and Hamblin, C. 1998. Immunohistochemical demonstration of African horse sickness antigen in tissues of experimentally infected equines. *Arch. Virol. Suppl.* 14:57–65.

144. Zientara, S., Sailleau, C., Moulay, S. and Cruciere, C. 1993. Diagnosis and molecular epidemiology of the African horse sickness virus by the polymerase chain reaction and restriction patterns. *Vet. Res.* 24:385–395.

145. Zientara, S., Sailleau, C., Moulay, S., Crucière, C., el-Harrak, M., Laegreid, W. W. and Hamblin, C. 1998. Use of reverse transcriptase-polymerase chain reaction (RT-PCR) and dot-blot hybridisation for the detection and identification of African horse sickness virus nucleic acids. *Arch. Virol. Suppl.* 14:317–27.

2. Borna Disease in Horses

R. V. S. Pawaiya, K. Dhama, S. Kapoor, and P. Bhatt

Introduction

A "disease of the head" affecting horses, as described in the seventeenth century, is now known as Borna disease (BD). It is a sporadic, transmissible, progressive neurologic disease primarily of horses but also occurs in cats, cattle, and sheep. Natural infections have been reported in other equines, rabbits, rodents, and ostriches (Carbone et al., 1987; Lipkin et al., 1993; Bode et al., 1994; Malkinson et al., 1995; Staeheli et al., 2000; Richt et al., 2007). BD was first described more than 240 years ago in 1766 and recognized as a neurological syndrome with an infectious basis in horses (Gellert, 1995); and it owes its name to the town Borna in Saxony, Germany, where a large number of horses, including a cavalry regiment, died during an epidemic in 1895 (Dürrwald and Ludwig, 1997). The virus etiology of BD was proven in the early 1900s when Zwick and White (1931, 1932) in Giessen, Germany, successfully transmitted brain homogenates from infected horses to experimental animals. Borna disease virus (BDV) has been experimentally transmitted to a very wide range of species, from chickens to nonhuman primates. The virus has now been isolated in several other countries and in many warm-blooded animal species, including humans (Chalmers et al., 2005), where it may be responsible for psychiatric disorders such as schizophrenia, autism, chronic fatigue syndrome, or chronic depression (Hornig et al., 2003).

Borna disease virus (BDV) is a unique RNA virus, whose organs of manifestation are the brain and blood of animals as well as humans. The infection disrupts certain cell functions but does not damage the cell structure. The infection with BDV can exist without associated clinical symptoms. Furthermore, the majority of natural BDV infections occur unnoticed without causing symptoms particularly those in connection with only a slight BDV infection. The questions of whether BDV infects humans and causes psychiatric diseases, as well as the issue of a possible worldwide distribution of BDV, have become highly controversial, and the debate is continued (Richt et al., 1997; Staeheli et al., 2000; Carbone, 2001). Recently the BD infection has been detected in children, cats, and horses in Sicily, Italy (Pisoni et al., 2007; Patti et al., 2008). The BDV is also suspected to cause disease in cattle, goat, and other ruminants (Ludwig and Bode, 2000). In horses, BD is characterized by a disseminated, nonpurulent meningoencephalomyelitis with infiltration of mononuclear cells and a predilection for the gray matter of the cerebral hemispheres and the brain stem (Richt et al., 1992; Rott and Becht, 1995). After an incubation period lasting a few weeks to several months, BDV infection causes locomotor and sensory dysfunctions followed by paralysis and death. Natural infections seem to be subclinical in most cases (Richt and Rott, 2001).

EPIDEMIOLOGY

Sero-epizootiological studies have shown that BDV is geographically more widely distributed and is also present at higher rates in animals than previously thought. It is difficult to know whether this is due to a larger BDV dissemination or merely to a higher interest for the virus, associated with an improvement in the diagnostic methods (Jordan and Lipkin, 2001; Richt and Rott, 2001). Moreover, the reason for the restricted BDV geographic distribution, despite all animal trades around the world, is still unknown. Natural BD has been well-known as a fatal behavioral and movement disorder of horses and sheep in endemic areas of Central Europe for more than a century (Ludwig et al., 1988). Outbreaks of severe disease are infrequent; however, through blood testing, evidence of infection has been found in clinically normal horses and other animal species in Japan, Austria, Iran, Italy, Israel, Luxembourg, the Netherlands, Poland, Russia, Sweden, the United Kingdom, and the United States (Kao et al., 1993; Lundgren et al., 1993; Malkinson et al., 1993; Caplazi et al., 1994; Nakamura et al., 1995, 1996; Bahmani et al., 1996; Reeves et al., 1998; Galabru et al., 2000; Dauphin et al., 2002; Hagiwara et al., 1996, 1997a, 1997b, 2002; Yilmaz et al., 2002; Pisoni et al., 2007; Richt et al., 2007; Patti et al., 2008). Enhanced case ascertainment due to surging interest in BDV and the introduction of sensitive serologic and nucleic acid–based diagnostic assays for infection almost certainly contribute to these findings; however, dissemination of the virus has not been excluded comparing archived materials to more recently collected specimens. With a few notable exceptions—including reports of disease in Japan in horses (Hagiwara et al., 2002; Weissenböck et al., 2002), domestic cats, (Nakamura et al., 1999) and dogs (Okamoto et al., 2002); and in Austria and France in horses and dogs (Weissenbock et al., 1998a, 1998b; Galabru et al., 2000)—investigators reporting infection in new regions have hardly studied virus isolation, experimental infection, or detailed neuropathology.

Sequence comparisons revealed that BDV strains from various host species seemed to lack species specificity. Viruses from horses did not show a higher degree of similarity to one another than to viruses from sheep, donkeys, or other hosts. If BDV mainly spread from horse to horse and from sheep to sheep, species-specific patterns of nucleotide exchanges would be expected.

Since this was not observed, the data rather seem to point toward a single source from which the various farm animals acquired the virus. It was speculated that persistently infected rodents or other wild animals might serve as a virus reservoir and that farm animals might contract the BDV infection by feed, which is contaminated with rodent urine. Several BDV strains were isolated from infected horses, sheep, and other animals, and their sequences have been determined either partly or completely. Furthermore, sequences of BDV genome fragments amplified by RT-PCR from the brains of horses, sheep, donkeys, dogs, and cats have been published (Binz et al., 1994) or deposited in the EMBL GenBank database. These sequence comparisons revealed that most strains are highly related to one another, and their genomes differed by less than 5%. It is more likely that some unrecognized functional constraints, including secondary or tertiary RNA, structures restricted sequence alterations to certain hot spots.

The only BDV strain known to date whose sequence differs markedly from viruses of the classical European group is strain No/98. This strain originated from a diseased horse in eastern Austria where no cases of BD had previously been recognized. No/98 differs from all other strains by about 15% at the nucleotide level (Nowotny et al., 2000). Interestingly, conservation at the amino acid level is very high (93–98%) for all viral proteins except for p10 (also designated protein X), which is only about 81% identical to its counterparts in other BDV strains. From an epidemiological point of view, the discovery of No/98 is of great importance. It shows that some natural variants of BDV may easily escape detection by RT-PCR when standard primer sets derived from sequences of classical European strains are used. It is possible, therefore, that infections with BDV are more frequent than previously believed. If, as in the case of No/98, the major antigens of other, yet unidentified, BDV strains are also conserved, those viruses could be identified by immunohistochemical methods using a cocktail of monoclonal antibodies rather than by RT-PCR technology.

The work with No/98 further suggested that additional BDV variants with distinct structural and possibly biological features might be present outside Central Europe. Unexpectedly, however, recent reports have indicated that BDV strains in horses, sheep, cats, and humans of Japan, Taiwan, Iran, the United Kingdom, and the United States of America are almost identical to laboratory strains derived from Central European isolates (Kishi et al., 1995, 1996; Bahmani et al., 1996; Berg et al., 1999; Czygan et al., 1999; Hagiwara et al., 1997b; Iwata et al., 1998; Reeves et al., 1998). These reports possibly mean that classical European BDV strains are predominantly present in horse breeds that are traded most extensively worldwide. It is of interest to note that a variant of a Central European BDV isolate adapted to grow in rabbits had been in use as an attenuated live vaccine (Zwick and Witte, 1931; Zwick, 1939) in some parts of Germany. Because its efficacy was questionable (Durrwald, 1993), the use of this vaccine was discontinued around 1980 in West Germany and a few years later in East Germany. Thus, remote possibility exists that nonpathogenic vaccine strain gave rise to present-day field isolates in the above-mentioned countries. However, since there is no clear evidence that transmission of BDV from horse to horse does occur, this scenario seems quite unlikely. Other possibility is that the reports on the detection of BDV in animals and people from non-European countries represent artifacts resulting from accidental contamination of samples with laboratory virus strains. It is also conceivable that complex mixtures of strains do indeed exist worldwide, but because everyone uses the same techniques to detect the virus, only a few strains become visible.

ETIOLOGY

The first reference strain of BDV (strain V) was isolated in 1929 and obtained from a brain homogenate of a diseased horse, after a series of passages on the rabbit (Dürrwald and Ludwig, 1997). BDV is the only prototype of Bornaviridae family within the nonsegmented negative-strand (NNS) RNA viruses under Mononegavirales order (de la Torre, 1994; Schneemann et al., 1995). Two BDV isolates (reference strains V and He/80) are completely sequenced (Dauphin et al., 2002). The Mononegavirales order also includes Filoviridae (Marburg and Ebola viruses), Paramyxoviridae (measle and mumps viruses), and Rhabdoviridae (rabies and vesicular stomatitis viruses). The BDV genome is very compact (8.9 kb) as compared to the other RNA NNS virusesc (11.0–15.0 kb), but its genomic organization is similar (Briese et al., 1994; Cubitt and de la Torre, 1994). Its genome encodes six major open reading frames (ORFs) (I, II, III, IV, V, X1) (de la Torre, 1994; Schneemann et al., 1995), which are divided into three transcription units: the first transcription unit encodes the nucleoprotein N (p40), the second one encodes the phosphoprotein P (p24) (cofactor of polymerase) and the protein X (p10) in overlapping ORFs, and the third transcription unit encodes the matrix protein M (p16), the membrane protein GP (p56) and the RNA polymerase L (p180 or p190). Although similar in genomic organization to other NNS RNA viruses, BDV is distinctive in its nuclear localization of replication and transcription (Carbone et al., 1991; Briese et al., 1994; Cubitt and de la Torre, 1994). This feature is shared with plant nucleorhabdoviruses; it is, however, unique among NNS RNA animal viruses. The molecular biology of BDV is complex, and includes overlap of ORFs and transcription units, transcriptional read-through of termination signals, and differential use of initiation codons (Briese et al., 1994; Schneemann et al., 1995). BDV uses cellular-splicing machinery to generate some of its mRNAs (Cubitt et al., 1994; Schneider et al., 1994), an aspect consistent with its nuclear localization of transcription and replication. Although splicing is also found in Orthomyxoviridae (segmented, negative-strand RNA viruses), it is unprecedented in Mononegavirales.

TRANSMISSION

Routes of transmission are unproven but thought to be via excreta or nasal, saliva, and conjunctival secretions, either directly or indirectly through contaminated food and water. BDV RNA has been detected in secretions from horses by reverse transcriptase polymerase chain reaction (RT-PCR), both in the presence and absence of clinical illness (Richt et al., 1993; Herzog et al., 1994;). The detection of viral markers, including BDV nucleic acid and proteins in peripheral blood mononuclear cells (PBMC), raises the possibility of blood-borne transmission (Bode, 1995; Nakaya et al., 1996). Neither the reservoir nor the mode of transmission of natural infection is known. However, it is likely that subclinically infected animals may represent potential virus reservoirs. In two groups of Swedish racing horses, one clinically healthy and one consisting of horses with diffuse neurological signs, the BDV seroprevalence was 24.5% and 57.7%, respectively (Berg et al., 1999). An olfactory route for transmission has been proposed because intranasal infection is efficient, and the olfactory bulbs of naturally infected horses show inflammation and edema early in the course of disease (Gosztonyi and Ludwig, 1995; Morales et al., 1988). Experimental infection of rodents results in virus persistence and is associated with the presence of viral gene products in saliva, urine, and feces (Nakaya et al., 1996). Thus, the rodent provides the potential for both a natural reservoir and vector; however, because natural BDV infection has not been reported in rodents, their role in BDV transmission to other domesticated animals and humans remains speculative. Recently, the bicolored, white-toothed shrew, *Crocidura leucodon*, has been detected as a BDV reservoir species in an area in Switzerland with endemic Borna disease (Hilbe et al., 2006).

CLINICAL SIGNS

In field outbreaks, the incubation period is about four weeks, which may extend up to six months or possibly years (Metzler et al., 1979; Rott and Becht, 1995; Richt and Rott, 2001; Richt et al., 2007). Symptomatic infection manifests itself with agitated and aggressive changes, often progressing to inanition and death in one to three weeks after the first appearance of clinical signs (Lipkin et al., 1995). The characteristic clinical signs of Borna disease are the result of disturbances in motor and sensory functions and changes in behavior. Clinically affected horses develop a slight fever, followed by a course of three to four weeks of lethargy or restlessness, resulting ataxia, circling, paralysis, and death in most animals (Jones et al., 1997). In a study, experimentally infected ponies developed ataxia, torticollis, postural unawareness, rhythmic repetitive motor activities, muscle fasciculation, and cutaneous hyperesthesia and hypoesthesia over several body surfaces (Katz et al., 1998). Initially, affected animals may display incoordination (ataxia), yawning, chewing movements, hypersensitivity to stimuli (hyperesthesia), loss of appetite, mild colic, and muscle contractions. The severity of signs progresses to severe depression, blindness, sawhorse stance, and leaning against objects. Terminal cases exhibit rapid, involuntary eye movement (nystagmus). The duration of clinical illness is normally one to three weeks. The case fatality rate ranges between 60 and 95% for horses and greater than 50% for sheep. Animals that survive may remain neurologically impaired permanently. Infection can occur without leading to overt clinical manifestations, but it usually results in a career state.

PATHOGENESIS AND PATHOLOGY

BDV is primarily a neurotropic virus. The virus appears to enter the body by intranasal infection through olfactory nerves endings (Ritch et al., 1993) or oral infection through trigeminal nerve (Bilzer et al., 1996). Having entered the axons of peripheral nerves, the virus spreads centripetally toward the central nervous system through peripheral nerves or the olfactory bulb (Bode, 1995). In brain, the virus replicates in neurons, astrocytes, and oligodendrocytes and has a predilection for gray matter of cerebral hemispheres and brain stem. The virus may also spread centrifugally to peripheral nerves, including along the optic nerve into the retina to cause retinal degeneration and progressive blindness (Krey et al., 1979b).

Once inside the host cell, mechanisms for BDV pathogenicity remain poorly defined. Most of the information available on the pathogenesis of BD has been derived from the studies in laboratory animal and tissue culture models (Herden et al., 2000). Virus infection is usually noncytopathic and persistent. Mechanisms of pathogenicity in the brain may include direct interaction with intracellular signaling and function, or interference with intercellular communication essential to brain function, probably through soluble factors such as cytokines, neurotrophins, and/or neurotransmitters (Gosztonyi and Ludwig, 1995; Hornig et al., 2003). The best-studied systems for BD pathogenesis are the adult—and the neonatally infected Lewis rat models.

The pathologic alterations or lesion development in BD are preceded by virus-induced immunopathologic reaction. Lesions result from an immune system response to the virus, which can be demonstrated using immunocompromised animals. Rats that are newborn, experimentally immunocompromised, or have had the thymus removed do not develop clinical signs of the disease despite productive BDV replication in the CNS (Stitz et al., 1995). Such animals do not experience any interference with their vital functions since the disease itself is the result of a virus-induced, cell-mediated response by the host. The infection of adult Lewis rats produces a prominent neurobehavioral disorder, being characterized by pronounced immunopathology. In the acute phase (four to eight weeks postinfection), cellular infiltrates (CD4$^+$ and CD8$^+$ T cells, natural killer [NK] cells and macrophages) and Th$_1$-type cytokines are prominent in perivascular and parenchymal regions of the central nervous system (CNS), while in the chronic phase (fifteen weeks postinfection and beyond), a decline in infiltrates is accompanied by an increase in Th$_2$-type cytokines and a shift to a humoral immune response (Hatalski et al., 1998). CD8$^+$ T cells mediate destruction of virus-infected cells in the CNS, whereas CD4$^+$ T cells promote production of antiviral antibodies. Although antibodies to N and P generated during the acute phase of disease are nonneutralizing (Furrer et al., 2001), antibodies with neutralizing capacity increase dramatically after the acute phase (Hatalski et al., 1995) and likely participate in restriction of virus to neural tissues (Stitz et al., 1998). Mechanisms contributing to viral persistence are as yet uncertain. Modulation of immune responses as BD progresses to the chronic phase may exert some influence on BDV persistence. BDV-specific Th$_1$ tolerance appears to be induced; as rats progress to the chronic stage of infection, the capacity of lymphocytes isolated from acute phase CNS to lyse BDV-specific target cells is lost (Sobbe et al., 1997). These changes in BDV-specific tolerance during chronic infection may result from presentation of BDV antigens in brain without essential costimulatory signals (Schwartz, 1992; Karpas et al., 1994; Khoury et al., 1995), allowing Th$_1$ cells to become anergic or undergo apoptosis. Indeed, apoptosis of perivascular inflammatory cells is most apparent at five to six weeks postinfection, corresponding with the onset of the chronic phase and the decline in encephalitis (Hatalski et al., 1997).

The distinct clinical and behavioral manifestations in adult rat model closely match the CNS pathology of the acute and chronic phases. In the acute phase, coinciding with monocyte infiltration in CNS regions of early viral burden—such as hippocampus, amygdala, and other limbic structures (Carbone et al., 1987)—animals demonstrate exaggerated startle responses and hyperactivity. As animals enter the chronic phase of infection, high-grade stereotyped motor behaviors (continuous repetition of behavioral elements, including sniffing, chewing, scratching, grooming, and self-biting), dyskinesias, dystonias, and flexed seated postures appear (Solbrig et al., 1994), in parallel with the spread of virus throughout limbic and prefrontal circuits. Movemental and behavioral disorders in infected adult rats are associated with dysfunction in dopamine (DA) circuits (Solbrig et al., 1998) as seen in human neuropsychiatric disorders (Anderson, 1994; Hamner and Diamond, 1996; Kelsoe et al., 1996; Partonen, 1996; Ernst et al., 1997), and may be further linked to serotonin (5HT) abnormalities (Solbrig et al., 1995). Increased gene expression of neurotrophic factors that support growth of DA-producing cells in vitro—including brain-derived neurotrophic factor, neurotrophin (NT)-3, NT-4, and ciliary neurotrophic factor—may also contribute to the sensitivity to DA agonist action in adult BD (Solbrig et al., 2000).

Neonatal rats when infected within the first twelve hours of life do not show overt immunopathology rather develop a mild behavioral syndrome and limited neuropathology despite high virus load in the brain and lifelong persistence. Direct viral effects on morphogenesis of the hippocampus and cerebellum have been attributed to cause CNS dysfunction in neonatally infected animals. In brain, granule cells of dentate gyrus (Hornig et al., 1999; Rubin et al., 1999) and Purkinje cells of cerebellum (Eisenman et al., 1999; Hornig et al., 1999) are lost through apoptosis. The extent of neuronal loss in dentate gyrus is correlated with the severity of spatial learning and memory deficiencies in neonatally infected Lewis rats (Rubin et al., 1999).

Effects of BDV infection at the cellular level are only beginning to be unveiled. Inhibition of cell-to-cell spread of BDV by a MAP kinase/extracellular signal-regulated kinase (ERK, MEK) inhibitor in cell culture (Planz et al., 2001) and analyses of neuronal differentiation of PC12 cells (Hans et al., 2001) indicate an interaction of BDV with cellular MAP kinase signaling pathways. Infected PC12 cells demonstrate constitutive phosphorylation of MEK, ERK, and the transcriptional activator, Elk-1 but fail to differentiate with nerve-growth factor (NGF) treatment. Inhibition of neurite outgrowth is also reported in other infected cell lines and has been ascribed to interference by P protein with the normal interaction between the neurite outgrowth factor, amphoterin, and its receptor, RAGE (Receptor for Advanced Glycation End-products). BDV-infected cells show altered intracellular distribution of amphoterin, with reduced levels of amphoterin, and of RAGE activation at growth cones of extending cells (Kamitani et al., 2001). BDV phosphoprotein has been found to interfere with protein kinase C-dependent signaling in neurons, thus contributing to neurobehavioral disorders (Prat et al., 2008). Distinct BDV-dependent reduction in the expression of the neuronal gap junction protein connexin36 (Cx36) has been observed very recently in the Lewis rat hippocampal formation and cerebellar cortex at four and eight weeks after neonatal infection by semiquantitative RT-PCR, suggesting altered neuronal network properties to be an important feature of persistent viral brain infections (Köster-Patzlaff et al., 2009).

PATHOLOGICAL CHANGES

There are no specific gross lesions. The most severe lesions are found in the olfactory bulbs, caudate nucleus, and hippocampus. The cerebellum is spared. Microscopic lesions are characterized by severe nonpurulent poliomeningoencaphalomylitis with massive perivascular and parenchymal infiltration with mononuclear inflammatory cells, consisting predominantly of macrophages, T lymphocytes ($CD4^+$ and $CD8^+$), plasma cells, and gliosis (Bilzer et al., 1995, Jones et al., 1997). Neuronophagic nodules may be encountered, but neuronal necrosis is not a prominent feature. However, a loss of pyramidal cells of the hippocampus might be observed, and a reactive astrocytosis can often be observed in all areas with inflammatory lesions. Besides the gray matter of the olfactory bulb, basal cortex, caudate nucleas, thalamus, and hippocampus, the periventricular areas, mainly in the medulla oblongata, can also be affected. In infected neurons, intranuclear eosinophilic *Joest-Degen inclusion bodies* may also be seen, preferentially in the hippocampus. These inclusion bodies were first described by Joest and Degen (1911) and termed as "Joest bodies" or "Joest-Degen bodies." When present, Joest-Degen inclusion bodies are considered as pathognomonic for BD (Jones et al., 1997; Dietzel et al., 2007; Sellon, 2007). Immunohistochemical, ultrastructural, and virological studies on the brain tissue of eight horses died of natural BD revealed highest viral titers in the hippocampus and piriform cortex and the lowest in the cerebellum on regional assessment of the infectivity (Gosztonyi and Ludwig, 1984). Immunohistochemically, the highest amounts of BDV-specific antigen was demonstrated in the nuclei of neurons followed by those in the perikarya, dendrites, and axons, where smaller amounts of antigen were found. The locations of viral antigenic distribution and inflammatory reaction were highly correlated. At ultrastructural level, stacks of fine filaments adhering closely to cytoplasmic cisterns, which were thought to be related to virus components or virus morphogenesis, were observed. Presence of virus-specific antigen seemed to trigger the exudation of inflammatory cells, which reflected the extension of the infectious process. Heavy inflammatory exudates in the white matter underlying diseased cortical areas can be explained by the axonal presence of virus-specific antigen. Virus particles could not be demonstrated with the electron microscope (Gosztonyi and Ludwig, 1984).

Experimental BDV infection in rats and rabbits involves pathological changes in the retina, resulting in nonpurulent chorioretinitis with degeneration of rods and cones (Krey et al., 1979a; Narayan et al., 1983; Kacza et al., 2001).

Similarly, histopathologic changes in the retinal tissue of BD-infected horses have also exhibited various stages of neurodegeneration of retina, with severity of neurodegeneration increasing with the duration of infection (Dietzel et al., 2007). This loss of neurons leads to blindness observed occasionally as clinical signs in horses. Blindness could also be caused by the severe inflammation observed in the optic region of the thalamus (Bilzer et al., 1996; Herden et al., 1999).

DIAGNOSIS

The diagnosis of Borna disease is difficult, mainly because of low viral replication and excretion rates. Several features of its molecular biology are remarkable, and some are relevant to questions regarding the detection and spread of the virus and the epidemiology of disease. For example, the virus replicates at lower levels than many other viruses, producing low numbers of infectious particles, although cell-to-cell transmission of incomplete particles may occur (Cubitt and de la Torre, 1994). Although a wide variety of tools have been developed for BDV diagnosis, standards have yet not been established, and large differences and contradictions have been observed between the published results (particularly serological surveys) (Hatalski et al., 1997; Staeheli, 2000; Richt and Rott, 2001). Borna disease can be diagnosed by serology, viral isolation, antigen detection, RT-nested-PCR, but none of these methods is yet sensitive and specific enough to be used alone for a sure diagnosis (Richt et al., 2007). Sensitive methods are therefore required for virus detection and identification. Detection of antigen markers in peripheral white blood cells, combined with nucleic acid amplification, is more convenient. Comparative RNA studies reveal an unusually high genetic homology of viruses. Isolates recovered from humans and equines suggest species specificity (Ludwig and Bode, 2000).

In human, demonstration of BDV antigens in populations of peripheral blood mononuclear cells (PBMCs) from hospitalized psychiatric patients (Bode et al., 1994) and the detection of BDV RNA in PBMCs of neonatally infected rats (Sierra-Honigmann et al., 1993) stimulated investigations and detection in psychiatric patients (Bode et al., 1995). The detection of antibodies in humans was first reported in 1985, in patients with depression and psychiatric disorders (Amsterdam et al., 1985). The s-antigen (p40 and p24 complex) initiates the major humoral response and has been the main target for serological studies (Ludwig et al., 1993).

1. *Clinical diagnosis.* Animals exhibit a variety of clinical nonspecific symptoms. Therefore, clinical diagnosis alone cannot be sufficient to diagnose the disease. Hematologic and biochemical parameters are usually within normal limits in affected horses. Hyperbilirubinemia is

frequently observed but is a nonspecific change related to decreased food intake. In late stages of BD when convulsions occur, a high concentration of lactate may be present in the plasma (Bilzer et al., 1996). In acute disease, cerebrospinal fluid (CSF) quantity, and the CSF proteins concentration (86.3±14.8 mg/dL) may be increased, and characteristic lymphomonocytic pleocytosis (56.4±32.8 cells/μL) is seen in the CSF during acute and subacute course of disease, which is consistent with the presence of nonpurulent encephalitis (Uhlig and Kinne, 1998; Grabner et al., 2002). However, in chronic disease, CSF parameters remain in the normal range, except the CSF lactate concentration, which is usually increased. These indicators are, however, nonspecific; therefore, Borna disease must be confirmed by serologic or molecular tests.

2. *Serological diagnosis.* The serological diagnosis can be applied to living animals by antibody detection in blood and/or cerebrospinal fluid (CSF). Western blot (Herzog et al., 1994), enzyme-linked immunosorbent assay (ELISA) (Dürrwald and Ludwig, 1997; Dieckhofer, 2008), and immunofluorescence assay (IFA) (Herzog and Rott, 1980) can be used. Detection of antibodies to BDV in sera and CSF samples from infected animals and humans has mainly relied on the use of IFAs (Rott et al., 1985). Many seroepidemiological studies have used a modified IFA that is based on double staining of BDV-infected cells using serum or CSF samples being tested and a monoclonal antibody (MAb) to the BDV 'N' (p40) or 'P' (p24) antigen (Bode et al., 1992). However, several investigators have indicated that this IFA is highly unreliable and prone to produce false positives (Waltrip et al., 1995), especially when analyzing human sera, which frequently exhibit only very modest titers of BDV antibodies. Antibody titers are usually very low in BDV-infected animals, and their detection requires particularly sensitive techniques (Katz et al., 1998; Staeheli, 2000). Increased sensitivity and specificity in BDV serology have been achieved with the introduction of Western blot (WB) assays using BDV-infected cell extracts (Waltrip et al., 1995); BDV proteins have been purified by affinity chromatography from infected rat brains (Kao et al., 1993) or from infected rabbit kidney (RK) cells (Fu et al., 1993) and/or recombinantly expressed BDV proteins (Briese et al., 1995; Sauder et al., 1996) as antigens. The expression and purification of large amounts of recombinant BDV antigens has also facilitated the establishment of ELISA for detection of BDV antibodies in biological samples (Briese et al., 1995). The use of ELISA allows a rapid and quantitative analysis of BDV antibody titers in large number of samples, facilitating the epidemiological survey of BDV. Another serological techniques such as reverse-type (RT)-ELISA (Horimoto et al., 1997) and electrochemiluminescence immunoassay (ECLIA)

2. BORNA DISEASE IN HORSES

(Yamaguchi et al., 1999) have been developed for the detection of BDV antibodies by the use of recombinant BDV proteins, for which even synthetic BDV peptides were also useful (Yamaguchi et al., 2001). These techniques also remain for consideration as standard diagnostic tools for BDV infection. Interplay of BDV-specific circulating immune complexes (CICs) with free antibodies and plasma antigens may give rise to detection "gaps" (Bode et al., 2001). Antibodies in human sera mainly recognize BDV 'P' protein, whereas animal sera preferentially recognize the 'N' protein. Sensitivity tests of immunoglobulins in up to 3 M urea suggest that antibodies in animals have high avidity to BDV, whereas reactive antibodies in human sera have low avidity (Allmang et al., 2001). Antibodies are detectable in 100% cases during the acute phase of the disease, but they are hardly detectable in a subacute or chronic disease.

3. *Histopathological diagnosis.* In BDV infection, various degrees of encephalomyelitis are observed, particularly with lymphocytic infiltrations in perivascular and parenchymal regions. Presence of intranuclear Joest-Degen inclusion bodies in the infected neurons have been used as BDV-specific pathognomic lesions; however, they are not always observed (Gosztonyi and Ludwig, 1995). Sensitivity of virus detection can be enhanced by immunohistochemistry, which permits to visualize the major BDV antigens p40 (nucleoprotein) and p24 (phosphoprotein) using monoclonal or polyclonal antibodies (Richt et al., 1997) and/or by additional RNA detection by in situ hybridization technique using nucleic acid probes (Herden et al., 1999). However, BDV-infected cells are not uniformly distributed in the brain tissue, and sometimes BD cases may escape detection (Caplazi and Ehrensperger, 1998).

4. *Virological diagnosis by viral isolation.* In vitro virus isolation from animals and humans has not yet achieved diagnostic importance because of difficulties in recovering the agent from infected animals and humans. Classical viral isolation methods from brain tissues are tedious and poorly sensitive due to the low number of infectious particles (Hatalski et al., 1997; Staeheli, 2000). BDV can be easily cultivated on Vero (monkey kidney cells) and MDCK (dog kidney cells) cells. BDV persistently infects cells without cytopathic effects.

5. *Molecular diagnosis.* Molecular characterization of the BDV genome (Briese et al., 1994; Cubitt et al., 1994) permits the development of specific and sensitive reverse transcriptase-polymerase chain reaction (RT-PCR) procedures to detect BDV RNA in biological samples. The RT-PCR was first used to detect BDV RNA in the brains and organs of experimentally infected rats (Shankar et al., 1992; Sierra-Honigmann

50   *Tropical viral diseases of large domestic animals*   *Thankam Mathew*

et al., 1993; Rubin et al., 1995). Thereafter, it has been instrumental in detecting viral RNA in tissues such as brains from naturally infected animals including horses, donkeys, sheep, cattle, and cats (Binz et al., 1994; Zimmermann et al., 1994; Lundgren et al., 1995; Sorg and Metzler, 1995; Hagiwara et al., 1996, 1997a; Richt et al., 1993, 2007). Although BDV was initially believed to have exclusive tropism for brain cells, it also has been detected in nonneural tissues as well as body secretions from infected animals (Richt et al., 1993). BDV RNA can be detected by RT-PCR in PBMCs, bone marrows (Sierra-Honigmann et al., 1993), and thymic stromal cells (Rubin et al., 1995) from neonatally infected rats. RT-PCR to examine the prevalence of BDV RNA in PBMCs from humans (Briese et al., 1995; Sauder et al., 1996; Nowotny and Kolodziejek, 2000; Tsuji et al., 2000) and domestic animals (Hagiwara et al., 1996; 1997a; Reeves et al., 1998; Nakamura et al., 1995, 1996, 1999; Vahlenkamp et al., 2000) have been applied to study molecular epidemiology of BDV infection. This technique can be used for brain or blood samples. However, this extremely sensitive technique is prone to cross-contamination between samples as well as laboratory contamination. Moreover, RT-PCR (using BDV standard primers) is not able to detect variant strains that have altered sequences in the target gene. This was the case with the new genotype identified by Nowotny et al. (2000). RT-nested-PCR detects sequences encoding the two major BDV-proteins p24 and p40 (Sauder et al., 1996). The amplified BDV-products after the two successive PCR are 528 bp for the p40 gene and 391 bp for the p24 gene. In order to control RT-nested-PCR in each reaction sample and to avoid the use of a BDV-positive control reaction that could induce contamination, internal RNA standard molecules (named "mimics") have been produced (Legay et al., 2000). These standards can be easily discriminated from the BDV fragments by agarose gel electrophoresis.

6. **Differential diagnosis.** It is important to make the distinction between Borna disease and other infections in horses, including tetanus, listeriosis, rabies, pseudorabies, hypomagnesemia, hypocalcemia, acute lead poisoning, and toxic plants.

TREATMENT AND CONTROL MEASURES

Two approaches have been applied to cope with BD in the past, namely, hygienic measures and vaccination. Long-term empirical data collected in the endemic areas predicted that separation of sheep and horses would prevent the spread of BD. Furthermore, the sanitary situation seemed to be a critical factor. Severe losses were mostly observed in farms where several animal species were kept together in one stable. Therefore, the recommendation to improve hygiene and prevent contact between susceptible species had some effect but did not lead to elimination of BD. Threatened by the severe losses of horses in rural areas of Saxony, Bavaria, and Hessia, in Germany, at the turn of the twentieth century, vaccination was envisaged (Ernst and Hahn, 1926; Zwick and Witte, 1932). When killed vaccines were shown to be ineffective, filtered brain suspensions from diseased horses with living virus were applied subcutaneously. Only when lapinized live vaccine became available (Zwick vaccine, based on strain V) (Zwick and Witte, 1932) and later a vaccine based on strain Dessau (Möhlmann and Maas, 1960) in some areas, especially the former German Democratic Republic, was rigorous vaccination made compulsory (from 1962 to 1992). Due to the change in political situation and progress of knowledge on the ineffectiveness of the vaccine, these campaigns were ceased. From a modern perspective, any vaccination against this persistent infection located in the nervous system cannot be recommended.

The possibility of antiviral treatment has been explored and appears to be quite encouraging. Researchers in France in the 1920s introduced hexamethylenetetramine treatment of BD in horses with some success (Moussu and Marchand, 1924). Recent in vitro studies with the antiviral substance amantadine sulphate (a chemical relative of hexamine) highlighted treatment of BDV infection. A BDV-infected patient who also suffered from Parkinson's disease, with underlying mood disorder, improved and returned to a state of good health after treatment with amantadine sulphate (AS), even clearing the BDV genome, although the Parkinsonism remained (Bode et al., 1997). Despite variable results on the effectiveness of the drug (Cubitt and de la Torre, 1997; Stitz et al., 1998), the AS has shown effectively inhibiting all wild-type BDV strains from humans and horses, whereas in vitro studies clarified that the laboratory strains (vaccine strains) are insensitive to the drug (Bode et al., 1997). Some human isolates are sensitive to AS (Bode et al., 1997; Ferszt et al., 1999; Dietrich et al., 2000), while other isolates appear to be resistant to this drug in vitro and in vivo (Cubitt and de la Torre, 1997; Stitz et al., 1998). A guanosine analogue, ribavirin, considered to be a universal antiviral drug, has also exhibited inhibitory effects on the transcription of BDV in persistently infected cells (Jordan et al., 1999; Mizutani et al., 1998). A likely mechanism for its activity is the reduction of the intracellular GTP pool, resulting in the inhibition of transcription and capping of BDV mRNA's (Jordan et al., 1999). However, there has been no report on its clinical trial in BDV associated diseases.

CONCLUSION
Borna disease is a sporadic, transmissible, progressive neurologic disease of horses, cats, cattle, and sheep. Natural infections have been reported in

other equines, rabbits, and ostriches. Borna disease virus (BDV) has been experimentally transmitted to a very wide range of species. Evidence in recent years indicates that BDV also infects humans, where it may be associated with various neuropsychiatric disorders, including schizophrenia.

The disease is a subacute viral encephalomyelitis. Historically, the Borna disease has been reported in horses, and occasionally in sheep, in endemic areas in Germany and Switzerland. The evidence of infection has been found in clinically normal horses and other animal species in Israel, Luxembourg, the Netherlands, Poland, Russia, Sweden, the United Kingdom, and the United States. In cases of natural infection in horses and sheep, the incubation period is usually two to three months. The characteristic clinical signs of Borna disease are the result of disturbances in motor and sensory functions and changes in behavior. Initially, affected animals may display incoordination (ataxia), yawning, chewing movement, hypersensitivity to stimuli (hyperesthesia), loss of appetite, mild colic, and muscle contraction. Terminal cases exhibit rapid, involuntary eye movement (nystagmus). The duration of clinical illness is normally one to three weeks. The case fatality rate ranges between 60 and 95% for horses and greater than 50% for sheep. Animals that survive may remain neurologically impaired permanently.

The cause of Borna disease is an enveloped, negative-strand RNA virus that has yet to be fully characterized. It only affects the nervous system and is disseminated from the site of infection through the nerves (intra-axonal transport). BDV appears in the brain and cerebral spinal fluid in three days in animals infected by the intracerebral or intranasal route. Less commonly, the virus can be isolated from salivary and mammary glands and the nasal mucous membrane. The virus can be grown in cell culture in which it produces no detectable cellular changes. It is currently believed that transmission of BDV in cases of natural infection occurs through direct contact with infective nasal secretions and saliva or via contaminated food and water. Based on detailed laboratory examination of nervous tissue from horses affected with Borna disease, evidence suggests that BDV enters the central nervous system (CNS) through nerve endings in the nose and throat area. The CNS of an animal affected with Borna disease does not develop changes visible to the naked eye. But histopathologically, there is generalized intense mononuclear perivascular cuffing, glial nodule formation, and astrocytosis in brain. Confirming a diagnosis of Borna disease is difficult and perhaps best accomplished using a combination of the clinical, serologic, and histopathologic indicators of this unusual disease supported by positive reverse transcription–polymerase chain reaction (RT-PCR) findings.

REFERENCES

1. Allmang, U., Hofer, M., Herzog, S., Bechter, K. and Staeheli, P. 2001. Low avidity of human serum antibodies for Borna disease virus antigens questions their diagnostic value. *Mol. Psychiatry* 6:329–333.
2. Amsterdam, J. D., Winokur, H., Dyson, W., Herzog, S., Rott, R. and Koprowski, H. 1985. Borna disease virus: A possible etiologic factor in human affective disorders *Arch. Gen. Psychiatry* 42:1093–1096.
3. Anderson, G. M. 1994. Studies on the neurochemistry of autism. In *The neurobiology of autism*, ed. M. L. Bauman and T. L. Kemper, 227–242. Baltimore: Johns Hopkins University Press.
4. Bahmani, M. K., Nowrouzian. I., Nakaya, T., Nakamura, Y., Hagiwara, K., Takahashi, H., Rad, M. A. and Ikuta, K. 1996. Varied prevalence of Borna disease virus infection in Arabic, thoroughbred and their cross-bred horses in Iran. *Virus Res.* 45:1–13.
5. Berg, A. L., Dorries, R. and Berg, M. 1999. Borna disease virus infection in racing horses with behavioral and movement disorders. *Arch. Virol.* 144:547–559.
6. Bilzer, T., Planz, O., Lipkin, W. I. and Stitz, L. 1995. Presence of CD4+ and CD8+ T cells and expression of MHC class I and MHC class II antigen in horses with Borna disease virus-induced encephalitis, *Brain Pathol.* 5:223–230.
7. Bilzer, T., Grabner, A. and Stitz, L. 1996. Immunpathologie der Borna-Krankheit beim Pferd: Klinische, virologische und neuropathologische Befunde. *Tierärztl Prax.* 24:567–576.
8. Binz, T., Lebelt, J., Niemann, H. and Hagenau, K. 1994. Sequence analyses of the p24 gene of Borna disease virus in naturally infected horse, donkey and sheep. *Virus Res.* 34:281–289.
9. Bode, L. 1995. Human infections with Borna disease virus and potential pathologic implications. *Curr. Top. Microbiol. Immunol.* 190:103–30.
10. Bode, L., Riegel, S., Lange, W. and Ludwig, H. 1992. Human infections with Borna disease virus: Seroprevalence in patients with chronic diseases and healthy individuals. *J. Med. Virol.* 36:309–315.
11. Bode, L. Durrwald, R. and Ludwig, H. 1994. Borna virus infections in cattle associated with fatal neurological disease. *Vet. Rec.* 135:283–284.
12. Bode, L., Zimmermann, W., Ferszt, R., Steinbach, F. and Ludwig, H. 1995. Borna disease virus genome transcribed and expressed in psychiatric patients. *Nat. Med.* 1:232–236.
13. Bode, L., Dietrich, D. E., Stoyloff, R., Emrich, H. M. and Ludwig, H. 1997. Amantadine and human Borna disease virus *in vitro* and *in vivo* in an infected patient with bipolar depression. *Lancet* 349:178179.
14. Bode, L., P. Reckwald, W. E. Severus, R. Stoyloff, R. Ferszt, D. E. Dietrich and H. Ludwig 2001. Borna disease virus specific circulating immune complexes, antigenemia, and free antibodies: The key marker triplet determining infection and prevailing in severe mood disorders. *Mol Psychiatry* 6:481–491.
15. Briese, T., Schneemann, A., Lewis, A. J., Park, Y. S., Kim, S., Ludwig, H. and Lipkin, W. I. 1994. Genomic organization of Borna disease virus. *Proc. Natl. Acad. Sci. U.S.A.* 91:4362–4366.
16. Briese, T., Hatalski, C. G., Kliche, S., Park, Y. S. and Lipkin, W. I. 1995. Enzyme-linked immunosorbent assay for detecting antibodies to Borna disease virus-specific proteins. *J. Clin. Microbiol.* 33:348–351.
17. Caplazi, P., Waldvogel, A., Stitz, L., Braun, U. and Ehrensperger, F. 1994. Borna disease in naturally infected cattle. *J. Comp. Pathol.* 111:65–72.
18. Caplazi, P. and Ehrensperger, F. 1998. Spontaneous Borna disease in sheep and horses: Immunophenotyping of inflammatory cells and detection of MHC-I and MHC-II antigen expression in Borna encephalitis lesions. *Vet. Immunol. Immunopathol.* 61:203–220.
19. Carbone, K. M., Duchala, C. S., Griffin, J. W., Kincaid, A. L. and Narayan, O. 1987. Pathogenesis of Borna disease in rats: Evidence that intraaxonal spread is the major route for virus dissemination and the determinant for disease incubation. *J. Virol.* 61:3431–3440.

20. Carbone, K. M., Moench, T. R. and Lipkin, W. I. 1991. Borna disease virus replicates in astrocytes, Schwann cells and ependymal cells in persistently infected rats: Location of viral genomic and messenger RNAs by in situ hybridization. *J. Neuropathol. Exp. Neurol.* 50:205–214.

21. Carbone, K. M. 2001. Borna disease virus and human disease. *Clin. Microbiol. Rev.* 14:513–527.

22. Chalmers, R. M., Thomas, D. R. and Salmon, R. L. 2005. Borna disease virus and the evidence for human pathogenicity: A systematic review. *Q. J. Med.* 98:255–274.

23. Cubitt, B. and de la Torre, C. 1994. Borna Disease virus (BDV) a nonsegmented RNA virus, replicates in the nuclei of infected cells where infectious BDV ribonucleoproteins are present. *J. Virol.* 68:1371–1381.

24. Cubitt, B., Oldstone, C. and de la Torre, J. C. 1994. Sequence and genome organization of Borna disease virus. *J. Virol.* 68:1382–1396.

25. Cubitt, B. and de la Torre, J. C. 1997. Amantadine does not have antiviral activity against Borna disease virus. *Arch. Virol.* 142:2035–2042.

26. Czygan, M., Hallensleben, W., Hofer, M., Pollak, S., Sauder, C., Bilzer, T., Blu$ mcke, I., Riederer, P., Bogerts, B., Falkai, P., Schwarz, M. J., Masliah, E., Staeheli, P., Hufert, F. T. and Lieb, K. 1999. Borna disease virus in human brains with a rare form of hippocampal degeneration but not in brains of patients with common neuropsychiatric disorders. *J. Infect. Dis.* 180:1695–1699.

27. Dauphin, G., Legay, V., Pitel, P. H. and Zientara, S. 2002. Borna disease: Current knowledge and virus detection in France. *Vet. Res.* 33:127–138.

28. de la Torre, J. C. 1994. Molecular biology of Borna disease virus: Prototype of a new group of animal viruses. *J. Virol.* 68:7669–75.

29. Dieckhofer, R. 2008. Infections in horses: Diagnosis and therapy. *APMIS Suppl.* 124:40–43.

30. Dietrich, D. E., Bode, L., Spannhuth, C. W., Lau, T., Huber, T. J., Brodhun, B., Ludwig, H. and Emrich, H. M. 2000. Amantadine in depressive patients with Borna disease virus (BDV) infection: An open trial. *Bipolar Disord.* 2:65–70.

31. Dietzel, J., Kuhrt, H., Stahl, T., Kacza, J., Seeger, J., Weber, M., Uhlig, A., Reichenbach, A., Grosche, A. and Pannicke, T. 2007. Morphometric analysis of the retina from horses infected with the Borna disease virus. *Vet Pathol.* 44:57–63.

32. Dürrwald, R. 1993. Die naturliche Borna-Virus-Infektion der Einhufer und Schafe. Untersuchungen zur Epidemiologie, zu neueren diagnostischen Methoden (ELISA, PCR) und zur Antiko rperkinetik bei Pferden nach Vakzination mit Lebendimpfstoff. Inaugural dissertation (Dr. Med. Vet.), Freie Universitast, Berlin, Germany.

33. Dürrwald, R. and Ludwig, H. 1997. Borna disease virus (BDV), a (zoonotic?) worldwide pathogen. A 136 G. Dauphin et al. review of the history of the disease and the virus infection with comprehensive bibliography. *J. Vet. Med. Series B.* 44:147–184.

34. Eisenman, L. M., Brother, R., Tran, M. H., Kean, R. B., Dickson, G. M., Dietzschold, B. and Hooper, D. C. 1999. Neonatal Borna disease virus infection in the rat causes a loss of Purkinje cells in the cerebellum. *J. Neuro. Virol.* 5:181–189.

35. Ernst, M., Zametkin, A. J., Matochik, J. A., Pascualvaca, D. and Cohen, R. M. 1997. Low medial prefrontal dopaminergic activity in autistic children. *Lancet* 350:638.

36. Ernst, W. and Hahn, H. 1926. Bestehen Aussichten, gegen die seuchenhafte Gehirn-Rückenmarksentzündung der Pferde (Borna'sche Krankheit) zu immunisieren *Berl. Münch. tierärztl. Wochenschr.* 77:477–478.

37. Ferszt, R., Kuhl, K. P., Bode, L., Severus, E. W., Winzer, B., Berghofer, A., Beelitz, G., Brodhun, B., Muller-Oerlinghausen, B. and Ludwig, H. 1999. Amantadine revisited: An open trial of amantadinesulfate treatment in chronically depressed patients with Borna disease virus infection. *Pharmacopsychiatry* 32:142–147.

38. Fu, Z. F., Amsterdam, J. D., Kao, M., Shankar, V., Koprowski, H. and Dietzschold, B. 1993. Detection of Borna disease virus-reactive antibodies from patients with affective disorders by western immunoblot technique. *J. Affective Disorders* 27:61–68.

39. Furrer, E., Bilzer, T., Stitz, L. and Planz, O. 2001. Neutralizing antibodies in persistent borna disease virus infection: Prophylactic effect of gp94-specific monoclonal antibodies in preventing encephalitis. *J. Virol.* 75:943–951.

40. Galabru, J., Saron, M. F., Berg, M., Berg, A. L., Herzog, S., Labie, J. and Zientara, S. 2000. Borna disease virus antibodies in French horses. *Vet Rec.* 147:721–722.

41. Gellert, M. 1995. In the beginning the horse is sad: A historical abstract of Borna Disease. *Tierarztl Prax* 23:207–16.

42. Gosztonyi, G. and Ludwig, H. 1984. Borna disease of horses. An immunohistological and virological study of naturally infected animals. *Acta Neuropathologica* (Berlin) 64:213–221.

43. Gosztonyi, G. and Ludwig, H. 1995. Borna disease neuropathology and pathogenesis. *Curr. Top. Microbiol. Immunol.* 190:39–73.

44. Grabner, A., Herzog, S., Lange-Herbst, H. and Frese, K. 2002. Die intra-vitam-Diagnose der Bornaschen Krankheit bei Equiden. *Pferdeheilkunde* 18:579–586.

45. Hagiwara, K., Nakaya, T., Nakamura, Y., Asahi, S., Takahashi, H., Ishihara, C. and Ikuta, K. 1996. Borna disease virus RNA in peripheral blood mononuclear cells obtained from healthy dairy cattle. *Med. Microbiol. Immunol.* 185:145–151.

46. Hagiwara, K., Kawamoto, S., Takahashi, H., Nakamura, Y., Nakaya, T., Hiramune, T., Ishihara, C. and Ikuta, K. 1997a. High prevalence of Borna disease virus infection in healthy sheep in Japan. *Clin. Diag. Lab. Immunol.* 4:339–344.

47. Hagiwara, K., Momiyama, N., Taniyama, H., Nakaya, T., Tsunoda, N., Ishihara, C. and Ikuta, K. 1997b. Demonstration of Borna disease virus (BDV) in specific regions of the brain from horses positive for serum antibodies to BDV but negative for BDV RNA in the blood and internal organs. *Med. Microbiol. Immunol.* 186:19–24.

48. Hagiwara, K., Okamoto, M., Kamitani, W., Takamura, S., Taniyama, H., Tsunoda, N., Tanaka, H., Iwai, H. and Ikuta, K. 2002. Nosological study of Borna disease virus infection in race horses. *Vet Microbiol.* 84:367–374.

49. Hamner, M. B. and Diamond, B. I. 1996. Plasma dopamine and norepinephrine correlations with psychomotor retardation, anxiety, and depression in non-psychotic depressed patients: A pilot study. *Psychiatry Res.* 64:209–211.

50. Hans, A., Syan, S., Crosio, C., Sassone-Corsi, P., Brahic, M. and Gonzalez-Dunia, D. 2001. Borna disease virus persistent infection activates mitogen-activated protein kinase and blocks neuronal differentiation of PC12 cells. *J. Biol. Chem.* 276:7258–7265.

51. Hatalski, C. G., Kliche, S., Stitz, L. et al. 1995. Neutralizing antibodies in Borna disease virus infected rats. *J. Virol.* 69:741–747.

52. Hatalski, C. G., Lewis, A. J. and Lipkin, W. I. 1997. Borna disease. *Emerg. Infect. Dis.* 3:129–135.

53. Hatalski, C. G., Hickey, W. F. and Lipkin, W. I. 1998. Evolution of the immune response in the central nervous system following infection with Borna disease virus. *J. Neuroimmunol.* 90:137–142.

54. Herden, C., Herzog, S., Richt, J. A., Nesseler, A., Christ M., Failing, K. and Frese, K. 2000. Distribution of Borna disease virus in the brain of rats infected with an obesity-inducing virus strain. *Brain Pathol.* 10:39–48.

55. Herden, C., Herzog, S., Wehner, T., Zink, C., Richt, J. A. and Frese, K. 1999. Comparison of different methods of diagnosing Borna disease in horses post mortem. *Equine Infect. Dis.* 8:286–290.

56. Herzog, S. and Rott, R. 1980. Replication of Borna disease virus in cell cultures. *Med Microbiol. Immunol.* (Berl) 173:153–158.

57. Herzog, S., Frese, K., Richt, J. A. and Rott, R. 1994. Ein beitrag zur epizootiologie der Bornaschen krankheit blim Pferd. *Wien Tierarztl Mschr.* 81:374–379.

58. Hilbe, M., Herrsche, R., Kolodziejek, J., Nowotny, N., Zlinszky, K. and Ehrensperger, F. 2006. Shrews as reservoir hosts of Borna disease virus. *Emerging Infect. Dis.* 12:675–677.

59. Horimoto, T., Takahashi, H., Sakaguchi, M., Horikoshi, K., Iritani, S., Kazamatsuri, H., Ikeda, K. and Tashiro, M. 1997. A reverse-type sandwich enzyme-linked immunosorbent assay for detecting antibodies to Borna disease virus. *J. Clin. Microbiol.* 35:1661–1666.

60. Hornig, M., Weissenbock, H., Horscroft, N. and Lipkin, W. I. 1999. An infection-based model of neurodevelopmental damage. *Proc. Natl. Acad. Sci. U.S.A.* 96:12102–12107.

61. Hornig, M., Briese, T. and Lipkin, W. I. 2003. Borna disease virus. *J. NeuroVirol.* 9:259–273.

62. Iwata, Y., Takahashi, K., Peng, X., Fukuda, K., Ohno, K., Ogawa, T., Gonda, K., Mori, N., Niwa, S. I. and Shigeta, S. 1998. Detection and sequence analysis of Borna disease virus p24 RNA from peripheral blood mononuclear cells of patients with mood disorders or schizophrenia and of blood donors. *J. Virol.* 72:10044–10049.

63. Joest, E. and Degen, K. 1911. Untersuchungen über die pathologische Histologie, Pathogenese und postmortale Diagnose der seuchenhaften Gehirn-Rückenmarksentzündung (Bornaschen Krankheit) des Pferdes, *Ztschr. f. Infectionskrankh, parasit. Krankh. u. Hyg. d. Haustiere* 9:1–98.

64. Jones, T. C., Hunt, R. D. and King, N. W. 1997. *Veterinary pathology*, 6th ed. Blackwell Publishing. 369–370.

65. Jordan, I., Briese, T., Averett, D. R. and Lipkin, W. I. 1999. Inhibition of Borna disease virus replication by ribavirin. *J. Virol.* 73:7903–7906.

66. Jordan, I. and Lipkin, W. I. 2001. Borna disease virus. *Rev Med Virol.* 11:37–57.

67. Kacza, J., Mohr, C., Pannicke, T., Kuhrt, H., Dietzel, J., Fluss, M., Richt, J. A., Vahlenkamp, T. W., Stahl, T., Reichenbach, A. and Seeger, J. 2001. Changes of the organotypic retinal organization in Borna virus-infected Lewis rats. *J. Neurocytol.* 30:801–820.

68. Kamitani, W., Shoya, Y., Kobayashi, T., Watanabe, M., Lee, B. J., Zhang, G., Tomonaga, K. and Ikuta, K. 2001. Borna disease virus phosphoprotein binds a neurite outgrowth factor, amphoterin/HMG-1. *J. Virol.* 75:8742–8751.

69. Kao, M., Hamir, A. N., Rupprecht, C. E., Fu, Z. F., Shankar, V., Koprowski, H. and Dietzschold, B. 1993. Detection of antibodies against Borna disease virus in sera and CSF of horses in the USA. *Vet. Rec.* 132:241–244.

70. Karpas, W. J., Peterson, J. D. and Miller, S. D. 1994. Anergy in vivo: Downregulation of antigen-specific CD4C Th1 but not Th2 cytokine responses. *Int. Immunol.* 6:721–730.

71. Katz, J. B., Alstad, D., Jenny, A. L., Carbone, K. M., Rubin, S. A. and Waltrip, R. W. II. 1998. Clinical, serologic, and histopathologic characterization of experimental Borna disease in ponies. *J. Vet. Diag. Invest.* 10:338–343.

72. Kelsoe, J. R., Savodnick, A. D., Kristbjarnarson, H., Bergesch, P., Mroczkowski-Parker, Z., Drennan, M., Rapaport, M. H., Flodman, P., Spence, M. A. and Remick, R. A. 1996. Possible locus for bipolar disorder near the dopamine transporter on chromosome 5. *Am. J. Med. Genet.* 67:533–540.

73. Khoury, S. J., Akalin, E., Chandraker, A., Turka, L. A., Linsley, P. S., Sayegh, M. H. and Hancock, W. W. 1995. CD28-B7 costimulatory blockade by CTLA4Ig prevents actively induced experimental autoimmune encephalomyelitis and inhibits Th1 but spares Th2 cytokines in the central nervous system. *J. Immunol.* 155:4521–4524.

74. Kishi, M., Nakaya, T., Nakamura, Y., Zhong, Q., Ikeda, K., Senjo, M., Kakinuma, M., Kato, S. and Ikuta, K. 1995. Demonstration of human Borna disease virus RNA in human peripheral blood mononuclear cells. *FEBS Letters* 364:293–297.

75. Kishi, M., Arimura, Y., Ikuta, K., Shoya, Y., Lai, P. K. and Kakinuma, M. 1996. Sequence variability of Borna disease virus open reading frame II found in human peripheral blood mononuclear cells. *J. Virol.* 70:635–640.

76. Köster-Patzlaff, C., Hosseini, S. M. and Reuss, B. 2009. Loss of connexin36 in rat hippocampus and cerebellar cortex in persistent Borna disease virus infection. *J. Chem. Neuroanat.* 37:118–127.

77. Krey, H. F., Ludwig, H. and Boschek, C. B. 1979a. Multifocal retinopathy in Borna disease virus infected rabbits. *Am. J. Ophthalmol.* 87:157–164.

78. Krey, H. F., Ludwig, H. and Rott, R. 1979b. Spread of infectious virus along the optic nerve into the retina in Borna disease virus-infected rabbits. *Arch. Virol.* 61:283–288.

79. Legay, V., Sailleau, C., Dauphin, G. and Zientara, S. 2000. Construction of an internal standard used in RT nested PCR for Borna disease virus RNA detection in biological samples. *Vet Res.* 31:565–572.

80. Lipkin, W. I., Schneeman, A. and Solbrig, M. L. 1995. Borna disease virus: Implications for human neuropsychiatric illness. *Trends Microbiol.* 3:64–69.

81. Ludwig, H., Bode, L. and Gosztonyi G. 1988. Borna disease: A persistent virus infection of the central nervous system. *Prog. Med. Virol.* 35:107–151.

82. Ludwig, H., Furuya, K., Bode, L. et al. 1993. Biology and neurobiology of Borna disease virus (BDV) defined by antibodies, neutralizability, and their pathogenic potential. *Arch. Virol. Suppl.* 7:111–133.

83. Ludwig, H. and Bode, L. 2000. Borna disease virus: New aspects on infection, disease, diagnosis and epidemiology. *Rev. Sci. Tech. Off. Int. Epiz.* 19:259–288.

84. Lundgren, A. L., Czech, G., Bode, L. and Ludwig, H. 1993. Natural Borna disease in domestic animals other than horses and sheep. *J. Vet. Med. Series* B 40:298–303.

85. Lundgren, A. L., Zimmermann, W., Bode, L., Czech, G., Gosztonyi, G., Lindberg, R. and Ludwig, H. 1995. Staggering disease in cats: Isolation and characterization of the feline Borna disease virus. *J. Gen. Virol.* 76:2215–2222.

86. Malkinson, M., Weisman, Y., Ashash, E., Bode, L. and Ludwig, H. 1993. Borna disease in ostriches. *Vet. Rec.* 133:304.

87. Malkinson, M., Weisman, Y., Perl, S. and Asash, E. 1995. A Bornalike disease of ostriches in Israel. Borna Disease. *Curr. Top. Microbiol. Immunol.* 190:31–8.

88. Metzler, A., Ehrensperger, F. and Danner, K. 1979. Bornavirus-Infektion bei Schafen: Verlaufsuntersuchungen nach spontaner Infektion, unter besonderer Beru cksichtigung der Antiko rperkinetik im Serum und Liquor cerebrospinalis. *Schweizer Archiv fuXr Tierheilkunde* 121:37–48.

89. Mizutani, T., Inagaki, H., Araki, K., Kariwa, H., Arikawa, J. and Takashima, I. 1998. Inhibition of Borna disease virus replication by ribavirin in persistently infected cells. *Arch. Virol.* 143:2039–2044.

90. Möhlmann, H. and Maas, A. 1960. Wertigkeitsprüfung des Borna-Trockenimpfstoffes "Dessau" bei Pferden unter den Verhältnissen der Praxis. *Arch. Experim. Vet Med.* 14:1267–1280.

91. Morales, J. A., Herzog, S., Kompter, C., Frese, K. and Rott, R. 1988. Axonal transport of Borna disease virus along olfactory pathways in spontaneously and experimentally infected rats. *Med. Microbiol. Immunol.* 177:51–68.

92. Moussu, R. and Marchand, L. 1924. L'encéphalite enzootique du cheval (maladie de Borna). *Rec. Méd. Vét.* 100:5–44, 65–90.

93. Nakamura, Y., Kishi, M., Nakaya, T., Asahi, S., Tanaka, S., Sentsui, H., Ikeda, K. and Ikuta, K. 1995. Demonstration of Borna disease virus RNA in peripheral blood mononuclear cells from healthy horses in Japan. *Vaccine* 13:1076–1079.

94. Nakamura, Y., Asahi, S., Nakaya, T., Bahmani, M. K., Saitoh, S., Yasui, K., Mayama, H., Hagiwara, K., Ishihara, C. and Ikuta, K. 1996. Demonstration of Borna disease virus RNA in peripheral blood mononuclear cells derived from domestic cats in Japan. *J. Clin. Microbiol.* 34:188–191.

95. Nakamura, Y., Watanabe, M., Kamitani, W., Taniyama, H., Nakaya, T., Nishimura, Y., Tsujimoto, H., Machida, S. and Ikuta, K. 1999. High prevalence of Borna disease virus in domestic cats with neurological disorders in Japan. *Vet. Microbiol.* 70:153–169.

96. Nakaya, T., Takahashi, H., Nakamura, Y., Asahi, S., Tobiume, M., Kuratsune, H., Kitani, T., Yamanishi, K. and Ikuta, K. 1996. Demonstration of Borna disease virus RNA in peripheral blood mononuclear cells derived from Japanese patients with chronic fatigue syndrome. *FEBS Letters* 378:145–149.

97. Narayan, O., Herzog, S., Frese, K., Scheefers, H. and Rott, R. 1983. Pathogenesis of Borna disease in rats: Immune-mediated viral ophthalmoencephalopathy causing blindness and behavioral abnormalities, *J. Infect. Dis.* 148:305–315.

98. Nowotny, N. and Kolodziejek, J. 2000. Demonstration of Borna disease virus nucleic acid in a patient suffering from chronic fatigue syndrome. *J. Infect. Dis.* 181:860–1861.

99. Nowotny, N., Kolodziejek, J., Jehle, C. O., Suchy, A., Staeheli, P. and Schwemmle, M. 2000. Isolation and characterization of a new subtype of Borna disease virus. *J. Virol.* 74:5655–5658.

100. Okamoto, M., Kagawa, Y., Kamitani, W., Hagiwara, K., Kirisawa, R., Iwai, H., Ikuta, K. and Taniyama, H. 2002. Borna disease in a dog in Japan. *J. Comp. Pathol.* 126:312–317.

101. Partonen, T. 1996. Dopamine and circadian rhythms in seasonal affective disorder. *Med. Hyp.* 47:191–192.

102. Patti, A. M., Vulcano, A., Candelori, E. and Travali, S. 2008. Serological evidence for Borna disease virus infection in children, cats and horses in Sicily (Italy). *APMIS Suppl.* 124:77–79.

103. Pisoni, G., Nativi, D., Bronzo, V. and Codazza, D. 2007. Sero-epidemiological study of Borna disease virus infection in the Italian equine population. *Vet. Res. Commun. Suppl.* 1:245–148.

104. Planz, O., Pleschka, S. and Ludwig, S. 2001. MEK-specific inhibitor U0126 blocks spread of Borna disease virus in cultured cells. *J. Virol.* 75:4871–4877.

105. Prat, C., Schmid, S., Schwemmle, M. and Gonzalez-Dunia, D. 2008. Borna disease virus phosphoprotein interferes with neuronal function and contributes to neurobehavioral disorders. *BMC Proc. 2 (Suppl. 1): P56.*

106. Reeves, N. A., Helps, C. R., Gunn-Moore, D. A., Blundell, C., Finnermore, P. L., Pearson, G. R. and Harbour, D. A. 1998. Natural Borna disease virus infection in cats in the United Kingdom. *Vet. Rec.* 143:523–526.

107. Richt, J. A., Vande Woude, S., Zink, M. C., Clements, J. E., Herzog, S. and Stitz, L. 1992. Infection with Borna disease virus: Molecular and immunobiological characterization of the agent. *Clin. Inf. Dis.* 14:1240–50.

108. Richt, J. A., Herzog, S., Haberzettl, K. and Rott, R. 1993. Demonstration of Borna disease virus-specific RNA in secretions of naturally infected horses by the polymerase chain reaction. *Med. Microbiol. Immunol.* 182:293–304.

109. Richt, J. A., Alexander, R. C., Herzog, S., Hooper, D. C., Kean, R., Spitsin, S., Bechter, K., Schuttler, R., Feldmann, H., Heiske, A., Fu, Z. F., Dietzschold, B., Rott, R. and Koprowski, H. 1997. Failure to detect Borna disease virus infection in peripheral leucocytes from humans with psychiatric disorders. *J. Neurovirol.* 3:174–178.

110. Richt, J. A. and Rott, R. 2001. Borna disease virus: A mystery as an emerging zoonotic pathogen. *Vet. J.* 161:24–40.

111. Richt, J. A., Grabner, A., Herzog, S., Garten, W. and Herden, C. 2007. Borna disease. In *Equine infectious diseases*, ed. D. C. Sellon and M. T. Long, chapter 22, 207–213. Philadelphia, USA: Saunders, Elsevier Inc.

112. Rott, R., Herzog, S., Fleischer, B., Winokur, A., Amsterdam, J., Dyson, W. and Koprowski, H. 1985. Detection of serum antibodies to Borna disease virus in patients with psychiatric disorders. *Science* 228:755–756.

113. Rott, R. and Becht H. 1995. Natural and experimental Borna disease in animals. *Curr. Top. Microbiol. Immunol.* 190:17–30.

114. Rubin, S. A., Sierra-Honigmann, A. M., Lederman, H. M., Waltrip, R. W. II, Eiden, J. J. and Carbone, K. M. 1995. Hematologic consequences of Borna disease virus infection of rat bone marrow and thymus stromal cells. *Blood* 85:2762–2769.

115. Rubin, S. A., Sylves, P., Vogel, M., Pletnikov, M., Moran, T. H., Schwartz, G. J. and Carbone, K. M. 1999. Borna disease virusinduced hippocampal dentate gyrus damage is associated with spatial learning and memory deficits. *Brain Res. Bull.* 48:23–30.

116. Sauder, C., Muller, A., Cubitt, B., Mayer, J., Steinmetz, J., Trabert, W., Ziegler, B., Wanke, K., Mueller-Lantzsch, N., de la Torre, J. C. and Grasser, F. A. 1996. Detection of Borna disease virus (BDV)

antibodies and BDV RNA in psychiatric patients: Evidence for high sequence conservation of human blood-derived BDV RNA. *J. Virol.* 70:7713–7724.

117. Schneemann, A., Schneider, P. A., Lamb, R. A. and Lipkin, W. I. 1995. The remarkable coding strategy of Borna disease virus: A new member of the nonsegmented negative strand RNA viruses. *Virol.* 210:1–8.

118. Schneider, P. A., Briese, T., Zimmermann, W., Ludwig, H. and Lipkin, W. I. 1994. Sequence conservation in field and experimental isolates of Borna disease virus. *J. Virol.* 68:63–68.

119. Schwartz, R. H. 1992. Costimulation of T lymphocytes: The role of CD28, CTLA-4 and B4/BB1 in interleukin-2 production and immunotherapy. *Cell* 71:1065–1068.

120. Sellon, D. C. 2007. Papillomavirus Infections. In *Equine infectious diseases*, ed. D. C. Sellon and M. T. Long, chapter 25, 226–232. Philadelphia, USA: Saunders, Elsevier Inc.

121. Shankar, V., Kao, M., Hamir, A. N., Sheng, H., Koprowski, H. and Dietzschold, B. 1992. Kinetics of virus spread and changes in levels of several cytokine mRNAs in the brain after intranasal infection of rats with Borna disease virus. *J. Virol.* 66:992–998.

122. Sierra-Honigmann, A. M., Rubin, S. A., Estafanous, M. G., Yolken, R. H. and Carbone, K. M. 1993. Borna disease virus in peripheral blood mononuclear and bone marrow cells of neonatally and chronically infected rats. *J. Neuroimmunol.* 45:31–36.

123. Sobbe, M., Bilzer, T., Gommel, S., Noske, K., Planz, O. and Stitz, L. 1997. Induction of degenerative brain lesions after adoptive transfer of brain lymphocytes from Borna disease virus-infected rats: Presence of CD8C T cells and perforin mRNA. *J. Virol.* 71:2400–2407.

124. Solbrig, M. V., Koob, G. F., Fallon, J. H. and Lipkin, W. I. 1994. Tardive dyskinetic syndrome in rats infected with Borna disease virus. *Neurobiol. Dis.* 1:111–119.

125. Solbrig, M. V., Fallon, J. H. and Lipkin, W. I. 1995. Behavioral disturbances and pharmacology of Borna disease virus. *Curr. Top. Microbiol. Immunol.* 190:93–102.

126. Solbrig, M. V., Koob, G. F. and Lipkin, W. I. 1998. Cocaine sensitivity in Borna disease virus-infected rats. *Pharmacol. Biochem. Behav.* 59:1047–1052.

127. Solbrig, M. V., Koob, G. F., Parsons, L. H., Kadota, T., Horscroft, N., Briese, T. and Lipkin, W. I. 2000. Neurotrophic factor expression after CNS viral injury produces enhanced sensitivity to psychostimulants: Potential mechanism for addiction vulnerability. *J. Neurosci.* 20:RC104.

128. Sorg, I. and Metzler, A. 1995. Detection of Borna disease virus RNA in formalin-fixed, paraffin-embedded brain tissues by nested PCR. *J. Clin. Microbiol.* 33:821–823.

129. Staeheli, P., Sauder, C., Hausmann, J., Ehrensperger, F. and Schwemmle, M. 2000. Epidemiology of Borna disease virus. *J. Gen. Virol.* 81:2123–2135.

130. Stitz, L., Dietzschold, B. and Carbone, K. M. 1995. Immunopathogenesis of Borna disease. *Curr. Top. Microbiol. Immunol.* 190:75–92.

131. Stitz, L., Planz, O. and Bilzer, T. 1998. Lack of antiviral effect of amantadine in Borna disease virus infection. *Med. Microbiol. Immunol.* 186:195–200.

132. Tsuji, K., Toyomasu, K., Imamura, Y., Maeda, H. and Toyoda, T. 2000. No association of borna disease virus with psychiatric disorders among patients in northern Kyushu, Japan. *J. Med. Virol.* 61:336–340.

133. Uhlig, A. and Kinne, J. 1998. Neurologische Befunde bei Pferden mit Bornascher Krankheit. *Prakt. Tierärztl. Coll. Vet.* XXVIII:33.

134. Vahlenkamp, T. W., Enbergs, H. K. and Muller, H. 2000. Experimental and natural Borna disease virus infections: Presence of viral RNA in cells of the peripheral blood. *Vet. Microbiol.* 76:229–244.

135. Waltrip, I. I., Buchanan, R. W., Summerfelt, A., Breier, A., Carpenter, W. T., Bryant, N. L., Rubin, S. A. and Carbone, K. M. 1995. Borna disease virus and schizophrenia. *Psychiatry Res.* 56:33–44.

136. Weissenböck, H., Bilzer, T., Ehrensperger, F., Gosztonyi, G., Herden, C., Staehli, P., Hausmann, J. and Pagenstecher, A. 2002. Equine borna disease in Japan. *Vet Rec.* 151:712.

137. Weissenbock, H., Nowotny, N., Caplazi, P., Kolodziejek, J. and Ehrensperger, F. 1998a. Borna disease in a dog with lethal meningoencephalitis. *J. Clin. Microbiol.* 36:2127–2130.

138. Weissenbock, H., Suchy, A., Caplazi, P., Herzog, S. and Nowotny, N. 1998b. Borna disease in Austrian horses. *Vet. Rec.* 143:21–22.

139. Yamaguchi, K., Sawada, T., Naraki, T., Igata-Yi, R., Shiraki, H., Horii, Y., Ishii, T., Ikeda, K., Asou, N., Okabe, H., Mochizuki, M., Takahashi, K., Yamada, S., Kubo, K., Yashiki, S., Waltrip, R. W. and Carbone, K. M. 1999. Detection of Borna disease virus-reactive antibodies from patients with psychiatric disorders and from horses by electrochemiluminescence immunoassay. *Clin. Diag. Lab. Immunol.* 6:696–700.

140. Yamaguchi, K., Sawada, T., Yamane, S., Haga, S., Ikeda, K., Igata-Yi, R., Yoshiki, K., Matsuoka, M., Okabe, H., Horii, Y., Nawa, Y., Waltrip, R. W. II and KM Carbone 2001. Synthetic peptide-based electrochemiluminescence immunoassay for anti-Borna disease virus p40 and p24 antibodies in rat and horse serum. *Ann. Clin. Biochem.* 38:348–355.

141. Yilmaz, H., Helps, C. R., Turan, N., Uysal, A. and Harbour, D. A. 2002. Detection of antibodies to Borna disease virus (BDV) in Turkish horse sera using recombinant p40. Brief report. *Arch Virol.* 147:429–345.

142. Zimmermann, W., Durrwald, R. and Ludwig, H. 1994. Detection of Borna disease virus RNA in naturally infected animals by a nested polymerase chain reaction. *J. Virol. Methods* 46:133–143.

143. Zwick, W. 1939. Bornasche Krankheit und Enzephalomyelitis der Tiere. In *Handbuch der Viruskrankheiten*, 2nd ed., E. Gildenmeister, E. Haagen and O. Waldmann, 254–354. Jena, Fischer.

144. Zwick, W. and Witte, J. 1931. Ueber die Widerstandsfahigkeit des Virus der Bornaschen Krankheit gegen Trocknung und u ber Schutzimpfungsversuche mit getrockneter virushaltiger Gehirnsubstanz. *Berliner TieraXrztliche Wochenschrift* 47:33–35.

145. Zwick, W. and Witte, J. 1932. Zur Frage der Schutzimpfung und der Inkubationsfrist bei der Bornaschen Krankheit. *Arch. Tierheilkd.* 64:116–124.

3. EQUINE ADENOVIRUSES

S. KAPOOR, K. DHAMA, R. V. S. PAWAIYA, AND D. K. GUPTA

INTRODUCTION

Contagious respiratory infections in horses can occur as a result of infection with many different viruses, mycoplasma, and bacteria. The viruses that can result in equine respiratory disease are the following: equine influenza virus type A, subtypes 1 and 2, equine herpesviruses type 1, 2 and 4, equine rhinitis viruses type 1, 2 and 3, equine arteritis virus; equine reoviruses; and equine adenoviruses (Mayr and Thein, 1984; Jolly et al., 1986; Mayr, 1987; Herbst et al., 1992; Powell, 1991; Carman et al., 1997; Dunowska et al., 2002a, b). The severity of clinical disease due to these viruses is influenced by the virulence of the viral isolate, dose, management, environmental conditions, and host defenses. Subclinical infections are common and occur in association with partial immunity as a result of maternal antibody, vaccination, or previous infection. These viruses produce similar clinical signs, with no clinical sign being characteristic of any one virus infection. Therefore, isolation and identification of virus is essential for confirmation of diagnosis.

Serologic surveys for equine adenovirus indicate that infection is widespread; however, the majority of infections do not result in clinical disease (Harasawa et al., 1977; Jolly et al., 1986; *Adeyefa* and *Durojaiye,* 1992; Herbst et al., 1992; Cullinane et al., 2006; Studdert, 2007). Adenovirus pneumonia is well documented in Arabian foals, and the virus has been isolated from foals of other breeds with respiratory disease and from clinically normal foals. The virus was first reported in Australia and has been isolated in 1970 and thereafter in the USA from Arabian foals suffering from respiratory diseases (Johnston and Hutchins, 1967; Todd, 1969; McChesney et al., 1970; Sherrod, 1973; Thompson et al., 1976; Moorthy and Spradbrow, 1978), as well as from clinically normal foals (Harden et al., 1972). Adenovirus infection does not appear to be a significant problem in adult horses, but it has occasionally been associated with upper respiratory disease, ocular discharge, and soft feces in race horses. Adenoviruses cause dominant infections in immunocompromised horses. Equine adenoviruses do not affect humans and/or cause any public health implications (Studdert, 2007).

Recently, adenoviruses have driven attention of the scientific community by possessing the beneficial potential to be used as vectors for the delivery of foreign genes for many genetically engineered recombinant vaccines against numerous infectious agents ranging from malaria to HIV-1.

Additionally, recombinant adenoviruses (rAd) are being explored as vaccines against a multitude of tumor-associated antigens and for the correction of defective genes in humans and the in vivo gene delivery for therapeutic purposes for the deadliest maladies like cancers and other diseases. However, at times these have resulted in untoward and unexpected often-dangerous consequences, which implies that caution must be exercised in promoting adenoviruses as generally insignificant pathogens and hence their applicability as vaccine vectors or gene therapy purposes (Studdert, 2000; Jooss and Chirmule, 2003; Tatsis and Ertl, 2004; Gabrilovich, 2006; Ghosh et al., 2006; Hartman et al., 2008; Tucker et al., 2008; Patterson et al., 2009).

ETIOLOGY

Equine adenoviruses are classified under genus *Mastadenovirus* of family Adenoviridae. Historically, two serotypes of equine adenoviruses were identified, viz, equine adenovirus serotype 1 and equine adenovirus serotype 2. The serologically distinguishable serotypes (synonym of types, designated by Arabic numbers) of genus *Mastadenovirus* have now been grouped into species. Species name reflects the first described host complemented by a letter if there are more than one adenovirus species bearing the same host name. The lack of cross-neutralization combined with a calculated phylogenetic distance of more than 10% separates two serotypes into different species. Currently, there are nineteen species within the genus *Mastadenovirus*. The viruses previously classified as serotypes of equine adenovirus have been reclassified as two separate species infecting equines within this genus (Benco et al., 2005). Therefore, equine adenovirus A is synonym for equine adenovirus serotype 1, commonly known as equine adenovirus 1 (EAdV-1), and equine adenovirus B is synonym for equine adenovirus serotype 2, commonly known as equine adenovirus 2 (EAdV-2).

The biophysical properties of equine adenoviruses (EAdVs) are similar to those of adenoviruses of other species. Adenovirus virions are nonenveloped, 70–80 nm in diameter with icosahedral symmetry. The capsid has a total of 252 capsomers consisting of 12 pentons present on the 12 apices, and 240 hexons occupy the 20 faces and 12 edges of the icosahedron. The fibers with terminal knob project from each of the 12 pentons. The EAdV1 fibers are reported to be the longest among adenoviruses (Fatemie et al., 1979). These fibers contain genus and type-specific determinants and cause hemagglutination. Type-specific antigenic determinants defined by serum neutralization (SN) and hemagglutination (HI) assays are located on the outward surface of the hexamers.

Only the EAdV1, and not the EAdV2, causes hemagglutination of equine and human blood group O erythrocytes (Wilks and Studdert, 1972; Studdert and Blackney, 1982). Virus infectivity is inactivated after heating at 56°C for more than ten minutes. The virus has a buoyant density of 1.31–1.34 g/ml in cesium chloride (Ardans et al., 1973). The genome consists of double-stranded DNA. The sequence data reveals the size of Mastadenovirus genomes to be in the range of 30,288 and 36,521 bp. The G+C content of the DNA varies between 40.8 and 63.8%. The inverted terminal repeats (ITRs) of Mastadenoviruses are considerably longer and consist of a variety of cellular-factor binding sites, making them more complex as compared to members of the other genera. The size of genome of EAdV1 is 34.4 kilobase pair (kbp), with inverted terminal repeats (Sheppard et al., 1992). Therefore, the genome size of EAdV1 is slightly smaller than human adenoviruses but larger than the murine or canine adenoviruses (Temple et al., 1981; Jouvenne et al., 1987). The genome is linked to a 55k protein at each 5' terminus making the genome infectious.

Only limited studies have been conducted on the molecular characterization, genome organization, and genomic sequence data of EAdV1 and EAdV2 (Shinagawa et al., 1983; Higashi and Harasawa, 1989; Sheppard et al., 1992; Reubel and Studdert, 1997a; 1997b). The hexon gene EAdV1 was identified on the basis of sequence homology with human adenovirus 2 (HAdV2). HindIII restriction fragments containing the hexon and other viral genes of EAdV1 were cloned into the plasmids pUC19 and pBlueScript SK(-) and sequenced. The complete nucleotide sequence of the hexon gene of EAdV1 was determined, and partial sequence was obtained for seven other genes. The genes for the IIIa, penton, pVII, pVI, endopeptidase, DNA binding, and 100K proteins were identified by comparing derived amino acid sequences with published adenovirus proteins. Two highly conserved regions at the N—and C-termini that flank intermediate variable and hypervariable regions in EAdV1 hexon gene were similar to the other members of the genus Mastadenovirus. The residue differences between EAdV1 and other adenovirus hexons have mostly been found in two loops, L1 and L2, that protrude from the surface of the capsid. Amino acid comparisons with other adenovirus hexons revealed highest homology with human adenovirus 12 hexon with 72% identical and 83% functionally similar residues, followed by bovine adenovirus 3 hexon with 71% identical and 82% functionally similar residues (Reubel and Studdert, 1997a).

The complete sequence of the genes of EAdV2 encoding the hexon and the 23K proteinase and the partial sequence of genes encoding E1B/19K, IVa2, DNA polymerase, terminal protein, pVI, DNA binding, and 100K proteins were determined. The EAdV2 hexon was more closely related to the human AdV48 hexon with 71.6% identical and 82.7% functionally similar amino acids than to the EAdV1 hexon gene with 69.3% amino acid identity and 80.7% functional similarity. The deduced amino acid sequence of the EAdV2 23K proteinase gene was most closely related to bovine adenovirus—3 23K proteinase with 59.7% identity and 75.0% similarity. Phylogenetic analysis of the hexon and 23K proteinase genes indicated that EAdV2 does not share an immediate common ancestor with EAdV1 and other adenoviruses. The eight identified EAdV1 genes and nine EAdV2 genes were found to be in the same relative order as the homologous genes of other adenoviruses (Reubel and Studdert, 1997a, 1997b). The proteins of human adenoviruses have been studied extensively and are well characterized. The capsid contains two major proteins, hexon and penton, and many minor proteins: IIIa, VI, VIII and IX. There are six other structural proteins situated in the virus core, five are associated with the double-stranded DNA genome (V, VII, Mu, IVa2, and the terminal protein [TP]), the remaining component is the 23K virion protease, which plays a vital role in the assembly of the virion (Vellinga et al., 2005, Russell, 2009). More work is required for the characterization of the proteins of EAdVs.

EPIDEMIOLOGY

Adenovirus infection in foals is worldwide in occurrence (Todd, 1969; McChesney and England, 1975; Harasawa et al., 1977; Kamada et al., 1977; Mayr and Thein, 1984; Jolly et al., 1986; Adeyefa and Durojaiye, 1992; Herbst et al., 1992 ; Dunowska et al., 2002a, b ; Cullinane et al., 2006; Studdert, 2007). There are two species of equine adenoviruses. The EAdV1 is mainly associated with respiratory infections (Studdert, 1996) and EAdV2 with diarrhea (Studdert and Blackney, 1982). EAdV1 causes acute respiratory disease, follicular conjunctivitis, bronchopneumonia, and infection of gastrointestinal tract; and it is an overriding pathogen to the fatal disorder known as primary, severe, combined immunodeficiency disease (PSCID), which affects certain Arabian foals. Adenovirus can usually be isolated from lung tissue (Cullinane et al., 2006). Latent carrier status and shedding of the virus appear to follow all the adenovirus infections (Studdert, 2007).

The fifty-one human adenovirus serotypes classified originally on the basis of their ability to be neutralized by specific animal antisera have now been subdivided into six species (A to F) based on their capacity to agglutinate erythrocytes of human, rat, and monkey as well as on their oncogenicity in rodents. Sequence availability has also allowed more detailed phylogenetic analysis to be employed in classification (Fauquet et al., 2005). There is some correlation between the human adenovirus species and their tissue tropism and clinical properties. Thus species B1, C, and E mainly cause respiratory disease, whereas species B, D, and E can induce ocular disease. Species

F is responsible for gastroenteritis, and B2 viruses infect the kidneys and urinary tract (Russell, 2009). Whether similar analogous situation observed in equines by EAdV1 and EAdV2 also occur need more detailed studies.

The EAdVs are transmitted through oral and nasopharyngeal routes. Healthy adult horses suffer only on rare occasions from adenoviral-associated respiratory disease, whereas immunocompetent foals show subclinical or asymptomatic infection (Wilks and Studdert, 1972; Studdert et al., 1974; Whitlock et al., 1975) when the maternal antibodies decline to a certain critical level. EAdV1 was detected in the nasal secretions of two healthy postparturient mares with adenovirus-positive offspring, but not in young racehorses (Bell et al., 2006). These differences in prevalence could be the result of age-related and/or gestational influences on immunity or viral persistence (Veenstra van Nieuwenhoven et al., 2003; Adkins et al., 2004). The adenoviruses can establish persistent, possibly latent, infections in other species (Mahr and Gooding, 1999). Studies in a pony herd in UK indicated that EAdV1 may persist in nasopharyngeal mucus up to sixty-eight days after exposure (Burrows et al., 1978). Therefore, origin of these viruses in postparturient mares can also be due to recrudescence of maternal EAdV1 infections (Bell et al., 2006). EAdV 1 has been isolated from a foal, without showing clinical signs at the time of isolation, at three days of age (Wilks and Studdert, 1972). It appears that foals may acquire infection from their dams or other horses in cohort during the suckling period, even in the presence of detectable levels of maternal antibody. Thus, if there is persistent or repeated EAdV infection, the passive immunity of the foals would be converted to an active immunity, probably without significant clinical signs (Studdert, 2007).

Arabian foals with primary, severe, combined immunodeficiency (PSCID) are highly susceptible to infection with equine adenovirus 1 (Whitlock et al., 1975; McGuire et al., 1974; Thompson et al., 1976; Perryman, 2000). The foals are very susceptible to adenovirus in this case, as well as to bacteria—such as *Streptococcus*, *Corynebacterium pyogenes*, *Escherichia coli*, *Staphylococcus aureus*, *Actnobacillus equuli*, *Psedomonas* spp., *Bacillus* spp., and to the protozoan *Pneumocystis carinii*—and usually die before reaching three to five months of age (Cullinane et al., 2006). Progressive infection followed by mortality within three months occurs in these foals in which the maternally derived antibodies have waned. The EAdV1 has also been speculated to be a cause of fatal pneumonia in Fell pony foals with an undefined immunodeficiency (Richards et al., 2000). Normal immunocompetent Thoroughbred foals may occasionally suffer from adenovirus-induced severe or fatal bronchopneumonia (Webb et al., 1981). In a single report, the virus has also been isolated from the spinal cord of a few horses suffering from cauda equina neuritis (Edington et al., 1984). Though unsubstantiated, EAdV1 was reported as a probable cause of abortion in mares (McChesney and England, 1978). Both EAdV2 and rotavirus were isolated from foals with severe diarrhea (Studdert et al., 1978).

Various serological surveys have found that antibodies to EAdV1 are very common, with incidence rates varying from <2–100% (Studdert, 2007). This wide variation in the incidence rate was found to be due to the influence of various factors such as serological test used and age, breed, activity, and size of the population sampled (Timoney, 1971; Harden et al., 1974; Studdert et al., 1974; Kamada, 1978). However, the association between the clinical respiratory disease and presence of adenovirus or seroconversion could not be established in many of the structured studies done in foals (Dunowska et al., 2002a, b) and young Throughbred racehorses (Christley et al., 2001; Newton et al., 2003; Wood et al., 2005). EAdV2 has been isolated from Australia and New Zealand (Horner and Hunter, 1982; Studdert and Blackney, 1982). Of the 339 serum samples collected from various parts of Australia, neutralizing antibodies to EAdV1 and EAdV2 were found in 86% and 77% of the samples, respectively. Besides these, only 51 serum samples were positive for EAdV1 and 19 only for EAdV2 neutralizing antibodies (Studdert and Blackney, 1982).

PATHOGENESIS AND PATHOLOGY
Since the adenovirus infection in normal healthy foals is self-limiting, little information is available about pathogenesis and pathology in them. EAdV1 presumably is frequently acquired as a droplet or close-contact respiratory or ocular infection (Studdert, 2007). The virus replicates in epithelial cells throughout the respiratory tract, producing lysis and sloughing of these cells and a hyperplastic response in underlying noninfected cells. In partial or total maternal antibody–transfer failure cases of foals, respiratory disease is more severe with presence of pneumonitis. In immuonocompetent horses, recovery occurs within a week to ten days due to development of antibodies, and generally virus is not recoverable from these horses by day 10 after infection. However, mixed infection with other pathogens (viruses and bacteria) may exacerbate the disease condition (Burrows and Goodridge, 1978). Reinfection by EAdV1 has been observed to occur frequently in mares and foals, even in the presence of high levels of circulating antibodies (McChesney and England, 1978). Rapidly declining levels of IgA (nasal antibody, the protective local immunoglobulin) after an infection could soon render the horse susceptible to reinfection. EAdV may infect cells of the gastrointestinal tract and may be shed in feces, and presumably it may also be transmitted through a fecal-oral route. Adenovirus in the intestinal epithelium of a foal with prolonged diarrhea has been reported (Corrier et al., 1982).

Experimental infection can occur in both immunocompetent and immunodeficient Arabian and non-Arabian foals. Experimentally, the colostrum-deprived, specific-pathogen-free (SPF) foal showed gross and microscopic evidence of pneumonia, indicating that the virus can cause respiratory disease characterized by nasal discharge, conjunctivitis, rhinitis, tracheitis, bronchitis, bronchopneumonia and interstitial pneumonia, and atelectasis (McChesney et al., 1974; Pascoe et al., 1974; Gleeson et al., 1978). Bronchi may contain thick mucoid exudate. Duodenal villous atrophy and idiopathic glomerular hyperplasia can also be observed. The lymph nodes may show serous inflammation with indistinguishable germinal centers. The virus can also cause cell lysis in the tissues of pancreas, salivary glands, kidney, urinary bladder, and gastrointestinal tract. Typical intranuclear inclusion bodies are present in epithelial cells of respiratory tract. In colostrum-receiving foal, gross and histologic picture of EAdV1 was generally similar but less severe than compared with colostrums-deprived foal (Gleeson et al., 1978).

EAdV infection has been associated with the production of soft feces in adult horses (Powell et al., 1974; Studdert and Blackney, 1982). The replication of EAdV1 in cells of the gastrointestinal tract following experimental intranasal infection further confirmed this observation (Gleeson et al., 1978).

The inherited autosomal defect in PSCID foals causes total absence of both T and B lymphocytes, resulting in immune incompetence. An interesting and intriguing aspect of adenovirus pathogenesis in PSCID foals is that why only adenovirus 1 is able to take advantage of immune incompetence and cause disease in them among all the potential opportunistic pathogens.

CLINICAL SIGNS AND POSTMORTEM LESIONS

Most of the adenovirus infections do not result in clinic disease. Several virus challenge studies have revealed that immunocompetent foals exposed to adenovirus by the respiratory route develop respiratory disease. Colostrum-deprived foals are most susceptible to pneumonia. Immunocompetent foals exposed to adenovirus by natural infection may develop conjunctivitis, dyspnea, fever, cough, and diarrhea. Uncomplicated adenovirus is rarely fatal, but deaths due to combined infections of adenovirus and various bacteria have been reported (Cullinane et al., 2006).

Foals with immunodeficiency develop generalized disease characterized by intermittent fever (pyrexia), nasal discharge, rhinitis, conjunctivitis, pneumonia, coughing after exercise, dyspnea, and less frequently diarrhea (Perryman, 2000; Sellon, 2000; Cullinane et al., 2006; Studdert, 2007;

Crisman and Scarratt, 2008). The submandibular lymph nodes are enlarged, and the delivery of soft and loose feces may be observed. Foals appear normal at birth but develop clinical signs between two and six weeks of age and usually die within two weeks. Lymphopenia is seen on hematologic examination (Cullinane et al., 2006).

In experimental intranasal infection studies on SPF foals, colostrum-deprived foals showed clinical signs that included mucopurulent nasal discharge, severe follicular conjunctivitis, transient anorexia and pyrexia, and sustained polypnea. The colostrum-fed foal showed clinical signs similar to colostrum-deprived foal, except that the severity and duration of fever and conjunctivitis were less, and nasal discharge was minimal. (Gleenson et al., 1978). EAdV1 was readily isolated from both categories of foals from nasal and conjunctival swabs and from lung and trachea. In addition, EAdV1 could also be isolated from rectal swabs, small intestine, or bronchial lymph nodes in the colostrum-deprived foal only when the foals were sacrificed and postmortem conducted six days postinfection. Contrary to these findings, experimental infection of horses with an EAdV1 did not produce clinical disease. Although these animals seroconverted, virus could not be isolated from their nasal swabs (Pascoe et al., 1974). Lesions in colostrum-deprived foals are similar to those in severe combined immunodeficiency disease as described earlier, but their lymphoid systems are normal.

Postmortem findings include necrotizing bronchitis, bronchiolitis, interstitial pneumonia, as well as fibrin and hyaline membranes within the alveoli. Because of bacterial infection, foci of abscess formation are frequently present. The lymph nodes, spleen, and thymus becomes atrophied/smaller with virtually no germinal centers. Large basophilic intranuclear inclusion bodies occur in respiratory epithelial cells and sometimes in the epithelial cells of the salivary glands and ducts, the conjunctivas, the pancreas, the bladders, and the small intestines (Cullinane et al., 2006).

DIAGNOSIS

The diagnosis of any viral respiratory disease relies on laboratory procedures to isolate the virus and demonstrate a significant rise in serum antibody titers. Since adenoviruses do not produce clinical disease, therefore, confirmatory diagnosis of the disease requires isolation of the virus. Virus can be isolated from nasal, ocular or rectal swabs, and infective tissues in equine fetal kidney or equine dermis cell cultures (Studdert et al., 1974; Dutta, 1975; Studdert and Blackney, 1982; Bell et al., 2006) and subsequently confirmed by virus neutralization or hemagglutination tests (Wilks and Studdert, 1972; Studdert et al., 1974; Studdert and Blackney, 1982). Choice for virus isolation is the primary equine kidney cells. EAdV1 isolated from rectal swabs need to be differentiated from EAdV2.

Virus can also be identified in infected tissues by light microscopy, electron microscopy (EM), immunofluorescent, immunohistochemical staining, and polymerase chain reaction (PCR) assay (Vassall, 1974; Shahrabadi et al. 1977; Dynon et al., 2001; Bell et al., 2006). Intranuclear inclusion bodies, the well-known feature of the cytopathology of adenovirus infected cells, can be examined by light microscopy and hematoxylin-eosin (HE) staining of the tissue sections and exfoliated epithelial cells in respiratory system. Crystalline aggregates of virions assembled in the nucleus can be observed on thin-section EM. Seroconversion of animals can be detected by virus neutralization (VN), immune precipitation, complement fixation, or hemagglutination inhibition (HI) tests (Wilks and Studdert, 1972; Studdert et al., 1974; Studdert and Blackney, 1982), which have all been extensively used for diagnosis and seroepidemiologic studies of adenoviruses. For testing of precipitating antibodies to adenovirus, the counterimmunoelectrophoresis method was observed to be about three times more sensitive than the agar gel precipitation test and thus has been suggested to be used to screen a large number of serum samples within a short period (Adeyefa and Durojaiye, 1992). Adenoviruses are typed on the basis of SN assays. HI test is probably the most widely used serological assay for the detection of equine adenovirus. EAdV1 possesses the common group-specific Mastadenovirus antigen (Wilks and Studdert, 1972). HI antibody to EAdV1 is type specific. Extensive analysis of adenoviruses recovered from horses with respiratory disease indicated that on SN and HI assays, all were a single-antigenic type designated as EAdV1 (Studdert et al., 1974; Studdert, 1978). On SN assay, EAdV2 is unrelated to EAdV1 (Studdert et al., 1982).

PREVENTION AND CONTROL

Adenoviral infection in normal healthy horses is a self-limiting disease. There are no specific therapies for adenovirus infections in horses. Commercial vaccines against equine adenoviruses are not available at present (Studdert, 2007). High antibody titers in rabbits, mice, and foals were induced by an experimental inactivated EAdV1 vaccine (Lew et al., 1970). Intramuscular immunization with live EAdV1 has shown to induce the development of high serum antibody levels in a SPF foal, and the foal proved resistant to intranasal challenge, with no development of any clinical disease; and greater than twofold increases in serum-neutralizing antibody was observed after challenge (Gleeson et al., 1978).

The stimulation indices of horses vaccinated with experimental vaccine compared to unvaccinated horses in response to EAdV1 antigen were found to be significantly higher in the in vitro lymphoblast assays (Campbell and Studdert, 1982). The Arabian foals found positive for PSCID by genetic tests are nowadays not allowed to take birth. Adenoviruses were isolated from the respiratory tract of 90% (9/10) foals that had not been given serum or blood from their dams as compared to only 34% (one-third) foals that received serum or blood from their dam (McChesney and England, 1973). Colostrum and hyperimmune sera may be given parentally to foals that are at high risk and in which the transfer of maternal antibodies has failed partially or completely. The colostral antibodies from mare may provide immunity to young foals for about three months.

CONCLUSION

Among all infectious diseases affecting horses, respiratory disease pose the greatest threat to horses kept in stables, horses used for breeding, and race horses. Based on seroepidemiologic studies, equine adenovirus infection has been reported worldwide, but the majority of infections do not produce clinical disease. Adenovirus infection does not appear to be a noteworthy problem in adult horses but has infrequently been associated with respiratory disease in race horses. Adenoviruses do not generally cause a fatal disease in equines but dominant adenoviral infections occurring in immunocompromised horses could be fatal. Equine adenoviruses do not cause any public health implications.

Equine adenoviruses (EAdVs) have two species—viz, equine adenovirus 1 (EAdV1), mainly associated with respiratory disease, and equine adenovirus 2 (EAdV2), associated with diarrhea. EAdV1 is an overriding pathogen in cases of primary, severe, combined immunodeficiency disease (PSCID) affecting certain Arabian foals in which it is the most prevalent pathogen causing fatal bronchopneumonia. The virus is transmitted mainly through oral and nasopharyngeal routes and presumably may also be transmitted through a fecal-oral route. Adenovirus infection in normal, healthy foals is self-limiting, and recovery occurs within a week or so, but in cases of mixed infection with other pathogens, the disease condition deteriorates. Experimentally, the respiratory disease is characterized by nasal discharge, conjunctivitis, dyspnea, fever, rhinitis, tracheitis, bronchitis, cough, and pneumonia. Colostrum-deprived and immunosuppressed foals are most susceptible to pneumonia. Foals with immunodeficiency mostly develop generalized disease. Clinical disease not seen generally—therefore, confirmatory diagnosis of the EAdVs infection—requires isolation of the virus from clinical samples and subsequent confirmation by virus identification employing various laboratory tests, viz, light microscopy, electron microscopy, and immunofluorescent/immunohistochemical staining.

Intranuclear inclusion bodies are very characteristic of the cytopathology of adenovirus-infected cells. Molecular tool of PCR has also been developed for detecting the viral DNA in clinical samples. Serological tests comprise of serum neutralization, immune precipitation, complement fixation, or hemagglutination-inhibition tests.

Specific therapies are not available for treating adenovirus infections in horses. Also, commercial vaccines against equine adenoviruses are not available till date. Good management practices along with following strict hygiene and sanitation measures should be followed to prevent the adenovirus infection and avoiding the infection of other pathogens and limiting the immunosuppressive and stressful conditions of horses. Vaccinations of horses against other important respiratory infectious could limit the chances of mixed infections accordingly. Colostrum and hyperimmune sera may be given parentally to foals that are at high risk. The colostral antibodies from mare may provide passive immunity to young foals for about three months. Despite common infection of horses with EAdVs, they are generally unable to cause any significant clinical condition, particularly in adult horses. Also, the Arabian foals found positive for PSCID by genetic tests are nowadays not allowed to take birth, which further reduces the importance of equine adenoviruses.

Adenoviruses have the potential to be used as recombinant vaccine vectors, and recombinant adenoviruses are also being explored for gene therapy purposes in humans. More research is needed to be conducted in understanding EAdVs in a better way and controlling the respiratory pathogens of horses in an effective manner.

REFERENCES

1. Adeyefa, C. A. and Durojaiye, O. A. 1992. Detection of adenovirus precipitating antibodies in the sera of Polo horses in Nigeria. *Rev. Elev. Med. Vet. Pays. Trop.* 45:21–22.
2. Adkins, B., Leclerc, C. and Marshall-Clarke, S. 2004. Neonatal adaptive immunity comes of age. *Nat. Rev. Immunol.* 4:890–896.
3. Ardans, A. A., Pritchett, R. F. and Zee, Y. C. 1973. Isolation and characterization of an equine adenovirus. *Infect. Immunity* 7:673–677.
4. Bell, S. A., Leclere, M., Gardener, I. A. and MacLachlan, N. J. 2006. Equine adenovirus 1 infection of hospitalised and healthy foals and horses. *Equine Vet. J.* 38:379–381.
5. Benko, M., Harrach, B., Both, G. W., Russell, W. C., Adair, B. M., Adám, E., de Jong, J. C., Hess, M., Johnson, M., Kajon, A., Kidd, A. H., Lehmkuhl, H. D., Li, Q.-G., Mautner, V., Pring-Akerblom, P. and Wadell, G. 2005. Family *Adenoviridae*. In *Virus taxonomy. VIIIth report of the International Committee on Taxonomy of Viruses*, ed. C. M. Fauquet, M. A. Mayo, J. Maniloff, U. Desselberger, and L. A. Ball, 213–228. New York: Elsevier.

6. Burrows, R. and Goodridge, D. 1978. Observations of picornavirus, adenovirus, and equine herpesvirus infections in the Pirbright pony herd. In *Fourth International Conference on Equine Infectious Diseases*, ed. J. T. Bryans and H. Gerber, 155–164. Princeton, NJ: Veterinary Publications.

7. Campbell, T. M. and Studdert, M. J. 1982. In vitro blastogenesis of equine lymphocytes by inactivated equine adenovirus type 1 antigen. *Am. J. Vet. Res.* 43:1922–1925.

8. Carman, S., Rosendal, S., Huber, L., Gyles, C., McKee, S., Willoughby, R. A., Dubovi, E., Thorsen, J. and Lein, D. 1997. Infectious agents in acute respiratory disease in horses in Ontario. *J. Vet. Diagn. Invest.* 9:17–23.

9. Christley, R. M., Hodgson, D. R., Rose, R. J., Wood, J. L., Reids, S. W., Whitear, K. G., and Hodgson, J. L. 2001. A case-control study of respiratory disease in Thoroughbred race-horses in Sydney, Australia. *Equine Vet. J.* 33:256–264.

10. Corrier, D. E., Montgomery, D. and Scutchfield, W. L. 1982. Adenovirus in the intestinal epithelium of a foal with prolonged diarrhea. *Vet. Pathol.* 19:564–567.

11. Crisman, M. V. and Scarratt, W. K. 2008. Immunodeficiency disorders in horses. *Vet. Clin. North Am. Equine Pract.* 24:299–310, vi.

12. Cullinane, A. A., Barr, B., Bernard, W., Duncan, J. L., Mulcahy, G., Smith, M. and Timoney, J. E. 2006. Infectious diseases (Chapter 1): Equine adenovirus. In *The Equine Manual*, 2nd ed., ed. A. J. Higgins and J. R. Snyder, 18–19. USA: Saunder, Elsevier Ltd.

13. Dunowska, M., Wilks, C. R., Studdert, M. J. and Meers, J. 2002a. Viruses associated with outbreaks of equine respiratory disease in New Zealand. *N. Z. Vet. J.* 50:132–139.

14. Dunowska, M., Wilks, C. R., Studdert, M. J. and Meers, J. 2002b. Equine respiratory viruses in foals in New Zealand. *N. Z. Vet. J.* 50:140–147.

15. Dutta, S. K. 1975. Isolation and characterization of an adenovirus and isolation of its adenovirus-associated virus in cell culture from foals with respiratory tract disease. *Am. J. Vet. Res.* 36:247–250.

16. Dynon, K., Varrasso, A., Ficorilli, N., Holloway, S. A., Reubel, G. H., Li, F., Hartley, C. A., Studdert, M. J. and Drummer, H. E. 2001. Identification of equine herpesvirus 3 (equine coital exanthema virus), equine gammaherpesviruses 2 and 5, equine adenoviruses 1 and 2, equine arteritis virus and equine rhinitis A virus by polymerase chain reaction. *Aust. Vet. J.* 79:695–702.

17. Edington, N., Wright, J. A., Patel, J. R., Edwards, G. B. and Griffiths, L. 1984. Equine adenovirus 1 isolated from cauda equina neuritis. *Res. Vet. Sci.* 37:252–254.

18. Fatemie, N. S. and Marusyk, R. 1979. Biophysical and serologic comparison of four equine adenovirus isolates. *Am. J. Vet. Res.* 40:521–528.

19. Fauquet, C. M., Mayo, M. A., Maniloff, J., Desselberger, U. and Ball, L. A. 2005. *Virus taxonomy: Seventh report of the International Committee of Viruses*. San Diego: Academic Press.

20. Gabrilovich, D. I. 2006. INGN 201 (Advexin): Adenoviral p53 gene therapy for cancer. *Expert Opin. Biol. Ther.* 6:823–832.

21. Ghosh, S. S., Gopinath, P. and Ramesh, A. 2006. Adenoviral vectors: A promising tool for gene therapy. *Appl. Biochem. Biotechnol.* 133:9–29.

22. Gleeson, L. J., Studdert, M. J. and Sullivan, N. D. 1978. Pathogenicity and immunologic studies of equine adenovirus in specific-pathogen-free foals. *Am. J. Vet. Res.* 39:1636–1642.

23. Harasawa, R., Konishi, S. and Ogata, M. 1977. Detection of antibody against adenovirus in horses imported into Japan. *Nippon Juigaku Zasshi.* 39:451–454.

24. Harden, T. J., Pascoe, R. R. and Spradbrow, P. B. 1972. Isolation of an adenovirus from an Arabian foal. *Aust. Vet. J.* 48:478.

25. Harden, T. J., Pascoe, R. R., Spradbrow, P. B. and Johnston, K. G. 1974. The prevalence of antibodies to adenoviruses in horses from Queensland and New South Wales. *Aust. Vet. J.* 50:477–482.

26. Hartman, Z. C., Appledorn, D. M. and Amalfitano, A. 2008. Adenovirus vector induced innate immune responses: Impact upon efficacy and toxicity in gene therapy and vaccine applications. *Virus Res.* 132:1–14.

27. Herbst, W., Görlich, P. and Danner, K. 1992. Virologico-serologic studies in horses with respiratory tract diseases. *Berl. Munch. Tierarztl. Wochenschr.* 105:49–52.

28. Higashi, T. and Harasawa, R. 1989. DNA restriction analysis of equine adenovirus serotype 1. *J. Vet. Med. Ser. B.* 36:473–476.

29. Horner, G. W. and Hunter, R. 1982. Isolation of two serotypes of equine adenovirus from horses in New Zealand. *N. Z. Vet. J.* 30:62–6.

30. Johnston, K. G. and Hutchins, D. R. 1967. Suspected adenovirus bronchitis in Arab foals. *Aust. Vet. J.* 43:600.

31. Jolly, P. D., Fu, Z. F. and Robinson, A. J. 1986. Viruses associated with respiratory disease of horses in New Zealand: An update. *N. Z. Vet. J.* 34:46–50.

32. Jooss, K. and Chirmule, N. 2003. Immunity to adenovirus and adeno-associated viral vectors: Implications for gene therapy. *Gene Ther.* 10:955–963.

33. Jouvenne, P., Dion, M. and Hamelin, C. 1987. Cloning, physical mapping, and cross-hybridization of the canine adenovirus types 1 and 2 genomes. *Gene* (Amst.) 60:21–28.

34. Kamada, M., Akiyama, Y., Sato, K. and Kodera, S. 1977. Isolation of adenovirus from adult thoroughbred horses. *Nippon Juigaku Zasshi.* 39:661–664.

35. Kamada, M. 1978. Comparison of the four serological tests for detecting antibodies against equine adenovirus. *Exp. Rep. Equine Health Lab.* 15:91–96.

36. Lew, A. M., Smith, H. V. and Studdert, M. J. 1979. Development and preliminary testing of an inactivated equine adenovirus vaccine. *Am. J. Vet. Res.* 40:1707–1712.

37. Mahr, J. A. and Gooding, L. R. 1999. Immune evasion by adenoviruses. *Immunol. Rev.* 168:121–130.

38. Mayr, A. 1987. Respiratory infectious diseases in horses. *Tierarztl Prax Suppl.* 2:1–4.

39. Mayr, A. and Thein, P. 1984. Current virus diseases in horses. Diseases in foals and respiratory tract infections. *Tierarztl. Prax.* 12:481–488.

40. McChesney, A. E., England, J. J., Adcock, J. L., Stackhouse, L. L. and Chow, T. L. 1970. Adenoviral infection in suckling Arabian foals. *Pathol. Vet.* 7:547–565.

41. McChesney, A. E. and England, J. J. 1973. Adenoviral infection in foals. *J. Am. Vet. Med. Assoc.* 162:545–549.

42. McChesney, A. E., England, J. J., Whiteman, C. E., Adcock, J. L., Rich, L. J. and Chow, T. L. 1974. Experimental transmission of equine adenovirus in Arabian and non-Arabian foals. *Am. J. Vet. Res.* 35:1015–1023.

43. McChesney, A. E. and England, J. J. 1975. Adenoviral infection in foals. *J. Am. Vet. Med. Assoc.* 166:83–85.

44. McChesney, A. E. and England, J. J. 1978. Equine adenoviral infection: Pathogenesis of experimentally and naturally transmitted infection. In *Equine infectious diseases*, ed. J. T. Bryans and H. Gerber, 144–145. Princeton, New Jersey: Vet Publications Inc.

45. McGuire, T. C., Poppie, M. J. and Banks, K. L. 1974. Combined (B—and T-lymphocyte) immunodeficiency: A fatal genetic disease in Arabian foals. *J. Am. Vet. Med. Assoc.* 164:70–76.

46. Moorthy, A. R. and Spradbrow, P. B. 1978. Adenoviral infection of Arab foals with respiratory tract disease. *Zentralbl. Veterinarmed. B.* 25:469–477.

47. Newton, J. R., Wood, J. I. and Chanter, N. 2003. A case control study of factors and infections associated with clinically apparent respiratory disease in UK Throughbred racehorses. *Preventive Vet. Med.* 60:107–132.

48. Pascoe, R. R., Harden, T. J. and Spradbrow, P. B. 1974. Experimental infection in a horse with an equine adenovirus. *Aust. Vet J.* 50:278–279.

49. Patterson, S., Papagatsias, T. and Benlahrech, A. 2009. Use of adenovirus in vaccines for HIV. *Handb. Exp. Pharmacol.* 188:275–293.

50. Perryman, L. E. 2000. Primary immunodeficiencies of horses. *Vet. Clin. North. Am. Equine Pract.* 16:105–116.

51. Powell, D. G., Burrows, R. and Goodridge, D. 1974. Respiratory viral infections among Thoroughbred horses in training during 1972. *Equine Vet. J.* 6:19–24.

52. Powell, D. G. 1991. Viral respiratory disease of the horse. *Vet. Clin. North Am. Equine Pract.* 7:27–52.

53. Reubel, G. H. and Studdert, M. J. 1997a. Identification, cloning and sequence analysis of the equine adenovirus 1 hexon gene. *Arch. Virol.* 142:1193–1212.

54. Reubel, G. H. and Studdert, M. J. 1997b. Sequence analysis of equine adenovirus 2 hexon and 23K proteinase genes indicates a phylogenetic origin distinct from equine adenovirus 1. *Virus Res.* 50:41–56.

55. Richards, A. J., Kelly, D. F., Knottenbelt, D. C., Cheeseman, M. T. and Dixon, J. B. 2000. Anemia, diarrhoea and opportunistic infections in Fell ponies. *Equine Vet. J.* 32:386–391.

56. Russell, W. C. 2009. Adenoviruses: Update on structure and function. *J. Gen. Virol.* 90:1–20.

57. Sellon, D. C. 2000. Secondary immunodeficiencies of horses. *Vet. Clin. North Am. Equine Pract.* 16:117–130.

58. Shahrabadi, M. S., Marusyk, R. G. and Crawford, T. B. 1977. Electron-microscopic study of the development of an equine adenovirus in cultured fetal equine kidney cells. *Can J Microbiol.* 23:497–509.

59. Sheppard, M., Drysdale, S. M. and Studdert, M. J. 1992. Restriction enzyme maps for equine adenovirus 1 genome. *Vet. Microbiol.* 31:343–349.

60. Sherrod, W. W. 1973. A practitioner's experiences with adenoviral infection in Arabian foals. *Vet. Med. Small Anim. Clin.* 68:793–795.

61. Shinagawa, M., Ishiyama, T., Padmanabhan, R., Fujinaga, K., Kamada, M. and Sato G. 1983. Comparative sequence analysis of the inverted terminal repetition in the genomes of animal and avian adenoviruses. *Virology* 125:491–495.

62. Studdert, M. J., Wilks, C. R. and Coggins, L. 1974. Antigenic comparisons and serologic survey of equine adenoviruses. *Am. J. Vet. Res.* 35:693–699.

63. Studdert, M. J. 1978. Antigenic homogeneity of equine adenoviruses. *Aust. Vet. J.* 54:263–264.

64. Studdert, M. J. and Blackney, M. H. 1982. Isolation of an adenovirus antigenically distinct from equine adenovirus type 1 from diarrheic foal feces. *Am. J. Vet. Res.* 43:543–544.

65. Studdert, M. J. 1996. Equine adenoviruses. In *Virus infections of vertebrates*. Vol. 6 *Virus infections of equines*, ed. M. J. Studdert, 67–80. Amsterdam:Elsevier.

66. Studdert, M. J. 2000. Veterinary perspective on gene therapy with adenoviruses. *Science* 287:973–974.

67. Studdert, M. J. 2007. Miscellaneous viral respiratory diseases: Equine adenoviruses. In *Equine infectious diseases*, ed. D. C. Sellon and M. T. Long, chapter 16, 171–174. Philadelphia, USA: Saunders, Elsevier Inc.

68. Studdert, M. J., Mason, R. W. and Patten, B. E. 1978. Rotavirus diarrhoea of foals. *Aust. Vet. J.* 54:363–364.

69. Tatsis, N. and Ertl, H. C. 2004. Adenoviruses as vaccine vectors. *Mol. Ther.* 10:616–629.

70. Temple, M., Antonie, G., Delius, H., Stahl, S. and Winnacker, E. L. 1981. Replication of mouse adenovirus strain FL DNA. *Virology* 109:1–12.

71. Thompson, G. B., Spradborw, P. B. and Studdert, M. J. 1976. Isolation of an adenovirus from an Arab foal with a combined immunodeficiency disease. *Aust. Vet. J.* 52:435–437.

72. Timoney, P. J. 1971. Adenovirus precipitating antibodies in the serums of some domestic animal species in Ireland. *Brit. Vet. J.* 127:567–571.

73. Todd, J. D. 1969. Comments on rhinovirus and parainfluenza viruses of horses. *J. Am. Vet. Med. Ass.* 155:387–390.

74. Tucker, S. N., Tingley, D. W. and Scallan, C. D. 2008. Oral adenoviral-based vaccines: Historical perspective and future opportunity. *Expert Rev. Vaccines* 7:25–31.

75. Vassall, J. H. II 1974. Serotyping of adenoviruses using immune electron microscopy. *Appl. Microbiol.* 28:623–627.

76. Veenstra van Nieuwenhoven, A. L., Heineman, M. J. and Faas, M. M. 2003. The immunology of successful pregnancy. *Hum. Reprod. Update* 9:347–357.

77. Vellinga, J., Van der Heijdt, S. and Hoeben, R. C. 2005. The adenovirus capsid: Major progress in minor proteins. *J. Gen. Virol.* 86:1581–1588.

78. Webb, R. F., Knight, P. R., and Walker, K. H. 1981. Involvement of adenovirus in pneumonia in a Thoroughbred foal. *Aust. Vet. J.* 57:142–143.

79. Whitlock, R. H., Dellers, R. W. and Shively, J. N. 1975. Adenoviral pneumonia in foal. *Cornell Veterinarian* 65:393–401.

80. Wilks, C. R., and Studdert, M. J. 1972. Isolation of an equine adenovirus. *Aust. Vet. J.* 48:580–581.

81. Wood, J. L., Newton, J. R., Chanter, N. and Mumford J. A. 2005. Association between respiratory disease and bacterial and viral infections in British racehorses. *J. Clin. Microbiol.* 43:120–126.

4. Equine Coital Exanthema

S. Kapoor, K. Dhama, R. V. S. Pawaiya, and P. Bhatt

Introduction

Equine coital exanthema (ECE), as a clinical disease but without known etiology, has been documented in the European literature in nineteenth century (Studdert, 1974). The ECE has been described under many names such as genital horse pox, eruptive venereal disease, equine venereal vulvitis or balanitis, and coital vesicular exanthema (Allen and Umphenour, 2004). The etiological agent of ECE, a relatively innocuous genital disease, was isolated independently in the United States (Bryans, 1968), in Canada (Girard et al., 1968), and in Australia (Pascoe et al., 1968). There are no international restrictions on the export/import of horses from countries or from horse populations in which ECE is known to occur as ECE is endemic in most horse-breeding areas. Equine herpesvirus type 3 (EHV-3), which causes equine coital exanthema, is the only equine herpesvirus that neither affects the respiratory tract nor is spread by airborne particles or nasal secretions. Rather, EHV-3 spreads from horse to horse via skin-to-skin contact, usually between stallions and mares during coitus. Transmission of the virus can also occur through shared breeding equipment or people handling different horses without washing. Poxlike lesions appear on the external genitals of the affected mare or stallion that erupt within a few days and in about two weeks heal completely in uncomplicated cases. The disease can also cause eye infections and lesions on the muzzle if one horse rubs against another horse with the disease, and sometimes lesions appear on a mare's teats as well as on the muzzle of her nursing foal. The internal reproductive organs are not affected by EHV-3. However, EHV-3 lesions can make affected horses, particularly stallions, reluctant to breed during an outbreak. Sexual rest is recommended while the horse heals. These may have economic consequences due to disruption of a busy breeding season.

Etiology

The ECE virus belongs to species Equine herpesvirus 3, genus *Vericellovirus*, subfamily Alphaherpesvirinae, family Herpesviridae, order Herpesvirales

(Davison et al., 2009). It is a typical herpesvirus on the basis of size, virion architecture, genome structure, and grouped under alphaherpes viruses based on biological properties (Ludwig et al., 1971; Bryans and Allen, 1973; Atherton et al., 1982; Sullivan et al., 1984; Jacob et al., 1985). The virus, equine herpesvirus 3 (EHV-3) is antigenically, genetically, and pathogenetically different from other herpesviruses (EHV-1, EHV-2, EHV-4, and EHV-5) isolated from equines (Bryans and Allen, 1973; Allen et al., 1977; Gutekunst et al., 1978; Baumann et al., 1986; Staczek et al., 1983). EHV-3 shows no cross-protection or serological cross-reactivity with other equine herpesviruses by neutralization tests, but shares antigens with EHV-1 in CFT and immunofluorescence tests (Wilks and Studdert, 1976; Allen et al., 1977; Staczek et al., 1983).

The virion has a size of about 150 nm in diameter and a buoyant density of 1725 g/cm^3 (Ludwig et al., 1971). Its icosahedral nucleocapsid is surrounded by globular tegument and envelope, which has numerous small surface glycoprotein spikes. The genome is single-linear dsDNA molecule with high G+C (66%) content. Complete nucleotide sequence of both EHV-1 (Telford et al., 1992) and EHV-4 (Telford et al., 1998) has been determined. The genome organization and the seventy-six genes are encoded by them, and their temporal expression are also known for both (EHV-1 and EHV-4) viruses (Caughman et al., 1985; Telford et al., 1992; 1998; Albrecht et al., 2005). The EHV-3 genome, though yet to be sequenced completely, is often compared, in parts, with EHV-1 and EHV-4. The fragments obtained from digestion of DNA of EHV-3 by various restriction endonucleases are different from the DNAs of EHV-1, EHV-2, EHV-4, and EHV-5. (Kamada and Studdert, 1983; Sullivan et al., 1984; Jacob et al., 1985; Bouchey et al., 1987).

The transcription of equine herpesvirus type 3 has been found to be temporally regulated into three classes: immediate early (IE), early (E), and late (L) (Sullivan et al., 1990). There is a single IE transcript, approximately 5.7 kb, which is derived exclusively from the inverted repeat segments (IRs) of the viral genome, while E and L transcripts are produced from various regions of the genome. This type of temporal regulation is similar to that seen in EHV-1 and EHV-4 (Caughman et al., 1985). The homology of EHV-1 and EHV-3 IE RNA species reflects colinearity of the genomes of these two related viruses.

The arrangement and location of homologous DNA sequences within the genomes of EHV-1 and EHV-3 were investigated by using Southern blot hybridization. Recombinant plasmid libraries comprising 95% and 84% of the EHV-1 and EHV-3 genomes, respectively, radiolabeled with ^{32}P-deoxynucleotides, were used as probes. The DNA homology between the EHV-1 and EHV-3 genomes was spread throughout the genomes in a colinear arrangement. Significant hybridization was detected between the EHV-1 short-region inverted repeat sequences, which are known to encode immediate early transcripts, and the corresponding EHV-3 inverted repeat sequences. The probes derived from the EHV-1 heterogeneous region, which is adjacent to the EHV-1 short region, hybridized strongly to EHV-3 DNA sequences within a similar genomic location. Surprisingly, these did not show any corresponding heterogeneity within the EHV-3 genome (Baumann et al., 1986).

Determination of complete nucleotide sequence of glycoprotein G (gG) gene of the EHV-3 revealed that this virus is most closely related to other two equine herpesvirus species, EHV-1 and EHV-4, within the genus *Vericellovirus*. The conserved and variable regions present in EHV-3 gG are homologous to those previously defined for EHV-1 and EHV-4 gG proteins. Similar to the EHV-1 and EHV-4 gG, experimental and natural infection of horses with EHV-3 induced a strong antibody response against the variable region of EHV-3 gG (Hartley et al., 1999). The gG encoded by EHV-3 demonstrated chemokine-binding activity. The finding of chemokine-binding activity secreted from cells infected with EHV-3 suggests that gG from these viruses is also proteolytically cleaved and secreted (Bryant et al., 2003).

Replication of EHV-3 is restricted to cell of equine origin only (Bryans and Allen, 1973), producing cytopathic effect (CPE) very rapidly. Under in vitro conditions, the EHV-3 replication gives maximum titers at 34°C in comparison to 39°C, where the virus yield is drastically reduced (Jacob, 1986; Bouchey et al., 1987; Jacob et al., 1990). EHV-3 has so far failed to grow in laboratory animals. This virus has one antigenic type; however, small and large plaque variants arise during passage in cell culture, indicating that variation may occur in the severity of field outbreaks (Bouchey et al., 1987; Bryans and Allen, 1973; Kamada and Studdert, 1983).

EPIDEMIOLOGY

The ECE caused by EHV-3 in horses has been isolated from many countries of the world such as Australia (Pascoe et al., 1968, 1969; Feilen et al., 1979), Canada (Girard et al., 1968), Denmark (Bitsch, 1972), England (Gibbs et al., 1970; 1972), India (Uppal et al., 1989), Japan (Seki et al., 2004), Norway (Krogsrud and Onstad, 1971), and the United States (Bryans and Allen, 1973; Crandall and Davis, et al., 1985).

The ECE is a venereal disease, primarily transmitted through direct skin-to-skin contact during coitus (Pascoe et al., 1969; Bagust et al., 1972; Studdert, 1996). Outbreaks have been reported in which noncoital transmission occurred through contaminated shared supplies and equipment or through people handling different horses without washing (Craig and Kehoe, 1921; Krogsrud and Onstad, 1971; Bryans and Allen, 1973; Burki et al., 1974; Pascoe and Bagust, 1975, Crandell and Davis, 1985; Couto and Hughes,

1993; Studdert, 1996). It is probably for this reason that EHV-3 has also been isolated from animals that have not been bred. Equine coital exanthema virus is the only equine herpesvirus that is not spread by airborne particles or nasal secretions. The role of stable flies in mechanical transmission has also been suggested (Gibbs et al., 1972). The virus may be transmitted from subclinically infected animals that have no visibly noticeable skin lesions to their breeding partners (Bitsch, 1972; Gibbs et al., 1972; Burrows and Goodridge, 1984,). Horses that have recovered from infection and those that showed no recognizable signs of typical skin lesions may become latent carriers of EHV-3. The most common source of infection for ECE is considered to be the periodic recrudescence and shedding of virus from a latently infected carrier animal that does not have clinical signs (Burrows and Goodridge, 1984; Seki et al., 2004). The seroprevalence of infection is low in young horses, which increase slowly with age in breeding animals when 18–52% horses of breeding age have EHV-3–specific antibodies (Bagust et al., 1972; Pascoe and Bagust, 1975; Aurich et al., 2003).

PATHOGENESIS AND PATHOLOGY

Transmission of EHV-3 mainly occurs through coitus, although noncoital transmission through contaminated inanimate objects and personnel has also been reported. Infection by EHV-3 requires genital or nongenital cutaneous contact. The infection can be established even in intact epidermis (Krogsrud and Onstad, 1971; Pascoe et al., 1972; Bryans and Allen, 1973; Wilks and Studdert, 1976). The replication of virus is restricted to the stratified squamous epithelium of epidermal tissue present within the skin or transitional epithelium covering the mucocutaneous margins (Allen and Umphenour, 2004). This restricted nature of replication may represent true tissue tropism or may reflect temperature-sensitive nature of the virus (Jacob, 1986; Bouchey et al., 1987; Jacob et al., 1990). The typical lesions of ECE results from localized inflammatory response to virus-induced epithelial destruction. The nature, severity, duration of EHV-3–induced lesions and course of recovery from them may be influenced by secondary bacterial infection. The systemic disease has not been reported in EHV-3 infection as the virus is unable to invade dermal stroma or the tissue within the blood vessels (Allen and Umphenour, 2004). The lesions do not affect the internal reproductive organs, and EHV-3 has never been linked to infertility. Ulcerations of the nasal mucosa, fever, and nasal discharge in foals have been reported after experimental intranasal inoculation of EHV-3 (Bryans and Allen, 1973; Burki et al., 1974; Wilks and Studdert, 1976).

The EHV-3 may have oncogenic potential. Infection of nonpermissive primary hamster embryo cells with EHV-3 caused an abortive infection and development of several hundred foci of rapidly growing cells with altered morphology. Five of these randomly chosen independent foci for the establishment of transformed cell lines, designated EVD-1 (equine venereal disease) through 5, have been characterized. These transformed cell lines exhibited altered biological properties typical of transformed cells, including immortality, growth to high-saturation density, ability to form colonies in soft agar or methylcellulose, reduced serum requirements, aneuploid karyotype, and oncogenicity in syngeneic animals. The hamsters, when inoculated with these transformed cells, rapidly developed tumors that metastasized to different organs, and these tumors were transplantable (Atherton et al., 1980, 1981). Subsequently, five corresponding tumor cell lines (EVD-1T through 5T) with similar biological properties were established. The EHV-3–specific proteins were expressed by all EHV-3 transformed and tumor cell lines that were detected by indirect immunofluorescence assays. Various treatments of the transformed cell lines such as cocultivation with permissive equine cells, growth at different temperatures, could not detect or induce infectious virus or viral particles or both in any of these cells (Sullivan et al., 1986).

Both complement-fixing (CF) and serum-neutralizing (SN) antibodies produced in response to infection reach maximum levels at two to three weeks postinfection. The complement-fixing antibodies decline rapidly and are usually not detectable by sixty days after infection, whereas serum-neutralizing antibody can be detected for about a year. This disparity in the kinetics of CF and SN antibodies has been used for the diagnosis of recent infections and estimation of the temporal incidence of infection in groups of mares (Pascoe et al., 1972; Bryans and Allen, 1973; Pascoe and Bagust, 1975; Burrows and Goodridge, 1984). Both stallions and mares can develop the disease in consecutive breeding seasons as immunity to reinfection by EHV-3 is short-lived.

The gG encoded by EHV-3 possess chemokine-binding activity. Chemokines are chemo-attractant cytokines that regulate trafficking and effector functions of leukocytes and play an important role in host defense against invading microbes and in the pathogenesis of inflammatory diseases (Baggiolini, 1998). The critical role of chemokines in antiviral defense has been highlighted by the discovery that poxviruses and herpesviruses encode proteins that mimic chemokines or chemokine receptors and secreted chemokine-binding proteins (Lalani et al., 2000; Murphy, 2001). Therefore, further studies are required to determine the role of EHV-3 gG in pathogenesis and protection.

The gross lesions occur sequentially in the form of papules, vesicles, pustules, erosions, or frank ulcers. In histopathology, ballooning degeneration, lysis, and sloughing of necrotic epithelium covering the erosions or ulcers are observed. The ulcers are then left filled with a fibrin and acute exudate containing polymorphonuclear and mononuclear leukocytes. The transition from necrotic tissue to normal epithelium at the edges of the erosions/ulcers is sharply defined. Typical eosinophilic herpesvirus intranuclear inclusion bodies are usually present in epithelial cells at the margins of the erosions/ulcers (Pascoe et al., 1969; Evermann et al., 1983; Allen and Umphenour, 2004).

CLINICAL FEATURES

The incubation period varies from two to ten days. The disease is characterized by the formation of pustular and ulcerative lesions on the external genitalia of both mares and stallions. Initially the lesions appear as small vesicles or papules and rapidly progress to pustules and which ultimately become raw or encrusted skin erosion or frank ulcers due to epidermal sloughing. The individual ulcers have pocklike appearance in the beginning and are surrounded by an erythematic zone. The lesions may merge to form extensive epidermal erosions or ulcers, which may be as large as 2 cm in diameter and 0.5 cm in depth. The number of lesions and their clinical stage, as well as the severity and duration of the disease varies considerably among individual horses (Girard et al., 1968; Bitsch, 1972; Gibbs et al., 1972; Bryans and Allen, 1973; Studdert, 1974; Pascoe and Bagust, 1975; Bryans, 1980; Kleiboeker and Chapman, 2004; Seki et al., 2004). Edema can develop in the perineum and may extend to between the thighs. Occasionally, ulcers may be found on the lips, muzzle, nostrils, and teats (Krogsrud and Onstad, 1971; Crandall and Davis et al., 1985). A noncoital form of EHV-3 infection may occasionally occur in maiden colts and fillies. It causes fever and very painful coalescing skin lesions around the anus and vulva in fillies, over the perineum, scrotum, and between the hind legs in colts. Complete healing usually occurs within ten to fourteen days in uncomplicated cases, although white depigmentation spots are often present at the site of lesions for the life of the horse. However, secondary infection with bacteria will delay healing and prolong the recovery. Secondary bacterial infection causes the ulcers to enlarge and exude a mucopurulent discharge, and the animal may becomes pyrexic. The stallion sometimes is unable/unwilling to copulate/ejaculate particularly when painful lesions are present on the urethral process. Both mares and stallions may become latently infected carrier.

The infection in breeding horses does not cause immediate or longer-term direct effect on the fertility of stallions or mares (Pascoe and Bagust, 1975; Pascoe, 1981). Reduced pregnancy rates may be an indirect consequence of missed mating opportunities where infection occurs toward the end of the breeding season. Abortions caused by natural EHV-3 infection of the fetus have not been reported (Leon et al., 2008). Although experimental in utero inoculation of pregnant mare with EHV-3 may cause abortion. The inoculation of EHV-3, strain 65/61, into the amniotic cavity of a mare six to seven months pregnant resulted in abortion eleven days later. Typical ECE lesions or isolation of virus from the aborted mare were not observed. However, the infection of this mare with EHV-3 following inoculation was confirmed due to its seroconversion. Grossly, the fetal disease was characterized by placentitis, focal ulcerative dermatitis, focal necrosis of the lungs, and diptheritic gastritis. Histological findings were interstitial pneumonia, diffuse hepatitis, generalized myositis, extensive vascular necrosis, and degeneration of a range of epithelial cells. EHV-3 was isolated from the placenta and placental fluids, stomach fluid, pooled thoracic and abdominal fluid, skin, lung, spleen, and small intestine of the fetus (Gleeson et al., 1976).

DIAGNOSIS

A tentative diagnosis of ECE can be made on the basis of typical genital lesions in both mares and stallions. Potential carriers may be identified by the presence of depigmented white spots in genital areas particularly when the skin of vulva, penis, and prepuce is black. However, sometimes the ECE lesions may also appear on lips, nostrils, muzzle, and teats. Therefore, these cases need to be differentiated from vesicular stomatitis virus, true horse pox, and contagious equine metritis (CEM) and EHV-1. There is copious mucopurulent vulvar discharge in CEM. The EHV-1 occasionally can cause exanthemous lesions on the external genitalia of mares (Petzoldt, 1970; Turner et al., 1970; Bryans and Allens, 1973). Virus isolation and identification, seroconversion, and detection of EHV-3 specific DNA by polymerase chain reaction (PCR) have been used for the laboratory confirmation of the diagnosis. Typical intranuclear herpesvirus inclusion bodies can also be seen in cytological or histological preparations.

The EHV-3 can grow only on cells of equine origin (Bryans and Allen, 1973) with the exception of rabbit kidney cells (Girard et al., 1968). The virus can be isolated in equine dermal (E-derm), fetal equine kidney (FEK), equine testis (ET), or equine embryonic lung (EEL) cells (Pascoe et al., 1969; Bryans and Allen, 1973; Studdert, 1996; Kleiboeker and Chapman, 2004; Seki et al., 2004) using scraping or swabs from the edges of fresh active lesions. The cytopathic effect is seen within twenty four to forty-eight hours in these cells, and the virus can be identified by virus neutralization test (Evermann et al., 1983; Seki et al., 2004) or PCR (Dynon et al., 2001).

Serum neutralization (Seki et al., 2004) or complement fixation (CF) tests have been used on acute and convalescent samples for detection of antibodies against EHV-3 infection, but these tests must be interpreted carefully because EHV-1 and EHV-4 have also been isolated from genital lesions. Seroconversion of less than fourfold is not considered as evidence for the absence of infection because the antibody response of an animal to infection with EHV-3 may be minimal (Gibbs et al., 1972). The presence of CF antibody to EHV-3 in the serum indicates that the viral infection has been acquired within the previous sixty days (Pascoe et al., 1972).

Molecular detection of EHV-3 by PCR is the most sensitive, specific, and accurate tool in assessing the infectivity of an affected horse (Dynon et al., 2001; Kleiboeker and Chapman, 2004; Seki et al., 2004). A sensitive and specific PCR assay was developed to amplify a region of the highly conserved DNA polymerase gene using novel EHV3 sequences (Kleiboeker and Chapman, 2004). Amplification of serial tenfold dilutions of DNA extracted from the skin lesions demonstrated that the analytical sensitivity of the EHV3 DNA polymerase assay was slightly greater than the EHV-3 gC-targeted PCR assay (Dynon et al., 2001; Kleiboeker and Chapman, 2004). The PCR was used for the diagnosis of EHV-3 in pastured draft stallion and mares by amplification of gG (Seki et al., 2004). The PCR was able to detect EHV-3 even in those cases where virus isolation results were negative (Kleiboeker and Chapman, 2004; Seki et al., 2004). This was speculated to be due to desiccation of the samples that might have inactivated any viable virus present in them (Kleiboeker and Chapman, 2004).

PREVENTION AND CONTROL

Commercial vaccines against ECE are not available. The immediate stoppage of mating activities of clinically affected stallions and mares, until they have recovered completely, is considered to be the most effective method for restricting the transmission of EHV-3 infection. All animals should be examined carefully before they are allowed to breed. Carrier animals can sometimes be identified by spots of pigment loss on black skin in the genital region. The infected horses should be isolated until all lesions have healed. The genitalia should be cleansed daily. Antibiotic ointments should be applied on the lesions to prevent secondary bacterial infections and quicken the healing process (Pascoe, 1981; Evermann et al., 1983). An antiviral compound, acyclovir, has been used locally to treat coital exanthema in both stallions and mares (Cullinane et al., 1994). During cleansing or topical application of drugs, it is important to take proper care to avoid accidental, traumatic removal of the crusts of healing sores. Stallions and mares given sexual rest and palliatively treated are usually ready for resumption of mating by ten to fourteen days. However, this period of ten to fourteen days may vary and depends on many factors such as extent and severity of lesions, secondary bacterial infection, and the healing process. Therefore, the decision to reengage the EHV-3–infected animal to mating and breeding activity should be based on freedom from clinical signs of infective genital lesions rather than the predefined time limits. Trained personnel, who are sensitized to the importance of hygiene and can recognize and identify the lesions of ECE, should be employed to prepare the mares and stallions for mating. The mechanical spread of EHV-3 during an ECE outbreak should be prevented by taking strict hygienic measures. The iatrogenic transmission of the virus through contaminated equipment such as rectal sleeves, vaginal specula, insemination utensils, etc., can be prevented by the use of disposable materials as far as possible. The premises, where the animals are prepared and mated, should be disinfected after every use to prevent cross-infection.

It is not advisable to use even the prized commercial stallion for mating before they have fully healed. This is because of a number of reasons such as unwillingness of the stallion to mate/ejaculate, increased chances of development of secondary complications, the healing and recovery process of the stallion may be delayed, which will increase the numbers of mares infected resulting in increased numbers of latently infected carriers in the horse population. If a stallion that has serviced a number of mares is found to be positive for ECE infection at a later date, then owners of all the mares mated by and booked to that stallion should be asked to examine them for any signs of infection. Similarly, when a mare that has been mated within three weeks is diagnosed to be ECE positive, the mating stallion should be stopped from further breeding activity and examined thoroughly for signs of infection. The owners/managers of other mares mated by that stallion within the previous three to four weeks should be informed for examination of these mares for the signs of infection. Mating should only recommence when the stallion as well as other mares that he has mated are found to be free from signs of infection. The Horserace Betting Levy Board, UK (*www.hblb.org.uk*) publishes a Codes of Practice recommending precautions to prevent or limit about some equine diseases, including equine coital exanthema. The recommendations within the Codes of Practice are not mandatory but adhered to in the Thoroughbred industries in France, Germany, Ireland, Italy, and the United Kingdom.

Conclusions

Equine coital exanthema is caused by equine herpesvirus 3 (EHV-3). The size, symmetry and architecture, and genome organization of EHV-3 virion resemble a characteristic herpesvirus, which belongs to subfamily alphaherpesvirinae due to its biological properties. EHV-3 is antigenically, genetically, and pathogenetically distinct from other herpesviruses (EHV-1,

EHV-2, EHV-4, and EHV-5) isolated from equines. It does not grow in laboratory animals and can be isolated in cell cultures of equine origin, where it produces rapid CPE and typical eosiophilic intranuclear inclusions. The ECE is generally a venereal disease transmitted by genital or nongenital skin contact. It normally has an acute, mild clinical course characterized by the formation of pustular and ulcerative lesions on the external genitalia of both mares and stallions. Uncomplicated skin lesions typically heal rapidly, although white depigmentation spots are often present at the site of lesions for the life of the horse. The diagnosis is confirmed in the laboratory by virus isolation and identification, seroconversion, and detection of specific DNA in PCR assays. Commercial vaccines for ECE are not available. Topical antibiotics are applied to prevent and treat secondary bacterial contamination. The lesions do not affect the internal reproductive organs, and EHV-3 has never been linked to infertility. EHV-3 lesions can be a nuisance, however, making affected horses, especially stallions, reluctant to breed during an outbreak. Rest is recommended while the horse heals; therefore, an outbreak can disrupt a busy breeding season. Barring a popular stallion from the breeding shed even for ten days at the height of the breeding season may have a considerable economic impact on the stallion station as well as the broodmare owner, who either has to short-cycle his mare's estrus or wait another month to breed. Equine genital herpesvirus is not a reportable disease. There are no international restrictions on the export/import of horses from countries or from horse populations in which ECE is known to occur as ECE is endemic in most horse-breeding areas.

REFERENCES

1. Albrecht, R. A., Kim, S. K., O'Callaghan, D. J. 2005. The EICP27 protein of equine herpesvirus 1 is recruited to viral promoters by its interaction with the immediate-early protein. *Virology* 333:74–87.
2. Allen, G. P., O'Callaghan, D. J. and Randall, C. C. 1977. Genetic relatedness of equine herpesvirus types 1 and 3. *J. Virol.* 24:761–767.
3. Allen, G. P. and Umphenour, N. W. 2004. Equine coital exanthema. In *Infectious diseases of livestock*, ed. J. A. W. Coetzer and R. C. Tustin, 860–867. Cape Town: Oxford Press.
4. Aurich, C., Achmann, R. and Aurich, J. E. 2003. Semen parameters and level of microsatellite heterozygosity in Noriker draught horse stallions. *Theriogenology* 60:371–378.
5. Atherton, S. S., Robinson, R. A. and O'Callaghan, D. J. 1980. Equine herpes virus type 3 (EHV-3) genomic structure and transforming potential. Fifth International Herpesvirus Workshop, Cold Spring Harbor Laboratory, 53.
6. Atherton, S. S., Robinson, R. A. and O'Callaghan, D. J. 1981. Genomic structure and oncogenic potential of equine coital exanthema virus (equine herpesvirus type 3 EHV-3). *Abstr. Annu. Meeting Am. Soc. Microbiol.* 226.
7. Atherton, S. S., Sullivan, D. C., Dauenhauer, S. A., Ruyechan, W. T. and O'Callaghan, D. J. 1982. Properties of the genome of equine herpesvirus type 3. *Virology* 120:18–32.
8. Baggiolini, M. 1998. Chemokines and leukocyte traffic. *Nature* 392:565–568.

9. Bagust, T. J., Pascoe, R. R. and Harden, T. J. 1972. Studies on equine herpes viruses. 3. The incidence in Queensland of three different equine herpesvirus infections. *Aust. Vet. J.* 48:47–53.

10. Baumann, R. P., Sullivan, D. C., Staczek, J. and O'Callaghan, D. J. 1986. Genetic relatedness and colinearity of genomes of equine herpesvirus types 1 and 3. *J. Virol.* 57:816–825.

11. Bitsch, V. 1972. Cases of equine coital exanthema in Denmark. *Acta. Veterinaria Scandinavica* 13:281–283.

12. Bryans, J. T. 1968. The herpesvirus in disease of horse. Proceedings of the 14th Annual Convention of the American Association of Equine Practitioners, Philadelphia, 119–125.

13. Bryans, J. T. and Allen, G. P. 1973. *In vitro* and *in vivo* studies of equine "coital" exanthema. In *Proceedings of the Third International Conference on Equine Infectious Diseases*, ed. J. Bryans and H. Gerber, 322–342. Paris (1972): Karger.

14. Bryans, J. T. 1980. Herpesviral diseases affecting reproduction in the horse. *Vet. Clin. N. Am. Large Anim. Pract.* 2:203–212.

15. Bryant, N. A., Davis-Poynter, N., van der Plasschen, A. and Alcami, A. 2003. Glycoprotein G isoforms from some alphaherpes viruses function as broad-spectrum chemokine binding proteins. *The EMBO J.* 22:833–846.

16. Bouchey, D., Evermann, J. and Jacob, R. J. 1987. Molecular pathogenesis of equine coital exanthema (ECE): Temperature sensitivity (TS) and restriction endonuclease (RE) fragment profiles of several field isolates. *Arch. Virol.* 92:293–299.

17. Burki, F., Lorin, D., Sibalin, M., Ruttner, O. and Arbeiter, K. 1974. Experimental genital and nasal infection of horses with the equine coital exanthema virus. *Zentralblatt für Veterinärmedizin, Reihe* B 21:362–375.

18. Burrows, R. and Goodridge, D. 1984. Studies of persistent and latent equid herpes virus 1 and herpes virus 3 infections in the Pirbright pony herd. In *Latent herpes virus infections in veterinary medicine*, ed. G. Wittmann, R. M. Gaskell, and Rziha, H.-J., 307–319. Boston: Martinus Nijhoff.

19. Caughman, G. B., Staczek, J., O'Callaghan, D. J. 1985. Equine herpesvirus type 1 infected cell polypeptides: Evidence for immediate early/early/late regulation of viral gene expression. *Virology* 145:49–61.

20. Couto, M. A. and Hughes, J. P. 1993. Sexually transmitted (venereal) diseases of horses. In *Equine reproduction*, ed. A. O. McKinnon and J. O. Voss, 845–854. Philadelphia: Lea and Febiger.

21. Craig, J. F. and Kehoe, D. 1921. Horse pox and coital exanthema. *J. Comp. Pathol. Therapeutics* 34:126–129.

22. Crandall, R. A. and Davis, E. R. 1985. Isolation of equine coital exanthema virus (equine herpesvirus 3) from the nostril of a foal. *J. Am. Vet. Med. Assoc.* 187:503–504.

23. Cullinane, A., McGing, B. and Naughton, C. 1994. The use of acyclovir in the treatment of coital exanthema and ocular disease caused by equine herpesvirus 3. In *Equine infectious diseases VII*, ed. W. Plowright and H. Nakajima, 55. Newmarket, Suffolk: R&W Publications.

24. Davison, A. J., Eberle, R., Ehlers, B., Hayward, G. S., McGeoch, D. J., Minson, A. C., Pellett, P. E., Roizman, B., Studdert, M. J., Thiry, E. 2009. The order Herpesvirales. *Arch Virol.* 154:171–7.

25. Dynon, K., Varrasso, A., Ficorilli, N., Holloway, S., Reubel, G., Li, F., Hartley, C., Studdert, M. and Drummer, H. 2001. Identification of equine herpesvirus 3 (equine coital exanthema virus), equine gammaherpesviruses 2 and 5, equine adenoviruses 1 and 2, equine arteritis virus and equine rhinitis A virus by polymerase chain reaction. *Aust. Vet. J.* 79:695–702.

26. Evermann, J. F., Bergstrom, P. K., Cornell, D. B., Morgan, W. D. and Whitlatch, L. D. 1983. Equine coital exanthema virus infection. *Equine Practice* 5:39–47.

27. Feilen, C. P., Walker, S. T. and Studdert, M. J. 1979. Equine herpesvirus type 3 (equine coital exanthema) in New South Wales. *Aust. Vet. J.* 55:443–444.

28. Gibbs, E. P., Roberts, M. C. and Morris J. M. 1970. Equine coital exanthema in the UK, *Vet. Rec.* 87:91.

4. EQUINE COITAL EXANTHEMA

29. Gibbs, E. P., Roberts M. C. and Morris J. M. 1972. Equine coital exanthema in the United Kingdom. *Equine Vet. J.* 4:74–80.

30. Girard, A., Greig, A. S. and Mitchell, D. 1968. A virus associated with vulvitis and balantitis in the horse. A preliminary report. *Can. J. Comp. Med.* 32:603–604.

31. Gleeson, L. J., Sullivan, N. D. and Studdert M. J. 1976. Equine herpesviruses: Type 3 as an abortigenic agent. *Aust. Vet. J.* 52:349–354.

32. Gutekunst, D. E., Malmquist, W. A. and Becvar, C. S. 1978. Antigenic relatedness of equine herpes virus types 1 and 3. *Arch. Virol.* 56:33–45.

33. Hartley, C. A., Drummer, H. E. and Studdert, M. J. 1999. The nucleotide sequence of the glycoprotein G homologue of equine herpesvirus 3 (EHV3) indicates EHV3 is a distinct equid alphaherpesvirus. *Arch. Virol.* 144:2023–2033.

34. Jacob, R. J. 1986. Molecular pathogenesis of equine coital exanthema: Temperature-sensitive function(s) in cells infected with equine herpesviruses. *Vet. Microl.* 11:221–237.

35. Jacob, R. J., Price, R. and Allen, G. P. 1985. Molecular pathogenesis of equine coital exanthema: Restriction endonuclease digestions of EHV-3 DNA and indications of a unique XbaI cleavage site. *Intervirology* 23:172–180.

36. Jacob, R. J., Price, R., Bouchey, D., Davis, T. and Borchelt, J. 1990. Temperature sensitivity of equine herpesvirus isolates: A brief review. *SAAS Bulletin: Biochem. Biotech.* 3:124–128.

37. Kamada, M. and Studdert, M. J. 1983. Analysis of small and large plaque variants of equine herpesvirus type 3 by restriction endonucleases. Brief report. *Arch. Virol.* 77:259–264.

38. Kleiboeker, S. B. and Chapman, R. K. 2004. Detection of equine herpesvirus 3 in equine skin lesions by polymerase chain reaction. *J. Vet. Diagn. Invest.* 16:74–79.

39. Krogsrud, J. and Onstad, O. 1971. Equine coital exanthema. Isolation of a virus and transmission experiments. *Acta Veterinaria Scandinavica* 12:1–14.

40. Lalani, A. S., Barrett, J. W. and McFadden, G. 2000. Modulating chemokines: More lessons from viruses. *Immunol. Today* 21:100–106.

41. Leon, A. Fortier, G., Fortier, C., Freymuth, F., Tapprest, J., Leclercq, R. and Pronost, S. 2008. Detection of equine herpesviruses in aborted foetuses by consensus PCR. *Vet. Microbiol.* 126:20–29.

42. Ludwig, H., Biswal, N., Bryans, J. T. and McCombs, R. M. 1971. Some properties of the DNA from a new equine herpesvirus. *Virology* 45:534–537.

43. Murphy, P. M. 2001. Viral exploitation and subversion of the immune system through chemokine mimicry. *Nat. Immunol.* 2:116–122.

44. Pascoe, R. R. 1981. The effect of equine coital exanthema on the fertility of mares covered by stallions exhibiting the clinical disease. *Aust. Vet. J.* 57:111–114.

45. Pascoe, R. R., Spradbrow, P. B. and Bagust, T. J. 1968. Equine coital exanthema. *Aust. Vet. J.* 44:485.

46. Pascoe, R. R., Spradbrow, P. B. and Bagust, T. J. 1969. An equine genital infection resembling coital exanthema associated with a virus. *Aust. Vet. J.* 45:166–170.

47. Pascoe, R. R., Bagust, T. J. and Spradbrow, P. B. 1972. Studies on equine herpes viruses. Infection of horses with a herpesvirus recovered from equine coital exanthema. *Aust. Vet. J.* 48:99–104.

48. Pascoe, R. R. and Bagust, T. L. 1975. Coital exanthema in stallions. *J. Reprod. Fertil. Suppl.* 23:147–150.

49. Petzoldt, K. 1970. Equine coital exanthema. *Berliner und Münchener Tierärztliche Wochenschrift* 83:93–95.

50. Seki, Y., Seimiya, Y. M., Yaegashi, G., Kumagai, Shin-hi., Sentsui, H., Nishimori, T. and Ishihara, R. 2004. Occurrence of equine coital exanthema in pastured draft horses and isolation of equine herpesvirus 3 in progenital lesions. *J. Vet. Med. Sci.* 66:1503–1508.

51. Staczek, J., Atherton, S. S. and O'Callaghan, D. J. 1983. Genetic relatedness of the genomes of equine herpesvirus types 1, 2, and 3. *J. Virol.* 45:855–858.

52. Studdert, M. J. 1974. Comparative aspects of equine herpesviruses. *Cornell Vet.* 64:94–122.

53. Studdert, M. J. 1996. Equine coital exanthema (Equine herpesvirus 3). In *Virus infections of equines*, ed. M. J. Studdert, 39–46. Amsterdam: Elsevier.

54. Sullivan, D. C., Atherton, S. S., Staczek, J. and O'Callaghan, D. J. 1984. Structure of the genome of equine herpesvirus type 3. *Virology* 132:352–367.

55. Sullivan, D. C., Atherton, S. S., Caughman, G. B., Staczek, J. and O'Callaghan, D. J. 1986. Oncogenic transformation of primary hamster embryo cells by equine herpesvirus type 3. *Virus Research* 5:201–212.

56. Sullivan, D. C., Gray, W. L., Caughman, G. B., Robertson, A. T. and O'Callaghan, D. J. 1990. Temporal regulation of equine herpesvirus type 3 transcription. *Virus Research* 15:135–148.

57. Telford, E. A., Watson, M. S., McBride, K. and Davison, A. J. 1992. The DNA sequence of equine herpesvirus-1. *Virology* 189:304–316.

58. Telford, E. A., Watson, M. J., Perry, J., Cullinane A. A. and Davison A. J. 1998. The DNA sequence of equine herpesvirus-4. *J. Gen. Virol.* 79:1197–1203.

59. Turner, A. J., Studdert, M. J. and Peterson, J. E. 1970. Equine herpesviruses. 2. Persistence of equine herpesviruses in experimentally infected horses and the experimental induction of abortion. *Aust. Vet. J.* 46:90–98.

60. Uppal, P. K., Yadav, M. P., Singh, B. K. and Prasad, S. 1989. Equine coital exanthema (EHV-3 virus) infection in India. *Zentralblatt für Veterinärmedizin, Reihe* B 36:786–788.

61. Wilks, C. R. and Studdert, M. J. 1976. Equine herpesviruses. 6. Sequential infection of horses with types 2, 3 and 1. *Aust. Vet. J.* 52:199–203.

5. EASTERN, WESTERN, AND VENEZUELAN EQUINE ENCEPHALOMYELITIS
(EEE, WEE, VEE)

S. KAPOOR, K. DHAMA, R. V. S. PAWAIYA, M. MAHENDRAN, AND THANKAM MATHEW

INTRODUCTION

Among the arthropodborne viruses that cause neurologic disease in equines, humans, and other vertebrates, there are three important diseases caused by viruses that belong to family Togaviridae and genus *Alphavirus*: eastern equine encephalomyelitis (EEE), western equine encephalomyelitis (WEE), and Venezuelan equine encephalomyelitis (VEE) (Del Piero et al., 2001; Estrada-Franco et al., 2004; Hachiya et al., 2007; Aguilar et al., 2008a; Zhang et al., 2009). Viruses belonging to the genus *Alphavirus* have been classified into seven complexes based on serological cross reactivity (Calisher and Karabatsos, 1988) and are transmitted between invertebrate insect vectors and vertebrate reservoir hosts (Griffin, 1998). There are at least twenty-nine species and many more subtypes of alphaviruses among which some are considered potential bioweapons too (Eshoo et al., 2007). One or more species are found within each alphavirus complex, and multiple subtypes and/or varieties have been reported in several species. They are also classified as old-world alphaviruses and New World alphaviruses that cause rash and arthritis or encephalitis, respectively, in humans. New World members of three alphavirus complexes—viz, EEE, WEE, and VEE—cause encephalitis in equines. They have been clustered along with *Sindbis virus* based on genetic analysis (Levinson et al., 1990). Because alphaviruses are transmitted by arthropod vectors, clinical disease occurs during the arbovirus season of late summer and early fall in temperate zones, with year-round transmission possible in the tropics and subtropics. Epidemics and epizootics occur sporadically in temperate regions occur in warmer months and with increased rainfall (Armstrong et al., 2008).

These three diseases are caused by viruses that are related, but antigenically distinct. Interestingly, they occur only in the American continent and maintain sylvatic cycles of infection involving birds or rodents and mosquitoes (Minke et al., 2004). The encephalitogenic alphaviruses—including VEEV, EEEV, and WEEV—constitute a continuing public health threat in the United States by circulating in Central, South, and North America, causing fatal disease in humans, horses, and other domestic animals (Garmashova et al.,

2007). EEE has a significant public health concern due to the high mortality rates observed in infected humans, equines, and game birds (Platteborze et al., 2005). Therefore, alphaviruses should be handled only, using certified biosafety cabinets in a biocontainment (biosafety level III) facility, by immunized personnels. Postmortem examinations of horses suspected to have died of encephalomyelitis should be performed taking full precautions to prevent human infection. Horses are considered dead-end hosts for WEE, but may serve as amplifying hosts for VEE and occasionally for EEE. They cause sporadic epidemics with high case-fatality rates in horses. Besides equines, in canines and South American camelids the EEEV and VEEV have been reported to cause clinical signs/diseases (Farrar et al., 2005; Nolen-Walston et al., 2007). EEE has been diagnosed in deer also (Tate et al., 2005).

Etiology

EEE, WEE, VEE viruses are positive-strand RNA viruses (9.7–11.8 kb) characterized by mutations and evolutionary stability and classified within the genus *Alphavirus* under the family Togaviridae (Rico-Hesse, 2000; Del Piero et al., 2001; Minke et al., 2004). Very recently, it was identified that a VEE virus isolated from a boy with severe febrile disease contained two mutations within the PE2 region (Vilcarromero et al., 2009). The EEE, WEE and, VEE viruses are divided into three antigenic complexes, which are further classified into species, subtypes, and varieties. The VEE viruses are classified into six subtypes (I–VI), with subtype I having six variants (IA–IF). The variants IAB and IC have been associated with epizootics in equids and humans (Minke et al., 2004).

The alphavirus virion is enveloped, having a diameter of 60–65 nm, with icosahedral symmetry. The nucleocapsid is enclosed in a lipid envelope derived from areas of the host cell plasma membrane, which had previously been modified, viral-coded glycoproteins, E1 and E2, forming heterodimers that group further into trimers to form short spikes on the virion surface (Rice and Strauss, 1982; Anthony and Brown, 1991). The genome is linear and nonsegmented, single-stranded RNA with methylated cap at 3' end and a poly A tail at 5' end (Strauss and Strauss, 1986, 1994). The genome is organized to contain structural proteins and nonstructural proteins at the 5'-end and 3'-end, respectively. The 5' proximal two-thirds of the genome encode a 220 kD precursor polypeptide, which is proteolytically processed to produce four nonstructural proteins, two of which form the viral RNA polymerase that utilizes viral genome for the synthesis of a negative-stranded 49S RNA, which subsequently serves as a template for the synthesis of additional genomic RNA, as well as for transcription of a capped and polyadenylated 26S subgenomic mRNA that is identical to the 3' third of the genome. The

26S mRNA encodes for five structural polypeptides including nucleocapsid protein (30–33 kD) and two envelope glycoproteins E1 and E2 (45–58 kD) (Strauss and Strauss, 1994). The nonstructural protein 2 (nsp2) encoded by alphaviruses is a multifunctional enzyme that is essential for viral replication and maturation. Its 39-kDa, C-terminal domain (nsp2pro) is a cysteine protease that is responsible for cleaving viral polyprotein at three sites to generate nonstructural proteins 1, 2, 3, and 4 (Zhang et al., 2009).

The replication takes place in the cytoplasm, and maturation of the virus occurs via budding from the plasma membrane of the infected cells. The nucleocapsid contains group-specific antigenic determinants, and the envelope contains virus-specific/subgroup (complex) antigens. The production of neutralization or hemagglutinating antibodies is associated with E2 (Roehrig and Mathew, 1985). The virus readily grows in continuous cell lines (Vero, BHK-21) and primary chicken and duck embryo cells, producing severe cytopathic effect (CPE) due to complete shutdown of host-cell protein and nucleic acid synthesis. These viruses can also be propagated in mosquito (C6/36) cells but without any apparent CPE (Calisher et al., 1988). Many laboratory animals can be experimentally infected, with suckling mice being the most susceptible to these viruses. These viruses are not very stable in the environment and are sensitive to lipid solvents, chlorine, phenol, and acidic pH and heating to 60°C for thirty minutes.

EPIDEMIOLOGY

Epidemics of equine encephalitis have been identified during earlier times; an outbreak occurred in the first half of the nineteenth century in Massachusetts, USA, being a notable one. Epizootics due to EEEV have been described along the Atlantic seaboard of USA and in the Pampas regions of South America (Tenbroeck and Merrill, 1933; Scott and Weaver, 1989). In the western region of North America, similar disease was described almost at the same time in which about six thousand cases of equine encephalitis occurred. However, it was caused by a distinct virus, the western equine encephalomyelitis virus (WEEV) (Meyer et al., 1931). The WEEV (Meyer et al., 1931) and EEEV (Tenbroeck et al., 1935) were isolated from brain of horses suffering from encephalitis in these outbreaks. The WEEV was further shown to be transmitted by mosquitoes (Kelser, 1933). Another antigenically distinct virus from an outbreak of equine encephalomyelitis was isolated from Venezuela in 1936 and named Venezuelan equine encephalomyelitis virus (VEE) (Kubes and Rios, 1939).

Two antigenic subtypes of EEEV have been recognized that can be distinguished readily by hemagglutination inhibition and plaque-reduction neutralization tests. One antigenic subtype comprises strains from North America and some from the Caribbean, and the other strains are found in Central and South America (Brault et al., 1999; Casals, 1964; Roehrig et al., 1990). These subtypes exhibit differences in their transmission cycles and virulence. In addition, the North American and South American subtypes differ by 25–38% at the nucleotide level too (Brault et al., 1999).

The first human EEE outbreak was recognized in Massachusetts in 1938, and thirty-four cases with twenty-five fatalities were recorded (Fothergill et al., 1938). In general, EEEV strains from Central and South America appear to be less virulent for humans than North American strains (Aguilar et al., 2007). The South American strains can occasionally cause disease and death in horses, but human infections are rarely recognized and seldom result in neurologic disease (Adams et al., 2008; Aguilar et al., 2008b). Enzootic transmission of EEE virus along the eastern coast of the United States occurs almost exclusively between passerine birds and the ornithophilic mosquito *Culiseta melanura* (Griffin, 1998; Hachiya et al., 2007; Dhama et al., 2008). The infection among humans and horses is most likely incidental and occurs when the virus circulates widely and expands from the enzootic cycle (Hachiya et al., 2007). Because of the strict ornithophilic feeding behavior of this mosquito, the less-host-restricted bridging vectors, such as *Aedes vexans* and *Coquillettidia* species, transmit EEE from birds to humans and horses. Mosquito vectors belonging to *Culex* species are involved in EEE transmission in Mexico, Central America, and southward to Argentina strains (Weaver et al., 1991, 1994). The *Culex pedroi* may serve as a primary enzootic vector of EEEV (Turell et al., 2008). Small rodents are also involved in the primary virus life cycle in South America. EEE virus causes sporadic human disease in the Eastern parts of the United States (Harvala et al., 2009). Recent studies have indicated that EEE is rare, but the most severe of the mosquitoborne encephalitis in the United States with a case fatality rate of 30% (Harvala et al., 2009).

WEE is found in western Canada, states in the USA west of the Mississippi, and in Mexico and South America. Western equine encephalomyelitis complex consist of two subtypes, viz, WEE and Highlands J virus. The Highlands J (HJ) present in east of Mississippi river in USA has been isolated from cases of equine encephalitis, and it has been found pathogenic for turkey and pheasants. The HJ virus is transmitted among passerine birds in eastern North American freshwater swamps by *Culiseta melanura.* The transmission cycle of HJ virus is nearly identical to that EEEV in geographic distribution, seasonality, and habitat. VEE viruses are likely to remain viable for many days after release into water, snow, or even chlorinated tap water (Fitzgibbon and Sagripanti, 2008).

The enzootic and epidemic/epizootic mosquito vector of WEE in western North America is *Culex tarsalis* that transmits virus among passerine birds in agroecosystems (Reissen and Monath, 1988). Several antigenic variants of WEE subtype are responsible for majority of the WEE infections in western USA, and there is variation in infectivity of the WEEV strains (Nagata et al., 2006). Fort Morgan and Buggy Creek viruses, antigenic variants of WEE subtype, are transmitted among the colonies of nestling songbirds by the swallow nest bug *Oeciacus vicarious*, which are not considered pathogenic for horses or humans (Weaver et al., 1992). Due to changes in ecological factors, the incidence of WEE in humans and equids, which peaked during the mid-twentieth century, has declined to fewer cases during the past two decades (Forrester et al., 2008).

Viruses in the Venezuelan equine encephalomyelitis (VEE) complex are serologically classified into six distinct antigenic subtypes (I to VI). Viruses of subtypes I and III are further differentiated into five (IA to IF) and three (IIIA to IIIC) antigenic varieties, respectively (Young and Johnson, 1969; Young et al., 1969; Young, 1972; Kinney et al., 1983; Walton and Grayson, 1988; Minke et al., 2004). The distribution of VEE is limited primarily to Central and South America (Anishchenko et al., 2006a). Ecological and epidemiological factors probably constrain the frequency of VEE epidemics more than the generation, via mutation, of amplification-competent virus strains in equines (Anishchenko et al., 2006b). Also, the persistence of IC strains suggest the possibility of a cryptic transmission cycle involving survival through the dry season in infected vectors or persistently infected vertebrates (Navarro et al., 2005). Antigenic variant Everglades virus (EVE) from subtype II and Bijou Bridge virus from subtype III are the two exceptions that are found in Florida and Colorado, respectively. EVE is antigenically classified as a subtype II virus (Young and Johnson 1969), but it is genetically more closely related to the epizootic subtype IAB and IC viruses than the VEE-IE virus strain.

VEE epizootics, which were caused by subtype IAB and IC viruses, frequently occurred in South America, including a 1969 to 1972 pandemic, which spread from Central America to Texas in the United States. Following a period of inactivity from 1973–1991, VEE reemerged in South America and Mexico (Weaver et al., 2004b). After an absence of twenty years, epizootic VEE (IC) reemerged in Venezuela in 1993 (Rico-Hesse et al., 1995) and has caused concern because of two epidemics affecting the southern Mexican horse population in 1993 and 1996 (Oberste et al., 1998). Both outbreaks in Mexico were caused by VEE strains of subtype-variety IE, considered enzootic and not pathogenic for horses (Walton et al., 1973). Considerable variation is revealed in the ability of equine-virulent, epizootic strains to exploit horses as efficient amplification hosts. Subtype IC strains amplify efficiently in equines, with a correlation between maximum viremia titers and the extent of the outbreak from which the virus strain was isolated. Horses are efficient amplifiers of virus especially in a VEE epidemic, which is in contrast to EEE and WEE. Mutations in the E2 envelope glycoprotein gene are major determinants of adaptation to both equines and mosquito vectors (Weaver et al., 2004b).

Subtypes II, III, IV, V, and VI and varieties ID and IF are referred to as the enzootic (or endemic) strains of VEEV. Mutations in the E2 glycoprotein allow relatively viremia-incompetent, enzootic subtype strains to adapt for equine replication, leading to VEE emergence (Greene et al., 2005b). The enzootic strains may cause disease in humans, but they differ from the epizootic strains in their lack of virulence for equines. The enzootic cycle revolves around sylvatic rodents and birds, which develop viremia and can transmit VEE to mosquitoes. The mosquitoes that serve as the primary vectors for the bird or rodent-mosquito life cycle are *Culex* mosquitoes of the *Melanoconion* subgenus (Ferro et al., 2008). Mosquitoes such as *Psorophora confinnis, P. columbiae, Ochlerotatus taeniorhynchus, Culex* species, and *Aedes aegypti* can transmit the virus during VEE epizootics (Weaver et al., 2004b; Moncayo et al., 2008; Ortiz et al., 2008).

The epidemiology of equine alphavirus encephalitis depends on various species, subtypes, and varieties present in three antigenic complexes, viz, EEE, WEE, VEE; their virulence; and presence of the transmission vectors (Griffin, 1998). The transmission of alphaviruses in endemically infected areas is by wild birds, which serve as the reservoir, and mosquitoes, which are mainly vectors (Del Piero et al., 2001). Interactions between arthropod vectors and avian populations play a significant role in the transmission dynamics of alphaviruses (Unnasch et al., 2006). Geographical and seasonal distribution of the infection also affects disease occurrences in the natural and incidental host species. Epidemics and epizootics of EEEV occur sporadically in temperate regions, where transmission occurs from late summer to early fall (Armstrong et al., 2008). The enzootic, equine avirulent, serotype ID VEEV strains appear to alter their serotype to IAB or IC and their vertebrate/nonvertebrate host range to mediate repeated VEE emergence via mutations in the E2 envelope glycoprotein representing convergent evolution (Weaver et al., 2004a). Further, it has been identified that the VEEV is highly infectious when transmitted by aerosol (Phillpotts, 2006; Sharma et al., 2008). VEEV is of high concern regarding its use in bioterrorism (Schlesinger, 2001; Weaver et al., 2004a; Anishchenko et al., 2006a; Kirsch et al., 2008).

PATHOGENESIS AND PATHOLOGY

The mosquito bite facilitates the virus entry into the host cells, and virus replication occurs in cells near the entry sites and regional lymph nodes. The primary viremia is followed by invasion of extraneural tissue where virus replication leads to high secondary viremia, a key to further infection of mosquitoes and also invasion of central nervous system (CNS). The virus replicates primarily in muscles, connective tissues, and reticuloendothelial system. In CNS, infection involves neurons, choroid plexus, ependyma, and meninges. The VEE virus also infects the upper respiratory tract, pancreas, and liver. WEEV infects the central nervous system with severe complications and even death (Wu et al., 2007a).

Both structural and nonstructural genes of alphaviruses are important for virulence (Davis et al., 1991; Grieder et al., 1995; White et al., 2001; Greene, et al, 2005b; Aguilar et al., 2008b). The capsid protein of EEEV is a potent inhibitor of host cell gene expression and helps in the protection of EEEV from the antiviral effects of interferons (IFNs) (Aguilar et al., 2008a). The avirulent South American strain was sensitive to human IFN, in contrast to North American strains that were highly resistant (Aguilar et al., 2008b). Mutations in the E1 and E2 glycoproteins to virulence of VEEV have been well characterized in mice (Davis et al., 1991; Grieder et al., 1995). Two viral determinants (glycoproteins and the 5' UTR) were responsible for the IFN-resistant phenotype of the TrD strain (Spotts et al., 1998). A virus carrying a single mutation at nucleotide position 3 in 5' UTR in VEEV resulted in avirulence in mice and reduced replication in cell culture (White et al., 2001).

The alphaviruses have developed the ability to interfere with cellular transcription and downregulate cellular antiviral response and produce cytopathic effect provided by the N-terminal, approximately 35-aminoacid-long peptide of capsid proteins (Garmashova et al., 2007). The E2 glycoprotein defines the enzootic and epizootic VEEV subtypes as well as mosquitoborne virus infectivity (Weaver et al., 2004a, b; Greene et al., 2005b). Both structural and nonstructural protein genes of VEEV have also been implicated as determinants of viral virulence in guinea pigs (Greene et al., 2005a). Genes related to important immune pathways such as antigen presentation, inflammation, apoptosis, and response to virus are upregulated as a result of VEE infection (Sharma et al., 2008).

Very little is known about the role of structural and nonstructural genes in EEEV pathogenesis. Both VEEV and EEEV cause encephalitis in the murine model. However, the diseases are different: EEEV is primarily neurotropic, whereas VEEV begins with a lymphotropic phase that progress to a neurotropic phase. EEEV replicates poorly in lymphoid tissues and preferentially infect osteoblasts. EEEV has affinity for myeloid lineage cells. Inhibition of genome translation restricts EEEV infectivity for myeloid lineage cells in vitro and in vivo (Gardner et al., 2008). VEEV infects dendritic cells (DCs) and macrophages in lymphoid tissues, fueling a serum viremia and facilitating neuroinvasion (Gardner et al., 2008). VEEV also causes systemic infection with pathological lesions in the lung, lymphoid tissues of the gastrointestinal tract, spleen, and peripheral lymph nodes (Jackson et al., 1991). The mechanisms by which these viruses enter the central nervous system appear to differ. VEEV invades the murine brain via the olfactory bulb (Charles et al., 1995), whereas EEEV may cross the blood-brain barrier by passive transfer or within infected leukocytes (Vogel et al., 2005). Recently, viruslike replicon particles (VRP) packaged with VEE-derived glycoproteins have been produced, and this can be used in future for studying the cellular tropism events (Kamrud et al., 2008).

A murine model for VEEV-induced encephalitis and lymphotropism is well established, with the infection of the CNS results in an acute meningoencephalitis, which causes death of large numbers of neuronal cells and 100% lethality (Kundin, 1961; Dal Canto and Rabinowitz. 1981; Davis et al., 1994). Subcutaneous infection of mice leads to biphasic disease with initial replication in lymphoid tissues, followed by viremia and penetration into the CNS (Ryzhikov et al., 1991), where the virus replicates until death of the animal (Jackson et al., 1991; Ryzhikov et al., 1995).

In experimentally infected mice, EEEV produces neurologic disease that resembles the human and equine infections. Virus is detected in the brain as early as day 1 postinfection (PI), and signs of disease are evident as early as days 3 to 4 PI. Clinical signs of murine disease include ruffled hair, anorexia, vomiting, lethargy, posterior limb paralysis, convulsions, and coma. Histopathological studies can reveal extensive involvement of the brain, including neuronal degeneration, cellular infiltration, and perivascular cuffing; these are similar to the pathological changes of the central nervous system that are described in naturally infected humans (Vogel et al., 2005).

The horses that die due to EEE, WEE, or VEE do not show any consistent gross lesions. However, of the three viruses, most extensive and severe lesions are caused by EEE. Lesions in the brain results from direct replication and are characterized by necrotizing encephalitis and neuronal malfunction. The affected neurons show degenerative changes such as tigrolysis, chromatolysis and neuronaphagia, marked perivascular cutting. The leukocytes and glial cells form small nodules around the injured neurons, which may persist.

More lesions are seen in the cerebral cortex, thalamus, and hypothalamus as compared to spinal cord. Neurologic defects may be asymmetric as the lesions are not necessarily symmetrically distributed.

CLINICAL MANIFESTATIONS

The clinical manifestations produced by the three virus complexes differ widely, which may be due to differences in their virulence. Infection may range from subclinical to encephalitis and death. The incubation period varies from three to four days to an occasional three weeks. Endemic VEE and WEE viruses produce less severe signs of the disease than EEE and epidemic VEE. Neurologic disease is most severe in EEE. EEEV cause polioencephalitis with lymphocytic perivascular cuffing, neutrophil infiltration, gliosis, neuron satellitosis, necrosis, and edema, with intracytoplasmic inclusions within neurons and glial cells (Nolen-Walston et al., 2007). In VEE, there is progressive systemic disease leading to death with minor neurologic manifestations. Initially, there may be a rise in body temperature, signs of drowsiness, and incoordination of movements. The disease progresses rapidly, and clinical signs include partial or complete blindness, aimless wandering, head pressing, circling, grinding of teeth, inability to swallow due to esophageal paralysis, irregular ataxic gait, paresis and paralysis, convulsions, and death. Animals with severe ataxia may stand against walls or other objects and occasionally with their hind legs crossed. In terminal stages of the disease, the animal shows signs of paralysis, unresponsiveness and occasional convulsions, loss of awareness to the surroundings, aimless wandering, walking in circles, collision with objects, and succumbing. Mortality in horses showing clinical signs varies 50–90% in EEE, 20–50% in WEE, and 50–75% in VEE. Horses usually die within two to three days after onset of clinical signs. Horses with clinical neurologic signs from alphavirus infection that recover have a high incidence of residual neurologic deficiencies such as dullness and dementia.

DIAGNOSIS

No specific treatment exists for infections by alphaviruses, but a specific and rapid diagnosis will help to prevent the further spread of the disease by movement control and quarantine of horses, trade restriction, vaccination, and vector control. This is of particular importance in countries such as Mexico, where all three equine encephalitis viruses circulate simultaneously. The diagnosis of the disease is based upon the geographical distribution of the virus, seasonal vector activity, and clinical signs and symptoms. The clinical signs of EEE-, WEE-, or VEE-infected horses are nonspecific and resemble with many nonviral and noninfectious agents. Brain or cerebrospinal fluid (CSF) is more suitable for virus isolation as viremia is usually low in horses affected by equine encephalomyelitis viruses. Detection of the viral antigen or its nucleic acid in serum is only successful if the blood is collected during the viremic phase of the infection, which lasts for three to five days. Virus isolation by intracerebral inoculation of suckling mice or various cell cultures is the "gold standard" for virus detection (OIE, 2008), but this has been considered to be very time-consuming. Confirmation of the isolates is done by neutralization test using reference monoclonal antibodies and also by partial genome sequencing.

The disease can also be confirmed by detection of specific antibodies by serological tests, viz, hemagglutination inhibition (HI), enzyme-linked immunosorbent assay (ELISA), or plaque-reduction neutralization (PRN). EEE viruses are traditionally divided into North America and South America antigenic varieties based on HI tests. Because virus-neutralizing antibodies appear at the end of viremia and may precede the appearance of neurologic signs, paired samples may not show a fourfold increase in horses with neurologic signs. Antibody capture ELISA for IgM, and IgG has also been used as possible adjuncts to HI and PRN tests to differentiate between recent exposure and those due to vaccination. The IgM antibodies of EEE virus have been found to be monospecific, which did not cross-react with WEE and VEE (Sahu et al., 1994). Epitope-blocking enzyme immunoassay (EIA) have been used to differentiate the antibody responses to endemic (IE and ID) and epidemic (IAB and IC) strains of VEE virus (Wang et al., 2005). Recently, Hu et al. (2008) revealed the potential of recombinant antigens, E1 and E2, expressed in bacteria, to be used as antigens in immunoassays to detect anti-WEEV antibodies.

Nucleic acid amplification has been used for direct virus detection and identification in field and clinical samples (Lambert et al., 2003). A sensitive and specific colorimetric dot assay following polymerase chain reaction (PCR) amplification method has been developed to detect EEEV RNA (Armstrong et al., 1995). EEE can be confirmed by viral detection using immunohistochemistry (IHC) and PCR and by serological tests (Nolen-Walston et al., 2007). Reverse transcriptase–polymerase chain reaction (RT-PCR)—a fast, sensitive, and specific alternative for the diagnosis—has been described for the detection of EEEV, WEEV, and VEEV (Vodkin et al., 1993, 1994; Monroy et al., 1996; Brightwell et al., 1998; Farrar et al., 2005). However, these assays fail to distinguish closely related heterologous alphaviruses (Linssen et al., 1999).

The use of a RT-PCR with ELISA (RT-PCR-ELISA), with combined sensitivity of PCR, detection simplicity of ELISA, and specificities of DNA probes could better identify pathogenic alphaviruses (Wang et al., 2006). A multilocus RT-PCR followed by electrospray ionization mass spectrometry (RT-PCR/ESI-MS) to detect and identify alphaviruses like VEEV and EEEV could provide a rapid, accurate, and high-throughput assay for surveillance of alphaviruses (Eshoo et al., 2007). TaqMan real-time RT-PCR assay has also been recently developed for the detection of EEE virus (Hull et al., 2008). Recently, the use of recombinant antibodies (r-Ab) for the detection of VEEV has been exploited, which will improve the fast identification of VEEV in case of a biological warfare or a natural outbreak (Kirsch et al., 2008).

Reverse genetics can also be used to detect E2 gene mutations that mediated emergence of VEEV strains (Anishchenko et al., 2006b). Further, by sequence analysis, the phylogenetic relationships of various alphavirus isolates can be obtained, which helps in grouping them into discrete clades (Luers et al., 2005; Armstrong et al et al., 2008; Young et al., 2008). Sequence analysis of EEE pathogenic strains also favor the production of infectious clone that can be used to create live, attenuated vaccine candidates (Platteborze et al., 2005).

As part of differential diagnosis, the disease caused by equine alphaviruses need to be differentiated from rabies, hepatic encephalopathy, leukoencephalomalacia, equine protozoal encephalomyelitis, equine herpesvirus 1, botulism, and ataxia as a result of cervical vertebral malformation.

PREVENTION AND CONTROL

The prevention of equine encephalomyelitis can be effectively achieved by pest management programs since perpetuation of these viruses involve arthropod vector, which can be achieved through eliminating mosquito-breeding sites by using larvicides or insecticides (Sudia and Newhouse, 1975). Timely mosquito testing and infection-rate calculation are critical for disease-risk estimation of EEE and outbreak control efforts (Hachiya et al., 2007). Use of sentinel surveillance system, quarantine, and prohibition of the movements of the horses are used to control the encephalitis epidemics. For birds, the use of insectproof rearing pens is also recommended.

Safe and efficacious vaccines are available for VEE, EEE, and WEE. The killed vaccines against EEE, WEE, and VEE are derived from formaldehyde or ethylene imine-inactivated cell cultures. Limitations with inactivated vaccines include low immunogenicity, multiple injections required to provide adequate protection, require growing large quantities of virus, are subject to manufacturing issues including adequate biosafety and may have possible detrimental effects following incomplete virus inactivation (Minke et al., 2004).

A modified live vaccine against VEE is available in North and South America, using the vaccine strain TC-83 derived from the Trinidad donkey strain (TrD-variant IAB) (Berge et al., 1961; Minke et al., 2004). In horses, the vaccine induces long-lasting neutralizing antibodies and had proven to be very efficacious in controlling the epidemics of VEE in Central America. However, several biosafety issues are associated with the use of this vaccine. It should be used with caution as low level of viremia and leukopenia has been observed in some vaccinated horses, but neutralizing antibody responses to homologous (serotype IA) virus eventually developed in 90% of these animals (Monlux et al., 1972; Walton et al., 1972; Jochim, et al., 1973). The vaccine is reactogenic in horses and man, and concerns remain about its potential to revert to virulence and introduction of the strain into the mosquito population. In addition, these current VEE vaccines do not seem to fully protect against enzootic viruses (Rico-Hesse, 2000). A live, attenuated IE1150K strain of VEEV can be used to elicit protection against challenge with virulent VEEV (Reed et al., 2005). V3526, a live-attenuated virus, intended for human use, was found safe and efficacious in protecting horses against a virulent VEEV IA/B TrD virus challenge (Fine et al., 2007). V3526, a strain of VEEV, was found immunogenic and essentially nonneurovirulent when administered via the clinically relevant subcutaneous route (Fine et al., 2008).

The horses are vaccinated with monovalent, divalent, or trivalent vaccine depending upon the epidemiology. Two doses of the vaccine are given at the interval of thirty days in the spring of each year. To raise colostral antibodies, mares should be vaccinated about a month before foaling. However, colostral antibodies at a titer >1:10 interfere with vaccination in foals. Therefore, in areas of high mosquito activities, foals should be vaccinated at three, four, and six months of age followed by annual vaccination program. It was observed that no VEE-related deaths occurred in horses known to have been vaccinated at least two weeks before any disease occurrence in the area, whereas up to 60% mortality occurred in unvaccinated animals (Burke et al., 1977). The transmission of vaccine virus between horses by mosquitoes and reversion to virulence is also possible. However, it has been reported that prior vaccination against one alphavirus can interfere with the development of neutralizing antibody to subsequent alphavirus vaccine (Calisher et al., 1973; McClain et al., 1998). There is some cross-protection between EEE and WEE, EEE and VEE, but not between WEE and VEE.

Future vaccines against equine encephalitis should be based on immunogens derived from enzootic viruses, the development of infectious cDNAs and their attenuation by genomic modifications, and recombinant DNA vaccines including the DNA vaccines (Rico-Hesse, 2000; Minke et al., 2004; Wu et al., 2007a, b; Volkova et al., 2008). Several experimental vaccines, including recombinant *Vaccinia*, baculovirus and adenovirus vectors, chimeric recombinants, deletion mutants, and DNA vaccines have been evaluated in animal models and equines as potential vaccine candidates against these encephalitis viruses (Minke et al., 2004; Nagata et al., 2005; Perkins et al., 2006; Das et al., 2007; Wu et al., 2007a, b; Perkins et al., 2008). Thompson et al. (2008) suggested that strongest mucosal immune responses can be induced by mucosal Ag delivery of VEEV replicon particles (VRP). A novel genetic vaccine induced an efficient prime to a VEE VRP boost, increasing both humoral and cellular immunity (Ljungberg et al., 2007).

Besides, the use of iodonaphthylazide (INA) for virus inactivation in developing vaccine (Sharma et al., 2007), RNA interference mechanism mediated by the short interfering RNAs (siRNAs) possessing activity against the virus (O'Brien, 2007), and peptide-conjugated phosphorodiamidate morpholino oligomers (PPMO) inhibiting VEEV replication through sequence-specific steric blockade of viral RNA (Paessler et al., 2008) have also been indicated to strategically counter these viruses.

CONCLUSION

Eastern, western, and Venezuelan equine encephalomyelitis (EEE, WEE, VEE) are mosquitoborne viral infections that can cause severe encephalitis in horses and humans, which occur especially in North, Central, and Southern parts of the American continent. As a result of vaccination, severe outbreaks of eastern and western equine encephalomyelitis no longer occur regularly in the United States, but sporadic cases and small outbreaks are still seen. Although mosquito control and immunization have significantly reduced the incidence of EEE in horses, small and large epidemics still occur, particularly in the Southern states. This could be attributed to the short duration of vaccine immunity and the long vector season. Hence, determining the amount of an arbovirus transmitted by a mosquito is important to design transmission and pathogenesis studies simulating natural infection to assess vector competence. To understand the impact of continuing circulation of alphaviruses on human and animal populations, serologic and viral isolation studies should also be conducted. The EEE epidemics underscore our still-limited knowledge of the pathogenesis and epidemiology of alphaviruses. Human EEE is relatively rare, but the disease produces significant morbidity and mortality and profound neurologic complications in majority of the survivors. Additionally, human EEE outbreaks have caused significant public concern, probably because of their intensity and infrequency.

Considering its serious consequences and social and economic impact, EEE is of public health importance, and accurate human risk estimation and outbreak prevention measures are needed, aside from the preventive and control programs implemented among equine populations. Also, the bioterrorism potential of VEE virus should be kept in mind.

REFERENCES

1. Adams, A. P., Aronson, J. F., Tardif, S. D., Patterson, J. L., Brasky, K. M., Geiger, R., de la Garza, M., Carrion, R. Jr. and Weaver, S. C. 2008. Common marmosets (*Callithrix jacchus*) as a nonhuman primate model to assess the virulence of eastern equine encephalitis virus strains. *J. Virol.* 82:9035–9042.

2. Aguilar, P. V., Robich, R. M., Turell, M. J., O'Guinn, M. L., Klein, T. A., Huaman, A., Guevara, C., Rios, Z., Tesh, R. B., Watts, D. M., Olson, J. and Weaver, S. C. 2007. Endemic eastern equine encephalitis in the Amazon region of Peru. *Am. J. Trop. Med. Hyg.* 76:293–298.

3. Aguilar, P. V., Leung, L. W., Wang, E., Weaver, S. C. and Basler, C. F. 2008a. A five-amino-acid deletion of the eastern equine encephalitis virus capsid protein attenuates replication in mammalian systems but not in mosquito cells. *J. Virol.* 82:6972–6983.

4. Aguilar, P. V., Adams, A. P., Wang, E., Kang, W., Carrara, A., Anishchenko, M., Frolov, I. and Weaver, S. C. 2008b. Structural and nonstructural protein genome regions of eastern equine encephalitis virus are determinants of interferon sensitivity and murine virulence. *J. Virol.* 82:4920–4930.

5. Anishchenko, M., Alekseev, V. V. and Lipnitskii, A. V. 2006a. Venezuelan equine encephalitis: State-of-the-art. *Vopr. Virusol.* 51:10–13.

6. Anishchenko, M., Bowen, R. A., Paessler, S., Austgen, L., Greene, I. P. and Weaver, S. C. 2006b. Venezuelan encephalitis emergence mediated by a phylogenetically predicted viral mutation. *Proc. Natl. Acad. Sci. USA.* 103:4994–4999.

7. Anthony, R. P. and Brown, D. T. 1991. Protein-protein interactions in an alphavirus membrane. *J. Virol.* 65:1187–1194.

8. Armstrong, P., Borovsky, D., Shope, R. E., Morris, C. D., Mitchell, C. J., Karabatsos, N., Komar, N. and Spielman, A. 1995. Sensitive and specific colorimetric dot assay to detect eastern equine encephalomyelitis viral RNA in mosquitoes (Diptera: Culicidae) after polymerase chain reaction amplification. *J. Med. Entomol.* 32:42–52.

9. Armstrong, P. M., Andreadis, T. G., Anderson, J. F., Stull, J. W. and Mores, C. N. 2008. Tracking eastern equine encephalitis virus perpetuation in the northeastern United States by phylogenetic analysis. *Am. J. Trop. Med. Hyg.* 79:291–296.

10. Berge, T. O., Banks, I. S., Tigertt, W. D. 1961. Attenuation of Venezuelan equine encephalomyelitis vaccine by in vitro cultivation in guinea-pig heart cells. *Am. J. Hyg.* 73:209–218.

11. Brault, A. C., Powers, A. M., Chavez, C. L., Lopez, R. N., Cachon, M. F., Gutierrez, L. F., Kang, W., Tesh, R. B., Shope, R. E. and Weaver, S. C. 1999. Genetic and antigenic diversity among Eastern equine encephalitis viruses from North, Central, and South America. *Am. J. Trop. Med. Hyg.* 61:579–586.

12. Brightwell, G., Brown, J. M. and Coates, D. M. 1998. Genetic targets for the detection and identification of Venezuelan equine encephalitis viruses. *Arch. Virol.* 143:731–742.

13. Burke, D. S., Ramsburg, H. H. and Edelman, R. 1977. Persistence in humans of antibody to subtypes of Venezuelan equine encephalomyelitis (VEE) virus after immunization with attenuated (TC-83) VEE virus vaccine. *J. Infect. Dis.* 136:354–359.

14. Calisher, C. H. and Karabatsos, N. 1988. Arbovirus serogroups: Definition and geographic distribution. In *The arboviruses: Epidemiology and ecology*, vol. 5., ed. T. P. Monath, 19–57. Boca Raton: CRC Press.

15. Calisher, C. H., Sasso, D. R. and Sather, G. E. 1973. Possible evidence of interference with Venezuelan equine encephalitis vaccination of equines by pre-existing antibody to eastern or western equine encephalitis virus or both. *Applied Microbiol.* 26:485–488.

16. Calisher, C. Shope, R. and Walton, T. 1988. Cell culture for the diagnosis of arbovirus infections in livestock and wildlife. *J. Tissue Culture Methods* 11:157–163.

17. Casals, J. 1964. Antigenic variants of Eastern equine encephalitis virus. *J. Exp. Med.* 119:547–565.

18. Charles, P. C., Walters, E. Margolis, F. and Johnston, R. E. 1995. Mechanism of neuroinvasion of Venezuelan equine encephalitis virus in the mouse. *Virology* 208:662–671.

19. Dal Canto, M. C. and Rabinowitz, S. G. 1981. Central nervous system demyelination in Venezuelan equine encephalomyelitis infection. *J. Neurol. Sci.* 49:397–418.

20. Das, D., Nagata, L. P. and Suresh, M. R. 2007. Immunological evaluation of Escherichia coli expressed E2 protein of western equine encephalitis virus. *Virus Res.* 128:26–33.

21. Davis, N. L., Powell, N., Greenwald, G. F., Willis, L. V., Johnson, B. J., Smith, J. F. and Johnston, R. E. 1991. Attenuating mutations in the E2 glycoprotein gene of Venezuelan equine encephalitis virus: Construction of single and multiple mutants in a full-length cDNA clone. *Virology* 183:20–31.

22. Davis, N. L., Grieder, F. B. Smith, J. F., Greenwald, G. F., Valenski, M. L., Sellon, D. C., Charles, P. C. and Johnston, R. E. 1994. A molecular genetic approach to the study of Venezuelan equine encephalitis virus pathogenesis. *Arch. Virol.* 9:99–109.

23. Del Piero, F., Wilkins, P. A., Dubovi, E. J., Biolatti, B. and Cantile, C. 2001. Clinical, pathologic, immunohistochemical and virologic findings of Eastern equine encephalomyelitis in two horses. *Vet. Pathol.* 38:451–456.

24. Dhama, K., Mahendran, M. and Tomar, S. 2008. Pathogens transmitted by migratory birds: Threat perceptions to poultry health and production. *Int. J. Poult. Sci.* 7:516–525.

25. Eshoo, M. W., Whitehouse, C. A., Zoll, S. T., Massire, C., Pennella, T. T., Blyn, L. B., Sampath, R., Hall, T. A., Ecker, J. A., Desai, A., Wasieloski, L. P., Li, F., Turell, M. J., Schink, A., Rudnick, K., Otero, G., Weaver, S. C., Ludwig, G. V., Hofstadler, S. A. and Ecker, D. J. 2007. Direct broad-range detection of alphaviruses in mosquito extracts. *Virology* 368:286–295.

26. Estrada-Franco, J. G., Navarro-Lopez, R., Freier, J. E., Cordova, D., Clements, T., Moncayo, A., Kang, W., Gomez-Hernandez, C., Rodriguez-Dominguez, G., Ludwig, G. V. and Weaver, S. C. 2004. Venezuelan equine encephalitis virus, southern Mexico. *Emerg. Infect. Dis.* 10:2113–2121.

27. Farrar, M. D., Miller, D. L., Baldwin, C. A., Stiver, S. L. and Hall, C. L. 2005. Eastern equine encephalitis in dogs. *J. Vet. Diagn. Invest.* 17:614–617.

28. Ferro, C., Olano, V. A., Ahumada, M. and Weaver, S. 2008. Mosquitos (Diptera: Culicidae) in the small village where a human case of Venezuelan equine encephalitis was recorded. *Biomedica* 28:234–244.

29. Fine, D. L., Roberts, B. A., Teehee, M. L., Terpening, S. J., Kelly, C. L., Raetz, J. L., Baker, D. C., Powers, A. M. and Bowen, R. A. 2007. Venezuelan equine encephalitis virus vaccine candidate (V3526) safety, immunogenicity and efficacy in horses. *Vaccine* 25:1868–1876.

30. Fine, D. L., Roberts, B. A., Terpening, S. J., Mott, J., Vasconcelos, D. and House, R. V. 2008. Neurovirulence evaluation of Venezuelan equine encephalitis (VEE) vaccine candidate V3526 in nonhuman primates. *Vaccine* 26:3497–3506.

31. Fitzgibbon, J. E. and Sagripanti, J. L. 2008. Analysis of the survival of Venezuelan equine encephalomyelitis virus and possible viral simulants in liquid suspensions. *J. Appl. Microbiol.* 105:1477–1483.

32. Forrester, N. L., Kenney, J. L., Deardorff, E., Wang, E. and Weaver, S. C. 2008. Western equine encephalitis submergence: Lack of evidence for a decline in virus virulence. *Virology* 380:170–172.

33. Fothergill, L. D., Dingle, J. H., Farber, S. and Connerley, M. L. 1938. Human encephalitis caused by the virus of the eastern variety of equine encephalomyelitis. *N. Engl. J. Med.* 219:411.

34. Gardner, C. L., Burke, C. W., Tesfay, M. Z., Glass, P. J., Klimstra, W. B. and Ryman, K. D. 2008. Eastern and Venezuelan equine encephalitis viruses differ in their ability to infect dendritic cells and macrophages: Impact of altered cell tropism on pathogenesis. *J. Virol.* 82:10634–10646.

35. Garmashova, N., Atasheva, S., Kang, W., Weaver, S. C., Frolova, E. and Frolov, I. 2007. Analysis of Venezuelan equine encephalitis virus capsid protein function in the inhibition of cellular transcription. *J. Virol.* 81:13552–13565.

36. Greene, I. P., Paessler, S. Anishchenko, M., Smith, D. R., Brault, A. C., Frolov, I. and Weaver, S. C. 2005a. Venezuelan equine encephalitis virus in the guinea pig model: Evidence for epizootic virulence determinants outside the E2 envelope glycoprotein gene. *Am. J. Trop. Med. Hyg.* 72:330–338.

37. Greene, I. P., Paessler, S., Austgen, L., Anishchenko, M., Brault, A. C., Bowen, R. A. and Weaver, S. C. 2005b. Envelope glycoprotein mutations mediate equine amplification and virulence of epizootic Venezuelan equine encephalitis virus. *J. Virol.* 79:9128–9133.

38. Grieder, F. B., Davis, N. L., Aronson, J. F., Charles, P. C., Sellon, D. C., Suzuki, K. and Johnston, R. E. 1995. Specific restrictions in the progression of Venezuelan equine encephalitis virus-induced disease resulting from single amino acid changes in the glycoproteins. *Virology* 206:994–1006.

39. Griffin, D. E. 1998. A review of alphavirus replication in neurons. *Neurosci. Biobehav. Rev.* 22:721–723.

40. Hachiya, M., Osborne, M., Stinson, C. and Werner, B. G. 2007. Human eastern equine encephalitis in Massachusetts: Predictive indicators from mosquitoes collected at 10 long-term trap sites, 1979–2004. *Am. J. Trop. Med. Hyg.* 76:285–292.

41. Harvala, H., Bremner, J., Kealey, S., Weller, B., McLellan, S., Lloyd, G., Staples, E., Faggian, F. and Solomon, T. 2009. Case report: Eastern equine encephalitis virus imported to the UK. *J. Med. Virol.* 81:305–308.

42. Hu, W. G., Chau, D., Wong, C., Masri, S. A., Fulton, R. E. and Nagata, L. P. 2008. Cloning, expression and purification of envelope proteins E1 and E2 of western equine encephalitis virus and potential use of them as antigens in immunoassays. *Vet. Microbiol.* 128:374–379.

43. Hull, R., Nattanmai, S., Kramer, L. D., Bernard, K. A. and Tavakoli, N. P. 2008. A duplex real-time reverse transcriptase polymerase chain reaction assay for the detection of St. Louis encephalitis and eastern equine encephalitis viruses. *Diagn. Microbiol. Infect. Dis.* 62:272–279.

44. Jackson, A. C., SenGupta, S. K. and Smith, J. F. 1991. Pathogenesis of Venezuelan equine encephalitis virus infection in mice and hamsters. *Vet. Pathol.* 28:410–418.

45. Jochim, M. M., Barber, T. L. and Luedke, A. J. 1973. Venezuelan equine encephalomyelitis: Antibody response in vaccinated horses and resistance to infection with virulent virus. *J. Am. Vet. Med. Assoc.* 162:280–283.

46. Kamrud, K. I., Alterson, K. D., Andrews, C., Copp, L. O., Lewis, W. C., Hubby, B., Patel, D., Rayner, J. O., Talarico, T. and Smith, J. F. 2008. Analysis of Venezuelan equine encephalitis replicon particles packaged in different coats. *PLoS One* 3:e2709.

47. Kelser, R. A. 1933. Mosquitoes as vectors of the virus of equine encephalomyelitis. *J. Am. Vet. Med. Assoc.* 82:767–771.

48. Kinney, R. M., Trent, D. W. and France, J. K. 1983. Comparative immunological and biochemical analyses of viruses in the Venezuelan equine encephalitis complex. *J. Gen. Virol.* 64:135–147.

49. Kirsch, M. I., Hulseweh, B., Nacke, C., Rulker, T., Schirrmann, T., Marschall, H. J., Hust, M. and Dubel, S. 2008. Development of human antibody fragments using antibody phage display for the detection and diagnosis of Venezuelan equine encephalitis virus (VEEV). *BMC Biotechnol.* 8:66.

50. Kubes, V. and Rios, F. A. 1939. Causative agent of infectious equine encephalomyelitis in Venezuela. *Science* 90:20–21.

51. Kundin, W. D. 1966. Pathogenesis of Venezuelan equine encephalomyelitis virus. II. Infection in young adult mice. *J. Immunol.* 96:49–58.

52. Lambert, A. J., Martin, D. A. and Lanciotti R. S. 2003. Detection of North American eastern and western equine encephalitis viruses by nucleic acid amplification assays. *J. Clin. Microbiol.* 41:379–385.

53. Levinson, R. S., Strauss, J. H. and Strauss, E. G. 1990. Complete sequence of genomic RNA of O'nyong-nyong virus and its use in the construction of alphavirus phylogenetic trees. *Virology* 175:110–123.

54. Linssen, B., Kinney, R. M., Kaaden, O. R. and Pfeffer, M. 1999. Specific detection of equine encephalitis viruses by RT-PCR. In *Equine infectious diseases VIII*, ed. U. Wernery, J. F. Wade, J. A. Mumford, and O. R. Kaaden, 280–285. Newmarket, United Kingdom: R&W Publications, Ltd.

55. Ljungberg, K., Whitmore, A. C., Fluet, M. E., Moran, T. P., Shabman, R. S., Collier, M. L., Kraus, A. A., Thompson, J. M., Montefiori, D. C., Beard, C. and Johnston, R. E. 2007. Increased immunogenicity

of a DNA-launched Venezuelan equine encephalitis virus-based replicon DNA vaccine. *J. Virol.* 81:13412–13423.

56. Luers, A. J., Adams, S. D., Smalley, J. V. and Campanella, J. J. 2005. A phylogenomic study of the genus alphavirus employing whole genome comparison. *Comp. Funct. Genomics* 6:217–227.

57. McClain, D. J., Pittman, P. R., Ramsburg, H. H., Nelson, G. O., Rossi, C. A., Mangiafico, J. A., Schmaljohn, A. L. and Malinoski, F. J. 1998. Immunologic interference from sequential administration of live attenuated alphavirus vaccines. *J. Infect. Dis.* 177:634–641.

58. Meyer, K. F., Haring, C. M. and Howitt, B. 1931. The etiology of epizootic encephalomyelitis of horses in the San Joaquin Valley. *Science* 74:227–228.

59. Minke, J. M., Audonnet, J. C. and Fischer, L. 2004. Equine viral vaccines: The past, present and future. *Vet. Res.* 35:425–43.

60. Moncayo, A. C., Lanzaro, G., Kang, W., Orozco, A., Ulloa, A., Arredondo-Jimenez, J. and Weaver, S. C. 2008. Vector competence of eastern and western forms of Psorophora columbiae (Diptera: Culicidae) mosquitoes for enzootic and epizootic Venezuelan equine encephalitis virus. *Am. J. Trop. Med. Hyg.* 78:413–421.

61. Monlux, W. S., Luedke, A. J. and Bowne, J. 1972. Central nervous system response of horses to Venezuelan equine encephalomyelitis vaccine (TC-83). *J. Am. Vet. Med. Assoc.* 161:265–269.

62. Monroy, A. M., Scott, T. W. and Webb, B. A. 1996. Evaluation of reverse transcriptase polymerase chain reaction for the detection of eastern equine encephalomyelitis virus during vector surveillance. *J. Med. Entomol.* 33:449–457.

63. Nagata, L. P., Hu, W. G., Masri, S. A., Rayner, G. A., Schmaltz, F. L., Das, D., Wu, J., Long, M. C., Chan, C., Proll, D., Jager, S., Jebailey, L., Suresh, M. R. and Wong, J. P. 2005. Efficacy of DNA vaccination against western equine encephalitis virus infection. *Vaccine* 23:2280–2283.

64. Nagata, L. P., Hu, W. G., Parker, M., Chau, D., Rayner, G. A., Schmaltz, F. L. and Wong, J. P. 2006. Infectivity variation and genetic diversity among strains of western equine encephalitis virus. *J. Gen. Virol.* 87:2353–2361.

65. Navarro, J. C., Medina, G., Vasquez, C., Coffey, L. L., Wang, E., Suarez, A., Biord, H., Salas, M. and Weaver, S. C. 2005. Postepizootic persistence of Venezuelan equine encephalitis virus, Venezuela. *Emerg. Infect. Dis.* 11:1907–1915.

66. Nolen-Walston, R., Bedenice, D., Rodriguez, C., Rushton, S., Bright, A., Fecteau, M. E., Short, D., Majdalany, R., Tewari, D., Pedersen, D., Kiupel, M., Maes, R. and Del Piero, F. 2007. Eastern equine encephalitis in 9 South American camelids. *J. Vet. Intern. Med.* 21:846–852.

67. Oberste, M. S., Fraire, M., Navarro, R., Zepeda, C., Zarate, M. L., Ludwig, G. V., Kondig, J. F., Weaver, S. C., Smith, J. F. and Rico-Hesse, R. 1998. Association of Venezuelan equine encephalitis virus subtype IE with two equine epizootics in Mexico. *Am. J. Trop. Med. Hyg.* 59:100–107.

68. O'Brien, L. 2007. Inhibition of multiple strains of Venezuelan equine encephalitis virus by a pool of four short interfering RNAs. *Antiviral Res.* 75:20–29.

69. OIE 2008. Venezuelan equine encephalomyelitis. In *Manual of standards for diagnostic tests and vaccines*, chapter 2.5.14, 931–935. Paris, France: OIE.

70. Ortiz, D. I., Kang, W. and Weaver, S. C. 2008. Susceptibility of *A. aegypti* (Diptera: Culicidae) to infection with epidemic (subtype IC) and enzootic (subtypes ID, IIIC, IIID) Venezuelan equine encephalitis complex alphaviruses. *J. Med. Entomol.* 45:1117–1125.

71. Paessler, S., Rijnbrand, R., Stein, D. A., Ni, H., Yun, N. E., Dziuba, N., Borisevich, V., Seregin, A., Ma, Y., Blouch, R., Iversen, P. L. and Zacks, M. A. 2008. Inhibition of alphavirus infection in cell culture and in mice with antisense morpholino oligomers. *Virology* 376:357–370.

72. Perkins, S. D., O'Brien, L. M. and Phillpotts, R. J. 2006. Boosting with an adenovirus-based vaccine improves protective efficacy against Venezuelan equine encephalitis virus following DNA vaccination. *Vaccine* 24:3440–3445.

73. Perkins, S. D., Williams, A. J., O'Brien, L. M., Laws, T. R. and Phillpotts, R. J. 2008. CpG used as an adjuvant for an adenovirus-based Venezuelan equine encephalitis virus vaccine increases the immune response to the vector, but not to the transgene product. *Viral Immunol.* 21:451–457.

74. Phillpotts, R. J. 2006. Venezuelan equine encephalitis virus complex-specific monoclonal antibody provides broad protection, in murine models, against airborne challenge with viruses from serogroups I, II and III. *Virus Res.* 120:107–112.

75. Platteborze, P. L., Kondig, J. P., Schoepp, R. J. and Wasieloski, L. P. 2005. Comparative sequence analysis of the eastern equine encephalitis virus pathogenic strains FL91–4679 and GA97 to other North American strains. *DNA Seq.* 16:308–320.

76. Reed, D. S., Lind, C. M., Lackemeyer, M. G., Sullivan, L. J., Pratt, W. D. and Parker, M. D. 2005. Genetically engineered, live, attenuated vaccines protect nonhuman primates against aerosol challenge with a virulent IE strain of Venezuelan equine encephalitis virus. *Vaccine* 23:3139–3147.

77. Reisen, W. K., and Monath, T. P. 1988. Western equine encephalomyelitis. In *The arboviruses: Epidemiology and ecology*, vol. 5., ed. T. P. Monath, 89–137. Boca Raton: CRC Press.

78. Rice, C. M. and Strauss, J. H. 1982. Association of sindbis virion glycoproteins and their precursors. *J. Mol. Biol.* 154:325–348.

79. Rico-Hesse, R. 2000. Venezuelan equine encephalomyelitis. *Vet. Clin. North Am. Equine Pract.* 16:553–563.

80. Rico-Hesse, R., Weaver, S. C., De Singer, J., Medina, G. and Salas, R. A. 1995. Emergence of a new epidemic/epizootic Venezuelan equine encephalitis virus in South America. *Proc. Natl. Acad. Sci. USA* 92:5278–5281.

81. Roehrig, J. T. and Mathew, J. H. 1985. The neutralization site on the E2 glycoprotein of Venezuelan encephalomyelitis virus is composed of multiple conformationally-stable epitopes. *Virology* 142:347–356.

82. Roehrig, J. T., Hunt, A. R., Chang, G. J., Sheik, B., Bolin, R. A., Tsai, T. F. and Trent, D. W. 1990. Identification of monoclonal antibodies capable of differentiating antigenic varieties of Eastern equine encephalitis viruses. *Am. J. Trop. Med. Hyg.* 42:394–398.

83. Ryzhikov, A. B., Tkacheva, N. V., Sergeev, A. N. and Ryabchikova, E. I. 1991. Venezuelan equine encephalitis virus propagation in the olfactory tract of normal and immunized mice. *Biomed. Sci.* 2:607–614.

84. Ryzhikov, A. B., Ryabchikova, E. I., Sergeev, A. N. and Tkacheva, N. V. 1995. Spread of Venezuelan equine encephalitis virus in mice olfactory tract. *Arch. Virol.* 140:2243–2254.

85. Sahu, S. P., Alstad, A. D., Pedersen, D. D. and Pearson, J. E. 1994. Diagnosis of Eastern equine encephalomyelitis virus infection in horses by immunoglobulin M and G capture enzyme linked-immunosorbent assay. *J. Vety. Diagn. Invest.* 6:34–38.

86. Schlesinger, S. 2001. Alphavirus vectors: Development and potential therapeutic applications. *Expert Opin. Biol. Ther.* 1:177–191.

87. Scott, T. W. and Weaver, S. C. 1989. Eastern equine encephomyelitis virus: Epidemiology and evolution of mosquito transmission. *Adv. Virus Res.* 37:277–328.

88. Sharma, A., Raviv, Y., Puri, A., Viard, M., Blumenthal, R. and Maheshwari, R. K. 2007. Complete inactivation of Venezuelan equine encephalitis virus by 1,5-iodonaphthylazide. *Biochem. Biophys. Res. Commun.* 358:392–398.

89. Sharma, A., Bhattacharya, B., Puri, R. K. and Maheshwari, R. K. 2008. Venezuelan equine encephalitis virus infection causes modulation of inflammatory and immune response genes in mouse brain. *BMC Genomics* 9:289.

90. Spotts, D. R., Reich, R. M., Kalkhan, M. A., Kinney, R. M. and Roehrig, J. T. 1998. Resistance to alpha/beta interferons correlates with the epizootic and virulence potential of Venezuelan equine encephalitis viruses and is determined by the 5' noncoding region and glycoproteins. *J. Virol.* 72:10286–10291.

91. Strauss, E. G. and Strauss, J. H. 1986. Structure and replication of the alphavirus genome. In *The togaviridae and flaviviridae*, ed. S. Schlesinger and M. J. Schlesinger, 350–390. New York, NY: Plenum Press.

92. Strauss, J. H. and Strauss, E. G. 1994. The alphaviruses: Gene expression, replication, and evolution. *Microbiol. Rev.* 58:491–562.

93. Sudia, W. D. and Newhouse, V. G. 1975. Epidemic Venezuelan equine encephalitis in North America: A summary of virus-vector-host relationships. *Am. J. Epidemiol.* 101:1–13.

94. Tate, C. M., Howerth, E. W., Stallknecht, D. E., Allison, A. B., Fischer, J. R. and Mead, D. G. 2005. Eastern equine encephalitis in a free-ranging white-tailed deer (*Odocoileus virginianus*). *J. Wildl. Dis.* 41:241–245.

95. Tenbroeck, C. and Merrill, M. H. 1933. A serological difference between eastern and western equine encephalomyelitis virus. *Proc. Soc. Exp. Biol. Med.* 31:217–220.

96. Tenbroeck, C., Hurst, E. W. and Traub, E. 1935. Epidemiology of equine encephalomyelitis in the eastern United States. *J. Exp. Med.* 62:677–685.

97. Thompson, J. M., Nicholson, M. G., Whitmore, A. C., Zamora, M., West, A., Iwasaki, A., Staats, H. F. and Johnston, R. E. 2008. Nonmucosal alphavirus vaccination stimulates a mucosal inductive environment in the peripheral draining lymph node. *J. Immunol.* 181:574–585.

98. Turell, M. J., O'Guinn, M. L., Dohm, D., Zyzak, M., Watts, D., Fernandez, R., Calampa, C., Klein, T. A. and Jones, J. W. 2008. Susceptibility of Peruvian mosquitoes to eastern equine encephalitis virus. *J. Med. Entomol.* 45:720–725.

99. Unnasch, R. S., Sprenger, T., Katholi, C. R., Cupp, E. W., Hill, G. E. and Unnasch, T. R. 2006. A dynamic transmission model of eastern equine encephalitis virus. *Ecol. Modell.* 192:425–440.

100. Vilcarromero, S., Laguna-Torres, V. A., Fernandez, C., Gotuzzo, E., Suarez, L., Cespedes, M., Aguilar, P. V. and Kochel, T. J. 2009. Venezuelan equine encephalitis and upper gastrointestinal bleeding in child. *Emerg. Infect. Dis.* 15:323–325.

101. Vodkin, M. H., McLaughlin, G. L., Day, J. F., Shope, R. E. and Novak R. J. 1993. A rapid diagnostic assay for eastern equine encephalomyelitis viral RNA. *Am. J. Trop. Med. Hyg.* 49:772–776.

102. Vodkin, M. H., Streit, T. Mitchell, C. J. McLaughlin, G. L. and Novak, R. J. 1994. PCR-based detection of arboviral RNA from mosquitoes homogenized in detergent. *BioTechniques* 17:114–116.

103. Vogel, P., Kell, W. M., Fritz, D. L., Parker, M. D. and Schoepp, R. J. 2005. Early events in the pathogenesis of Eastern equine encephalitis virus in mice. *Am. J. Pathol.* 166:159–171.

104. Volkova, E., Frolova, E., Darwin, J. R., Forrester, N. L., Weaver, S. C. and Frolov, I. 2008. IRES-dependent replication of Venezuelan equine encephalitis virus makes it highly attenuated and incapable of replicating in mosquito cells. *Virology* 377:160–169.

105. Walton, T. E. and Grayson, M. A. 1988. Venezuelan equine encephalomyelitis. In *The arboviruses: Epidemiology and ecology*, vol. 4, ed. T. P. Monath, 203–231. Boca Raton, FL: CRC Press.

106. Walton, T. E., Alvarez, O. Jr., Buckwalter, R. M. and Johnson, K. M. 1972. Experimental infection of horses with an attenuated Venezuelan equine encephalomyelitis vaccine (strain TC-83). *Infect. Immunol* 5:750–756.

107. Walton, T. E., Alvarez, O. Jr., Buckwalter, R. M. and Johnson, K. M. 1973. Experimental infection of horses with enzootic and epizootic strains of Venezuelan equine encephalomyelitis virus. *J. Infect. Dis.* 128:272–282.

108. Wang, E., Paessler, S., Aguilar, P. V., Smith, D. R., Coffey, L. L., Kang, W., Pfeffer, M., Olson, J., Blair, P. J., Guevara, C., Estrada-Franco, J. and Weaver, S. C. 2005. A novel, rapid assay for detection and differentiation of serotype-specific antibodies to Venezuelan equine encephalitis complex alphaviruses. *Am. J. Trop. Med. Hyg.* 72:805–810.

109. Wang, E., Paessler, S., Aguilar, P. V., Carrara, A. S., Ni, H., Greene, I. P. and Weaver, S. C. 2006. Reverse transcription-PCR-enzyme-linked immunosorbent assay for rapid detection and differentiation of alphavirus infections. *J. Clin. Microbiol.* 44:4000–4008.

110. Weaver, S. C., Scott, T. W. and Rico-Hesse, R. 1991. Molecular evolution of eastern equine encephalomyelitis virus in North America. *Virology* 182:774–784.

111. Weaver, S. C., Ricp-Hesse, R. and Scott, T. W. 1992. Genetic diversity and slow rates of evolution in New World alphaviruses. *Current Topics Microbiol. Immunol.* 176:99–117.

112. Weaver, S. C., Hagenbaugh, A., Bellew, L. A., Gousset, L., Mallampalli, V., Holland, J. J. and Scott. T. W. 1994. Evolution of alphaviruses in the eastern equine encephalomyelitis complex. *J. Virol.* 68:158–169.

113. Weaver, S. C., Ferro, C., Barrera, R., Boshell, J. and Navarro, J. C. 2004a. Venezuelan equine encephalitis. *Annu. Rev. Entomol.* 49:141–174.

114. Weaver, S. C., Anishchenko, M., Bowen, R., Brault, A. C., Estrada-Franco, J. G., Fernandez, Z., Greene, I., Ortiz, D., Paessler, S. and Powers, A. M. 2004b. Genetic determinants of Venezuelan equine encephalitis emergence. *Arch. Virol.* 18:43–64.

115. White, L. J., Wang, J. G., Davis, N. L. and Johnston, R. E. 2001. Role of alpha/beta interferon in Venezuelan equine encephalitis virus pathogenesis: Effect of an attenuating mutation in the 5' untranslated region. *J. Virol.* 75:3706–3718.

116. Wu, J. Q., Barabe, N. D., Huang, Y. M., Rayner, G. A., Christopher, M. E. and Schmaltz, F. L. 2007a. Pre—and post-exposure protection against western equine encephalitis virus after single inoculation with adenovirus vector expressing interferon alpha. *Virology* 369:206–213.

117. Wu, J. Q., Barabe, N. D., Chau, D., Wong, C., Rayner, G. R., Hu, W. G. and Nagata, L. P. 2007b. Complete protection of mice against a lethal dose challenge of western equine encephalitis virus after immunization with an adenovirus-vectored vaccine. *Vaccine* 25:4368–4375.

118. Young, N. A. 1972. Serologic differentiation of viruses of the Venezuelan encephalitis (VE) complex. In *Proceedings of the Workshop-Symposium on Venezuelan Encephalitis Virus, Scientific Publ. 243*, 84–89. Washington, D.C.: Pan American Health Organization.

119. Young, N. A. and Johnson, K. M. 1969. Antigenic variants of Venezuelan equine encephalitis virus: Their geographic distribution and epidemiologic significance. *Am. J. Epidemiol.* 89:286–307.

120. Young, D. S., Kramer, L. D., Maffei, J. G., Dusek, R. J., Backenson, P. B., Mores, C. N., Bernard, K. A. and Ebel, G. D. 2008. Molecular epidemiology of eastern equine encephalitis virus, New York. *Emerg. Infect. Dis.* 14:454–460.

121. Young, N. A., Johnson, K. M. and Gauld, L. W. 1969. Viruses of the Venezuelan equine encephalomyelitis complex. Experimental infection of Panamanian rodents. *Am. J. Trop. Med. Hyg.* 18:290–296.

122. Zhang, D., Tozser, J. and Waugh, D. S. 2009. Molecular cloning, overproduction, purification and biochemical characterization of the p39 nsp2 protease domains encoded by three alphaviruses. *Protein Expr. Purif.* 64:89–97.

6. EQUINE HERPESVIRUSES

S. KAPOOR, K. DHAMA, R. V. S. PAWAIYA, AND THANKAM MATHEW

INTRODUCTION

Equids are host to eleven taxonomically grouped herpesviruses (EHV), six of which (EHV-1,—3,—4,—6,—8,—9) are alphaherpesviruses and five (EHV-2,—5,—7,—10,—11) are gammaherpesviruses (Agius and Studdert, 1994; Crabb and Studdert, 1995; Kleiboeker et al., 2002). Asinine herpesvirus—1,—2,—3,—4,—5 are synonymous for EHV-6,—7,—8,—10,—11, respectively and have been isolated from donkeys. Two novel herpesviruses, designated asinine herpesvirus 4 (AHV-4 or EHV-10) and asinine herpesvirus 5 (AHV-5 or EHV-11), were consistently detected in lung tissue from donkeys in which the histopathology was characterized by interstitial pneumonia (Kleiboeker et al., 2002). Equine herpesvirus (EHV) 9 is most closely related to the recently emergent neurotropic pathogen, EHV-1, but was first described in an outbreak of disease in Thomson's gazelles (Gazella thomsoni), subsequently in a giraffe, and very recently in a polar bear (Schrenzel et al., 2008). Recently, EHV-7 has been detected from healthy mules (Bell et al., 2008).

Five herpesviruses (EHV-1 to EHV-5) can infect the domestic horse. Equine herpesviruses (EHVs) can affect the respiratory, reproductive, and nervous systems causing a wide variety of diseases. Equine herpesviruses 1 and 4 (EHV-1 and EHV-4) are important and widespread pathogens in horse population. EHV-1 infections result in respiratory disease, abortion, stillbirth, neonatal foal mortality, and myoencepathalopathy. The EHV-4 is mainly, but not exclusively, involved in the respiratory infections. It causes equine rhinopneumonitis characterized by upper respiratory tract infection of horses during the first two years of life and on rare occasions is associated with abortion (Allen and Bryans, 1986; Crabb and Studdert, 1995). Equine herpesvirus 2 has been isolated from domestic horses with various clinical signs and from clinically healthy horses. Its involvement in keratoconjunctivitis and respiratory disease, mainly in foals, has been reported (Collinson et al., 1994; Kershaw et al., 2001). Exposure to EHV-2 was detected in a number of captive wild equine species (Borchers et al., 1999), and detection of a high-neutralizing antibody titer in one of twenty-one free-ranging mountain zebras from Namibia (Borchers and Frölich, 1997) indicate that EHV-2 infections are not restricted to domestic horses. The EHV-5 has repeatedly been isolated from healthy horses (Dunowska et al.,

1999, Nordengrahn et al., 2002). Both EHV-2 and EHV-5 have been reported to be involved in equine abortion (Leon et al., 2008). The EHV-3 causes coital exanthema (Hartley et al., 1999), a venereal disease characterized by ulcerative lesion of vaginal mucosa of mare and in the mucosa of penis in stallions (described in a separate chapter). The focus of this chapter is on EHV-1 and EHV-4.

ETIOLOGY

Recently, the International Committee on Taxonomy of Viruses (ICTV) has split the former family Herpesviridae into three families, which have been incorporated into the new order Herpesvirales (Davison et al., 2009). The revised family Herpesviridae retains the mammal, bird, and reptile viruses, the fish and frog viruses have been incorporated in the new family Alloherpesviridae, and the new family Malacoherpesviridae contains a bivalve virus. Three new genera have been created in the family Herpesviridae, namely, Proboscivirus in the subfamily Betaherpesvirinae and Macavirus and Percavirus in the subfamily Gammaherpesvirinae (Davison et al., 2009).

The species equine herpesvirus 1, equine herpesvirus 3, equine herpesvirus 4, equine herpesvirus 8, equine herpesvirus 9 have been put under the genus Varicellovirus, subfamily Alphaherpesvirinae, family Herpesviridae of a new order Herpesvirales. The species equid herpervirus 2 and equine herpesvirus 5 have been put under a new genus Percavirus, subfamily Gamaherpesvirinae, family Herpesviridae of a new order Herpesvirales.

The equine herpes virions are about 150 nm in diameter. They have icosahedral nucleocapsid surrounded by a layer of globular tegument, which is enclosed in an envelope having numerous small surface glycoprotein spikes. The genome is single linear dsDNA molecule with 57% G+C ratio. Both EHV-1 and EHV-4 have been sequenced completely (Telford et al., 1992, 1998). The genome of EHV-4 is about 145 kilobase pairs (kbp). The Ab4 strain of EHV-1 has been sequenced and found to be composed of 150,223 base pairs (bp). These two viruses (EHV-1 and EHV-4) have considerable sequence homology, and each code for seventy-six genes. The genomes EHV-1 and EHV-4 are composed of a unique long (U_L) region attached to a unique short (U_S) region. The U_S is flanked by a set of indirect repeat sequences termed internal and terminal sequences (IRS and TRS). Out of the total seventy-six genes of EHV-1 and EHV-4, sixty-three, nine, and four genes are located in U_L U_S and IRS, respectively. These genes are expressed in a very controlled way that may be divided into three distinct phases, viz, immediate early (IE), early (E), and late (L) (Caughman et al.,

1985, Albrecht et al., 2005). The virus encodes a single IE gene, fifty-five E genes and twenty L genes. The regulation of the sequential cascade of viral genes into these three phases (Caughman et al., 1985) is controlled by six viral proteins encoded by one IE gene (gene 64), four E genes (EICP 22, 27, 0, and TR2), and one L gene (ETIF). The envelope of EHV-1 has eleven glycoproteins (gB, gC gD, gE, gG, gH, gI, gK, gL, gM, and gp300), which have role in its pathogenesis (Turtinen and Allen, 1982). The gB, gC, and gD glycoprotein are immunodominant proteins and main candidates for vaccine development. The gE, gI, gK, and gM glycoproteins are involved in cell-to-cell spread. The gM is also involved in cell penetration while gK is responsible for virus egress (Rudolph and Osterrieder, 2002). The EHV-2 genome is 184 kbp long and contains seventy-nine ORFs encoding seventy-seven proteins (Telford et al., 1995).

EPIDEMIOLOGY

The natural host range and reservoir of infection with EHV-1 and EHV-4 are primarily restricted to members of equids. Both the viruses are endemic in the horse populations throughout the world. The foals get infected within the first few weeks or months of their life around the time of weaning from adult mares, which asymptomatically shed the virus. The lactating mares act as a source of EHV-1 from which their foals get infected, and these foals then infect other foals by close contact (Crabb and Studdert, 1995; Gilkerson et al., 1999a, 1999b; Foote et al., 2004). During the first twelve to eighteen months of life, the animals may get reinfected, or there may be reactivation of the latent infection.

The virus is transmitted directly from horse to horse and indirectly by inanimate objects and personnel. It is mainly transmitted by inhalation of the infected droplets or by the ingestion of material contaminated with nasal secretions, aborted fetuses, and placental membranes (Crabb and Studdert, 1995).

Latency and reactivation have an important role in the epidemiology of EHV-1 abortion and neurologic disease. Infection with EHV-1 and EHV-4 may result in the establishment of latency, which usually is lifelong and through periodic reactivations results in persistence of infection in horse populations (Edington et al., 1994). EHV-1 and EHV-4 establish latent infections in sensory ganglia such as the trigeminal ganglion (Borchers et al., 1997; Slater et al., 1994) and lymphoreticular system, both in circulating and lymph node CD8+ T lymphocytes (Welch et al., 1992). EHV-2 and EHV-5 can establish latent infection in foals in B lymphocytes and PBMCs (Drummer et al., 1996; Bell et al., 2006). Foals were found to shed both

EHV-2 and EHV-5 in nasal secretions, but their presence was not related with the occurrence of any disease. However, infection of foals with EHV-2 occurred earlier than with EHV-5 (Dunowska et al., 2002a; Nordengrahen et al., 2002; Bell et al., 2006). Recently, both EHV-2 and EHV-5 have been reported to be involved in equine abortion (Leon et al., 2008). Periodic reactivation of EHV-1 and EHV-4 may result in viremia and thus putting the affected horse at risk of abortion or EHM, and/or shedding of infectious virus in nasal secretion may lead to infection of susceptible animals. The transport of the horses for racing, handling, rehousing, weaning, illness, or any other kind of stress in field situations has many a time leads to the reactivation of both these viruses. Clinically normal animals in which the reactivation of the virus result only in shedding of the virus but not disease become silent shedders of the virus and, therefore, provide an important mechanism for maintenance of endemic infection cycle.

PATHOGENESIS

Various factors—including the age and physical condition of the host; type of infection whether primary, a reinfection, or a reactivation of latent virus; the immune status of the host; and the virulence of the strain involved—influence the severity of disease resulting from EHV-1 infection. The cell-associated viremia; reactivation of the latent virus and subsequent vascular endothelial damage, thrombosis, and ischemia; and immune evasion strategies have roles in the pathogenesis of EHV-1.

Following infection, both EHV-4 and EHV-1 replicate in the epithelial cells of the upper respiratory tract. During the initial phase, there is rapid amplification and proliferation of the virus in the nasal, pharyngeal, and tonsillar mucosae and subsequent penetration and infection of local blood vessels. The virus becomes intracellular and spreads quickly infecting different type of cells, including endothelial cells (Edington et al., 1986), lymphocytes (Scott et al., 1983) and monocytes, and dendritic cells (Kydd et al., 1994a, 1994b). The infection of lymphocytes by EHV-1 leads to the development of CD8+ T cell–associated viremia (Bryans, 1969, Scott et al., 1983), which ultimately disseminates the virus widely to sites of secondary replication, including the vascular endothelium of pregnant uterus and central nervous system (Edington et al., 1986; Gibson et al., 1992). During the same time, EHV-1 also reaches the trigeminal ganglion through the neurons of the trigeminal nerve by forty-eight hours postinfection where it establishes latency (Slater et al., 1994).

Infection of endothelial cells is associated with vasculitis and thrombosis, restricted blood flow leading to ischemic damage at the uteroplacental junction. This may cause "typical" EHV-1 abortions if both placenta and fetus are virus positive (Edington et al., 1991; Smith et al., 1992, 1993; Smith and Borchers, 2001) or "atypical" EHV-1 abortions due to endometrial damage without the establishment of detectable fetus infection (Smith et al., 1992, 2004; Mukaiya et al., 2000; Gerst et al., 2003; Szeredi et al., 2004).

The EHV-1 endotheliotropism is central to the neurological disease. The vasculitis and thrombosis with resultant ischemia and hemorrhage occur as a consequence of endothelial cell infection in small blood vessels of brain and/or spinal cord. Impairment of blood flow results in secondary hypoxic degeneration of adjacent neural tissue (Edington et al., 1986). This is in direct contrast to the neurologic disease associated with herpesvirus in other species as neurons are not directly infected (Jackson et al., 1977; Studdert et al., 2003).

The virulence of EHV-1 field isolates may show great variation. The Ab4 strain of EHV-1 is endotheliotropic, abortigenic, and a neuropathogenic strain that causes efficient viremia, whereas V592, a less virulent nonneuropathogenic strain, is associated with low-level viremia and has reduced endotheliotropism and abortigenic potential. The comparison of Ab4 and V592 EHV-1 strains revealed only 0.1% difference in nucleotide sequence (150 bases in 150,000) that was spread in thirty-one genes. There was no evidence of a relationship between the pathogenic potential and phylogentic groups generated even in gene sixty-eight, which showed highest (2.0%) variation (Tearle et al., 2003; Smith et al., 2000). However, it has been shown that variation of a single amino acid of the DNA polymerase is strongly associated with neurological versus nonneurological disease outbreaks. A single nucleotide polymorphism (SNP) within the EHV-1 gene encoding the viral DNA polymerase (ORF30) has been identified that is highly associated with the neuropathogenicity of the virus for horses. Of the thirty-two investigated outbreaks of EHV-1 neurological disease that occurred in the United States and the United Kingdom between 2001 and 2006, thirty (94%) were caused by the ORF30 mutant strain of EHV-1. The paralytic potential correlated with two single-base changes. The majority of the nonparalytic strains were having A at position 2254, whereas in the paralytic strains A was substituted with G at this position (Nugent et al., 2006).

The EHV-1 has developed a wide variety of immune-evasion strategies, which allow the virus to evade recognition and elimination. This helps the EHV-1 to cause viremia in the presence of virus-specific antibodies and CTL precursors. However, these immune evasion-strategies of EHV-1 appear to be effective only after six months following a previous infection. The peripheral blood mononuclear cells (PBMC) carry the EHV-1 to various locations during cell-associated viremia. It has been demonstrated that EHV-1 interferes with the expression of viral proteins on the surface of PBMC. The absence of viral antigens on the surface of EHV-1–infected PBMC makes them insensitive to antibody-dependent complement-mediated cell lysis and antibody-dependent cell-mediated cytotxicity (van der Meulen et al., 2003, 2006). Specific but incomplete downregulation of MHC class I expression in EHV-1–infected equine cell lines has been reported. This downregulation may be due to enhanced endocytosis of MHC class I molecules from the cell surface resulting in (Rappocciolo et al., 2003) or interference with the peptide translocation by transporter associated with antigen processing (Ambagala et al., 2004).

The gG gene sequences of EHV-1 isolated from horses were 99.9–100% identical and 98, 98, and 97.8% similar to gG from onager, zebra, and gazelle isolates, respectively. Hamsters inoculated with onager, zebra, and gazelle isolates had severe weight loss, compared with hamsters inoculated with horse isolates. The results indicated that EHV-1 isolates from onager, zebra, and gazelle differ from horse EHV-1 and are much more virulent in hamsters (Ibrahim et al., 2007).

The pathogenesis of EHV-4 infection and disease during the initial mucosal phase appears to be similar to EHV-1 with infection of the respiratory tract and adjoining lymph nodes. The genome of EHV-4 may persist in the trigeminal ganglion (Borchers et al., 1997) and circulating lymphocytes (Welch et al., 1992) after recovery from infection. EHV-4 rarely causes abortion, neonatal septicemia, or neurological disease due to its low endotheliotropism and less ability to cause viremia (Kydd et al., 1994a, Tearle et al., 2003; Gerst et al., 2003).

EHV Lesions

Gross lesions of viral rhinopneumonitis are hyperemia and ulceration of the respiratory epithelium and multiple tiny plum-colored foci in the lungs. Histologically, there is evidence of inflammation, necrosis, and intranuclear inclusions in the respiratory epithelium and lymph nodes. Lung lesions are characterized by neutrophilic infiltration of the terminal bronchioles, peribronchiolar and perivascular mononuclear cell infiltration, and serofibrinous exudate in the alveoli. Postmortem findings in fetuses aborted before six months show widespread cell necrosis. It is evident that the virus after crossing the placenta is carried viremically to the fetus. The fetuses that abort after six months may show jaundice and petechial hemorrhages on the visible mucus membranes. Excessive pleural fluid, pulmonary edema, and spleenomegaly with prominent lymphoid follicles and white—to cream-colored foci of necrosis in the liver can also be seen. Microscopic lesions include bronchiolitis, pneumonitis in lungs, severe necrosis of the white pulp, and focal hepatic necrosis. Typical herpesvirus acidophilic intranuclear inclusion bodies may be present in these lesions of liver, lung, and adrenals. Gross pathologic findings in horses with neurologic syndrome are often minimal. Hemorrhage around the spinal root ganglion is a common finding. The arteries and arterioles of the CNS show vasculitis, thrombosis, with secondary hypoxic degeneration of adjacent neural tissues in EHM (Crab and Studdert, 1995).

CLINICAL FINDINGS

The EHV-1 infection in horses is manifested with any or all the following disease syndromes: respiratory disease, abortion, neonatal foal mortality, myeloencephalopathy paralysis. EHV-4 primarily causes rhinopneumonitis (Patel and Heldens, 2005).

The incubation period is of two to ten days. Primary infection in neonatal and naive foals results in clinically apparent respiratory disease. Susceptible horses develop fever of 39.0–41.5°C and show serous nasal discharge, inappetence, depression, mild cough, neutropenia and lymphopenia, pharyngitis, and/or progressive lymphadenopathy of submandibular or retropharyngeal lymph nodes. Cell-associated viremia observed in EHV-1 infection generally coincides with the second temperature peak of biphasic fever. Majority of such respiratory infections by EHV-1 are subclinical or mild and of short duration in previously infected and immunologically sensitized horses (Allen and Bryans, 1986; Gibson et al., 1992; Kydd et al., 1996).

Abortion in mares due to EHV1 usually occurs between seven and eleven months of gestation (Gleeson and Coggins, 1980; Matsumra et al., 1992). The incubation period is highly variable with abortions occurring from ten days to twelve weeks after virus infection. EHV-1 abortion occurs without premonitory signs, and the fetus is expelled sometimes still covered with the placenta (Smith et al., 1992), and evidence of the previous respiratory tract infection is usually not observed. Aborted fetuses are fresh or minimally autolyzed. The incidences of most abortions associated with EHV-1 infection involve only one or two mares in a group. However, abortion storms may occur in poor hygiene and management conditions (Mumford et al., 1987). There is no evidence of damage to the mare's reproductive tract, and subsequent conception is unimpaired. Most mares conceive successfully shortly after abortion and foal normally the following year. Abortion in successive years in EHV-1–infected mares is rare. However, they may eventually abort again due to reinfection or reactivation of the latent virus. Highly virulent strains of EHV-4 may occasionally cause abortion (Studdert et al., 1984).

Neonatal foal mortality is usually caused by EHV-1 (Murray et al., 1998), or occasionally by EHV-4 (O'Keefe et al., 1995). Mares infected in late pregnancy may give birth to weak foals that show signs of respiratory distress, pyrexia, lethargy, and poor nursing ability. These foals usually die within hours or a few days of life (Giles et al., 1993). Congenital EHV-1 infection can be epidemic in nature and may be present either in association with an outbreak of abortion or without concurrent abortion or obvious respiratory disease in the dams. It is uncertain whether such foals are infected in utero with EHV-1 or acquire a rapid postparturient infection from their dams. These prenatal foal mortalities may be the dominant manifestation of the disease when majority of mares in a group are infected close to term (Dixon et al., 1977).

Neurological disease associated with equine herpesvirus type—1 was first confirmed by Saxegaard (1966). Equine herpesvirus myeloencephalopathy (EHM), an inflammation of the blood vessels that supply the brain and spinal cord, is caused by some virulent strains of EHV-1. The incidence of EHM in recent years has been observed with increasing and alarming frequency (Henninger et al., 2007). The signs of EHM develop in many horses in about two weeks after disease becomes obvious in an index case. The onset of the neurologic signs is sudden and reaches their maximum intensity within two to three days of onset. The signs can vary from mild incoordination and posterior paresis to severe posterior paralysis with recumbency, altered gaits, staggering, the inability to rise from the sitting position (typical "dog sitting position"), loss of bladder tone and anal tone, and urinary incontinence. In exceptional cases, the paralysis may progress to quadriplegia and death. Prognosis depends on severity of signs and the period of recumbency (Kohn and Fenner, 1987; McCartan et al., 1995; van Maanen et al., 2001; Studdert et al., 2003; Goehring et al., 2005).

DIAGNOSIS

Equine herpersvirus 1 and/or 4 can cause a variety of disorders such as respiratory disease, abortion, neonatal foal pneumonitis, or myeloencephalopathy. The clinical signs observed in these disorders are not diagnostic as they are present in many other diseases. Equine viral rhinopneumonitis cannot be clinically differentiated from equine influenza, equine viral arteritis, or other equine respiratory infections. The abortions caused by EHV need to be differentiated from those caused by equine viral arteritis, leptospira, *Salmonella abortusequi*. The clinical signs similar to that associated with EHV-1 myeloencephalopathy can also be seen in rabies, equine protozoal myeloencephalitis, equine polyneuritis, and equine alphavirus infections.

Unambiguous diagnosis of EHV-1 or EHV-4 is done by virus isolation and identification, detection of viral antigens and nucleic acid, and serology. Naso7uld be collected in cold sterile viral transport medium at febrile stage of respiratory disease. Lung, liver, spleen, and thymus samples of aborted fetuses or spinal cord or brain of horses with nervous are sent in viral transport medium for virus isolation, detection of viral antigen in tissues by fluorescent antibody testing, or by polymerase chain reaction (PCR).

Both EHV-1 and EHV-4 can be isolated in primary equine fetal kidney cells or cell strains of equine fibroblasts derived from dermal (E-Derm) or lung tissue and primary lamb kidney cell culture (LKCC). A number of cell lines—viz, rabbit kidney (RK-13), baby hamster kidney (BHK-21), Madin-Darby bovine kidney (MDBK), pig kidney (PK-15), equine skin fibroblast cell line (NBL-6), equine embryonic lung cell line (EEL)—have been used for isolation of EHV-1 from the tissues of aborted fetuses or from postmortem cases of neurological disease, but equine-derived cell cultures are most sensitive. Specific identification of an isolate is done by immunofluorescence in the infected cell culture (Gunn, 1992), immunoperoxidase (Schultheiss et al., 1993), or by the PCR (Lawrence et al., 1994; Varraso et al., 2001).

Direct immunofluorescence test has been used to demonstrate EHV-1 antigens in nasal or nasopharyngeal swabs and postmortem tissues samples collected from aborted equine fetuses (Gunn, 1992). The EHV-1 antigen in paraffin-embedded tissues of aborted equine fetuses or neurologically affected horses has been detected by an immunohistochemical technique (immunoperoxidase) (Whitwell et al., 1992; Schultheiss et al., 1993). The PCR has been used for rapid amplification and diagnostic detection of EHV-1 and—4 DNA in nasopharyngeal swabs (Sharma et al., 1992), clinical specimens, paraffin-embedded archival tissue or from stained tissue sections from histopathological slides (O'Keefe et al., 1994), or inoculated cell cultures (Kirisawa et al., 1993; Lawrence et al., 1994; Varrasso et al., 2001). Various type-specific PCR primers have been employed to distinguish between the presence of EHV-1 and EHV-4. Multiplex PCR assay for simultaneous detection of both EHV-1 and EHV-4 (Wagner et al., 1992) or seminested PCR detection and differentiation of EHV-1 or EHV-4 (Borchers and Slater, 1993; Varrasso et al., 2001) in clinical or pathological specimens (nasal secretions, blood leukocytes, fetal tissues, etc.) has been described. The correlation between PCR and virus isolation techniques for diagnosis of EHV-1 or EHV-4 is high (Varrasso et al., 2001). A real-time polymerase chain reaction (PCR)-based assay that uses EHV-1 pathotype-specific TaqMan reporter probes for discrimination between neuropathogenic and nonneuropathogenic strains of EHV-1 in equine blood or nasal swabs has recently been developed and applied in field (Allen, 2007). The ability to rapidly identify horses infected with neuropathogenic strains of EHV-1 using a single-step, PCR-based method has significant implications for future diagnostic evaluation of suspect animals. The effect of intramuscular vaccination of healthy adult horses with a killed or a modified live equine herpesvirus type 1 (EHV-1) vaccine to induce transient positive PCR results in either blood or nasopharyngeal swab was investigated. It was demonstrated that detection of EHV-1 DNA by PCR in vaccinated and unvaccinated healthy horses is uncommon (Pusterla et al., 2007). The real-time PCR was found to be a sensitive and quantitative test for EHV-1 nasal shedding and viremia that provides a valuable tool for EHV-1 surveillance, diagnosis of clinical disease, and investigation of vaccine efficacy (Hussey et al., 2006). Recently, the viral loads, strain (neuropathogenic versus nonneuropathogenic), and state (lytic, nonreplicating, and latent) of equine herpesvirus 1 (EHV-1) was determined by real-time polymerase chain reaction (PCR) in the blood and nasopharyngeal secretions of adult horses following natural exposure (Pusterla et al., 2009). The contribution of these five different EHVs (EHV-1, EHV-2, EHV-3, EHV-4, or EHV-5) to equine abortion in a variety of biological tissues using a consensus polymerase chain reaction (PCR) was analyzed. Specimens from 407 fetuses, stillbirths, and premature foals were collected over a period of thirty months. The positive results obtained with this assay were compared to other EHV type-specific PCR or by sequencing. EHV-1 was identified as the major cause of abortion in French mares (59/407 cases). Surprisingly, EHV-2 (in three cases) and EHV-5 (in one case) were also found to have a role in abortion. The presence of viral DNA from EHV-3 or EHV-4 strains was not detected in the specimens studied. The consensus herpesvirus PCR is, therefore, an efficient screening tool as it allows the identification of herpesviruses other than the EHV-1 strain (Leon et al., 2008). The isolation and preliminary characterization of a mule gammaherpesvirus tentatively identified as asinine herpesvirus 2 (AHV-2, also designated equine herpesvirus 7 [EHV-7]) from the nasal secretions (NS) of a healthy mule in Northern California was reported recently. A 913-nucleotide sequence of the DNA polymerase gene was amplified using degenerate primers, and comparison of this sequence with those of various other herpesviruses showed that the mule herpesvirus was most closely related to EHV-2 (AHV-2 sequences were not available for comparison). The sequence of a shorter portion (166 nucleotides) of the mule herpesvirus DNA polymerase gene was identical to that of the published sequence of an asinine gammaherpesvirus, previously designated as AHV-4-3 (AY054992). AHV-2 was detected by real-time polymerase chain reaction assay in the NS of approximately 8% of a cohort of 114 healthy mules and 13 donkeys (Bell et al., 2008).

The serological diagnosis of EHV-1 and EHV-4 usually require paired serum samples. Antibodies can be detected in virus neutralization, complement fixation, counterimmunoelectrophoresis, radial immunodiffusion, agar gel precipitation, indirect immunoflorescence tests, indirect ELISA and blocking ELISA (Doll and Bryans, 1962; Thompson et al., 1976; Dutta et al., 1983; Hohdatsu et al., 1986; Crabb and Studdert, 1993; Sinclair et al., 1993; Crabb et al., 1995; Van Maanen et al., 2000; Singh et al., 2004). The virus-neutralizing antibodies (VN) are long lived, persisting for up to one year after infection. These largely type-specific (EHV-1 and EHV-4) antibodies are directed mainly against the major enveloped glycoproteins B (gB) and C (gC) (Allen et al., 1992). Unlike VN antibodies, the complement-fixing (CF) antibodies are short-lived and can be detected up to three months postinfection (Thompson et al., 1976). The CF test is, therefore, a useful indicator of recent infection when applied to paired sera collected two weeks apart. Commonly used routine laboratory tests cannot unequivocally differentiate polyclonal serum antibodies after field infection with EHV-1 and EHV-4. It occurs because most of the glycoproteins, except gG, of EHV-1 and EHV-4 have both type-common and type-specific antigens (Allen and Bryans, 1986; Crabb and Studdert, 1990, 1993). Type-specific ELISAs based on variable regions of C terminus of gG that can distinguish between antibodies to EHV-1 and EHV-4 have been developed (Crabb and Studdert, 1993; Crabb et al., 1995; Van Maanen et al., 2000; Hartley et al., 2005) and extensively applied to epidemiological studies of EHV-1 and EHV-4 infection (Gilkerson et al., 1999a, 1999b; Foote et al., 2004). However, it must be kept in mind that interpretation of serological results can be confounded by previous vaccination and maternal-derived antibodies.

Histopathological examination of sections of formalin-fixed, paraffin-embedded tissues from aborted fetuses or from horses with neurological disease is a useful aid for the laboratory diagnosis of these two clinical manifestations. In aborted fetuses, typical herpetic, acidophilic intranuclear inclusion bodies present within bronchiolar epithelium or in cells at the periphery of areas of hepatic necrosis are considered to be pathognomonic lesions for EHV-1. Microscopic lesion associated with EHM is a degenerative thrombotic vasculitis of small blood vessels in the brain or spinal cord. Perivascular cuffing and infiltration by inflammatory cells, endothelial proliferation and necrosis, and thrombus formation may be observed. The increased protein concentration and breakdown of erythrocytes in cerebrospinal fluid (CSF) may cause xanthochromia of CSF.

PREVENTION AND CONTROL

The basis of protective immunity to EHVs is not fully known. The protection against EHVs may require three types of immune responses (Allen et al., 1999; Kydd et al., 2006). Both virus-neutralizing antibodies and CTLs at mucosal and systemic compartments are believed to be involved in protection. Since both EHV-1 and EHV-4 replicate extensively in the epithelial cells of upper respiratory tract (Kydd et al., 1994a, 1994b), therefore, mucosal IgA antibody with neutralizing activity is believed to represent the first line of defense. While the mucosal antibody is protective, it is short-lived (Breathnach et al., 2001). Systemically produced virus-neutralizing antibodies are IgG type, long-lived, largely type-specific (i.e., EHV-1 or EHV-4), and primarily directed against gB, gC, and gD (Crabb et al., 1991; Allen et al., 1992). The role of these VN antibodies is restricted to the clearance of limited amounts of extracellular progeny virus from the bloodstream. The systemic virus-neutralizing (VN) antibody titers do not correlate with protection from viremia and abortion (Burki et al., 1990; Mumford et al., 1987; Hannant et al., 1993). The CD8+ MHC class I—restricted CTLs are primarily involved in the clearance of viremic lymphocytes (Allen et al., 1995, 1999; O'Neill et al., 1999). The limiting dilution analysis studies have demonstrated that the frequency of circulating CTL precursors (CTLp) correlates with protection from EHV-1 infection and disease (Kydd et al., 2003). The IE protein was found to have the CTL epitope. However, the ability of this protein to induce CTL responses varies with MHC haplotypes. Only the horses with ELA-A3.1 haplotype showed efficient CTL responses (Soboll et al., 2003). Approximately eighteen haplotypes of equine MHC class I have been identified by serological typing (Antczak, 1992). Protective immunity to EHV-1 infection was also characterized by polarized IFN-γ–dependent immunoregulatory cytokine response (Coombs et al., 2006). An assay that measures EHV-1–specific interferon gamma synthesis (IFN_γ), a cytokine produced following the activation of memory T lymphocytes and therefore a measure of cell mediated immunity, has been developed. The frequency of EHV-1–specific IFN_γ^+ PBMC among the sample Thoroughbred population was diverse but lowest in unvaccinated young horses in training. The frequency of EHV-1-specific lymphocytes synthesizing IFN_γ may be associated with the susceptibility to infection with this virus. The antigenicity of vaccines and their effectiveness at stimulating cellular immunity against EHV-1 may be monitored by this technique (Luce et al., 2007).

Control programs for EHV disease rely on a combination of good hygiene measures and management practices along with vaccination. The EHV-1 disease control programs are aimed at reducing the risk of introduction and transmission and spread of virus in susceptible horse populations. Small groups of horse of similar age and reproductive status should be maintained on a farm to minimize the chance of spread of infection (Dunowska et al., 2002b). Introduction of the virus into a susceptible group of horses from an exogenous source should be avoided. All horses, both new arrivals and those returning to a farm from events, should be isolated from the resident population for twenty-one to twenty-eight days before coming with resident horses, especially with pregnant mares. Pregnant mares and mares with nursing foals should be kept isolated from all other horses, both resident and new arrivals. This is especially relevant with respect to pregnant mares, which if possible should be maintained in a group away from weanlings, yearlings, and horses out of training. In an outbreak of respiratory disease or abortion or neurologic disease, affected horses should be isolated and measures taken for disinfection of contaminated premises, equipments, and vehicle. Equine herpesvirus 1 can survive on fomites for up to three days. Appropriate steps such as cleaning, disinfecting, and not sharing equipment should be taken to control the spread of EHV-1. If EHV-1 is confirmed as the cause of abortion; then the aborted mare and the in-contact horses should be kept isolated for four weeks and not mixed with other pregnant mares for eight weeks. The pregnant in-contact mares should be allowed to leave the premises only after foaling. No horse should leave the premises for three weeks after recovery of the last clinical case. Management-related stress-inducing circumstances (such as crowding, poor nutritional state, heavy parasite infestation, lengthy transport, disruption of established social groups, inclement weather, en masse weaning, etc.) should be avoided to prevent reactivation of latent virus. The spread of the disease to adjacent stud farms can be limiting by informing the common veterinarian or attendants, farm owners, or other owners of horses that have come into contact with the animals on the affected premises (Allen and Bryans, 1986; Dunowska et al., 2002b; Irwin et al., 2007).

The Horserace Betting Levy Board, UK (*www.hblb.org.uk*) publishes a Codes of Practice recommending precautions to prevent or limit the disease due to EHV. The recommendations within the Codes of Practice are not mandatory but adhered to in the Thoroughbred industries in France, Germany, Ireland, Italy, and the United Kingdom. Similar management practices are used in North America (Ostlund, 1993).

Vaccination against EHVs started about seven decades back. The first vaccines against EHV-1 were prepared from virus grown in the equine fetal tissues or hamsters' adapted live virus (Doll et al., 1959) but were abandoned because of unacceptable local and systemic adverse reactions and poor immunogenicity. Subsequently, a hamster-adapted modified live vaccine against EHV-1 was developed for use in a "planned infection" control program for immunizing mares against abortion (Doll and Bryans, 1963a, 1963b). It was recommended to use the vaccine during early stages of pregnancy as it contained some residual virulence, which could cause abortion if given later during gestation. During the next decade, the incidence of abortion in 9,480 vaccinated pregnant mares was found to be 0.93% as compared to 15.00% in unvaccinated animals.

A modified live EHV-1 vaccine derived from the RacH strain grown on porcine embryonic kidney cells was developed (Mayr and Pette, 1968, Mayr et al., 1968), which later on was found to have a deletion in U_S region of the genome (Neubauer et al., 1999). However, with earlier reports on the efficacy of this vaccine in preventing viremia, abortion could not be substantiated (Bürki et al., 1990). The RacH vaccine strain was further passaged in rabbit kidney cells and equine dermal cells to reach a final passage of p265. This resultant vaccine (Rhinomune) was marketed in North America and parts of Europe. However, abortion occurred in 50% of the pony mares experimentally challenged with this vaccine virus (Dutta and Shipley, 1975). Another modified live vaccine against EHV-1 produced on Vero cells had to be withdrawn from the market after being associated with postvaccinal myeloencephalitis (Liu and Castleman, 1977).

The safety problems associated with live-virus vaccines led to the development of a fomalin-inactivated whole-virus adjuvanted vaccine, Pneumoabort K. This vaccine reduced the incidence of abortion from 0.68% (140/20,732) in unvaccinated mares as compared to 0.18% (14/6,806) vaccinated mares during a three-year study period in USA (Bryans and Allen, 1982). However, no difference in the occurrence of abortion between Pneumoabort K vaccinated and unvaccinated controls in two-year-old pregnant pony mares in UK was found (Burrows et al., 1984), though it reduced the viremia in them. Vaccination with a commercially inactivated combined EHV-1 and EHV-4 vaccine was reported to reduce the shedding of virus in nasal secretions and incidence of abortion but did not decrease viremia or clinical signs of respiratory disease (Heldens et al., 2004). The efficacy studies on a modified live vaccine, containing a temperature-sensitive abortion isolate, have been conducted in a randomized, controlled respiratory and abortion challenge studies in pregnant mares, young stock, and foals (Patel et al., 2003a, 2003b, 2004). However, virus shedding and cell-associated viremia occurred among vaccinated animals. Recombinant vaccines—including gene deletion mutants, vector, and DNA vaccines—are still in experimental stage. Vaccination trials with gE/gI gene deleted EHV-1 mutant was found to be safe for horses but only gave partial clinical protection against an

EHV-1 challenge (Matsumura et al., 1998). An experimental vaccine based on a thymidine kinase–negative (TK–) mutant did not prevent viremia after EHV-1 challenge (Slater et al., 1993; Tewari et al., 1993). A canary pox recombinant expressing the gB, gC, and gD genes of EHV-1 significantly decreased virus excretion after challenge but could not protect against cell-associated viremia (Audonnet et al., 1998; Minke et al., 2006). The efficacy of inactivated combination and modified live virus vaccines against challenge infection with neuropathogenic equine herpesvirus type 1 (EHV-1) was investigated. Based on data from neurological signs, rectal temperatures, virus isolation from nasal swabs, and immune response specificity, it was concluded that protection induced by the modified live virus vaccine is superior to that induced by the inactivated combination vaccine (Goodman et al., 2006).

The aim of vaccination against EHV-1 and EHV-4 is to protect horses against respiratory disease and to prevent abortion. No current commercial vaccine has been demonstrated to protect against the neurological manifestation of EHV-1 infection. Ten inactivated and two live commercially manufactured vaccines are currently marketed. These commercial EHV vaccines induce high titers of neutralizing antibodies and give only partial clinical and virological protection against respiratory infections with EHV-1 or EHV-4 but do not prevent cell-associated viremia or fully protect against abortion. The highly variable results on protection obtained in the different studies on the same vaccine may be due to the difference in the immunological status of the animals, the use of EHV primed animals and mares at different stages of pregnancy, or may be related to breed differences. Nevertheless, the widespread use of intramuscular vaccines and/or improved methods of managing herds of breeding stock appear to have decreased the incidence of EHV-1–related abortion storms in the United States by 75% (Ostlund, 1993).

CONCLUSION

The equine herpesvirus 1 (EHV-1) and equine herpesvirus 4 (EHV-4) are alphaviruses that cause serious loss to the equine industry throughout the world. EHV-4 predominantly causes respiratory disease, whereas EHV-1 infection can result in abortion, neonatal foal mortality, paralysis, and respiratory disease. Economic losses due to respiratory disease are related not only to the lost training days and with veterinary care cost during the acute stage of infection, but also to the longer-term effects on the athletic performance. The role of cell-associated viremia, latency, and immune evasion in pathogenesis and epidemiology has been elucidated. The epidemiological picture of equine herpesviruses is quite dynamic as they are being isolated from new host species and new locations. Also, EHV-2 and EHV-5 have been reported to be associated with abortions. The correlates of protective immunity for EHV-1 are not fully understood. The current commercial vaccines stimulate some, but not all, of the desired components of the immune responses against EHV-1. None of them consistently prevent infection in a vaccinated animal or provide complete protection against disease associated with EHV-1. Vaccination against EHV-1 is an important part of most equine herd health programs, despite the incomplete protection given by vaccines. To be effective, the future vaccines will need a safe and efficient delivery route that induces both mucosal and systemic cellular as well as humoral immunity in the horses. It should also be kept in mind that the MHC haplotype, virus virulence, latency, and immune status of the animal are likely to influence the response to vaccination. The hygienic measures and good management along with vaccination has greatly reduced the incidence of abortion. However, the incidence of EHM is on the rise, and the currently marketed vaccines do not afford protection against the neurological disease.

REFERENCES

1. Agius, C. T. and Studdert, M. J. 1994. Equine herpesviruses 2 and 5: Comparisons with other members of the subfamily gammaherpesvirinae. *Adv. Virus Res.* 44:357–379.
2. Albrecht, R. A., Kim, S. K. and O'Callaghan, D. J. 2005. The EICP27 protein of equine herpesvirus 1 is recruited to viral promoters by its interaction with the immediate-early protein. *Virology* 333:74–87.
3. Allen, G. P. and Bryans, J. T. 1986. Molecular epidemiology, pathogenesis and prophylaxis of equine herpesvirus-1 infections. In Progress in veterinary microbiology and immunology, vol. 2, ed. R. Pandey, 78–144. Basel, Switzerland, and New York, USA: Karger.
4. Allen, G. P., Coogle, L. D., Ostlund, E. N. and Yeargan, M. R. 1992. Molecular dissection of two major equine herpesvirus glycoprotein antigens (gB and gC) that elicit humoral immune responses in horse. In Equine infectious diseases VI, ed. W. Plowright, P. D. Rossdale, and J. F. Wade, 181–193. Newmarket, UK: R&W Publications.
5. Allen, G., Yeargan, M., Costa, L. R. and Cross, R. 1995. Major histocompatibility complex class I-restricted cytotoxic T-lymphocyte responses in horses infected with equine herpesvirus 1. *J. Virol.* 69:606–612.
6. Allen, G. P., Kydd, J. K., Slater, J. D. and Smith, K. C. 1999. Advances in understanding of the epidemiology, pathogenesis and immunological control of equid herpesvirus-1 abortion. In Equine infectious diseases VIII, ed. U. Wernery, J. Wade, J. Mumford, and O. R. Kaaden, 129–146. Newmarket, UK: R&W Publications.
7. Allen, G. P. and Breathnach, C. C. 2006. Quantification by real-time PCR of the magnitude and duration of leucocyte-associated viraemia in horses infected with neuropathogenic vs. non-neuropathogenic strains of EHV-1. *Equine Vet. J.* 38:252–257.
8. Allen, G. P. 2006. Antemortem detection of latent infection with neuropathogenic strains of equine herpesvirus-1 in horses. *Am. J. Vet. Res.* 67:1401–1405.
9. Allen, G. P. 2007. Development of a real-time polymerase chain reaction assay for rapid diagnosis of neuropathogenic strains of equine herpesvirus-1. *J. Vet. Diagn. Invest.* 19:69–72.
10. Ambagala, A. P. N., Gopinath, R. S. and Srikumaran, S. 2004. Peptide transport activity of the transporter associated with antigen processing (TAP) is inhibited by an early protein of equine herpesvirus-1. *J. Gen. Virol.* 85:349–353.

6. EQUINE HERPESVIRUSES

11. Antczak, D. F. 1992. The major histocompatibility complex of the horse. In Equine infectious diseases VI, ed. W. Plowright, D. Rossdale, and J. F. Wade, 99–112. Newmarket, UK: R&W Publications.

12. Audonnet, J. C., Mumford, J. A., Jessett, D. M., Pardo, M. C., Taylor, J., Tartaglia J. and Minke, J. M. 1998. Safety and efficacy of a canarypox-EHV recombinant in horses. In Equine infectious diseases VIII, ed. U. Wernery, J. F. Wade, J. A. Mumford, and O. R. Kaaden, 418–419. Newmarket: R&W Publications Ltd.

13. Bell, S. A., Balasuriya, U. B. R., Gardner, I. A., Barry, P. A., Wilson, D. A., Ferraro, G. L. and MacLachlan, N. J. 2006. Temporal detection of equine herpesvirus infections of a cohort of mares and their foals. *Vet. Microbiol.* 116:249–257.

14. Bell, S. A., Pusterla, N., Balasuriya, U. B. R., Mapes, S. M., Nyberg, N. L. and MacLachlan, N. J. 2008. Isolation of a gammaherpesvirus similar to asinine herpesvirus-2 (AHV-2) from a mule and a survey of mules and donkeys for AHV-2 infection by real-time PCR. *Vet. Microbiol.* 130:176–183.

15. Borchers, K. and Slater, J. 1993. A nested PCR for the detection and differentiation of EHV-1 and EHV-4. *J. Virol. Methods* 45:331–336.

16. Borchers, K. and Frolich, K. 1997. Antibodies against equine herpesviruses in free-ranging mountain zebras from Namibia. *J. Wildl. Dis.* 33:812–817.

17. Borchers, K., Wolfinger, U., Lawrenz, B., Schellenbach, A. and Ludwig, H. 1997. Equine herpesvirus 4 DNA in trigeminal ganglia of naturally infected horses detected by direct in situ PCR. *J. Gen. Virol.* 78:1109–1114.

18. Borchers, K., Frolich, K. and Ludwig, H. 1999. Detection of equine herpesvirus types 2 and 5 (EHV-2 and EHV-5) in Przewalski's wild horses, *Arch. Virol.* 144:771–780.

19. Breathnach, C. C., Yeargan, M. R., Sheoran, A. S. and Allen, G. P. 2001. The mucosal humoral immune response of the horse to infective challenge and vaccination with equine herpesvirus-1 antigens. *Equine Vet. J.* 33:651–657.

20. Bryans, J. T. 1969. On immunity to disease caused by equine herpesvirus-1. *J. Am. Vet. Med. Assoc.* 155:294–300.

21. Bryans, J. T. and Allen, G. P. 1982. Application of a chemically inactivated, adjuvanted vaccine to control abortigenic infection of mares by equine herpesvirus 1. *Dev. Biol. Stand.* 52:493–498.

22. Bürki, F., Rossmanith, W., Nowotny, N., Pallan, C., Möstl, K. and Lussy, H. 1990. Viraemia and abortions are not prevented by two commercial equine herpesvirus 1 vaccines after experimental challenge of horses. *Vet. Q.* 12:80–86.

23. Burrows, R., Goodridge, D. and Denyer, M. S. 1984. Trials of an inactivated equid herpes virus vaccine: Challenge with a subtype 1 virus. *Vet. Rec.* 114:369–374.

24. Collinson, P. N., O'Rielly, J. L., Ficorilli, N. and Studdert, M. J. 1994. Isolation of equine herpesvirus 2 (equine gamaherpes virus 2) from foals with keratoconjunctivitis. *J. Am. Vet. Med. Assoc.* 205:329–331.

25. Caughman, G. B., Staczek, J. and O'Callaghan, D. J. 1985. Equine herpesvirus type 1 infected cell polypeptides: Evidence for immediate early/early/late regulation of viral gene expression. *Virology* 145:49–61.

26. Coombs, D. K., Patton, T., Kohler, A. K., Soboll, G., Breathnach, C., Townsend, H. G. G. and Lunn, D. P. 2006. Cytokine responses to EHV-1 infection in immune and non-immune ponies. *Vet. Immunol. Immunopathol.* 111:109–116.

27. Crabb, B. S. and Studdert, M. J. 1990. Comparative studies of the proteins of equine herpesviruses 4 and 1 and asinine herpesvirus 3: Antibody response in the natural hosts. *J. Gen. Virol.* 71:2033–2041.

28. Crabb, B. S., Allen, G. P. and Studdert, M. J. 1991. Characterization of major glycoproteins of equine herpesviruses type 4 and 1 and asinine herpesvirus 3 using monoclonal antibodies. *J. Gen. Virol.* 72:2075–2082.

29. Crabb, B. S. and Studdert, M. J. 1993. Epitopes of glycoprotein G of equine herpesvirus 4 and 1 located near the C termini elicit type-specific antibody responses in the natural hosts. *J. Virol.* 67:6332–6338.

30. Crabb, B. S. and Studdert, M. 1995. Equine herpesviruses 4 (rhinopneumonitis virus) and 1 (equine abortion virus). *Adv. Virus Res.* 45:153–190.

31. Crabb, B. S., MacPherson, C. M., Reubel, G. H., Browning, G. F., Studdert, M. J. and Drummer, H. E. 1995. A type-specific serological test to distinguish antibodies to equine herpesviruses 4 and 1. *Arch. Virol.* 140:245–258.

32. Davison, A. J., Eberle, R., Ehlers, B., Hayward, G. S., McGeoch, D. J., Minson, A. C., Pellett, P. E., Roizman, B., Studdert, M. J. and Thiry, E. 2009. The order Herpesvirales. *Arch Virol.* 154:171–177.

33. Dixon, R. J., Hartley, W. J., Hutchins, D. R., Lepherd, E. E., Feilen, C., Jones, R. F., Love, D. N., Sabine, M. and Wells, A. L. 1977. Perinatal foal mortality associated with a herpesvirus. *Aust. Vet. J.* 54:103–105.

34. Doll, E. R., Bryans, J. T. and McCollum, W. H. 1959. A procedure for evaluating the antigenicity of killed virus vaccines for equine rhinopneumonitis. *Cornell Vet.* 49:212–220.

35. Doll, E. R. and Bryans, J. T. 1962. Development of complement-fixing and viral-neutralizing antibodies in viral rhinopneumonitis of horses. *Am. J. Vet. Res.* 23:843–846.

36. Doll, E. R. and Bryans, J. T. 1963a. Immunization of young horses against viral rhinopneumonitis. *Cornell Vet.* 53:24–41.

37. Doll, E. R. and Bryans, J. T. 1963b. A planned infection program for immunizing mares against viral rhinopneumonitis. *Cornell Vet.* 53:249–262.

38. Drummer, H. E., Reubel, G. H. and Studdert, M. J. 1996. Equine gamaherpesvirus 2 (EHV2) is latent in B lymphocytes. *Arch. Virol.* 141:495–504.

39. Dunowska, M., Meers, J. and Wilks, C. R. 1999. Isolation of equine herpes virus type 5 in New Zealand. *N. Z. Vet. J.* 47:44–46.

40. Dunowska, M., Wilks, C. R., Studdert, M. J. and Meers, J. 2002a. Equine respiratory viruses in foals in New Zealand. *N. Z. Vet. J.* 50:140–147.

41. Dunowska, M., Wilks, C. R., Studdert, M. J. and Meers, J. 2002b. Viruses associated with outbreaks of equine respiratory disease in New Zealand. *N. Z. Vet. J.* 50:132–139.

42. Dutta, S. K., Talbot, N. C. and Myrup, A. C. 1983. Detection of equine herpesvirus-1 antigen and the specific antibody by enzyme-linked immunosorbent assay. *Am. J. Vet. Res.* 44:1930–1934.

43. Dutta, S. K. and Shiply, W. D. 1975. Immunity and levels of neutralization antibodies in foals and mares vaccinated with a modified live-virus rhinopneumonitis vaccine. *Am. J. Vet. Res.* 36:445–448.

44. Edington, N., Bridges, C. G. and Patel, J. R. 1986. Endothelial cell infection and thrombosis in paralysis caused by equid herpesvirus-1: Equine stroke. *Arch. Virol.* 90:111–124.

45. Edington, N., Smyth, B. and Griffiths, L. 1991. The role of endothelial cell infection in the endometrium, placenta and foetus of equid herpesvirus 1 (EHV-1) abortions. *J. Comp. Pathol.* 104:379–387.

46. Edington, N., Welch, H. M. and Griffiths, L. 1994. The prevalence of latent equid herpesviruses in the tissues of 40 abattoir horses. *Equine Vet. J.* 26:140–142.

47. Foote, C. E., Love, D. N., Gilkerson, J. R. and Whalley, J. M. 2004. Detection of EHV-1 and EHV-4 DNA in unweaned Thoroughbred foals from vaccinated mares on a large stud farm. *Equine Vet. J.* 36:341–345.

48. Gerst, S., Borchers, K., Gower, S. M. and Smith, K. C. 2003. Detection of EHV-1 and EHV-4 in placental sections of naturally occurring EHV-1—and EHV-4-related abortions in the UK: Use of the placenta in diagnosis. *Equine Vet. J.* 35:430–433.

49. Gibson, J. S., Slater, J. D., Awan, A. R. and Field, H. J. 1992. Pathogenesis of equine herpesvirus-1 in specific pathogen-free foals: Primary and secondary infections and reactivation. *Arch. Virol.* 123:351–366.

50. Giles, R. C., Donahue, J. M., Hong, C. B., Tuttle, P. A., Petrtes-Murphy, M. B., Pooncha, K. B., Roberts, A. W., Tramotin, R. R., Smith, B. and Swerczek, T. W. 1993. Causes of abortion, stillbirth, and perinatal death in horses: 3,527 cases (1986–1991). *J. Am. Vet. Med. Assoc.* 203:1170–1175.

51. Gilkerson, J. R., Walley, J. M., Drummer, H. E., Studdert, M. J. and Love D. N. 1999a. Epidemiology of EHV-1 and EHV-4 in the mare and foal populations on a Hunter Valley stud farm: Are mares the source of EHV-1 for unweaned foals. *Vet. Microbiol.* 68:27–34.

52. Gilkerson, J. R., Walley, J. M., Drummer, H. E., Studdert, M. J. and Love D. N. 1999b. Epidemiological studies of equine herpesvirus 1 (EHV-1) in Thoroughbred foals: A review of studies conducted in the Hunter Valley of New South Wales between 1995 and 1997. *Vet. Microbiol.* 68:15–25.

53. Gleeson, L. J. and Coggins, L. 1980. Response of pregnant mares to equine herpesvirus 1 (EHV1). *Cornell Vet.* 70:391–400.

54. Goehring, L. S., van Maanen, C., Sloet van Oldruitenborgh and Oosterbaan, M. M. 2005. Neurological syndromes among horses in the Netherlands: A 5 year retrospective survey (1999–2004). *Vet. Q.* 27:11–20.

55. Goodman, L. B., Wagner, B., Flaminio, M. J., Sussman, K. H., Metzger, S. M., Holland, R. and Osterrieder, N. 2006. Comparison of the efficacy of inactivated combination and modified-live virus vaccines against challenge infection with neuropathogenic equine herpesvirus type 1 (EHV-1). *Vaccine* 24:3636–3645.

56. Gunn, H. M. 1992. A direct fluorescent antibody technique to diagnose abortion caused by equine herpesvirus. *Irish Vet. J.* 44:37–40.

57. Hannant, D., Jessett, D. M., O'Neill, T., Dolby, C. A., Cook, R. F. and Mumford, J. A. 1993. Responses of ponies to equid herpesvirus-1 ISCOM vaccination and challenge with virus of the homologous strain. *Res. Vet. Sci.* 54:299–305.

58. Hartley C. A., Drummer, H. E. and Studdert, M. J. 1999. The nucleotide sequence of the glycoprotein G homologue of equine herpesvirus 3 (EHV3) indicates that EHV3 is a distinctive equid alphaherpesvirus. *Arch. Virol.* 144:2023–2033.

59. Hartley, C. A., Wilks, C. R., Studdert, M. J. and Gilkerson, J. R. 2005. Comparison of antibody detection assays for the diagnosis of equine herpesvirus 1 and 4 infections in horses. *Am. J. Vet. Res.* 66:921–928.

60. Heldens, J. G., Pouwels, H. G. and van Loon, A. A. 2004. Efficacy and duration of immunity of a combined equine influenza and equine herpesvirus vaccine against challenge with an American-like equine influenza virus (A/equi-2/Kentucky/95). *Vet. J.* 167:150–157.

61. Henninger, R. W., Reed, S. M., Saville, W. J., Allen, G. P., Hass, G. F., Kohn, C. W. and Sofaly, C. 2007. Outbreak of neurologic disease caused by equine herpesvirus-1 at a university equestrian center. *J. Vet. Intern. Med.* 21:157–165.

62. Hohdatsu, T., Eiki, T., Ide, S. and Yamagishi, H. 1986. Enzyme-linked immunosorbant assay for the detection of antibodies to equid herpesvirus type 1 (EHV1). *Jpn. J. Vet. Sci.* 48:1045–1048.

63. Hussey, S. B., Clark, R., Lunn, K. F., Breathnach, C., Soboll, G., Whalley, J. M. and Lunn, D. P. 2006. Detection and quantification of equine herpesvirus-1 viremia and nasal shedding by real-time polymerase chain reaction. *J. Vet. Diagn. Invest.* 18:335–342.

64. Ibrahim, E. S., Kinoh, M., Matsumura, T., Kennedy, M., Allen, G. P., Yamaguchi, T. and Fukushi, H. 2007. Genetic relatedness and pathogenicity of equine herpesvirus 1 isolated from onager, zebra and gazelle. *Arch. Virol.* 152:245–255.

65. Irwin, V. L., Traub-Dargatz, J. L., Newton, J. R., Scase, T. J., Davis-Poynter, N. J., Nugent, J., Creis, L., Leaman, T. R. and Smith, K. C. 2007. Investigation and management of an outbreak of abortion related to equine herpesvirus type 1 in unvaccinated ponies. *Vet. Rec.* 160:378–380.

66. Jackson, T. A., Osburn, B. I., Cordy, D. R. and Kendrick, J. W. 1977. Equine herpesvirus 1 infection of horses: Studies on the experimentally induced neurologic disease. *Am. J. Vet. Res.* 38:709–719.

67. Kershaw, O., von Oppen, T., Glitz, F., Deegen, E., Ludwig, H. and Borchers, K. 2001. Detection of equine herpes virus 2 (EHV-2) in horses with keratoconjunctivitis. *Virus Res.* 80:93–99.

68. Kirisawa, R., Endo, A., Iwai, H. and Kawakami, Y. 1993. Detection and identification of equine herpesvirus-1 and—4 by polymerase chain reaction. *Vet Microbiol.* 36:57–67.

69. Kleiboeker, S. B., Schommer, S. K., Johnson, P. J., Ehlers, B., Turnquist, S. E., Boucher, M. and Kreeger, J. M. 2002. Association of two newly recognized herpesviruses with interstitial pneumonia in donkeys (*Equus asinus*). *J. Vet. Diagn. Invest.* 14:273–280.

70. Kohn, C. W. and Fenner, W. R. 1987. Equine herpes myeloencephalopathy. *Vet. Clin. North Am. Equine Pract.* 3:405–419.

71. Kydd, J. H., Smith, K. C., Hannant, D., Livesay, G. L. and Mumford, J. A. 1994a. Distribution of equid herpesvirus-1 (EHV-1) in the respiratory tract of ponies: Implications for vaccination strategies. *Equine Vet. J.* 26:466–469.

72. Kydd, J. H., Smith, K. C., Hannant, D., Livesay, G. L. and Mumford, J. A. 1994b. Distribution of equid herpesvirus-1 (EHV-1) in respiratory tract associated lymphoid tissue: Implications for cellular immunity. *Equine Vet. J.* 26:470–473.

73. Kydd, J. H., Hannant, D. and Mumford, J. A. 1996. Residence and recruitment of leucocytes to the equine lung after EHV-1 infection. *Vet. Immunol. Immunopathol.* 52:15–26.

74. Kydd, J. H., Wattrang, E. and Hannant, D. 2003. Pre-infection frequencies of equine herpesvirus-1 specific, cytotoxic T lymphocytes correlate with protection against abortion following experimental infection of pregnant mares. *Vet. Immunol. Immunopathol.* 96:207–217.

75. Kydd, J. H., Townsend, H. G. and Hannant, D. 2006. The equine immune response to equine herpesvirus-1: The virus and its vaccines. *Vet. Immunol. Immunopathol.* 111:15–30.

76. Lawrence, G. L., Gilkerson, J., Love, D. N., Sabine, M. and Whalley, J. M. 1994. Rapid, single-step differentiation of equid herpesvirus 1 and 4 from clinical material using the polymerase chain reaction and virus-specific primers. *J. Virol. Methods* 47:59–72.

77. Leon, A. Fortier, G., Fortier, C., Freymuth, F., Tapprest, J., Leclercq, R. and Pronost, S. 2008. Detection of equine herpesviruses in aborted foetuses by consensus PCR. *Vet. Microbiol.* 126:20–29.

78. Liu, I. K. M. and Castleman, W. 1977. Equine posterior paresis associated with equine herpesvirus 1 vaccine in California: A preliminary report. *J. Equine Med. Surg.* 1:397–401.

79. Luce, R., Shepherd, M., Paillot, R., Blacklawst, B., Wood, J. L. and Kydd, J. H. 2007. Equine herpesvirus-1-specific interferon gamma (IFNgamma) synthesis by peripheral blood mononuclear cells in thoroughbred horses. *Equine Vet. J.* 39:202–209.

80. Matsumura, T., Sugiura, T., Imagawa, H., Fukunaga, Y. and Kamada, M. 1992. Epizootological aspects of type 1 and type 4 equine herpesvirus infections among horse populations. *J. Vet. Med. Sci.* 54:207–211.

81. Matsumura, T., Kondo, T., Sugita, S., Damiani A. M., O'Callaghan, D. J. and Imagawa, H. 1998. An equine herpesvirus type 1 recombinant with a deletion in the gE gene and gI genes is avirulent in young horses. *Virology* 242:68–79.

82. Mayr, A. and Pette, J. 1968. First experiments concerning the vaccination of horses against rhinopneumonia (viral abortion of mares) with a live vaccine from cell cultures. *Bull. Off. Int. Epizoot.* 70:133–140.

83. Mayr, A., Pette, J., Petzoldt, K. and Wagener, K. 1968. Studies on the development of a live vaccine against rhinopneumonitis (mare abortion) of horses. *Zentralbl. Veterinaermed.* B 15:406–418.

84. McCartan, C. G., Russell, M. M., Wood, J. L. and Mumford, J. A. 1995. Clinical, serological and virological characteristics of an outbreak of paresis and neonatal foal disease due to equine herpesvirus-1 on a stud farm. *Vet. Rec.* 136:7–12.

85. Minke, J. M., Fischer, L., Baudu, P., Guigal, P. M., Sindle, T., Mumford, J. A. and Audonnet, J. C. 2006. Use of DNA and recombinant canarypox viral (ALVAC) vectors for equine herpes virus vaccination. *Vet. Immunol. Immunopathol.* 111:47–57.

86. Mukaiya, R., Kimura, T., Ochiai, K., Wada, R. and Umemura, T. 2000. Demonstration of equine herpesvirus-1 gene expression in the placental trophoblasts of naturally aborted fetuses. *J. Comp. Pathol.* 123:119–125.

87. Mumford, J. A., Rossdale, P. D., Jessett, D. M., Gann, S. J., Ousey, J. and Cook, R. F. 1987. Serological and virological investigations of an equid herpesvirus 1 (EHV-1) abortion storm on a stud farm in 1985. *J. Reprod. Fertil. Suppl.* 35:509–518.

88. Murray, M. J., del Piero, F., Jeffrey, S. C., Jeffrey, S. C., Davis, M. S., Furr, M. O., Dubovi, E. J. and Mayo, J. A. 1998. Neonatal equine herpesvirus type 1 infection on a thoroughbred breeding farm. *J. Vet. Intern. Med.* 12:36–41.

89. Neubauer, A., Meindl, A. and Osterrieder, N. 1999. Mutations in the US2 and glycoprotein B genes of the equine herpesvirus 1 vaccine strain RacH have no effects on its attenuation, *Berl. Muench. Tieraerztl. Wochenschr.* 112:351–354.

90. Nordengrahn, A., Merza, M., Ros, C., Lindholmc, A., Palfl, V., Hannat, D. and Belak, S. 2002. Prevalence of equine herpesvirus types 2 and 5 in horse populations by using type-specific PCR assays. *Vet. Res.* 33:251–259.

91. Nugent, J., Birch-Machin, I., Smith, K. C., Mumford, J. A., Swann, Z., Newton, J. R., Bowden, R. J., Allen, G. P. and Davis-Poynter, N. 2006. Analysis of equid herpesvirus 1 strain variation reveals a point mutation of the DNA polymerase strongly associated with neuropathogenic versus nonneuropathogenic disease outbreaks. *J. Virol.* 80:4047–4060.

92. O'Keefe, J. S., Julian, A., Moriarty, K., Murray, A. and Wilks, C. R. 1994. A comparison of the polymerase chain reaction with standard laboratory methods for the detection of EHV-1 and EHV-4 in archival tissue samples. *N. Z. Vet. J.* 42:93–96.

93. O'Keefe, J. S., Alley, M. R., Jones, D. and Wilks, C. R. 1995. Neonatal mortality due to equid herpesvirus 4 (EHV-4) in a foal. *Aust. Vet. J.* 72:353–354.

94. O'Neill, T., Kydd, J. H., Allen, G. P., Wattrang, E. Mumford, J. A. and Hannat, D. 1999. Determination of equid herpesvirus1-specific, CD8+, cytotoxic T lymphocyte precursor frequencies in ponies. *Vet. Immunol. Immunopathol.* 70:43–54.

95. Ostlund, E. N. 1993. The equine herpesviruses. *Vet. Clin. North Am. Equine Pract.* 9:283–294.

96. Patel, J. R., Bateman, H., Williams, J. and Didlick, S. 2003a. Derivation and characterization of a live equid herpesvirus-1 (EHV-1) live vaccine to protect against abortion and respiratory disease due to EHV types 1. *Vet. Microbiol.* 91:23–39.

97. Patel, J. R., Földi, J., Bateman, H., Williams, J., Didlick, S. and Stark, R. 2003b. Equid herpesvirus (EHV-1) live vaccine strain C147: Efficacy against respiratory disease following EHV types 1 and 4 challenges. *Vet. Microbiol.* 92:1–17.

98. Patel, J. R., Didlick, S. and Bateman, H. 2004. Efficacy of a live equine herpes virus-1 (EHV-1) strain C147 vaccine in foals with maternally derived antibody: Protection against EHV-1 infection. *Equine Vet. J.* 36:447–451.

99. Patel, J. R. and Heldens, J. 2005. Equine herpesviruses 1 (EHV-1) and 4 (EHV-4): Epidemiology, disease and immunoprophylaxis: A brief review. *Vet. J.* 170:14–23.

100. Pusterla, N., Chaney, K. P., Maes, R., Wise, A. G., Holland, R. and Schott, H. C. 2nd. 2007. Investigation of the molecular detection of vaccine-derived equine herpesvirus type 1 in blood and nasal secretions from horses following intramuscular vaccination. *J. Vet. Diagn. Invest.* 19:290–293.

101. Pusterla, N., Wilson, W. D., Mapes, S., Finno, C., Isbell, D., Arthur, R. M. and Ferraro, G. L. 2009. Characterization of viral loads, strain and state of equine herpesvirus-1 using real-time PCR in horses following natural exposure at a racetrack in California. *The Vet. Journal* 179:230–239.

102. Rappocciolo, G., Birch, J. and Ellis, S. A. 2003. Down-regulation of MHC class I expression by equine herpesvirus-1. *J. Gen. Virol.* 84:293–300.

103. Rudolph, J. and Osterrieder, N. 2002. Equine herpesvirus type 1 devoid of gM and gp2 is severely impaired in virus egress but not direct cell-to-cell spread. *Virology* 293:356–367.

104. Saxegaard, F. 1966. Isolation and identification of equine rhinopneumonitis virus (equine abortion virus) from cases of abortion and paralysis. *Nord. Vet. Med.* 18:504–512.

105. Schrenzel, M. D., Tucker, T. A., Donovan, T. A., Busch, M. D. M., Wise, A. G., Maes, R. K. and Kiupel, M. 2008. New hosts for equine herpesvirus 9. *Emerg. Infect. Dis.* 14:1616–1619.

106. Schultheiss, P. C., Collins, J. K. and Carman, J. 1993. Use of an immunoperoxidase technique to detect equine herpesvirus-1 antigen in formalin-fixed paraffin-embedded equine fetal tissues. *J. Vet. Diagn. Invest.* 5:12–15.

107. Scott, J. C., Dutta, S. K. and Myrup, A. C. 1983. In vivo harbouring of equine herpesvirus-1 in leukocyte populations and subpopulations and their Quantitation from experimentally infected ponies. *Am. J. Vet. Res.* 44:1344–1348.

108. Sharma, P. C., Cullinane, A. A., Onion, D. E. and Nicolson, L. 1992. Diagnosis of equid herpesvirus1 and—4 by polymerase chain reaction. *Equine Vet. J.* 24:20–25.

109. Singh, B. K., Ahuja, S. and Gulati, B. R. 2004. Development of a neutralizing monoclonal antibody-based blocking ELISA for detection of equine herpes virus-1 antibodies. *Vet. Res. Commun.* 28:437–446.

110. Sinclair, R., Binns, M. M., Chirnside, E. D. and Mumford, J. A. 1993. Detection of antibodies against equine herpesvirus types 1 and 4 by using recombinant protein derived from an immunodominant region of glycoprotein B. *J. Clin. Microbiol.* 31:265–271.

111. Slater, J. D., Gibson, J. S. and Field, H. J. 1993. Pathogenicity of a thymidine kinase-deficient mutant of equine herpesvirus 1 in mice and specific pathogen-free foals. *J. Gen. Virol.* 74:819–828.

112. Slater, J. D., Borchers, K., Thackray, A. M. and Field, H. J. 1994. The trigeminal ganglion is a location for equine herpesvirus 1 latency and reactivation in the horse. *J. Gen. Virol.* 75:2007–2016.

113. Smith, K. C., Whitwell, K. E., Binns, M. M., Dolby, C. A., Hannant, D. and Mumford. J. A. 1992. Abortion of virologically negative foetuses following experimental challenge of pregnant pony mares with equid herpesvirus 1. *Equine Vet. J.* 24:256–259.

114. Smith, K. C., Whitwell, K. E., Mumford, J. A., Gower, S. M., Hannant, D. and Tearle, J. P. 1993. An immunohistological study of the uterus of mares following experimental infection with equid herpes virus-1. *Equine Vet. J.* 25:36–40.

115. Smith, K. C., Whitwell, K. E., Mumford, J. A., Hannant, D., Blunden, A. S. and Tearle, J. P. 2000. Virulence of the V592 isolate of equid herpesvirus type 1 in ponies. *J. Comp. Pathol.* 122:288–297.

116. Smith, K. C. and Borchers, K. 2001. A study of the pathogenesis of equid herpesvirus-1 (EHV-1) abortion by DNA in-situ hybridization. *J. Comp. Pathol.* 125:304–310.

117. Smith, K. C., Whitwell, K. E., Blunden, A. S., Bestbier, M., Scase, T. J., Geraghty, R. J., Nugent, J., Davis-Poynter, N. J. and Cardwell, J. M. 2004. Equine herpesvirus-1 abortion: Atypical cases with lesions largely or wholly restricted to the placenta. *Equine Vet. J.* 36:79–82.

118. Soboll, G., Whalley, J. M., Koen, M. T., Allen, G. P., Fraser, D. G., Macklin, M. D., Swain, W. F. and Lunn, D. P. 2003. Identification of equine herpesvirus-1 antigens recognized by cytotoxic T lymphocytes. *J. Gen. Virol.* 84:2625–2634.

119. Studdert, M. J., Fitzpatrick, D. R., Horner, G. W., Westbury, H. A. and Gleeson, L. J. 1984. Molecular epidemiology and pathogenesis of some equine herpesvirus type 1 (equine abortion virus) and type 4 (equine rhinopneumonitis virus) isolates. *Aust. Vet. J.* 61:345–348.

120. Studdert, M. J., Hartley, C. A., Dynon, K., Sandy, J. R., Slocombe, R. F., Charles, J. A., Milne, M. E., Clarke, A. F. and El Hage, C. 2003. Outbreak of equine herpesvirus type 1 myeloencephalitis: New insights from virus identification by PCR and the application of an EHV-1-specific antibody detection ELISA. *Vet. Rec.* 153:417–423.

121. Szeredi, L., Aupperle, H. and Steiger, K. 2003. Detection of equine herpesvirus-1 in the fetal membranes of aborted equine fetuses by Immunohistochemical and in-situ hybridization techniques. *J. Comp. Pathol.* 129:1147–153.

122. Tearle, J. P., Smith, K. C., Platt, A. J., Hannat, D., Davis-Poynter, N. J. and Mumford, J. A. 2003. In vitro characterisation of high and low virulence isolates of equine herpesvirus-1 and—4. *Res. Vet. Sci.* 75:83–86.

123. Telford, E. A., Watson, M. S., McBride, K. and Davison, A. J. 1992. The DNA sequence of equine herpesvirus-1. *Virology* 189:304–316.

124. Telford, E. A., Watson, M. S., Aird, H. C., Perry, J. and Davison, A. J. 1995. The DNA sequence of equine herpesvirus 2. *J. Mol. Biol.* 249:520–528.

125. Telford, E. A., Watson, M. J., Perry, J., Cullinane, A. A. and Davison A. J. 1998. The DNA sequence of equine herpesvirus-4. *J. Gen. Virol.* 79:1197–1203.

126. Tewari, D., Gibson, J. S., Slater, J. D., O'Neill, T., Hannant, D., Allen, G. P. and Field, H. J. 1993. Modulation of the serological response of specific pathogen-free (EHV-free) foals to EHV-1 by previous infection to EHV-4 or a TK-deletion mutant of EHV-1. *Arch. Virol.* 132:101–120.

127. Thomson, G. R., Mumford, J. A., Campbell, J., Griffiths, L. and Clapham P. 1976. Serological detection of equid herpesvirus 1 infections of the respiratory tract. *Equine Vet. J.* 8:58–65.

128. Turtinen, L. W. and Allen, G. P. 1982. Identification of the envelope surface glycoproteins of equine herpesvirus type 1. *J. Gen. Virol.* 63:481–485.

129. Van der Meulen, K. M., Nauwynck, H. J. and Pensaert, M. B. 2003. Absence of viral antigens on the surface of equine herpesvirus-1-infected peripheral blood mononuclear cells: A strategy to avoid complement-mediated lysis. *J. Gen. Virol.* 84:93–97.

130. Van der Meulen, K. M., Favoreel, H. W., Pensaert, M. B. and Nauwynck, H. J. 2006. Immune escape of equine herpesvirus 1 and other herpesviruses of veterinary importance. *Vet. Immunol. Immunolpathol.* 111:31–40.

131. Van Maanen, C., de Boer-Luijtze, E. and Terpstra, C. 2000. Development and validation of a monoclonal antibody blocking ELISA for the detection of antibodies against both equine herpesvirus type 1 (EHV1) and equine herpesvirus type 4 (EHV4). *Vet. Microbiol.* 71:37–51.

132. Van Maanen, C., Sloet van Oldruitenborgh-Oosterbaan, M. M., Damen, E. A. and Derksen, A. G. 2001. Neurological disease associated with EHV-1-infection in a riding school: Clinical and virological characteristics. *Equine Vet. J.* 33:191–196.

133. Varrasso, A., Dynon, K., Ficorilli, N., Hartley, C. A., Studdert, M. J. and Drummer, H. E. 2001. Identification of equine herpesviruses 1 and 4 by polymerase chain reaction. *Aust. Vet. J.* 79:563–569.

134. Wagner, W. N., Bogdan, J., Haines, D., Townsend, H. G. G. and Misra V. 1992. Detection of equine herpesvirus and differentiation of equine herpesvirus type 1 from type 4 by the polymerase chain reaction. *Can. J. Microbiol.* 38:1193–1196.

135. Welch, H. M., Bridges, C. G., Lyon, A. M., Griffiths, L. and Edington, N. 1992. Latent equid herpesviruses 1 and 4: Detection and distinction using the polymerase chain reaction and co-cultivation from lymphoid tissues. *J. Gen. Virol.* 73:261–268.

136. Whitwell, K. E., Gower, S. M. and Smith, K. C. 1992. An immunoperoxidase method applied to the diagnosis of equine herpesvirus abortion, using conventional and rapid microwave techniques. *Equine Vet. J.* 24:10–12.

7. Equine Influenza

Thankam Mathew, K. Dhama, R. V. S. Pawaiya, and M. Mahendran

Introduction

Equine influenza is a highly contagious disease of horses caused by influenza A virus. Enlisted among OIE list B diseases, it has a worldwide distribution among equines, especially in young horses, and causes respiratory distress and flulike symptoms (Wilson, 1993; van Maanen and Cullinane, 2002; Newton and Mumford, 2005; Cullinane et al., 2006; Landolt et al., 2007; OIE, 2008). A detailed chapter of influenza in equine is described by Mathew et al. (2006). The disease, which is present throughout Europe, North America, and parts of Asia, evinces fever with dry cough and may sometimes exacerbate due to secondary bacterial infections (Wood and Mumford, 1992; Timoney, 1996; Daly et al., 2004; Smyth, 2007). It is understood that two subtypes of influenza A virus cause equine influenza in horses, viz, H7N7 and H3N8 designated as A/equine 1 and A/equine 2, respectively are responsible for the infection. Initially, H7N7 was identified as the etiological factor for various outbreaks, but in recent years, H3N8 subtype causes majority of the disease outbreaks worldwide. Also, it is reported that H3N8 viruses are undergoing "antigenic drift" to generate distinct lineages designated as "European" and "American" (Wilson, 1993; Daly et al., 1996; Purzycka et al., 2004; Daly et al., 2004; Oxburgh and Klingeborn, 1999). As a result of variations in the genetic makeup of the H3N8 subtype of influenza virus, the vaccines currently used against this disease have not been completely successful. This is evident from the fact that the disease is still prevalent in regions where vaccination programs have been regularly practiced. Nowadays, efforts are being made to develop appropriate control measures and newer immunoprohylactic agents against equine influenza to ensure its complete wipe out.

In countries where there is extensive horse breeding and racing industries, equine influenza is still considered to be the most economically important respiratory disease of horses (Holland, 2003; Smyth, 2007). Infection of zebras, dogs, and humans has also been reported. In contrast to avian influenza, the equine influenza has till date not shown any zoonotic implications. This may be due to the fact that mutational changes occurring in the viral genome is due to antigenic drift and not antigenic shift, the latter being commonly present in case of avian influenza virus (AIV). But there have been reports of interspecies transmission of equine influenza virus (EIV) as the genomic analysis of three influenza viruses isolated from outbreaks of severe respiratory disease of racing greyhounds in United States revealed that they are closely related to H3N8 equine influenza viruses (Crawford et al., 2005). Serological evidence of infection in human has been described. Although these are not genuine human pathogens, humans can become infected with equine influenza virus subtypes. Such infections are unusual and subclinical, but may represent a potential biohazard to laboratory personnel (Alexander and Brown, 2000; OIE, 2008).

EPIDEMIOLOGY

Equine influenza was first recognized in 1956, when influenza was recovered during a widespread epidemic of respiratory disease among horses in Eastern Europe (Sovinova et al., 1958). Equine influenza is present in almost all countries except Iceland and New Zealand (Waddell et al., 1963; Gerber, 1970; Uppal et al., 1987; Wood and Mumford, 1992; Wilson, 1993; Timoney, 1996; van Maanen and Cullinane, 2002; Radostits et al., 2003; Purzycka et al., 2004; Newton and Mumford, 2005; Mathew et al., 2006; Smyth et al., 2007; Landolt et al., 2007; Foord et al., 2008). The disease is endemic in most countries with substantial equine populations, viz, Europe, Canada, USA, Scandinavia, and South America. Periodic epidemics in other areas are associated with import of infected horses, like the one being in South Africa in 2003. EIV (H3N8) infection has only recently been identified in the Australian horse population for the first time in 2007 (Foord et al., 2008) and reintroduced into South Africa and Japan (Ito et al., 2008; Yamanaka et al., 2008a; OIE, 2008).

During a study of acute viral respiratory disease in horses, equine influenza virus was found in 72% of cases for which the cause was identified (Mumford et al., 1998). A study of the respiratory diseases at a race track in Canada gave similar results, with equine influenza virus identified in 76% of the cases (Morley et al., 2000). Explosive outbreaks have been seen in susceptible equine populations following the import of infected horses from endemic areas. Distinct prototype strains of influenza virus have been isolated from horses since 1956, viz, influenza A/equine/Prague/1/56 (H7N7), influenza A/equine/Miami/ 1/63 (H3N8), and influenza A/equine/Jilin/1/89 (H3N8). The emergence of the new H3N8 EIV in China in 1989 (influenza A/equine/ Jilin/1/89) is thought to have occurred through transspecies infection from birds (Chambers, 1992; Guo et al., 1992). Isolation of H7N7 subtype has only been reported twice since 1977, first in Malaysia (1977) and later in India (1987). The last reported H7N7 outbreak occurred in India during the year 1987 (Uppal and Yadav, 1987; Uppal et al., 1987; Webster, 1993). Since then, only influenza subtype H3N8 has been isolated in the world. H3N8 viruses, which have evolved from the influenza A/equine/Miami/1/63 isolate, are currently circulating in horse populations. Presently, there are no reports of serological or virological evidence of H7N7 subtype viruses circulating among equine population.

Evolution of equine influenza H3N8 viruses has been studied by antigenic and genetic analysis of different isolates, which suggested that antigenic and genetic variants of equine H3N8 viruses cocirculates in Europe and the USA that are distinguishable by hemagglutinin (HA) gene sequencing and hemagglutination inhibition (HI) tests. These two distinct lineages of equine influenza H3N8 viruses have adversely affected the vaccine strain selection (Daly et al., 1996, 2004). Further, there is increasing evidence from field studies that antigenic drift in the HA gene, which is the major surface protein of these influenza A strains, eventually renders vaccine strains obsolete (Mumford and Wood, 1993; Wilson, 1993). Lai et al. (2001) reported diverged evolution of equine-2 influenza (H3N8) viruses in the Western Hemisphere and suggested that the evolution of equine-2 influenza virus resembled the multiple evolution pathways of influenza B virus.

Major outbreaks of equine influenza that occurred throughout the world are enlisted below with the subtypes of virus in brackets: 1956, Czech Republic (H7N7 or A/equine-1); 1963, USA (H3N8 or A/equine-2); 1977, Malaysia (H7N7); 1978, Bulgaria (H7N7 and H3N8); 1979, Italy (H7N7); 1986, South Africa (H3N8); 1987, India (H7N7); 1989, China (H3N8); 1992, Sweden (H3N8); 1993, China (H3N8) and Croatia (H3N8); 1995, Czech Republic and UK (H3N8); 1998, UK (H3N8) and Tunisia (H3N8); 2000, Germany (H3N8); 2001, Quebec (H3N8); 2002, Canada, France, Germany, Israel, Italy, Sweden, USA, and UK (H3N8); 2003, UK (H3N8); 2004, Argentina, Croatia, Denmark, Greece, Ireland, Italy, Hungary, UK, and USA (H3N8); 2007, Australia (H3N8) (Sovinova et al., 1958; Waddell et al., 1963; Uppal et al., 1987, 1989; Wood and Mumford, 1992; Guo et al., 1995; Guthrie et al., 1999; Newton et al., 2000; Daly et al., 2004; Smyth, 2007; Reeve-Johnson, 2007; Patterson-Kane et al., 2008; Virmani et al., 2008; Barbic et al., 2009).

Damiani et al. (2008) reported, while genetically characterizing equine influenza viruses, that the Italian isolates were closely related to other recent strains isolated in America as well as in Europe, including the latest-recommended American lineage vaccine prototype, A/eq/ SouthAfrica/4/2003. Phylogenetic analysis conducted by Ito et al. (2008) for a H3N8 influenza virus isolate in Japan indicated that Kanazawa/07 was classified into the American sublineage Florida. Their finding also suggests that Japanese commercially inactivated vaccine contributed to reducing the morbidity rate and manifestation of the clinical signs of horses infected with Kanazawa/07 that may be antigenically different from the vaccine strains.

ETIOLOGY

There are three basic types of influenza viruses that are differentiated as A, B, and C based on their highly conserved internal proteins, viz, matrix and nucleoproteins. Type A viruses have been isolated from horses, humans, pigs, seals, whales, and birds, but the host range of types B and C is predominantly restricted to humans. Equine influenza virus (EIV), causing an acute and highly contagious disease of horses, belongs to the genus *Influenza A* within the family Orthomyxoviridae. The virus is generally having a diameter of 80–120 nm with segmented RNA genome and a lipid envelope (Timoney, 1996). Influenza virion, having about 1% RNA, 70% protein, 20% lipid, and 9% carbohydrate, is relatively sensitive to lipid solvents such as detergents (Easterday et al., 1997).

The genome of influenza A viruses consists of eight unique segments of single-stranded RNA of negative polarity and are subtyped according to their surface proteins, hemagglutinin (HA), and neuraminidase (NA) (Webby et al., 2007). The EIV genome is capable of coding for ten viral proteins, eight being virion associated and two nonstructural proteins (NS1 and NS2). Virion-associated proteins are hemagglutinin (HA), neuraminidase (NA), nucleoprotein (NP), matrix proteins (M1 and M2), and minor proteins PB1, PB2, and PA. The glycoproteins HA and NA, which project as "spikes" from the surface of the envelope, are important for the entry of virus into the host respiratory tract and their release from host cells, respectively (Timoney, 1996; Easterday et al., 1997). Majority of neutralizing antibodies are produced against the HA molecule, which are important targets for antibodies generated in response to infection or vaccination. Accumulation of amino acid changes in the HA result in novel emergent strains by antigenic drift. This can result in new strains that are no longer susceptible to antibodies developed against previous strains.

DISEASE TRANSMISSION

All equidae (horses, donkeys, and mules) are susceptible to EIV. The virus can easily spread from one animal to the other as a result of droplets released into the air by virtue of coughing and also from nasal discharge and fomites (Timoney, 1996; Easterday et al., 1997). The disease is spread between premises and internationally by movement of infected horses. The virus can survive in the environment for up to thirty-six hours so spread by fomites—e.g., people, contaminated equipment, and transport vehicles—are also important. The disease is rapidly spread by close direct contact between horses via the respiratory route. Coughing may project the virus, and under favorable conditions wind can spread the virus. Human beings can also function as carriers for it as well. The incubation period of EIV may be as short as one to three days, and horses can remain infective and shed virus through their nasal secretions for up to ten days (Daly et al., 2004).

Sporadic outbreaks of equine influenza can occur via aerosol or droplet infection. Outbreaks are most likely when horses are congregated together. Equines in barns, with a lot of in-and-out traffic, will have frequent contacts with a large number of horses and are therefore more likely to come in contact with the virus. Contaminated transport vehicles and other equipments can also spread infection as the virus can survive in the environment for thirty-six hours or longer (Daly et al., 2004). The disease is highly contagious, and there is almost 100% infection rate in an unvaccinated or unexposed population. Infected horses excrete the virus in their exhaled air before they show any signs, but recovered horses do not become carriers. Horses of one to five years of age, with no previous exposure to the field or vaccine strains of the virus, will have a lower immune status and are found more susceptible to the disease. The severity of disease depends on the degree of existing immunity. Horses that are partially immune can become subclinically infected and shed virus. Immunity to homologous strain of virus following natural infection persists for approximately one year. Further, the immunity following vaccination with inactivated influenza vaccines can be short-lived, allowing recently vaccinated horses to become infected and shed virus, thereby contributing to maintenance and spread of infection within equine population. Regarding the interspecies jump, the molecular and antigenic analyses of three influenza viruses isolated from outbreaks of severe respiratory disease in racing greyhounds revealed that they are closely related to H3N8 EIV (Crawford et al., 2005). The dogs may have been infected by eating horse meat. Recently, it has been confirmed that there occurs a transmission of influenza virus from horses to canines (Newton et al., 2007). Further, Daly et al. (2008) demonstrated that canine respiratory tissue possesses the relevant receptors for infection with equine influenza virus. Also, when genetically characterized H3N8 influenza viruses were isolated from domestic ducks in northern China, the sequence analysis showed that HA, NA, and M genes of all the isolates had a close relationship with those of Equine/Jilin/1/89 (H3N8) virus, which once caused outbreak in equine populations in northern China (Pu et al., 2009).

CLINICAL MANIFESTATIONS
Equine influenza is a common disease of the horse, causing significant morbidity worldwide. Disease outbreaks are characterized by sudden onset and rapid spread. Clinical signs most commonly noticed are fever, dry, and harsh cough, depression, loss of appetite, weakness, watery eyes, enlarged lymph nodes, edema with stiffness of legs, labored breathing, mucopurulent nasal discharge that becomes yellow with secondary bacterial infection,

and pneumonia (Gerber, 1970; Radostits, 2003; Newton and Mumford, 2005; Cullinane et al., 2006; Landolt et al., 2007). The fever, having body temperature about 103–106°F, may last for two to three days. Equine influenza can cause explosive outbreaks of fever with persistent coughing and nasal discharge, depression, and anorexia in unvaccinated horse populations. Signs in vaccinated horses are less severe. The incubation period is generally one to fifteen days, and horses remain infectious for about eight days. There is no long-term carrier state, but mild or subclinical disease in recently infected horses, which are vaccinated, may escape notice. While morbidity is high, mortality is usually low unless horses are stressed or sick for other reasons. Occasional deaths occur in young foals. Secondary complications like strangles, purpura hemorrhagica, chronic bronchiolitis, and chronic alveolar pulmonary emphysema could be observed. Horses with relatively mild cases of equine influenza usually recover in a week or two, but severely ill and rest-deprived horses may require weeks or months to recover completely. Clinical signs associated with infection in dogs also include fever and a cough; occasionally, infection results in suppurative bronchopneumonia and peracute death. Even though equine influenza appears similar to other viral respiratory diseases—including equine herpesvirus, equine rhinovirus, and equine adenovirus infections—most of these viruses differ in their manifestations by evincing rather mild respiratory signs. Pneumonia in young foals and donkeys and neurological signs like encephalitis in horses have been reported to be rare in equine influenza (Gerber, 1970; Daly et al., 2006).

PATHOGENESIS AND PATHOLOGY

In horses, EIV is a leading cause of respiratory disease. The virus largely infects and damages the ciliated epithelial cells of the upper and lower respiratory tracts, which lead to their decreased ability to clear bacteria and other foreign substances. The HA glycoprotein attaches its spikes to respiratory epithelial cell receptors and enters the cell by endocytosis (Radostits, 2003). The abundance of the Neu5Gc2-3Gal moiety in epithelial cells of horse trachea supports that the recognition of Neu5Gc2-3Gal moiety is critical for the replication of EIV in horses (Suzuki, 2000). Apoptosis may represent a general mechanism of cell death in hosts infected with influenza viruses (Hinshaw et al., 1994). It has been identified that caspase activation and cleavage of its cellular targets play a critical role in virus-mediated cytotoxicity (Lin et al., 2002).

Viral replication occurs, and new viral particles are released into the airway to infect other cells or become aerosolized that augments the rapid spread of the virus. In a couple of days, this invasion causes necrosis and desquamation of respiratory epithelial cells, exudation of protein-rich fluid into airways, clumping of cilia, and impairment of the mucociliary apparatus. Exudate accumulates, and this predisposes to secondary bacterial infections. Proliferation by opportunistic bacteria such as *Streptococcus zooepidemicus* often exacerbates the inflammation to bronchopneumonia (Radostits, 2003). Lesions most commonly observed are bronchiolitis with abundant bilateral serous discharge. During the outbreak in Australia (2007), gross pathological lesions noticed were diffuse or extensive pulmonary consolidation, and histological changes were bronchiolar and alveolar necrosis, neutrophilic infiltration, hyaline membrane formation, hyperplasia, and squamous metaplasia of airway epithelium (Patterson-Kane et al., 2008). Recently, it has been reported that equines possess a preventive defence, consisting of the secretion of a mucous layer at nasal level, which could specifically inactivate the hemagglutinins of equine influenza virus, and in addition, it expresses other sialo receptors, which can mask the influenza-specific ones (Scocco and Pedini, 2008).

DIAGNOSIS

Diagnosis is based on observing the clinical signs in affected horses, virus isolation, antigen and/or genome detection from horses with acute respiratory illness, or on the demonstration of a serological response to infection. Various immunodiagnostic and molecular biology–based techniques have been employed for diagnosing equine influenza (Mumford, 1990; Chambers et al., 1994; Gupta et al., 2003; Cullinane et al., 2006; Landolt et al., 2007; OIE, 2008). Signs like fever and dry hacking cough can be considered as indicative of the disease in horses. Blood picture may show mild to moderate normocytic normochromic anemia, leucopenia, and lymphopenia during earlier stages of the disease. Recovering horses may show monocytosis, neutrophilia if secondary infection is present. Serum enzyme levels of creatine kinase (CK), aspartate transaminase (AST), and lactate dehydrogenase (LDH) may be elevated if myositis occurs (Radostits, 2003). The disease should be differentially diagnosed from other diseases that cause respiratory infection in horses such as equine rhinopneumonitis, equine herpesvirus infections, equine adenoviral infections, equine viral arteritis, travel sickness (pleuropnemonia), and strangles (Radostits, 2003).

Virus isolation can be performed in suitable cell cultures and chicken embryos (Ilobi et al., 1994; OIE, 2008). Nasal swab samples are obtained by passing a swab into the nasopharynx to absorb respiratory secretions. It is important to obtain samples immediately after the onset of clinical signs. The swabs should be transferred to a container with suitable virus-transport medium on ice. If samples are kept for more than two days, they should be frozen at—60°C or below. Traditionally, eggs have been preferred for isolation of equine influenza. Isolation is carried out in embryonated chicken eggs by amniotic cavity route. Cultures of the Madin-Darby canine kidney (MDCK) cell lines are considered best to isolate influenza viruses (Easterday et al., 1997). It is important to obtain samples (nasopharyngeal swabs and nasal or tracheal washings) as soon as possible after the onset of clinical signs, preferably within three to five days. Samples that yield negative results should be repassaged; up to five passages may be necessary to isolate viruses from vaccinated horses. Serological techniques such as enzyme-linked immunosorbent assay (ELISA), hemagglitination inhibition (HI), single radial immunodiffusion (SRID), and single radial hemolysis (SRH) are used to detect the viral antigen in suspected samples (OIE, 2008). In situations where laboratory facilities for virus isolation are unavailable, influenza virus antigen in nasal secretions can be detected directly by an antigen-capture ELISA for the H3N8 virus using a monoclonal antibody (MAb) against the nucleoprotein (Cook et al., 1988; Livesay et al., 1993). Isolates can be characterized by hemagglutination inhibition (HI) using strain-specific antisera. The HA subtype of new isolates of EIVs is best determined by HI test using H7N7—and H3N8-specific antisera. SRID tests can provide a great improvement on the chick cell agglutination test as it is not susceptible to wide test variation and measures immunologically active hemagglutinin (Wood et al., 1983). An acute and convalescent serum sample should be taken two weeks apart for serological detection and analyzed if there is a change in antibody levels in the serum. A four times increase in specific antibody titer means that the horse is infected with influenza virus. Vila-Roza et al. (2000) have developed an indirect ELISA for screening equine influenza in horses. An easy and rapid diagnostic system for equine influenza in the field is strongly required for minimizing the spread of EIV among horses when disease occurs. The use of rapid antigen-detection kits for human influenza has been suggested for the diagnosis of equine influenza too (Chambers et al., 1994; Yamanaka et al., 2008b).

Apart from these, molecular biology tools such as reverse transcriptase–polymerase chain reaction (RT-PCR) and real-time PCR can be used for the rapid diagnosis of the viral genome in suspected samples and studying the molecular epidemiology of the disease (Donofrio et al., 1994; Foord et al., 2008). Typing of neuraminidase requires specific antisera, and no routine technique is available. Typing can be done using specific PCR primers. Detection of the EIV genome by RNA-DNA hybridization has also been reported (Gupta et al., 2003). Nested RT-PCR assay for the rapid diagnosis and characterization of the virus from clinical samples was proved to be useful in ascertaining the infection (Oxburgh and Hagstrom, 1999). Ozaki et al. (2000) reported the diagnosis of the nonstructural protein (NS1) by using a rapid and highly sensitive immuno-PCR technique, which was found to be more sensitive than viral detection by RT-PCR. TaqMan-based real-time PCR assay has been developed for the detection of the virus in samples (Sugita and Matsumura, 2003). Real-time LightCycler RT-PCR technology has been shown to be more sensitive for the detection of positive samples than virus culture in eggs or detection of nucleoprotein using ELISA technology (Quinlivan et al., 2005b). Recently, a one-step RT-PCR assay followed by sequencing has been developed for the detection and subtyping of different neuraminidases from a range of host species and from different geographical locations (Alvarez et al., 2008). Developing a new EI H3–specific TaqMan real-time RT-PCR assay targeting the HA gene of all recent EI H3 strains, Foord et al. (2008) have recently reported the incidence of equine influenza virus (H3N8) for the first time Australian horse population. The EI H3 TaqMan assay was the most sensitive of the assays, able to detect EI from day 1 or 2 postchallenge, as early as virus isolation, and before clinical signs of disease were observed.

PREVENTION AND CONTROL

Vaccination against equine influenza has been practiced since the 1960s, but there are continued problems regarding its efficacy under field conditions (Bryans et al., 1966; Minke et al., 2004; Mathew et al., 2006; Els et al., 2007). Vaccine breakdown has been attributed to inadequate vaccine potency, inappropriate vaccination schedules, and outdated vaccine viruses that have become irrelevant as a result of antigenic drift. Use of a recent strain of EIV in vaccines is often suggested as a measure to control equine influenza outbreaks (Barbic et al., 2009). Also, vaccinated dams give protective immunity to the ponies for the initial period, but by one to two months, it declines, so it is essential to protect the young ones using vaccines developed from strains similar to those circulating in the region (Townsend et al., 1999; Els et al., 2007). Vaccination may not completely prevent influenza, but the disease severity will be lessened in vaccinated horses (Daly et al., 2004; Yamanaka et al., 2008a). The duration of protection provided by current vaccines is limited, and they have less ability to control infection (Nelson et al., 1998), but if booster vaccinations are given, then the disease occurrence and severity can be minimized. Recently, the serological studies conducted, along with the low morbidity rate and the existence of numbers of asymptomatically infected racehorses, suggested that the cross-reactivity of the antibodies provided by vaccination against the epidemic strain contributed to reducing the morbidity rate and duration of epidemic (Yamanaka et al., 2008a).

The vaccination strategies do differ among horses of different classes and age groups. Performance horses are vaccinated regularly with timely boosters as such horses will be exposed to the virus in a constant manner. Breeding horses should be vaccinated in the late stages of pregnancy—i.e., usually within two weeks prior to foaling—and this will ensure that the foal receives sufficient amount of maternal antibodies via colostrum. These maternal antibodies are the first line of defense, and they begin to wane by about one to two months. However, the maternal antibodies can interfere with the vaccination in foals and render commercial vaccines ineffective. So vaccination of foals is commonly done at the age of six months after maternal antibody titers have declined to negligible levels. If the dam is nonimmunized, then the foal should be vaccinated earlier.

Previously, the conventional vaccine against equine influenza was inactivated one with suitable adjuvants. Recently, live vaccine that can be given intranasally to the horses is gaining much popularity. Equine influenza vaccines containing inactivated virus were first developed in the 1960s, and despite their intensive use, equine influenza outbreaks still continue to occur, and therefore new strategies of vaccination are necessary to improve vaccine efficacy (Paillot et al., 2006a). Continued antigenic drift of field virus has compromised the efficacy of vaccines (Wilson, 1993) by which vaccination against H3N8 has been reported to be less effective. Inactivated vaccines for EIV need to be continuously adapted to contain the appropriate serotypes. The most important equine subtypes are H7N7 and H3N8, although H7N7 has not been detected for several decades and is no longer included in vaccines, at least in Europe and the United States (Minke et al., 2004).

Inactivated vaccines have been shown to be efficacious in providing protection against clinical disease and viral shedding. They use multiple strains of EIV A2 representing the major circulating strains. Majority of these vaccines require two-dose priming regimens, although a three-dose priming regimen is recommended and required for at least one of the most effective inactivated vaccines. These vaccines are best suited to vaccinate dams to increase colostral antibody levels against influenza virus. Killed-virus vaccines are commonly administered three to six weeks apart starting at six months of age. Revaccination should be at intervals of three to twelve months depending on age and risk of exposure. Most of the licensed EIV vaccines available are inactivated whole virus of subtypes H7N7 and H3N8 vaccines or subunit vaccines (Park et al., 2003). It has been recommended that modern equine influenza vaccines should contain an A/equi-1 strain and A/equi-2 strains of the American and European-like subtype (Heldens et al., 2004). The formalin-inactivated aluminium hydroxide gel vaccine containing partially purified HA protein can also be used at a dose of 1 ml (Daly et al., 2004). As there are no reports of H7N7 infection in the past twenty years nowadays, it is recommended that vaccines to be used should contain the following virus strains of H3N8 subtype like A/eq/Newmarket/1/93 or A/eq/Kentucky/94 viruses (American lineage) or A/eq/Newmarket/2/93 virus (European lineage) as per OIE (2008). Recently, Damiani et al. (2008) reported that all the most recent outbreaks of equine influenza, occurring between 1999 and 2005, in Italy have been caused by the currently circulating American-like strains, even in vaccinated populations, confirming that vaccines should contain an updated representative strain of this lineage.

Live vaccine includes the modified live, cold-adapted equine influenza A2 vaccine that is administered intranasally (Chambers et al., 2001; Townsend et al., 2001). It is proven to be very safe, phenotypically stable, and able to reduce the frequency, severity, and duration of outbreaks among horse populations. A single administration to naive horses is protective for about twelve months. Local protection at the level of nasal mucosa is enhanced by this vaccine, even though the circulating antibody titers were found to be low. Similarly, the vaccine is protective when administered to foals six months of age or older. The vaccine is not recommended for vaccination of mares in late pregnancy as there is no considerable increase in the circulating antibody responses. Likewise, a canary pox vector vaccine has also been recently used, which could be administered by intramuscular injection (Minke et al., 2007). It has been shown to provide protection of at least six months, and a two-dose priming regimen is recommended, with boosters at a six-month interval. The onset of immunity has been documented at fourteen days after administration of the first dose of vaccine. The vaccine is safe to be used in foals as young as four months of age, and there is some evidence of efficacy in the face of maternal immunity. Because this vaccine generates high levels of antibody response, it is suitable for generating colostral antibodies to protect neonates (Daly et al., 2004).

In horses, natural infection confers long lasting protective immunity characterized by mucosal IgA and humoral IgGa and IgGb responses. However, conventional inactivated or subunit vaccines against EIV induce a short-lived antibody-based immunity to infection. Alternative strategies of vaccination, like the immune-stimulating complex (ISCOM)–based vaccines, have been subsequently developed to mimic the long-term protection induced by natural infection. Crouch et al. (2004) demonstrated that intramuscularly administered ISCOM-based vaccine containing A/eq/Kentucky/98 provides strong protective immunity against challenge with an "American lineage" H3N8 reference virus. Later, Crouch et al. (2005) reported the use of a systemic prime/mucosal boost strategy to induce protective immunity in horses. Their results indicated that the intranasal administration of ISCOM-based vaccine primes the mucosal system for an enhanced IgA response following exposure to live influenza virus. The use of these vaccines induces a strong antibody response and protection against influenza in horses, humans, and a mouse model. Cell-mediated immunity (CMI) has been demonstrated in humans and mice after ISCOM vaccination but rarely investigated in the horse. Evidence of type 1 immunity induced by an ISCOM-based vaccine has been recently described for the first time in horses (Paillot et al., 2007, 2008). The vaccinated ponies were significantly protected as there were no evidence on clinical signs and virus excretion on challenge studies.

The advent of recombinant technology has stimulated the development of second-generation vaccines, including gene-deleted mutants, live vectored vaccines, and DNA vaccines (Minke et al., 2004; OIE, 2008; Dhama et al., 2008). DNA vaccines are a novel alternative to conventional vaccination strategies and offer many of the potential benefits of live-virus vaccines without their risks. DNA vaccination offers a radical alternative to conventional vaccines, with the potential to generate the same protective immune responses seen following viral infection (Lunn et al., 1999). Studies have focused on gene gun delivery of DNA vaccines against equine influenza viruses in mice and ponies, including studies employing coadministration of interleukin-6 DNA as an approach for modulating and adjuvanting influenza virus hemagglutinin-specific immune responses and is an effective method for priming and/or inducing virus-specific immune responses and for providing partial to complete protection from challenge infection in mice, horses, and pigs (Olsen, 2000). Studies conducted on the use of a DNA vaccine, incorporating the HA gene of influenza virus, revealed satisfactory elicitation of both the humoral and cell-mediated immune responses by eliciting IgG antibodies and lymphoproliferative changes with γ-interferon (IFN) mRNA production; however, the vaccine failed to induce IgA response (Soboll et al., 2003). A recombinant vaccine was constructed using the modified vaccinia Ankara vector (MVA) expressing the HA and NP genes. Marked rise in the influenza-virus-specific antibodies was noticed in the serum following the administration of MVA. Both the HA and NP genes incorporated in the vector were able to elicit the γ-IFN mRNA production significantly (Breathnach et al., 2004). During the protective efficacy study of recombinant strains of modified vaccinia Ankara (rMVA) strains in ponies, the advantage of combining rMVA vaccination with a DNA priming dose was identified, contributing as an effective means of inducing protective immunity to influenza virus infection (Breathnach et al., 2006). Another recombinant equine influenza vaccine has been tested and found to be efficacious in ponies that were given intramuscularly in two doses five weeks apart. There was complete suppression of the virus excretion in the study group, which the conventional vaccines were unable to do (Toulemonde et al., 2005).

Improved adjuvants and antigenic presentation systems that extend the duration of immunity induced by inactivated-virus vaccines and live-attenuated or vectored equine influenza vaccines to mimic the immunity generated by influenza infection than the inactivated-virus vaccines are now available (Daly et al., 2004; Minke et al., 2004; Els et al., 2007). The most recent is the cold-adapted influenza virus and poxvirus-based vaccines. There is also considerable progress in the development of a novel vaccination strategy against equine influenza using reverse genetics (Paillot et al., 2006a). Recently, recombinant mutant viruses, impaired in their ability to inhibit IFN production in vitro and not replicating efficiently as the parental recombinant strain, have been developed. These attenuated mutant NS1 viruses encoding carboxy-terminally truncated NS1 proteins, generated utilizing plasmid-based reverse genetics system, may have potential as candidates for a live equine influenza vaccine (Quinlivan et al., 2005b). Paillot et al. (2006b) reported the development of a recombinant vaccine derived from the canary pox virus vector expressing HA genes of EIV (subtype H3N8) and demonstrated the induction of protective antibody and IFN-gamma responses. Their study also provided the evidence for increased IFN-gamma protein synthesis in vaccinated ponies following challenge infection with EIV. A canary pox–vectored recombinant vaccine against EIV H3N8 has also been developed, which was able to efficiently prime foals in the presence of maternally derived immunity (Minke et al., 2007). These newer vaccines are also designed to protect horses against the highly virulent N/5/03 American strain of EIV and to prevent the virus from spreading through the elimination of viral shedding. Live, attenuated virus and canary pox–vectored vaccines have recently become available commercially in some countries.

Similar to preventive measures, infection control entails minimizing exposure to infectious agents or optimizing resistance to infection at the individual or population levels (Traub-Dargatz et al., 2004). The development of equine isolation facilities and improved methods of barn cleaning and use of disinfectant hand wipes are essential to prevent the spread of infectious diseases (Smith, 2004). Due to its rapid transmission, once a horse infected with equine influenza is detected, prompt isolation of the horse from other healthy horses is required. As equine influenza is one of the most economically important contagious respiratory diseases of horses, it should be effectively controlled by sound management principles, including quarantine of new stock (van Maanen and Cullinane, 2002; Daly et al., 2004; Twentyman, 2008; OIE, 2008). Vaccinated horses may continue to shed the virus for up to seven days after exposure, which underlines the importance of quarantine measures. One has to strictly follow quarantining new horses up to six weeks as a precautionary measure. Stress-free environment has to be provided, and good hygienic and sanitary practices have to be followed in barns. During disease outbreaks, additional precautionary measures should be followed in order to minimize the disease spread. The precautions for the control of disease comprises of stoppage of movement of all equines for a period of one month from the infected to healthy farm, premises, state, or region and ban on the holding of equine fairs, horse shows, and race events (Daly et al., 2004). Affected animals should be given complete rest for three weeks along with isolation of sick animals and their attendants. Supportive treatment should be given as per clinical condition of animals. Stalls, equipments, and transport vehicles should be thoroughly cleaned and disinfected. Bad ventilation, excessive dust, and poor supportive care can exacerbate the condition, leading to secondary infections.

TREATMENT

As equine influenza is a viral disease, there are no drugs that can control the infection. But antiviral drugs such as amantadine can be tried (Radostits, 2003). An early initiation of antiviral treatment for horses infected with EI by neuraminidase inhibitor is required to obtain a satisfactory outcome. However, damage to the respiratory tract epithelium means that many horses develop secondary bacterial infections, which can lead to pneumonia and dry hacking cough. Treatment with antibiotics to lessen the impact of secondary infections is recommended when fever persists or when purulent nasal discharges or pulmonary involvement are present. Antibiotic-sensitivity test is recommended while prescribing antibiotics (Radostits, 2003). Good nursing, care, and rest are important parts of treatment. Rest should be complete and for a sufficient time, even after clinical signs have gone, to prevent long-term lung or myocardial damage. Resting the horses will reduce the severity of the clinical signs, reduce the recovery period, and minimize virus shedding.

CONCLUSION

Equine influenza is one among the most common infectious diseases of the respiratory tract of horses. The disease is endemic in most parts of the world, except New Zealand and Iceland. For past three decades, it has caused many casualties in equine population all over the world. Strategies for controlling the spread of this highly contagious disease among continents has been devised that included strong biosecurity and quarantine methods and timely vaccination programs. Despite vaccination, equine influenza still exists in an endemic form in many European countries. It is largely due to the evolution of different strains of the H3N8 virus as a result of antigenic drift.

Intercontinental exchanges of horses have led to the transfer of American strains to other regions of the world, including UK and Scandinavian countries. It is advisable to update the influenza vaccine strains regularly so that they contain similar strains to variants that are circulating in the field. Moreover, improvements should be made to enhance the efficacy of the inactivated-virus vaccines using improved adjuvants and antigenic presentation systems that extends the duration of immunity. Live and attenuated, or vector vaccines that could better mimic the immunity generated by influenza infection should be popularized after the required clinical trials. Similarly, the development in the field of molecular biology has revolutionized the field of immunoprophylaxis, enabling researchers to venture into production of more effective and reliable strategies such as DNA and recombinant vaccines. More stress should be given to the development of new-generation vaccines that are safer and can give adequate protection against this economically important disease affecting continents. Rapid and reliable diagnostic techniques like real-time PCR should be efficiently exploited, especially during disease outbreaks, to detect the equine influenza in field conditions.

REFERENCES

1. Alexander D. J. and Brown I. H. 2000. Recent zoonoses caused by influenza A viruses. *Rev. Sci. Tech. Off. Int. Epiz.* 19:197–225.
2. Alvarez, A. C., Brunck, M. E., Boyd, V., Lai, R., Virtue, E., Chen, W., Bletchly, C., Heine, H. G. and Barnard, R. 2008. A broad spectrum, one-step reverse-transcription PCR amplification of the neuraminidase gene from multiple subtypes of influenza A virus. *Virol. J.* 5:77.
3. Barbic, L., Madic, J., Turk, N. and Daly, J. 2009. Vaccine failure caused an outbreak of equine influenza in Croatia. *Vet. Microbiol.* 133:164–171.
4. Breathnach, C. C., Rudersdorf, R. and Lunn, D. P. 2004. Use of recombinant modified vaccinia Ankara viral vectors for equine influenza vaccination. *Vet. Immunol. Immunopathol.* 98:127–136.
5. Breathnach, C. C., Clark, H. J., Clark, R. C., Olsen, C. W., Townsend, H. G. and Lunn, D. P. 2006. Immunization with recombinant modified vaccinia Ankara (rMVA) constructs encoding the HA or NP gene protects ponies from equine influenza virus challenge. *Vaccine* 24:1180–1190.
6. Bryans, J. T., Doll, E. R., Wilson, J. C., and McCollum, W. H. 1966. Immunization for equine influenza. *J. Am. Vet. Med. Assoc.* 148:413–417.
7. Chambers, T. M. 1992. Cross reactivity of existing influenza vaccine with a new strain of equine influenza virus from China. *Vet. Rec.* 31:388.
8. Chambers, T. M., Shortridge, K. F., Li, P., H., Powell, D. G. and Watkins, K. L. 1994. Rapid diagnosis of equine influenza by the directigen FLU-A enzyme immunoassay. *Vet. Rec.* 135:275–279.
9. Chambers, T. M., Holland, R. E., Tudor, L. R., Townsend, H. G. G., Cook, A., Bogdan, J., Lunn, D. P., Hussey, S., Whitaker-Dowling, P., Youngner, O. S., Sebring, R. W., Penner, S. J. and Stiegler, G. L. 2001. A new modified live equine influenza virus vaccine: Phenotypic stability, restricted spread and efficacy against heterologous virus challenge. *Equine Vet. J.* 33:630–636.
10. Cook, R. F., Sinclair, R. and Mumford, J. A. 1988. Detection of influenza nucleoprotein antigen in nasal secretions from horses infected with A/equine influenza (H3N8) viruses. *J. Virol. Methods* 20:1–12.
11. Crawford, P. C., Dubovi, E. J., Castleman, W. L., Stephenson, I., Gibbs, E. P., Chen, L., Smith, C., Hill, R. C., Ferro, P., Pompey, J., Bright, R. A., Medina, M. J., Johnson, C. M., Olsen, C. W., Cox, N.

J., Klimov, A. I., Katz, J. M. and Donis, R. O. 2005. Transmission of equine influenza virus to dogs. *Science* 310:482–485.

12. Crouch, C. F., Daly, J., Hannant, D., Wilkins, J. and Francis, M. J. 2004. Immune responses and protective efficacy in ponies immunized with and equine influenza ISCOM vaccine containing an "American lineage" H3N8 virus. *Vaccine* 23:418–425.

13. Crouch, C. F., Daly, J., Henley, W., Hannant, D., Wilkins, J. and Francis, M. J. 2005. The use of a systemic prime/mucosal boost strategy with an equine influenza ISCOM vaccine to induce protective immunity in horses. *Vet. Immunol. Immunopathol.* 108:345–355.

14. Cullinane, A. A., Barr, B., Bernard, W., Duncan, J. L., Mulcahy, G., Smith, M. and Timoney, J. E. 2006. Infectious diseases (Chapter 1): Equine influenza. In *The equine manual*, 2nd ed., A. J. Higgins and J. R. Snyder, 13–18. USA: Saunder, Elsevier Ltd.

15. Daly, J. M., Lai, A. C., Binns, M. M., Chambers, T. M., Barrandeguy, M. and Mumford, J. A. 1996. Antigenic and genetic evolution of equine H3N8 influenza A viruses. *J. Gen. Virol.* 77:661–671.

16. Daly, J. M., Newton, J. R. and Mumford, J. A. 2004. Current perspectives on control of equine influenza. *Vet. Res.* 35:411–423.

17. Daly, J. M., Whitwell, K. E., Miller, J., Dowd, G., Cardwell, J. M. and Smith, K. C. 2006. Investigation of equine influenza cases exhibiting neurological disease: Coincidence or association? *J. Comp. Pathol.* 134:231–135.

18. Daly, J. M., Blunden, A. S., Macrae, S., Miller, J., Bowman, S. J., Kolodziejek, J., Nowotny, N. and Smith, K. C. 2008. Transmission of equine influenza virus to English foxhounds. *Emerg. Infect. Dis.* 14:461–464.

19. Damiani, A. M., Scicluna, M. T., Ciabatti, I., Cardeti, G., Sala, M., Vulcano, G., Cordioli, P., Martella, V., Amaddeo, D. and Autorino, G. L. 2008. Genetic characterization of equine influenza viruses isolated in Italy between 1999 and 2005. *Virus Res.* 131:100–105.

20. Dhama, K., Mahendran, M., Gupta, P. K. and Rai, A. 2008. DNA vaccines of veterinary importance: Current perspectives. *Vet. Res. Commun.* 32:341–356.

21. Donofrio, J. C., Coonrod, J. D. and Chambers, T. M. 1994. Diagnosis of equine influenza by the polymerase chain reaction. *J. Vet. Diagn. Invest.* 6:39–43.

22. Easterday, B. C., Hinshaw, V. S. and Halvorson, D. A. 1997. Influenza. In *Diseases of poultry*, 10th ed., B. W. Calnek, H. J. Barnes, C. W. Beard, L. R. McDougald, and Y. M. Saif, 583–605. Mosby-Wolfe.

23. Els, N. T. Walker, M. J., Peters, A., Pastoret, P. P. and Jungersen, G. 2007. Current status of veterinary vaccines. *Clin. Microbiol. Rev.* 20:3489–3510.

24. Foord, A. J., Selleck, P., Colling, A., Klippel, J., Middleton, D. and Heine, H. G. 2008. Real-time RT-PCR for detection of equine influenza and evaluation using samples from horses infected with A/equine/Sydney/2007 (H3N8). *Vet. Microbiol.* 2008 Dec 11 [Epub ahead of print].

25. Gerber, H. 1970. Clinical features, sequelae and epidemiology of equine influenza. In *Proceedings of the 2nd International Conference on Equine Infectious Diseases*, ed. J. T. Bryans, 63–80. Paris (1969) and New York (1970): Karger Basel.

26. Guo, Y., Wang, M. and Kaqaoka, Y. 1992. Characterization of new avian like influenza A virus from horses in China. *Virology* 188:245.

27. Guo, Y., Wang, M., Zheng, G. S., Li, W. K., Kawaoka, Y. and Webster, R. G. 1995. Sero-epidemiological and molecular evidence for the presence of two H3N8 equine influenza viruses in China in 1993–94. *J. Gen. Virol.* 76:2009–2014.

28. Gupta, A. K., Anita, A. and Vandanajay, B. 2003. Detection of equine influenza viral genome by RT-PCR and RNA-DNA hybridization. *Indian J. Biotech.* 2:214–219.

29. Guthrie, A. J., Stevens, K. B. and Bosman, P. P. 1999. The circumstances surrounding the outbreak and spread of equine influenza in South Africa. *Rev. Sci. Tech.* 8:179–185.

30. Heldens, J. G., Pouwels, H. G. and van Loon, A. A. 2004. Efficacy and duration of immunity of a combined equine influenza and equine herpesvirus vaccine against challenge with an American-like equine influenza virus (A/equi-2/Kentucky/95). *Vet. J.* 167:150–157.

31. Hinshaw, V. S., Olsen, C. W., Dybdahl-Sissoko, N. and Evans, D. 1994. Apoptosis: A mechanism of cell killing by influenza A and B viruses. *J. Virol.* 68:3667–3673.

32. Holland, R. E. 2003. Equine influenza. Art. no. 4584. www.thehorse.com.

33. Ilobi, C. P., Henfrey, R., Robertson, J. S., Mumford, J. A., Erasmus, B. J. and Wood, J. M. 1994. Antigenic and molecular characterisation of host-cell mediated variants of equine H3N8 influenza viruses. *J. Gen. Virol.* 75:669–673.

34. Ito, M., Nagai, M., Hayakawa, Y., Komae, H., Murakami, N., Yotsuya, S., Asakura, S., Sakoda, Y. and Kida, H. 2008. Genetic analyses of an H3N8 influenza virus isolate, causative strain of the outbreak of equine influenza at the Kanazawa Racecourse in Japan in 2007. *J. Vet. Med. Sci.* 70:899–906.

35. Lai, A. C., Chambers, T. M., Holland, R. E. Jr., Morley, P. S., Haines, D. M., Townsend, H. G. and Barrandeguy, M. 2001. Diverged evolution of recent equine-2 influenza (H3N8) viruses in the Western Hemisphere. *Arch. Virol.* 146:1063–1074.

36. Landolt, G. A., Townsend, H. G. G. and Lunn, D. P. 2007. Equine influenza infection. In *Equine infectious diseases*, ed. D. C. Sellon and M. T. Long, chapter 12, 124–134. Philadelphia, USA: Saunders, Elsevier Inc.

37. Lin, C., Holland, R. E. Jr., Donofrio, J. C., McCoy, M. H., Tudor, L. R. and Chambers, T. M. 2002. Caspase activation in equine influenza virus induced apoptotic cell death. *Vet. Microbiol.* 84:357–365.

38. Livesay, G. J., O'Neill, T., Hannant, D., Yadav, M. P. and Mumford, J. A. 1993. The outbreak of equine influenza (H3N8) in the United Kingdom in 1989: Diagnostic use of an antigen capture ELISA. *Vet. Rec.* 133:515–519.

39. Lunn, D. P., Soboll, G., Schram, B. R., Quass, J., McGregor, M. W., Drape, R. J., Macklin, M. D., McCabe, D. E., Swain, W. F. and Olsen, C. W. 1999. Antibody responses to DNA vaccination of horses using the influenza virus hemagglutinin gene. *Vaccine* 17:2245–2258.

40. Mathew, T., Mahendran, M. and Dhama, K. 2006. Equine influenza (Chapter VII). In *Influenza and its public health significance*, ed. M. Tripthi and T. Mathew, 112–129. USA: Thajema Publishers.

41. Minke, J. M., Audonnet, J. C. and Fischer, L. 2004. Equine viral vaccines: The past, present and future. *Vet. Res.* 35:425–443.

42. Minke, J. M., Toulemonde, C. E., Dinic, S., Cozette, V., Cullinane, A. and Audonnet, J. C. 2007. Effective priming of foals born to immune dams against influenza by a canarypox-vectored recombinant influenza H3N8 vaccine. *J. Comp. Pathol.* 137:76–80.

43. Morley, P. S., Townsend, H. G. G., Bogdan, J. R. and Haines, D. M. 2000. Descriptive epidemiologic study of disease associated with influenza virus infections during three epidemics in horses. *J. Am. Vet. Med. Assoc.* 216:535–544.

44. Mumford, J. A. 1990. The diagnosis and control of equine influenza. *Proc. Am. Assoc. Equine Pract.* 36:377.

45. Mumford, J. A. and Wood, J. 1993. Conference report on WHO/OIE meeting: Consultation on newly emerging strains of equine influenza. *Vaccine* 11:1172–1175.

46. Mumford, E. L., Traub-Dargatz, J. L., Salman, M. D., Collins, J. K., Getzy, D. M. and Carman, J. 1998. Monitoring and detection of acute viral respiratory tract disease in horses. *J. Am. Vet. Med. Assoc.* 213:385–390.

47. Nelson, K. M., Schram, B. R. and McGregor, M. W. 1998. Local and systemic isotype-specific antibody responses to equine influenza virus infection versus conventional vaaccination. *Vaccine* 16:1306–1313.

48. Newton, J. R., Townsend, H. G., Wood, J. L., Sinclair, R., Hannant, D. and Mumford, J. A. 2000. Immunity to equine influenza: Relationship of vaccine-induced antibody in young Thoroughbred racehorses to protection against field infection with influenza A/equine-2 viruses (H3N8). *Equine Vet. J.* 32:65–74.

49. Newton, J. R. and Mumford, J. A. 2005. Equine influenza. In *Infectious diseases of livestock*, vol. 1, ed. J. A. W. Coetzer and R. C. Tustin, 766–774. Oxford: Oxford University Press.

50. Newton, R., Cooke, A., Elton, D., Bryant, N., Rash, A., Bowman, S., Blunden, T., Miller, J., Hammond, T. A., Camm, I. and Day, M. 2007. Canine influenza virus: Cross-species transmission from horses. *Vet. Rec.* 161:142–143.

51. OIE. 2008. Equine influenza. *Manual of diagnostic tests and vaccines for terrestrial animals*, chapter 2.5.7, 871–883, www.oie.int.

52. Olsen, C. W. 2000. DNA vaccination against influenza viruses: A review with emphasis on equine and swine influenza. *Vet. Microbiol.* 74:149–164.

53. Oxburgh, L. and Hagstrom, A. 1999. A PCR based method for the identification of equine influenza virus from clinical samples. *Vet. Microbiol.* 67:161–174.

54. Oxburgh, L. and Klingeborn, B. 1999. Cocirculation of two distinct lineages of equine influenza virus subtype H3N8. *J. Clin. Microbiol.* 37:3005–3009.

55. Ozaki, H., Sugita, S. and Kida, H. 2000. A rapid and sensitive method for diagnosis of equine influenza by antigen detection using immuno-PCR. *Jap. J. Vet. Res.* 48:187–195.

56. Paillot, R., Hannant, D., Kydd, J. H. and Daly, J. M. 2006a. Vaccination against equine influenza: *Vaccine* 24:4047–4061.

57. Paillot, R., Kydd, J. H., Sindle, T., Hannant, D., Edlund Toulemonde, C., Audonnet, J. C., Minke, J. M. and Daly, J. M. 2006b. Antibody and IFN-gamma responses induced by a recombinant canarypox vaccine and challenge infection with equine influenza virus. *Vet. Immunol. Immunopathol.* 112:225–233.

58. Paillot, R., Kydd, J. H., MacRae, S., Minke, J. M., Hannant, D. and Daly, J. M. 2007. New assays to measure equine influenza virus-specific type 1 immunity in horses. *Vaccine* 25:7385–7398.

59. Paillot, R., Grimmett, H., Elton, D. and Daly, J. M. 2008. Protection, systemic IFN gamma, and antibody responses induced by an ISCOM-based vaccine against a recent equine influenza virus in its natural host. *Vet. Res.* 39:21.

60. Park, A. W., Wood, J. L. N., Newton, J. R., Daly, J., Mumford, J. A. and Grenfell, B. T. 2003. Optimizing vaccination strategies in equine influenza. *Vaccine* 21:2862–2870.

61. Patterson-Kane, J. C., Carrick, J. B., Axon, J. E., Wilkie, I. and Begg, A. P. 2008. The pathology of bronchointerstitial pneumonia in young foals associated with the first outbreak of equine influenza in Australia. *Equine Vet. J.* 40:199–203.

62. Pu, J., Liu, Q. F., Xia, Y. J., Fan, Y. L., Brown, E. G., Tian, F. L. and Liu, J. H. 2009. Genetic analysis of H3 subtype influenza viruses isolated from domestic ducks in northern China during 2004–2005. *Virus Genes* 38:136–142.

63. Purzycka, M., Rozek, W. and Zmudzinski, J. F. 2004. Global distribution of equine influenza. *Med. Weter.* 60:675–679.

64. Quinlivan M., Dempsey E., Ryan F., Arkins, S. and Cullinane A. 2005a. Real-time reverse transcription PCR for detection and quantitative analysis of equine influenza virus. *J. Clin. Microbiol.* 43:5055–5057.

65. Quinlivan, M., Zamarin, D., Garcia-Sastre, A., Cullinane, A., Chambers, T. and Palese P. 2005b. Attenuation of equine influenza viruses through truncations of the NS1 protein. *J. Virol.* 79:8431–8439.

66. Radostits, O. M., Gay, C. C., Blood, D. C. and Hinchcliff, K. W. 2003. Equine influenza. In *Veterinary medicine: A textbook of diseases of cattle, sheep, pigs, goats and horses*, 9th ed., 1144–1147. ELBS.

67. Reeve-Johnson, L. 2007. Equine influenza in Australia. *Vet. Rec.* 161:635.

68. Scocco, P. and Pedini, V. 2008. Localization of influenza virus sialoreceptors in equine respiratory tract. *Histol. Histopathol.* 23:973–978.

69. Smith, B. P. 2004. Evolution of equine infection control programs. *Vet. Clin. North Am. Equine Pract.* 20:521–530.

70. Smyth, B. 2007. Equine influenza: An update. *Aust. Vet. J.* 85:14-16.

71. Soboll, G., Horohov, D. W., Aldridge, B. M., Olsen, C. W., McGregor, M. W., Drape, R. J., Macklin, M. D., Swain, W. F. and Lunn, D. P. 2003. Regional antibody and cellular immune responses to equine influenza virus infection, and particle mediated DNA vaccination. *Vet. Immunol. Immunopathol.* 94:47–62.

72. Sovinova, O., Tumova, B., Pouska, F. and Nemec, J. 1958. Isolation of a virus causing respiratory disease in horses. *Acta Virol.* 2:51–61.

73. Sugita, S. and Matsumura, T. 2003. Detection of equine-2 influenza virus by real-time PCR. *J. Equine Sci.* 14:111–117.

74. Suzuki, Y. 2000. Receptor sialylsugar chains as determinants of host range of influenza viruses. *Nippon Rinsho.* 58:2206–2210.

75. Timoney, P. J. 1996. Equine influenza. *Comp. Immunol. Microbiol. Infect. Dis.* 19:205–211.

76. Toulemonde, C. E., Daly, J., Sindle, T., Guigal, P. M., Audonnet, J. C. and Minke, J. M. 2005. Efficacy of a recombinant equine influenza vaccine against challenge with and American lineage H3N8 virus responsible for the 2003 outbreak in United Kingdom. *Vet. Rec.* 156:367–371.

77. Townsend, H. G. G., Cook, A. and Watts, T. C. 1999. Efficacy of a cold-adapted, modified-live virus influenza vaccine: A double-blind challenge trial. *Pro. Am. Assoc. Equine Pract.* 45:41–42.

78. Townsend, H. G. G., Penner, S. J., Watts, T. C., Cook, A., Bogdan, J., Haines, D. M., Griffin, S., Chambers, T., Holland, R. E., Whitaker-Dowling, P., Youngner, J. S. and Sebring, R. W. 2001. Efficacy of a cold-adapted, intranasal, equine influenza vaccine-challenge trials. *Equine Vet. J.* 33:637–643.

79. Traub-Dargatz, J. L., Dargatz, D. A., Morley, P. S. and Dunowska M. 2004. An overview of infection control strategies for equine facilities, with an emphasis on veterinary hospitals. *Vet. Clin. North Am. Equine Pract.* 20:507–520.

80. Twentyman, B. 2008. Equine influenza: A team effort. *Aust. Vet. J.* 86: N4.

81. Uppal, P. K. and Yadav, M. P. 1987. Outbreak of equine influenza in India. *Vet. Rec.* 121:569–570.

82. Uppal, P. K., Yadav, M. P. and Sharma, S. N. 1987. Occurrence of equine influenza outbreaks in India. *Indian J. Comp. Microbiol. Immunol. Infect. Dis.* 8:91–94.

83. Uppal, P. K., Yadav, M. P. and Oberoi, M. S. 1989. Isolation of A/Equi-2 virus during 1987 equine influenza epidemic in India. *Equine Vet. J.* 21:364–366.

84. van Maanen, C. and Cullinane, A. 2002. Equine influenza virus infections: An update. *Vet. Q.* 24:79–94.

85. Vila-Roza, M. V., Galosi, C. M., Olivia, G. A., Echeverria, M. G., Pecoraro, M. R., Corva, S. and Etcheverrigaray, M. E. 2000. Indirect ELISA for rapid diagnosis of equine influenza. *Rev. Arg. Microbiol.* 32:39–43.

86. Virmani, N., Singh, B. K., Gulati, B. R. and Kumar, S. 2008. Equine influenza outbreak in India. *Vet. Rec.* 163:607–608.

87. Webby, R. J., Webster, R. G. and Richt, J. A. 2007. Influenza viruses in animal wildlife populations. *Curr. Top. Microbiol. Immunol.* 315:67–83.

88. Webster, R. G. 1993. Are equine 1 influenza viruses still present in horses? *Equine Vet. J.* 25:537–538.

89. Wilson, W. D. 1993. Equine influenza. *Vet. Clin. North Am. Equine Pract.* 9:257–282.

90. Waddell, G. H., Teigland, M. B. and Sigel, M. M. 1963. A new influenza virus associated with equine respiratory disease. *J. Am. Vet. Med. Assoc.* 143:587–590.

91. Wood, J. and Mumford, J. 1992. Epidemiology of equine influenza. *Vet. Rec.* 130:126.

92. Wood, J. M., Schild, G. C., Folkers, C., Mumford, J. and Newman, R. W. 1983. The standardisation of inactivated equine influenza vaccines by single-radial immunodiffusion. *J. Biol. Standard.* 11:133–136.

93. Yamanaka, T., Niwa, H., Tsujimura, K., Kondo, T. and Matsumura, T. 2008a. Epidemic of equine influenza among vaccinated racehorses in Japan in 2007. *J. Vet. Med. Sci.* 70:623–625.

94. Yamanaka, T., Tsujimura, K., Kondo, T. and Matsumura, T. 2008b. Evaluation of antigen detection kits for diagnosis of equine influenza. *J. Vet. Med. Sci.* 70:189–192.

8. Equine Infectious Anemia

K. Dhama, R. V. S. Pawaiya, P. Bhatt, and S. Kapoor

Introduction

Equine infectious anemia (EIA) is a contagious viral disease affecting horses and other equids (ponies, donkeys, mules, and zebras) worldwide, caused by the equine infectious anemia virus (EIAV) of *Lentivirus* (Lignee, 1843; Coggins and Auchnie, 1977; Uppal and Yadav, 1989; Sellon, 1993; Leroux et al., 2004; Cullinane et al., 2006; Mealey, 2007; Brangan et al., 2008). Affected animals remain viremic and often suffer irregularly recurring disease episodes and develop into lifelong carriers of the virus. Disease occurs as an acute, subacute, or chronic illness and may terminate in death. Immune mechanisms play important role in the development of clinical disease. EIA was first described in France by Lignee (1843). It is also known as swamp fever as disease spreads most actively in summer and in warm, wet, marshy areas where hematophagous insects that transmit the virus are abundant. Once infected, a horse remains as a carrier even though it may not show any signs of illness, and its blood is infectious for susceptible horses throughout its life time (Stein et al., 1955) Its ability to evade host's immune defenses by lying dormant in apparently healthy animals and by rapidly changing its antigenic determinants is a major obstacle to vaccine development. The EIAV does not possess any public health implications as it only infects Equidae.

Etiology

The causative agent equine infectious anemia virus (EIAV) belongs to genus *Lentivirus*, family Retroviridae that also includes the human immunodeficiency virus (HIV) or AIDS virus (Leroux et al., 2004; Cullinane et al., 2006; Mealey, 2007). EIAV has a ribonucleic acid (RNA) genome of 8 kb in length and includes three principal genes (gag, pol, env) and three regulatory genes. EIAV encodes four regulatory/accessory genes (tat, rev, ttm, and S2) and is the least genetically complex of all known lentiviruses. It contains two envelope glycoproteins, gp90 and gp45, and four internal proteins, p26, p15, p11 and p9. EIA virus binds to specific receptor like the equine lentivirus receptor-1 on the target host cell surface via gp90 glycoprotein (Zhang et al., 2005). EIAV receptor-mediated productive entry into target cells is low-pH-dependent, and the virus entry occurs through clathrin-mediated endocytosis (Jin et al., 2005; Brindley and Maury, 2008). The virus envelope fuses with host cell membrane, virion gets internalized, uncoating occurs, and viral replication begins. Double-stranded DNA copy of genomic RNA is translocated to the nucleus and inserted into the host cell genome as provirus, which is a principal mechanism of EIA virus persistence within the host. Virus is released by budding from the host cell.

Persistent replication of the virus within the host leads to the periodic emergence of novel antigenic strains of EIAV. EIAV envelope variation produces newly dominant quasi-species with each sequential disease cycle; new populations arise in response to ongoing immune pressures, and previous plasma quasi-species, including the original inoculum, become undetectable (McGuire et al., 1987; Leroux et al., 1997, 2001; Craigo et al., 2006). A number of antigenically different, serologically identifiable serotypes of EIAV, with marked difference in virulence among them, have been identified. Integration as provirus, antigenic variation, and immune escape are the major contributing factors to EIAV persistence. Recently, during an outbreak of EIA in Ireland, comparison of the gag gene of EIAV(Ire) strain with North American and Asian strains of the virus showed that the gag gene is less well conserved than previously believed, and that EIAV strains can have similar phenotypes despite considerable variations in genotype (Quinlivan et al., 2007).

The EIA virus is not infectious for the common laboratory animals. The virus has been used to produce the disease experimentally in horses and possibly in pigs and sheep, but the disease occurs naturally only in Equidae. EIA can be transmitted through blood, saliva, milk, and body secretions. All lentiviruses cause slowly progressive disease that frequently results in death. On the contrary, EIAV infection results in acute phase followed by recurrent clinical disease episodes that eventually subside in most horses. These horses become persistently infected and remain inapparent carriers for whole life (Coggins, 1984; Cullinane et al., 2006; Mealey, 2007). The virus can be cultivated/propagated in horse cell cultures, viz, equine leukocytes and tissue culture (equine fibroblasts, kidney cells). The virus is stable in refrigerated serum but is inactivated at 56°C and is readily destroyed by sunlight, boiling, and by most chemical disinfectants, detergents, and organic solvents such as ether. The severity of the disease caused by the EIAV depends on the dose of the virus, susceptibility of the horse, and the virulence of the virus strain (Kemeny et al. 1971). Kono (1973) reported after conducting challenge studies and neutralization studies in horses and in tissue culture that there is immunological difference in EIA virus isolates.

EPIDEMIOLOGY

Equine infectious anemia (EIA) occurs in horse populations worldwide. EIA infection was first recorded in France in 1843 by Lignee, then reported by Dreguss and Lombard, 1954. Afterward, it has been reported in horses, mules, and donkeys in Asia, Africa, North and South America, Australia, and occasionally in many European countries, including the UK, France, and Italy (Lignee, 1843; Coggins and Auchnie, 1977; Lepherd, 1978; Thomas and Elder, 1978; Bamigboye and da Silva, 1981; Uppal and Yadav, 1989; Loftin et al., 1990; Montelaro et al., 1993; Leroux et al., 2004; Cullinane et al., 2006; Mealey, 2007). Nusbaum (1975), in his serological survey in New York State, reported that greater than 75% of positive horses had no observable signs of illness. Recently, Bicout et al. (2006) reported the distribution of EIA in horses in Brazil; and also an outbreak of EIA occurred in Ireland in 2006 (Cullinane et al., 2007; Quinlivan et al., 2007; Brangan et al., 2008). Because disease is often transmitted by insect vectors, the prevalence is higher in regions with warm climates. The morbidity rate in EIA can be 100% in a group of horses with mortality as high as 30%.

A reliable serological test, agar gel precipitation (immunodiffusion), for EIA was developed in the early 1970s (Coggins and Norcross, 1970; Coggins et al., 1972), which became the basis for the EIA control program implemented by the U.S. Department of Agriculture (USDA) in 1972. Consequently, the prevalence of EIA in the USA has declined from 3.09% in 1972 to 0.01% in 2003 and in Gulf Coast region from 11.08–0.03%. Since testing were being done on high-quality horses competing in events, entering exhibitions, moving interstate, during import/export, and marketing, which all require negative results, the majority of horses like in the USA are therefore not tested; hence, the true EIA prevalence is unknown. Although statistics of prevalence of the disease are unreliable because of failure to diagnose and report the disease, it is of major importance and appears to be increasing in incidence (Radostits et al., 2000). Large-scale movements of horses during wartime have been responsible for extensive dissemination of the disease. It is suggested that the rapid expansion of "pleasure horse" activity in affluent countries causes greater movement and hence opportunities for spread of the infection from relatively few donors (Coggins, 1984).

Horses, ponies, mules, and donkeys are the only known natural hosts of EIA virus. Diseased horses, once infected, carry the virus for life regardless of the severity of symptoms, and also serums of some inapparent carriers of EIA are infectious; thus, all horses positive for EIA are potential spreaders of EIAV infection. The predominant means of natural transmission is via blood-feeding insects as blood of an infected horse is the most important source of EIAV transmission to other susceptible horses. Insects serve only as mechanical vectors, and the virus is carried on their mouthparts. The most important insect vectors for natural transmission are horseflies (*Tebanus* spp.)

and deerflies (*Chryosomyia* spp.), both of which are members of Tabanidae family. Stable flies (*Stomoxys calcitrans*) have also been reported to transmit the virus but less efficiently (Foil et al., 1983; Issel and Foil, 1984). There are several factors involved that could prove crucial in the transmission of the virus—viz, compared to inapparent carriers with very low levels of virus in the blood, horses with a high titer viremia, or pyrexic—and clinical disease are much more likely to transmit EIAV; the population of vectors and their feeding behavior; and the distance between infected and susceptible horses (Radostitis et al., 2000; Cullinane et al., 2006; Mealey, 2007). There is evidence that foals have become infected in utero and from nursing have infected dams after ingestion of virus-contaminated colostrum or milk. When the mare develops acute clinical disease and high titer viremia during gestation, transplacental transmission can occur; however, this mode of transmission appears to be a rare event. Veneral transmission is also feasible. Contaminated or unsterile needles, stomach tubes, and other surgical equipments that may cause abrasion can also transmit the EIAV mechanically. Foals born to infected dams may carry a maternal antibody titer for two to six months after birth.

CLINICAL PICTURE

EIA manifests acute, subclinical, or chronic course. The incubation period varies from a few days to more than three months. The clinical course of EIA is variable, and the form it takes is influenced by the dose and virulence of the virus strain, the susceptibility of the horse, presence or absence of antibody in the donor horse, and the physical stress the animal is under at the time. Compared to horses, clinical disease may be less severe in donkeys and mules (Montelaro et al., 1993; Cook et al., 2001). The initial illness is commonly acute or subacute with definite clinical signs, and lasts from 3 to twenty days followed by cycles of febrile periods and death or apparent recovery. The introduction of the virus into a susceptible herd is usually associated with the acute form. However, the emergence of a newantigenic variant can give rise to acute clinical signs in a carrier.

In acute form, pronounced viremia can develop characterized by a sudden onset of a high fever (104–108°F), thrombocytopenia, severe depression, lethargy, depressed appetite, and a rapid loss in physical condition. The initial feverish episode usually subsides within a few days; however, few horses can build up a severe and lethal form of the disease characterized by persistent viremia, severe anemia, hemorrhagic diarrhea, and elevated viral loads in many organs (Crawford et al., 1978). A profound weakness may result in incoordination, recumbency, or prostration. Jaundice and edema of the dependent parts like the ventral abdomen, sheath, and limbs may develop, with or without petechial hemorrhages of the mucous membranes at the base of the tongue and on the conjunctivae. The heart rate and intensity of heart sounds are greatly increased, especially with moderate exercise. A yellowish or bloody nasal discharge may be present. An enlarged spleen may be palpated on rectal examination. Anemia is characterized by a low hematocrit, low hemoglobin value, low red blood cell count, and a high sedimentation rate. However, immature red cells are usually not observed; the white blood cell picture may show a leucopenia or may be normal. Death is usually related to the severity of the anemia and may also be associated with intravascular clotting of blood and thrombus formation. The acute form of the disease may develop at the initial attack or at any subsequent attack of a virulent strain of EIAV and often terminates in the death of the horse within three to fourteen days (Cullinane et al., 2006; Mealey, 2007).

After the initial disease episode, the majority of horses experience recurrent episodes of acute clinical disease, but a few horses may develop an inapparent infection. An antigenically distinct virus isolate is associated with each episode, defined by neutralizing antibody. In subacute form of EIA, the signs are similar to the acute form but not as severe, and death seldom occurs. Most horses with this form of the disease appear to recover after seven to twenty days and remain free of symptoms for weeks or months, after which another subacute episode may occur. The relapses often develop during periods of stress and result in weakness if repeated at frequent intervals, loss of weight, marked unthriftiness, and anemia. With the drop in viral load, clinical signs, including thrombocytopenia, resolve rapidly as each episode ends; between the episodes, the infected horses appear normal.

Chronic form of the disease produces progressive anemia, loss of condition, weakness, and tachycardia after exercise; the affected horse suffers recurrent episodes of fever, anemia, weight loss, and edema that may last only a few days or persist for weeks. Recurrences are often aggravated by stress factors—viz, malnutrition, overloaded work, or surgery—and the majority occur within the first three months after initial infection. If clinical disease episodes become frequent and severe, the horse develops the classical signs of chronic disease (a "swamper"). Horses develop anemia, thrombocytopenia, weight loss, and dependent edema. Pale mucus membranes, petechiation, icterus, and epistaxis linked with more severe hemolytic anemia and thrombocytopenia can also be exhibited. Occasionally, neurologic signs develop and can include ataxia and encephalitis (McClure et al., 1982; Oaks et al., 2004). The severity as well as frequency of clinical episodes usually decreases with time factor, and for the majority of infected horses, clinical disease episodes subside within a year of initial infection, and these horses become inapparent carriers of the EIAV. Inapparent carriers are infected for life, though these horses have very low plasma viral loads and appear clinically normal. Although the risk of EIAV transmission from such carriers is low, they serve as virus reservoirs and can transmit it under field situation. Environmental stress could provoke a clinical episode in these carriers.

PATHOLOGICAL FINDINGS AND PATHOGENESIS

In the acute stages, necropsy findings in horses can include gross lesions of splenomegaly, hepatomegaly, generalized lymphadenopathy, ventral subcutaneous edema, anemia, jaundice, emaciation, vessel thrombosis, petechial or ecchymotic subserous hemorrhages, mucosal and visceral hemorrhages (Sellon et al., 1994; Cullinane et al., 2006; Mealey, 2007). The most characteristic microscopic lesions are interstitial mononuclear cell infiltrations in the liver, kidney, and spleen. Nonsuppurative hepatitis with infiltrates of macrophages and lymphocytes, primarily in the periportal areas, are the characteristic tissue lesions (McGuire et al., 1990). The Kupffer cells become enlarged and laden with hemosiderin. Glomerulonephritis, characterized by thickened basement membranes with inflammatory cell infiltrates, is associated with immune-complex deposition. In neurologic disease, lesions include lymphohistiocytic periventricular leukoencephalitis, nonsuppurative granulomatous ependymitis, encephalitis, meningitis, and plasmocytic-lymphocytic infiltration of the brain and spinal cord (McClure et al., 1982; Oaks et al., 2004). Necropsy results are usually normal in inapparent carriers, and if present, then the tissue lesions are usually mild or absent (Montelaro et al., 1993; Sellon et al., 1994). In the chronic stages, emaciation and pallor of tissues are the only gross findings. Virus is present in greatest concentration in the spleen, liver, bone marrow, and abdominal lymph nodes.

The virus appears to have a predilection for macrophages and monocytes that present a means of transportation and dissemination to a variety of vital organs, including the liver, kidney, adrenal, brain, and heart. The anemia results from hemolysis of erythrocytes and from impairment of bone marrow functions. EIAV infects macrophages, with viral replication primarily occurring in mature tissue macrophages and most infected macrophages detected in the spleen. In EIA, immune mechanisms involving destruction of macrophages and formation of immune complexes are implicated in the development of clinical disease and the lesions (Cheevers and McGuire, 1985; McGuire et al., 1972, 1990; Oaks et al., 1998, 1999; Sellon et al., 1992, 1994; Harrold et al., 2000). The induction and elevation of macrophage proinflammatory cyokines like TNF- , interleukin-1 (IL-1) and IL-6 are upregulated by virulent EIAV, which most likely contributes to the fever, lethargy, and inappetance during acute EIA cases (Costa et al., 1997; Tornquist et al., 1997; Sellon et al., 1999; Lim et al., 2005). Predominant mechanism of EIAV-induced thrombocytopenia includes impairment of platelet production; platelets become activated and hypofunctional, which may result in platelet aggregation that are removed from the circulation; and immune-complex deposition and subsequent degradation by mononuclear phagocytes (Oaks et al., 1999; Russell et al., 1999; Clabough et al. 1991; Sellon et al., 1994). A nonimmune-mediated mechanism may be involved during EIAV-associated platelet destruction and/or thrombocytopenia. Elevation of TNF and TGF has been described in horses during EIAV infection in days preceding the onset of thrombocytopenia.

Pathogenesis of anemia is also multifactorial, including immune-mediated erythrocyte destruction/hemolysis and suppression of erythropoiesis (Cheevers and McGuire, 1985; McGuire et al., 1969, 1990). Anemia due to the hemolysis is exacerbated by depression of bone marrow activity and erythropoiesis. TNF suppresses erythropoiesis in vitro and may participate in the observed hemolytic anemia in EIAV-infected animals (Sentsui and Kono, 1987; Dufour et al., 2003). Damage to the vascular endothelium is followed by inflammatory changes in the parenchymatous organs, particularly the liver. Similar changes occur in nervous tissue and result in the ataxia and spinal leptomeningitis and encephalomyelitis, which are characteristic of the disease (McClure et al., 1982). Glomerulonephritis in acute EIA results from the deposition of circulating viral antigen and antibody immune complexes in the kidney, which may also be responsible for damage to the reticuloendothelial system leading to hemorrhage and edema. The hepatitis and lymphadenopathy probably have the same basis. Cytoplasmic inclusions in EIAV infection of cells (equine dermal, ED) have been reported (Weiland and Matheka, 1984). Differential effects of virulent and avirulent EIAV on macrophage cytokine expression show a direct correlation between cytokine dysregulation and EIAV pathogenesis (Lim et al., 2005).

The severity of disease correlates with virus load, and the frequency and duration of febrile episodes correlates with the severity of anemia. The virus disappears from tissues during periods between attacks. During subclinical infection of EIAV, tissue macrophages are the primary cellular reservoir for the virus, and replication occurs in a restricted way (Oaks et al., 1998). Termination of viremia is the result of specific immune responses. Recurrences of viremia are associated with antigenic variation of neutralization-sensitive epitopes (E:/sites/entrez). Factors other than the host's cell permissiveness mediate the clinical differences observed between horses and donkeys infected with EIAV (Cook et al., 2001).

DIAGNOSIS

The clinical diagnosis of EIA presents many difficulties no matter what form of the disease is present. EIA should be ruled out in horses showing clinical signs, including recurrent fever, thrombocytopenia, anemia, petechiation, weight loss, or ventral edema. However, many infected horses show no clinical symptoms and have no history of clinical signs. A history of illness following shipping, advance training, foaling, surgery, or other recent stress often provides a clue. Abnormalities in the blood count and serum biochemistry can include monocytosis, leukopenia or leukocytosis, hyperbilirubinemia, hemoglobinemia, hypergammaglobulinemia, and elevation of liver enzyme levels; but these findings are reported to be inconsistent of EIA (Mealey, 2007). A marked drop in blood platelet count is the first detectable abnormality of the blood. In the acute form, the packed cell volume (PCV) is low (14–20%), there is a leucopenia (down to 2000/µl) with a marked neutropenia and a lymphopenia. The anemia is normocytic and normochromic. The affected horse rarely releases immature erythrocytes to the circulation in response to severe hemolytic or blood-loss anemia. Hematological tests such as a platelet count, a differential white blood cell count, the determination of PCV value, and a sideroleukocyte count may be helpful indicators in EIA diagnosis but are not pathognomonic. A single hematological examination is of less value in diagnosis than serial tests matched with a temperature curve because the blood picture gradually returns to near normal between attacks.

The only available in vitro assay for field strains of the virus is a cumbersome leukocyte culture system, and the horse is the only experimental animal available so that the level of infectivity of animals is very difficult to measure. Currently, four approved serologic tests include the agar gel immunodiffusion (AGID) test, the competitive enzyme-linked immunosorbent assay (cELISA), the Vira-CHEK ELISA, and the synthetic antigen ELISA (SA-ELISA II) (Shane et al. 1984; Thomas et al., 1992; Issel and Cook, 1993; Lew et al., 1993; Cullinane et al., 2006; Mealey, 2007). The virus can be isolated in equine macrophages or equine dermal cells or detected by polymerase chain reaction (PCR), but the Coggins test, an agar gel immunoprecipitation test has, since its development in 1970, formed the basis of most control programs for EIA (Langemeier et al., 1996; Cullinane et al., 2006; Mealey, 2007). Since EIAV is a hemagglutinating virus, the indirect hemagglutination test has also been documented as a very sensitive serological test for EIA (Bürki et al., 1992). Development of a rapid fluorescence polarization-based diagnostic assay for EIAV has also been reported, which have been claimed to have field applicability (Tencza et al., 2000).

Definitive diagnosis of EIA is made with serological testing. The AGID test is the most widely accepted procedure for diagnosis of EIA and is highly specific; however, false negative results could occur with low levels of antibody. Although the precipitating antibodies detected by Coggins (AGID) test are usually present at the time of onset of symptoms, sometimes they may not be at a detectable level until up to initial few days; thus, serologic tests for EIAV can be negative ten to fourteen days postinfection, and therefore, early diagnosis may be difficult (Coggins et al., 1972). However, by forty-five days, most horses seroconvert (Crawford et al., 1978; Sellon et al., 1994). AGID detects antibody against the EIAV gag p26 protein/ antigen, which is very stable and reacts with serum from horses infected with different variants. The cELISA and Vira-CHEK ELISA also detect antibody against p26. They are more sensitive than the AGID but less specific. The SA-ELISA II detects antibody to the EIAV envelope gp45 or the p26 protein. The AGID test procedure requires a minimum of twenty-four hours; however, cELISA and Vira-CHEK ELISA provide EIAV diagnosis within an hour. But the positive results with these three ELISA systems must be confirmed by the AGID test. Although some countries will accept a negative ELISA, most countries require a horse to have a negative Coggins test result prior to importation.

Laboratory tests detecting EIAV in blood include animal inoculation, virus titration, and PCR/RT-PCR assays, which are sensitive and specific. Animal inoculation test is performed by intravenous inoculation of blood from the suspect horse to a susceptible pony, then monitoring the test animal for the development of clinical signs, and seroconversion (Coggins et al., 1972). This test is extremely sensitive for detecting infection as well as the inapparent carrier stage. Detection of EIA viral RNA in plasma samples from recently infected and long-term inapparent carrier animals can also be achieved by employing molecular tools of PCR assays, including reverse transcriptase–nested PCR (RT-nPCR) assay and multiplex real-time RT-PCR (Langemeier et al., 1996; Nagarajan and Simard 2001; Cook et al., 2002). Quantitation of infectious virus in plasma can be performed by titration in cell culture (O' Rourke et al., 1988) and of viral RNA by real-time quantitative RT-PCR (Cook et al., 2002; Mealey et al., 2003). PCR assays effectively detect EIAV and are more sensitive for detection of early stages of infection (Cullinane et al., 2007). The nested PCR assay have been reported to detect more EIAV-positive animals and found as specific as the AGID (Coggins) assay and offers great potential as a diagnostic test for the detection of EIAV infections in field horses (Nagarajan and Simard, 2001). Recently, highly sensitive, specific, and quantitative real-time RT-PCR and PCR assays have been developed and used to quantify the EIAV nucleic acid in postmortem tissues, plasma, and secretions of infected horses, which can be very useful for the epidemiological studies (Quinlivan et al., 2007).

Western blot (WB) test, detecting EIAV-specific antibodies, has been reported to be used as a supplemental test to reach a consensus in case when contradictory results are obtained with other diagnostic tests since it is a highly sensitive and specific assay (Rossmanith and Horvath, 1989). A novel confirmatory single-band WB test has been recently developed and validated for EIAV antibody detection based on the use of recombinant p26 (rp26) antigen and was shown to be a reliable diagnostic tool that can be used as a follow-up test after a doubtful, discordant, or inconclusive ELISA or AGID test result (Alvarez et al., 2007a). Serological method, using recombinant S2 protein, has been applied to differentiate EIAV-infected and EIAV-vaccinated horses (Jin et al., 2004). Recently, the development of an AGID test possessing an excellent EIAV diagnostic sensitivity and specificity employing a rp26 antigen has also been reported, which could be adopted as an official test method for the diagnosis and control of EIA (Alvarez et al., 2007b; Piza et al., 2007). EIAV rp26 has proven to be a reliable reagent for both AGID and ELISA (Archambault et al., 1989; Sentsui et al., 2001; Alvarez et el., 2007b) and is currently included in some commercial tests (EIA AGID test kit [VMRD Inc.] and Vira-CHEK/EIA [Synbiotics Corp.]).

DIFFERENTIAL DIAGNOSIS
Equine infectious anemia should be differentiated from equine babesiosis, leptospirosis, severe strongylosis (blood-worm infection) and purpura hemorrhagica.

TREATMENT
As for other viral diseases, no specific treatment for EIA is available. Good management practices and supportive treatment may facilitate clinical recovery (Mealey, 2007). Infected horse need to be isolated from other horses, and stress should be minimized by following good nursing care. Nonsteroidal anti-inflammatory drugs (NSAIDs), leg wraps, hydrotherapy, fluid therapy, blood transfusions, and hematinic drugs may assist in recovery from clinical disease. Corticosteroids are contraindicated. Though EIAV cause only transient immunosuppression, antimicrobial drugs may be prescribed to help prevent secondary bacterial infections, especially during febrile episodes. Recently, some alternative approaches are also being explored to treat EIAV infection, including extracts of *Prunella vulgaris,* displaying antilentiviral activity, which may function as promising microbicides against lentiviruses (Brindley et al., 2009), and a structural model of the rev regulatory protein of EIAV with antiviral prospectives may also provide a basis for the design of new therapies for lentiviral diseases (Ihm et al., 2009).

PREVENTION AND CONTROL

No approved vaccine exists for EIA. EIA is a reportable/notifiable disease in many countries, including those in the EU, Sweden, Canada, and certain states in Australia. Seropositive horses are destroyed in some countries, and interstate travel or the movement of infected animals is prohibited with a requirement for a negative test for horses prior to interstate movements; except few circumstances where AGID or c-ELISA test positive, horses are allowed to move only under specified conditions. In countries where the incidence is high, it is usual to control horse movement by a system of permits and certificates of freedom from the disease and to insist on skin branding or lip tattooing of horses. If it is absolutely necessary to keep an infected horse, the animal should be isolated from others on the farm and must be permanently identified as positive horses with a brand or lip tattoo. Prior to introduction of horses into the premises, horse owners should be advised to have horses tested. The prevention of EIA is based primarily on the detection of infected horses by the Coggins test and their isolation from other horses. Since infected horses are the only known reservoir of the virus, it is quite feasible to eradicate EIA from an area by testing and slaughter of reactors. The testing of all incoming horses will help to maintain the disease-free status (Issel et al. 1990; Cullinane et al., 2006; Mealey, 2007; Brangan et al., 2008).

Detection and removal of EIAV-infected horses decreases the likelihood of transmission. Horses must be tested when being imported, while entering into competitive events or exhibitions, being moved interstate, changing of ownerships, and during auctions or sales markets. The horse is to be quarantined on obtaining a positive result and retested for confirmation. Confirmed EIA-positive cases are called reactors. Quarantined horses are tested at thirty—to sixty-day intervals, and any additional reactors are removed. The quarantine is lifted if all exposed horses are negative at least sixty days after the removal of the last reactor.

Procedures for minimizing the risk of EIAV transmission need to be given due attention and priority. All horses should be tested annually, especially in areas with increased prevalence; purchase only horses known to be negative for EIAV; blood and plasma donors should be screened for EIAV infection; and use any instruments or equipment only after thorough cleaning, disinfecting, and sterilizing properly between each use (Cullinane et al., 2006; Mealey, 2007). A rigorous environmental hygiene and sanitation program supported with suitable vector-control strategies should be executed for minimizing natural transmission of EIAV. Biting flies—especially horseflies, deerflies, and stable flies—and other insects should be controlled through good sanitation, drainage of swampy areas, and by the strategic and judicious use of insecticides/pesticides; these altogether may help to limit the spread of the disease. Although strict adherence to sanitary regulations will minimize the likelihood of epizootics, the existence of a large reservoir of untested horses with occasional contact with uninfected test-negative horses will ensure the continued transmission of EIAV. The change of this transmission occurring as a result of human intervention can be eliminated, but it is not possible to eliminate the threat posed by blood-feeding insects.

IMMUNITY, INFECTION CONTROL, AND PROSPECTS FOR VACCINE DEVELOPMENT

Adaptive immune response are required to terminate plasma viremia, especially the EIAV-specific B lymphocytes for virus-neutralizing activity and T (cytotoxic T lymphocytes, CTLs) lymphocytes critical for providing protection against EIAV (Issel et al., 1992; McGuire et al., 2002, 2004; Travis et al., 2004; Mealey et al., 2004, 2005). Maturation of the cellular and humoral immune responses to persistent infection in horses by EIAV is a complex and lengthy process with humoral immune response requiring a six—to eight-month period to fully mature. During acute EIAV infection, the initial plasma viremia is terminated before the appearance of neutralizing antibody but coincides with the appearance of CTLs (Hammond et al., 1997; McGuire et al., 1994, 2002). Gag, pol, env, rev proteins, and S2 open reading frame–encoded protein comprises the CTL epitopes for EIA virus (Zhang et al., 1998; Lonning et al., 1999; McGuire et al., 2000; Chung et al., 2004; Mealey et al., 2003, 2004). Responses to these peptides in immunized horses are needed to be enhanced. However, other problems in inducing protection against lentiviruses remain, the most significant of them being EIAV variants that can escape both CTL and neutralizing antibody. A possible solution to CTL escape variants is the induction of high-avidity CTL to multiple EIAV epitopes. In inapparent carriers, the virus replication is ultimately controlled likely by the result of a broad CTL and neutralizing-antibody response, and the most frequently CTL-recognized proteins are gag p15 and gag p26, which possibly serve as vital targets for protective CTL responses. Thus, a vaccine for EIAV needs to induce effective CTL responses.

It is suggested that the epitope specificity of high—and moderate-avidity memory CTL (CTLm) is an important determinant for disease outcome in the EIAV-infected horses (Mealey et al., 2003). Epitope specificity is very crucial as the control of EIAV replication and clinical disease is associated with sustained CTL recognition of gag-specific epitopes (Mealey et al., 2005). Soutullo et al. (2005) reported that synthetic peptides of gp45 and p26 could be included in an effective vaccine design. A single amino acid difference within the alpha-2 domain of two naturally occurring equine MHC class I molecules alters the recognition of gag and rev epitopes EIAV-specific CTL, which can result in significantly different patterns of epitope recognition by lentivirus-specific CTL (Mealey et al., 2006). It is hypothesized that the EIAV envelope (Env) proteins gp90 and gp45 are major determinants of vaccine efficacy. Envelope-specific T-helper and cytotoxic T-lymphocyte responses are associated with protective immunity to EIAV. Recently, Tagmyer et al. (2007) reported a comprehensive mapping of EIAV Env-specific cellular regions as potential cellular immune determinants of protective immunity. The high levels of EIAV-specific cytokines induced by the attenuated EIAV vaccine may contribute to the protective immune response against EIA disease (Zhang et al., 2007). Neutralizing antibody exerts selective pressure throughout infection, and virus strategically adapts immune-evasion mechanisms and persistence change in the face of an evolving and maturing host immune response (Sponseller et al., 2007).

No vaccine of proven efficacy is currently available. Unfortunately, EIAV-vaccine development has only been moderately successful, and classical vaccines based on inactivated or attenuated whole virus and on viral recombinant protein failed to elicit a broadly protective immune response. The antigenic variation of the virus presents a major obstacle to the development of an efficacious vaccine. In the early 1970s, the Chinese EIAV live, attenuated vaccine, EIAV (DLA), was developed through successive passages of a wild-type virulent virus EIAV (L) in donkey leukocyte cells (Shen and Wang, 1985). Both inactivated whole virus and envelope glycoprotein subunit vaccines protected horses from challenge with homologous EIAV strain, but not heterologous virus, and subunit vaccine even appeared to have a high potential to enhance the disease induced by heterologous infection (Issel et al., 1992; Raabe et al., 1998). An experimental live, attenuated vaccine for EIAV, based on mutation of the viral S2 accessory gene (EIAV [UK] deltaS2]), elicited protection from detectable infection by virulent virus challenge (Li et al., 2003). Jin et al. (2004) reported the development of a S2-based diagnostic ELISA having the potential to accurately differentiate horses infected with EIAV from horses inoculated with an attenuated EIAV vaccine strain with a mutant S2 gene.

Discerning an effective balance between EIAV attenuation and vaccine efficacy is of prime importance (Craigo et al., 2005). The neutralizing epitopes of EIAV Env proteins and the effects of sequence variation on viral neutralization properties have been examined in detail (Ball et al., 1992; Craigo et al., 2002; Howe et al., 2002). Lipopeptide immunization with MHC class I–restricted CTL epitopes from the surface glycoprotein proved to have a protective effect against EIAV-induced disease (Ridgely and McGuire, 2002; Ridgely et al., 2003). The characterization of Th and CTL peptides of EIAV gp90 and gp45 provide a comprehensive mapping of EIAV Env-specific cellular regions that can be used to examine the development of protective immunity (Tagmyer et al., 2007). The Chinese EIAV donkey-leukocyte attenuated vaccine (DLV) provides a unique natural model system to study the attenuation mechanism and immunological control of lentivirus replication. Critical consensus mutations occur during the viral passages in vitro and in vivo, particularly in the envelope (env) region, which accounts for virus pathogenicity loss and are being studied to help understand the protective mechanism of EIAV vaccine (Liang et al., 2006; Shen et al., 2006; Wang et al., 2008; Wei et al., 2009). EIAV attenuation and cell tropism adaptation are associated with changes in both envelope and long terminal repeat (LTR)*http://www.ncbi.nlm.nih.gov/sites/entrez?Db=pubmed&Cm d=Search&Term=%22Issel%20CJ%22%5BAuthor%5D&itool=EntrezSy stem2.PEntrez.Pubmed.Pubmed_ResultsPanel.Pubmed_DiscoveryPanel. Pubmed_RVAbstractPlus* (Zhou et al., 2007). Studies with a highly effective attenuated EIAV vaccine (EIAV [D9]) capable of protecting 100% of horses from disease induced by a homologous Env challenge strain revealed an inverse correlation between challenge strain Env variation and vaccine protection from disease (Craigo et al., 2007a). Relatively minor Env variation can pose a substantial challenge to lentiviral vaccine immunity, even when attenuated vaccines are used that, to date, achieve the highest levels of vaccine protection.

Tagmyer et al. (2008) identified potential Env determinants of EIAV vaccine efficacy and demonstrated the profound effects of defined Env variation on immune recognition. Eight CTL peptides were found to associate closely with vaccine protection. Studies have highlighted the utility of postchallenge immune suppression for evaluating persistent viral vaccine protective efficacy (Craigo et al., 2007b). DNA vaccine is also being developed for EIAV (Mealey et al., 2007). EIAV vaccines trials are encouraging, but correlates of protection remain to be clearly defined. Protection against disease seems to be a reachable goal for which continuous efforts are being made.

CONCLUSION

Equine infectious anemia (EIA) is caused by Equine infectious anemia virus (EIAV), which is a macrophage-tropic lentivirus that persistently infects horses producing disease characterized by periodic episodes of fever, thrombocytopenia, and high levels of viremia. EIAV infects and persists in the macrophage populations, wherein its periodic replication leads to an immunologically mediated acute disease. In EIA, morbidity can approach 100% while mortality figures around 30%. The frequency and severity of clinical episodes of EIA decrease in most horses with time, leading to an inapparent carrier state where the virus persists in infected animals for life. Recrudescence of acute EIA is the result of antigenic variation of the surface glycoprotein of EIAV. Confirmatory diagnostic tests include serologic tests, viz, AGID and ELISA. Western blot test can be used to resolve any discordant results. PCR assays—including PCR, RT-PCR, nested PCR, multiplex and real-time RT-PCR—are also being employed for sensitive/ specific virus detection. Recombinant proteins have also been recently exploited to be used in serological diagnostic assays with good reliability. EIA has been managed in most countries by the imposition of testing and quarantine regulations, primarily on the identification and elimination of seropositive horses, predominantly by AGID assay in centralized reference laboratories. The recent developments made in EIAV diagnostics would be an adjunct to the AGID test. Currently, approved EIAV vaccines are not available. Utilizing new-generation molecular tools, scientists worldwide are focusing their researches on two areas: elimination of the virus from carriers and development of a vaccine to protect against this infection. Uniform active surveillance measures and improved documentation of EIA status of horses would improve the EIA control program. EIAV infection of horses provides a valuable model for examining the natural immunological control of lentivirus infection and disease and the mechanisms of protective and enhancing vaccine immunity. Lentiviral envelope antigenic variation, and associated immune evasion are believed to present major obstacles to effective vaccine development, which remains a high priority area in veterinary medicine. Strengthening the research studies on EIAV would also help evolve understanding the mechanisms of controls for other lentiviruses like the deadly AIDS (HIV) virus of human beings.

REFERENCES

1. Alvarez, I., Gutierrez, G., Ostlund, E., Barrandeguy, M. and Trono, K. 2007a. Western blot assay using recombinant p26 antigen for detection of equine infectious anemia virus-specific antibodies. *Clin. Vaccine Immunol.* 14:1646–1648.
2. Alvarez, I., Gutierrez, G., Vissani, A., Rodriguez, S., Barrandeguy, M. and Trono, K. 2007b. Standardization and validation of an agar gel immunodiffusion test for the diagnosis of equine infectious anemia using a recombinant p26 antigen. *Vet. Microbiol.* 121:344–351.
3. Archambault, D., Wang, Z. M., Lacal, J. C., Gazit, A., Yaniv, A., Dahlberg, J. E. and Tronick, S. R. 1989. Development of an enzyme-linked immunosorbent assay for equine infectious anemia virus detection using recombinant Pr55*gag*. *J. Clin. Microbiol.* 27:1167–1173.
4. Ball, J. M., Rushlow, K. E., Issel, C. J. and Montelaro, R. C. 1992. Detailed mapping of the antigenicity of the surface unit glycoprotein of equine infectious anemia virus by using synthetic peptide strategies. *J. Virol.* 66:732–742.

5. Bamigboye, O. and da Silva, R. M. 1981. Prevalence of equine infectious anaemia (swamp fever) in Guyana. *Br. Vet. J.* 137:538–40.

6. Bicout, D. J., Carvalho, R., Chalvet-Monfray, K. and Sabatier, P. 2006. Distribution of equine infectious anemia in horses in the north of Minas Gerais State, Brazil. *J. Vet. Diagn. Invest.* 18:479–482.

7. Brangan, P., Bailey, D. C., Larkin, J. F., Myers, T. and More, S. J. 2008. Management of the national programme to eradicate equine infectious anaemia from Ireland during 2006: A review. *Equine Vet. J.* 40:702–704.

8. Brindley, M. A. and Maury, W. 2008. Equine infectious anemia virus entry occurs through clathrin-mediated endocytosis. *J. Virol.* 82:1628–1637.

9. Brindley, M. A., Widrlechner, M. P., McCoy, J. A., Murphy, P., Hauck, C., Rizshsky, L., Nikolau, B. and Maury, W. 2009. Inhibition of lentivirus replication by aqueous extracts of Purnella vulgaris. *Virol J.* 20:6–8.

10. Bürki, F., Rossmanith, W. and Rossmanith, E. 1992. Equine lentivirus, comparative studies on four serological tests for the diagnosis of equine infectious anaemia. *Vet. Microbiol.* 33:353–360.

11. Cheevers, W. P. and McGuire, T. C. 1985. Equine infectious anemia virus: Immunopathogenesis and persistence. *Rev. Infect. Dis.* 7:83–88.

12. Chung, C., Mealey, R. H. and McGuire, T. C. 2004. CTL from EIAV carrier horses with diverse MHC class I alleles recognize epitope clusters in Gag matrix and capsid proteins. *Virology* 327:144–154, 2004.

13. Clabough, D. L., Gebhard, D., Flaherty, M. T., Whetter, L. E., Perry, S. T., Coggins, L., Fuller and F. J. 1991. Immune-mediated thrombocytopenia in horses infected with equine infectious anemia virus. *J. Virol.* 65:6242–6251.

14. Coggins, L. and Norcross, N. L. 1970. Immunodiffusion reaction in equine infectious anemia. *Cornell Vet.* 60:330–335.

15. Coggins, L., Norcross, N. L. and Nusbaum, S. R. 1972. Diagnosis of equine infectious anemia by immunodiffusion test. *Am. J. Vet. Res.* 33:11–18.

16. Coggins, L. and Auchnie, J. A. 1977. Control of equine infectious anemia in horses in Hong Kong. *J. Am. Vet. Med. Assoc.* 170:1299–1301.

17. Coggins, L. 1984. Carriers of equine infectious anemia virus. *J. Am. Vet. Med. Assoc.* 184:279–281.

18. Cook, S. J., Cook, R. F., Montelaro, R. C. and Issel, C. J. 2001. Differential responses of *Equus caballus* and *Equus asinus* to infection with two pathogenic strains of equine infectious anemia virus. *Vet. Microbiol.* 79:93–109.

19. Cook, R. F., Cook, S. J., Li, F. L., Montelaro, R. C. and Issel, C. J. 2002. Development of a multiplex real-time reverse transcriptase-polymerase chain reaction for equine infectious anemia virus (EIAV). *J. Virol. Methods* 105:171–179.

20. Costa, L. R., Santos, I. K., Issel, C. J. and Montelaro, R. C. 1997. Tumor necrosis factor-alpha production and disease severity after immunization with enriched major core protein (p26) and/or infection with equine infectious anemia virus. *Vet. Immunol. Immunopathol.* 57:33–47.

21. Craigo, J. K., Leroux, C., Howe, L., Steckbeck, J. D., Cook, S. J., Issel, C. J. and Montelaro, R. C. 2002. Transient immune suppression of inapparent carriers infected with a principal neutralizing domaindeficient equine infectious anaemia virus induces neutralizing antibodies and lowers steady-state virus replication. *J. Gen. Virol.* 83:1353–1359.

22. Craigo, J. K., Feng Li, F., Steckbeck, J. D., Durkin, S., Howe, L., Cook, S. J., Charles Issel, C., Ronald, C. and Montelaro, R. C. 2005. Discerning an effective balance between equine infectious anemia virus attenuation and vaccine efficacy. *J. Virol.* 79:2666–2677.

23. Craigo, J. K., Sturgeon, T. J., Cook, S. J., Issel, C. J., Leroux, C. and Montelaro, R. C. 2006. Apparent elimination of EIAV ancestral species in a long-term inapparent carrier. *Virology* 344:340–353.

24. Craigo, J. K., Zhang, B., Barnes, S., Tagmyer, T. L., Cook, S. J., Issel, C. J., Montelaro, R. C. 2007a. Envelope variation as a primary determinant of lentiviral vaccine efficacy. *Proc. Natl. Acad. Sci. USA* 104:15105–15110.

25. Craigo, J. K., Durkin, S., Sturgeon, T. J., Tagmyer, T., Cook, S. J., Issel, C. J. and Montelaro, R. C. 2007b. Immune suppression of challenged vaccinates as a rigorous assessment of sterile protection by lentiviral vaccines. *Vaccine* 25:834–845.

26. Crawford, T. B., Cheevers, W. P., Klevjer-Anderson, P. et al. 1978. Equine infectious anemia: Virion characteristics, virus-cell interaction and host responses. *ICN-UCLA Symp. Mol. Cell. Biol.* 11:727–749.

27. Cullinane, A. A., Barr, B., Bernard, W., Duncan, J. L., Mulcahy, G., Smith, M. and Timoney, J. E. 2006. Infectious diseases (Chapter 1): Equine infectious anemia. In *The equine manual*, 2nd ed., A. J. Higgins and J. R. Snyder, 29–32. USA: Saunder, Elsevier Ltd.

28. Cullinane, A., Quinlivan, M., Nelly, M., Patterson, H., Kenna, R., Garvey, M., Gildea, S., Lyons, P., Flynn, M., Galvin, P., Neylon, M. and Jankowska, K. 2007. Diagnosis of equine infectous anaemia during the 2006 outbreak in Ireland. *Vet Rec.* 161:647–652.

29. Dufour, C., Corcione, A., Svahn, J., Haupt, R., Poggi, V., Beka'ssy, A. N., Scime, R., Pistorio, A. and Pistoia, V. 2003. TNF-alpha and IFN-gamma are overexpressed in the bone marrow of Fanconi anemia patients and TNF-alpha suppresses erythropoiesis in vitro. *Blood* 102:2053–2059.

30. Foil, L. D., Meek, C. L., Adams, W. V. and Issel, C. J. 1983. Mechanical transmission of equine infectious anemia virus by deer flies (*Chrysops flavidus*) and stable flies (*Stomoxys calcitrans*). *Am. J. Vet. Res.* 44:155–156.

31. Hammond, S. A., Cook, S. J., Lichtenstein, D. L., Issel, C. J. and Montelaro, R. C. 1997. Maturation of the cellular and humoral immune responses to persistent infection in horses by equine infectious anemia virus is a complex and lengthy process. *J. Virol.* 71:3840–3852.

32. Harrold, S. M., Cook, S. J., Cook, R. F., Rushlow, K. E., Issel, C. J. and Montelaro, R. C. 2000. Tissue sites of persistent infection and active replication of equine infectious anemia virus during acute disease and asymptomatic infection in experimentally infected equids. *J. Virol.* 74:3112–3121.

33. Howe, L., Leroux, C., Issel, C. J. and Montelaro, R. C. 2002. Equine infectious anemia virus envelope evolution in vivo during persistent infection progressively increases resistance to in vitro serum antibody neutralization as a dominant phenotype. *J. Virol.* 76:10588–10597.

34. Ihm, Y., Sparks, W. O., Lee, J. H., Cao, H., Carpenter, S., Wang, C. Z., Ho, K. M. and Dobbs, D. 2009. Structural model of the Rev regulatory protein from equine infectious anemia virus. *PLoS ONE* 4:ed. 4178.

35. Issel, C. J. and Foil L. D. 1984. Studies on equine infectious anemia virus transmission by insects. *J. Am. Vet. Med. Assoc.* 184:293–297.

36. Issel, C. J., McManus, J. M., Hagius, S. D., Foil, L. D., Adams, W. V. Jr. and Montelaro, R. C. 1990. Equine infectious anemia: Prospects for control. *Dev. Biol. Stand.* 72:49–57.

37. Issel, C. J., Horohov, D. W., Lea, D. F., Adams, W. V. J., Hagius, S. D., McManus, J. M., Allison, A. C. and Montelaro, R. C. 1992. Efficacy of inactivated whole-virus and subunit vaccines in preventing infection and disease caused by equine infectious anemia virus. *J. Virol.* 66:3398–3408.

38. Issel, C. J. and Cook, R. F. 1993. A review of techniques for the serologic diagnosis of equine infectious anemia. *J. Vet. Diagn. Invest.* 5:137–141.

39. Jin, S., Issel, C. J. and Montelaro, R. C. 2004. Serological method using recombinant S2 protein to differentiate equine infectious anemia virus (EIAV)-infected and EIAV-vaccinated horses. *Clin. Diagn. Lab. Immunol.* 11:1120–1129.

40. Jin, S., Zhang, B., Weisz, O. A. and Montelaro, R. C. 2005. Receptor-mediated entry by equine infectious anemia virus utilizes a pH-dependent endocytic pathway. *J. Virol.* 79:14489–14497.

41. Kemeny, L. J., Mott, L. O. and Pearson, J. E. 1971. Titration of equine infectious anemia virus: Effect of dosage on incubation time and clinical signs. *Cornell Veterinarian* 61:687–695.

42. Kono, Y. 1973. Development of immunity after immunization and infection with avirulent, attenuated and virulent equine infectious anemia virus. In *Proceedings Third International Equine Infectious Diseases*, ed. J. T. Bryans and H. Gerber, 242–254. Basel: S. Karger.

43. Langemeier, J. L., Cook, S. J., Cook, R. F., Rushlow, K. E., Montelaro, R. C. and Issel, C. J. 1996. Detection of equine infectious anemia viral RNA in plasma samples from recently infected and long-term inapparent carrier animals by PCR. *J. Clin. Microbiol.* 34:1481–1487.

44. Lepherd, E. E. 1978. Equine infectious anaemia and the Australian horse industry. *Aust. Vet. J.* 54:42–43.

45. Leroux, C., Issel, C. J. and Montelaro, R. C. 1997. Novel and dynamic evolution of equine infectious anemia virus genomic quasispecies associated with sequential disease cycles in an experimentally infected pony. *J. Virol.* 71:9627–9639.

46. Leroux, C., Craigo, J. K., Issel, C. J. and Montelaro, R. C. 2001. Equine infectious anemia virus genomic evolution in progressor and nonprogressor ponies. *J. Virol.*75:4570–4583.

47. Leroux, C., Cadoré, J. L. and Montelaro, R. C. 2004. Equine infectious anemia virus (EIAV): What has HIV's country cousin got to tell us? *Vet. Res.* 35:485–512.

48. Lew, A. M., Thomas, L. M. and Huntington, P. J. 1993. A comparison of ELISA, FAST-ELISA and gel diffusion tests for detecting antibody to equine infectious anaemia virus. *Vet. Microbiol.* 34:1–5.

49. Lignee, M. 1843. Mémoire et observations sur une maladie de sang, connue sous le nom d'anhémie hydrohémie, cachexie acquise du cheval. *Rec. Med. Vet. Ec. Alfort.* 30–44.

50. Li, F., Craigo, J. K., Howe, L., Steckbeck, J. D., Cook, S., Issel, C. and Montelaro, R. C. 2003. A live attenuated equine infectious anemia virus proviral vaccine with a modified S2 gene provides protection from detectable infection by intravenous virulent virus challenge of experimentally inoculated horses. *J. Virol.* 77:7244–7253.

51. Liang, H., He, X., Shen, R. X., Shen, T., Tong, X., Ma, Y., Xiang, W. H., Zhang, X. Y. and Shao, Y. M. 2006. Combined amino acid mutations occurring in the envelope closely correlate with pathogenicity of EIAV. *Arch. Virol.* 151:1387–403.

52. Lim, W. S., Payne, S. L., Edwards, J. F., Kim, I. and Ball, J. M. 2005. Differential effects of virulent and avirulent equine infectious anemia virus on macrophage cytokine expression. *Virology* 332:295–306.

53. Loftin, M. K., Levine, J. F., McGinn, T., Coggins, L. 1990. Distribution of equine infectious anemia in equids in southeastern United States. *J. Am. Vet. Med. Assoc.* 197:1018–1020.

54. Lonning, S. M., Zhang, W., Leib, S. R. and McGuire, T. C. 1999. Detection and induction of equine infectious anemia virus-specific cytotoxic T-lymphocyte responses by use of recombinant retroviral vectors. *J. Virol.* 73:2762–2769.

55. McClure, J. J., Lindsay, W. A., Taylor, W., Ochoa R., Issel, C. J. and Coulter, S. J. 1982. Ataxia in four horses with equine infectious anemia. *J. Am. Vet. Med. Assoc.* 180:279–283.

56. McGuire, T. C., Henson, J. B., Quist, S. E. 1969. Viral-induced hemolysis in equine infectious anemia. *Am. J. Vet. Res.* 30:2091–2097.

57. McGuire, T. C., Crawford, T. B., Henson, J. B. 1972. Equine infectious anemia: Detection of infectious virus-antibody complexes in the serum. *Immunol. Commun.* 1:545–551.

58. McGuire, T. C., O'Rourke, K. and Cheevers, W. P. 1987. A review of antigenic variation by the equine infectious anemia virus. *Contrib. Microbiol. Immunol.* 8:77–89.

59. McGuire, T. C., O'Rourke, K. I. and Perryman, L. E. 1990. Immunopathogenesis of equine infectious anemia lentivirus disease. *Dev. Biol. Stand.* 72:31–37.

60. McGuire, T. C., Tumas, D. B., Byrne, K. M., Hines, M. T., Leib, S. R., Brassfield, A. L., O'Rourke, K. I. and Perryman, L. E. 1994. Major histocompatibility complex-restricted CD8+ cytotoxic T lymphocytes from horses with equine infectious anemia virus recognize Env and Gag/PR proteins. *J. Virol.* 68:1459–1467.

61. McGuire, T. C., Leib, S. R., Lonning, S. M., Zhang, W., Byrne, K. M. and Mealey, R. H. 2000. Equine infectious anaemia virus proteins with epitopes most frequently recognized by cytotoxic T lymphocytes from infected horses. *J. Gen. Virol.* 81:2735–2739.

62. McGuire, T. C., Fraser, D. G. and Mealey, R. H. 2002. Cytotoxic T lymphocytes and neutralizing antibody in the control of equine infectious anemia virus. *Viral. Immunol.* 15:521–531.

63. McGuire, T. C., Fraser, D. G. and Mealey, R. H. 2004. Cytotoxic T lymphocytes in protection against equine infectious anemia virus. *Anim. Health Res. Rev.* 5:271–276.

64. Mealey, R. B. 2007. Equine infectious anemia. In *Equine infectious diseases*, ed. D. C. Sellon and M. T. Long, chapter 23, 213–219. Philadelphia, USA: Saunders, Elsevier Inc.

65. Mealey, R. H., Zhang, B., Leib, S. R., Littke, M. H. and McGuire, T. C. 2003. Epitope specificity is critical for high and moderate avidity cytotoxic T lymphocytes associated with control of viral load and clinical disease in horses with equine infectious anemia virus. *Virology* 313:537–552.

66. Mealey, R. H., Leib, S. R., Pownder, S. L. and McGuire, T. C. 2004. Adaptive immunity is the primary force driving selection of equine infectious anemia virus envelope SU variants during acute infection. *J. Virol.* 78:9295–9305.

67. Mealey, R. H., Sharif, A., Ellis, S. A., Littke, M. H., Leib, S. R. and McGuire, T. C. 2005. Early detection of dominant Env-specific and subdominant Gag-specific CD8+ lymphocytes in equine infectious anemia virus-infected horses using major histocompatibility complex class I/peptide tetrameric complexes. *Virology* 339:110–126.

68. Mealey, R. H., Lee, J. H., Leib, S. R., Littke, M. H. and McGuire, T. C. 2006. A single amino acid difference within the alpha-2 domain of two naturally occurring equine MHC class I molecules alters the recognition of Gag and Rev epitopes by equine infectious anemia virus-specific CTL. *J. Immunol.* 177:7377–7390.

69. Mealey, R. H., Stone, D. M., Hines, M. T., Alperin, D. C., Littke, M. H., Leib, S. R., Leach, S. E. and Hines, S. A. 2007. Experimental Rhodococcus equi and equine infectious anemia virus DNA vaccination in adult and neonatal horses: Effect of IL-12, dose, and route. *Vaccine* 25:7582–7597.

70. Montelaro, R. C., Ball, J. M. and Rushlow, K. E. 1993. Equine retroviruses. In *The retroviridae*, ed. J. A. Levy. New York: Plenum Press.

71. Nagarajan, M. M. and Simard, C. 2001. Detection of horses infected naturally with equine infectious anemia virus by nested polymerase chain reaction. *J. Virol. Methods* 94:97–109.

72. Nusbaum, S. R. 1975. Survey findings of equine infectious anemia positive horses in New York State. Proceedings Seventy-ninth Annual Meeting of United State Animal Health Association, 201–209.

73. Oaks, J. L., McGuire, T. C., Ulibarri, C. and Crawford, T. B. 1998. Equine infectious anemia virus is found in tissue macrophages during subclinical infection. *J. Virol.* 72:7263–7269.

74. Oaks, J. L., Ulibarri, C. and Crawford, T. B. 1999. Endothelial cell infection in vivo by equine infectious anaemia virus. *J. Gen. Virol.* 80:2393–2397.

75. Oaks, J. L., Long, M. T. and Baszler, T. V. 2004. Leukoencephalitis associated with selective viral replication in the brain of a pony with experimental chronic equine infectious anemia virus infection. *Vet. Pathol.* 41:527–532.

76. O'Rourke, K., Perryman, L. E. and McGuire, T. C. 1988. Antiviral, anti-glycoprotein and neutralizing antibodies in foals with equine infectious anaemia virus. *J. Gen. Virol.* 69:667–674.

77. Piza, A. S., Pereira, A. R., Terreran, M. T., Mozzer, O., Tanuri, A., Brandão, P. E. and Richtzenhain, L. J. 2007. Serodiagnosis of equine infectious anemia by agar gel immunodiffusion and ELISA using a recombinant p26 viral protein expressed in *Escherichia coli* as antigen. *Prev. Vet. Med.* 78:239–245.

78. Quinlivan, M., Cook, R. F. and Cullinane, A. 2007. Real-time quantitative RT-PCR and PCR assays for a novel European field isolate of equine infectious anaemia virus based on sequence determination of the gag gene. *Vet. Rec.* 160:611–18.

79. Raabe, M. L., Issel, C. J., Cook, S. J., Cook, R. F., Woodson, B. and Montelaro, R. C. 1998. Immunization with a recombinant envelope protein (rgp90) of EIAV produces a spectrum of vaccine efficacy ranging from lack of clinical disease to severe enhancement. *Virology* 245:151–162.

80. Radostits, O. M., Gay, C. C., Blood, D. C. and Hinchcliff, K. W. 2000. Equine infectious anaemia. In *Veterinary medicine*, 9th ed., 1032–1036. W. B. Saunders Co.

81. Ridgely, S. L. and McGuire, T. C. 2002. Lipopeptide stimulation of MHC class I-restricted memory cytotoxic T lymphocytes from equine infectious anemia virus-infected horses. *Vaccine* 20:1809–1819.

82. Ridgely, S. L., Zhang, B. and McGuire, T. C. 2003. Response of ELA-A1 horses immunized with lipopeptide containing an equine infectious anemia virus ELA-A1-restricted CTL epitope to virus challenge. *Vaccine* 21:491–506.

83. Rossmanith, W. and Horvath, E. 1989. A western blot test for the serological diagnosis of equine infectious anemia. *Zentralbl Veterinarmed* B 36:49–56.

84. Russell, K. E., Perkins, P. C., Hoffman, M. R., Miller, R. T., Walker, K. M., Fuller, F. J. and Sellon, D. C. 1999. Platelets from thrombocytopenic ponies acutely infected with equine infectious anemia virus are activated in vivo and hypofunctional. *Virology* 259:7–19.

85. Sellon, D. C. 1993. Equine infectious anemia. *Vet. Clin. North Am. Equine Pract.* 9:321–336.

86. Sellon, D. C., Perry, S. T., Coggins, L. et al. 1992. Wild-type equine infectious anemia virus replicates in vivo predominantly in tissue macrophages, not in peripheral blood monocytes. *J. Virol.* 66:5906–5913.

87. Sellon, D. C., Fuller, F. J. and McGuire, T. C. 1994. The immunopathogenesis of equine infectious anemia virus. *Virus Res.* 32:111–138.

88. Sellon, D. C., Russell, K. E., Monroe, V. L. and Walker K. M. 1999. Increased interleukin-6 activity in the serum of ponies acutely infected with equine infectious anaemia virus. *Res. Vet. Sci.* 66:77–80.

89. Sentsui, H. and Kono, Y. 1987. Complement-mediated hemolysis of horse erythrocytes treated with equine infectious anemia virus. *Arch. Virol.* 95:53–66.

90. Sentsui, H., Inoshima, Y., Murakami, K., Akashi, H., Purevtseren, B., Pagmajav, O. and Sugiera, T. 2001. Cross reaction of recombinant equine infectious anemia virus antigen to heterologous strains and application for serological survey among horses in the field. *Microbiol. Immunol.* 45:45–50.

91. Shane, B. S., Issel, C. J. and Montelaro, R. C. 1984. Enzyme-linked immunosorbent assay for detection of equine infectious anemia virus p26 antigen and antibody. *J. Clin. Microbiol.* 19:351–355.

92. Shen, R. and Wang, Z. M. 1985. Development and use of an equine infectious aneamia donkey leukocyte attenuated vaccine. In *Equine infectious anemia: A national review of policies, programs, and future objectives*, ed. R. Tashjian, 135–148. Amarillo, Texas.

93. Shen, T., Liang, H., Tong, X., Fan, X., He, X., Ma, Y., Xiang, W., Shen, R., Zhang, X. and Shao, Y. 2006. Amino acid mutations of the infectious clone from Chinese EIAV attenuated vaccine resulted in reversion of virulence. *Vaccine* 24:738–749.

94. Soutullo, A., García, M. I., Bailat, A., Racca, A., Tonarelli, G. and Malan Borel. I. 2005. Antibodies and PMBC from EIAV infected carrier horses recognize gp45 and p26 synthetic peptides. *Vet. Immunol. Immunopathol.* 108:335–43.

95. Sponseller, B. A., Sparks, W. O., Wannemuehler, Y., Li, Y., Antons, A. K., Oaks, J. L. and Carpenter, S. 2007. Immune selection of equine infectious anemia virus env variants during the long-term inapparent stage of disease. *Virology* 363:156–165.

96. Stein, C. D., Mott, L. O. and Gates, D. W. 1955. Some observations on Carriers of Equine infectious anemia. *J. Am. Vet. Med. Association* 126:277–287.

97. Tagmyer, T. L., Craigo, J. K., Cook, S. J., Issel, C. J. and Montelaro, R. C. 2007. Envelope-specific T-helper and cytotoxic T-lymphocyte responses associated with protective immunity to equine infectious anemia virus. *J. Gen. Virol.* 88:1324–1336.

98. Tagmyer, T. L., Craigo, J. K., Cook, S. J., Even, D. L., Issel, C. J. and Montelaro, R. C. 2008. Envelope determinants of equine infectious anemia virus vaccine protection and the effects of sequence variation on immune recognition. *J. Virol.* 82:4052–4063.

99. Tencza, S. B., Islam, K. R., Kalia, V., Nasir, M. S., Jolley, M. E. and Montelaro, R. C. 2000. Development of a fluorescence polarization-based diagnostic assay for equine infectious anemia virus. *J. Clin. Microbiol.* 38:1854–1859.

100. Thomas, R. J. and Elder, J. K. 1978. Equine infectious anaemia in Queensland. *Aust. Vet. J.* 54:456–457.

101. Thomas, L. M., Huntington, P. J., Mead, L. J., Wingate, D. L., Rogerson, B. A. and Lew, A. M. 1992. A soluble recombinant fusion protein of the transmembrane envelope protein of equine infectious anaemia virus for ELISA. *Vet. Microbiol.* 31:127–137.

102. Tornquist, S. J., Oaks, J. L. and Crawford, T. B. 1997. Elevation of cytokines associated with the thrombocytopenia of equine infectious anaemia. *J. Gen. Virol.* 78:1997.

103. Travis, C., McGuire, Darrilyn, G. Fraser and Robert H. Mealey. 2004. Cytotoxic T lymphocytes in protection against equine infectious anemia virus. *Anim. Hlth. Res. Rev.* 5:271–276.

104. Uppal, P. K. and Yadav, M. P. 1989. Occurrence of equine infectious anaemia in India. *Vet. Rec.* 124:514–515.

105. Wang, X. F., Jiang, C. G., Guo, W., Xiang, W., Lv X. L., Zhao, L. P., Wang, F. L., Kong, X. G., Zhang, X. Y., Shao, Y. M. and Zhou, J. H. 2008. Comparision of proviral genomes between the Chinese EIAV donkey leukocyte-attenuated vaccine and its parental virulent strain. *Bing Du Xue Bao.* 24:443–450.

106. Wei, L., Fan, X., Lu, X., Zhao, L., Xiang, W., Zhang, X., Xue, F., Shao, Y., Shen, R. and Wang, X. 2009. Genetic variation in the long terminal repeat associated with the transition of Chinese equine infectious anemia virus from virulence to avirulence. *Virus Genes* 2009 Jan 7 [Epub ahead of print].

107. Weiland, F. and Matheka, H. D. 1984. Cytoplasmic inclusions in cells infected with the virus of equine infectious anemia (EIAV). *Eur. J. Cell Biol.* 33:294–299.

108. Zhang, W., Lonning, S. M. and McGuire, T. C. 1998. Gag protein epitopes recognized by ELA-A-restricted cytotoxic T lymphocytes from horses with long-term equine infectious anemia virus infection. *J. Virol.* 72:9612–9620.

109. Zhang, B., Jin, S., Jin, J., Li, F. and Montelaro, R. C. 2005. A tumor necrosis factor receptor family protein serves as a cellular receptor for the macrophage-tropic equine lentivirus. *Proc. Natl. Acad. Sci. USA* 102:9918–9923.

110. Zhang, X., Wang, Y., Liang, H., Wei, L., Xiang, W., Shen, R. and Shao, Y. 2007. Correlation between the induction of Th1 cytokines by an attenuated equine infectious anemia virus vaccine and protection against disease progression. *J. Gen. Virol.* 88:998–1004.

111. Zhou, T., Yuan, X. F., Hou, S. H., Tu, Y. B., Peng, J. M., Wen, J. X., Qiu, H. J., Wu, D. L., Chen, H. C., Wang, X. J. and Tong, G. Z. 2007. Long terminal repeat sequences from virulent and attenuated equine infectious anemia virus demonstrate distinct promoter activities. *Virus Res.* 128:58–64.

9. Equine Papillomatosis

R. V. S. Pawaiya, K. Dhama, S. Kapoor, and D. K. Gupta

Introduction

Papilloma refers to a benign epithelial tumor growing exophytically (outwardly projecting) in fingerlike fronds. Papilloma, usually caused by a species-specific papillomavirus (PV), may arise from skin, conjunctiva, mucous membranes, or glandular ducts and varies from keratinized to fibrovascular and squamous. Papillomaviruses are small nonenveloped, double-stranded DNA viruses of the Papovaviridae family (Lowy and Howley, 2002). All domestic animals, including whales (turtles also) and humans, are affected by papillomaviruses (de Villiers et al., 2004). Some mammals have several distinct papilloma viruses: humans have more than 120; cattle, 6; dogs, 3; equine, 2; and rabbits, 2 (Lancaster and Olson, 1982; Coggins et al., 1985; Antonsson and Hansson, 2002; Christensen, 2005; Fakhry and Gillison, 2006). Different papillomaviruses have considerable species, site, and histologic specificity (Hargis and Ginn, 2007). Many papillomaviruses that infect animal species, including humans and equines, have been characterized (O'Banion et al., 1986). There are five different papilloma viruses suspected to be involved in horse warts. They are EPV1, EPV2, BPV1, BPV2, and EPV—the last one isolated from penile papilloma and characterized to be a distinct one from EPV1 and 2, but it has not been given name like EPV3.

Horses can be infected by at least five different papilloma viruses: *two equine-specific papilloma viruses, EPV-1 and EPV-2,* cause *various presentations of warts,* including *aural plaques* in horses (Castro et al., 1992; Williams, 1997; Scott and Miller, 2003); a third EPV may be associated with *penile papillomas* (O'Banion et al., 1986); and two bovine-specific papilloma viruses, BPV-1 and BPV-2, especially BPV-2, have been found associated with the development of *equine sarcoids,* a form of nonmetastatic cutaneous fibrosarcoma (Amtmann et al., 1980; Carr et al., 2001b; Chambers et al., 2003; Nixon et al., 2005; Kasperowicz et al., 2006; Bogaert et al., 2007). In a recent survey of equine cutaneous neoplasia in the Pacific Northwest, equine sarcoid constituted the highest (51.4%) numbers among 536 cutaneous neoplasias, whereas papillomas were 4.3% (Valentine, 2006). Histopathology, immunohistochemistry, and molecular studies involving identification of EPV DNA and/or PV antigen in thirty-eight cases of equine papillomas, nine cases of aural plaques, and ten cases of sarcoids could detect EPV DNA and/ or PV antigen in 68.0% (twenty-six cases) of papilloma cases, whereas only

PV antigen could be detected immunohistochemically in four cases of aural plaques and only one case of sarcoid was positive for EPV DNA by polymerase chain reaction (PCR) test (Postey et al., 2007). The authors hypothesized that EPV had a direct involvement in the pathogenesis of papillomas, whereas aural plaques may have the involvement of distinctively different PV.

EQUINE CUTANEOUS PAPILLOMA (WARTS)

Cutaneous papillomatosis or equine viral papillomatosis or more commonly known as warts (grass warts) are small lumps on the skin caused by an infectious virus. They affect the skin, particularly on the muzzle and lower part of the head of young horses usually less than three years old, most commonly in horses between six months and a year old and occasionally very old horses (in their twenties) as well (Fulton et al., 1970; Pascoe et al., 1999; Scott and Miller, 2003). Any breed and both sexes are equally affected. The EPV responsible for these warts is highly contagious, and horses become infected either through direct contact with one another or through fomites.

ETIOLOGY

Papillomaviruses are nonenveloped, meaning that the outer shell or capsid of the virus is not covered by a lipid membrane. A single viral protein, known as L1, is necessary and sufficient for formation of a 60-nm capsid composed of seventy-two star-shaped capsomers. Like most nonenveloped viruses, the capsid is geometrically regular and presents icosahedral symmetry. The papillomavirus genome is a double-stranded circular DNA molecule of about eight thousand base pairs in length. It is packaged within the L1 shell along with cellular histone proteins, which serve to wrap and condense DNA. The papillomavirus capsid also contains a viral protein known as L2, which is less abundant. Although not clear how L2 is arranged within the virion, it is known to perform several important functions, including facilitating the packaging of the viral genome into nascent virions as well as the infectious entry of the virus into new host cells (Lowy and Howley, 2002).

Cook and Olson (1951) demonstrated that intradermal or subcutaneous injection of bacteria-free filtrates of equine papilloma tissues resulted in growth of typical papilloma lesions within sixty to seventy days, establishing the infectious viral nature of the etiological agent. However, calves, lambs, dogs, rabbits, and guinea pigs remained resistant to the inoculations with known active suspensions of equine cutaneous papilloma, suggestive of species specificity of the viral agent. Later, *Equus caballus* papillomavirus type 1 (EcPV-l) has been isolated, characterized, and cloned from equine warts (O'Banion et al., 1986). Papillomaviruses are associated with epithelial proliferations in many vertebrate species. Recently, the complete nucleotide sequence of *Equus caballus papillomavirus type 1* (EcPV-1), obtained from an equine cutaneous papilloma, has been published, and studies on phylogenetic analysis have shown that EcPV-1 is a close-to-root papillomavirus, with only distant relationships to the fibropapillomaviruses and the benign cutaneous papillomaviruses (Ghim et al., 2004). A second mucosotropic equine papillomavirus, designated as EcPV-2, has been isolated from papillomas affecting the genital area of horses. EcPV-2 differs from EcPV-l in restriction endonuclease digestion pattern (O' Banion et al., 1986).

Epidemiology

The EPV appears to be species specific—as calves, lambs, dogs, rabbits, and guinea pigs were found resistant on experimental inoculations with known active suspensions of equine cutaneous papilloma (Cook and Olson, 1951). Most horses with cutaneous papillomatosis (warts) are usually less than three years of age. There are no breed or gender predilections. Disease can be spread by fomites or by close contact with affected horses. Spread is common when young horses are brought together in large groups for show, sale, or kept together in the breeding stud (Sellon, 2007).

Transmission

The EcPV is highly contagious and may spread from one infected horse in the herd to others either through direct contact with each other or via fomites, although some horses appear more susceptible than others. Natural infections are thought to require contact of virus with damaged skin, which could be due to environmental trauma, ectoparasites, or ultraviolet light damage (Williams, 1997; Scott and Miller, 2003). The incubation period is estimated at approximately sixty days and may be influenced by the dose of virus, route of exposure, and immunity of the host (Postey et al., 2007).

Clinical Signs

Equine papilloma virus has an incubation period of about sixty days, and the warts reach maturity after a growth period of four to eight weeks and usually disappear spontaneously about three to four months and sometimes even up to nine months later. In horses, small scattered papillomas develop on the nose, lips, eyelids, distal legs, penis, vulva, mammary glands, and inner surfaces of the pinnae, often secondary to mild abrasions (Cook and Olson, 1951). Generally, multiple warts are found singly and in clumps; often the clumps may look like one big wart. They may vary in size from 0.1–2.0 cm in diameter. They may be round smooth bumps or appear cauliflower-like. They are pink to gray in color, often depending on the horse's skin pigmentation in the area such as darker warts on darker skin (Williams, 1997; Scott and Miller, 2003). They can be a herd problem, especially when young horses are kept together, but regress in a few months as a foal's immune system matures. When they develop in older horses, they often persist for more than one year.

Pathogenesis and Pathology

Warts affect various cutaneous sites, as well as oral, ocular, and genital mucous membranes, and can be problematic depending on physical location and esthetics, although spontaneous regression is usual in one to nine months (Cook and Olson, 1951). Papillomaviruses cause lesions by two different mechanisms. In some cells, infection elicits increased activity, mitosis, and proliferation, which result in gross and histopathological changes of hyperplasia and hyperkeratosis (nonproductive infection), wherein hyperplastic cells are considered neoplastically transformed. In other cells, infection causes virion production within the cell nucleus, degeneration, and eventual cell death (productive infection). The effect exerted by papillomaviruses on the cell (proliferation or death by virion production) is dependent on the way the viral genome is inserted into the host cell genome and on the stage of cell cycle of the host cell at the time of infection (Hargis and Ginn, 2007).

Histopathologically, stratified squamous epithelium is covered by thickened orthokeratotic or parakeratotic keratin, is acanthotic, and has elongated epidermal-dermal interdigitations. The epidermis rests on collagenous core. In some papillomas, keratinocytes, and spinous cells in upper layer are swollen with amphophilic cytoplasm and have an eccentric nucleus and a perinuclear halo; such keratinocytes are termed as "koilocytes" (meaning hollow or concave). Keratohyalin granules are irregular. Pale basophilic intranuclear inclusion bodies are seen in some papillomas located in the degenerating cells in the outer spinous and granular cell layers in which virion production is taking place. Since papillomas regress spontaneously, in regressing stages, there is decreased epidermal hyperplasia, increased fibroblastic proliferation, collagen deposition, and infiltration of T lymphocytes at the epidermal-dermal junction (Hamada et al., 1990). In warts, PV virions have been observed in nuclei of cells of the stratum granulosum, corneum, and spinosum by electron microscopy (Fulton et al., 1970), and PV antigen has been identified with immunohistochemical (IHC) techniques (Sundberg et al., 1984; O' Banion et al., 1986).

Diagnosis

The diagnosis of equine warts is usually obvious based on history, clinical signs, and age of the affected horse. When lesions of equine papillomas are multiple, they may be sufficiently characteristic to confirm the diagnosis. Additional diagnostic testing is rarely performed. However, there are many simulants of warts, and a definitive diagnosis requires identification of the virus or its cytopathic effects on individual cells such as characteristic koilocytic atypia or koilocytosis. Equine papillomas are disfiguring, but benign. They need to be distinguished from verrucous equine sarcoid. Verrucous sarcoid resembles warts in their gross appearance and predilection for the face. Proliferative lesions in older horses should be considered sarcoids until proved otherwise.

TREATMENT AND CONTROL

Equine papillomas rarely need any treatment as they usually clear up within a few months; however, if warts are stressful physically and bothering the horse, they can be removed by surgical excision, ligation, or cryosurgery. Previously warts were treated by crushing one or two with pliers or hemostats in an attempt to stimulate the animals' immune system to help clear the wart virus faster. However, this can result in infection and may even prolong the disease (Pascoe et al., 1999; Carter and Wise, 2005). A variety of therapies have been proposed for equine warts. Since most lesions resolve spontaneously within a few months of appearance, it is difficult to ascertain the true efficacy of any therapeutic intervention. If lesions persist beyond six to nine months, an underlying immune deficiency should be suspected.

As most horses with warts do not require treatment, in case of esthetic exigencies, cryosurgery—with a two-cycle, freeze-thaw-freeze technique—is a valid treatment. Chemical cautery with trifluoroacetic acid is also considered safe and effective. A solution of 25 g anhydrous trifluoroacetic acid, 3 g water, and 20 g glacial acetic acid is applied to the affected tissues only. Adjacent tissues should be protected with petroleum jelly. Applications are repeated on the fourth and seventh days after initial treatment (Logas and Barbet, 1999). Topical treatment with podophyllin (50% podophyllin, 20% podophyllin in 95% ethyl alcohol, 2% podophyllin in 25% salicylic acid) and undiluted medical-grade dimethyl sulfoxide (DMSO) may be used once daily until remission occurs. There is no scientific evidence to support the theory that surgical excision of some lesions enhances or hastens regression of remaining lesions. Recurrence after surgical excision has been reported (Logas and Barbet, 1999; Scott and Miller, 2003). A variety of immunomodulatory drugs, including mycobacterial cell wall extracts and *Propionibacterium* extracts, have also been recommended for treatment of equine warts. EqStim (immunostimulant) given intravenously has had reported success in both prevention and treatment of equine warts. Any treatment of warts that creates an inflammatory response may increase the risk of white hair and skin depigmentation.

There is also information supporting the use of wart vaccines in the treatment of equine warts. The vaccines are made using excised wart tissue from an affected animal to create a vaccine specifically for use on that individual; this is called an autogenous vaccine. However, its efficacy to treat the warts is controversial. In addition, there are numerous topical products emerging as potential treatments, but to date, there are no studies confirming that any are effective. Bovine papilloma vaccines are not efficacious in equine (Borzacchiello and Roperto, 2008; Nasir and Campo, 2008).

PREVENTION

Because the EPV is so highly contagious, prevention is very difficult if one horse in the herd is infected. Spread of warts can be controlled by keeping a closed herd, restricting entry of new horses, isolating infected animals, and not sharing equipment between horses; however, this is not practically possible at most breeding stables. Skin trauma from the environment or ectoparasites should be minimized. Disinfection of premises and equipment with formaldehyde is recommended after exposure to a horse with warts (Logas and Barbet, 1999; Scott and Miller, 2003).

CONGENITAL PAPILLOMATOSIS

Congenital papillomatosis, also known by common name "baby warts," is the condition where warts are present on the foal skin at birth (http://homepage. usask.ca/~vim458/virology/studpages2007/Kahuna/definitions.html). When a mare is infected with EPV during pregnancy, the virus can cross the placenta and infect the foal in utero. This, however, does not mean that the warts are inherited; warts are an infectious disease that may affect any breed or sex. (Pascoe et al., 1999; White et al., 2004) (*http://homepage.usask.ca/~vim458/ virology/studpages2007/Kahuna/definitions.html*). Most of the time the foal will have a single wart; sizes can vary from very small (a few millimeters in diameter) to quite a large size, even up to 20 cm and may be located anywhere in the body, including rib cage, head, hind legs, and forehead (Garma-Aviña et al., 1981; Atwell and Summers, 1977). They are usually gray or grayish pink in color and may be flat or look like flattened cauliflower (Pascoe et al., 1999; Scott and Miller, 2003). Unlike other equine warts, congenital warts do not usually regress spontaneously and are required to be treated. They are removed by surgical excision or ligation.

AURAL PLAQUES

Aural plaques—also known as ear or pinnal papilloma, papillary acanthosis, hyperplastic dermatitis of the ear, or more commonly ear fungus—can occur in horses of any age, breed, or sex, manifesting as well-demarcated raised, depigmented, hyperkeratotic plaques of 1–3 cm in diameter on the inner surface of the ear pinnae. Similar lesions may be present around the anus and external genitalia (Binninger and Piper, 1968; Scott and Miller,

2003). Black flies (*Simulium* sp.) are likely the mechanical vectors, which are active at dawn and dusk, when they attack the head, ears, and ventral abdomen of horses. Usually both ears are affected, and the lesions may be worse in the summer. Aural plaques rarely, if ever, spontaneously resolve and are susceptible to fly bites and secondary infection.

ETIOLOGY

Equine aural plaques are caused by a papillomavirus. Black flies (*Simulium* sp.) may act as the mechanical vector. These flies are active at dawn and dusk, when they attack the head, ears, and ventral abdomen of horses. Equine papilloma viral (EPV) particles have been demonstrated in these lesions by electron microscopy and immunohistochemistry (Fairley and Haines, 1992; Williams, 1997; Scott and Miller, 2003); however, EPV DNA for definitive identification of the virus could not be detected in the aural plaques cases (Postey et al., 2007).

CLINICAL SIGNS

Aural plaques are clinically recognized as different from warts. Clinically, the lesions are characterized by flat desquamated, depigmented, hyperkeratotic coalescing papules and plaques localized to the concave aspect of the pinna. Sometimes they look roundish, raised coalescence of small papules giving a cauliflower-like appearance like other warts (Pascoe et al., 1999; Sousa et al., 2008). Usually horses over one year of age are affected. Often both pinnae are affected. In addition to the ears, the anus and external genitalia can also be affected. The plaques can be limited to just a few and remain static for some time, or the condition can progress to involve the entire inner surface of the ear. The ear plaques do not spontaneously regress as the facial warts do. The flat smooth lesions develop a waxy coating that can appear flaky, which can be misleading when making a diagnosis. Because of this, the condition has often been referred to as ear fungus, but there is no fungal infection. Plaques are not sensitive, pruritic, or painful but may be considered esthetically displeasing by owners. Similar lesions may occur around the anus and vulva (Williams, 1997; Scott and Miller, 2003).

PATHOGENESIS AND PATHOLOGY

The pathogenesis of aural plaques in horses is unclear. Lesions often appear worse in the summer and fall, possibly because of fly irritation. Aural plaque lesions are usually asymptomatic, but in some cases the direct effect of the fly bite causes dermatitis and discomfort. Histologically, the lesions are characterized by mildy papillated epidermal hyperplasia and marked hyperkeratosis. Increased size of keratohyalin granules, poikilocytosis, and hypomelanosis may also be present in the epidermis with abrupt change between the normal and the affected epithelium (Sousa et al., 2008). Intranuclear viral particles have been seen in electron microscopic studies.

DIAGNOSIS

Diagnosis of aural plaques is usually based on the clinical signs, history, and appearance. Biopsy is usually not indicated, but if the diagnosis is in question, a biopsy specimen may be collected for histologic diagnosis. The lesions appear histologically identical to *verruca plana*, a wartlike disease of humans, with epithelial proliferation and epidermal hypomelanosis (Sousa et al., 2008).

TREATMENT AND CONTROL

There is no documented treatment for aural plaques. There are anecdotal reports on a variety of topical preparations, but there are no controlled studies confirming effectiveness. Treatment with a soothing ointment, like Mentholatum, to the inner surface of the ear can be helpful. Even various corticosteroid/antibiotic ointments may be tried with some extent of success. These ointments will relieve the inflammation, but the plaques remain. The product tretinoin (Retin-A) has been reported to effectively treat this condition (Olsen et al., 1992). It is recommended to keep the inner surface of the ear clean, provided with fly protection, and to leave the lesions completely alone. However, in severe cases where the lesions coalesce into a rather large mass, which usually result in the horse to become severely head shy and painful, the lesions may be excised by cryosurgery—that is, freezing with liquid nitrogen—although aural plaques often return after surgery (Pascoe et al., 1999; Scott and Miller, 2003). The main complication or risk with using cryotherapy in this area is causing damage to the thin cartilage within the ear, which can cause disfigurement as the ear heals and scar tissue forms. Use of fly repellents is recommended to minimize secondary irritation or infection of lesions. Also horses should be stabled during the fly's feeding times.

EQUINE SARCOIDS

Equine sarcoids are most common (accounting for up to 30% of tumors), locally aggressive fibroblastic dermatologic neoplasm of horses, donkeys, and mules with a high rate of recurrence after surgical removal (Ragland et al., 1970; Goldschmidt and Hendrick, 2002; Ackermann, 2007; Postey et al., 2007). They may be single or multiple and can occur at any location, although they have a predilection for the head, neck, legs, and ventral abdomen. They frequently occur at sites of previous injury and scarring (Marti et al., 1993; Scott and Miller, 2003). Sarcoids can have the typical cauliflower-like appearance of warts; they can be flattened or a combination, with many sarcoids, may ulcerate, and bleed causing discomfort and attracting flies (Postey et al., 2007; Radostits et al., 2007). Young adult horses three to six years of age are most commonly affected. These tumors are seldom life threatening but may cause esthetic and performance-limiting problems, depending on their location, size, and rate of growth. Some sarcoids resemble equine papillomas; however, the spontaneous regression that is common with equine papillomas is rarely seen with sarcoids (Brostrom, 1995; Ragland and Spencer, 1969; Sellon, 2007).

Equine sarcoids are therefore considered to be the result of a nonproductive BPV infection, the viral DNA persisting episomally (Amtmann et al., 1980). However, a direct causal relationship has not been established (Chambers et al., 2003), and involvement of other PVs has not been investigated. Fibromatous lesions exhibiting histologic characteristics similar to those of dermal sarcoids and bovine fibropapillomas were identified in the dermis of ten spontaneous and experimentally induced equine warts, suggesting that fibropapillomas in horses may be induced by EPV (Hamada et al., 1990).

ETIOLOGY
The viral cause of the equine sarcoid was suggested as early as in 1936 based on tumor's pattern of spread (Jackson, 1936). Later on, successful transmission of tumor in healthy horses by inoculation with cell-free supernatant from minced sarcoid tissue evidenced its viral etiology (Voss, 1969), although unlike natural sarcoids, experimentally induced sarcoids showed spontaneous regression. Then, after several futile attempts by several workers, Olson and Cook (1951) demonstrated that intradermal inoculation of horses with cell-free extracts from bovine papilloma tissue containing bovine papillomavirus (BPV) caused lesions resembling equine sarcoids. Equine cutaneous papillomaviruses, the etiologic agent of equine warts, are not causally related to equine sarcoids (O' Banion et al., 1986). Most equine sarcoids examined employing molecular hybridization, restriction enzyme analysis, PCR, and in situ hybridization (ISH) techniques have revealed demonstrable *Bovine papillomavirus* (BPV) DNA sequences (Amtmann et al., 1980; Angelos et al., 1991; Teifke et al., 1994). However, the reported detection rate varied between study groups, ranging from 73% (Bloch et al., 1994) to 88–91% (Martens et al., 2001a, b) and 96–100% (Carr et al., 2001a, b; Otten et al., 1993), which is attributed to the differences in tumor collection and preservation methodology as the lowest rates of detection are seen in studies using tumors preserved in formaldehyde for long periods of time. Of at least six distinct BPV, BPV types 1, 2, and 5 are frequently identified in association with equine sarcoid (Jarrett, 1985).

BPV is very resistant to physical and chemical inactivation. It remains viable after thirty minutes at 67°C (152.5°F), is stable at a pH between 4 and 8, is stable in ether, and survives in 50% glycerol when frozen or lyophilized. Because of these properties, the BPV may be able to survive for a long time in the environment (Bogaert et al., 2005, 2008).

Despite the consistent finding of papillomavirus DNA in the sarcoid lesions, papillomavirus particles have not been demonstrated, and the disease is, therefore, considered to be a nonproductive infection in which viral DNA exists episomally (Amtmann et al., 1980; Lancaster, 1981; Yuan et al., 2007). Carr et al. (2001b) analyzed twenty-three sarcoids by Western blot and demonstrated the presence of the BPV E5 protein in all tumors (including one in which the amount of viral DNA was too low for detection), whereas E5 was absent in all the nonsarcoid samples. However, sequence analysis of BPV DNA extracted from sarcoids has revealed two minor differences in the sequence of the BPV E5 open reading frame in donkey sarcoids compared with the published bovine sequences (Reid et al., 1994). Yet another report suggested absolute identity between the BPV E5 sequences in sarcoids and the published BPV sequences (Carr et al., 2001a), indicating the possibility of equine sarcoid-specific variants of BPV. Bogaert et al. (2008) have detected high prevalence of bovine papillomaviral DNA in the normal skin of equine sarcoid-affected (57% positive) and healthy horses (30% positive), suggesting latent infection and a widespread occurrence of BPV in the horse population. In yet another study, screening of peripheral blood mononuclear cell (PBMC) DNA derived from horses with and without BPV-1/2–induced sarcoid lesions demonstrated the exclusive presence of E5, but not L1, in PBMCs of BPV-1/2–infected equines (Brandt et al., 2008). This suggested deletion or interruption of L1 gene in PBMCs of BPV-1/2–infected equines and role of PBMCs to serve as host cells for BPV-1/2 DNA and contribute to virus latency.

EPIDEMIOLOGY

The incidence of sarcoid tumors in the general equine population is not known. Studies on the epidemiology of the equine sarcoid have been hampered by a lack of population data and the low prevalence of disease in animals usually kept as individuals or in small groups (Chambers et al., 2003). Ragland et al. (1966) described an outbreak of sarcoids in a small group of horses while postulating on the virus etiology of the disease, and Reid et al. (1994) estimated an incidence of 0.6 cases per 100 animal years in a population of donkeys. In a retrospective study, sarcoids accounted for 0.7% of all equine cases presented to the Cornell University Veterinary Hospital between 1975 and 1987 and to the Ohio State University between 1976 and 1985 (Marti et al., 1993). Similarly, the occurrence of disease has been described in association with equine leucocyte antigens within particular breeds and bloodlines (more frequently in Quarter Horses and less frequently in Standardbred horses) (Lazary et al., 1985; Meredith et al., 1986; Angelos et al., 1988; Brostrom et al., 1988). Risk factors are confounding, although MHC type, age, and sex are of significance. Overall, young males appear to be at more risk of disease (Mohammed et al., 1992; Reid et al., 1994; Torrontegui and Reid, 1994; Reid and Mohammed, 1997). Surveys have estimated the prevalence of sarcoid at 20% of all equine neoplasms and 36% of all skin tumors (Bolin, 1999).

TRANSMISSION

Although there is strong evidence that BPV types 1 and 2 are the principal causative agent of sarcoids, there is currently no clear evidence of a mode of transmission. Since sarcoids frequently develop in areas subjected to trauma or at sites of wounds six to eight months after wound healing, it has been proposed to be due to flies acting as a vector as they move between wound sites on different horses. One study has reported the detection of BPV viral DNA sequences in face flies, which are commonly seen around wounds and which tend to frequent the head and neck area, one of the most common areas in which sarcoids occur (Kemp-Symonds, 2000). Furthermore, the same viral DNA sequences were detected in the horses from which the flies were removed. Alternatively, BPV infection may be transmitted via stable management practices, such as the sharing of contaminated tack or passed into existing wounds from contaminated pasture.

CLINICAL SIGNS

Sarcoids are typically found on adult horses of three to six years of age and are common on or around the ears, face, head, ventral abdomen, groin, axillae, limbs, sheath, genitals, between the front legs, and behind the elbow, but they can be anywhere on the body (Goodrich et al., 1998). Approximately 30–50% of affected horses have multiple lesions (Scott and Miller, 2003). Lesions are usually firm on palpation because of fibroblastic proliferation. The overlying epidermis may be thick, tough, and hyperkeratotic or ulcerated. Sarcoid tumors may occur in the subcutaneous tissues as firm, movable masses with an intact covering of grossly normal skin (Piscopo, 1999). Many times a sarcoid will remain static and relatively insensitive, but they can become locally invasive in their growth and, depending on their location on the body, become quite painful.

The tumors are classified according to their gross appearance as verrucous, fibroblastic, mixed verrucous and fibroblastic, or occult (Hargis and Ginn, 2007). The verrucous type is a small wartlike growth usually measuring less than 6 cm in diameter with a dry, rough, horny, cauliflower-like surface, and variable alopecia. They can remain static in size and shape for years but may undergo transformation and become fibroblastic if traumatized (Tarwid, 1985). Verrucous sarcoids appear more frequently around the face, body, groin, and sheath areas. The fibroblastic type of sarcoid is more variable in appearance and can range from firm nodules within the dermis with intact dermis to a large mass, greater than 25 cm in diameter, with an ulcerated surface prone to hemorrhage and resembling exuberant granulation tissue. The mixed type is a transitional form in which verrucous sarcoid becomes a fibroblastic type as a result of trauma or biopsy. The occult form consists of a slow-growing, slightly thickened area of skin with slight surface roughening and alopecia that remain static for a long period. This presentation is partially or totally devoid of hair and seems to favor areas of the body with sparse hair growth, including the skin around the mouth, eyes, neck, and medial aspects of the forearm and thigh.

PATHOGENESIS
In addition to epitheliotropism, some papilloma virus, including BPV types 1 and 2, can also infect fibroblasts and induce fibroepithelial tumors, causing benign fibropapillomas in cattle. BPV 1 and 2 have a genome of 7900 bp of ds DNA, with at least nine potential reading frames, and can be divided into two major regions. The early (E) region encodes the transforming proteins (E5, E6, and E7) and the replication and transcription regulatory proteins (E1 and E2). The late (L) region encodes the viral structural proteins, L1 and L2. During acute virus infection, replication of the virus genome is linked strictly to the state of differentiation of the infected cell. In papilloma formation, for example, the virus infects initially the basal epithelial cells, where E region genes are expressed in undifferentiated basal and suprabasal layers. The viral DNA is replicated in differentiating spinous and granular layers, whereas the expression of L region genes is limited to the terminally differentiated cells of the squamous layer, where the new virus particles are encapsidated and released into the environment as the cells die. Initiation of malignant transformation is linked to the deregulated expression of the early (E) virus genes, resulting in uncontrolled proliferation of the infected cells (Campo, 1997, 2002).

The major BPV transforming protein, E5, binds to and constitutively activates the platelet-derived growth factor- receptor (PDGF-R) in transformed cells by forming a stable complex with the receptor, causing its dimerization and transphosphorylation. This, in turn, activates a receptor signalling cascade, resulting in an intracellular growth stimulatory signal (DiMaio and Mattoon, 2001). E5 also interacts with 16K ductin/subunit c, a component of gap junctions and vacuolar ATPase, leading to the downregulation of gap junction intracellular communication with the consequent isolation of the infected cell from its neighbors (Faccini et al., 1996). Interaction with 16K also leads to alkalinization of the endosomes and the Golgi apparatus (Straight et al., 1995; Schapiro et al., 2000), with consequent intracellular retention of MHC class I molecules (Ashrafi et al., 2002; Marchetti et al., 2002). The absence of MHC class I from the cell surface helps the infected cells to evade host immunosurveillance (Ackermann, 2007). Furthermore, E5 activates numerous kinases, including cyclin A-cdk2, MAP, JNK, PI3, and c-Src—thus interfering with proper cell cycle control and signal transduction cascades (Venuti and Campo, 2002).

The actions and interactions of E6 protein with ERC-55/E6BP, a calcium-binding protein (Chen et al., 1995), CBP/p300, a transcriptional coactivator (Zimmermann et al., 2000), paxillin, focal adhesion protein (Tong and Howley, 1997; Tong et al., 1997; Vande Pol et al., 1998), and c subunit of the clathrin adaptor complex AP-1 (Tong et al., 1998) result in disruption of cytoskeleton and vesicular traffic pathways, which are vital for the maintenance of cellular morphology, motility, division and cell-cell and cell-matrix interactions and cell proliferation and differentiation.

In contrast to malignant progression of human papillomavirus-induced lesions that result due to the integration of the viral DNA into the host genome with consequent loss of regulated expression of the transforming viral genes, BPV genomes are maintained episomally during transformation of cells of a nonhost species. As only the early genes are transcribed in order to maintain viral copy number and cellular growth, virus capsids are not formed, probably because the expression of capsid proteins requires the cellular milieu found only in the well-differentiated keratinocytes of the host species (Sousa et al., 1990). Although BPV DNA has been detected widely (Otten et al., 1993; Bogaert et al., 2007; Nasir and Campo, 2008) and mRNA expression for L1 has been shown in equine sarcoids (Nasir and Reid, 1999; Postey et al., 2007; Brandt et al., 2008), there is little evidence for expression of the BPV structural proteins or for virus capsid formation as evidenced by failure of sarcoid extracts to induce warts in cattle in an experimental study (Ragland and Spencer, 1969). Thus, BPV infection of equine fibroblasts appears to be nonproductive. Detection of distinct equine sarcoid–specific variants of BPV in BPV DNA isolates extracted from sarcoids (Otten et al., 1993; Reid et al., 1994), which may affect the functional expression of early virus proteins, have been suggested to be responsible for the different pathogenesis in the sarcoids compared to the papillomas induced by BPV in cattle. In addition to BPV infection, significant association has been found between the MHC class II haplotypes and predisposition to sarcoids, particularly in the Thoroughbred population (Meredith et al., 1986), Swedish halfbreds

(Brostrom et al., 1988) and Swiss Warmbloods (Gerber et al., 1988). Thus, specific MHC class II alleles may be associated with an impaired immune response to BPV and/or other tumor-associated sarcoid antigens.

Pathology

Histopathologically, sarcoids are typically biphasic tumors characterized by fibroblastic and epidermal proliferation; however, epithelial (epidermal) component may be minimal or absent in some tumors, which have extensive ulceration. The lesions of hyperkeratosis, parakeratosis, and with deep extension of thin rete pegs in the dermis are common when the epidermis is intact (Hargis and Ginn, 2007). The dermis contains collagen fibers and fibroblasts in variable proportions. The fibroblasts have plump nuclei and usually prominent nucleoli. The mitotic index is usually low. Fibroblasts at the dermal-epidermal junction are frequently oriented perpendicular to the basement membrane in a "picket fence" pattern, which is a distinctive histologic feature seen in most sarcoids (Martens et al., 2000a). The cells are arranged in a classic whorled interlacing bundles or haphazard arrays of variable density. Tumor margins are typically indistinct, making it very difficult to determine the adequacy of the excision. Occult sarcoids may exhibit only focal epidermal hyperplasia and hyperkeratosis with underlying junctional fibroblastic proliferation (Tarwid, 1985; Martens et al., 2000a; Scott and Miller, 2003; Hargis and Ginn, 2007).

Diagnosis

The diagnosis of equine sarcoid is usually done on the basis of characteristic clinical signs. However, the gross lesions may resemble papillomas, granulation tissue, fungal or bacterial granuloma, habronemiasis, solar keratosis, squamous cell carcinoma, neurofibroma, melanoma, and fibrosarcoma; therefore, histolopathogic examination of biopsy specimens should be performed for a definitive diagnosis. Biopsy of static verrucous and occult sarcoids is usually not indicated because intervention may elicit transformation into an aggressive fibrosarcoma-like lesion. Partial removal of a sarcoid tumor may incite aggressive regrowth of tissue. If possible, wide excision of the entire mass should be performed at biopsy to decrease the likelihood of recurrence. Because autotransplantation of an equine sarcoid tumor may occur, surgical instruments that contact the tumor should not be used on healthy adjacent skin (Tarwid, 1985).

The application of BPV testing in the diagnosis of sarcoids has been examined recently, resulting in a detection rate of 88–91% (Martens et al., 2001a, b). However, the presence of a large amount of connective tissue in some types of sarcoid may affect the ability of PCR amplification to detect viral DNA

(Carr et al., 2001b). Further, detection of viral protein expression in samples apparently negative for viral DNA (Postey et al., 2007) raises the question on the sensitivity of PCR-based tests for BPV DNA in sarcoid lesions. As of now, the PCR detection of BPV DNA would result in a proportion of false negatives. Hence, the application of BPV DNA as a diagnostic test for sarcoids would need to be carefully evaluated and validated.

TREATMENT AND CONTROL

Because of its frequency, equine sarcoid presents a significant problem for horse owners and breeders. Although slow-growing sarcoids often cause minimal trouble to a horse, if they appear in an area where tack or equipment might rub against them (near the mouth where a bit would rest, or on the girth-line), they can crack and bleed frequently, causing significant discomfort. Larger masses are even more troublesome, sometimes splitting and becoming infected by flies and maggots. There's always the possibility that a sarcoid tumor can interfere with normal functions, like when one grows on an eyelid or ear. Spontaneous regression of equine sarcoids is a very rare event. In view of these troubles, a proper treatment of sarcoids is warranted.

Currently, there is no effective therapy available for equine sarcoids, although a wide range of methods are used for the treatment, including surgical excision, autologous vaccination, immune modulation injection of Bacille Calmette-Guérin (BCG), chemotherapy, homeopathy, and cryotherapy (Goodrich et al., 1998; Mattil-Fritz et al., 2008). The specific treatment selected should be determined after consideration of the tumor site, size, type, and aggressiveness; clinical experience of the attending veterinarian; and the availability of services, equipment, and facilities (Bertone and McClure, 1990; McConaghy et al., 1994). Static verrucous and occult sarcoids are usually not treated because intervention may kindle transformation to an aggressive fibroblastic type of sarcoid. The efficacy of these treatments is difficult to assess because of the large variation in tumor size, location, and treatment methods. Most studies have not been controlled and are based on referral populations of horses treated at major clinics or veterinary hospitals, which may not be the overall tumor population in the field but a subset of fast-growing, recurrent, or multiple tumors that have not been successfully treated by field veterinarians. On the other hand, successfully treated sarcoids by private veterinary clinicians may again represent a specific small population of sarcoids that remain quiescent or the rare spontaneous regressors (Goodrich et al., 1998). Frequently, veterinarians will use more than one of these methods in combination, depending on the size and location of the sarcoid and whether it is benign or rapidly growing.

1. **Surgical resection.** Surgical excision is probably the most common approach, although it works best with flat wartlike sarcoids. Vigorously active tumors are more difficult to remove surgically as they have a tendency to recur at the same site. Sarcoids frequently display hyperproliferation or recurrence when treated by surgical excision, which has led some to speculate that this could be due to activation of latent BPV in apparently normal tissue surrounding the lesion. Martens et al. (2001a) used PCR to test for BPV in sarcoids removed by surgery and also tested apparently normal skin around the sarcoids. They found BPV in all the sarcoids and also in the surrounding normal skin. The frequency of detection of BPV in the normal skin decreased as the resection margin was increased. They also found that animals with a surgical margin containing BPV had a greater probability to show local recurrence. These observations confirmed the results of an earlier study where simple scratching induced papillomas in latent papillomavirus containing normal skin (Siegsmund et al., 1991). Surgical resection, even with wide margins of normal tissue, is not generally recommended as a sole therapy for equine sarcoids because of a recurrence rate estimated at 50–64%, mostly within six months (Ragland et al., 1970; McConaghy et al., 1994). Often, surgery is used in combination with other treatment methods. Large tumors might need to be "debulked" (surgically reduced in size) before other methods (adjunctive therapies) can be applied successfully; for example, the visible parts of the tumor might be surgically trimmed as much as possible, and then cryosurgery could be used to freeze the margins of the tumor site (the goal being to kill any remaining tumor cells).

2. **Cryotherapy.** Cryotherapy with liquid nitrogen is a common adjunctive therapy for equine sarcoids after surgical debulking of lesions. One-year cure rates for cryotherapy are estimated at 70–100% (Krahwinkel, 1976; Goodrich et al., 1998). Horses are sedated or anesthetized to facilitate restraint during the procedure. Lesions are frozen two or three times to $-20°-30°C$, with complete thawing to room temperature between each freeze Tissue temperature is monitored with cryoprobes to avoid any unintended damage to sensitive normal tissues in the area and ensure complete freezing of the tumor. Treated tissues undergo necrosis, with local swelling and inflammation. Healing occurs by secondary intention or delayed closure, which may result in scarring or regrowth of white hair from damage to hair follicles (McConaghy et al., 1994). The mean time taken for complete healing is 2.4 months (range, 1.0–3.5 months). Adverse consequences of cryotherapy are usually related to damage adjacent normal tissues, and facial nerve paralysis, septic arthritis, loss of the upper eyelid, and evisceration of the globe have been described

(Lane, 1977; Fretz and Barber, 1980). However, some reports suggested that cryotherapy may enhance the immune response of the horse, leading to spontaneous regression of multiple sarcoids (Lane, 1977).

3. *Carbon dioxide laser therapy.* Equine sarcoid can be treated with carbon dioxide (CO_2) laser therapy with a success rate (of 62–81%), without any recurrence at the same site for six to twelve months (Carstanjen et al., 1997). However, about 58% of equids developed new sarcoid lesions elsewhere on the body after laser therapy. Swelling is minimal after laser resection, and the horse exhibits minimal pain to palpation of the surgical wound. If sufficient normal skin is available, primary closure of the surgical site can be performed (Goodrich et al., 1998). Treatment with CO_2 laser requires specialized equipment and training.

4. *Irradiation.* Radiation therapy (brachytherapy) is another modality to treat sarcoids with success rates of up to 95% (Goodrich et al., 1998; Turrel and Koblik, 1983; Theon and Pascoe, 1995), particularly those that are very large or difficult to excise because of their location. To the owners, radiation may appear daunting as the horse is required to remain absolutely still for the treatments (which only last a couple of minutes each) by placing under general anesthesia. The usual regime is six treatments over a three-week period. Brachytherapy provides continuous delivery of a high radiation dose directly to the tumor while sparing adjacent healthy tissue. Isotopes used for interstitial brachytherapy of equine sarcoids include permanently implantable seeds of radon[222] or gold[198]; removable needles of radium[226], cobalt[60], or iridium[192]; and iridium[192] seeds. Response rates range from 50–100% (Goodrich et al., 1998). Hyperthermia may be combined with brachytherapy for synergistic tumor killing (Turrel et al., 1985). In a study of 155 horses treated with iridium[192] interstitial brachytherapy for periocular tumors, adverse effects included palpebral fibrosis (10.4%), cataract (7.8%), keratitis and corneal ulceration (6.9%), permanent hair loss (21.7), and hair dyspigmentation (78.3%) (Theon and Pascoe, 1995).

5. *Photodynamic therapy.* Photodynamic therapy involves the administration of a photosensitizer to a patient. The drug accumulates in tumor tissue and is activated by visible light to a higher energy state from which free radicals and reactive oxygen are formed. Intratumoral injections of the photodynamic agent hypericin into three sarcoid tumors on a donkey resulted in an 81% reduction in tumor volume at the end of twenty-five days therapy and a 90% reduction after two months (Martens et al., 2000b).

6. *Immunotherapy.* Injection with immune-stimulant drugs is a useful approach with sarcoids that are in locations (like eyelid) difficult to approach surgically or when multiple tumors are involved. Cosmetically,

this approach has the advantage of far less visible scarring than surgery, but its success rate varies from horse to horse. One approach that has been used over the past couple of decades is the injection of BCG (Bacille Calmette-Guréin) vaccine, also used to combat tuberculosis in humans. BCG serves as an immunostimulant, enhancing the body's response to tumor-specific antigens. Its usefulness seems to be limited to small tumors, and occasionally the treatment seems to stimulate sarcoids to become aggressive. As a result, BCG has fallen out of favor as a sarcoid treatment in recent years. Treatments are administered by intralesional injection every two to three weeks for an average of four treatments. (Scott and Miller, 2003). Debulking before initiating intralesional therapy is recommended. Reported response rates for treatment of periorbital sarcoids with BCG range from 69–100%, with best results for treatment of fibroblastic and nodular lesions (Lavach et al., 1985; Owen and Jagger, 1987; Knottenbelt and Kelly, 2000). Remission rate with BCG therapy of sarcoid lesions elsewhere on the body is approximately 48%, with the poorest response for lesions on the legs and in the axillary region. Occasional reports of anaphylactic reactions after repeated use of BCG have led to recommendations that horses be medicated with flunixin meglumine and corticosteroids before BCG injection (Vanselow et al., 1988; Scott and Miller, 2003). Autogenous vaccines, prepared from surgically debulked and resected tumor tissue, have also been used as immunotherapeutic agents for equine sarcoid tumors with various degrees of success (Page and Tiffany, 1967; Brostrom, 1995; Kinnunen et al., 1999). The major viral structural protein L1 has the intrinsic ability to assemble into viruslike particles (VLPs) in a wide range of experimental systems, which resemble infectious virions, by inducing virus-neutralizing antibodies and by mounting strong cytolytic T cell response against the L1 protein (Rudolf et al., 2001; Schiller and Lowy, 2001; Ohlschlager et al., 2003). Chimeric viruslike particles (CVLPs) of BPV 1 L1–E7 has been developed and tried for the immunotherapy of equine sarcoid, which induced a robust anti-L1 antibody response in sarcoid-affected horses with a clear improvement of the clinical status after treatment in terms of the reduction of tumor numbers per horse and regression of sarcoids (Mattil-Fritz et al., 2008). However, further clinical trials and evaluations are needed for their usefulness in field conditions.

7. *Chemotherapy.* A variety of topical and intralesional chemotherapy protocols have been described for treatment of equine sarcoids. These therapies are usually applied after surgical debulking of a lesion but may be efficacious as a sole therapy for small tumors. Administration of chemotherapeutic agents should be undertaken with caution to avoid human contact with potentially toxic agents. Daily topical application of 5-fluorouracil, a fluorinated

pyrimidine antimetabolite that interferes with DNA biosynthesis, or podophyllin, an irritant cathartic, has been used successfully to treat some sarcoid lesions (McConaghy et al., 1994; Piscopo, 1999; Foy et al., 2002). Treatment may be continued for up to ninety days. Topical 5-fluorouracil cream applied daily to occult and verrucose periorbital lesions (not directly on margin of eyelid) was successful in eliminating lesions in six of nine horses (Knottenbelt and Kelly, 2000). The other three horses improved, but lesions recurred in a fibroblastic form over the next three to thirty-six months. An experimental topical ointment, containing a variety of heavy metals and the antimitotic compound 5-fluorouracil and thiouracil, was described by Knottenbelt and Kelly (2000). The ointment is applied daily or every other day for three to five treatments. A response is anticipated in five to ten weeks with necrosis and sloughing of sarcoid tissue.

Intralesional injections or implants or chemotherapeutic agents result in a high local drug concentration for extended periods. Implants may consist of a high-molecular-weight collagen matrix that contains a chemotherapeutic agent (cisplatin or 5-fluorouracil) and a vasoactive modifier such as epinephrine (McConaghy et al., 1994; Foy et al., 2002). Alternatively, sterilized sesame oil may be used to slow drug release and increase tumor/ plasma drug concentration ratio. Intratumoral treatment of nineteen horses with cisplatin resulted in a one-year disease-free period for 87% of horses (Page and Tiffany, 1967). Theon et al. (1994) also reported a 92% and 77% relapse-free survival rate at one and four years, respectively, after surgical debulking combined with perisurgical wound injection of cisplatin sesame oil injections. Perioperative cisplatin in sesame oil injections are recommended when surgical debulking results in a site that cannot be surgically closed and an open wound that is less than 5 cm in largest diameter. The first treatment is administered at surgery. Tumor dosage is planned as 1 mg of cisplatin per cubic centimeter of tissue to be injected. All visible tumor tissue and a margin of normal tissue of 1–2 cm should be injected. The target volume is injected through multiple sites using a parallel-row or field-block technique. Rows of injections should be 0.6–0.8 cm apart. Number and frequency of treatments vary with differing protocols. A standard therapy may include four intratumoral treatment sessions at two-week intervals (Theon, 1997).

8. Electrochemotherapy. Electrochemotherapy (ECT) is a treatment modality that uses a combination of chemotherapeutic drug administration with the direct application of electric pulses to skin tumors using a technique called electropermeabilization, which is a method that uses electric field pulses to induce an electrically mediated reorganization of the plasma membrane of cells. Since some chemotherapy drugs such as bleomycin or cisplatin have poor membrane permeability, they cannot enter certain types of cells, including skin cells. When electric pulse is applied to the tumor, the membranes of the cancer cells become permeable (electropermeabilization), allowing the exogenous drugs to enter and kill the abnormal tumor cells (Cemazar et al., 2008). ECT has been found to be a highly effective, affordable, and simple procedure that might prove to be the cure for equine skin tumors, including sarcoids (Sersa et al., 2002; Cemazar et al., 2008). In addition, ECT functions to keep the drug at the site of the lesion and prevents cancer cell dissemination. Preclinical studies have demonstrated excellent antitumor effectiveness of electrochemotherapy on different animal models and various tumor types, minimal toxicity, and safety of the procedure. Based on results of preclinical studies, clinical studies were conducted in human patients, which demonstrated pronounced antitumor effectiveness of electrochemotherapy with 80–85% objective responses of the treated cutaneous and SC tumors (Cemazar et al., 2008). ECT has shown a 100% response rate on small equine sarcoid tumors (less than 5 cm) and 98% on tumors of all sizes for more than twenty-four months duration of response (Rols et al., 2002; Tamzali et al., 2001, 2003, 2007).

PREVENTION

There are no known management strategies or treatment techniques to prevent development of sarcoid tumors in horses.

CONCLUSION

The common wart occurs in horses less than three years of age (most commonly in those less than one year of age). The lesions are classically wartlike with multiple frondlike projections growing from the infected skin. The most commonly affected areas of the body are the lips and muzzle, and less commonly the eyelids, genitalia, and lower legs. These warts, being of viral etiology (equine and bovine papilloma viruses), are very contagious to susceptible horses, and the spread can be limited by isolating affected animals and carefully disinfecting contaminated equipment. These warts typically undergo a spontaneous remission within two to three months with virtually no scarring of the affected tissue.

Ear papillomas (aural plaques) are typically roundish raised, depigmented lesions on the inside surface of the ears. The condition usually occurs in horses over one year of age. In addition to the ears, the anus and external genitalia can also be affected. Unlike common warts, the aural plaques do not spontaneously regress. Black fly may contribute to the condition by causing the predisposing skin damage that allows viral invasion, and the black fly also plays a role in transmitting the virus from horse to horse. There is no documented treatment for aural plaques. The compound tretinoin (Retin-A) has been reported to effectively treat this condition. The best way is to keep the inner ear clean, provide fly protection, and to leave the lesions completely alone.

Sarcoids are one of the most common skin tumors in the horse. They usually occur in younger horses but have been known to occur in horses of any age. Common locations for sarcoids include the legs, eyelids, and ears. Sarcoids are known to occur in areas of prior trauma and may grow in areas where there was previously a wound. There are several different types of sarcoids, which have variable appearances and different growth patterns and behaviors. The most common types of sarcoids include verrucous, fibroblastic, mixed, and occult. Quarter Horses appear to be the ones most commonly affected with sarcoids, whereas Standardbreds are rarely affected. The cause of sarcoids has been investigated and both genetic, and viral components may play a role in their occurrence. Bovine papilloma virus (BPV) types 1 and 2 have been shown to be present in sarcoids and normal horse skin but is changed to a tumor-producing form in sarcoids.

There have been many different treatments described for equine sarcoids. The multiplicity of treatments reported reflects the lack of a simple and effective treatment. The probability of recurrence after any treatment increases with both the increasing size of tumor and if it has been treated previously without success. Surgical excision is commonly acknowledged to have a high rate of recurrence (50–64% failure rate). Wide margins (or removing a lot of normal skin around the sarcoid) are recommended, but may not be possible due to the location (next to a joint) or may result in an unacceptable cosmetic outcome (around the eye or ear). Other therapies include cryotherapy (freezing) and laser-assisted excision, which have variable success. Some therapies aimed at enhancing the immune response to the tumor, such as a BCG (an immune stimulant) injection and autogenous vaccines, have been tried, but are not proven. These often require repeated injections and have variable success rates. Radiation therapy has been described as a successful long-term treatment for sarcoids, most frequently in the form of brachytherapy. Injecting the sarcoid with chemotherapy drugs (such as cisplatin and 5-flourouracil) has been described and is moderately successful. Treatments are given in a variety of ways but often at two-week intervals for a total of four or more injections. Side effects that have been observed include significant local skin reactions. Recent development of electrochemotherapy, a combination of chemotherapy and electropermeabilization, appears to be quite promising in successful treatment of sarcoids.

REFERENCES

1. Ackermann, M. R. 2007. Chronic inflammation and wound healing. In *Pathologic basis of veterinary diseases*, 4th ed., M. D. McGavin and J. F. Zachary, 161–162. St. Louis, Missouri: Mosby Elsevier.

2. Amtmann, E., Muller, H. and Sauer, G. 1980. Equine connective tissue tumors contain unintegrated bovine papilloma virus DNA. *J. Virol.* 35:962–964.

3. Angelos, J. A., Oppenheim, Y., Rebhun, W., Mohammed, H. and Antczak, D. F. 1988. Evaluation of breed as a risk factor for sarcoid and uveitis in horses. *Anim. Genet.* 19:417–425.

4. Angelos, J. A., Marti, E., Lazary, S. and Carmichael, L. E. 1991. Characterization of BPV-like DNA in equine sarcoids. *Arch. Virol.* 119:95–109.

5. Antonsson, A. and Hansson, B. G. 2002. Healthy skin of many animal species harbors papillomaviruses which are closely related to their human counterparts. *J. Virol.* 76:12537–12542.

6. Ashrafi, G. H., Tsirimonaki, E., Marchetti, B., O'Brien, P. M., Sibbet, G. J., Andrew, L. and Campo, M. S. 2002. Down-regulation of MHC class I by bovine papillomavirus E5 oncoproteins. *Oncogene* 21:248–259.

7. Atwell, R. B. and Summers, P. M. 1977. Congenital papilloma in a foal. *Aust. Vet. J.* 53:299.

8. Bertone, A. L. and McClure, J. J. 1990. Therapy for sarcoids. *Compr. Contin. Educ. Pract. Vet.* 12:262–265.

9. Binninger, C. E. and Piper, R. C. 1968. Hyperplastic dermatitis of the equine ear. *J. Am. Vet. Med. Assoc.* 153:69–75.

10. Bloch, N., Breen, M. and Spradbrow, P. B. 1994. Genomic sequences of bovine papillomaviruses in formalin-fixed sarcoids from Australian horses revealed by polymerase chain reaction. *Vet. Microbiol.* 41:163–172.

11. Bogaert, L., Martens, A., De Baere, C. and Gasthuys, F. 2005. Detection of bovine papillomavirus DNA on the normal skin and in the habitual surroundings of horses with and without equine sarcoids. *Res. Vet. Sci.* 79:253–258.

12. Bogaert, L., Martens, A., Van Poucke, M., Ducatelle, R., De Cock, H., Dewulf, J., De Baere, C., Peelman, L. and Gasthuys, F. 2008. High prevalence of bovine papillomaviral DNA in the normal skin of equine sarcoid-affected and healthy horses. *Vet Microbiol.* 129:58–68.

13. Bogaert, L., Van Poucke, M., De Baere, C., Dewulf, J., Peelman, L., Ducatelle, R., Gasthuys, F. and Martens, A. 2007. Bovine papillomavirus load and mRNA expression, cell proliferation and p53 expression in four clinical types of equine sarcoid. *J. Gen. Virol.* 88:2155–2161.

14. Bolin, D. C. 1999. Equine sarcoid. *Equine Dis. Quart.* 7:1.

15. Borzacchiello, G. and Roperto, F. 2008. *Bovine papillomaviruses*, papillomas and cancer in cattle. *Vet. Res.* 39:1–19.

16. Brandt, S., Haralambus, R., Schoster, A., Kirnbauer, R. and Stanek, C. 2008. Peripheral blood mononuclear cells represent a reservoir of bovine papillomavirus DNA in sarcoid-affected equines. *J. Gen. Virol.* 89:1390–1395.

17. Brostrom, H., Fahlbrink, E., Dubath, M. L. and Lazary, S. 1988. Association between equine leucocyte antigens (ELA) and equine sarcoid tumours in the population of Swedish halfbreds and some of their families. *Vet. Immunol. Immunopathol.* 19:215–223.

18. Brostrom, H. 1995. Equine sarcoids. A clinical and epidemiological study in relation to equine leucocyte antigens (ELA). *Acta Vet. Scand.* 36:223–236.

19. Campo, M. S. 1997. Bovine papillomavirus and cancer. *Vet. J.* 154:175–188.

20. Campo, M. S. 2002. Animal models of papillomavirus pathogenesis. *Virus Res.* 89:249–261.

21. Carr, E. A., Théon, A. P., Madewell, B. R., Hitchcock, M. E., Schlegel, R. and Schiller, J. T. 2001a. Expression of a transforming gene (E5) of bovine papillomavirus in sarcoids obtained from horses. *Am J Vet Res.* 62:1212–217.

22. Carr, E. A., Theon, A. P., Madewell, B. R., Griffey, S. M. and Hitchcock, M. E. 2001b. Bovine papillomavirus DNA in neoplastic and nonneoplastic tissues obtained from horses with and without sarcoids in the western United States. *Am. J. Vet. Res.* 62:741–744.

23. Carstanjen, B., Jordan, P. and Lepage, O. M. 1997. Carbon dioxide laser as a surgical instrument for sarcoid therapy: A retrospective study on 60 cases. *Can. Vet. J.* 38:773–776.

24. Carter, G. R. and Wise, D. J. 2005. Papillomaviridae: A concise review of veterinary virology. International Veterinary Information Service, Ithaca, NY (www.ivis.org). Last updated: 9-Jun-2005; A3412.0605 (accessed on 22 February, 2009).

25. Castro, A. E. and Heuschele, W. P. 1992. *Veterinary diagnostic virology: A practitioners guide.* Mosby-year Book Inc. 171–177.

26. Cemazar, M., Tamzali, Y., Sersa, G., Tozon, N., Mir, L. M., Miklavcic, D., Lowe, R. and Teissie, J. 2008. Electrochemotherapy in veterinary oncology. *J. Vet. Int. Med.* 22:826–831.

27. Chambers, G., Ellsmore, V. A., O'Brien, P. M., Reid, S. W. J., Love, S., Campo, M. S. and Nasir, L. 2003. Association of bovine papillomavirus with the equine sarcoid. *J. Gen. Virol.* 84:1055–1062.

28. Chen, J. J., Reid, C. E., Band, V. and Androphy, E. J. 1995. Interaction of papillomavirus E6 oncoproteins with a putative calcium-binding protein. *Science* 269:529–531.

29. Christensen, N. D. 2005. Cottontail rabbit papillomavirus (CRPV) model system to test antiviral and immunotherapeutic strategies. *Antivir. Chem. Chemother* 16:355–362.

30. Coggins, L. W., Ma, J. Q., Slater, A. A. and Campo, M. S. 1985. Sequence homologies between bovine papillomavirus genomes mapped by a novel low-stringency heteroduplex method. *Virology* 143:603–611.

31. Cook, R. H. and Olson, C. 1951. Experimental transmission of cutaneous papilloma of the horse. *Am. J. Pathol.* 27:1087–1097.

32. de Villiers, E. M., Fauquet, C., Broker, T. R., Bernard, H. U. and zur Hausen, H. 2004. Classification of papillomaviruses. *Virol.* 324:17–27.

33. DiMaio, D. and Mattoon, D. 2001. Mechanisms of cell transformation by papillomavirus E5 proteins. *Oncogene* 20:7866–7873.

34. Faccini, A. M., Cairney, M., Ashrafi, G. H., Finbow, M. E., Campo, M. S. and Pitts, J. D. 1996. The bovine papillomavirus type 4 E8 protein binds to ductin and causes loss of gap junctional intercellular communication in primary fibroblasts. *J. Virol.* 70:9041–9045.

35. Fairley, R. A. and Haines, D. M. 1992. The electron microscopic and immunohistochemical demonstration of a papillomavirus in equine aural plaques. *Vet. Pathol.* 29:79–81.

36. Fakhry, C. and Gillison, M. L. 2006. Clinical implications of human papillomavirus in head and neck cancers. *J. Clin. Oncol.* 24:2606–2611.

37. Foy, J. M., Rashmir-Rave, A. M. and Brashier, M. K. 2002. Common equine skin tumors. *Compr. Contin. Educ. Pract. Vet.* 24:242–254.

38. Fretz, P. B. and Barber, S. M. 1980. Prospective analysis of cryosurgery as the sole treatment for equine sarcoids. *Vet. Clin. North. Am. Small Anim. Clin.* 10:847.

39. Fulton, R. E., Doane, F. W. and Macpherson, L. W. 1970. The fine structure of equine papillomas and the equine papillomavirus. *J. Ultrastruct. Res.* 30:328–343.

40. Garma-Aviña, A., Valli, V. E. and Lumsden, J. H. 1981. Equine congenital cutaneous papillomatosis: A report of 5 cases. *Equine Vet. J.* 13:59–61.

41. Gerber, H., Dubath, M. L. and Lazary, L. 1988. Association between predisposition to equine sarcoid and MHC in multiple-case families. In *Equine infectious diseases: Proceedings of the Fifth International Conference*, ed. D. G. Powel, 272–277. Kentucky: University Press.

42. Ghim, S. J., Rector, A., Delius, H., Sundberg, J. P., Jenson, A. B. and Van Ranst, M. 2004. Equine papillomavirus type 1: Complete nucleotide sequence and characterization of recombinant virus-like particles composed of the EcPV-1 L1 major capsid protein. *Biochem. Biophys. Res. Commun.* 324:1108–1115.

9. EQUINE PAPILLOMATOSIS

43. Goldschmidt, M. H. and Hendrick, M. J. 2002. Equine sarcoid. In *Tumours in domestic animals*, 4th ed., D. J. Meuten, 88–89. Iowa: Iowa State University Press.

44. Goodrich, L., Gerber, H., Marti, E. and Antczak, D. F. 1998. Equine sarcoids. *Vet. Clin. North. Am. Equine Pract.* 14:607–623.

45. Hamada, M., Oyamada, T., Yoshikawa, H., Yoshikawa, T., and Itakura, C. 1990. Histopathological development of equine cutaneous papillomas. *J. Comp. Pathol.* 102:393–403.

46. Hargis, A. M. and Ginn, P. E. 2007. The integument. In *Pathologic basis of veterinary diseases*, 4th ed., ed. M. D. McGavin and J. F. Zachary, 1177–1179. St. Louis, Missouri: Mosby Elsevier.

47. Jackson, C. 1936. The incidence and pathology of tumours of domesticated animals in South Africa. Onderstepoort. *J. Vet. Sci. Anim. Ind.* 6:378–385.

48. Jarrett, W. F. H. 1985. The natural history of bovine papilloma-virus infections. In *Advances in viral oncology*, ed. G. Klein. New York: Raven Press.

49. Kasperowicz, B., Rotkiewicz, T. and Otrocka-Domagała, I. 2006. Pathomorphological and immunohistochemical study of selected markers of tumour cell proliferation in equine sarcoids. *Pol. J. Vet. Sci.* 9:109–119.

50. Kemp-Symonds, J. G. 2000. The detection and sequencing of bovine papillomavirus type 1 and 2 DNA from Musca autumnalis (Diptera: Muscidae) face flies infesting sarcoid-affected horses. MSc thesis, Royal Veterinary College, London, UK.

51. Kinnunen, R. E., Tallberg, T., Stenback, H. and Sarna S. 1999. Equine sarcoid tumour treated by autogenous tumour vaccine. *Anticancer Res.* 19:3367–3374.

52. Klein, W. R., Bras, G. E., Misdorp, W., Steerenberg, P. A., de Jong, W. H., Tiesjema, R. H., Kersjes, A. W. and Ruitenberg, E. J. 1986. Equine sarcoid: BCG immunotherapy compared to cryosurgery in a prospective randomised clinical trial. *Cancer Immunol. Immunother* 21:133–140.

53. Knottenbelt, D. C. and Kelly, D. F. 2000. The diagnosis and treatment of periorbital sarcoid in the horse: 445 cases from 1974 to 1999. *Vet. Ophthalmol.* 3:169–191.

54. Krahwinkel, D. J. 1976. Cryosurgical treatment of cancerous and noncancerous diseases of dogs, horses and cats. *J. Am. Vet. Med. Assoc.* 169:201.

55. Lancaster, W. D. 1981. Apparent lack of integration of bovine papillomavirus DNA in virus-induced equine and bovine tumor cells and virus-transformed mouse cells. *Virology* 108:251–255.

56. Lancaster, W. D. and Olson, C. 1982. Animal papillomaviruses. *Microbiol. Rev.* 46:191–207.

57. Lane, L. G. 1977. The treatment of equine sarcoids by cryosurgery. *Equine Vet. J.* 9:127–133.

58. Lavach, J. D., Sullins, K. E., Roberts, S. M., Severin, G. A., Wheeler, C. and Lueker, D. C. 1985. BCG treatment of periocular sarcoid. *Equine Vet. J.* 17:445–448.

59. Lazary, S., Gerber, H., Glatt, P. A. and Straub, R. 1985. Equine leucocyte antigens in sarcoid-affected horses. *Equine Vet. J.* 17:283–286.

60. Logas, D. B. and Barbet, J. L. 1999. Inflammatory, infectious, and immune diseases. In *Equine medicine and surgery*, ed. P. T. Colahan, I. G. Mayhew, A. M. Merritt et al., 1874–1875. St. Louis: Mosby.

61. Lowy, D. and Howley, P. 2002. Papillomaviruses. In *Fields virology*, 4th ed., D. M. Knipe and P. M. Howley, 2231–2264. Philadelphia, PA: Lippincott Williams and Willkins.

62. Marchetti, B., Ashrafi, G. H., Tsirimonaki, E., O'Brien, P. M. and Campo, M. S. 2002. The papillomavirus oncoprotein E5 retains the major histocompatibility class I in the Golgi apparatus and prevents its transport to the cell surface. *Oncogene* 21:7808–7816.

63. Martens, A., De Moor, A. Demeulemeester, J. and Ducatelle, R. 2000a. Histopathological characteristics of five clinical types of equine sarcoid. *Res. Vet. Sci.* 69:295–300.

64. Martens, A., De Moor, A., Waelkens, E., Merlevede, W. and De Witte, P. 2000b. *In vitro* and *in vivo* evaluation of hypericin for photodynamic therapy of equine sarcoids. *Vet. J.* 159:77–84.

65. Martens, A., De Moor, A., Demeulemeester, J. and Peelman, L. 2001a. Polymerase chain reaction analysis of the surgical margins of equine sarcoids for bovine papilloma virus DNA. *Surg.* 30:460–467.

66. Martens, A., De Moor, A. and Ducatelle, R. 2001b. PCR detection of bovine papilloma virus DNA in superficial swabs and scrapings from equine sarcoids. *Vet. J.* 161:280–286.

67. Marti, E., Lazary, S., Antczak, D. F. and Gerber, H. 1993. Report of the first international workshop on equine sarcoid. *Equine Vet. J.* 25:397–407.

68. Mattil-Fritz, S., Scharner, D., Piuko, K., Thones, N., Gissmann, L., Muller, H. and Muller, M. 2008. Immunotherapy of equine sarcoid: Dose-escalation trial for the use of chimeric papillomavirus-like particles. *J. Gen. Virol.* 89:138–147.

69. McConaghy, F. F., Davis, R. E. and Hodgson, D. R. 1994. Equine sarcoid: A persistent therapeutic challenge. *Compr. Contin. Educ. Pract. Vet.* 7:1022–1030.

70. Meredith, D., Elser, A. H., Wolf, B., Soma, L. R., Donawick, W. J. and Lazary, S. 1986. Equine leukocyte antigens: Relationships with sarcoid tumors and laminitis in two pure breeds. *Immunogenetics* 23:221–225.

71. Mohammed, H. O., Rebhun, W. C. and Antczack, D. F. 1992. Factors associated with the risk of developing sarcoid tumours in horses. *Equine Vet. J.* 24:165–168.

72. Nasir, L. and Campo, M. S. 2008. Bovine papillomaviruses: Their role in the aetiology of cutaneous tumours of bovids and equids. *Vet. Dermatol.* 19:243–254.

73. Nasir, L. and Reid, S. W. 1999. Bovine papillomaviral gene expression in equine sarcoid tumours. *Virus Res.* 61:171–175.

74. Nixon, C., Chambers, G., Ellsmore, V., Campo, M. S., Burr, P., Argyle, D. J., Reid, S. W. and Nasir, L. 2005. Expression of cell cycle associated proteins cyclin A, CDK-2, p27kip1 and p53 in equine sarcoids. *Cancer Lett.* 221:237–245.

75. O'Banion, M. K., Reichmann, M. E. and Sundberg, J. P. 1986. Cloning and characterization of an equine cutaneous papillomavirus. *Virology* 152:100–109.

76. Ohlschlager, P., Osen, W., Dell, K., Faath, S., Garcea, R. L., Jochmus, I., Muller, M., Pawlita, M., Schafer, K. Sehr, P., Staib. C., Sutter, G. and Gissmann L. 2003. Human papillomavirus type 16 L1 capsomeres induce L1-specific cytotoxic T lymphocytes and tumor regression in C57BL/6 mice. *J. Virol.* 77:4635–4645.

77. Olsen, E. A., Katz, H. I., Levine, N., Shupack, J., Billys, M. M., Prawer, S., Gold, J., Stiller, M., Lufrano, L. and Thorne, E. G. 1992. Tretinoin emollient cream: A new therapy for photodamaged skin. *J. Am. Acad. Dermatol.* 26:215–224.

78. Olson, C. and Cook, R. H. 1951. Cutaneous sarcoma-like lesions of the horse caused by the agent of bovine papilloma. *Proc. Soc. Exp. Biol. Med.* 77:281–284.

79. Otten, N., Von Tscharner, C., Lazary, S., Antczak, D. F. and Gerber, H. 1993. DNA of bovine papillomavirus type 1 and 2 in equine sarcoids: PCR detection and direct sequencing. *Arch. Virol.* 132:121–131.

80. Owen, R. A. and Jagger, D. W. 1987. Clinical observations on the use of BCG cell wall fraction for treatment of periocular and other equine sarcoids. *Vet. Rec.* 120:548–552.

81. Page, E. and Tiffany, L. W. 1967. Use of an autogenous equine fibrosarcoma vaccine. *J. Am. Vet. Med. Assoc.* 150:177.

82. Pascoe, R. R. R., Knottenbelt, D. C., and Saunders, W. B. 1999. *Manual of equine dermatology.* Harcourt and Brace Company Ltd.

83. Piscopo, S. E. 1999. The complexities of sarcoid tumors. *Equine Pract.* 21:14–18.

84. Postey, R. C., Appleyard, G. D. and Kidney, B. A. 2007. Evaluation of equine papillomas, aural plaques, and sarcoids for the presence of *equine papillomavirus* DNA and *papillomavirus* antigen. *Can. J. Vet. Res.* 71:28–33.

85. Radostits, O. M., Gay, C. C., Hinchcliff, K. W. and Constable, P. D. 2007. *Veterinary medicine: A textbook of the diseases of cattle, horses, sheep, pigs, and goats*, 10th ed. Saunders Elsevier.

86. Ragland, K. W. L., Keown, G. F. H. and Spencer, G. R. 1970. Equine sarcoids. *Equine Vet. J.* 2:2–11.

87. Ragland, W. L. and Spencer, G. R. 1969. Attempts to relate bovine papilloma virus to the cause of equine sarcoid: Equidae inoculated intradermally with bovine papilloma virus. *Am. J. Vet. Res.* 30:743–752.

88. Ragland, W. L., Keown, G. H. and Gorham. 1966. An epizootic of equine sarcoid. *Nature* 210:1399.

89. Reid, S. W. J., Smith, K. T. and Jarrett, W. H. F. 1994. Detection, cloning and characterisation of papillomaviral DNA present in sarcoid tumours of Equus asinus. *Vet. Rec.* 135:430–432.

90. Reid, S. W. J. and Mohammed, H. O. 1997. Longitudinal and cross-sectional studies to evaluate the risk of sarcoid associated with castration. *Can. J. Vet. Res.* 61:89–93.

91. Rols, M. P., Tamzali, Y. and Teissie, J. 2002. Electrochemotherapy of horses. A preliminary clinical report. *Bioelectrochem.* 1–2:101–105.

92. Rudolf, M. P., Fausch, S. C., Da Silva, D. M. and Kast, W. M. 2001. Human dendritic cells are activated by chimeric human papillomavirus type-16 virus-like particles and induce epitope-specific human T cell responses in vitro. *J. Immunol.* 166:5917–5924.

93. Schapiro, F., Sparkowski, J., Adduci, A., Suprynowicz, F., Schlegel, R. and Grinstein, S. 2000. Golgi alkalinization by the papillomavirus E5 oncoprotein. *J. Cell Biol.* 148:305–315.

94. Schiller, J. T. and Lowy, D. R. 2001. Papillomavirus-like particle vaccines. *J. Natl. Cancer Inst. Monogr.* 50–54.

95. Scott, D. W. and Miller, W. H. 2003. Epithelial neoplasms. In *Equine dermatology*, 700–731. St. Louis: Saunders.

96. Sellon, D. C. 2007. Papillomavirus infections. In *Equine infectious diseases*, ed. D. C. Sellon and M. T. Long, chapter 25, 226–232. Philadelphia, USA: Saunders, Elsevier Inc.

97. Sersa, G., Miklavcic, D., Cemazar, M., Rudolf, Z., Pucihar, G. and Snoj, M. 2002. Electrochemotherapy in treatment of tumours. *Euro. J. Surg. Oncol.* 34:232–240.

98. Siegsmund, M., Wayss, K. and Amtmann, E. 1991. Activation of latent papillomavirus genomes by chronic mechanical irritation. *J. Gen. Virol.* 72:2787–2789.

99. Sousa, R., Dostatni, N. and Yaniv, M. 1990. Control of papillomavirus gene expression. *Biochim. Biophys. Acta* 1032:19–37.

100. Sousa, N. R., Adorno, V. B., Marcondes, J. S., Oliveira Filho, J. P., Conceicao, L. G., Amorim, R. L. and Borges, A. S. 2008. Clinical and histopathological characteristics of the aural plaque in Mangalarga and Quarter Horses. *Pesq. Vet. Bras.* 28:279–284.

101. Straight, S. W., Herman, B. and McCance, D. J. 1995. The E5 oncoprotein of human papillomavirus type 16 inhibits the acidification of endosomes in human keratinocytes. *J. Virol.* 69:3185–3192.

102. Sundberg, J. P., Junge, R. E. and Lancaster, W. D. 1984. Immunoperoxidase localization of papillomaviruses in hyperplastic and neoplastic lesions of animals. *Am. J. Vet. Res.* 45:1441–1446.

103. Tamzali, Y., Teissie, J. and Rols, M. P. 2001. Cutaneous tumor treatment by electrochemotherapy: Preliminary clinical results in horse sarcoids. *Revue Med. Vet.* 152:605–609.

104. Tamzali, Y., Teissie, J. and Rols, M. P. 2003. First horse sarcoid treatment by electrochemotherapy: Preliminary experimental results. *AEEP Proc.* 49:381–384.

105. Tamzali, Y., Teissie, J., Golzio, M. and Rols, M. P. 2007. Electrochemotherapy of equids cutaneous tumors: A 57 case retrospective study 1999–2005. In *IFBME Proceedings*, ed. T. Jarm, P. Kramar, and A. Zupanic, 16:610–613. New York: Springer.

106. Tarwid, J. N. 1985. Equine sarcoids: A study with emphasis on pathologic diagnosis. *Compr. Contin. Educ. Pract. Vet.* 7:S293–301.

107. Teifke, J. P., Hardt, M. and Weiss, E. 1994. Detection of bovine papillomavirus DNA in formalin-fixed and paraffin-embedded equine sarcoids by polymerase chain reaction and nonradioactive in situ hybridization. *Eur. J. Vet. Pathol.* 4:5–10.

108. Theon, A. P. 1997. Cisplatin treatment for cutaneous tumors. In *Current therapy in equine medicine*, 4th ed., N. E. Robinson, 372–377. Philadelphia: Saunders.

109. Theon, A. P. and Pascoe, J. R. 1995. Iridium[192] interstitial brachytherapy for equine periocular tumours: Treatment results and prognostic factors in 115 horses. *Equine Vet. J.* 27:117–121.

110. Theon, A. P., Pascoe, J. R. and Meagher, D. M. 1994. Perioperative intratumoral administration of cisplatin for treatment of cutaneous tumors in Equidae. *J. Am. Vet. Med. Assoc.* 205:1170.

111. Tong, X. and Howley, P. M. 1997. The bovine papillomavirus E6 oncoprotein interacts with paxillin and disrupts the actin cytoskeleton. *Proc. Natl. Acad. Sci. USA* 94:4412–4417.

112. Tong, X., Salgia, R., Li, J. L., Griffin, J. D. and Howley, P. M. 1997. The bovine papillomavirus E6 protein binds to the LD motif repeats of paxillin and blocks its interaction with vinculin and the focal adhesion kinase. *J. Biol. Chem.* 272:33373–33376.

113. Tong, X., Boll, W., Kirchhausen, T. and Howley, P. M. 1998. Interaction of the bovine papillomavirus E6 protein with the clathrin adaptor complex AP-1. *J. Virol.* 72:476–482.

114. Torrontegui, B. O. and Reid, S. J. 1994. Clinical and pathological epidemiology of the equine sarcoid in a referral population. *Equine Vet. Educ.* 6:85–88.

115. Turrel, J. M. and Koblik, P. D. 1983. Techniques of afterloading iridium-192 interstitial brachytherapy in veterinary medicine. *Vet. Radiol.* 24:278.

116. Turrel, J. M., Stover, S. M. and Gyorgyfalvy, J. 1985. Iridium-192 interstitial brachytherapy of equine sarcoid. *Vet. Radiol.* 26:20.

117. Valentine, B. A. 2006. Survey of equine cutaneous neoplasia in the Pacific Northwest. *J. Vet. Diag. Invest.* 18:123–126.

118. Vande Pol, S. B., Brown, M. C. and Turner, C. E. 1998. Association of bovine papillomavirus type 1 E6 oncoprotein with the focal adhesion protein paxillin through a conserved protein interaction motif. *Oncogene* 16:43–52.

119. Vanselow, B. A., Abetz, I. and Jackson, A. R. 1988. BCG emulsion immunotherapy of equine sarcoid. *Equine Vet. J.* 20:444–447.

120. Venuti, A. and Campo, M. S. 2002. The E5 protein of papillomaviruses. In *Progress in medical virology: Papillomaviruses*, ed. D. J. McCance, 141–162. Iowa: Iowa State Press.

121. Voss, J. L. 1969. Transmission of equine sarcoid. *Am. J. Vet. Res.* 30:183–191.

122. White, K. S., Fuji, R. N., Valentine, V. A. and Bildfell, R. J. 2004. Equine congenital papilloma: Pathological findings and results of papillomavirus immunohistochemistry in five cases. *Vet. Dermatol.* 15:240–244.

123. Williams, M. A. 1997. Papillomatosis: Warts and aural plaques. In *Current therapy in equine medicine*, 4th ed., N. E. Robinson, 389–399. Philadelphia: WB Saunders.

124. Yuan, Z., Philbey, A. W., Gault, E. A., Campo, M. S. and Nasir, L. 2007. Detection of bovine papillomavirus type 1 genomes and viral gene expression in equine inflammatory skin conditions. *Virus Res.* 124:245–249.

125. Zimmermann, H., Koh, C. H., Degenkolbe, R., O'Connor, M. J., Muller, A., Steger, G., Chen, J. J., Lui, Y., Androphy, E. and Bernard, H. U. 2000. Interaction with CBP/p300 enables the bovine papillomavirus type 1 E6 oncoprotein to down regulate CBP/p300-mediated transactivation by p53. *J. Gen. Virol.* 81:2617–2623.

10. Equine Rabies

R. V. S. Pawaiya, K. Dhama, and S. Kapoor

Introduction

Rabies is a fatal infection of the central nervous system acquired through the bite of a rabid animal. The 100% fatality rate of this infection when left untreated, and its near-global distribution, makes rabies one of the most significant and dread diseases (Beran, 1993; Green, 1997; Radostits et al., 2000; Bender and Schulman, 2004; Arai, 2005; Fooks, 2007; Gruzdev, 2008). It is a viral *zoonosis* that causes approximately fifty thousand to one hundred thousand deaths per year worldwide (Leung et al., 2007). "Rabies" is a word derived from the Latin expression *rabere*, which means "to be mad," and is a highly fatal neurologic disease of mammals caused by a neurotropic virus of the genus *Lyssavirus* of the family Rhabdoviridae. It is an acute viral encephalomyelitis that mainly affects carnivores and bats, although it can affect any mammal, including humans and several wildlife species, which act as predominant natural reservoir for infection. The vast majority of rabies cases reported each year occur in wild animals like raccoons, skunks, bats, and foxes. While endemic dog rabies is of major concern worldwide, rabies control programs have reduced the number of dog rabies cases in countries like USA. However, a large reservoir of rabies exists in the wildlife animals. Domestic animals account for less than 10% of the reported rabies cases, with cats, cattle, and dogs most often reported as rabid.

Rabies in the horse is a relatively uncommon disease but is still of a serious nature as is invariably fatal, and there is often significant potential for human exposure (Weese, 2002). Equine rabies is a severe, rapidly progressive neurological disease. Horses get rabies from the saliva of an infected animal, either through a bite or by the saliva contaminating an open wound (Baer, 1991; Green, 1993). Rabid skunks are responsible for the majority of rabies cases in horses; however, foxes, raccoons, bats, and unimmunized dogs and cats have also been known to transmit the disease. Horses being very curious, especially foals and yearlings, naturally tend to probe the roaming wildlife in the pasture, which make them likely to get bitten, especially on the nostrils or lips. Symptoms can appear in as little time as two weeks but can take up to one year for clinical signs to appear.

On the average, symptoms will be seen four to eight weeks after the exposure. Death usually occurs within two to four days after the horse begins to show clinical signs, although death may not occur until up to two weeks later with supportive care.

In 2007 (the most current year with reported incidence), there were only forty-two positive cases of equine rabies reported in the United States (Blanton et al., 2008). The number of rabies cases in both wildlife and domestic animals has increased over the last twenty years with reported cases in wild and domestic animals generally exceeding nine thousand annually. With the continued increase in the number of rabies cases, the threat and potential exposure to the horse is also likely to increase. With the increased urbanization of areas in which the disease is endemic in wildlife populations, the risk of exposure continues to be a concern for horse owners and veterinarians. Rarely is the exposure to the wild animal observed, and bite wounds on the horse are rarely found. In one retrospective study of twenty-one horses with rabies, bite wounds were not found on any of the horses (Green et al., 1992). Because the rabid animal has a high concentration of rabies virus in its saliva, its bite inoculates the bite victim. The virus then replicates and travels up the peripheral nerves to the central nervous system. The incubation period averages two to nine weeks but may be as long as fifteen months.

EPIDEMIOLOGY

Rabies, an acute progressive encephalitis, is an ancient zoonosis recognized for centuries. It wasn't until the 1880s when work done by Louis Pasteur identified a virus as the cause of the disease. Its distribution encompasses all continents, except Antarctica (Radostits et al., 2000; Rupprecht et al., 2008). Agents consist of at least eleven species orgenotypes of rhabdoviruses, in the genus *Lyssavirus*. Primary reservoirs reside in the orders Carnivora and Chiroptera. A plethora of variants, maintained by a diversity of abundant hosts, presents a challenge to a strict concept of true eradication (Rupprecht et al., 2008). Rabies virus is the most cosmopolitan member, with primary reservoirs within dogs and mongoose, but other wildlife vectors are important in viral maintenance, such as jackals (Nel and Rupprecht, 2007). Globally, the domestic dog remains the most significant species for viral transmission, responsible for millions of suspect human exposures and tens of thousands of fatalities.

Rabies is found throughout the world, but a few countries claim to be free of the disease due either to successful elimination programs and/or to their island status and enforcement of rigorous quarantine regulations (Arai, 2005; Cleaveland et al., 2006; Cleaveland et al., 2007; Nel and Rupprecht, 2007; Leung et al., 2007; Gruzdev, 2008; Seimenis, 2008; Blancou, 2008;

Blanton et al., 2008). In some of the countries, there is a considerable death rate due to rabies. Dogs are the main source of human infection, while cats constitute the second most important group of domestic animals followed by cattle, sheep, goats, camels, donkeys, and then wild animals.

Equine rabies is a sporadic but highly fatal zoonotic disease (Weese, 2002). With the continued increase in the number of wildlife rabies cases reported, this disease will remain a threat to the horse as the potential for exposure to infected wildlife and other domestic animals is likely to also increase (Green, 1993, 1997; Meltzer and Rupprecht, 1998; Tamashiro et al., 2007). Thus, it remains a threat to all domestic species, including the horse (Hamir et al., 1992; Green et al., 1992; Hudson et al., 1996; Fooks, 2007; Matouch, 2008). Carrieri et al. (2006) reported that equine rabies transmitted by the vampire bat (*Desmodus rotundus*) has increased gradually in the state of São Paulo.

The causal *Lyssaviruses* are usually confined to one major reservoir species in a given geographic area, although spillover to other species is common (Arai, 2005). Generally, each virus variant is responsible for rabies transmission between members of same species in a given geographic area. Rabies maintained by dog-to-dog transmission is termed canine rabies, whereas rabies in a dog as a result of infection with a variant from a different reservoir, e.g., skunk (or fox), is referred to as skunk (or fox, etc.) rabies (Cliquet and Picard-Meyer, 2004).

In North America, distinct virus variants are responsible for rabies in dogs and coyotes in Mexico and south Texas, red and Arctic foxes in Canada and Alaska, raccoons along the eastern seaboard, gray foxes in Texas and a closely related variant in gray foxes in the southwestern USA (Griego et al., 1995; Blanton et al., 2008). Two different variants are responsible for rabies in striped skunks, one in south central states and other in north central states. Another skunk rabies virus variant is seen in California (McColl et al., 2000). The epidemiology of rabies in bats is complex, but in general, each variant found in bats may be assigned to a predominant bat species. Spillover from bats to terrestrial animals is seen infrequently (van der Poel et al., 2006).

Reservoirs of rabies vary throughout the world. Canine rabies predominates in Africa, Asia, Latin America, and Middle East (David et al., 2007). In North America and Europe, where canine rabies has been practically eliminated, rabies is maintained in wildlife. For many years, skunks were the most commonly reported rabid animal in USA, but since 1990, rabid raccoons have been the most numerous. Canine rabies became established in coyotes (*Canis latrans*) in southern Texas and Mexico, with the potential to spread throughout much of the USA and Canada. Skunk, raccoon, and fox rabies are each found in fairly distinct geographic regions of North America, although some overlap occurs. Bat rabies is distributed throughout the USA and Central and South America. In Europe, red fox rabies predominates. In parts of northern and eastern Europe, rabies in raccoon dogs is of increasing concern (Matouch, 2008). Rabies in insectivorous bats may be widely distributed in Europe. The vampire bat is an important reservoir in Mexico, Central and South America, and is the source of outbreaks in cattle. Other wild species play an important role in the transmission of rabies in certain areas, including mongooses in the Caribbean, southern Africa, and parts of Asia; dogs and monkeys in India; jackals in certain parts of Africa; wolves in parts of northern Europe; and red fox, steppe fox and raccoon dogs in Russia and Eurasia (Bhargava et al., 1996; Kuzmin et al., 2004; Diop et al., 2007; Tamashiro et al., 2007; Nel and Rupprecht, 2007; Blancou, 2008; Chhabra et al., 2004; Gruzdev, 2008; Ichhpujani et al., 2008; Smreczak et al., 2008).

ETIOLOGY

Rabies is caused by a neurotropic virus of the genus *Lyssavirus* of the family Rhabdoviridae, and is transmissible to all mammals (Green, 1997; Radostits et al., 2000; Rupprecht et al., 2008). Seven distinct genetic lineages can be distinguished within the genus *Lyssavirus* by cross-protection tests and molecular biological analysis (Fekadu et al., 1988; Baer, 1991; Bourhy et al., 1993)—namely, the classical rabies virus itself (RABV: genotype 1, serotype 1), Lagos bat virus (LBV: genotype 2, serotype 2), Mokola virus (MOKV: genotype 3, serotype 3), and Duvenhage virus (DUVV: genotype 4, serotype 4). The European bat *Lyssaviruses* (EBLV), subdivided into two biotypes (EBLV1, genotype 5; and EBLV2, genotype 6), and the Australian bat *Lyssavirus* (ABLV, genotype 7), isolated in Australia (Hooper et al., 1997), are also members of the *Lyssavirus* genus, but are not yet classified into serotypes. Viruses of serotypes 2–4, EBLV, and ABLV are known as rabies-related viruses. The use of monoclonal antibodies directed against viral nucleocapsid or glycoprotein antigens and the sequencing of defined genomic areas have made possible the definition of numerous subtypes within each serotype. *Lyssaviruses* cause a clinical disease indistinguishable from classical rabies (Nel and Rupprecht, 2007). Conserved antigenic sites on the nucleocapsid proteins permit recognition of all *Lyssaviruses* with modern commercial preparations of antirabies antibody conjugates used for diagnostic tests on brain tissue. There exist two *Lyssavirus* phylogroups with distinct pathogenicity and immunogenicity (Badrane et al., 2001). For RABV, DUVV, EBLV, and ABLV, conserved antigenic sites on the surface glycoproteins allow cross-neutralization and cross-protective immunity to be elicited by rabies vaccination. Little or no cross-protection against infection with MOKV or LBV is elicited by rabies vaccination, and most antirabies virus antisera do not neutralize these *Lyssaviruses*. Four new rabies-related viruses (Aravan, Khujand, Irkut, and West Caucasian bat viruses) have been isolated recently from Eurasian bats and are described as new putative *Lyssavirus* species (Cliquet and Picard-Meyer, 2004). There are no differences between different rabies strains (Arctic fox, raccoon, and bat rabies) as far as their ability to kill their carrier species, other animals, and possibly humans.

VIRUS STRUCTURE

Rabies virus belongs to the order Mononegavirales, viruses with nonsegmented, negative-stranded RNA genomes (Green, 1997). Viruses with a distinct "bullet" shape are classified in the *Rhabdoviridae* family, which includes at least three genera of animal viruses, *Lyssavirus*, *Ephemerovirus*, and *Vesiculovirus*. The genus *Lyssavirus* includes rabies virus, Lagos bat, Mokola virus, Duvenhage virus, European bat virus 1 and 2, and Australian bat virus. Rhabdoviruses are approximately 180 nm long and 75 nm wide. Rabies virions are bullet shaped with 10-nm spikelike glycoprotein peplomers covering the surface (Wunner, 1991). The ribonucleoprotein is composed of RNA encased in nucleoprotein, phosphorylated or phosphoprotein, and polymerase. The viral genome is single-stranded, antisense, nonsegmented, RNA of approximately 12 kb (Tordo et al., 1986; 1988). There is a leader sequence (LDR) of approximately fifty nucleotides, followed by N, P, M, G, and L genes (Finke et al., 2003). The rabies genome encodes five proteins, namely, nucleoprotein (N), phosphoprotein (P), matrix protein (M), glycoprotein (G), and polymerase (L). All rhabdoviruses have two major structural components: a helical ribonucleoprotein core (RNP) and a surrounding envelope. In the RNP, genomic RNA is tightly encased by nucleoprotein (Albertini et al., 2006). Two other viral proteins, the phospoprotein and the large protein (L-protein or polymerase), are associated with RNP. The glycoprotein forms approximately four hundred trimeric spikes, which are tightly arranged on the virus surface. The M protein is associated both with the envelope and the RNP and may be the central protein of rhabdovirus assembly (*http://www.cdc.gov/Ncidod/dvrd/rabies/images/spacer.gif*).

VIRAL REPLICATION

The fusion of rabies virus envelope to the host cell membrane (adsorption) initiates the infection process. The interaction of the G protein and specific cell surface receptors may be involved. After adsorption, the virus penetrates the host cell and enters the cytoplasm by pinocytosis (via clathrin-coated pits). The virions aggregate in the large endosomes (cytoplasmic vesicles). The viral membranes fuse to the endosomal membranes, causing the release of viral RNP into the cytoplasm (uncoating). Because lyssaviruses have a linear single negative-stranded ribonucleic acid (RNA) genome, messenger RNAs (mRNAs) must be transcribed to permit virus replication (*http://www.cdc.gov/Ncidod/dvrd/rabies/the_virus/images/genome.gifhttp://www.cdc.gov/Ncidod/dvrd/rabies/the_virus/images/cycbig.jpg*.) A viral-encoded polymerase (L gene) transcribes the genomic strand of rabies RNA into leader RNA and five capped and polyadenylated mRNAs, which are translated into proteins. Translation (which involves the synthesis of the N, P, M, G, and L proteins) occurs on free ribosomes in the cytoplasm. Although G protein synthesis is initiated on free ribosomes, completion of synthesis and glycosylation (processing of the glycoprotein), occurs in the endoplamsic reticulum (ER) and Golgi apparatus. The intracellular ratio of leader RNA to N protein regulates the switch from transcription to replication. When this switch is activated, replication of the viral genome begins. The first step in viral replication is synthesis of full-length copies (positive strands) of the viral genome. When the switch to replication occurs, RNA transcription becomes "nonstop" and stop codons are ignored. The viral polymerase enters a single site on the 3' end of the genome and proceeds to synthesize full-length genome copies. These positive strands of rabies RNA serve as templates for synthesis of full-length negative strands of the viral genome.

During the assembly process, the N-P-L complex encapsulates negative-stranded genomic RNA to form RNP core, and the M protein forms a capsule, or matrix, around the RNP. The RNP-M complex migrates to an area of the plasma membrane containing glycoprotein inserts, and the M-protein initiates coiling, thus regulating the balance of virus transcription and replication (Finke et al., 2003). The M-RNP complex binds with the glycoprotein, and the completed virus buds from the plasma membrane. Within the central nervous system (CNS), there is preferential viral budding from plasma membranes. Conversely, virus in the salivary glands buds primarily from cell membrane into the acinar lumen. Viral budding into the salivary gland and aggressive virus-induced biting behavior in the host animal maximize chances of viral infection of a new host.

HOST RANGE AND DISEASE TRANSMISSION

Rabies affects both animals and humans. All warm-blooded animals can be infected with rabies, but it is most often transmitted by foxes, jackals, mongoose, raccoons, skunks, and bats (Green, 1997; Radostits et al., 2000; Weese, 2002; Fooks et al., 2003; Rupprecht et al., 2006).

The disease persists in wildlife populations throughout the world (Rupprecht et al., 2004). Wildlife infected with rabies may show no fear of man, be aggressive, or be incoordinated. Animals that are normally nocturnal may be active during the day. Variation in susceptibility is noticeable. Foxes, rats, and coyotes are extremely susceptible; cattle, rabbits, and cats are highly susceptible; dogs, sheep, and goats are moderately susceptible; and opossums little, if at all (Rupprecht et al., 2004). Transmission of rabies virus usually begins when infected saliva of a host is passed to an uninfected animal. Various routes of transmission have been documented and include contamination of mucous membranes (i.e., eyes, nose, mouth), aerosol transmission, and corneal transplantations. The most common mode of rabies virus transmission is through the bite and virus-containing saliva of an infected host (Carrieri et al., 2006; Dendle and Looke, 2008; Ichhpujani et al., 2008). Horses frequently come in contact with these wild animals in barns and pastures. The horse is one of the most susceptible domestic animals and is usually infected via a bite wound from a rabid wild animal. Horses, being curious creatures, are apt to investigate a wild animal that is acting strangely and may be bit on the muzzle, face, and/or lower legs, which generally go unnoticed. Veterinary exposure to rabies is less likely in equine practice than small animal or wildlife practice. Despite the low incidence of disease, veterinary personnel must remain vigilant because of the severity of disease (Weese, 2002).

PATHOGENESIS

Following primary infection, the rabies virus enters an eclipse phase in which it cannot be easily detected within the host, which may last for several days or months. During this phase, the host immune defenses may confer cell-mediated immunity against viral infection because rabies virus is a good antigen. Investigations have shown both direct entry of virus into peripheral nerves at the site of infection and indirect entry after viral replication in nonnervous tissue (i.e., muscle cells). The uptake of virus into peripheral nerves is important for progressive infection to occur, after which the virus is transported to the central nervous system (CNS) via retrograde axoplasmic flow (Larsen et al., 2008), which typically occurs via sensory and motor nerves at the initial site of infection. The incubation period varies from two weeks to six years (average two to three months), depending on the amount of virus in the inoculum and site of inoculation. The proximity of the site of virus entry to the CNS increases the likelihood of a short incubation period. Axonal transport of virus to the CNS is at a rate of 3 mm/hour or the estimated speed of virus migration ranges from 15–100 mm/day (WHO, 2005). In the brain, the virus infects neurons in almost all regions, where it continues replication. Neuronal virus transmission from the periphery of the body to the brain is called centripetal virus spread. Possible receptors for the virus are the following: acetylcholine receptors, gangliosides, and phospholipids. The virus then moves from the CNS via anterograde axoplasmic flow within peripheral nerves, leading to infection of some of the adjacent nonnervous tissues: for example, secretory tissues of salivary glands. The virus is widely disseminated throughout the body at clinical onset, and at this time can be found in salivary glands, taste buds, nasal cavities, tears, skin, the adrenal glands, pancreas, kidney, heart muscle, brown fat, hair follicles, retina, and cornea. (The virus has never been detected in blood or blood cells.) The first clinical symptom is usually neuropathic pain at the wound site, which is caused by virus replication in dorsal root ganglia and ganglionitis. Major clinical signs are related to the virus-induced encephalomyeloradiculitis. Two major clinical presentations are observed: furious and paralytic forms that cannot be correlated with any specific anatomical localization of rabies virus in the CNS (Radostits et al., 2000). Nevertheless, peripheral nerve dysfunction is responsible for weakness in paralytic rabies. In furious rabies, electrophysiological studies indicate anterior horn cell dysfunction even in the absence of clinical weakness. Without intensive care, death occurs within a few days (one to five days) of the development of neurological signs. Rabies is inevitably fatal diseases.

It has been suggested that death from rabies is not a result of structural damage caused by the virus, but rather a result of functional alteration of neurons. The rabies RNA most likely competes with hosts RNA, impairing neural functions (Finke et al., 2003; Mavrakis et al., 2006). Neurologic damage is exacerbated by the production of certain cytokines, such as tumor necrosis factor-alpha. In addition, the immune response to rabies includes the production of nitric oxide, which may act as a toxin to the CNS. One of the determining factors of rabies virulence is the glycoprotein (G), which makes up the viral membrane. A single amino acid change in rabies virus glycoprotein peptide, especially when arginine at 194 position, is replaced with lysine residue, enhanced viral pathogenicity due to increased viral spread, faster internalization of the pathogenic virus into cells, and a shift in the pH threshold for membrane fusion (Faber et al., 2005; Gaudin, 2000). Viral glycoprotein is the target for most rabies virus-neutralizing antibodies and has been a strong inducer of apoptosis in infected cells, which is evidently an immunogenic process in rabies (Consales and Bolzan, 2007).

CLINICAL SIGNS AND SYMPTOMS
Clinical signs in the horse include behavior changes ranging from aggression, ataxia (incoordination), paresis (partial paralysis, ascending), convulsions, restlessness, hyperesthesia (hypersensitivity to stimuli-increased sensitivity

to touch or other stimulation), muscle spasms of the third eyelid, fever, colic, dysphagia, lameness, depression, loss of appetite, blindness, urinary incontinence, and recumbency (Meyer et al., 1986; Green et al., 1992; Green, 1997; Radostits et al., 2000; Leung et al., 2007). The "paralytic" and "dumb" forms are most common in horses, whereas the "furious" form is not as common as in other species (Green et al., 1992; Green, 1997; Weese, 2002). Behavioral signs in dumb form are mainly depression/stupor while in furious form mania develops, and these horses are extremely dangerous.

Early symptoms may include an intense scratching, licking, biting, and even tearing of tissue around the bite wound as a result of paresthesia. Bizarre hypersensitivity to touch (hyperesthesia) is an early sign. Other obscure signs such as lameness or colic may be the only abnormalities evident early in disease. Lameness due to sudden weakness or paralysis of a limb has been seen in many cases. This can appear as a front leg knuckling or dragging, but there is no tenderness or lack of mobility as would be expected in lameness. Affected animals usually die of cardiorespiratory failure within 2 to 5 days of onset of clinical signs; however, progression can be slower (up to two weeks) in some cases (Green, 1997) in which case horses may survive up to 15 days. Horses pose a serious threat to humans because they may bite one another and their handlers. In a study, the average incubation period for a horse infected with rabies was 12.3 days, and the time period from first signs to death was 5.5 days (Hudson et al., 1996). Those animals that had no previous vaccination history had significantly shorter incubation periods and died sooner. Muzzle tremors were the most frequently observed (81%) and most common initial sign. Other common signs included the following: difficulty in swallowing (71%), incoordination or paralysis (71%), weakness or drowsiness (71%). The furious form was noted in 43% of rabid horses and clinical signs in some of these animals initially appeared as the dumb form. The paralytic form was not observed. Horses that develop the furious form show excitement, become vicious, bite, kick, exhibit blind staggers, suddenly fall, and may chew themselves or foreign objects.

Equine rabies can have many different clinical manifestations and a wide variety of nonspecific and confusing clinical signs. For this reason, the disease is frequently initially misdiagnosed. It is often stated that rabies can "look like anything." Because of the extreme variability in clinical signs, it is difficult to make generalizations. However, most horses exhibit some degree of hyperesthesia, fever, neurological signs of ataxia (incoordination), and/or paralysis at some point during the course of the disease. While some horses exhibit intermittent or continuous signs of aggression, affected horses are more typically depressed or stuporous. Some horses may become anorectic and refuse to drink while others will continue to eat and drink until shortly before death. Hydrophobia (fear of water) is not a frequent sign in the horse. Occasionally, horses exhibit signs of ptyalism (grinding of the teeth). Obscure lameness and posterior ataxia (incoordination) are relatively common early signs. In most horses, the progression of the disease is rapid with death in three to five days following onset of clinical signs. Prior to death, most horses become recumbent with convulsions and/or a comatose state and violent thrashing. Rabies infection in the unvaccinated horse is invariably fatal.

PATHOLOGY

Gross lesions of rabies in central nervous tissue are limited. Microscopic lesions are typically nonsuppurative and include a variable meningitis and perivascular cuffing with lymphocytes, macrophages, and plasma cells; microgliosis, which is sometimes predominant; variable neuronal degeneration; and ganglioneuritis. Negri body formation within neurons of the CNS and even in the peripheral ganglia has long been the hallmark of rabies infection (Perl, 1975). The inclusions are intracytoplasmic and initially develop as an aggregation of strands of viral nucleocapsid, which rather quickly transforms into an ill-defined granular matrix (Murphy et al., 1973). Mature rabies virions, which bud from the nearby endoplasmic reticulum, may also be located around the periphery of the matrix. With time, the inclusion body becomes larger and detectable by light microscopy. Classically, the Negri body has one or more very small light, clear areas in hematoxylin and eosin staining called inner bodies, which result from the invagination of cytoplasmic component into the matrix of the inclusion (Matsumoto, 1975). Inclusions that do not possess inner bodies have been referred to as lyssa bodies, but they are Negri bodies without cytoplasmic indentation (Perl, 1975). It should also be noted that both fixed viruses (adapted to CNS by passage) and street viruses (that produce naturally occurring disease) produce the same ultrastructural features, except that fixed viral strains generally cause severe neuronal degeneration precluding the development and detection of Negri bodies. Also, Negri body formation generally occurs more frequently in large than in small neurons and are often present in neurons that are not located in areas of inflammation (Perl, 1975). However, some authors observed that Negri bodies are not frequently formed in equine nervous tissue (Silva et al., 1974).

DIAGNOSIS

One of the problems with the diagnosis of equine rabies is the impressive array of clinical signs it can produce (Green et al., 1992; Weese, 2002). A history of exposure to a rabid animal is not commonly reported, and absence of visible wounds does not preclude rabies. Further, a history of vaccination does not completely rule out the possibility of rabies because one study reported that five of twenty-one affected horses had been previously vaccinated (Green et al., 1992).

Rabies should be high on the list of differential diagnosis for any horse exhibiting obscure neurological signs like acute encephalitis especially if the horse is in an endemic area. Currently, there are no diagnostic tests that can be performed on a live animal that are accurate enough to be of practical use. The highly variable, nonspecific clinical signs of equine rabies along with the lack of accurate diagnostic tests make the diagnosis of rabies in the live horse very difficult. Since rabies typically is rare in horses, a veterinarian should attempt to rule out other diagnoses before diagnosing rabies. Other diseases with clinical symptoms similar to rabies are tetanus, equine herpesvirus, the various causes of encephalomyelitis, botulism, lead poisoning, moldy corn poisoning, protozoal myelitis, and trauma to the brain or spinal cord. Rabies, therefore, remains a disease in which the diagnosis is most often made only after death during postmortem examination of the brain and spinal cord. For postmortem diagnosis, the intact head should be submitted to a designated diagnostic laboratory. In transit, the head should be refrigerated by wet ice but not frozen. Because of the rapid progression of the disease, if undiagnosed neurological disease in the horse has not rapidly progressed by day 5 after the onset of clinical signs, rabies can probably be considered less likely to be the infective agent. However, because of the serious threat to human life, any suspected case of equine rabies should be handled as if it were a positive until proven otherwise. Clinical observation may only lead to a suspicion of rabies because signs of the disease are not characteristic and may vary greatly from one animal to another. The only way to perform a reliable diagnosis of rabies is to identify the virus or some of its specific components using laboratory tests, which are essential to confirm suspected cases of equine rabies (Meslin and Kaplan, 1996; World Health Organization, 1996; Green, 1997; Carrieri et al., 2006; Consales and Bolzan, 2007; Leung et al., 2007).

LABORATORY TEST FOR RABIES

The standard test for rabies testing is direct fluorescent antibody test (FAT), which has been thoroughly evaluated for more than forty years and is recognized as the most rapid and reliable of all the tests available for routine use. Almost all rabies laboratories in the world perform this test postmortem on animals suspected to have died of rabies. Other tests for diagnosis and research—such as electron microscopy (EM), histological examination, immunohistochemistry (IHC), reverse transcription–polymerase chain reaction (RT-PCR), and isolation in cell culture—are useful tools for studying the virus structure, histopathology, molecular typing, and virulence of rabies viruses (Bourhy and Sureau, 1991; Meslin and Kaplan, 1996; World Health Organization, 1996; Carrieri et al., 2006). Molecular detection using PCR and nucleic acid sequence-based amplification techniques shows the highest level of sensitivity but can produce false positive or false negative results and should only be used in combination with other conventional techniques. However, in laboratories with strict quality control procedures in place and demonstrable experience and expertise, these molecular techniques have been successfully applied for confirmatory diagnosis and epidemiological surveys. Virus identification using molecular techniques is of epidemiological importance (Consales and Bolzan, 2007). The amplified portion of the viral genome can be sequenced to confirm the origin of the virus and which can prove useful for molecular epidemiological and evolutionary studies. For detailed procedures for sample collection, shipment, and other essential procedures required for dispatching the biological material to diagnostic laboratories for diagnosis of rabies, one may refer to the rabies chapter of *OIE Terrestrial Manual 2008* available on the official Web site of OIE (*www.oie.int*).

1. *Direct fluorescent antibody test (FAT).* It is based on the observation that animals infected by rabies virus have specific viral proteins (antigen) present in their tissues (Umoh and Blenden, 1981; Warner et al., 1997; Carrieri et al., 2006). Recommended by both WHO and OIE, FAT is the most widely used test for rabies diagnosis. FAT gives reliable results on fresh specimens within a few hours in more than 95–99% of cases. FAT may be used directly on a smear and can also be used to confirm the presence of rabies antigen in cell culture or in brain tissue of experimental mice that have been inoculated for diagnosis. Because rabies is present in nervous tissue, the ideal tissue to test for rabies antigen is brain. The sensitivity of the FAT depends on the specimen, the degree of autolysis, and how the brain is sampled on the type of *Lyssavirus* and on the proficiency of the diagnostic staff (Aubert, 1982; Barrat and Aubert, 1995). The most important part of a FAT is fluorescent-labeled antirabies antibody, primarily directed against the nucleoprotein (antigen) of the virus, which when is incubated with rabies-suspect brain tissue will bind to rabies antigen (Rudd et al., 2005). Unbound antibody can be washed away, and areas where antigen is present can be visualized as fluorescent apple green areas using a fluorescence microscope. If rabies virus is absent, there will be no staining. Rabies virus replicates in the cytoplasm of cells, and infected cells may contain large round or oval inclusions containing collections of nucleoprotein (N) or smaller

collections of antigen that appear as dustlike fluorescent particles if stained by the direct fluorescent antibody procedure.

2. *Histopathology.* Histological examination of biopsy or autopsy tissues is occasionally useful in diagnosing unsuspected cases of rabies that have not been tested by routine methods. When brain tissue from rabies-virus-infected animals are stained with a histologic stain, such as hematoxylin and eosin, evidence of encephalomyelitis may be recognized by a trained veterinary pathologist. This method is nonspecific and not considered diagnostic for rabies. Before current diagnostic methods were available, rabies diagnosis was made using this method and clinical case history (Hamir et al., 1992). After Louis Pasteur's successful experiments with rabies vaccination, scientists were motivated to identify the pathologic lesions of rabies virus. In fact, most of the significant histopathologic features of rabies infection were described in the last quarter of nineteenth century. Evidence of rabies-induced nonsuppurative encephalomyelitis in brain tissue includes the following: mononuclear infiltration, perivascular cuffing of predominantly lymphocytes (seldom polymorphonuclear cells), lymphocytic foci, Babès' nodules consisting of glial cells, and Negri bodies.

3. *Negri bodies.* In 1903, most of the histopathologic signs of rabies were recognized, but rabies inclusions had not yet been detected. At this time, Dr. Adelchi Negri reported the identification of what he believed to be the etiologic agent of rabies, the Negri bodies are round or oval inclusions within the cytoplasm of nerve cells of animals infected with rabies (Murphy et al., 1973; Perl, 1975; Tierkel et al., 1996). Negri bodies may vary in size from 0.25–27.00 μm and are found most frequently in the pyramidal cells of Ammon's horn and the Purkinje cells of cerebellum. They are also found in the cells of the medulla and various other ganglia and in the neurons of the salivary glands, tongue, or other organs. Staining with Mann's, Giemsa, or Sellers stains can permit differentiation of rabies inclusions from other intracellular inclusions, where Negri bodies appear magenta in color and have small (0.2 μm–0.5 μm) dark blue interior basophilic granules. The presence of Negri bodies is variable, and they are quite infrequent particularly in equine nervous tissue (Silva et al., 1974). Histologic staining for Negri bodies is neither as sensitive nor as specific as other tests. Some experimentally infected cases of rabies display Negri bodies in brain tissue; others do not (Perl, 1975). Histologic examination of tissues from clinically rabid animals show Negri bodies in about 50% of the samples; in contrast, the FAT shows rabies antigen in nearly 100% of the samples. Green et al. (1992) found 53% of equine rabies cases negative for Negri bodies, whereas Peixoto et al. (2000) found both Negri bodies observation and FAT less

sensitive in equine rabies (36.9% and 76.6%, respectively) compared to bovine rabies (79.5% and 94.1%, respectively).

4. *Immunohistochemistry.* Immunohistochemical methods for rabies detection provide sensitive and specific means to detect rabies in formalin-fixed tissues. These methods are more sensitive than histologic staining methods, such as H and E and Sellers stains. Like the FAT, these procedures use specific antibodies to detect rabies virus inclusions (Genovese and Andral, 1978). The techniques use enzyme-labeling systems that increase sensitivity. In addition, monoclonal antibodies may be used to detect rabies virus variants.

5. *Ultrastructure.* The ultrastructure of viruses can be examined by electron microscopy. Using this method, the structural components of viruses and their inclusions can be observed in detail. When viewed with an electron microscope, Rhabdoviruses are seen as bullet-shaped particles.

6. *Amplification methods.* Samples containing small amounts of rabies virus may be difficult to confirm as rabies positive by routine methods. Amplification methods should be used if the FAT gives an uncertain result or when the FAT is negative. Virus isolation in cell cultures increases the virus concentration because the virus replicates in cell cultures. Virus-isolation tests such as the rabies tissues culture inoculation test (RTCIT) involve infecting neuroblastoma cells with rabies-positive brain material. Mouse neuroblastoma cells (MNA) and baby hamster kidney (BHK) cells provide an excellent environment for amplification of rabies virus without the use of animals (Barrat et al., 1986; Rudd and Trimachi, 1987).

7. In *Mouse inoculation test* three to four weeks old (12–14 g) or a litter of two-day-old newborn mice are inoculated intracerebrally. The inoculum is the clarified supernatant of a 20% (w/v) homogenate of brain material (cortex, Ammon's horn, cerebellum, medulla oblongata) in an isotonic buffered solution containing antibiotics. The young adult mice are observed daily for twenty-eight days, and every dead mouse is examined for rabies using the FAT. For faster results in newborn mice, it is possible to check one baby mouse by FAT on days 5, 7, 9, and 11 postinoculation. Any deaths occurring during the first four days are regarded as nonspecific.

8. *Nucleic Acid Amplification:* Another method for amplifying the nucleic acid portion of rabies virus uses biochemical methods. With this procedure, rabies virus RNA can be enzymatically amplified as DNA copies. Rabies RNA can be copied into a DNA molecule using reverse transcriptase (RT). The DNA copy of can then be amplified

using polymerase chain reaction (PCR). This technique can confirm FAT results and can detect rabies virus in saliva and skin biopsy samples. These techniques would include the use of MAbs, nucleic acid probes, or the RT-PCR (Ito et al., 2001; Sato et al., 2005), followed by DNA sequencing of genomic areas for typing the virus (Bourhy and Sureau, 1991). This characterization enables a distinction to be made between vaccine virus and a field strain of virus and, possibly, the geographical origin of the latter. Vázquez-Morón et al. (2006) reported RT-PCR for detection of all seven genotypes of *Lyssavirus* genus and suggested that this method can be used to complement immunofluorescence for the diagnosis of rabies, enabling the detection of unexpected *Lyssaviruses* during rabies surveillance.

9. ***PCA(Passive Cutaneous anaphylaxis reaction).*** Another test for the quick diagnosis of rabies is by ***PCA (passive cutaneous anaphylaxis reaction)*** (Mathew, 1971). More details are given in chapter 13 on "Bovine Rabies" in this book.

10. ***Serological tests.*** Serological tests are rarely used in epidemiological surveys due to late seroconversion and the low percentage of animals surviving the disease and therefore having postinfection antibodies. Circulating antibodies appear slowly in the course of infection, but they are usually present by the time of onset of clinical symptoms. The most commonly used serological tests were the mouse infection neutralization test (MNT) or the rapid fluorescent focus inhibition test (RFFIT) (WHO, 1996). These tests have now been largely superseded by ELISAs. The main application of serology is to determine responses to vaccination, either in domestic animals prior to international travel or in wildlife populations following oral immunization of rabies reservoirs. For follow-up investigations in oral vaccination campaigns, virus neutralization (VN) tests in cell culture are preferred (Cliquet et al., 1998). However, if poor-quality sera are submitted, the VN tests in cell culture are sensitive to cytotoxicity, which could lead to false-positive results. For such samples, the use of an indirect ELISA with rabies glycoprotein-coated plates has been shown to be as sensitive and specific as the VN test on cells (Cliquet et al., 2000).

TREATMENT

Currently, there is no treatment for rabies, and infected horses invariably die. Since many rabies cases present as undiagnosed neurologic disease, supportive care and symptomatic treatment is often initiated. Horses that are known to have been exposed to rabies should have all wounds cleaned and irrigated with iodine or quaternary ammonium disinfectant. The virus is relatively fragile and is killed by most disinfectants (including 70% isopropyl alcohol, aldehydes, ethanol, lipid solvents, povidine iodine, quaternary ammonium compounds, bleach, etc.), ultraviolet light, and heat (1 h at 50°C). The virus dies in dried saliva within hours and will die in a carcass within twenty-four hours at 20°C (68°F) (Health Canada, Material Safety Data Sheet, 2002). However, the virus survives longer at colder temperatures, living for days in carcasses under cold conditions. In a known exposed horse, rabies antiserum, if available, should be infiltrated around the area of the bite would. Unfortunately, as mentioned previously, most exposures are not observed, and most bite wounds are not found. Because of the serious public health risk and the invariably fatal nature of the disease, if a horse is showing clinical signs and a diagnosis of rabies is made, treatment is not advocated, and euthanasia should be performed immediately.

PREVENTION AND CONTROL

1. *Preexposure vaccination and management.* Animal management is the keystone of any modern program for the prevention and control of rabies (Meltzer and Rupprecht, 1998; Larghi, 2004; Cleaveland et al., 2006; Rupprecht et al., 2006; Fooks, 2007; Leung et al., 2007; Rupprecht et al., 2008; Blancou, 2008). Certain countries of the Middle East region are facing increasing problems due to wildlife rabies, including Saudi Arabia, Oman, Yemen, Israel, Iran, and Turkey (Siemens, 2008). While control activities have traditionally focused upon certain Carnivora species, bats represent another worldwide rabies reservoir (van der Poel et al., 2006; Rupprecht et al., 2008). Animal rabies control primarily consists of the vaccination of dogs and cats, the elimination of stray animals, health education for the public, etc. Although there may be some differences of opinion with regard to vaccination of horses against rabies, the vaccination of companion animals, including the horse, cannot be overemphasized. Just like for dogs and cats, the potential for exposure to rabies for horses exists and generally justifies rabies protection through vaccination. Unfortunately, rabies vaccination in horses is often overlooked because a lot of clinical cases of equine rabies are not seen. However, the fact that the disease is invariably fatal, as well as the considerable human health significance, makes rabies vaccination in horses something that veterinarians and horse owners should strongly consider (Brun et al., 1980; Green, 1993, 1997; Weese, 2002; Monaco et al., 2006; *www.thehorse.com*, 2008).

All horses kept in areas where rabies is endemic in the wildlife population are at risk and should be vaccinated. Parenteral animal rabies vaccines should be administered only by or under the direct supervision of a veterinarian. Within twenty-eight days after initial vaccination, a peak rabies virus antibody titer is reached, and the animal can be considered immunized. Regardless of the age of the animal at initial vaccination, a booster vaccination should be administered one year later. There are several key points to consider regarding vaccination: (1) the incidence of rabies in both wild and domestic animals is on the increase; (2) it is not uncommon for pastured or stalled horses to be unknowingly exposed to wildlife; (3) most exposures are not noticed, and most bite wounds are no found; (4) there is a significant and serious potential for human exposure from an infected animal because horses are often kept in close contact with people; (5) vaccination of the horse may serve to establish an immune barrier between humans and wildlife, (6) equine rabies cases are invariably fatal, (7) vaccination of horses against rabies is safe and, although not 100% effective, is generally highly protective; and (8) when dealing with a horse showing neurological signs, the concern for rabies can be somewhat minimized in a horse known to have been properly immunized. Feeding and/ or housing of wild animals (as pets) should be discouraged.

Animals that have frequent contact with humans and horses traveling interstate should be currently vaccinated against rabies (Bender and Schulman, 2004). Manufacturers of the two rabies vaccines marketed in Canada, Rabvac 3 (Ayerst) and RM Imrab 3 (Merial), recommend that horses receive a single 2-ml dose of vaccine starting at three months of age and repeated at one year of age, followed by annual revaccination. Merial recommends that RM Imrab 3 be given by either intramuscular or subcutaneous injection. Ayerst recommends that Rabvac 3 be administered by intramuscular injection only. Neither vaccine has a caution for use in pregnant mares. Rabies vaccine can only be sold to a licensed veterinarian. Recently, EquiRab (Intervet/Schering-Plough Animal Health)—a new equine rabies vaccine aseptically injected intramuscularly, offering long-lasting protection against rabies in a single low-dose injection—has been introduced. Its annual revaccination is recommended (*www.thehorse.com*, 2008). Practitioners should consult with state or provincial authorities regarding the need for vaccination in their area. Since rabies have zoonotic significance, veterinary technicians, veterinarians, and other animal health workers should, therefore, be vaccinated against rabies (Green, 1993; Weese, 2002).

Rabies vaccines for use in animals contain either live virus attenuated for the target species (such as Flury low egg passage, Flury high egg passage, Street-Alabama-Dufferin, or Kelev) or virus inactivated by chemical or physical means or recombinant vaccines. The virus is cultivated in the CNS tissue of newborn animals, in embryonated eggs, or in cell cultures. Rabies vaccines are usually lyophilized, but inactivated-virus vaccines, preferably with an adjuvant, may be stored in liquid form (*www.oie.int*).

The advent of genetic engineering has influenced the development of vaccines, providing more opportunities for the production of inactivated antigens and the attenuation of different viruses through direct mutation. Several new strategies including the use of vectors, plasmid DNA, lipopeptide vaccines, and plant-virus-based rabies vaccines are also being explored. Also, the paucity of vaccine adjuvants, essentially limited to aluminum salts, is at last being corrected by the production of new oil-in-water emulsions, liposomes, tool-like receptor agonists, cytokines, CpG oligonucleotides, and other substances (Yusibov et al., 2002; Fischer et al., 2003; Consales and Bolzan, 2007; Dhama et al., 2008).

2. *Postexposure management.* Any animal exposed to a confirmed or suspected rabid animal should be placed in strict isolation for six months, which refers to confinement in an enclosure that precludes direct contact with people and other animals. Rabies vaccine should be administered upon entry into isolation or one month before release. There are currently no licensed biologicals for postexposure prophylaxis of previously unvaccinated domestic animals, and there is evidence that the use of vaccine alone will not reliably prevent the disease in these animals (Green, 1997; Hanlon et al., 2002). Animals overdue for a booster vaccination need to be evaluated on a case-by-case basis for severity of exposure, time elapsed since last vaccination, number of previous vaccinations, current health status, and local rabies epidemiology. All species of livestock are susceptible to rabies; cattle and horses are the most frequently reported infected species (Blanton et al., 2008). Livestock exposed to a rabid animal and currently vaccinated with a vaccine should be revaccinated immediately and observed for forty-five days. Unvaccinated livestock should be kept under close observation for six months. If signs suggestive of rabies develop, the animal should be euthanized and the head shipped for testing.

3. *Outbreak prevention and control.* The emergence of new rabies virus variants or the introduction of nonindigenous viruses poses a significant risk to humans, domestic animals, and wildlife.

A rapid and comprehensive response includes the following measures: a. Characterize the virus at a national or regional reference laboratory. b. Identify and control the source of the introduction. c. Enhance laboratory-based surveillance in wild and domestic animals. d. Increase animal rabies vaccination rates. e. Restrict the movement of animals. f. Evaluate the need for vector population reduction. g. Coordinate a multiagency response. h. Provide public and professional outreach and education.

Being a zoonotic disease, appropriate precautions should be taken while handling suspicious or confirmed rabies case; all veterinary personnel need to be adequately protected. All tissues of infected animals are potentially infectious, with highest titers in the central nervous system, saliva, and salivary glands (Health Canada, Material Safety Datasheet, 2002; Weese, 2002). Rabies virus is most commonly transmitted through contact of saliva with broken skin or mucous membranes. Personal hygiene and the use of barrier precautions when handling animals, body fluids, or postmortem specimens will greatly reduce the possibility of disease transmission. Veterinarians should notify the appropriate authorities and all in-contact individuals should be taken care of as to determine whether postexposure prophylaxis is required by observing the likelihood of rabies (Beran, 1993; Centers for Disease Control and Prevention, 1999; Weese, 2002; Bender and Schulman, 2004; Hankins and Rosekrans, 2004; Leung et al., 2007; Dendle and Looke, 2008). Persons more likely to be exposed to rabies should be suitably vaccinated and monitored for antibody titers every two years to ensure that adequate protection persists.

CONCLUSION

Rabies is a sporadic viral disease caused by a neurotropic Rhabdovirus. Rabies in the horse is a relatively uncommon disease. While the incidence of rabies in horses is low, the potential for human exposure is quite significant. Horses get rabies from the saliva of an infected animal, either through a bite or by the saliva contaminating an open wound. Rabid skunks are responsible for the majority of rabies cases in horses. Skunks are nocturnal, so if one is seen during the day, it should be suspected as being rabid. However, foxes, raccoons, bats, and unimmunized dogs and cats have also been known to transmit the disease to horses. Horses are very curious, especially foals and yearlings, and try to investigate wildlife roaming the pasture. This makes them more likely to get bitten, especially on the nostrils or lips. The incubation period for the disease is usually two to six weeks, although sometimes it may take up to three months before symptoms appear. Diagnosing rabies is difficult because of the wide range of clinical signs. The most common sign of rabies is behavioral changes. The majority of horses initially are dull and depressed. A low-grade fever usually is present along with convulsions, increased sensitivity at the site of injury, lameness, gnawing the affected area, and anorexia. Symptoms usually progress quickly over five to seven days resulting in recumbency and death.

In many cases, rabies is not diagnosed upon the initial onset of symptoms as the horse is still calm, alert, and eating. Once symptoms appear, rabies progresses rapidly. Since rabies typically is rare in horses, a veterinarian should attempt to rule out other diagnoses before diagnosing rabies. Other diseases that present clinical symptoms similar to rabies are tetanus, equine herpesvirus, the various causes of encephalomyelitis, botulism, lead poisoning, moldy corn poisoning, protozoal myelitis, and trauma to the brain or spinal cord. Diagnosis can be performed accurately and rapidly within hours using the FAT. A positive test means treatment should be started for anyone who has come in contact with the rabid animal. The FAT may be confirmed by mouse inoculation studies or virus isolation in tissue culture. Other useful diagnostic tests are EM, histological examination, VN, IHC, RT-PCR, PCA and ELISA.

At the present, there is no antiserum for the treatment of the rabies virus. Immediate cleansing of the affected wound area may prevent infection, but postexposure vaccination of the animal is not really useful as the horse will die before immunity has time to develop. If a horse has been previously immunized, an immediate booster vaccination should be given. Strict quarantine and observation for six months should be mandatorily followed in all cases. If clinical symptoms develop, the horse should be euthanasized. Horses can be vaccinated for rabies; therefore, immunization is recommended for horses in an endemic area. Vaccination should begin at three to four months of age with a booster shot given annually.

REFERENCES

1. Albertini, A. A., Wernimont, A. K., Muziol, T., Ravelli, R. B., Clapier, C. R., Schoehn, G., Weissenhorn, W. and Ruigrok, R. W. 2006. Crystal structure of the rabies virus nucleoprotein-RNA complex. *Science* 5785:360–363.
2. Arai, Y. T. 2005. Epidemiology of rabies virus and other lyssaviruses. *Nippon Rinsho.* 63:2167–2172.
3. Aubert, M. F. A. 1982. Une méthode simple de calcul des titres des suspensions virales, vaccinales ou séroneutralisantes: La méthode graphique. (A simple method for calculating titres of virus, vaccine or serumneutralising suspensions: The graphic method.) *Rev. Sci. Tech. Off. Int. Epiz.* 1:828–833.
4. Badrane, H., Bahloul, C., Perrin, P. and Tordo, N. 2001. Evidence of two lyssavirus phylogroups with distinct pathogenicity and immunogenicity. *J. Virol.* 75, 3268–3276.
5. Baer, G. M. 1991. *The natural history of rabies*, 2nd ed. Boca Raton, Florida, USA: CRC Press.
6. Barrat, J. and Aubert M. F. A. 1995. Diagnostic de la rage animale en France de 1991 à 1993, bilan de CNEVA laboratoire d'études sur la rage et la pathologie des animaux sauvages en France. *Revue Méd. Vét.* 146, 561–566.
7. Barrat, J., Barrat, M. J., Picard, M. and Aubert, M. F. A. 1986. Diagnostic de la rage sur culture cellulaire, comparaison des résultats de l'inoculation au neuroblastome murin et de l'inoculation à la souris. *Comp. Immunol. Microbiol. Infect. Dis.* 11, 207–214.

8. Bender, J. and Schulman, S. 2004. Reports of zoonotic disease outbreaks associated with animal exhibits and availability of recommendations for preventing zoonotic disease transmission from animals to people in such settings. *J. Am. Vet. Med. Assoc.* 224:1105–1109.

9. Beran, G. W. 1993. Zoonoses in practice. *Vet. Clin. North Am. [Small Anim. Pract.]* 23:1085–1097.

10. Bhargava, A., Deshmukh, R., Ghosh, T. K., Goswami, A., Prasannaraj, P., Marfatia, S. P., Sudarshan, M. K. 1996. Profile and characteristics of animals' bites in India. *J. Assoc. Physicians India* 44:37–38.

11. Blancou, J. 2008. The control of rabies in Eurasia: Overview, history and background. *Dev. Biol.* (Basel) 131:3–15.

12. Blanton, J. D., Palmer, D., Christian, K. A. and Rupprecht, C. E. 2008. Rabies surveillance in the United States during 2007. *J. Am. Vet. Med. Assoc.* 233:884–97.

13. Bourhy, H. and Sureau, P. 1991. Méthodes de laboratoire pour le diagnostic de la rage; Metodos de laboratorio para el diagnostics de la rabia; Laboratory methods for rabies diagnosis. Commission des Laboratoires de référence et d'Expertise de l'Institut Pasteur, Paris, France, 197.

14. Bourhy, H., Kissi, B. and Tordo, N. 1993. Molecular diversity of the lyssavirus genus. *Virology* 194:70–81.

15. Brun, A., Duret, C., Devaux, B. and Calmels, D. 1980. Simple, simultaneous or combined vaccinations of horses against equine influenza, rabies and tetanus (author's transl.). *Comp. Immunol. Microbiol. Infect. Dis.* 3:93–99.

16. Carrieri, M. L., Peixoto, Z. M., Paciencia, M. L., Kotait, I. and Germano, P. M. 2006. Laboratory diagnosis of equine rabies and its implications for human postexposure prophylaxis. *J. Virol. Methods* 138:1–9.

17. Centers for Disease Control and Prevention 1999. Human rabies prevention. *MMWR Morb. Mortal Wkly Rep.,* 1999, 48:RR1–RR17.

18. Chhabra, M., Ichhpujani, R. L., Tewari, K. N. and Lal, S. 2004. Human rabies in Delhi. *Indian J. Pediatr.* 71:217–220.

19. Cleaveland, S., Hampson, K. and Kaare, M. 2007. Living with rabies in Africa. *Vet. Rec.* 161:293–294.

20. Cleaveland, S., Kaare, M., Knobel, D. and Laurenson, M. K. 2006. Canine vaccination: Providing broader benefits for disease control. *Vet. Microbiol.* 117:43–50.

21. Cliquet, F., Aubert, M. and Sagne, L. 1998. Development of a fluorescent antibody virus neutralisation test (FAVN test) for the quantitation of rabies-neutralising antibody. *J. Immunol. Methods* 212, 79–87.

22. Cliquet, F., Sagne, L., Schereffer, J. L. and Aubert M. F. A. 2000. ELISA tests for rabies antibody titration in orally vaccinated foxes sampled in the fields. *Vaccine* 18:3272–3279.

23. Cliquet, F. and Picard-Meyer, E. 2004. Rabies and rabies-related viruses: A modern perspective on an ancient disease. *Rev. Sci. Tech.* 23:625–642.

24. Consales, C. A. and Bolzan, V. L. 2007. Rabies review: Immunopathology, clinical aspects and treatment. *J. Venom. Anim. Toxins Incl. Trop. Dis.* 13:5–38.

25. David, D., Hughes G. J., Yakobson, B. A., Davidson, I., Un, H., Aylan, O., Kuzmin, I. V. and Rupprecht, C. E. 2007. Identification of novel canine rabies virus clades in the Middle East and North Africa. *J. Gen. Virol.* 88:967–980.

26. Dendle, C. and Looke, D. 2008. Review article: Animal bites: An update for management with a focus on infections. *Emerg. Med. Australas.* 20:458–467.

27. Dhama, K., Mahendran, M., Gupta, P. K. and Rai, A. 2008. DNA vaccines of veterinary importance: Current perspectives. *Vet. Res. Commun.* 32:341–356.

28. Diop, S. A., Manga, N. M., Dia, N. M., Ndour, C. T., Seydi, M., Soumare, M., Diop, B. M. and Sow, P. S. 2007. The point on human rabies in Senegal from 1986 to 2005. *Med. Mal. Infect.* 37:787–791.

29. Faber, M., Faber, M. L., Papaneri, A., Bette, M., Weihe, E., Dietzschold, B. and Schnell, M. J. 2005. A single amino acid change in rabies virus glycoprotein increases virus spread and enhances virus pathogenicity *J. Virol.* 79:14141–14148.

30. Fekadu, M., Shaddock, J. H., Sanderlin, D. W. and Smith, J. S. 1988. Efficacy of rabies vaccines against Duvenhage virus isolated from European house bats *(Eptesicus serotinus)*, classic rabies virus and rabiesrelated viruses. *Vaccine* 6:533–539.

31. Finke, S., Mueller-Waldeck, R. and Conzelmann, K. K. 2003. Rabies virus matrix protein regulates the balance of virus transcription and replication. *J. Gen. Virol.* 84:1613–1621.

32. Fischer, L., Minke, J., Dufay, N., Baudu, Ph. and Audonnet, J. C. 2003. Rabies DNA vaccine in the horse: Strategies to improve serological responses. *Vaccine* 21:4593–4596.

33. Fooks, A. R., Brookes, S. M., Johnson, N., McElhinney, L. M. and Hutson, A. M. 2003. European bat lyssaviruses: An emerging zoonosis. *Epidemiol. Infect.* 131:1029–1039.

34. Fooks, A. R. 2007. Rabies: The need for a "one medicine" approach. *Vet. Rec.* 161:289–290.

35. Gaudin, Y. 2000. Rabies virus-induced membrane fusion pathway. *J. Cell Biol.* 150:601–611.

36. Genovese, M. A. and Andral L. 1978. Comparaison de deux techniques utilisées pour le diagnostic de la rage: L'immunofluorescence et l'immunoperoxydase. *Rec. Med. Vet.* 154 (7–8): 667–671.

37. Green, S. L. 1993. Equine rabies. *Vet. Clin. North. Am. Equine Pract.* 9:337–347.

38. Green, S. L. 1997. Rabies. *Vet. Clin. North Am. Equine Pract.* 13:1–11.

39. Green, S. L., Smith, L. L., Vernau, W. and Beacock, S. M. 1992. Rabies in horses: 21 cases (1970–1990). *J Am Vet Med Assoc.* 200:1133–1137.

40. Griego, R. D., Rosen, T., Orengo, I. F. and Wolf, J. E. 1995. Dog, cat, and human bites: A review. *J. Am. Acad. Dermatol.* 33:1019–1029.

41. Gruzdev, K. N. 2008. The rabies situation in Central Asia. *Dev. Biol* (Basel) 131:37–42.

42. Hamir, A. N., Moser, G. and Rupprecht, C. E. 1992. A five year (1985–1989) retrospective study of equine neurological diseases with special reference to rabies. *J. Comp. Pathol.* 106:411–421.

43. Hanlon, C. A., Niezgoda, M. N. and Rupprecht, C. E. 2002. Postexposure prophylaxis for prevention of rabies in dogs. *Am. J. Vet. Res.* 63:1096–1100.

44. Hankins, D. G. and Rosekrans, J. A. 2004. Overview, prevention and treatment of rabies. *Mayo. Clin. Proc.* 79:671–676.

45. Health Canada. Material Safety Data Sheet: Infectious substances: Rabies virus. Available online at http://www.hc-sc.gc.ca/pphb-dgspsp/msds-ftss/msds124e.html. Accessed on April 2, 2002. 8. Beran GW. Zoonoses.

46. Hooper, P. T., Lunt, R. A., Gould, A. R., Samaratunga, H., Hyatt, A. D., Gleeson, L. J., Rodwell, B. J., the?Rupprecht, C. E., Smith, J. S. and Murray, P. K. 1997. A new lyssavirus—first endemic rabies-related virus recognized in Australia. *Bull. Inst. Pasteur* 95:209–218.

47. Hudson, L. C., Weinstock, D., Jordan, T. and Bold-Fletcher, N. O. 1996. Clinical presentation of experimentally induced rabies in horses. *Zentralbl Veterinarmed* B 43:277–285.

48. Ichhpujani, R. L., Mala, C., Veena, M., Singh, J., Bhardwaj, M., Bhattacharya, D., Pattanaik, S. K., Balakrishnan, N., Reddy, A. K., Samnpath, G., Gandhi, N., Nagar, S. S. and Shiv, L. 2008. Epidemiology of animal bites and rabies cases in India. A multicentric study. *J. Commun. Dis.* 40:27–36.

49. Ito, M., Arai, Y. T., Itou, T., Sakai, T., Ito, F. H., Takasaki, T. and Kurane, I. 2001. Genetic characterization and geographic distribution of rabies virus isolates in Brazil: Identification of two reservoirs, dogs and vampire bats. *Virology* 284:214–222.

50. Kuzmin, I. V., Botvinkin, A. D., McElhinney, L. M., Smith, J. S., Orciari, L. A., Hughes, G. J., Fooks, A. R. and Rupprecht, C. E. 2004. Molecular epidemiology of terrestrial rabies in the former Soviet Union. *J. Wildlife Dis.* 40:617–631.

51. Larghi, O. P. 2004. Perspectives for rabies control and eradication from domestic species in developing countries. *Dev. Biol.* (Basel) 119:205–212.

52. Larsen, D. D., Wickersham, I. R. and Callaway, E. M. 2008. Retrograde tracing with recombinant rabies virus reveals correlations between projection targets and dendritic architecture in layer 5 of mouse barrel cortex. *Frontiers in Neural Circuits* 1:1–7.

10. EQUINE RABIES

53. Leung, A. K., Davies, H. D. and Hon, K. L. 2007. Rabies: Epidemiology, pathogenesis, and prophylaxis. *Adv. Ther.* 24:1340–1347.
54. Mathew, Z. 1971. Diagnosis of rabies infection by passive cutaneous anaphylaxis reaction, 53–95. PhD thesis, Haffkine Institute, University of Bombay.
55. Matouch, O. 2008. The rabies situation in Eastern Europe. *Dev. Biol.* (Basel) 131:27–35.
56. Matsumoto, S. 1975. Electron microscopy of central nervous system. In *The natural history of rabies*, vol. 1, ed. G. M. Baer, 217. New York: Academic Press.
57. Mavrakis, M., Mehouas, S., Real, E., Iseni, F., Blondel, D., Tordo, N. and Ruigrok, R. W. 2006. Rabies virus chaperone: Identification of the phosphoprotein peptide that keeps nucleoprotein soluble and free from non-specific RNA. *Virology* 2:422–429.
58. McColl, K. A., Tordo, N. and Aguilar Setién, A. A. 2000. Bat lyssavirus infections. *Rev Sci Tech.* 19:177–96.
59. Meltzer, M. I. and Rupprecht, C. E. 1998. Review of the economics of the prevention and control of rabies. Part 2: Rabies in dogs, livestock and wildlife. *Pharmacoeconomics* 14:481–498.
60. Meslin, F. X. and Kaplan, M. M. 1996. An overview of laboratory techniques in the diagnosis and prevention of rabies and in rabies research. In *Laboratory techniques in rabies*, 4th ed., F. X. Meslin, M. M. Kaplan and H. Koprowski, 9–16. Genebra: World Health Organization.
61. Meyer, E. E., Morris, P. G., Elcock, L. H. and Weil, J. 1986. Hind limb hyperesthesia associated with rabies in two horses. *J. Am. Vet. Med. Assoc.* 188:629–632.
62. Monaco, F., Franchi, P. M. and Lelli, R. 2006. Studies on an inactivated vaccine against rabies virus in domestic animals. *Dev. Biol.* (Basel) 125:233–239.
63. Murphy, F. A., Harrison, A. K., Win, W. C. and Baur, S. P. 1973. Comparative pathogenesis of rabies and rabies-like viruses. Infection of the central nervous system and centrifugal spread of virus to peripheral tissue. *Lab. Invest.* 29:1–16.
64. Nel, L. H. and Rupprecht, C. E. 2007. Emergence of lyssaviruses in the old world: The case of Africa. *Curr Top Microbiol Immunol.* 315:161–193.
65. Peixoto, Z. M. P., Cunha, E. M. S., Sacramento, D. R. V., Souza, M. C. A. M., da Silva, L. H. Q., Germano, P. L., Kroeff, S. S. and Kotait, I. 2000. Rabies laboratory diagnosis: Peculiar features of samples from equine origin. *Braz. J. Microbiol.* 31:72–75.
66. Perl, D. P. 1975. The pathology of rabies in the central nervous system. In *The natural history of rabies*, vol. 1, ed. G. M. Baer, 235. New York: Academic Press.
67. Radostits, O. M., Gay, C. C., Blood, D. C. and Hinchcliff, K. W. 2000. Rabies. In *Veterinary medicine*, 9th ed., 2000:1201–1208. Philadelphia, PA: W. B. Saunders Co. Ltd.
68. Rudd, R. J. and Trimachi, C. V. 1987. Comparison of sensitivity of BHK-21 and murine neuroblastoma cells in the isolation of a street strain rabies virus. *J. Clin. Microbiol.* 25:145–168.
69. Rudd, R. J., Smith, J. S., Yager, P. A. et al. 2005. A need for standardized rabies virus diagnostic procedures: Effect of cover-glass mountant on the reliability of antigen detection by the fluorescent antibody test. *Virus Res.* 111:83–88.
70. Rupprecht, C. E., Hanlon, C. A. and Slate, D. 2006. Control and prevention of rabies in animals: Paradigm shifts. *Dev. Biol.* (Basel) 125:103–111.
71. Rupprecht, C. E., Barrett, J., Briggs, D., Cliquet, F., Fooks, A. R., Lumlertdacha, B., Meslin, F. X., Muler, T., Nel, L. H., Schneider, C., Tordo, N. and Wandeler, A. I. 2008. Can rabies be eradicated? *Dev. Biol.* (Basel) 131:95–121.
72. Rupprecht, C. E., Hanlon, C. A., and Slate, D. 2004. Oral vaccination of wildlife against rabies: Opportunities and challenges in prevention and control. *Dev. Biol.* (Basel) 119:173–184.
73. Sato, G., Tanabe, H., Shoji, Y., Itou, T., Ito, F. H., Sato, T. and Sakai, T. 2005. Rapid discrimination of rabies viruses isolated from various host species in Brazil by multiplex reverse transcription-polymerase chain reaction. *J. Clin. Virol.* 33:267–273.
74. Seimenis A. 2008. The rabies situation in the Middle East. *Dev. Biol.* (Basel) 131:43–53.

75. Silva, R. A., Silva, N. M. and Menezes, P. R. V. 1974. Ocorrência do vírus da raiva na medula e no bulbo de eqüinos na doença natural e sua ausência nas diferentes regiões do sistema nervoso central e outro tecidos. *Pesq. Agrop. Bras.*, *Sér. Vet.* 9:29–31.

76. Smreczak, M., Trebas, P., Orłowska, A., Mudziński, J. F. 2008. Rabies surveillance in Poland (1992–2006). *Dev Biol* (Basel) 131:249–256.

77. Tamashiro, H., Matibag, G. C., Ditangco, R. A., Kanda, K. and Ohbayashi, Y. 2007. Revisiting rabies in Japan: Is there cause for alarm? *Travel Med. Infect. Dis.* 5:263–275.

78. Tierkel, E. S. and Atanasiu, P. 1996. Routine laboratory procedures: Rapid microscopic examination for Negri bodies and preparation of specimens for biological tests. In *Laboratory techniques in rabies*, 4th ed., F. X. Meslin, M. M. Kaplan and H. Koprowski, 55–65. Geneva World Health Organization.

79. Tordo, N., Poch, O., Ermine, A., Keith, G. and Rougeon, F. 1986. Walking along the rabies genome: Is the large G-L intergenic region a remnant gene? *Proc. Natl. Acad. Sci. USA* 11:3914–3918.

80. Tordo, N., Poch, O., Ermine, A., Keith, G. and Rougeon, F. 1988. Completion of the rabies virus genome sequence determination: Highly conserved domains among the L (polymerase) proteins of unsegmented negative-strand RNA viruses. *Virology.* 2:565–576.

81. Umoh, J. U. and Blenden, D. C. 1981. Immunofluorescent staining of rabies virus antigen in formalin fixed tissue after treatment with trypsin. *Bull. WHO* 59:737–744.

82. van der Poel, W. H., Lina, P. H. and Kramps, J. A. 2006. Public health awareness of emerging zoonotic viruses of bats: A European perspective. *Vector Borne Zoonotic Dis.* 6:315–324.

83. Vázquez-Morón, S., Avellón, A. and Echevarría, J. E. 2006. RT-PCR for detection of all seven genotypes of lyssavirus genus. *J. Virol. Methods* 135:281–287.

84. Warner, C. K., Whitfield, S. G., Fekadu, M. and Ho, H. 1997. Procedures for reproducible detection of rabies virus antigen mRNA and genome *in situ* in formalin-fixed tissues. *J. Virol. Methods* 67:5–12.

85. Weese, J. S. 2002. A review of equine zoonotic diseases: Risks in veterinary medicine. *Proceedings of the Annual Convention of the AAEP 2002*, 48:362–369.

86. World Health Organisation 1996. *Laboratory techniques in rabies*, 4th ed., ed. F. X. Meslin, M. M. Kaplan, and H. Koprowski. Geneva, Switzerland: WHO.

87. World Health Organization Expert Committee on Rabies, First Report. 2005. World Health Organisation, WHO Technical Report Series, 931, 1–87. Geneva, Switzerland: WHO,

88. Wunner, W. H. 1991. The chemical composition and molecular structure of rabies viruses. In *The natural history of rabies*, ed. G. M. Baer, 31–67. Boca Raton, FL: CRC Press.

89. www.oi.int. 2008. *Manual of diagnostic tests and vaccines for terrestrial animals.*

90. www.thehorse.com 2008. Intervet's Equirab Rabies Vaccine: New Equine Rabies Vaccine Introduced: Edited Press Release July 10, 2008, Article # 12253. http://www.thehorse.com/ViewArticle. aspx?ID=12253.

91. Yusibov V., Hooper, D. C., Stitsin, S. V., Fleysh, N., Kean, R. B., Mikheeva, T., Deka, D., Karasev, A., Cox, S., Randall, J. and Koprowski, H. 2002. Expression in plants and immunogenicity of plant virus-based experimental rabies vaccine. *Vaccine* 20:3155–3164.

11. Equine Rhinoviruses / Rhinitis Viruses

S. Kapoor, K. Dhama, R. V. S. Pawaiya, and P. Bhatt

Introduction

Equine rhinitis viruses, formerly named equine rhinoviruses, are known to cause clinical and subclinical upper respiratory infections in horses. Serologic studies indicate a high prevalence of these viruses worldwide, and it is likely that the majority of horses are exposed to rhinitis viruses at some stage in their lives (Plummer, 1962; Burrows, 1970; Becker et al., 1974; Thorsen, 1991; Studdert, 1996; Carman et al., 1997; Cullinane et al., 2006; Studdert, 2007). These viruses belong to family Picornaviridae, as do human rhinoviruses, frequently associated with common cold. Picornaviruses are recognized causes of acute upper respiratory and systemic diseases in horses. The clinical signs in horses are similar to that of common cold in humans. Serologic studies indicate a high prevalence of these viruses worldwide. Diagnosis of the disease is achieved by virus isolation, serological tools, and the application recent molecular tools. Vaccines have not been developed for equine rhinitis viruses; therefore, management practices need to be finely tuned for prevention and control of disease in horses.

Etiology

Several different types of equine rhinitis viruses have been identified. Among those viruses that were formerly called equine rhinoviruses (genus: *Rhinovirus*), three acid-labile virus serotypes were identified (Flammini and Allegri, 1970, 1971; Hofer et al., 1973; Newman et al., 1977; Steck et al., 1978). First isolated in 1960s, the biophysical properties of these viruses, like being acid labile (infectivity destroyed at pH3), indicated them to be in the genus *Rhinovirus* of Picornaviridae family, which includes the common cold viruses of humans. As per current classification, equine rhinitis viruses belong to the genera *Aphthovirus* or *Erbovirus* in the family Picornaviridae (Thorsen, 1991; Studdert, 1996; Black and Studdert, 2006; Cullinane et al., 2006; Studdert, 2007). Equine rhinitis A virus is a species within the genus *Aphthovirus* containing a single serotype while equine rhinitis B viruses (ERBV-1 and ERBV-2) are classified in the genus *Erbovirus*. The former ungrouped acid-stable equine picornavirus is now classified as equine rhinitis B virus 3 (ERBV-3).

Serotype 1 (equine rhinovirus 1, ERV-1), appearing to be the most clinically significant, has been renamed equine rhinitis A virus (ERAV); and on the basis of its close relationship to foot-and-mouth disease virus (FMDV), it has been reclassified (King et al., 2005) as a member (the only non-FMD virus) of genus *Aphthovirus*, although as a separate cluster. Many of the known physicochemical and biological properties of the virus (Plummer, 1963; Newman et al., 1973; Studdert and Gleeson, 1978) are consistent with its reclassification. The illness resembles the common cold brought about by rhinoviruses in humans; however, the presence of a viremia during ERV-1 infection, the occurrence of persistent infections, and the physical properties are all more reminiscent of FMDV (Wutz et al., 1996). The phylogenetic trees also confirmed the homology of the nucleotide sequence of the ERAV genome with that of FMDV, which suggested that ERAV may be a member, although very distant, of the *Aphthovirus* genus (Li et al., 1996; Wutz et al., 1996). Similarly, bovine rhinovirus 2 (BRV-2), a causative agent of respiratory disease in cattle, tentatively assigned to the genus *Rhinovirus* in the family Picornaviridae, has been only recently proposed to be considered as a new species within the genus *Aphthovirus*. Molecular and phylogenetic analyses of BRV-2 suggested it to be closely related to FMDV (Hollister et al., 2008).

The identity of a second serotype (prototype 1436/71) was confirmed by Newman et al. (1973). Equine rhinovirus serotype 2 (ERV-2) has been presently renamed equine rhinitis B virus (ERBV-1) and reclassified (King et al., 2005) as a member of the new genus *Erbovirus* (erb: equine rhinitis B) (Wutz et al., 1996; Stanway et al., 2002). The cDNA cloning and sequencing of the genomes of ERV-1 and ERV-2 between the poly(C) and poly(A) tracts showed that the serotypes are heterogeneous (Wutz et al., 1996). ERV-2 is most closely related to encephalomyocarditis virus, a member of the *Cardiovirus* genus (Wutz et al., 1996).

Existence of a third serotype was indicated by Steck et al. (1978), with prototype virus strain 313/75, formerly known as equine rhinovirus 3 (ERV-3) (Mumford and Thomson, 1978). Sequence comparison and phylogenic analysis suggest that ERBV strain P313/75 is most closely related to P1436/71. Thus, P313/75 was classified into as a new member of the genus *Erbovirus*, tentatively proposed to be designated ERBV-2. The genetically related and possessing similar physicochemical properties but antigenically/ serologically distinct ERBV-2.313/75 (Huang et al., 2001) is recognized as the only other member of this genus (Huang et al., 2001; King et al., 2005). Some ERBV-1 isolates have been shown to be stable at acid pH, distinguishable from acid-labile ERBV-1 by genomic sequence analysis (Black et al., 2005). Acid-stable picornaviruses (ASPs) were isolated from nasal swabs taken from horses with acute febrile respiratory disease in the UK and Japan and were placed in the group of unclassified picornaviruses. The nucleotide sequence of the P1 region, encoding the capsid proteins, of ASP isolates aligned with published sequences of ERBV, genus *Erbovirus*—including acid-labile ERBV-1 and ERBV-2 and the recently identified acid-stable ERBV-1—indicated that the ASPs belong to the same phylogenetic group, composed of acid-stable ERBV-1 isolates (Black and Studdert, 2006). This supported prior findings that ASPs are a distinct serotype, although cross-neutralizing weakly with ERBV-1 (Mumford and Thomson, 1978; Fukunaga et al., 1983). These ASPs formed the fourth serotype and named as ERBV-3. Based on sequence variation, existence of three distinct phylogenetic groups within equine rhinitis B viruses (erboviruses, ERBV) has been reported that correlate with serotype and acid-stability phenotypes (Black et al., 2005; Wesley et al., 2005). The genus *Erbovirus*, therefore, presently comprises three serotypes: ERBV-1 (prototype 1436/71), ERBV-2 (prototype 313/75), and the proposed ERBV-3 (prototype 4442/75) (Wutz et al., 1996; Huang et al., 2001; Black and Studdert, 2006; Studdert, 2007).

Equine rhinitis viruses are nonenveloped, 24–30 nm in diameter with icosahedral symmetry. Their genome is single-stranded, positive-sense RNA with a small oligopeptide, VPg (virus-protein-attached-to-the-genome) covalently linked to its 5' terminus, and a poly A sequence at 3' terminus. The transcription of the genome gives rise to a polyprotein that is furthermore processed and cleaved to give four structural/capsid proteins (VP1, VP2, VP3, and VP4), and several nonstructural proteins (2A, 2B, 2C, 3A [VPg], 3B, 3C, 3D) (Korant et al., 1970, 1972; Wutz et al., 1996; Hartley et al., 2001). The structural proteins (VP1-4) of erboviruses are not well described but are predicted by sequence to be 35, 29, 26, and 7kDa (Black et al., 2008). The VP1 protein has been shown to be a target of neutralizing antibodies, and neutralizing epitopes within VP1 are highly conformational (Hartley et al., 2001; Warner et al., 2001; Kriegshauser et al., 2003). N-terminal region of ERAV VP1, in particular, contains strong B cell epitopes (Stevenson et al., 2003). BetaE-betaF (EF) loop of VP1 is suggested to be involved in a neutralization epitope of ERAV (Stevenson et al., 2004a). Sialic acid acts as a receptor for ERAV binding and infection (Stevenson et al., 2004b). Sequence conservation and antigenic variation of the structural proteins (neutralization epitopes) of ERAV have been reported by Varrasso et al. (2001). Black et al. (2008) have recently suggested that the nonstructural 27kDa 3C(pro) copurifies with ERBV-1 virions.

The density of the ERAV in cesium chloride (CsCl) is 1.45g/ml. The ERBV-1.1436/71 virion has a heterogenous buoyant density in CsCl of 1.40–1.45g/ml (Newman et al., 1977). They are not inactivated by lipid solvents (ether or chloroform) or by nonionic detergents. The ERAV is inactivated at 50°C after sixty minutes and is not stabilized by 1M MgCl$_2$, whereas ERBV-1 and ERBV-3 are stabilized by 1M $MgCl_2$ (Ditchfield and Macpherson, 1965; Wilson et al., 1966; Flammini and Allegri, 1970; Newmann et al., 1977; Mumford and Thomson, 1978; Studdert and Gleeson, 1978). The ERAV, ERBV-1, ERBV-2 are acid labile, whereas ERBV-3 is acid stable surviving pH 3.6 for one hour at room temperature (Black et al., 2005; Black and Studdert, 2006). ERAV is nonhemagglutinating (human O, guinea pig, equine, and chicken RBCs).

EPIDEMIOLOGY

ERAV was first isolated and characterized in the United Kingdom (Plummer, 1962 and 1963; Plummer and Kerry, 1962). Thereafter, the virus has been isolated from many parts of world (Plummer and Kerry, 1962; Studdert, 1996 and 2007). The ERBV-1 and ERBV-2 have been isolated in Switzerland, UK, USA, Canada, Australia, and Japan over an approximately forty-five-year period (Plummer, 1962; Ditchfield et al., 1965; Teufel and Keller, 1970; Studdert and Gleeson, 1977, 1978; Mumford and Thomson, 1978; Steck et al., 1978; Fukunaga et al., 1983; McCollum and Timoney, 1992; Carman et al., 1997; Huang et al., 2001; Black et al., 2007b; Dynon et al., 2007; Studdert, 2007; Kriegshäuser et al., 2008). Generally, ERAV is most frequently isolated, whereas others (ERBV-1, ERBV-2, and ERBV-3) appear to be less frequently isolated. However, ERBV was isolated from twenty-eight of sixty-four (44%) samples from horses with acute febrile respiratory disease, of which six (21%) showed a significant rise to ERBV-2 antibody (Carman et al., 1997). Only one other isolation of ERBV-2 from a horse with febrile respiratory disease has been reported (Black et al., 2007b; Dynon et al., 2007).

The neutralizing antibodies to ERAV, ERBV-1, and ERBV-2 have been reported to be present in approximately 50–90% of horses in Switzerland, UK, Austria, Canada, Japan, New Zealand, the Netherlands, Australia, USA, and United Arab Emirates (Burrows, 1970; Holmes et al., 1978; Studdert and Gleeson, 1978; de Boer et al., 1979; Sugiura et al., 1987; McCollum and Timoney, 1991; Herbst et al., 1992; Carman et al., 1997; Wernery et al., 1998; Huang et al., 2001; Dunowska et al., 2002; Kriegshäuser et al., 2005; Black et al., 2007a; Dynon et al., 2007; Studdert, 2007). Despite high seroprevalence rates for ERAV, ERVB-1 and ERBV-2, these viruses are seldom specifically diagnosed as causes of respiratory diseases in horses; this is due to leading position of equine influenza and herpesviruses (EHV-1 and EHV-4) as causes of acute upper respiratory disease in horses and lack of sensitive, widely available, and adopted tests for rhinoviruses (Studdert, 2007). Maternal antibody for ERAV, ERBV-1, and ERBV-2 has been detected after twelve hours of suckling in foals born to antibody-positive mares. By ten to twelve months, however, ERAV SN antibodies were not be detected in any of the progeny, whereas ERBV-1 and ERBV antibodies were common (Black et al., 2007a).

Equine rhinitis viruses have been isolated mainly from the nasopharynx of horses with acute febrile respiratory disease. These are spread by contact through nasal secretions and aerosol inhalation (Burrows, 1970; Studdert and Gleeson, 1978). However, horses may carry and shed ERAV in their urine and feces for up to four weeks postinfection, and urine aerosol may also transmit the virus (McCollum and Timoney, 1991). The frequency of ERAV shedding in urine has been reported to be highest in two-year-old horses and appear to decline in older horses, although horses up to ten years of age shed virus. Virus shedding from urine is more long prolonged than shedding from the nasal cavity.

ERAV may remain infectious in the environment under favorable conditions for extended periods, perhaps months (Burrows, 1970). In general, Thoroughbred horses six to twenty-four months of age are serologically negative to ERAV and do not seroconvert until after entering training stables, which suggest that most horses are infected with ERAV during the period of training and racing (Burrows, 1970; Thorsen, 1991; Black et al., 2007a). ERAV enters the blood and elicits a very high serum antibody response that seems to then limit the spread of the virus by herd immunity, given that only approximately 40% of horses have detectable ERAV antibody (Black et al., 2007a). ERBVs infect most foals and weanlings, eliciting a low serum antibody response in sharp contrast to ERAVs, and appears to only infect horses once they begin training for racing (~two years old). The low serum antibody response of ERBV appears to allow the continual, seasonal reinfection of horses.

Recently, ERAV has been isolated from aborted dromedary (*Camelus dromedarius*) fetuses during an abortion storm in Dubai, United Arab Emirates (Wernery et al., 2008). The association of ERAV with abortion in dromedary was further confirmed as both aborted, and an identical virus was reisolated from the fetuses from two pregnant dromedaries that were experimentally infected with the camel virus isolate. The prevalence of antibody was very high (>90%), and the high titers recorded against ERAV in the dromedary herd clearly showed that dromedaries can be infected by ERAV. However, unlike horses, the target organ of ERAV in dromedaries appears to be the genital tract rather than the upper respiratory.

Natural and experimental infections with ERAV have been evidenced in humans. Natural infection of human with equine rhinitis A virus (ERAV) was reported about five decades ago. Severe pharyngitis and swelling of the pharyngeal lymph nodes accompanied by fever has been reported in experimentally infected person (Plummer, 1962, 1963). Virus has also been isolated from the blood from experimentally infected volunteer. Based on serological reports, persons working with horses can be infected with ERAV, but clinical symptoms have not been observed, and neither any human-to-human transmission of virus has been documented in such naturally occurring infections (Kriegshauser et al., 2005). High ERAV neutralizing antibodies in 3/9 (25%) stable workers as compared to 0% in nonstable workers have been reported (Plummer and Kerry, 1962). Out of 137 veterinary personnel's sera, only four (2.7%) and five (3.6%) human sera showed weak neutralizing activity to ERAV and ERBV-1, respectively, indicating that the risk of acquiring equine rhinoviruses as zoonotic infection from horses among veterinarians is low (Kriegshäuser et al., 2005).

PATHOGENESIS AND PATHOLOGY

The ERAV replication in the nasal epithelial cells leads to viremia. The virus is not detected in the blood after the appearance of antibodies. The virus has been speculated to cause persistent infection. It may persist in pharynx, bladder or lower gut cells (Plummer, 1963; Plummer and Kerry, 1962; McCollum and Timoney, 1991). The virus may be isolated from feces in small amounts for at least one month after infection. The cell-mediated immunity in Standardbred horses with decreased athletic performance, using lymphocyte proliferation assay and equine type 1 interferon bioassay, has been found to be suppressed. These horses also showed mild pharyngitis and intermittent fever (Jensen-Waern et al., 1998).

Infection with ERBVs is usually subclinical. The ERBV-1 and ERBV-2 may sometimes cause slight fever and mild respiratory signs (Steck et al., 1978). Experimental infection of gnotobiotic foals failed to produce signs of respiratory disease. However, these animals seroconverted as well as virus could be recovered from them (Mumford and Thompson, 1978).

The pathological studies of ERAV and ERBVs are very scanty. Organ cultures of equine fetal tracheal and nasal turbinate epithelium inoculated with ERAV appeared normal with the exception of rare island like lesions in infected nasal turbinate. Virus particles were not seen in thin sections of organ cultures infected with ERAV. Growth kinetics revealed that ERAV replicated in cell and organ cultures but was released almost exclusively from nasal turbinate epithelium (O'Niell and Issel, 1984; O'Niell et al., 1984). Studies are also required on the pathogenesis of abortion in dromedary (*Camelus dromedarius*) (Wernery et al., 2008) caused by equine rhinitis A virus (ERAV).

CLINICAL FEATURES

The equine rhinitis viruses have been isolated from horses with or without acute febrile respiratory disease. Most of the clinical information available concerns ERAV, which is spread by aerosols and direct contact. ERAV is generally considered to cause mild or severe respiratory disease with variable clinical symptoms, and nasal discharge is not invariably present (Burrows, 1970; Hofer et al., 1973). Subclinical disease is seen in many infections. The incubation period is two to eight days, and viremia is a regular feature. Viremia may last several days before dissipating with the appearance of circulating antibody (Plummer, 1963).

Equine rhinitis A virus (ERAV) infection of horses is characterized by fever ($41.0\pm5°C$) for up to four to five days and clinical signs such as copious nasal discharge that becomes mucopurulent, moist cough, anorexia, severe pharyngitis and lymphadenitis, and swelling of the retropharyngeal lymph nodes (Plummer and Kerry, 1962; Ditchfield and Macpherson, 1965; Klaey et al., 1998). Lymphadenitis and abscesses of the regional lymph nodes may result from secondary bacterial infection, usually with streptococci. During persistence phage of pharyngitis, coughing may continue for up to two to three weeks. Virus shedding for prolonged periods of time from the pharyngeal region, urine, and feces also accompany infection (Plummer and Kerry, 1962; Plummer, 1963). Urinary tract may become persistently infected, and thus urine aerosol is also considered an important mode of transmission (McCollum and Timoney, 1991; Powell, 1991). Though there may be prolonged infection, disease is not linked to nonrespiratory sites of infection; however, ERAV virus has been reported to cause abortion in dromedary (*Camelus dromedarius*) (Wernery et al., 2008).

Like in humans, there are greater incidences of colds in children compared to adults; similarly ERAV is more likely to cause disease in young horses (Cullinane et al., 2006). Upper respiratory tract disease due to ERAV infection is a significant problem in two-year-old horses in training. It is most prevalent in autumn/fall and winter months. The virus appears to circulate constantly in most racehorse populations, and the disease often occurs when horses are stressed by intensive work such as before their first race. Infection with other agents such as equine herpesvirus can also predispose a horse to ERAV infection. The virus spreads quite slowly, and active cases of disease may occur in training yard for several months. Lower respiratory tract is not very susceptible to rhinitis viruses, and horses usually recover from an uncomplicated ERAV infection within a week. Inadequate resting of horses with rhinitis (ERAV) disease increases their susceptibility to secondary bacterial pathogens that prolongs the recovery period. It is possible that virus infection may contribute to the development of sinusitis in the horse since rhinoviruses have been isolated from sinus fluids collected from persons with acute sinusitis. ERAV infection in older horses is often subclinical but may contribute to a loss of performance. A high incidence of ERAV antibody titers is a common finding in yards with loss of performance.

Equine rhinitis B virus 1 and 2 (ERBV-1 and ERB-2) have also been isolated from horses with acute febrile respiratory disease with clinical signs that include fever up to 41.0°C for one to three days, serous nasal discharge, anorexia, coughing, edema of legs, lethargy, pain and swelling of the lymph nodes of head and neck. These can also cause subclinical infection and subsequent seroconversion in horses (Steck et al., 1978; Black et al., 2007b). ERBV also cause persistent infection, and virus shedding occurs from the respiratory tract; however, unlike ERVA, the ERBVs are not shed in urine or feces. Recovery occurs as for rhinoviruses (Burrows, 1978; Mumford and Thomson, 1978; McCollum and Timoney, 1991; Thorsen, 1991; Carman et al., 1997).

DIAGNOSIS

Equine rhinitis viruses can be diagnosed by virus isolation in cell cultures, detection of viral RNA by reverse transcription–polymerase chain reaction (RT-PCR) from clinical samples (nasal swabs, etc.), serologic examination by complement fixation test (CFT), or demonstration of seroconversion using serum neutralization test (SNT) (Teufel and Becker, 1972; McCollum and Timoney, 1991; Li et al., 1997; Cullinane et al., 2006; Dynon et al., 2007; Mori et al., 2009).

For virus isolation, clinical material includes nasal swabs, blood, feces, or urine. ERAV replicates in primary cell cultures (equine fetal kidney, EFK) from horse; cell line of equine origin; cells of several other animal species—viz, dog, rabbit, hamster, and monkey; and cell lines (HeLa, Hep 2, LLC-MK2, RK-13, and Vero) (Burrows, 1970). Of these, RK-13 and Vero cell cultures have been found to be efficient for virus isolation of some ERAV strains (Plummer, 1963; Fukunaga et al., 1983; McCollum and Timoney, 1991; Huang et al., 2001; Kriegshäuser et al., 2005; Black et al., 2007a, 2007b; Dynon et al., 2007). Cytopathic effect (CPE) is quite similar to other picornaviruses, characterized by rounding up, shrinkage, and marked nuclear pyknosis of cells; and cells become refractile, degenerate, and then detach from the surface. The ERBV-1 produces cytopathic effect (CPE) on RK-13 but not on Vero cells (Fukunaga et al., 1983). It was reported that ERBV-2 did not produce plaques on confluent monolayer cell cultures of either Vero or RK-13 cells, whereas ERBV-1 produced plaques.

However, ERBV-2 was found to form plaques of irregular shape on about 60% confluent RK-13 monolayer cell cultures or when freshly seeded RK-13 cells were used (Huang et al., 2001). The addition of 20 mg/ml $MgCl_2$ to the cell culture medium enhanced the growth of the ERBV-2 isolated from a nasopharyngeal swab sample obtained from a horse with clinical signs of acute febrile respiratory disease (Black et al., 2007b). Viral antigen can be detected by immunofluorescence assay in the cytoplasm of cells infected with nasopharyngeal swab samples, indicating the presence and presumably replication of ERAV. The situation at the time of sample collection, variation in the susceptibility of the cell cultures used for isolation, or genetic variation in the viruses themselves could account for higher success rates of isolation in some studies compared with others (Studdert, 2007).

Serum neutralization test (SNT) has been used to detect antibodies against ERAV, and ERBV-1, and ERBV-2 (Mumford and Thompson, 1978; Studdert and Gleeeson, 1978; de Boer et al., 1979; McCollum and Timoney, 1991; Carman et al., 1997; Kriegshäuser et al., 2005; Black et al., 2007a; Dynon et al., 2007). Rising serum-neutralizing antibody titer in paired sera (between acute—and convalescent-phase sera) collected at about two-week time intervals, confirms diagnosis of ERAV or ERBV infection and that equine rhinovirus virus is causatively associated with disease outbreaks.

Equine rhinovirus 1 (ERAV) is a recognized cause of acute febrile respiratory disease in horse, although the virus is rarely isolated from such animals, despite seroprevalence rates generally as high as 50% in some horse populations. Attempts to isolate ERAV from nasopharyngeal swabs by conventional cell culture methods are many a time unsuccessful because of cytopathology not being observed. Relative importance of ERAV as a cause of acute febrile respiratory disease in horses has been underestimated due to failure in many instances to isolate virus by conventional cell culture methods (Li et al., 1997). Standard method for the detection of antibody against equine rhinoviruses is by serum neutralisation test; however, it is labor intensive and time consuming, require tissue culture facilities, and generally do not provide same-day results. Therefore, molecular assays should be considered as the method of choice to detect infection in symptomatic or apparently healthy horses.

The development of PCR as a diagnostic test for detecting rhinoviruses in clinical samples provided a major advancement in the rapid diagnosis of disease. The ERAV RNA can be detected in nasopharyngeal swabs or other clinical samples collected from horses during the acute phase of disease by RT-PCR (Li et al., 1997; Varrasso et al., 2001; Dynon et al., 2001, 2007).

Detection of virus by PCR in nasal swabs has proven to be more sensitive than virus isolation. Nucleotide sequencing of PCR-amplified products have revealed that within each outbreak, a single strain of ERAV was involved but that distinct viruses were involved in each outbreak (Li et al., 1997). Six out of twenty nasal swabs collected from horses with acute febrile upper respiratory disease were positive for equine rhinitis viruses by RT-PCR. Out of these six positive samples, ERBV was detected by RT-PCR singly in three samples and in the other three along with equine herpesvirus 4 or 5 (Dynon et al., 2007). A nested RT-PCR that amplified a product within the 3D(pol) and 3' nontranslated region of the genome of ERBV has been developed. The RT-PCR detected all twenty-four available ERBV-1 isolates and one available ERBV-2 isolate. The detection limit for the prototype strain ERBV-1.1436/71 was 0.1 $TCID_{50.}$ The RT-PCR was used to detect viral RNA in six of seventeen nasopharyngeal swab samples from horses that had clinical signs of acute febrile respiratory disease but from which ERBV was not initially isolated in cell culture (Black et al., 2007b). Initial PCR identification and subsequent virus isolation led to the isolation of ERBV-2 for the first time in Australia and the second time anywhere of ERBV-2 (Dynon et al., 2007). Thus, RT-PCR was found to be more sensitive as it detected viruses in clinical samples that were initially considered negative by conventional cell culture isolation (Li et al., 1997; Black et al., 2007b). Recently, Mori et al. (2009) have developed a real-time duplex TaqMan-PCR for detection of equine rhinitis A and B viruses in clinical specimens, which is a useful new diagnostic method for the rapid detection and differentiation of ERAV and ERBV.

Recombinant antigens from VP1 C-terminal and VP2 N-terminal of ERAV have been used to develop a diagnostic enzyme-linked immunosorbent assay (ELISA). The reactivity of these VP1 and VP2 recombinant (r) proteins in ELISAs correlated well with the results from a range of native antigen-based serological assays using field sera, and thus r-proteins could provide promising candidates for development of a diagnostic ERAV ELISA (Li et al., 2005). However, these did not show as significant a distinction between positive and negative field sera as is required for a diagnostic assay, despite the clear distinction with the experimentally infected horse sera noted. Further characterization of these important proteins and optimization of their antigenicities as well as ELISA conditions are in progress. Kriegshäuser et al. (2008) used denatured recombinant virion protein 1 (rVP1) as a coating antigen in a prototype ELISA for detection of ERBV-1 antibody present in horse serum and suggested that denatured rVP1 is a promising candidate for the development of an ELISA to be used in the routine laboratory diagnosis of ERBV-1 infection in horses.

PREVENTION AND CONTROL

Commercial vaccines for ERAV or ERBVs have not been developed till date. However, natural infection with ERAV generates strong clinical immunity. Immunization with an inactivated virus has been reported to induce production of neutralizing antibodies and provided protection against experimental infection (Burrows, 1970). An experimental ERAV-inactivated vaccine produced primary immune responses in horses, mice (including athymic nu/nu mice) and rabbits (Campbell et al., 1982). Natural immunity to ERBVs is considered to be poor as neutralizing antibodies and are not maintained at high levels, and prolonged excretion of the virus often occurs after natural infection (Fukunaga et al., 1983). Planned and controlled, deliberate infection programs in racehorses with ERAV have been suggested to ensure that they do not suffer from the disease shortly before important race events (Powell, 1975; Klaey et al., 1998). However, this method has not been widely implemented due to the fear of prolonged shedding of the ERAV in urine after primary infection (McCollum and Timoney, 1991).

ERAV is antigenically and genomically remarkable over time and geographic location (Varrasso et al., 2001); therefore, problem of multiple serotypes as that of FMDV does not occur. However, the occurrence of three serotypes of ERBV would need to be considered for any vaccine development. ERAV VP1, like its counterpart in FMDV, appears to be both a target of protective antibodies and involved directly in receptor binding, which reveals the potential of recombinant VP1 molecules to serve as vaccines and diagnostic reagents for the control of ERAV infections (Warner et al., 2001).

Like human rhinoviruses, equine rhinitis viruses are also quite stable and can survive for weeks on a variety of surfaces in the environment. Management of the disease should include attention to stable hygiene and use of a disinfectant with proven efficacy against rhinitis/rhinoviruses (Cullinane et al., 2006; Studdert, 2007). It is a common observation that the infection of horses with ERAV occurs when they enter the training stables. Therefore, proper hygienic and management measures should be taken to prevent and contain the disease. There is no specific antiviral therapy for rhinitis virus infection in horses. Symptomatic and supportive treatment should be given accordingly. Administration of reconstituted lyophilized serum orally has been suggested to be useful to protect newborn foals (Burton et al., 1981).

CONCLUSION

Equine rhinitis viruses, formerly called equine rhinoviruses (ERVs of genus *Rhinovirus*), belonging to the family Picornaviridae, are the causative agents of mild to severe upper respiratory infections in horses worldwide. These are small nonenveloped, single-stranded RNA viruses. Currently, four viral serotypes have been recognized including equine rhinitis A viruses (ERAV) (genus *Aphthovirus*) and B viruses (ERBV-1, ERBV-2, and ERBV-3) (genus *Erbovirus*). ERAV and ERBV-1 are the most frequent serotypes. ERAV is a significant respiratory pathogen of horses and is of additional interest because of its close relationship with foot-and-mouth disease virus (FMDV). ERAV spreads by contact through nasal secretions and aerosol inhalation. Also, urine aerosol may transmit the virus. The clinical symptoms in horses resemble that of common cold caused by rhinoviruses in humans: fever, nasal discharge, cough, anorexia, and pharyngitis. Disease is most prevalent in colder months. Serologic studies indicate a high prevalence of these viruses, and it is likely that the majority of horses are exposed to rhinitis viruses at some stage in their lives. The virus appears to circulate in most racehorse populations, where disease often occurs when animals are stressed by exhaustive workloads. Relative significance of ERAV in horses has been underestimated due to failure in many instances to isolate virus, foremost position of equine influenza and herpesviruses as causes of acute upper respiratory disease, and lack of sensitive and widely available diagnostic tools for rhinoviruses. The knowledge remains limited about the prevalence and pathogenesis of ERVs.

Diagnosis is achieved by virus isolation in cell cultures, detection of viral RNA by RT-PCR from clinical samples, serologic examination by CFT, or demonstration of seroconversion employing SNT. Viral antigen can be detected by immunofluorescence assay in infected cell cultures. PCR as a diagnostic test possesses the potential for rapidly detecting viruses in clinical samples. Real-time PCR has been suggested to be a useful new diagnostic tool for the rapid detection and differentiation of ERAV and ERBV. Recombinant (r) antigens could provide hopeful candidates for development of an ERAV ELISA. Virus isolation is often unsuccessful; therefore, molecular tools need to be explored to the full potential for detecting and characterizing ERVs. Commercial vaccines for equine rhinitis viruses have not been developed till date. The occurrence of three ERBV serotypes would need to be well thought-out for any vaccine-designing in the future. The potential of r-VP1 molecules to serve as effective vaccines for the prevention and control of ERAV infections could also be explored. Good management practices comprising of proper hygienic and biosecurity measures are very essential against rhinitis/rhinoviruses and to prevent and contain the disease. No specific antiviral therapy for rhinitis virus infection in horses is available. Recent studies reflecting dromedaries can be infected by rhinitis viruses and need to be further exploited for revealing the viral pathogenesis. The advancements in diagnosis of equine rhinoviruses would more clearly define the role of this important respiratory pathogen to cause disease incidences in horses.

REFERENCES

1. Black, W., Hartley, C., Ficorilli, N. and Studdert, M. 2005. Sequence variation divides equine rhinitis B virus into three distinct phylogenetic groups that correlate with serotype and acid stability. *J. Gen. Virol.* 86:2323–2332.

2. Black, W. D. and Studdert, M. J. 2006. Formerly unclassified, acid-stable equine picornaviruses are a third equine rhinitis B virus serotype in the genus *Erbovirus J. Gen. Virol.* 87:3023–3027.

3. Black, W. D., Wilcox, R. S., Stevenson, R. A., Hartley, C. A., Ficorilli, N. P., Gilkerson, J. R. and Studdert, M. J. 2007a. Prevalence of serum neutralising antibody to equine rhinitis A virus (ERAV), equine rhinitis B virus 1 (ERBV1) and ERBV2. *Vet. Microbiol.* 119:65–71.

4. Black, W. D., Hartley, C. A., Ficorilli, N. P. and Studdert, M. J. 2007b. Reverse transcriptase-polymerase chain reaction for the detection of equine rhinitis B viruses and cell culture isolation of the virus. *Arch. Virol.* 152:137–149.

5. Black, W. D., Hartley, C. A., Ficorilli, N. P. and Studdert, M. J. 2008. Virion associated proteins of equine rhinitis B virus 1 (ERBV1): The non-structural protein 3C(pro) co-purifies with virions. *Virus Res.* 2008 Dec 15 [Epub ahead of print].

6. Becker, W., Heller, H. and Teufel, P. 1974. Equine rhinovirus infection. *Berl Munch Tierarztl Wochenschr.* 87:305–308.

7. Burrows, R. 1970. Equine rhinovirus. In *Equine infectious diseases II*, ed. J. T. Bryans and H. Gerber, 154–164. Basel, Switzerland: S. Karger.

8. Burrows, R. 1978. Equine rhinovirus and adenovirus infections. *Proc. Am. Assoc. Equine Pract.* 24:299–306.

9. Burton, S. C., Hintz, H. F., Kemen, M. J. and Holmes, D. F. 1981. Lyophilized hyperimmune equine serum as a source of antibodies for neonatal foals. *Am. J. Vet. Res.* 42:308–310.

10. Campbell, T. M., Studdert, M. J. and Blackney, M. H. 1982. Immunogenicity of equine herpesvirus type 1 (EHV1) and equine rhinovirus type 1 (ERhV1) following inactivation by betapropiolactone (BPL) and ultraviolet (UV) light. *Vet. Microbiol.* 7:535–544.

11. Carman, S., Rosendal, S., Huber, L., Gyles, C., McKee, S., Willoughby, R. A., Dubovi, E., Thorsen, J. and Lein, D. 1997. Infectious agents in acute respiratory disease in horses in Ontario. *J. Vet. Diagn. Invest.* 9:17–23.

12. Cullinane, A. A., Barr, B., Bernard, W., Duncan, J. L., Mulcahy, G., Smith, M. and Timoney, J. E. 2006. Infectious diseases (Chapter 1): Equine rhino/rhinitis viruses. In *The equine manual*, 2nd ed., A. J. Higgins and J. R. Snyder, 18–19. USA: Saunder, Elsevier Ltd.

13. de Boer, G. F., Osterhaus, A. D., van Oirschot, J. T. and Wemmenhove, R. 1979. Prevalence of antibodies to equine viruses in the Netherlands. *Vet. Q.* 1:65–74.

14. Ditchfield, J. and Macpherson, L. W. 1965. The properties and classification of two new rhinoviruses recovered from horses in Toronto, Canada. *Cornell Vet.* 55:181–189.

15. Ditchfield, J., Macpherson, L. W. and Zbitnew, A. 1965. Upper respiratory disease in Thoroughbred horses: Studies of its viral etiology in the Toronto area, 1960 to 1963. *Can. J. Comp. Med. Vet. Sci.* 29:18–22.

16. Dunowska, M., Wilks, C. R., Studdert, M. J. and Meers, J. 2002. Viruses associated with outbreaks of equine respiratory disease in New Zealand. *N. Z. Vet. J.* 50:132–139.

17. Dynon, K., Varrasso, A., Ficorilli, N., Holloway, S., Reubel, G., Li, F., Hartley, C., Studdert, M. and Drummer, H. 2001. Identification of equine herpesvirus 3 (equine coital exanthema virus), equine gammaherpesviruses 2 and 5, equine adenoviruses 1 and 2, equine arteritis virus and equine rhinitis A virus by polymerase chain reaction. *Aust. Vet. J.* 79:695–702.

18. Dynon, K., Black, W. D., Ficorilli, N., Hartley, C. A. and Studdert, M. J. 2007. Detection of viruses in nasal swab samples from horses with acute, febrile, respiratory disease using virus isolation, polymerase chain reaction and serology. *Australian Vet. J.* 85:46–50.

19. Flammini, C. F. and Allegri, G. 1970. Rhinovirus strain as a possible cause of equine respiratory infection. *Arch. Vet. Ital.* 21:309–316.

20. Flammini, C. F. and Allegri, G. 1971. Serological identification of an equine Rhinovirus strain. *Arch. Vet. Ital.* 22:269–272.

21. Fukunaga, Y., Kumanomido, T., Kamada, M. and Wada, R. 1983. Equine picornavirus: Isolation of virus from the oral cavity of healthy horses. *Bull. Equine Res. Inst.* 20:103–109.

22. Hartley, C. A., Ficorilli, N., Dynon, K., Drummer, H. E., Huang, J. A., Studdert, M. J., Li, F., Browning, G. F. and Crabb, B. S. 2001. Equine rhinitis A virus: Structural proteins and immune response. *J. Gen. Virol.* 82:1725–1728.

23. Herbst, W., Görlich, P. and Danner, K. 1992. Virologico-serologic studies in horses with respiratory tract diseases. *Berl. Munch. Tierarztl. Wochenschr.* 105:49–52.

24. Hofer, B., Steck, F., Gerber, H., Lohrer, J., Nicholet, J. and Paccaud, M. F. 1973. An investigation of the etiology of viral respiratory disease in a remount depot. In *Third International Conference on Equine Infectious Diseases*, ed. J. T. Bryans and H. Gerber, 527–545. Basel (1973): Karger.

25. Hollister, J. R., Vagnozzi, A., Knowles, N. J. and Rieder, E. 2008. Molecular and phylogenetic analyses of bovine rhinovirus type 2 shows it is closely related to foot-and-mouth disease virus. *Virology* 373:411–425.

26. Holmes, D. F., Kemen, M. J. and Coggins, L. 1978. Equine rhinovirus infection-serologic evidence of infection in selected horse populations. In *Equine infectious diseases IV*, ed. J. T. Bryans and H. Gerber, 315–319. Basel: Karger.

27. Huang, J., Ficorilli, N., Hartley, C. A., Wilcox, R. S., Weiss, M. and Studdert, M. J. 2001. Equine rhinitis B virus: A new serotype. *J. Gen. Virol.* 82:2641–2645.

28. Jensen-Waern, M., Persson, S. G., Nordengrahn, A. et al. 1998. Temporary suppression of cell-mediated immunity in Standardbred horses with decreased athletic capacity. *Acta Vet. Scand.* 39:25–33.

29. King, A. M. Q., Brown, F., Christian, P., Hovi, T., Hyypia, T., Knowles, N. J., Lemon, S. M., Minor, P. D., Palmenberg, A. C., Skern, T. and Stanway, G. 2005. Family picornaviridae. In *Virus: Taxonomy of viruses*, ed. C. M. Fauquet, M. A. Mayo, J. Maniloff, U. Desselberger, and D. A. Ball, 757–778. Burlington, MA: Elsevier.

30. Klaey, M., Sanchez-Higgins, M., Leadon, D. P., Cullinane, A., Straub, R. and Gerber, H. 1998. Field case study of equine rhinovirus 1 infection: Clinical signs and clinicopathology. *Equine Vet. J.* 30:267–269.

31. Korant, B. D., Lonberg-Holm, K. K. and Halperen S. 1970. Structural polypeptides of three rhinoviruses. *Biochem. Biophys. Res. Commun.* 41:477–481.

32. Korant, B. D., Lonberg-Holm, K., Noble, J. and Stasny, J. T. 1972. Naturally occurring and artificially produced components of three rhinoviruses. *Virology* 48:71–86.

33. Kriegshauser, G., Wutz, G., Lea, S., Stuart, D., Skern, T. and Kuechler, E. 2003. Model of the equine rhinitis A virus capsid: Identification of a major neutralizing immunogenic site. *J. Gen. Virol.* 84:2365–2373.

34. Kriegshäuser, G., Deutz, A., Kuechler, E., Skern, T., Lussy, H. and Nowotny, N. 2005. Prevalence of neutralising antibodies to equine rhinitis A and B virus in horses and man. *Vet. Microbiol.* 106:293–296.

35. Kriegshäuser, G., Cullinane, A., Kuechler, E. and Skern, T. 2008. Denatured virion protein 1 of equine rhinitis B virus 1 contains authentic B-cell epitopes recognised in an enzyme-linked immunosorbent assay. *Acta Veterinaria Hungarica* 56:265–270.

36. Li, F., Browning, G. F., Studdert, M. J. and Crabb, B. S. 1996. Equine rhinovirus 1 is more closely related to foot-and-mouth disease virus than to other picornaviruses. *Proceedings of the National Academy of Sciences, USA* 93:990–995.

37. Li, F., Drummer, H. E., Ficorilli, N., Studdert, M. J. and Crabb, B. S. 1997. Identification of noncytopathic equine rhinovirus 1 as a cause of acute febrile respiratory disease in horses. *J. Clin. Microbiol.* 35:937–943.

38. Li, F., Stevenson, R. A., Crabb, B. S., Studdert, M. J. and Hartley, C. A. 2005. Several recombinant capsid proteins of equine rhinitis A virus show potential as diagnostic antigens. *Clin. & Diagn. Lab. Immunol.* 12:778–785.

39. McCollum, W. H. and Timoney, P. J. 1991. Studies on the seroprevalence and frequency of equine rhinovirus I and II infection in normal horse urine. In *Equine infectious diseases VI*, ed. W. Plowright, P. D. Rossdale, and J. F. Wade, 83–87. Newmarket, UK: R&W Publications.

40. Mori, A., De Benedictis, P., Marciano, S., Zecchin, B., Zuin, A., Zecchin, B., Capua, I. and Cattoli, G. 2009. Development of a real-time duplex TaqMan-PCR for the detection of equine rhinitis A and B viruses in clinical specimens. *J. Virol. Methods* 155:175–181.

41. Mumford, J. A. and Thomson, G. R. 1978. Studies on picornaviruses isolated from the respiratory tract of horses. In *Proceedings of the Fourth International Conference on Equine Infectious Diseases*, ed. J. T. Bryans and H. Gerber, 419–429. Princeton, NJ: Veterinary Publications.

42. Newman, J., Rowlands, D. J. and Brown, F. 1973. A physico-chemical sub-grouping of the mammalian picornaviruses. *J. Gen. Virol.* 18:171–180.

43. Newman, J. F. E., Rowlands, D. J., Brown, F., Goodridge, D., Burrows, R. and Steck, F. 1977. Physicochemical characterization of two serologically unrelated equine rhinoviruses. *Intervirology* 8:145–154.

44. O'Niell, F. D. and Issel, C. J. 1984. Growth kinetics of equine respiratory tract viruses in cell and organ cultures. *Am. J. Vet. Res.* 45:1961–1966.

45. O'Niell, F. D., Issel, C. J. and Henk, W. G. 1984. Electron microscopy of equine respiratory viruses in organ cultures of equine fetal respiratory tract epithelium. *Am. J. Vet. Res.* 45:1953–1960.

46. Plummer, G. 1962. An equine respiratory virus with enterovirus properties. *Nature* 195:519–520.

47. Plummer, G. and Kerry, J. B. 1962. Studies on an equine respiratory virus. *Vet. Rec.* 74:967–970.

48. Plummer, G. 1963. An equine respiratory enterovirus: Some biological and physical properties. *Arch. Virol.* 12:694–700.

49. Powell, D. G. 1975. Equine infectious respiratory disease. *Vet Rec.* 96:30–34.

50. Powell, D. G. 1991. Viral respiratory disease of the horse. *Vet. Clin. North Am. Equine Pract.* 7:27–52.

51. Stanway, G., Hovi, T., Knowles, N. J. and Hyypiä, T. 2002. Molecular and biological basis of picornavirus taxonomy. In *Molecular biology of picornaviruses*, ed. B. L. Semler and E. Wimmer, 17–24. Washington, D.C.: ASM Press.

52. Steck, F., Hofer, B., Schaeren, B., Nicolet, J. and Gerber, H. 1978. Equine rhinoviruses: New serotypes. In *Proceedings of the 4th International Conference on Equine Infectious Disease*, 312–328. Princetown: Veterinary Publication Inc.

53. Stevenson, R. A., Hartley, C. A., Huang, J. A., Studdert, M. J., Crabb, B. S. and Warner, S. 2003. Mapping epitopes in equine rhinitis A virus VP1 recognized by antibodies elicited in response to infection of the natural host. *J. Gen. Virol.* 84:1607–1612.

54. Stevenson, R. A., Huang, J. A., Studdert, M. J. and Hartley, C. A. 2004a. Identification of a neutralizing epitope in the betaE-betaF loop of VP1 of equine rhinitis A virus, defined by a neutralization-resistant variant. *J. Gen. Virol.* 85:2545–2553.

55. Stevenson, R. A., Huang, J. A., Studdert, M. J. and Hartley, C. A. 2004b. Sialic acid acts as a receptor for equine rhinitis A virus binding and infection. *J. Gen. Virol.* 85:2535–2543.

56. Studdert, M. J. 1996. Equine rhinovirus infections. In *Virus infections of equines*, vol. 6, ed. M. J. Studdert, 213–217. Amsterdam: Elsevier Science Publishers.

57. Studdert, M. J. 2007. Miscellaneous viral respiratory diseases: Equine rhinitis A viruses and equine rhinitis B viruses. In *Equine infectious diseases*, ed. D. C. Sellon and M. T. Long, chapter 16, 177–180. Philadelphia, USA: Saunders, Elsevier Inc.

58. Studdert, M. J. and Gleeson, L. J. 1977. Isolation of equine rhinovirus type 1. *Aust. Vet. J.* 53:452.

59. Studdert, M. J. and Gleeson, L. J. 1978. Isolation and characterisation of an equine rhinovirus. *Zentralbl Veterinarmed* B 25:225–237.

60. Sugiura, T., Matsumura, T., Fukunaga, Y. and Hirasawa, K. 1987. Sero-epizootiological study of racehorses with pyrexia in the training centers of the Japan Racing Association. *Nippon Juigaku Zasshi* 49:1087–1096.

61. Thorsen, J. 1991. Equine rhinoviruses. *Equine Pract.* 13:19–22.

62. Teufel, P. and Keller, H. 1970. Occurrence of neutralizing antibodies against equine rhinovirus (strain NM 11) in horse stocks in Berlin. *Berl Munch Tierarztl Wochenschr.* 83:466–467.

63. Teufel, P. and Becker, W. 1972. Demonstration of complement fixing antibodies in equine rhinovirus equine 1 infection. *Zentralbl Veterinarmed* B 19:840–847.

64. Varrasso, A., Drummer, H. E., Huang, J. A., Stevenson, R. A., Ficorilli, N., Studdert, M. J. and Hartley, C. A. 2001. Sequence conservation and antigenic variation of the structural proteins of equine rhinitis A virus. *J. Virol.* 75:10550–10556.

65. Warner, S., Hartley, C. A., Stevenson, R. A., Ficorilli, N., Varrasso, A., Studdert, M. J., Crabb, B. S., Dynon, K., Drummer, H. E., Huang, J. A., Li, F. and Browning, G. F. 2001. Evidence that equine rhinitis A virus VP1 is a target of neutralizing antibodies and participates directly in receptor binding. *J. Virol.* 75:9274–9281.

66. Wernery, U., Wernery, R., Zachariah, R. and Hayden-Evans, J. 1998. Serological survey of some equine infections in the United Arab Emirates. In *Proceedings of the Eighth International Conference on Equine Infectious Diseases*, ed. U. Wernery, J. F. Wade, J. A. Mumford, and O. R. Kaaden, 367–370. Dubai (1998), Newmarket, Suffolk: R&W Publications.

67. Wernery, U., Knowles, N. J., Hamblin, C., Wernery, R., Joseph, S., Kinne, J. and Nagy, P. 2008. Abortions in dromedaries (*Camelus dromedarius*) caused by equine rhinitis A virus. *J. Gen. Virol.* 89:660–666.

68. Wesley, D., Hartley, C. A., Ficorilli, N. P. and Studdert, M. J. 2005. Sequence variation divides equine rhinitis B virus into three distinct phylogenetic groups that correlate with serotype and acid stability. *J. Gen. Virol.* 86:2323–2332.

69. Wilson, J. C., Bryans, J. T., Doll, E. R. and Tudor, L. 1966. Isolation of a newly identified equine respiratory virus. *Cornell Vet.* 55:425–431.

70. Wutz, G., Auer, H., Nowotny, N., Grosse, B., Skern, T. and Kuechler, E. 1996. Equine rhinovirus serotypes 1 and 2: Relationship to each other and to aphthoviruses and cardioviruses. *J. Gen. Virol.* 77:1719–1730.

12. Equine Viral Arteritis

S. Kapoor, K. Dhama, M. Mahendran, and R. V. S. Pawaiya

Introduction

Equine viral arteritis (EVA), also known as epizootic lymphangitis, equine typhoid, epizootic cellulites, pink eye or *rotlaufseuche,* is a contagious viral disease of equines caused by equine arteritis virus (EAV). The disease is characterized by fever, depression, anorexia, edema (especially of limbs, scrotum, and prepuce in stallion), conjunctivitis, nasal discharges, urticarial type skin reaction, abortion in pregnant mares; and rarely pneumonia or pneumoenteritis in young foals (Jones et al., 1957; Timoney and McCollum, 1993; Glaser et al., 1997a; Del Piero, 2000; MacLachlan and Balasuriya, 2006). The disease was first recognized in nineteenth century, but the virus was isolated in 1953 from lung tissues of aborted fetuses during an epidemic/epizootic on a breeding farm near Bucyrus, Ohio, USA (Doll et al., 1957). The virus was identified as differed from etiological entity different to the equine rhinopheumonitis–caused influenza (Edison, 2005). Equine arteritis has not been widely reported in animals other than horses and donkeys. Although virus appears to be globally distributed, clinical outbreaks of EVA are rarely recognized. Epidemics of "abortion storms" occur during congregation of horses during sales, horse shows, races, and at breeding farms. Although infrequently reported in the past, confirmed outbreaks of EVA appear to be on the increase (OIE, 2008).

EVA has been confirmed in a variety of horse breeds, with the highest infection rate found in adult Standardbreds. Antibodies to this virus have also been identified in zebras. However, outbreaks have been confined to horses and ponies. Mortality, even though, is rare except in old, young, and debilitated horses; the economic losses can be of much significance, which include decreased demand for carrier stallions as breeders, deaths in young foals, and abortions in 10–50% of susceptible mare (Glaser et al., 1997a; Del Piero, 2000; Campbell, 2006). EVA can eliminate an entire breeding season by causing numerous mares to abort. In addition, horses that test positive for EVA antibodies and horse semen from EVA-infected horses can be barred from entering foreign countries. The import policies of nearly all major horse-breeding countries are including measures to reduce the risk of EVA. Virus does not present a human health hazard (Timoney and McCollum, 1993).

ETIOLOGY

Equine arteritis virus (EAV) is a positive-sense, single-stranded RNA virus (approx. 12.7 kb) and the prototype member of the genus *Arterivirus*, family Arteriviridae, order Nidovirales (Cavanagh, 1997; Glaser et al., 1997a; Del Piero, 2000; Deshpande et al., 2007; Wei and Yuan, 2008; Veit et al., 2008). The family also includes porcine reproductive and respiratory syndrome virus (PRRSV), lactate dehydrogenase elevating virus (LDV) of mice, and simian hemorrhagic fever virus (SHFV) (Balasuriya and MacLachlan, 2004). Only one major serotype of the virus has been identified so far. The EAV virion is 50–65 nm in diameter and has an icosahedral nucleocapsid (35 nm), which is surrounded by an envelope (Hyllseth, 1973; Balasuriya and MacLachlan, 2004). The genomic RNA is infectious, has a 5' cap and is polyadenylated at its 3' end. The leader sequence at 5' end of genome is followed by eight open reading frames (ORFs)-ORFs 1a and 1b and 2 to 7 (de Vries et al., 1997; Snijder and Meulenberg, 1998; Balasuriya et al., 1999; Deshpande et al., 2007). The ORFs 1a and 1b, occupying approximately 75% genome at 5' end, encode two replicase polyproteins (PP1a and pp1b). Three viral proteases—viz, nsp1, nsp2, and nsp4—act on these precursor polyproteins to form at least twelve nonstructural proteins (nsp1-nsp12) (Snijder and Meulenberg, 1998; Wei and Yuan, 2008).

The portion of the genome downstream of replicase gene contains six genes, which encode structural proteins and are translated from subgenomic viral mRNAs (Zientara, 1994; Wei and Yuan, 2008). These mRNAs have a 224-nucleotide long common leader sequence at 5' and a 3'-coterminal nested set sequences that overlap with neighboring genes (de Vries et al., 1990, 1997; Snijder and Meulenberg, 1998; Wei and Yuan, 2008). The ORFs 2a, 2b, and 3 to 7 located at 3' proximal quarter of the genome encode, respectively, six structural proteins present in envelope (viz, E, GP2b [GS], GP3, GP4, GP5 [GL], and M; and a nucleocapsid protein [N]) (Balasuriya et al., 1999). The nonglycosylated M protein is the most conserved structural protein, whereas greatest variation occurs in GP3 and GP5 proteins. Major neutralization determinants are present on GP5 protein (de Vries et al., 1992; Hedges et al., 1999; Stadejek et al., 1999; Wieringa et al., 2002; Veit et al., 2008; Wei and Yuan, 2008).

Recently, molecular characterization studies have enabled the comparative sequence analyzes of the entire structural protein genes, coupled with construction of chimeric viruses utilizing an infectious cDNA clone of EAV. This has confirmed that the alterations in neutralization phenotype of EAV were caused by amino acid changes in the GP5 protein encoded by ORF5. Also, site-directed mutagenesis confirmed that amino acid 98 in the GP5 protein was responsible for an altered neutralization phenotype of various EAV isolates (Zhang et al., 2008).

Regarding the physical features of EAV, the buoyant density of arteriviruses is 1.13–1.17 gm/ml in sucrose and the sedimentation coefficient varies from 214S-230S (Hyllseth, 1970; Glaser et al., 1997a; Del Piero, 2000). The virus particles are sensitive to common disinfectants and detergents, ether, chloroform, heat, low pH, and 1M $MgCl_2$. The virion can be inactivated at 56°C in thirty minutes but remains viable at-20°C for six hours and is also resistant to the action of trypsin. The virus is stable at low temperatures (-70°C). It multiplies in cell cultures of horse kidney, rabbit and baby hamster kidneys, and the cell culture–adapted virus produces plaques in BHK-21, Vero, RK-13, and equine kidney cell cultures (Timoney et al., 1996; Glaser et al., 1997a; Del Piero, 2000; Campbell, 2006). Laboratory animals and embryonated eggs have not been found suitable for virus propagation. Recently, Veit et al. (2008) suggested that there is evidence for EAV having hemagglutinating and hemolytic activity.

EPIDEMIOLOGY

Based on the findings of serologic surveys and reported outbreaks of EVA, the virus is present in horse populations in many countries throughout the world; disease outbreaks are infrequent but have been reported in the United States, Canada, Switzerland, Austria, the United Kingdom, Poland, and Hungary while Japan and Iceland are notable exceptions (Timoney and McCollum, 1993; Timoney et al., 1996; Glaser et al., 1996 and 1997b; Del Piero, 2000; Cardwell et al., 2002; Szeredi et al., 2005; Campbell, 2006). There has been an increase in the incidence of EVA as it has been linked to the greater frequency of movement of horses and use of transported semen (Timoney and McCollum, 1993; Del Piero, 2000). The EAV has only one serotype and one recognized strain (the Bucyrus strain); however, various isolates have different degrees of virulence (Glaser et al., 1997a; Del Piero, 2000; Campbell, 2006; Deshpande et al., 2007). Strains isolated from different geographical areas and at different times may also vary in their virulence and, in turn, in the severity of clinical signs and ability to cause abortion (Fukunaga and McCollum, 1977; Timoney and McCollum, 1988; Timoney et al., 1996). The field strains of EAV can be differentiated by their neutralization reactions with polyclonal antisera and monoclonal antibodies.

The epidemiology of EVA involves virus, host, and environment-related factors, including variability in pathogenicity among naturally occurring strains of the virus, routes of transmission, existence of the carrier state in the stallion, and the nature of acquired immunity to infection (Timoney et al., 1996; Glaser et al., 1997a). The natural and experimental host range appears to be restricted to equines, although very limited evidence would suggest it may also include New World camelids, viz alpacas and llama (Weber et al., 2006). The virus can infect many breeds of horses, the prevalence of infection varies widely, usually being highest in Standardbreds, and there is little evidence of infection in populations of wild equids. Outbreaks of EVA are usually linked to the movement of animals or the shipment of semen. Viral transmission can be widespread at horse shows, racetracks, or on breeding farms; such occurrences are not always associated with the appearance of clinical illness characteristic of EVA (Del Piero, 2000). In fact, the vast majority of cases of natural infection with the virus are asymptomatic.

The virus has been isolated from horses in USA (Doll et al., 1957; Timoney et al., 1986; Zientara, 1994), Canada (Clayton, 1987), Switzerland (Burki, 1970), Austria (Nowotny, 1991), Poland (Golnik et al., 1981), South Africa (Paweska et al., 1996; Guthrie et al., 2003), Sweden (Mittelholzer et al., 2006b), and England (Chirnside, 1992; Cardwell et al., 2002). In addition, serosurveys have identified EAV-antibody-positive animals from England, Japan, France, Yugoslavia, Spain, Ireland, Portugal, Senegal, Morocco, Egypt, Ethiopia, USSR, Australia, India, Sweden, and New Zealand (Akashi et al., 1976; Moraillon and Moraillon, 1978; Huntington et al., 1990a, 1990b; McKenzie, 1990; Singh et al., 1997; Mittelholzer et al., 2006b; OIE, 2008). The serological studies indicate that difference in the prevalence of EAV infection is not only among countries but also among horses of different breeds and age. Seroprevalence of EAV infection increases with age. Screening in USA and Australia showed positive incidence of up to 80% in Standardbred as compared to only 3% in Thoroughbred horses (Timoney and McCollum, 1985; Huntington et al., 1990b).

TRANSMISSION

EAV is most commonly introduced on to an equine establishment by the arrival of an acutely infected horse, introduction of a carrier stallion, or a shipment of infective fresh/frozen semen (Zientara, 1994; Glaser et al., 1997a; Del Piero, 2000). Secondary spread occurs by the respiratory route from the mare inseminated with the infective semen to other susceptible horses. Generally, the transmission of EAV infection can occur by respiratory, venereal, congenital, or indirect means (Balasuriya and Maclachlan, 2004). Aerosol transmission is the principal mode of spread by horses acutely infected with the virus, which predominates when horses are in close contact with one another such as at racetracks, sales, shows, and other events (Zientara, 1994; Timoney et al., 1996; Hullinger et al., 1998; Balasuriya et al., 1999; Guthrie et al., 2003; Campbell, 2006). The virus is present in nasal secretions in acutely infected horses for up to sixteen days. Aborted fetuses, fetal membranes and amniotic fluids of mares, and genital fluids of infected stallions are a potent source of aerosol transmission. Kidney is the most affected organ, and the virus is excreted in the urine and becomes the major source of infection (Zientara, 1994; Del Piero, 2000; Campbell, 2006).

The virus can be transmitted venereally by acutely infected mare and acutely or chronically by infected/carrier stallion (Glaser et al., 1997a; Hullinger et al., 1998; Del Piero, 2000; Samper and Tibary, 2006). Mares and geldings eliminate virus after acute infection, but 30–60% of stallions become persistently infected (Glaser et al., 1996 and 1997a; Guthrie et al., 2003). In stallions, EAV infection will cause a transient or permanent virus presence in the accessorial apparatus of the genital tract with transient or permanent shedding of the virus via seminal secretions (Klug and Sieme, 1999; Samper and Tibary, 2006). Mares can be infected by the venereal route either following natural service or artificial insemination with infective semen (Zientara, 1994; Timoney et al., 1996; Campbell, 2006). Unlike mares, geldings, or sexually immature colts, carrier stallions are viral reservoirs and are primarily responsible for persistence of the virus in horse populations throughout the world. The virus is shed constantly in the semen, and such animals transmit infection to susceptible mares to which they are bred. While the duration of the carrier state varies between individuals, the virus may persist in some clinically healthy stallions for years (Guthrie et al., 2003). Such stallions do not suffer any apparent decrease in fertility. Spontaneous resolution of the carrier state has been observed in persistently infected stallions. Venereal transmission is perhaps most important as virus has been isolated from semen of stallions (Timoney, 1984; Zientara, 1994; Glaser et al., 1997a; Guthrie et al., 2003). Venereal transmission from carrier stallions is particularly significant on breeding farms and may also be transmitted by the use of infective semen. In the Kentucky outbreak of 1984, a high percentage (34%) of stallions infected by the respiratory route continued to shed the virus in their semen after recovery (Timoney, 1985; Timoney et al., 1996). Such stallions led in transmission of infection to susceptible mares to which they were bred.

The impact of EAV-infected stallions on reproduction/fertility is a major concern to equine breeders. The role of semen shedder stallions in disease transmission has been reported (Timoney and McCollum, 1993 and 2000). A stallion may be seropositive but not necessarily a semen shedder. A semen-shedder stallion may disseminate the virus both to seronegative as well as seropositive mares. Seronegative mares serviced by semen shedders frequently seroconvert (Burki et al., 1992; Del Piero, 2000; Guthrie et al.,

2003). The carrier state, which has been shown to be androgen dependant, has been found in the stallion, but not in the mare, gelding, or sexually immature colt (Timoney and McCollum, 2000). Rise in antibody titer has been demonstrated in mares that already possessed anti-EAV antibodies before getting covered, indicating reinfection at service. The likelihood of older mares compared to young ones in getting repeated infection is more. Seronegative pregnant mares, if kept in contact with seropositive mares, may get infected and eventually abort (Cole et al., 1986; Guthrie et al., 2003). During late gestation, if infected, the pregnant mare transmits the virus into the fetus, and weak foal having EAV infection could be born. The virus can also be transmitted indirectly through the use of virus-contaminated fomites (shanks, twitches, head collars, and breeding shed equipment) and through the hands or clothing of animal handlers (Timoney and McCollum, 1988; Glaser et al., 1997a; Del Piero, 2000; Guthrie et al., 2003).

VIRAL PERSISTENCE IN STALLION

Clinical recovery is usually complete, but stallions can become long-term carriers of the virus and are regarded as playing a major epidemiological role in the dissemination and perpetuation of EAV (Timoney et al., 1986; Timoney and McCollum, 1993; Stadejek et al., 1999; Del Piero, 2000). Stallions appear to be the only carriers for the virus; carrier states have not been seen in mares, geldings, or sexually immature colts. Carrier stallion shed EAV in their semen and transmits the infection venereally to a high percentage of susceptible mares (Timoney et al., 1986; Glaser et al., 1997b; Del Piero, 2000). Vas deferens ampullae, seminal vesicle, prostate, and bulbourethral glands were found to be sites of EAV persistence in stallion (Timoney et al., 1986). The duration of virus excretion from persistently infected stallions has been used to divide the carrier status into three types—viz, short term, intermediate, and long term. The duration of short-term or convalescent carrier state is only for a few weeks after recovery. The intermediate-carrier state lasts for three to seven months after natural or experimental infection, whereas the long-term or chronic carrier status can be for even lifelong in infected stallion (Timoney et al., 1986, 1987a, 1987b). Carrier state in twenty-five naturally infected stallions was studied by using "test" cover of seronegative mares and by isolation of virus from semen. Each seropositive stallion was bred to two "test" mares. The mares were mated twice a day for two to four days during same estrus period, kept in isolation, and observed clinically for fourteen days. Clinical signs of EVA were observed in most of the mares with difference in severity. The establishment and maintenance of viral persistence in stallions is testosterone dependent, and high serum titers of neutralizing antibodies are not able to clear the virus from persistently infected stallions (Timoney and McCollum,

1993; Balasuriya and Maclachlan, 2004). The virus will not persist after castration of an infected stallion.

The asymptomatic, persistently infected carrier stallion is essential natural reservoir, which not only maintains EAV between breeding seasons but also leads to the generation of variants. These variants have sequence variation in ORF5 gene leading to altered neutralization phenotype that correlate with specific regions on GP5 glycoprotein. However, evasion of immune responses is not the mechanism for establishment of viral persistence as these variants are neutralized by high-titer polyclonal antiserum. It has been reported that neither defective interfering particles nor immune evasion from B-cell responses are involved in persistence (Balasuriya et al., 2004).

CLINICAL FEATURES

Clinical signs mainly include respiratory illness, vasculitis, and abortion (Timoney et al., 1996; Del Piero, 2000; Campbell, 2006). The outcome of exposure to EAV depends on the interaction of factors such as virus strain, viral dose, age, and physical condition of the animal(s). The symptoms are generally more severe in old and young animals, pregnant mares, and in horses which are in poor condition. But most natural infections with EAV are asymptomatic and subclinical (Timoney et al., 1996). The onset of clinical signs is preceded by an incubation period of three to fourteen days when infection occurs by respiratory route while it is about a week after venereal exposure (Timoney et al., 1996; Campbell, 2006). The range and severity of clinical disease varies widely. Mild clinical disease with signs of edema of limbs and ventral abdomen, conjunctivitis, and transient anorexia is commonly seen. The clinical symptoms include fever up to 41 °C that may persist for three to nine days, leukopenia, seropurulent excessive ocular and nasal discharge, conjunctivitis (Pink eye), rhinitis, anorexia, depression and limb edema (particularly in the hind limbs), and edema of the prepuce and scrotum (Del Piero, 2000; Holyoak et al., 2008). Symptoms such as lacrimation, conjunctivitis, photophobia, periorbital or supraorbital edema, nasal discharge, rhinitis, and edema of the ventral body wall may be seen inconsistently (Campbell, 2006; Holyoak et al., 2008). Some horses develop urticaria; the hives are most often localized to the head or neck but are sometimes generalized. A stiff gait, ataxia, icterus, dyspnea, or diarrhea may also be seen (Doll et al., 1957; Clayton, 1987; Timoney et al., 1987a; Timoney et al., 1996; Del Piero, 2000). Most adult horses recover completely, but deaths can occur in both neonatal foals and yearlings as a result of rapidly progressive bronchointerstitial pneumonia or pneumoenteritis (Carman, 1988; Timoney and McCollum, 1988; Golnik, 1991; Glaser et al., 1997b). Death occurs within forty-eight to ninety-six hours of birth.

Abortion may occur late in the acute phase or early in the convalescent phase of the disease. In natural outbreaks, abortion rates can vary from 10–50% and can occur at any time between from three and seven months of gestation (Timoney and McCollum, 1985; Cole et al., 1986; Glaser et al., 1997b). Abortion usually does not result from a mare being bred to a carrier stallion or inseminated with infective semen. Mares that abort are already pregnant at time of exposure, which principally occurs by the respiratory route from an acutely infected animal. However, mares infected late in gestation may not abort, but give birth to a congenitally infected foal (Timoney et al., 1996; Campbell, 2006). Fertility problems after infection have not been observed in mares. But stallions affected with EVA may undergo a period of short-term temporary infertility, which could be due to increased intratesticular temperature caused by the high fever and severe scrotal edema (Timoney et al., 1996; Del Piero, 2000; Campbell, 2006).

PATHOGENESIS AND PATHOLOGY

The virus primarily replicates in alveolar macrophages, endothelial cells, and bronchial lymph nodes. In young and adult horses, following colonization of macrophages, the virus spreads systemically via circulating monocytes and enters the endothelium and tunica media of blood vessels, histiocytes, and dendritelike cells. Eventually, the virus multiplies within renal tubular cells (Del Piero, 2000; Campbell, 2006). Hematogenous spread leads to dissemination of the virus throughout the body, and it can be found in body fluids and tissues by third-day of infection. Except from the semen of carrier stallion, the virus is no longer detectable in most tissues/body fluids beyond twenty-eight days postinfection (PI). In carrier stallion, the virus is localized primarily in accessory sex glands (Timoney et al., 1987b).

The primary targets of EAV are the endothelium and mesothelium of vessels throughout the body, and the secondary multiplication sites include the epithelium of certain organs, viz, the thyroid and adrenal glands, kidneys, liver, and seminiferous tubules. At ten days PI, the most severe damage occurs to blood vessels (Del Piero, 2000). Characteristic vascular lesions include endothelial swelling and degeneration, neutrophil infiltration, and necrosis of the tunica media of affected vessels. The lesions progress to variety of changes in various major organs, viz, infarction and thrombosis of intestine, lung, and spleen (McCollum et al., 1971; McCollum, 1981; Mumford, 1985; Del Piero, 2000). The generation of chemotactic factors resulting from increased vascular permeability and lecukocyte infiltration lead to hemorrhage and fluid accumulation in peritoneal and pleural cavities. Besides endothelial cells, the macrophages from infected horses also support replication of EAV and produce cytokine mediators such as tumor necrosis factor alpha

(TNF-). Quantitative differences in the induction of cytokine mediators from endothelial cells and macrophages obtained from horses infected with virulent and avirulent strains of EAV have been reported (Moore et al., 2003). These cytokine mediators may have a prominent role in the pathogenesis of disease. The vascular lesions caused by EAV are responsible for many of the clinical signs. Vascular lesions do not appear to be the consequence of immune-mediated injury as neither IgG or complement component C3 is present in these lesions. Recently, St-Louis and Archambault (2007) reported that EAV induces apoptosis initiated by caspase-8 activation and subsequent mitochondria-dependent caspase-9 activation.

Clinical pathology findings reported in affected foals include hypoxia, hypercapnia, respiratory and metabolic acidosis, neutropenia/neutrophilia, lymphopenia/lymphocytosis, thrombocytopenia, and hyperfibrinogenemia (Del Piero et al., 1997). The abortion caused by equine arteritis virus may be due to a variety of reasons. The myometritis in the pregnant mare may lead to impairment of progesterone synthesis due to damage to placental and eventually death and expulsion of the fetus (Coignoul and Cheville, 1984; Johnson et al., 1991; Del Piero, 2000). However, the observations that the virus is present in higher titers in tissues of aborted fetuses as compared to dam indicates active replication in fetus, which could in turn may be another mechanism of EAV-induced abortion.

LESIONS

The gross and microscopic lesions have been described based on natural outbreaks of EVA or experimental infection of horses with prototype virulent Bucyrus strain. The observations with field strains may not be similar to that obtained with Bucyrus strain. The most important gross lesions are edema, congestion, and hemorrhages, especially in the subcutis of the limbs and abdomen along with fluid accumulation in peritoneal, pleural, and pericardial cavities. Infarctions in spleen, lungs, and intestine and segmental necrosis of small arteries throughout the body are observed in terminal stages of the disease. Pulmonary edema, emphysema and interstitial pneumonia, enteritis, panvasculitis with edema, thrombosis and hemorrhage, lymphoid necrosis, renal tubular necrosis, and infarcts in the spleen have been described in fatal cases of the disease in foals (Del Piero, 2000).

Aborted fetuses are partly autolyzed and are expelled with fetal membranes without premonitory clinical signs. The gross lesions, if present, are limited to an excess of fluid in body cavities, variable degree of interlobular pulmonary edema, petechial hemorrhages on the mucosal linings of respiratory and gastrointestinal tract and on the serosal linings of peritoneal and pleural cavities (Del Piero, 2000; Campbell, 2006). Vascular lesions are not prominent in aborted fetuses, but if present, they are mild, and EAV antigen is frequently not detectable within fetal tissues and placenta (Del Piero, 2000).

Severe necrotizing panvasculitis, involving primarily small arteries but also small veins, is the characteristic microscopic lesion. Histopathological changes can vary from vascular and perivascular edema, with occasional lymphocytic infiltration and endothelial cell hypertrophy in mild cases, to fibrinoid necrosis of the tunica media, extensive lymphocytic infiltration, necrosis and loss of endothelium, and thrombus formation in severe cases (Timoney et al., 1996; Campbell, 2006). Microscopic lesions are not a constant feature in abortions. Vasculitis may be present in placenta, brain, liver, spleen, and lungs of the fetus. Severe interstitial pneumonia can be seen in the lungs of the affected neonatal foals. Immunofluorescent and immunoperoxidase tests demonstrated the distribution of EAV antigen in endothelium lining of blood vessels, macrophages in lymph nodes, and many other organs (Del Piero, 2000).

DIAGNOSIS
Equine viral arteritis can be suspected in outbreaks of disease in equines that include fever, depression, edema, conjunctivitis, nasal discharges, and abortions. However, the clinical symptoms of this disease may be difficult to differentiate from other equine respiratory and nonrespiratory illnesses such as equine influenza; infection with equine herpesvirus 1 and 4, equine rhinitis A and B viruses; equine adenoviruses; streptococcal infections (purpura hemorrhagica); Getah virus infection; African horse sickness; and septic shock (Del Piero, 2000; Campbell, 2006).

The diagnosis can be confirmed in the laboratory by virus isolation, antigen detection, serology, histopathology immunohistochemistry, and nucleic acid–based techniques (Del Piero, 2000; Gerahty et al., 2003; Campbell, 2006; OIE, 2008). Reverse transcription–polymerase chain reaction (RT-PCR) or nested RT-PCR techniques can efficiently detect viral DNA in tissue samples, blood, and semen (St. Laurent et al., 1994; Belak et al., 1995; Sekiguchi et al., 1995; Gilbert et al., 1997; Starick, 1998; Ramina et al., 1999; Echeverria et al., 2003; Szeredi et al., 2005; Campbell, 2006; Mittelholzer et al., 2006b). Serologic tests include virus neutralization, complement fixation, agar gel immunodiffusion, indirect fluorescent antibody, immunoperoxidase test, and enzyme-linked immunosorbent (ELISA) assays (Crawford and Henson, 1973; Cook et al., 1989; Lopez et al., 1996; Kondo et al., 1998; Nugent et al., 2000; Cho et al., 2000; Del Piero, 2000; Echeverria et al.,

2003; Szeredi et al., 2005; Legrand et al., 2007). Immunocytochemical methods include indirect immunofluorescence or avidin-biotin-peroxidase techniques. Other serological tests such as plaque reduction and complement fixation (CF) test (Fukunaga and McCollum, 1977) have also been used to detect antibodies against EAV.

Virus neutralization tests are prescribed for international trade. The detection of seroconversion with virus neutralization performed using the Bucyrus strain in EAV-infected animals is a reliable method for identifying EAV infection in equines (Senne et al., 1985; Fukunaga et al., 1994; Del Piero, 2000; Horner, 2004). Microneutralization test carried out in the presence of guinea pig complement not only enhances the sensitivity of the test but is essential for some EAV strains and is the gold standard test as per OIE for detection of EAV antibodies in serum. Fourfold or greater increase in the neutralizing antibody titers in paired sera samples taken at twenty-one to twenty-eight days apart indicates seroconversion. ELISA utilizes purified EAV antigen to recognize EAV-positive horse sera. However, the major problem encountered by EAV ELISAs are their failure to give clear and sensitive results when the horse being tested has been previously vaccinated such as those used to prevent equine influenza and herpesvirus infections. The high background color development in such cases due to nonspecific binding of antibodies to tissue culture–derived antigen can mask the EAV ELISA results (Chirnside, 1992). Indirect ELISAs utilizing the major structural proteins of EAV expressed from recombinant baculoviruses have also been developed. M protein is the major target of the equine antibody response to EAV. Chirnside et al. (1995) reported the recombinant protein based on ELISA EAV detection. ELISA, based on these recombinant proteins, successfully detected antibodies in most equine sera that were positive in the standard SN assay following EAV infection (Hedges et al., 1998). Recently, recombinant chimeric N/G (L) protein was used to detect antibodies to EAV in horse sera (Turan et al., 2007).

Nasopharyngeal and conjunctival swabs, blood samples, placental and fetal fluids, together with placenta, lung, lymphoreticular, and other fetal tissues are used for virus isolation or detection by PCR (Timoney and McCollum, 1993; Del Piero, 2000; Campbell, 2006). Virus can be isolated in RK-13, horse kidney, Vero and BHK-21 cell lines, or primary cells of horse or rabbit origin (Golnik et al., 1981; Timoney et al., 1986, 1987b; Del Piero, 2000; Echeverria et al., 2003; Zhang et al., 2004). The identity of EAV isolates can be confirmed in a microneutralization test, RT-PCR assay (Chirnside and Spaan, 1990; Balasuriya et al., 1998, 2002; Gilbert et al., 1997) or by indirect immunofluorescence, or by avidin-biotin-peroxidase technique (Little et al.,

1995; Legrand et al., 2007). Carrier stallions are first identified by serology. The carrier state can be readily confirmed by demonstration of the virus in semen, either by virus isolation or PCR testing. It can also be confirmed by test breeding using seronegative mares and monitoring them for seroconversion to EAV after breeding. Histopathologic examination and immunohistochemical staining may also be useful for diagnosis of abortion.

The virus neutralization test is considered the gold standard serological screening test, but it is time consuming and labor intensive; consequently, there is a move toward more rapid screening methodology (Timoney et al., 1996; Del Piero, 2000; Campbell, 2006; Duthie et al., 2008). A single-tube, real-time TaqMan RT-PCR have been developed for the detection of EAV in seminal plasma and nasal secretions using primers and a fluorogenic TaqMan probe to amplify ORF7 (Balasuriya et al., 2002). Similarly, a real-time RT-PCR strategy with minor groove binder (MGB) technology for the detection of EAV from semen samples of stallions had better sensitivity and high specificity (Mankoc et al., 2007). However, Lu et al. (2008) have suggested the importance of evaluation and validation of real-time RT-PCR assays prior to their recommended use in a diagnostic laboratory.

Westcott et al. (2003) used an internal standard in a closed, one-tube RT-PCR for the detection of equine arteritis virus RNA with fluorescent probes. Regarding molecular characterization, exploiting the nucleotide sequencing of the ORF5 gene that encode the glycoprotein GP5, EAV isolates can be categorized into subgroups to identify their genetic diversity (Echeverria et al., 2007; Larska and Rola, 2008). Earlier, Chirnside et al. (1994) have reported the use of sequencing of M and N gene to identify variation among various EAV isolates; and later, a conclusive phylogeny of EAV from Italy, Austria, Hungary, Sweden, South Africa, and other parts of the world were derived by direct sequencing of ORF5, which evinced a clear division between European—and American-type viruses (Mittelholzer et al., 2006a). Also, phylogenetic analysis based on ORF5 sequences of French EAV isolates classified them into two distinct groups: North American and European, out of which the latter could be further divided into European subgroup 1 (EU-1) and European subgroup 2 (EU-2) (Zhang et al., 2007). Also, partial sequences of ORF5 enabled identification of mutations that clustered in antigenic neutralization site within variable region 1 of the GP5 (Liu et al., 2008).

PREVENTION AND CONTROL
The aim of most prevention and control programs is to prevent or curtail spread of equine arteritis virus in breeding populations, to minimize the

risk of virus-related abortion or death in young foals, the and establishment of the carrier state in stallions. Such programs are based on good breeding management practices, identification of any carrier stallions, and immunization of the noncarrier breeding stallion population (Timoney et al., 1996; Del Piero, 2000; Holyoak et al., 2008). During outbreaks, the virus spread can be controlled by restriction of movements in affected areas, isolation of infected animals on stud farms followed by a quarantine period of recovery, intense diagnostic surveillance, good hygiene and management practices, and use of modified live vaccine to immunize the animals at risk (Chirnside, 1992; Del Piero, 2000; Campbell, 2006; MacLachlan and Balasuriya, 2006).

There is no known specific antiviral treatment for EAV. Symptomatic treatment with antipyretic, anti-inflammatory, and diuretic agents are indicated only in severe cases. Very recently, in an attempt to develop novel and save therapies against the infection an RNA interference (RNAi) study has been conducted in an equine in vitro system (Heinrich et al., 2008). Application of small interfering RNA oligonucleotides (siRNAs) led to a significant protection of the cells, and virus titers decreased drastically, thus evolving as a therapeutic approach to combat EAV.

Blood samples from all horses should be collected before breeding for EVA testing. Semen, used for natural service or artificial insemination, should be tested for virus before use. Strict hygiene and disinfection of instruments and equipment are essential to minimize spread of the virus (Del Piero, 2000; Holyoak et al., 2008). The stables should be thoroughly cleaned and disinfected. EVA-negative mares should be bred only to EVA-negative, noncarrier stallions. SNT is performed on a serum sample to detect presence of antibodies against EAV. An antibody titer of ≥1:4 is considered a positive reaction, and the horse will be considered seropositive for exposure to EAV (Timoney et al., 1996). Antibodies that develop following natural exposure to the virus cannot be distinguished from antibodies that develop following vaccination. If blood test results are positive in a stallion, but there is no official documentation of negative EVA status prior to vaccination, the stallion must be tested for the presence of a carrier state. For this, semen from two separate ejaculations is processed for virus isolation. Alternately, two EVA-negative mares are mated with the stallion. Twenty-eight days after breeding, mare's blood should be tested for the development of the neutralizing antibodies to the EVA virus. Carrier stallions should be managed separately to avoid the risk of inadvertent viral spread to previously uninfected or unvaccinated horses on the premises (Holyoak et al., 2008). Carrier stallions should be bred only to EVA-positive mares or mares that are properly vaccinated. When breeding an EVA-positive or carrier stallion to an EVA-negative, vaccinated mare, isolate both horses for twenty-four hours after breeding to prevent mechanical spread of EVA from voided semen. If this is the first time the mare has been bred to a carrier stallion, she should be isolated from other horses for an additional twenty-one days due to potential virus shedding (Chirnside, 1992). Morrell and Geraghty (2006) have suggested the technique of double sperm processing for generating EAV-free sperm preparations, which included density gradient centrifugation and "swim-up" in protocols for the processing of equine semen.

One way for prevention and control of EVA is vaccination of all intact young colts and adult stallions. There are two commercial vaccines against EVA: one, a modified live virus (MLV) vaccine (Doll et al., 1968; McKinnon et al, 1986) is only available in North America; and the other, an inactivated vaccine (Fukunaga et al., 1990), is only approved for use in certain countries in Europe. MLV vaccine is not recommended for use in pregnant mares, especially in the last two months of gestation, or in foals of less than six weeks of age. Glaser et al. (1997a) reported the use of a live, attenuated (ARVAC), and a formalin-inactivated (ARTERVAC) vaccine for preventing EAV in equines. New-generation vaccines include MLVs with deletions and/ or mutations of critical genes, subunit vaccines that incorporate immunogenic proteins or expression vectors that produce these proteins as immunogens, and DNA vaccines (MacLachlan et al., 2007).

Traditional inactivated and live-attenuated (modified live virus) virus vaccines remain popular and efficacious, but recombinant vaccines are increasingly being developed and used in part because of the perceived deficiencies of some existing products (MacLachlan et al., 2007). Modified live EAV vaccine can be administered to foals at eight months old without risk of interference from maternal antibodies, regardless of serologic status of the dam (McCollum, 1970; Hullinger et al., 1998). Further, the prevention of the carrier state in stallions would eliminate the viral reservoir in the horse population (Timoney et al., 1996; MacLachlan and Balasuriya, 2006; Holyoak et al., 2008). Hence, most prevention and control programs are focused on preventing or curtailing dissemination of EAV in breeding populations to minimize the risk of virus-related abortion or death in young foals and establishment of the carrier state in stallions (Chirnside, 1992; MacLachlan and Balasuriya, 2006). Another way is to vaccinate mares that are to be bred to carrier stallions to reduce transmission of the virus. Mares should be vaccinated a minimum of twenty-one days prior to breeding to a carrier stallion to allow sufficient time for development of protective antibodies (Del Piero, 2000; Holyoak et al., 2008). Colostrum from immune mares can prevent arteritis in young foals. When neonates are not protected by passive maternal immunity, they may present with sudden death or severe respiratory distress followed by death (Del Piero, 2000). All vaccinated horses should receive yearly boosters to protect against infection and, for the stallions, to prevent the development of a carrier state. The humoral immune response plays an important role in recovery as production of neutralization antibodies in EAV-infected horses coincides with virus clearance. Much less is known about the cellular immune responses to the EAV infection. Studies in ponies experimentally infected with EAV have shown that cytotoxicity induced by EAV-stimulated PBMC was virus specific, genetically restricted, and mediated by CD8+ T cells, with the persistence of the precursors for at least one year after infection (Castillo-Olivares et al., 2003, Balasuriya and Maclachlan, 2004).

CONCLUSION

Although not frequently diagnosed as a cause of abortion, due to neonatal mortality and disease in adults, EVA is considered as an important and emerging disease that can incur severe economic losses to equine industry. The economic losses primarily arise due to direct losses from abortion and pneumonia in neonates and febrile disease in performance horses, while indirect losses are related to national and international trade regulations. Although infrequently reported in the past, confirmed outbreaks of EVA appear to be on the rise in recent years. More relevantly, it is important to appreciate the significance or the manner in which the horse-breeding countries ascribe to this disease as a significant percentage of stallions can become long-term carriers and constant semen shedders of EAV. Also to stress at this point is the importance of developing effective measures for the prevention and control of EVA through a clear understanding of the epidemiology of the disease. The major factors to consider in future are the following: modes of transmission of EAV during the acute and carrier stage; the carrier state in stallions, the potential to cause abortion by certain strains of EAV; and the nature and duration of immunity to natural infection. However, the current programs for the control of EVA are largely focused on minimizing the risk of introduction and dissemination of the virus on breeding farms to prevent EAV-related abortions through the carrier stallions. Also, based on the knowledge from current research trends regarding novel techniques to evolve rapid diagnostic agents and safe and effective new-generation vaccines, it has to be assumed that this disease that cause significant impact on the equine population could be successfully curtailed in the years to come.

REFERENCES

1. Akashi, H., Konishi, S. and Ogata, M. 1976. A-serological survey of equine viral arteritis in horses imported in 1973–74. *Jap. J. Vet. Sci.* 38:71.
2. Balasuriya, U. B. R., Evermann, J. F., Hedges, J. F., McKeirnan, A. J., Mitten, J. Q., Beyer, J. C., McCollum, W. H., Timoney, P. J. and MacLachlan, N. J. 1998. Serologic and molecular characterization of an abortigenic strain of equine arteritis virus isolated from infective frozen semen and an aborted equine fetus. *J. Am. Vet. Med. Assoc.* 213:1586–1589.
3. Balasuriya, U. B., Hedges, J. F., Nadler, S. A., McCollum, W. H., Timoney, P. J. and MacLachlan, N. J. 1999. Genetic stability of equine arteritis virus during horizontal and vertical transmission in an outbreak of equine viral arteritis. *J. Gen. Virol.* 80:1949–1958.
4. Balasuriya U. B. R., Leutenegger, C. M., Topol, J. B., McCollum, W. H., Timoney, P. J. and MacLachlan, N. J. 2002. Detection of equine arteritis virus by real-time TaqMan reverse transcription-PCR assay. *J. Virol. Methods* 101:21–28.
5. Balasuriya, U. B. and MacLachlan, N. J. 2004. The immune response to equine viral arteritis virus: Potential lessons for other arteriviruses. *Vet. Immunol. Immunopathol.* 102:107–129.
6. Balasuriya, U. B., Hedges, J. F., Smalley, V. L., Navarrette, A., McCollum, W. H., Timoney, P. J., Snijder, E. J. and MacLachlan, N. J. 2004. Genetic characterization of equine arteritis virus during persistent infections of stallions. *J. Gen. Virol.* 85:379–390.
7. Belak, S., Ballagi-Pordany, A., Timoney, P., McCollum, W. H., Little, T. V., Hyllseth, B. and Klingeborn, B. 1995. Evaluation of a nested PCR assay for the detection of equine arteritis virus infection. Proc. 7th Intl. Conf. Equine Infect. Dis., Tokyo, Japan, 1994, 33–38.
8. Burki, F. 1970. The virology of equine arteritis. Proceedings 2nd Int. Conf. Equine Infect. Dis., Paris. 1996,125.
9. Burki, F., Hofer, A. and Nowtny, N. 1992. Objective data plead to suspend import bans for seroreactors against equine arteritis virus except for breeder stallions. *J. Appl. Anim. Res.* 1:31.
10. Campbell, M. L. 2006. Equine viral arteritis. *Vet. Rec.* 158:455.
11. Cardwell, J. M., Wood, J. L., Mumford, J. A., Geraghty, R. J., Hillyer, L. L. and Pascoe, R. J. 2002. Equine viral arteritis in the UK. *Vet. Rec.* 150:819–820.
12. Carman, S. 1988. Equine arteritis virus isolated from a standard bred foal with pneumonia. *Can. Vet. J.* 29:937.
13. Castillo-Olivares, J., Tearle, J. P., Montesso, F., Westcott, D., Kydd, J. H., Davis-Poynter, N. J. and Hannant, D. 2003. Detection of equine arteritis virus (EAV)-specific cytotoxic CD8+ T lymphocyte precursors from EAV-infected ponies. *J. Gen. Virol.* 84:2745–2753.
14. Cavanagh, D. 1997. Nidovirales: A new order comprising Coronaviridae and Arteriviridae. *Arch. Virol.* 142:629–633.
15. Chirnside, E. D. and Spaan, W. J. M. 1990. Reverse transcription and cDNA amplification by the polymerase chain reaction of equine arteritis virus (EAV). *J. Virol. Methods* 30:133–40.
16. Chirnside, E. D. 1992. Equine arteritis virus: An overview. *Br. Vet. J.* 148:181–97.
17. Chirnside, E. D., Wearing, C. M., Binns, M. M. and Mumford, J. A. 1994. Comparison of M and N gene sequences distinguishes variation amongst equine arteritis virus isolates. *J. Gen. Virol.* 75:1491–1497.
18. Chirnside, E. D., Francis, P. M., de Vries, A. A. F., Sinclair, R. and Mumford, J. A. 1995. Development and evaluation of an ELISA using recombinant fusion protein to detect the presence of host antibody to equine arteritis virus (EAV). *J. Virol. Methods* 54:1–13.
19. Cho, H. J., Entz, S. C., Deregt, D., Jordan, L. T., Timoney, P. J. and McCollum, W. H. 2000. Detection of antibodies to equine arteritis virus by a monoclonal antibody-based blocking ELISA. *Can. J. Vet. Res.* 64:38–43.
20. Clayton, H. 1987. The 1986 outbreak of EAV in Alberta, Canada. *J. Equine Vet. Sci.* 7:101.

21. Coignoul, F. L. and Cheville, N. F. 1984. Pathology of the maternal genital tract, placenta and foetus in equine viral arteritis. *Vet. Pathol.* 21:333–340.

22. Cook, R. F., Gann, S. J. and Mumford, J. A. 1989. The effects of vaccination with tissue culture-derived viral vaccines on detection of antibodies to equine arteritis virus by enzyme-linked immunosorbent assay (ELISA). *Vet. Microbiol.* 20:181–189.

23. Cole, J. R., Hall, R. F., Gosser, M. S., Hendricks, J. B., Pursel, R., Senne, D. A., Pearson, J. E. and Gipson, C. A. 1986. Transmissibility and abortigenic effect of equine viral arteritis in mares. *J. Am. Vet. Med. Assoc.* 189:769–71.

24. Crawford, T. B. and Henson, J. B. 1973. Immunofluorescent, light microscopic and immunologic studies of equine viral arteritis. Proc. Third Intl. Conf. Equine Infect. Dis., Paris, 1972, 282–302.

25. Deshpande, A., Wang, S., Walsh, M. A. and Dokland, T. 2007. Structure of the equine arteritis virus nucleocapsid protein reveals a dimer-dimer arrangement. *Acta Crystallogr. D Biol. Crystallogr.* 63:581–586.

26. de Vries, A. A. F., Chirnside, E. D., Bredenbeek, P. J., Gravestein, L. A., Horzinek, M. C. and Spaan, W. J. M. 1990. All subgenomic mRNAs of equine arteritis virus contain a common leader sequence. *Nucleic Acids Res.* 18:3241–3247.

27. de Vries, A. A. F., Chirnside, E. D., Horzinek, M. C. and Rottier, P. J. M. 1992. Structural proteins of equine arteritis virus. *J. Gen. Virol.* 66:6294–6303.

28. de Vries, A. A. F., Horzinek, M. C., Rottier, P. J. M. and de Groot, R. J. 1997. The genome organization of the *Nidovirales*: Similarities and differences between arteri-, toro—and coronaviruses. *Seminars Virol.* 8:33–47.

29. Del Piero, F., Wilkins, P. A., Lopez, J. W., Glaser, A. L., Dubovi, E. J., Schlafer, D. H. and Lein, D. H. 1997. Equine viral arteritis in newborn foals: Clinical, pathological, serological, microbiological and immunohistochemical observations. *Equine Vet. J.* 29:178–185.

30. Del Piero, F. 2000. Equine viral arteritis. *Vet. Pathol.* 37:287–296.

31. Doll, E. R., Knappenberger, R. E. and Bryans, J. T. 1957. An outbreak of abortion caused by the equine arteritis virus. *Cornell Vet.* 47:69–75.

32. Doll, E. R., Bryans, J. T., Wilson, J. C. and McCollum, W. H. 1968. Immunisation against equine viral arteritis using modified live virus propagated in cell cultures of rabbit kidney. *Cornell Vet.* 48:497–524.

33. Duthie, S., Mills, H. and Burr, P. 2008. The efficacy of a commercial ELISA as an alternative to virus neutralisation test for the detection of antibodies to EAV. *Equine Vet. J.* 40:182–183.

34. Echeverria, M. G., Pecoraro, M. R., Galosi, C. M., Etcheverrigaray, M. E. and Nosetto, E. O. 2003. The first isolation of equine arteritis virus in Argentina. *Rev. Sci. Tech.* 22:1029–1033.

35. Echeverria, M. G., Diaz, S., Metz, G. E., Serena, M. S., Panei, C. J. and Nosetto, E. 2007. Genetic typing of equine arteritis virus isolates from Argentina. *Virus Genes* 35:313–320.

36. Edison, P. 2005. Equine viral arteritis: A review. *Rev. Fac. de Ciencias Veterinar* 46:74–86.

37. Fukunaga, Y. and McCollum, W. H. 1977. Complement fixation reactions in equine viral arteritis. *Am. J. Vet. Res.* 38:2043.

38. Fukunaga, Y., Wada, R., Matsumura, T., Sugiura, T. and Imagawa, H. 1990. Induction of immune response and protection from equine viral arteritis (EVA) by formalin inactivated-virus vaccine for EVA in horses. *J. Vet. Med.* 37:135–141.

39. Fukunaga, Y., Matsumura, T., Sugiura, T., Wada, R., Imagawa, H., Kanemaru, T. and Kamada, M. 1994. Use of the serum neutralisation test for equine viral arteritis with different virus strains. *Vet. Rec.* 136:574–576.

40. Gerahty, R. J., Newton, J. R., Castillo-Olivares, J., Cardwell, J. M. and Mumford, J. A. 2003. Testing for equine arteritis virus. *Vet. Rec.* 152:478.

41. Gilbert, S. A., Timoney, P. J., McCollum, W. H. and Deregt, D. 1997. Detection of equine arteritis virus in the semen of carrier stallions using a sensitive nested PCR assay. *J. Clin. Microbiol.* 35:2181–2183.

42. Glaser, A. L., de Vries, A. A., Rottier, P. J., Horzinek, M. C. and Colenbrander, B. 1996. Equine arteritis virus: A review of clinical features and management aspects. *Vet. Q.* 18:95–99.

43. Glaser, A. L., Chirnside, E. D., Horzinek, M. C. and de Vries, A. A. 1997a. Equine arteritis virus. *Theriogenology* 47:1275–1295.

44. Glaser, A. L., de Vries, A. A., Rottier, P. J., Horzinek, M. C. and Colenbrander, B. 1997b. Equine arteritis virus: Clinical symptoms and prevention. *Tijdsch. Diergeneeskd.* 122:2–7.

45. Golnik, W. 1991. Viruses isolated from aborted fetuses and still born foals. In *Proceedings of the Sixth Conference on Equine Infectious Disease, Cambridge, 1991*, ed. W. Plowright, P. D. Rossdale, and J. F. Wade. Newmarket: R&W Publications.

46. Golnik, W., Michalska, A. and Michalak, T. 1981. Natural equine viral arteritis in foals. *Schweiz Arch. Tierheilk.* 123:523.

47. Guthrie, A. J., Howell, P. G., Hedges, J. F., Bosman, A. M., Balasuriya, U. B., McCollum, W. H., Timoney, P. J. and MacLachlan, N. J. 2003. Lateral transmission of equine arteritis virus among Lipizzaner stallions in South Africa. *Equine Vet. J.* 35:596–600.

48. Hedges, J. F., Balasuriya, U. B., Ahmad, S., Timoney, P. J., McCollum, W. H., Yilma, T. and MacLachlan, N. J. 1998. Detection of antibodies to equine arteritis virus by enzyme linked immunosorbant assays utilizing G(L), M and N proteins expressed from recombinant baculoviruses. *J. Virol. Methods* 76:127–137.

49. Hedges, J. F., Balasuriya, U. B. and MacLachlan, N. J. 1999. The open reading frame 3 of equine arteritis virus encodes an immunogenic glycosylated, integral membrane protein. *Virology* 264:92–98.

50. Heinrich, A., Riethmuller, D., Gloger, M., Schusser, G. F., Giese, M. and Ulbert, S. 2008. RNA interference protects horse cells in vitro from infection with equine arteritis virus. *Antiviral Res.* [Epub ahead of print, NCBI.]

51. Holyoak, G. R., Balasuriya, U. B., Broaddus, C. C. and Timoney, P. J. 2008. Equine viral arteritis: Current status and prevention. *Theriogenology* 70:403–414.

52. Horner, G. W. 2004. Equine viral arteritis control scheme: A brief review with emphasis on laboratory aspects of the scheme in New Zealand. *NZ. Vet. J.* 52:82–84.

53. Hullinger, P. J., Wilson, W. D., Rossitto, P. V., Patton, J. F., Thurmond, M. C. and MacLachlan, N. J. 1998. Passive transfer, rate of decay, and protein specificity of antibodies against equine arteritis virus in horses from a Standardbred herd with high seroprevalence. *J. Am. Vet. Med. Assoc.* 213:839–842.

54. Huntigdon, P. J., Ellis, P. M., Forman, A. J. and Timoney, P. J. 1990a. Equine viral arteritis. *Aust. Vet. J.* 67:429.

55. Huntigdon, P. J., Forman, A. J. and Ellis, P. M. 1990b. The occurrence of equine arteritis virus in Australia. *Aust. Vet. J.* 67:432.

56. Hyllseth, B. 1970. Buoyant density studies on equine arteritis virus. *Arch. Ges. Virusforsch.* 30:97–104.

57. Hyllseth, B. 1973. Structural proteins of equine arteritis virus. *Arch. Ges. Virusforsch.* 40:177–188.

58. Johnson, B., Baldwin, C., Timoney, P. and Ely, R. 1991. Arteritis in equine fetuses aborted due to equine viral arteritis. *Vet. Pathol.* 28:248–250.

59. Jones, T. C., Doll, E. R. and Bryans, J. T. 1957. The lesions of equine viral arteritis. *Cornell Vet.* 47:52–68.

60. Klug, E. and Sieme, H. 1999. Veterinary recommendations for the handling of equine virus arteritis (EVA) in practical breeding care. *Tierarztl. Prax. Ausg. G Gross. Nutztiere.* 27:61–66.

61. Kondo, T., Fukunaga, Y., Sekiguchi, K., Sugiura, T. and Imagawa, H. 1998. Enzyme-linked immunosorbent assay for serological survey of equine arteritis virus in racehorses. *J. Vet. Med. Sci.* 60:1043–1045.

62. Larska, M. and Rola, J. 2008. Molecular epizootiology of equine arteritis virus isolates from Poland. *Vet. Microbiol.* 127:392–398.

63. Legrand, L., Pitel, P. H., Fortier, G., Pronost, S. and Vabret, A. 2007. Testing for antibodies to equine arteritis virus. *Vet. Rec.* 161:599–600.

64. Little, T. V., Deregt, D., McCollum, W. H., and Timoney, P. J. 1995. Evaluation of an immunocytochemical method for rapid detection and identification of equine arteritis virus in natural cases of infection. Proceedings of the Seventh International Conference on Equine Infectious Diseases, Tokyo, Japan, 1994, 27–31.

65. Liu, L., L., Castillo-Olivares, J., Davis-Poynter, N. J., Baule, C., Xia, H. and Belak, S. 2008. Analysis of ORFs 2b, 3, 4, and partial ORF5 of sequential isolates of equine arteritis virus shows genetic variation following experimental infection of horses. *Vet. Microbiol.* 129:262–268.

66. Lopez, J. W., Del Piero, F., Glaser, A. and Finazzi, M. 1996. Immunoperoxidase histochemistry as a diagnostic tool for detection of equine arteritis virus antigen in formalin fixed tissues. *Equine Vet. J.* 28:77–79.

67. Lu, Z., Branscum, A. J., Shuck, K. M., Zhang, J., Dubovi, E. J., Timoney, P. J. and Balasuriya, U. B. 2008. Comparison of two real-time reverse transcription polymerase chain reaction assays for the detection of equine arteritis virus nucleic acid in equine semen and tissue culture fluid. *J. Vet. Diagn. Invest.* 20:147–155.

68. MacLachlan, N. J. and Balasuriya, U. B. 2006. Equine viral arteritis. *Adv. Exp. Med. Biol.* 581:429–433.

69. MacLachlan, N. J., Balasuriya, U. B., Davis, N. L., Collier, M., Johnston, R. E., Ferraro, G. L. and Guthrie, A. J. 2007. Experiences with new generation vaccines against equine viral arteritis, West Nile disease and African horse sickness. *Vaccine* 25:5577–5582.

70. Mankoc, S., Hostnik, P., Grom, J., Toplak, I., Klobucar, I., Kosec, M. and Barlic-Maganja, D. 2007. Comparison of different molecular methods for assessment of equine arteritis virus (EAV) infection: A novel one-step MGB real-time RT-PCR assay, PCR-ELISA and classical RT-PCR for detection of highly diverse sequences of Slovenian EAV variants. *J. Virol. Methods* 146:341–354.

71. McCollum, W. H. 1970. Vaccination for equine viral arteritis. *Proc. Second Intl. Conf. Equine Infect. Dis.*, Paris, 1969, 143–151.

72. McCollum, W. H., Prickett, M. F. and Bryans, J. T. 1971. Temporal distribution of EAV in respiratory mucosa, tissue and body fluids of horses infected by inhalation. *Res. Vet. Sci.* 2:459.

73. McCollum, W. H. 1981. Pathological feature of horses given avirulent virus intramuscularly. *Am. J. Vet. Res.* 42:1218–1220.

74. McKenzie, J. 1990. Survey of stallions for equine viral arteritis. *Surveillance* 16:17–18.

75. McKinnon, A. O., Colbern, G. T., Collions, J. K., Bowen, R. A., Voss, J. L. and Umphenour, J. W. 1986. Vaccination of stallions with a modified live equine arteritis virus vaccine. *J. Equine Vet. Sci.* 6:66–69.

76. Mittelholzer, C., Stadejek, T., Johansson, I., Baule, C., Ciabatti, I., Hannant, D., Paton, D., Autorino, G. L., Nowotny, N. and Belak, S. 2006a. Extended phylogeny of equine arteritis virus: Division into new subgroups. *J. Vet. Med. Infect. Dis.* 53:55–58.

77. Mittelholzer, C., Johansson, I., Olsson, A. K., Roneus, M., Klingeborn, B. and Belak, S. 2006b. Recovery of Swedish equine arteritis viruses from semen by cell culture isolation and RNA transfection. *J. Virol. Methods* 133:48–52.

78. Moore, B. D., Balasuriya, U. B., Watson, J. L., Bosio, C. M., Mackay, R. J. and MacLachlan, N. J. 2003. Virulent and avirulent strains of equine arteritis virus induce different quantities of TNF-alpha and other proinflammatory cytokines in alveolar and blood-derived equine macrophages. *Virology* 314:662–670.

79. Moraillon, R. and Moraillon, A. 1978. Results of a serosurvey of viral arteritis in France and several European and African countries. In *Proceedings of the Fourth Conference on Equine Infectious Disease, Lyon, 1976*, ed. T. J. Bryans and H. Gerber, 467–74. Princeton, NJ: Veterinary Publications.

80. Morrell, J. M. and Geraghty, R. M. 2006. Effective removal of equine arteritis virus from stallion semen. *Equine Vet. J.* 38:224–229.

81. Mumford, J. A. 1985. Preparing for equine arteritis. *Equine Vet. J.* 17:6–11.

82. Nowotny, N. 1991. First isolation of equine arteritis virus from three aborted fetuses from three different premises in Austria. In *Proceedings of the Sixth Conference on Equine Infectious Disease, Cambridge, 1991*, ed. W. Plowright, P. D. Rossdale, and J. F. Wade. Newmarket: R&W Publications.

83. Nugent, J., Sinclair, R., de Vries, A. A. F., Eberhardt, R. Y., Castillo-Olivares, J., Davis Poynter, N., Rottier, P. J. M. and Mumford, J. A. 2000. Development and evaluation of ELISA procedures to detect antibodies against the major envelope protein (GL) of equine arteritis virus. *J. Virol. Methods* 90:167–183.

84. OIE. 2008. Equine viral arteritis. *Manual of diagnostic tests and vaccines for terrestrial animals*, chapter 2.5.10, 904–918. www.oie.int.

85. Paweska, J. T., Aitchison, H., Chirnside, E. D. and Barnard, B. J. 1996. Transmission of the South African asinine strain of equine arteritis virus (EAV) among horses and between donkeys and horses. *Onderstepoort J. Vet. Res.* 63:189–196.

86. Ramina, A., Dalla Valle, L., De Mas, S., Tisato, E., Zuin, A., Renier, M., Cuteri, V., Valente, C. and Cancellotti, F. M. 1999. Detection of equine arteritis virus in semen by reverse transcriptase polymerase chain reaction-ELISA. *Comp. Immunol. Microbiol. Infect. Dis.* 22:187–197.

87. Samper, J. C. and Tibary, A. 2006. Disease transmission in horses. *Theriogenology* 66:551–559.

88. Sekiguchi, K., Sugita, S., Fukunaga, Y., Kondo, T., Wada, R., Kamada, M. and Yamaguchi, S. 1995. Detection of equine arteritis virus (EAV) by the polymerase chain reaction (PCR) and differentiation of EAV strains by restriction enzyme analysis of PCR products. *Arch. Virol.* 140:1483–1491.

89. Senne, D. A., Pearson, J. E. and Cabrey, E. A. 1985. Equine viral arteritis: A standard procedure for the virus neutralisation test and comparison of results of a proficiency test performed at five laboratories. *Proc. U.S. Anim. Health Assoc.* 89:29–34.

90. Singh, B. K., Uppal, P. K., Yadav, M. P. and Gupta, A. K. 1997. Detection of equine viral arteritis specific antibody in Indian horses. XII Annual Convention Indian Virol. Soc. GAU. Anand, Gujarat, August 1–3, 1997.

91. Snijder, E. J. and Meulenberg, J. J. M. 1998. The molecular biology of arterivirus. *J. Gen. Virol.* 79:961–979.

92. Stadejek, T., Bjorklund, H., Ros Bascunana, C., Ciabatti, I. M., Scicluna, M. T., Amaddeo, D., McCollum, W. H., Autorino, G. L., Timoney, P. J., Paton, D. J., Klingeborn, B. and Belak, S. 1999. Genetic diversity of equine arteritis virus. *J. Gen. Virol.* 80:691–699.

93. Starick, E. 1998. Rapid and sensitive detection of equine arteritis virus in semen and tissue samples by reverse transcription-polymerase chain reaction, dot blot hybridization and nested polymerase chain reaction. *Acta Virol.* 42:333–339.

94. St. Laurent, G., Morin, G. and Archambault, D. 1994. Detection of equine arteritis virus following amplification of structural and nonstructural viral genes by reverse transcription-PCR. *J. Clin. Microbiol.* 32:658–665.

95. St. Louis, M. C. and Archambault, D. 2007. The equine arteritis virus induces apoptosis via caspase-8 and mitochondria-dependent caspase-9 activation. *Virology* 367:147–155.

96. Szeredi, L., Hornyak, A., Palfi, V., Molnar, T., Glavits, R. and Denes, B. 2005. Study on the epidemiology of equine arteritis virus infection with different diagnostic techniques by investigating 96 cases of equine abortion in Hungary. *Vet. Microbiol.* 108:235–242.

97. Timoney, P. 1984. Equine viral arteritis in Kentucky, 1984. Proc. Int. Equine Viral Arteritis. Se. Ireland, Grayson Foundation.

98. Timoney, P. J. and McCollum, W. H. 1993. Equine viral arteritis. *Vet. Clin. North Am. Equine Pract.* 9:295–309.

99. Timoney, P. J. 1985. Epidemiological features of the 1984 outbreak of equine viral arteritis in the thoroughbred population in Kentucky, USA. *Proc. Soc. Vet. Epid. and Preventive Med. Reading* 1985:84.

100. Timoney, P. J. and McCollum, W. H. 1985. The epidemiology of equine arteritis virus. *Proc. Am. Ass. Equine Pract.* 31:545–551.

101. Timoney, P. J., McCollum, W. H., Roberts, A. W. and Murphy, T. W. 1986. Demonstration of the carrier state in naturally acquired equine arteritis virus infection in the stallion. *Res. Vet. Sci.* 41:279.

102. Timoney, P. J., McCollum, W. H., Murphy, T. W., Roberts, A. W. Wilard, A. W. and Carlswell, J. G. 1987a. The carrier state in equine arteritis virus infection in the stallion with specific emphasis on the venereal mode of transmission. *J. Reprod. Fert. Suppl.* 35:95–102.

103. Timoney, P. J., McCollum, W. H., and Roberts, A. W. 1987b. Detection of the carrier state in stallions persistently infected with equine arteritis virus. *Proc. Am. Ass. Equine Pract.* 32:57–65.

104. Timoney, P. J. and McCollum, W. H. 1988. Equine viral arteritis, epidemiology and control. *J. Equine Vet Sci.* 8:54.

105. Timoney, P. J. and McCollum, W. H. 1993. Equine viral arteritis. *Vet. Clin. North Am. Equine Pract.* 9:295–309.

106. Timoney, P. J., Klingeborn, B. and Lucas, M. H. 1996. A perspective on equine viral arteritis (infectious arteritis of horses). *Rev. Sci. Tech.* 15:1203–1208.

107. Timoney, P. J. and McCollum, W. H. 2000. Equine viral arteritis: Further characterization of the carrier state in the stallion. *J. Reprod. Fertil. (Suppl.)* 56:3–11.

108. Turan, N., Ekici, H., Yilmaz, H., Kondo, T., Hasoksuz, M., Sato, I., Tuchiya, K. and Fukunaga, Y. 2007. Detection of antibodies to equine arteritis virus in horse sera using recombinant chimaeric N/G(L) protein. *Vet. Rec.* 161:352–354.

109. Veit, M., Kabatek, A., Tielesch, C. and Hermann, A. 2008. Characterization of equine arteritis virus particles and demonstration of their hemolytic activity. *Arch. Virol.* 153:351–356.

110. Weber, H., Beckmann, K. and Haas, L. 2006. Fallbericht. Equines arteritisvirus (EAV) als aborterreger bei alpacas? *Dtsch. Tierarztl. Wschr.* 113:162–163.

111. Wei, Z. Z. and Yuan, S. S. 2008. Molecular biological progression of equine arteritis virus. *Bing. Du. Xue. Bao.* 24:404–408.

112. Westcott, D. G., King, D. P., Drew, T. W., Nowotny, N., Kindermann, J., Hannant, D., Belak, S. and Paton, D. J. 2003. Use of an internal standard in a closed one-tube RT-PCR for the detection of equine arteritis virus RNA with fluorescent probes. *Vet. Res.* 34:165–176.

113. Wieringa, R., de Vries, A. A. F., Raamsman, M. J. B. and Rottier, P. J. M. 2002. Characterization of two new structural glycoproteins GP(3), and GP(4) of equine arteritis virus. *J. Virol.* 76:10829–10840.

114. Zhang, J., Shuck, K. M., McCollum, W. H. and Timoney, P. J. 2004. Comparison of virus isolation in cell culture and RT-PCR assays for detection of equine arteritis virus in cryopreserved semen. In *Proceedings of the International Workshop on the Diagnosis of Equine Arteritis Virus Infection*, M. H. Cluck Equine Research Center, October 2004, Lexington, Kentucky, USA, 41–42.

115. Zhang, J., Miszczak, F., Pronost, S., Fortier, C., Balasuriya, U. B. R., Zientara, S., Fortier, G. and Timoney, P. J. 2007. Genetic variation and phylogenetic analysis of 22 French isolates of equine arteritis virus. *Arch. Virol.* 152:1977–1994.

116. Zhang, J., Timoney, P. J., MacLachlan, N. J. and Balasuriya, U. B. 2008. Identification of an additional neutralization determinant of equine arteritis virus. *Virus Res.* 138:150–153.

117. Zientara, S. 1994. Equine infectious arteritis: Molecular biology, epidemiology and preventative measures. *Rev. Sci. Tech.* 13:845–854.

13. Equine Vesicular Stomatitis

R. V. S. Pawaiya, K. Dhama, S. Kapoor, and D. K. Gupta

Introduction

Vesicular stomatitis (VS) is a highly contagious viral disease (OIE list A disease) caused by vesicular stomatitis virus (VSV) belonging to *Vesiculovirus* genus of Rhabdoviridae family that affect horses, cattle, and swine and rarely camelids, sheep, goats, and other wild ungulates. Many species of wild animals can be affected wherein serological positivity for VSV antibodies is found. Humans are also susceptible. Guinea pigs, hamsters, mice, ferrets, and chickens can be infected experimentally (Anonymous, 1995; Geering et al., 1995; Letchworth et al., 1999; Lin and Kitching, 2000; Acha and Szyfres, 2003; Stallknecht et al., 2004; Gelberg, 2007). The disease is limited to the Western Hemisphere and is enzootic in parts of South and Central America and of the United States of America. Its most significant impact is on horses and their movement (Webb et al., 1987a; 1987b; Fletcher et al., 1991; Inch, 1998; McCluskey et al., 2003). The disease most commonly occurs during warm months in the southwest region of the United States, particularly along river ways and in valleys. Recent outbreaks in the southwest have occurred from May to December in 1995, 1998, and 2005 (Bridges et al., 1997; McCluskey et al., 1999; McCluskey, 2007; Rainwater-Lovett et al., 2007). This zoonotic viral disease is characterized by vesiculation, ulceration, and erosion of the oral and nasal mucosa and epithelial surface of the tongue, coronary bands, and teats along with crusting lesions of the muzzle, ventral abdomen, and sheath. Pain, anorexia, and secondary mastitis can cause decreased productivity in all species (Inch, 1998; Gelberg, 2007). The viruses are zoonotic and may cause influenza-like disease in people working in close contact with the virus and through laboratory exposure (Acha and Szyfres, 2003).

The horse owners with VS-infected animals may suffer economic losses in caring for sick animals. Infected horses also are not allowed to compete in most shows and other events, and VSV-positive horses, generally, are not allowed to move between states or countries (Anderson, 2005). Due to heavy economic losses the disease may incur (Mebus, 1998), and being easily confused with foot-and-mouth disease (FMD), significant economic repercussions of misdiagnosis in an animal population occurs. Also, wide range of possible vectors of VSV makes the disease difficult to eradicate.

ETIOLOGY

Vesicular stomatitis is caused by vesicular stomatitis viruses (VSV), which is a member of the genus *Vesiculovirus* in the family Rhabdoviridae. The VSVs are the prototypes of the *Vesiculovirus* genus. In general, VSV resembles rabies virus in its morphology, genome, and protein structure (Zee and MacLachlan, 2004). They are bullet-shaped, negative-sense RNA viruses and generally 180 nm long and 80 nm wide, composed of five genes N, P, M, G, and L, representing the nucleocapsid protein, phosphoprotein, matrix protein, glycoprotein, and the large protein, respectively (Zee and MacLachlan, 2004; McCluskey, 2007). The two major serotypes are New Jersey and Indiana. These two viruses are similar in size and morphology but generate distinct neutralizing antibodies in infected animals (Llewellyn et al., 2000; Martinez and Wertz, 2005). They have both been isolated in recent outbreaks in the USA. Currently, four viruses are known to cause vesicular stomatitis: vesicular stomatitis Indiana virus (VSV-IN, formerly known as the Indiana 1 subtype of VSV), vesicular stomatitis New Jersey virus (VSV-NJ), vesicular stomatitis Alagoas virus (VSV-AV, formerly Indiana 3), and Cocal virus (formerly Indiana 2). In addition to these two serotypes of VSV, there are other viruses within the genus Vesiculovirus including Piry, Chandipura, Isfahan, Jurona, Carajas, Maraba, Calchaqui, Yug Bogdanovac, Perinet, and Porton-s, of which Piry (first isolated from an opossum in Brazil), Chandipura (first isolated from a person in India), and Isfahan (isolated from sand flies and humans in Iran) can experimentally cause vesicular lesions in domestic animals and infect humans (Wilks and House, 1986; Wagner and Rose, 2001; Basak et al., 2007).

VSV is inactivated by pasteurization temperatures (50–60°C for thirty minutes) and by light, ultraviolet light, and lipid solvents. It is also sensitive to common disinfectants such as sodium hypochlorite (Clorox) and quaternary ammonium compounds (Roccal), phenol, and formalin; effective disinfectants are 2% sodium carbonate, 4% sodium hydroxide, 2% iodophore and chlorine dioxide disinfectants. The virus is more resistant to lye (NaOH); 2–3% lye fails to inactivate VSV after an exposure of two hours. Preservation of virus can be done for years at -70°C and by freeze-drying under vacuum (Zee and MacLachlan, 2004).

EPIDEMIOLOGY

Vesicular stomatitis disease is endemic in Mexico, Central America, northern South America, and eastern Brazil, as well as in limited regions of the southeastern and southwestern United States.

Occasional outbreaks are seen in other parts of the Western Hemisphere, both north and south of the endemic area. There are reports of endemic occurrence of VS in Brazil, Argentina, Columbia, and other South American countries (Astudillo et al., 1984; Calisher et al., 1987; Tesh et al., 1987). VSV-NJ and VSV-IN outbreaks occur in North, Central, and South America. In the United States, VSV-NJ was once endemic in a large part of the Southeast, but it may now exist only in limited areas such as Ossabaw Island, Georgia. VSV-IN is not thought to be endemic in the United States, but newly introduced viruses occasionally cause outbreaks. VSV-AV (Indiana-3) and Cocal virus (Indiana-2) have been seen only in parts of South America, with VSV-AV outbreaks occurring in parts of Brazil every one to two years and Cocal virus seen sporadically in Argentina and Southern Brazil. (Zee and MacLachlan, 2004; McCluskey, 2007; Rainwater-Lovett et al., 2007). This disease is usually seasonal, although particularly common at the end of the rainy season or early in the dry season. Disease epidemiology is complicated since VSV infection in horses is often inapparent or subclinical, and many cases would not be detected under existing surveillance strategies that are based on the detection of clinical signs (Mumford et al., 1998).

Disease outbreaks are sporadic and unpredictable. The first report of VS in USA was in 1916 (Hanson, 1952). The disease recurred extensively in 1926 in New Jersey, affecting about 750 cattle in thirty-three farms and few horses. The isolated causal virus was found to be distinct from the previously isolated Indiana strain and aptly named as VSV-New Jersey strain (Cotton, 1927). Until the early 1970s, VSV-NJ also affected animals in an endemic pattern in the southeast. This virus remains endemic in areas such as Ossabaw Island, Georgia, where feral pigs are infected. During the nineties, three outbreaks of VS occurred in southwestern United States in 1995, 1997, and 1998. The etiological viruses isolated and recognized from these outbreaks were VSV-NJ, both VSV-NJ and VSV-IN, and VSV-IN, respectively (Anonymous, 1997; Bridges et al., 1997; McCluskey et al., 1999; McCluskey, 2007). Most recent outbreaks recorded in United States were started in 2004 followed by in 2005 affecting the widest geographical area since 1980s, and then during August through December of 2006 in only a limited state (Anonymous, 2004; 2005; 2006; McCluskey, 2007). VSV-NJ was found to be responsible for all these outbreaks. Molecular epidemiologic studies indicate that each VS epidemic in North America is caused by a single genetic variant of VSV. A study suggested that strains causing U.S. outbreaks were closely related to strains causing outbreaks in Mexico (Rodriguez, 2002). Determining the phylogenetic relationships among VSV-NJ strains of 2004 outbreak and from endemic areas in Mexico demonstrated that VS outbreaks in the southwestern USA resulted from the introduction of viral strains from endemic areas in Mexico (Rainwater-Lovett et al., 2007). Multiple genetic lineages of VSVs occur in tropical regions of Americas (Zee and MacLachlan, 2004).

Outbreaks of VS typically occur at approximately every ten years in some areas of the United States. Recent outbreaks in the southwestern USA have resulted in clinical disease in greater proportions in horses than in cattle (McCluskey et al., 1999; McCluskey, 2007).

TRANSMISSION

VSV has a diversity of potential transmission routes, including biological vector, mechanical vector, and contact transmission, but their relative significance regarding outbreaks in horses is unknown. The spread of VS within the United States has been described as sporadic; however, only 4.5% of cattle and 45.0% of horses that seroconvert have had observable clinical signs in one study (Inch, 1998). Clinical spread among horses is commonly attributed to direct contact, insect vectors, mechanical transmission, and drinking water or feeds contaminated with saliva and vesicular fluids (Howerth et al., 2006). In areas where VS is endemic, the virus is transmitted by arthropod vectors (Brinson et al., 1992; Wagner and Rose, 2001; Zee and MacLachlan, 2004). Arthropods apparently transmit VS viruses in the southwestern USA (Tesh et al., 1987; Francy et al., 1988). *Simulium* spp. (black flies) and *Culicoides* spp. (midges) can transmit VS viruses biologically. Transovarian transmission has been demonstrated in sand flies and blackflies, and it may be possible in *Culicoides* (Tesh et al., 1972, 1987; Walton et al., 1987; Cupp et al., 1992; Mead et al., 1999; 2000; Nunamaker et al., 2000; Drolet et al., 2005; Perez de Leon and Tabachnick, 2006). The VSVs have been isolated from horsefly (*Tabanus* spp.), deerfly (*Chrysops* spp.), mosquitoes (*Aedes* spp., *Culex* spp.), biting midge (*Culicoides*), housefly (*Musca* spp.), eye gnats (*Hippelates* spp.), black fly (*Simulium* spp.), sand fly (*Lutzyomia* spp.), and stable fly (*Stomoxys* spp.), many of them found actively transmitting VSV during outbreaks (Francy et al., 1988; Brinson et al., 1992; Kramer et al., 1990; Cupp et al., 1992; Comer et al., 1993; 1994; 1995a; 1995b; McCluskey, 2007). *Aedes* mosquitoes, Chloropidae (eye gnats), and flies in the genus *Musca* or family Anthomyiidae may act as mechanical vectors. Grasshoppers (*Melanoplus sanguinipes*) can be infected experimentally, and cattle ingesting experimentally infected grasshoppers can develop clinical signs (Nunamaker et al., 2003; Mead et al., 2004a; 2004b). Biting insects become infected mostly from feeding on lesions rather than blood because viremia in animals, if present, is very transient (Stallknecht et al., 2001). It has also been suggested that the spread of VS occurs through transport of virus-infected or virus-carrying vectors by winds during appropriate climatic conditions (Sellers and Maarouf, 1990; McCluskey et al., 2003). There is also some speculation that VSV could be a plant virus found in pastures, with animals at the end of an epidemiological chain.

Infected animals shed VSV in vesicle material, saliva, and to a lesser extent, in nasal secretions (Zee and MacLachlan, 2004; Brown et al., 2007). Virus can spread from animal to animal by direct contact; broken skin or mucous membranes may facilitate entry of the virus. VSV has been found in the saliva of experimentally infected animals with or without oral lesions (Howerth et al., 2006). Fecal shedding has been reported occasionally in experimentally infected swine, but not in horses (Stallknecht et al., 2004). Contaminated fomites—including food, water, and milking machines—may also facilitate transmission; however, this virus is inactivated by sunlight and does not remain viable for long periods in the environment except in cool, dark places. Transplacental crossing of VSV or fetal seroconversion has not been reported.

The reservoir and amplifying hosts for VSV are unknown. Viremia sufficient to infect insect vectors has not been reported in animals; however, insects could become infected by feeding on lesion material or contaminated secretions. Experimentally, bats (*Myotis lucifugus*), Syrian hamsters, and deer mice (*Peromyscus maniculatus*) have been demonstrated to harbor the VSVs up to eight months (Donaldson, 1970; Fultz et al., 1982; Cornish et al., 2001). Overwintering has been reported in some but not all outbreaks in the United States. (McCluskey et al., 2003). Humans may be infected by contact with the lesions or secretions from infected animals and through aerosol during working in laboratories. Therefore, proper biosafety practices need to be followed during handling of affected animals and/or virus in the laboratory. Insect bites may also infect people (Tesh et al., 1987).

CLINICAL SIGNS

The incubation period for VS is usually two to eight days; however, longer or shorter incubation periods may occur (Knight and Messer, 1983; Bennett, 1986; Reif, 1994; Howerth, et al., 2006; Brown et al., 2007). Clinical signs include fever ranging from 104 to 106°F (40–4°C), and the lesions usually resemble those of FMD, except that horses are affected very severely with oral and coronary band vesicles (Howerth, et al., 2006; Gelberg, 2007). The most common early signs are excessive salivation and drooling. Vesicles, papules, erosions, and ulcers are seen in affected horses, especially around the mouth and most often on the upper surface of the tongue, the gums and lips, and around the nostrils and corners of the mouth, which may also be present in feet, udder, and prepuce (McCluskey et al., 2003). The vesicles are characteristically raised in the form of blisters and variably sized. The vesicles may go unnoticed in few horses, and there the disease appears as crusting scabs on the muzzle and lips. The VS lesions usually cause anorexia, dyspepsia, and lameness due to severe painfulness. Some animals may develop swelling on nostrils and muzzle and sloughing of epithelium over tongue or muzzle while others may exhibit catarrhal nasal discharge and blood-oozing ulcers, with foul mouth. Affected animals usually recover in about two to three weeks unless secondary bacterial complications occur (McCluskey and Mumford, 2000; Zee and MacLachlan, 2004; Brown et al., 2007). The morbidity rate for VS is variable, ranging from 5% to more than 90%, with typically 5–20% of the animals in a herd are symptomatic but up to 100% may be seroconvert (Reif, 1994; Rodríguez, 2002). Most cases occur in adults as young cattle and horses under one year of age are less commonly affected. Deaths are very rare in cattle and horses, but higher mortality rates have been seen in some pigs infected with VSV-NJ (McCluskey and Mumford, 2000; Stallknecht et al., 2004).

PATHOLOGY AND PATHOGENESIS

Gross lesions of vesicular stomatitis are epitheliotropic and usually indistinguishable from those of FMD. They begin as small raised, flattened pale pink to whitish papules in buccal mucosa, surface and margins of tongue and lips, and they rapidly become inflamed and hyperemic. In a day or so, lesions enlarge or coalesce to develop vesicles of 2–3 cm in diameter and may further coalesce to form bullae. These lesions easily rupture or may subsequently erode or ulcerate to create irregular patches of denuded red submucosa (Howerth, et al., 2006; Gelberg, 2007). The shallow erosions usually heal within one to two weeks unless secondary infections occur (Howerth, et al., 2006). There may also be similar changes in the nasal mucosa, particularly in swine or in esophagus and rumen. Oral lesions heal rapidly in swine, but coronary band lesions often become secondarily infected resulting into separation and sloughing of claw (Stallknecht et al., 2004; Brown et al., 2007).

Microscopic changes are observed in the deeper layers of the stratum spinosum (Green, 1993). Intercellular edema (spongiosis) is followed by cytoplasmic retraction; epithelial cells float freely in enlarging vacuoles loculated by strands of cytoplasmic debris (Brown et al., 2007). Inclusion bodies are not found in VS. With the epithelial necrosis, there is pleocellular inflammatory reaction in the mucosa and underlying lamina propria. Electron microscopic examination of epithelial cells adjacent to the vesicles confirms the intercellular edema and keratinocyte necrosis seen under the light microscope (Green, 1993; Rodriguez, 2002; Schmitt, 2002; Howerth, et al., 2006). The lesions in tongue are fully to partially reepithelialized or superficially ulcerated with a narrow underlying bed of neovascularization and submucosa revealing mild to moderate lesions characterized by perivascular infiltrations of mononuclear cells, predominantly of plasma cells and lymphocytes admixed with fewer neutrophils.

Little is known about the pathogenesis of vesicular stomatitis in livestock or other animals. Viremia associated with VSV-NJ or VSV-IN infection has not been demonstrated in animals, except the rodents in which a detectable viremia has been demonstrated (Comer et al., 1995a, 1995b; Cornish et al., 2001). Viremia associated with experimental infection has been demonstrated in deer mice (*Peromyscus maniculatus*), laboratory mice (*Mus musculus*), spiny rats (*Proechimys semispinosus*), and Syrian hamsters (*Mesocricetus auratus*) (Falke and Rowe, 1965; Tesh et al., 1970; Fultz and Holland, 1985; Webb et al., 1987b). The experimental pathologic studies in horses revealed that primary virus replication occurs in tonsils after oral inoculation or within the epithelium at the site of inoculation with subsequent spread to tonsils, possibly via low-titer viremia or via saliva in the presence of oral lesions. Viral replication in tonsils results in viral shedding into the oral cavity leading to the development of secondary lesions in the event of breach in the oral mucosa. Subsequent spread of the infection to lymph nodes of the head followed by rapid resolution of the lesions occurs probably due to development of neutralizing antibodies and local immunity (Howerth et al., 2006).

The molecular basis of pathogenicity of VSV is typical of viral infections. Entry of virus into host cells require virus binding to receptors at the host cell surface followed by fusion of the viral envelope with a cellular membrane (Roche et al., 2007). VSV glycoprotein (G) is involved in both receptor recognition and membrane fusion. Fusion is triggered by low-pH-induced structural rearrangements during which G shifts from a prefusion native state to a postfusion conformation (Roche and Gaudin, 2002; Weissenhorn et al., 2007). Penetration and uncoating of viral particles occur, and transcription and replication starts. Finally, new viral particles are assembled at the cellular plasma membrane. The M protein plays a specific role in the attachment of condensed nucleocapsids to the plasma membrane and to subsequent budding of the new virions (Blondel et al., 1990). Inhibition of cellular RNA, DNA, and protein synthesis occurs before cellular rounding that result from M protein–induced disruption in the cytoskeleton (Weck and Wagner, 1979). However, in swine, glycoprotein (G) has been implicated as a determinant of VSV virulence and pathogenicity (Martinez et al., 2003; Martinez and Wertz, 2005). The VSV, due to its short reproductive cycle followed by high viral titers in the host cell, is being explored to be used as a new therapeutic oncolytic virus candidate for cancer (Giedlin et al., 2003).

DIAGNOSIS
Diagnosis of VS is based on the presence of typical clinical signs and either antibody detection through serologic tests, viral detection through isolation, and/or detection of viral genetic material by molecular techniques

(Howerth, et al., 2006; Gelberg, 2007). Samples for viral isolation may include vesicular fluid, epithelial tags from lesions, or swabs of lesions. VSVs are easily propagated in cell culture. Serologic tests include competitive enzyme-linked immunosorbent assays (ELISA), virus neutralization (VN), and complement fixation (CF) tests (Rice, 1960; Blickwede et al., 2002). Polymerase chain reaction (PCR) may also be used to identify the virus (Magnuson et al., 2003; Rasmussen et al., 2005; Fernández et al., 2008). Vesicular stomatitis in cattle and swine is required to be differentiated accordingly from clinically indistinguishable diseases (including FMD, swine vesicular disease, and vesicular exanthema of swine) while toxic and mechanical causes of ulcers and erosions should be considered in horses (Green, 1993; Mebus, 1998; Brown et al., 2007; Gelberg, 2007). Since VS is often clinically indistinguishable from FMD, confirming a diagnosis with laboratory tests is critical (Mebus, 1998; WAHO, 2004).

Vesicular stomatitis is a zoonotic disease; therefore, samples should be collected properly and handled with all appropriate precautions and care. Vesicle fluids, the epithelium covering unruptured vesicles, epithelial flaps from freshly ruptured vesicles, or swabs of the ruptured vesicles are the preferred diagnostic samples. Other good specimen sources are oral, nasal, pedal, and mammary lesions. As the lesions are very painful, application of mild sedation may be helpful before sample collection. Samples should be sent refrigerated unless shipping will take longer than two days; in this case, they may be sent frozen with dry ice. Serum samples or paired serum samples taken one to two weeks apart may also be collected (Rice, 1960). Once an outbreak of vesicular stomatitis has been diagnosed in a state, an animal can be declared positive after a single positive test (Mebus, 1998; WAHO, 2004).

Detection of the virus or viral antigens is preferred for a definitive diagnosis. VSV can be isolated from vesicular fluids, epithelial tissue, and swabs in tissue culture, embryonated chicken eggs, or mice. Many cell lines are susceptible to this virus; however, VSV, FMD virus, and swine vesicular disease virus cause different cytopathic effects in African green monkey kidney (Vero), baby hamster kidney (BHK-21), and IB-RS-2 cells (WAHO, 2004). Inoculation of all three cell lines with the sample is helpful in the diagnosis. Electron microscopy can also be helpful in differentiating these three viruses. The identity of the virus is confirmed in cultures by immunofluorescence, complement fixation, ELISAs, and other tests.

Antibodies to VSV can be detected by VNT, CFT, or ELISA. All these tests are considered as standard serologic tests for VSV antibodies and have been prescribed by the World Animal Health Organization (OIE: Office of International Des Epizootis) for international trade (Rice, 1960; WAHO, 2004). There are several ELISAs developed for the detection and quantitation of VSV antibodies; however, the competitive (c) ELISA is considered as the test of choice for screening and trade purpose (Afshar et al., 1993; Eernisse, 1995; Hernández de Anda et al., 1992; Katz et al., 1995; Alvarado et al., 2002). Vernon and Webb (1985) developed an ELISA capable of detecting the IgM class of antibody to VSV (mcELISA) that facilitated the detection of fresh/recent exposure to VSV, which was further improved upon by Zhou et al. (2001) that provided relatively higher sensitivity for the detection of equine and swine IgM antibodies to VSV-NJ and VSV-IN. Serotype differentiation between VSV-NJ and VSV-IN can be done by employing staining with specific conjugated fluorescent antibodies (Carbrey, 1984). In clinical samples (vesicle fluid, epithelium, etc.), viral antigens also can be detected by employing ELISA, CFT, or VNT.

Presence of genomic sequences of VSV may be detected in the clinical samples by using PCR assays. Rodriguez et al. (1993) developed a PCR assay to detect P gene of VSV-NJ, but not VSV-IN serotype, which is claimed to be more sensitive in detecting positive tissue samples than virus isolation. Presence of both VSV-NJ and VSV-IN serotypes, even in unviable conditions, could be detected by targeting L gene sequence by heminested PCR method (Höfner et al., 1994). Simultaneous detections of VSV, FMDV, and swine vesicular disease virus can be made by a reverse transcriptase–PCR (RT-PCR) which can also distinguish between VSV-NJ and VSV-IN serotypes (Núñez et al., 1998). A more sensitive single-tube multiplex RT-PCR is able to detect as little as 20 fg (femtograms) of viral RNA of VSV-NJ and VSV-IN serotypes in macerated pool of mosquitoes (Magnuson et al., 2003). Rasmussen et al. (2005) have developed a quantitative RT-PCR assay for the detection, quantification, and differentiation of VSV-NJ and VSV-IN serotypes. The method is said to be a powerful tool for the rapid identification of VSV. A multiplex, real-time RT-PCR assay (Hole et al., 2006) and a highly sensitive and specific one-step multiplex RT-PCR assay (Fernández et al., 2008) for the simultaneous diagnosis of vesicular stomatitis, FMD, and swine vesicular disease as well as for rapid differentiation of VSV-NJ and VSV-IN have also been developed recently.

TREATMENT
There is no specific treatment for vesicular stomatitis, but symptomatic treatments can be provided. Cleansing the lesions with a mild antiseptic solution (1–2% solution of Lugol's iodine for oral ulcers, saturated solution of copper sulfate for feet lesions, and spray solutions of antibiotics and

anti-inflammatory drugs for teat ulcers) may help in rapid healing and reduce secondary bacterial infections. If secondary infection is present, antibiotics should be used. High-energy liquid gruel feed or electrolytes added to the water supply can be helpful for animals having difficulty eating or drinking. Animals with mouth lesions should be provided with softened feed such as silages and fresh grasses, which will decrease the anorectic period. Prognosis is good for VSV infection, but production losses can be permanent if the udder of cattle is affected (Mebus, 1998; WAHO, 2004).

PREVENTION AND CONTROL

U.S. Department of Agriculture licensed the production and sale of alive VSV-NJ lyophilized vaccine in 1967 (Lauerman and Hanson, 1968) that was subsequently discontinued in 1972. Attempts for prophylaxis against VSVs were made using biologically active defective interfering (DI) particles as well as glycoprotein subunit vaccines in mice and cattle (Jones and Holland, 1980; Yilma et al., 1985). During 1985 outbreak of VS in Colorado, a commercially available Killed-VSV-NJ vaccine was used (Gearhart et al., 1987). A killed-autogenous vaccine, produced from the isolate of VSV during 1995 VS outbreak in Colorado, showed good elicitation of serum-neutralizing antibodies to VSV-NJ (McCluskey, 1997). Using advances in modern biological tools and genomic manipulation, researchers have succeeded in attenuating the virulence of virus by translocation of the N gene, which reduced mortality in mice without compromising the ability of immunogenicity (Wertz et al., 1998). Recombinant DNA vaccines expressing the glycoprotein (G) genes of VSV-NJ as well as VSV-IN have been found to evoke neutralizing antibody responses in swine, horses, calves, and mice (Cantlon et al., 2000; Martinez et al., 2004). Attempts for development of recombinant vaccines against VSVs are in, being continuously made by researchers the world over (Gao et al., 2006; Stauffer et al., 2006). Since the vaccination is comprised of killed virus, a vaccinated horse's serum becomes positive for serological tests, rendering them to the similar limitations and restrictions/regulations to that of a VSV-infected horse. Therefore, maintenance of proof of identification and excellent vaccination records by the owner is must to avoid travel limitations of vaccinated horse. In view of these difficulties, horses are rarely vaccinated, except in the case where an outbreak has occurred in the vicinity.

Control of vesicular stomatitis spread is done through state quarantine of affected premises and control of movement of animals from affected areas. Management measures suggested to reduce the risk of exposure to the virus include limiting time on pasture, providing shelters or barns during insect feeding times, and implementing other procedures that reduce animal contact with insects, including application of insecticides (Hurd et al., 1999; WAHO, 2004; Kahn and Line, 2006). Good sanitation and disinfection can reduce the spread of the virus on fomites (Zee and MacLachlan, 2004; WAHO, 2004; Kahn and Line, 2006). Insect control also helps prevent occurrences of the disease on the premises. Insect breeding areas should be eliminated or reduced, and insecticide sprays or treated ear tags can be used on animals. Also, avoid hard or abrasive feeds to prevent oral abrasions and injuries that could facilitate infections (Hurd et al., 1999; McCluskey et al., 2003; WAHO, 2004). During outbreaks, uninfected livestock should be kept away from infected animals. When affected animals are identified, they should be isolated, and there should be no movement of animals from an infected premise for at least twenty-one days after all lesions are healed, except for slaughter. Horses appear to be most contagious for the first six days after infection; therefore, stable the animals if possible. Vesicular stomatitis is a reportable disease in most areas, including the USA, so animal health officials must be notified when it is suspected. Commercially produced vaccines are not available in the USA, but vaccines are available in some Latin American countries (Green, 1993; Mebus, 1998; Kahn and Line, 2006; Gelberg, 2007).

CONCLUSION

Vesicular stomatitis is a viral disease caused by two distinct serotypes of vesicular stomatitis virus (VSV) belonging to *Vesiculovirus* genus of Rhabdoviridae family that primarily affect cattle, horses, and swine and occasionally sheep, goats, llamas, and alpacas. Humans can be exposed to the virus when handling affected animals. Disease occurs only in the Western Hemisphere, with presence of endemic disease in the warmer regions of North, Central, and South America, but outbreaks in other temperate geographic parts of the hemisphere also occur sporadically. The southwestern and Western United States have experienced several VS outbreaks in recent years. The mechanisms of transmission of the VS are not fully known; insect vectors, especially sand flies and black flies, mechanical transmission, and movement of animals are probably responsible. Once introduced into a herd, the disease apparently moves from animal to animal by contact or exposure to saliva or fluid from ruptured lesions. Humans, though, rarely contract vesicular stomatitis but, when infected, the disease causes an acute influenza-like illness with symptoms such as fever, muscle ache, headache, and malaise.

In affected livestock, the incubation period for VSV ranges from two to eight days. Often, excessive salivation is the first sign of the disease. In affected livestock, VS causes blisterlike lesions in the mouth and on the dental pad, tongue, lips, nostrils, hooves, and teats. Animals usually recover within two weeks. In horses, vesicular lesions generally occur on the upper surface of the tongue, the lips, around nostrils, corners of the mouth, and gums. Lesions in horses may also be expressed as crusting scabs on the muzzle, lips, or ventral abdomen. The VS does not generally cause death in animals, but its occurrence can cause severe economic losses to livestock producers and owners. Clinical signs and pathological lesions produced by the VSV are not specific, and the disease can be confirmed only through laboratory tests.

Vesicular stomatitis is recognized internationally as a reportable disease (list A disease, OIE) having serious economic and regulatory repercussions associated with the diagnosis. There is no specific treatment or cure for VS. Owners can protect their animals from the disease by avoiding congregating animals in the vicinity where VS has broken out. Mild antiseptic mouthwashes may bring comfort and more rapid recovery to an affected animal. Good sanitation and quarantine practices on affected farms usually contain the infection until it subsides and soon ends. Commercial vaccines are not available for VSV. Newer strategies for designing recombinant VSV vaccines are being carried out. VSV is also being explored for its promising cancer gene therapy ability and novel utility for viral-vectored vaccines. Studies are needed further to elucidate various aspects of the virus and the disease it produces in detail, especially the molecular pathogenesis, relative significance of different transmission routes, and development of effective vaccines.

References

1. Acha, P. N. and Szyfres, B. 2003. In *Zoonoses and communicable diseases common to man and animals. Vol. 2. Chlamydioses, rickettsioses, and viruses. 3rd ed.* [Pan American Health Organization (PAHO)]. Washington, D.C. Scientific and Technical Publication No. 580. Vesicular stomatitis, 347–353.
2. Afshar, A., Shakarchi, N. H. and Dulac, G. C. 1993. Development of a competitive enzyme-linked immunosorbent assay for detection of bovine, ovine, porcine, and equine antibodies to vesicular stomatitis virus. *J. Clin. Microbiol.* 31:1860–1865.
3. Alvarado, J. F., Dolz, G., Herrero, M. V., Mccluskey, B. and Salman, M. 2002. Comparison of the serum neutralization test and a competitive enzyme-linked immunosorbent assay for the detection of antibodies to vesicular stomatitis virus New Jersey and vesicular stomatitis virus Indiana. *J. Vet. Diag. Invest.* 14:204–242.
4. Anderson, K. 2005. Vesicular stomatitis in horses. University of Nebraska–Lincoln Extension, Institute of Agriculture and Natural Resources. Document no. G1609. http://www.ianrpubs.unl.edu/epublic/pages/publicationD.jsp?publicationId=169 (accessed on March 8, 2009).
5. Anonymous. 1995. Notifiable Diseases: Special Issue of the State Veterinary Journal, vol. 5, no. 3, October 1995. Ministry of Agriculture, Fisheries and Food, United Kingdom ISSN: 0269 5545.
6. Anonymous. 1997. Vesicular stomatitis strikes more horses. *J. Am. Vet. Med. Assoc.* 211:401.
7. Anonymous. 2004. Vesicular stomatitis quarantines lifted in Texas remain in Colorado, New Mexico. *J. Am. Vet. Med. Assoc.* 225:1657.

8. Anonymous. 2005. Vesicular stomatitis cases identified. *J. Am. Vet. Med. Assoc.* 226:1961–1962.

9. Anonymous. 2006. Vesicular stomatitis surveillance–2006. Final Summary. APHIS, USDA. *http://www. aphis.usda.gov/vs/nahss/equine/vsv/vsv2006_final.htm* (accessed on March 10, 2009).

10. Astudillo, V. M., Estupinan, A. J., Rosenberg, F. J., da Silva, A. J. M. and Dora, J. F. P. 1984. Epidemiological study of vesicular stomatitis in South America. Proceedings of the International Conference on Vesicular Stomatitis, Mexico City, 23–83.

11. Basak, S., Mondal, A., Polley, S., Mukhopadhyay, S. and Chattopadhyay, D. 2007. *Reviewing chandipura: A vesiculovirus in human epidemics. Biosci. Rep.* 27:275–298.

12. Bennett, D. G. 1986. Vesicular stomatitis. *Proc. Am. Assoc. Equine Pract.* 32:399–403.

13. Blickwede, M., Dolz, G., Herrero, M. V., Tomlinson, S. M. and Salman, M. 2002. Neutralizing antibodies against vesicular stomatitis viruses (serotypes New Jersey and Indiana) in horses in Costa Rica. *J. Vet. Diag. Invest.* 14:438–441.

14. Blondel, D., Harmison, G. G. and Schubert, M. 1990. Role of matrix protein in cytopathogenesis of vesicular stomatitis virus. *J. Virol.* 64:1716–1725.

15. Bridges, V. E., McCluskey, B. J., Salman, M. D., Hurd, H. S. and Dick, J. 1997. Review of the 1995 vesicular stomatitis outbreak in the western United States. *J. Am. Vet. Med. Assoc.* 211:556–560.

16. Brinson, F. J., Hagan, D. V., Comer, J. A. and Strohlein, D. A. 1992. Seasonal abundance of *Lutzomyia shannoni* (Diptera: Psychodidae) on Ossabaw Island, Georgia. *J. Med. Entomol.* 29:178–182.

17. Brown, C. C., Baker, D. C. and Barker, I. K. 2007. Alimentary system. In *Jubb, Kennedy and Palmer's pathology of domestic animals*, 5th ed., M. G. Maxie, vol. 2, 1–296. Philadelphia, USA: Saunders, Elsevier Inc.

18. Calisher, C. H., Monath, T. P., Sabattini, M. S., Mitchell, C. J., Lazuick, J. S., Tesh, R. B. and Cropp, C. B. 1987. A newly recognized vesiculovirus, Calchaqui virus, and subtypes of Melao and Maguari viruses from Argentina, with serologic evidence for infections of humans and horses. *Am. J. Trop. Med. Hyg.* 36:114–119.

19. Cantlon, J. D., Gordy, P. W. and Bowen, R. A. 2000. Immune responses in mice, cattle and horses to a DNA vaccine for vesicular stomatitis. *Vaccine* 18:2368–2374.

20. Carbrey, E. A. 1984. Laboratory diagnosis of vesicular stomatitis. *In proceedings of the International Conference on Vesicular Stomatitis, Mexico City, 1984*, 446–456.

21. Comer, J. A., Irby, W. S. and Kavanaugh, D. M. 1994. Hosts of *Lutzomyia shannoni* (Diptera: Psychodidae) in relation to vesicular stomatitis virus on Ossabaw Island, Georgia, United States. *Med. Vet. Entomol.* 8:325–330.

22. Comer, J. A., Kavanaugh, D. M., Stallknecht, D. E., Ware, G. O., Corn, J. L. and Nettles, V. F. 1993. Effect of forest type on the distribution of *Lutzomyia shannoni* (Diptera: Psychodidae) and vesicular stomatitis virus on Ossabaw Island, Georgia. *J. Med. Entomol.* 30:555–560.

23. Comer, J. A., Stallknecht, D. E. and Nettles, V. F. 1995a. Incompetence of white-tailed deer as amplifying hosts of vesicular stomatitis virus for *Lutzomyia shannoni* (Diptera: Psychodidae). *J. Med. Entomol.* 32:738–740.

24. Comer, J. A., Stallknecht, D. E. and Nettles, V. F. 1995b. Incompetence of domestic pigs as amplifying hosts of vesicular stomatitis virus for *Lutzomyia shannoni* (Diptera: Psychodidae). *J. Med. Entomol.* 32:741–744.

25. Cornish, T. E., Stallknecht, D. E., Brown, C. C., Seal, B. S. and Howerth, E. W. 2001. Pathogenesis of experimental vesicular stomatitis virus (New Jersey serotype) infection in the deer mouse *(Peromyscus maniculatus)*. *Vet. Pathol.* 38:396–406.

26. Cupp, E. W., Mare, C. J., Cupp, M. S. and Ramberg, F. B. 1992. Biological transmission of vesicular stomatitis virus (New Jersey) by *Simulium vittatum* (Diptera: Simuliidae). *J. med. Entomol.* 29 (2): 137–140.

27. Donaldson, A. I. 1970. Bats as possible maintenance hosts for vesicular stomatitis virus. *Am. J. Epidemiol.* 92:132–136.

13. EQUINE VESICULAR STOMATITIS

28. Drolet, B. S., Campbell, C. L., Stuart, M. A. and Wilson, W. C. 2005. Vector competence of *Culicoides sonorensis* (Diptera: Ceratopogonidae) for vesicular stomatitis virus. *J. Med. Entomol.* 42:409–418.
29. Eernisse, K. 1995. Evaluation of a competitive ELISA in an outbreak of vesicular stomatitis. Proceedings of the American Association of Veterinary Laboratory Diagnosticians, Sparks, Nev, 124.
30. Falke, D. and Rowe, W. P. 1965. Die erkrankung der maus durch das virus der stomatitis vesicularis. *Arch. Gesamte Virusforschung* 17:550–559.
31. Fernández, J., Agüero, M., Romero, L., Sánchez, C., Belák, S., Arias, M. and Sánchez-Vizcaíno, J. M. 2008. Rapid and differential diagnosis of foot-and-mouth disease, swine vesicular disease, and vesicular stomatitis by a new multiplex RT-PCR assay. *J. Virol. Methods* 147:301–311.
32. Fletcher, W. O., Stallknecht, D. E. and Kearney, M. T. 1991. Antibodies to vesicular stomatitis New Jersey type virus in white-tailed deer on Ossabaw Island, Georgia, 1985–1989. *J. Wildl. Dis.* 27:675–680.
33. Francy, D. B., Moore, C. G., Smith, G. C., Jakob, W. L., Taylor, S. A. and Calisher, C. H. 1988. Epizootic vesicular stomatitis in Colorado, 1982: Isolation of virus from insects collected along the northern Colorado Rocky Mountain Front Range. *J. Med. Entomol.* 25:343–347.
34. Fultz, P., Shadduck, J. A., Kang, C. Y. and Streilein, J. W. 1982. Vesicular stomatitis virus can establish persistent infections in Syrian hamsters. *J. Gen. Virol.* 63:493–497.
35. Fultz, P. N. and Holland, J. J. 1985. Differing responses of hamsters to infection by vesicular stomatitis virus Indiana and New Jersey serotypes. *Virus Res.* 3:129–140.
36. Gao, Y., Whitaker-Dowling, P., Watkins, S. C., Griffin, J. A. and Bergman, I. 2006. Rapid adaptation of a recombinant vesicular stomatitis virus to a targeted cell line. *Brazil. J. Virol.* 80:8603–8612. *c:\citwww\paper\16912309.*
37. Gearhart, M. A., Webb, P. A., Knight, A. P., Salman, M. D., Smith, J. A. and Erickson, G. A. 1987. Serum neutralizing antibody titers in dairy cattle administered an inactivated vesicular stomatitis virus vaccine. *J. Am. Vet. Med. Assoc.* 191:819–822.
38. Geering, W. A., Forman, A. J. and Nunn, M. J. 1995. *Exotic diseases of animals: A field guide for Australian veterinarians.* Canberra: Australian Government Publishing Service. ISBN 0 644 335130.
39. Gelberg, H. B. 2007. Alimentary system. In *Pathologic basis of veterinary diseases*, 4th ed., M. D. McGavin and J. F. Zachary, 301–391. St. Louis, Missouri: Mosby Elsevier.
40. Giedlin, M. A., Cook, D. N. and Dubensky, T. W. Jr. 2003. Vesicular stomatitis virus: An exciting new therapeutic oncolytic virus candidate for cancer. *Cancer Cell* 4:241–243.
41. Green, S. L. 1993. Vesicular stomatitis in the horse. *Vet. Clin. North Am. Equine Pract.* 9:349–353.
42. Hanson, R. P. 1952. The natural history of vesicular stomatitis. *Bacteriol. Rev.* 16:179–204.
43. Hernández de Anda, J., Salman, M. D., Webb, P. A., Keefe, T. J., Arregín Arévalo, A. and Mason, J. 1992. Evaluation of an enzyme-linked immunosorbent assay for detection of antibodies to vesicular stomatitis virus in cattle in an enzootic region of Mexico. *Am. J. Vet. Res.* 53:440–443.
44. Höfner, M. C., Carpenter, W. C., Ferris, N. P., Kitching, R. P. and Ariza Botero, F. 1994. A hemi-nested PCR assay for the detection and identification of vesicular stomatitis virus nucleic acid. *J. Virol. Methods* 50:11–20.
45. Hole, K., Clavijo, A. and Pineda, L. A. 2006. Detection and serotype-specific differentiation of vesicular stomatitis virus using a multiplex, real-time, reverse transcription-polymerase chain reaction assay. *J. Vet. Diag. Invest.* 18:139–146.
46. Howerth, E. W., Mead, D. G., Mueller, P. O., Duncan, L., Murphy, M. D. and Stallknecht, D. E. 2006. Experimental vesicular stomatitis virus infection in horses: Effect of route of inoculation and virus serotype. *Vet. Pathol.* 43:943–955.
47. Hurd, H. S., McCluskey, B. J. and Mumford, E. L. 1999. Management factors affecting the risk for vesicular stomatitis in livestock operations in the western United States. *J. Am. Vet. Med. Assoc.* 215:1263–1268.

48. Inch, C. 1998. An overview of pseudorabies (Aujeszky's disease) and vesicular stomatitis from the Canadian Animal Health Network. *Can. Vet. J.* 39:23–32.

49. Jones, C. L. and Holland, J. J. 1980. *Requirements for DI particle prophylaxis against vesicular stomatitis virus infection in vivo. J. Gen. Virol.* 49:215–220.

50. Kahn, C. M. and Line, S. 2006. The Merck veterinary manual [online]. Whitehouse Station, NJ: Merck and Co; 2006. Vesicular stomatitis. *http://www.merckvetmanual.com/mvm/index.jsp?cfile=htm/bc/52500. htm (accessed 14 March 2009).*

51. Katz, J. B., Shafer, A. L. and Eernisse, K. A. 1995. Construction and insect larval expression of recombinant vesicular stomatitis nucleocapsid protein and its use in competitive ELISA. *J. Virol. Methods* 54:145–157.

52. Knight, A. P. and Messer, N. T. 1983. Vesicular stomatitis. *Compend. Cont. Educ. Equine Pract.* 5:2–6.

53. Kramer, W. L., Jones, F. R., Holbrook, F. R., Walton, T. E. and Calisher, C. H. 1990. Isolation of abroviruses from Culicoides midges (Diptera: Ceratopogonidae) in Colorado during an epizootic of vesicular stomatitis New Jersey. *J. Med. Entomol.* 27:487–493.

54. Lauerman, L. H. and Hanson, R. P. 1968. Live vesicular stomatitis virus vaccines. *Proc. US Livestock Sanitary Assoc.* 72:591–597.

55. Letchworth, G. J., Rodriguez, L. L. and Delcbarrera, J. 1999. Vesicular stomatitis. *Vet. J.* 157:239–260.

56. Lin, F. and Kitching, R. P. 2000. Swine vesicular disease: An overview. *Vet. J.* 160:192–201.

57. Llewellyn, Z. N., Ou, X., Chang, G. J., Schmitt, B., Salman, M. D. and Akkina, R. K. 2000. Genetic analysis of vesicular stomatitis virus: New Jersey from the 1995 outbreak in the western United States. *Am. J. Vet. Res.* 61:1358–1363.

58. Magnuson, R. J., Triantis, J., Rodriguez, L. L., Perkins, A., Meredith, C. O., Beaty, B., McCluskey, B. and Salman, M. 2003. A single-tube multiplex reverse transcription-polymerase chain reaction for detection and differentiation of vesicular stomatitis Indiana 1 and New Jersey viruses in insects. *J. Vet. Diag. Invest.* 15:561–567.

59. Martinez, I. and Wertz, G. W. 2005. Biological differences between vesicular stomatitis virus Indiana and New Jersey serotype glycoproteins: Identification of amino acid residues modulating pH-dependent infectivity. *J. Virol.* 79:3578–3585.

60. Martinez, I., Rodriguez, L. L., Jimenez, C., Pauszek, S. J. and Wertz, G. W. 2003. Vesicular stomatitis virus glycoprotein is a determinant of pathogenesis in swine, a natural host. *J. Virol.* 77:8039–8047.

61. Martinez, I., Barrera, J. C., Rodriguez, L. L. and Wertz, G. W. 2004. Recombinant vesicular stomatitis (Indiana) virus expressing New Jersey and Indiana glycoproteins induces neutralizing antibodies to each serotype in swine, a natural host. *Vaccine* 22:4035–4043.

62. McCluskey, B. J. 1997. Emerging animal diseases: Epidemiology and the role of vaccination. Proceedings of the Symposium on Veterinary Epidemiology and Economics, Fort Collins, Colo, 1997, 119–128.

63. McCluskey, B. J. 2007. Vesicular stomatitis. In *Equine infectious diseases*, ed. D. C. Sellon and M. T. Long, chapter 24, 219–225. Philadelphia, USA: Saunders, Elsevier Inc.

64. McCluskey, B. J. and Mumford, E. L. 2000. Vesicular stomatitis and other vesicular, erosive, and ulcerative diseases of horses. *Vet. Clin. North. Am. Equine Pract.* 16:457–469.

65. McCluskey, B. J., Beaty, B. J. and Salman, M. D. 2003. Climatic factors and the occurrence of vesicular stomatitis in New Mexico, United States of America. *Rev. Sci. Tech. Off. Int. Epiz.* 22:849–856.

66. McCluskey, B. J., Hurd, H. S. and Mumford, E. L. 1999. Review of the 1997 outbreak of vesicular stomatitis in the western United States. *J. Am. Vet. Med. Assoc.* 215:1259–1262.

67. Mead, D. G., Mare, C. J. and Ramberg, F. B. 1999. Bite transmission of vesicular stomatitis virus (New Jersey serotype) to laboratory mice by *Simulium vittatum* (Diptera: Simuliidae). *J. Med. Entomol.* 36:410–413.

13. EQUINE VESICULAR STOMATITIS

68. Mead, D. G., Gray, E. W., Noblet, R., Murphy, M. D., Howerth, E. W. and Stallknecht, D. E. 2004a. Biological transmission of vesicular stomatitis virus (New Jersey serotype) by *Simulium vittatum* (Diptera: Simuliidae) to domestic swine (*Sus scrofa*). *J. Med. Entomol.* 41:78–82.

69. Mead, D. G., Howerth, E. W., Murphy, M. D., Gray, E. W., Noblet, R. and Stallknecht, D. E. 2004b. Black fly involvement in the epidemic transmission of vesicular stomatitis New Jersey virus (Rhabdoviridae: Vesiculovirus). *Vector Borne Zoonotic Dis.* 4:351–359.

70. Mead, D. G., Ramberg, F. B., Besselsen, D. G. and Mare, C. J. 2000. Transmission of vesicular stomatitis virus from infected to noninfected black flies co-feeding on nonviremic deer mice. *Science* 287:485–487.

71. Mebus, C. A. 1998. Vesicular stomatitis. In *Foreign animal diseases. "The gray book."* 6th ed., part IV, ed. W. W. Buisch, J. L. Hyde, and C. H. Mebus, 394–397. Richmond, VA: United States Animal Health Association. *http://www.vet.uga.edu/VPP/gray_book02/fad/vst.php (accessed 14 March 2009)*.

72. Mumford, E. L., McCluskey, B. J., Traub-Dargatz, J. L., Schmitt, B. J. and Salman, M. D. 1998. Serologic evaluation of vesicular stomatitis virus exposure in horses and cattle in 1996. *J. Am. Vet. Med. Assoc.* 213:1265–1269.

73. Nunamaker, R. A., Perez de Leon, A. A., Campbell, C. L. and Lonning, S. M. 2000. Oral infection of *Culicoides sonorensis* (Diptera: *Ceratopogonidae*) by vesicular stomatitis virus. *J. Med. Entomol.* 37:784–786.

74. Nunamaker, R. A., Lockwood, J. A., Stith, C. E., Campbell, C. L., Schell, S. P., Drolet, B. S., Wilson, W. C., White, D. M. and Letchworth, G. J. 2003. Grasshoppers (Orthoptera: Acrididae) could serve as reservoirs and vectors of vesicular stomatitis virus. *J. Med. Entomol.* 40:957–963.

75. Núñez, J. I., Blanco, E., Hernández, T., Gómez-Tejedor, C., Martín, M. J., Dopazo, J. and Sobrino, F. 1998. A RT-PCR assay for the differential diagnosis of vesicular viral diseases of swine. *J. Virol. Methods* 72:227–235.

76. Perez de Leon, A. A. and Tabachnick, W. J. 2006. Transmission of vesicular stomatitis New Jersey virus to cattle by the biting midge *Culicoides sonorensis* (Diptera: Ceratopogonidae). *J. Med. Entomol.* 43:323–329.

77. Rainwater-Lovett, K., Pauszek, S. J., Kelley, W. N. and Rodriguez, L. L. 2007. Molecular epidemiology of vesicular stomatitis New Jersey virus from the 2004–2005 US outbreak indicates a common origin with Mexican strains. *J. Gen. Virol.* 88:2042–2051.

78. Rasmussen, T. B., Uttenthal, A., Fernández, J. and Storgaard, T. 2005. Quantitative multiplex assay for simultaneous detection and identification of Indiana and New Jersey serotypes of vesicular stomatitis virus. *J. Clin. Microbiol.* 43:356–362.

79. Reif, J. S. 1994. Vesicular stomatitis. In *Handbook of zoonoses*, ed. G. Beran. Boca Raton, Fla.: CRC Press.

80. Rice, C. E. 1960. The use of the complement-fixation test in the study and diagnosis of viral diseases in man and animals: A review. Part III. Vesicular viruses. *Can. J. Comp. Med. Vet. Sci.* 24:238–241.

81. Roche, S. and Gaudin, Y. 2002. Characterization of the equilibrium between the native and fusion-inactive conformation of rabies virus glycoprotein indicates that the fusion complex is made of several trimers. *Virology* 297:128–135.

82. Roche, S., Rey, F. A., Gaudin, Y. and Bressanelli, S. 2007. Structure of the prefusion form of the vesicular stomatitis virus glycoprotein G. *Science* 315:843–848.

83. Rodriguez, L. L. 2002. Emergence and re-emergence of vesicular stomatitis in the United States. *Virus Res.* 85:211–219.

84. Rodriguez, L. L., Letchworth, G. J., Spiropoulou, C. F. and Nichol, S. T. 1993. Rapid detection of vesicular stomatitis virus New Jersey serotype in clinical samples by using polymerase chain reaction. *J. Clin. Microbiol.* 31:2016–2020.

85. Schmitt, B. 2002. Vesicular stomatitis. *Vet. Clin. North Am. Food Anim. Pract.* 18:453–459.

86. Sellers, R. F. and Maarouf, A. R. 1990. Trajectory analysis of winds and vesicular stomatitis in North America, 1982–1985. *Epidemiol. Infect.* 104:313–328.

87. Stallknecht, D. E., Perzak, D. E., Bauer, L. D., Murphy, M. D. and Howerth, E. W. 2001. Contact transmission of vesicular stomatitis virus New Jersey in pigs. *Am. J. Vet. Res.* **62**:516–520.

88. Stallknecht, D. E., Greer, J. B., Murphy, M. D., Mead, D. G. and Howerth, E. W. 2004. Effect of strain and serotype of vesicular stomatitis virus on viral shedding, vesicular lesion development, and contact transmission in pigs. *Am. J. Vet. Res.* 65:1233–1239.

89. Stauffer, F., De Miranda, J., Schechter, M. C., Carneiro, F. A., Salgado, L. T., Machado, G. F. and Da Poian, A. T. 2006. Inactivation of vesicular stomatitis virus through inhibition of membrane fusion by chemical modification of the viral glycoprotein. *Antiviral Res.* 73:31–39. *c:\citwww\ paper\16934341.*

90. Tesh, R. B., Boshell, J., Modi, G. B., Morales, A. A., Young, D. G., Corredor, A. A., de Carrasquilla, C. F., de Rodriguez, C., Walters, L. L., and Gaitan, M. O. 1987. Natural infection of humans, animals, and phlebotomine sand flies with the Alagoas serotype of vesicular stomatitis virus in Colombia. *Am. J. Trop. Med. Hyg.* 36:653–661.

91. Tesh, R. B., Chaniotis, B. N. and Johnson, K. M. 1972. Vesicular stomatitis virus (Indiana serotype): Transovarial transmission by phlebotomine sandflies. *Science* 175:1477–1479.

92. Tesh, R. B., Peralta, P. H. and Johnson, K. M. 1970. Ecologic studies of vesicular stomatitis virus. II. Results of experimental infection in Panamanian wild animals. *Am. J. Epidemiol.* 91:216–224.

93. Vernon, S. D. and Webb, P. A. 1985. Recent vesicular stomatitis virus infection detected by immunoglobulin M antibody capture enzyme-linked immunosorbent assay. *J. Clin. Microbiol.* 22:582–586.

94. Wagner, R. R. and Rose, J. K. 2001. Rhabdoviridae. In *Fields virology*, 4th ed., ed. D. M. Knipe and P. M. Howley. Philadelphia: Lippincott, Williams & Wilkins.

95. WAHO, 2004. World Arabian Horse Organization Conference, 2004. Poland.

96. Walton, T. E., Webb, P. A., Kramer, W. L., Smith, G. C., Davis, T., Holbrook, F. R., Moore, C. G., Schiefer, T. J., Jones, R. H. and Janney, G. C. 1987. Epizootic vesicular stomatitis in Colorado, 1982: Epidemiologic and entomologic studies. *Am. J. Trop. Med. Hyg.* 36:166–176.

97. Webb, P. A., McLean, R. G., Smith, G. C., Ellenberger, J. H., Francy, D. B., Walton, T. E. and Monath, T. P. 1987a. Epizootic vesicular stomatitis in Colorado, 1982: Some observations on the possible role of wildlife populations in an enzootic maintenance cycle. *J. Wildlife Dis.* 23:192–198.

98. Webb, P. A., Monath, T. P., Reif, J. S., Smith, G. C., Kemp, G. E., Lazuick, J. S. and Walton, T. E. 1987b. Epizootic vesicular stomatitis in Colorado, 1982: Epidemiologic studies along the northern Colorado Front Range. *Am. J. Trop. Med. Hyg.* 36:183–188.

99. Weck, P. K. and Wagner, R. R. 1979. Transcription of vesicular stomatitis virus is required to shut off cellular RNA synthesis. *J. Virol.* 30:410–413.

100. Weissenhorn, W., Hinz, A. and Gaudin, Y. 2007. Virus membrane fusion. *FEBS Lett.* 581:2150–2155.

101. Wertz, G. W., Perepelitsa, V. P. and Ball, L. A. 1998. Gene rearrangement attenuates expression and lethality of a nonsegmented negative strand RNA virus. *Proc. Natl. Acad. Sci. USA* 95:3501–3506.

102. Wilks, C. R. and House, J. A. 1986. Susceptibility of various animals to the vesiculoviruses Isfahan and Chandipura. *J. Hyg.* (London) 97:359–368.

103. World Organization for Animal Health [OIE]. *Manual of diagnostic tests and vaccines for terrestrial animals* [online]. Paris: OIE; 2004. Vesicular stomatitis. http://www.oie.int/eng/normes/mmanual/ A_00025.htm (accessed 14 March 2009).

104. Yilma, T., Breeze, R. G., *Ristow*, S., Gorham, J. R. and Leib, S. R. 1985. Immune responses of cattle and mice to the G glycoprotein of vesicular stomatitis virus. *Adv. Exp. Med. Biol.* 185:101–115.

105. Zee, Y. C. and MacLachlan, N. J. 2004. Rhabdoviridae. In *Veterinary microbiology*, 2nd ed., D. C. Hirsh, N. J. MacLachlan, and R. L. Walker, 377–382. Ames, Iowa: Blackwell Publishing.

106. Zhou, E.-M., Riva, J. and Clavijo, A. 2001. Development of an immunoglobulin M (IgM) capture enzyme-linked immunosorbent assay for detection of equine and swine IgM antibodies to vesicular stomatitis virus. *Clin. Diag. Lab. Immunol.* 8:475–481.

14. GETAH VIRUS INFECTION IN HORSES

K. DHAMA, P. BHATT, R. V. S. PAWAIYA, AND M. MAHENDRAN

INTRODUCTION

Getah virus (GETV) is an arthropod-borne virus that can cause a mild, self-limiting illness in horses. Infection occurs through the bite of an infected mosquito (Kamada et al., 1980; Kono, 1988; Fukunaga et al., 2000; Hinchcliff, 2007). The first known outbreak occurred in Japan in 1978, which affected racehorses at two densely populated training stables (Kamada et al., 1980; Sentsui and Kono, 1980; Imagawa et al., 1981). A small number of cases were also reported in Japanese horses in 1983 (Sentsui and Kono, 1985). In 1990, clinical disease was reported outside Japan, at a Thoroughbred breeding farm in India (Brown and Timoney, 1998). GETV was first isolated in Malaysia in 1955 from *Culex gelidus* mosquitoes (Berge, 1975) and has since been found widely in many countries (Kono, 1988; Kamada et al., 1991a, b; Shortbridge et al., 1994; Brown and Timoney, 1998; Sugiura and Shimada, 1999; Fukunaga et al., 2000; Hinchcliff, 2007). Outbreaks of clinical disease due to Getah virus infection occur infrequently.

Getah virus does not cause disease in humans. Although antibodies to GETV have been found in humans, there are no reports of symptomatic infections, and thus Getah viruses probably do not represent a threat to the public health (Marchette et al., 1980; Kono, 1988; Li et al., 1992; Hinchcliff, 2007).

ETIOLOGY

Getah virus is a member of the Getah subgroup in the genus *Alphavirus* within the Semliki Forest complex of the family Togaviridae. It is a small spherical enveloped virus with a linear single-stranded, positive-sense ribonucleic acid (RNA) genome (Kono et al., 1980; Kono, 1988; Hinchcliff, 2007). Virus has a diameter of approximately 70 nm and a buoyant density of 1.22 g/ml. It can grow and produce cytopathic effects in a variety of cell cultures and is sensitive to organic solvents, heat, and low pH. Hemolytic activity of GETV has been demonstrated (Yoshinaka et al., 1979; Kono et al., 1980). *Alphavirus* genome encodes four nonstructural proteins (nsP) including nsP1, nsP2, nsP3, and nsP4, which mediate viral RNA synthesis, and five structural proteins including one nucleocapsid core protein C and three envelope glycoproteins—viz, E1, E2, and E3 (Srivastava and Igarashi, 1986; Strauss and Strauss, 1994). Getah virus has been suggested to be a potentially useful challenge virus for antiviral assay of human interferon (IFN) (Ogiso et al., 2005).

The phylogenetic analysis of the GETV strains significantly reflected the identification of phylogenetical groups within the Sempliki Forest serocomplex (Gur'ev et al., 2008a). Sagiyama virus (SAGV), which is found in Japan and causes identical symptoms in horses, is very closely related to Getah virus. The clinical signs in diseased racehorses caused by naturally acquired GETV infection are similar to those induced by experimental inoculation of SAGV in horses (Kamada et al., 1980; Sentsui and Kono, 1980; Kumanomido et al., 1988b). Serologic testing and biological characteristics have also indicated that SAGV is closely related to GETV. Some researchers consider SAGV to be a member of the GETV group or a strain of GETV (Kamada et al., 1980; Kono, 1988; Kumanomido et al., 1988b; Shirako and Yamaguchi, 2000; Chang et al., 2006). Based on the comparative genome analysis and phylogenetic studies, Wen et al. (2007) concluded that M-1 strain of *Alphavirus*, isolated in 1964 in China, can be considered as a strain of Getah-like virus and suggested that M-1 is genetically closely linked to SAGV with 98.0% identity and GATV with 97.8% identity. Recent results of genetic analysis suggested that SAGV is most closely related to GETV as opposed to its earlier/current classification (Weaver et al., 2000) as a subtype of Ross River virus (RRV) (Chang et al., 2006). Using the reverse transcription–polymerase chain reaction (RT-PCR) and direct sequencing, Wekesa et al. (2001) reported difference in the capsid region to be one of the useful markers in the genetic classification between these two viruses and that these genomic differences among the GETV strains may be due to time factor rather than geographical distribution. Ross River virus (RRV) has also similar cladistic classification, ecology, and clinical signs in horses as that of Getah virus (Hinchcliff, 2007). Considerable sequence homology exists between Getah and Ross virus genomes (Strauss and Strauss, 1994).

Getah virus causes disease in horses and pigs, whereas Ross virus causes disease in humans and, arguably, horses.

Oligonucleotide fingerprint analysis of strains of Getah virus isolated from mosquitoes, swine, and horses in Japan and Malaysia (1956 to 1981) suggested that the virus genome undergoes mutation frequently; however, there is a tendency for the isolates of the same year to show greater similarity. Thus, there is considerable variation in the strains of GETV-infecting mosquitoes in the wild, and also that the variants or mutants present in mosquitoes might be subject to selection during viral multiplication in the mammalian host (Morita and Igarashi, 1984). There are at least eight strains of this virus, which appears to mutate fairly often. In a recent study, molecular genetic study conducted by Gur'ev et al. (2008a), a genetic diversity of Getah virus strains in northeastern Asia has been discussed. However, molecular analysis of Getah viruses, isolated in China, has indicated that these viruses comprised a genetically highly conserved group (Zhai et al., 2007). Further molecular studies of Zhai et al. (2008), regarding sequence and phylogenetic analyses of the E2 gene of the Chinese GETV isolates, revealed nucleotide sequence identities of 98–100% compared with other GETV isolates, which also indicated that there is a relatively high degree of conservation among GETV isolates. Geographically, genetic variability has not been reported among isolates of Getah virus from Southeast Asia and Japan (Wekesa et al., 2001).

GEOGRAPHIC DISTRIBUTION

Serologic studies suggest that Getah virus is widely distributed from Eurasia (including Siberia and Mongolia) to southeast and far eastern Asia, the Pacific islands, and Australasia. It has been reported from Japan, Hong Kong, Southeast Asia, the Pacific islands, Korea, and India (Sentsui and Kono, 1980; Kono, 1988; Kamada et al., 1991a, b; Shortbridge et al., 1994; Brown and Timoney, 1998; Sugiura and Shimada, 1999; Fukunaga et al., 2000; Hinchcliff, 2007). Antibodies to Getah virus in animals have been reported in Australia, but the presence of the virus or the disease has not been confirmed.

Seroepizootiological survey of Japanese encephalitis virus and Getah virus in regional horse race tracks from 1991 to 1997 in Japan suggested that the viruses have spread among racehorses almost every year in Japan although, fortunately, there was no horse showing clinical illness due to these viruses was observed (Sugiura and Shimada, 1999). It was also suggested that surveillance of GETV should be continued in the future in Japan and that it is necessary to promote the wider use of vaccines to persons related to horseracing.

Many strains of GETV have been isolated in Japan from mosquitoes (Kumanomido et al., 1986a), swine (Nakamura et al., 1967), and racehorses (Kamada et al., 1980; Sentsui and Kono, 1985). Getah virus has been frequently isolated from mosquitoes from various countries (Simpson et al., 1975; Ksiazek et al., 1981; Takashima and Hashimoto, 1985; Kumanomido et al., 1986a; Leake et al., 1986; Li et al., 1992; Peiris et al., 1994; Turell et al., 2003; Bryant et al., 2005; Wang et al., 2006). Kumanomido et al. (1986b) reported the isolation of GETV from mosquitoes collected at two horse habitations in the western areas of Japan (Izumida et al., 1988; Kumanomido et al., 1988c). Li et al. (1992) isolated GETV from mosquitoes collected in China during 1964; the virus (strain M-1) replicated in laboratory-bred mosquitoes and was transmitted by to healthy newborn albino mice. L'vov et al. (2000) isolated fifteen strains of GETV for the first time from *Aedes* and *Culex* mosquitoes in different regions of the Russian Federation and

Mongolia and indicated that Getah virus is the only *Alphavirus* occurring under such severe climatic conditions. Isolation of Getah viruses from Korea indicated that these are actively circulating in Korea (Turell et al., 2003). Recently, Turell et al. (2006) reported the laboratory transmission of GETVs by mosquitoes (Diptera: Culicidae) in Korea, when allowed to feed on chickens with viremias induced by the virus.

Clinical signs have been reported only in horses, pigs, and experimentally infected mice. However, serologic studies suggest that asymptomatic GETV infections occur in many vertebrates, including horses (Fukunaga et al., 2000), pigs, cattle, water buffalo, kangaroos, wallabies, birds, reptiles, nonhuman primates, and humans (Li et al., 1992). Mice, rats, rabbits, hamsters, and guinea pigs can be infected experimentally. Antibody prevalence in humans and animals in China ranged from 10.3% by neutralization tests of samples from healthy people to 26.4% by complement fixation (CF) tests of samples from people with febrile illnesses in 1982. The high prevalence of antibody in pigs, horses, and goats (17.6–37.5%) indicated that infection with Getah or a closely related virus is relatively common in domestic animals (Li et al., 1992). The isolation of this virus from various provinces in China and also in Russia and Mongolia are an indication of changes in the world distribution of this reemerging virus (Zhai et al., 2007, 2008).

TRANSMISSION

Getah virus appears to be maintained in a natural cycle between mosquitoes and various vertebrate hosts, which is typical of arboviruses. This virus seems to be transmitted mainly by various species of *Aedes* and *Culex*; the specific vector varies with the climate and geographic region (Takashima et al., 1983; Kono, 1988). The amplifying hosts are thought to include horses, pigs, and possibly other species such as rodents. Horses and pigs become viremic and presumably can infect mosquitoes, although this does not appear to have been confirmed experimentally. In the enzootic cycle, interspecies transmission is possible, where pigs may play a role in amplifying GETV (Kumanomido et al., 1988c) before horses are infected (Kono et al., 1980). The virus is thus assumed to be maintained in a mosquito-pig-mosquito cycle in those areas with year-round mosquito activity (Simpson et al., 1976; Calisher and Walton, 1996; Hinchcliff, 2007).

The spread of GETV has been suspected by horse-to-horse contact, based on the rapidity of spread among horses during disease outbreaks, the short duration of the outbreak, and the lack of mosquito activity at the time some horses developed the disease (Sentsui and Kono, 1980; Brown and Timoney, 1998). Thus, Getah virus is also directly contagious between horses, probably via aerosols or direct contact with nasal secretions. This route is thought to be uncommon and is of limited importance in propagation of epidemics because high doses of virus are needed to establish disease in horses by intranasal route, but only small amounts of virus are found in the nasal/oral secretions of naturally infected horses (Kamada et al., 1991a). GETV has not been recovered from the feces or urine of horses; however, it was found in the feces of an experimentally infected piglet with diarrhea. Vertical transmission has been reported in pigs, as well as in experimentally infected mice, hamsters, guinea pigs, and rabbits (Yago et al., 1987; Kumanomido et al., 1988a; Asai et al., 1991). Transplacental transmission demonstrated in pregnant mice subcutaneously inoculated with GETV suggested that the virus may readily cross the placental barrier through hematogenous infection (Kumanomido et al., 1988a). There is no indication that vertical transmission occurs in horses.

CLINICAL SIGNS

Clinical signs of the disease are mild and nonlife threatening. In horses, Getah virus infection is a mild, self-limiting illness characterized by pyrexia with rectal temperatures ranging from 38.5°C to—40°C, urticarial rashes on various portions of the body, and exanthema/edema of the hind legs mainly in the fetlock and an abnormal gait, often described as "stiffness" (Sentsui and Kono, 1980; Kamada et al., 1980; Brown and Timoney, 1998; Hinchcliff, 2007). Swelling of the submandibular lymph nodes (submandibular lymphadenopathy), mild abdominal pain, depression, mild icterus, and scrotal edema have also been reported. Urticarial rash consists of 3–5 mm papules mainly on the neck from the shoulder to the forearm and over the hindquarters from the thigh to the gaskin. Serous nasal discharge has been reported in experimentally infected horses but not in natural cases. In some horses, the clinical signs are limited to one or two symptoms such as fever alone, fever and a skin rash, or fever and limb edema. GETV does not seem to cause abortions or birth defects in horses; pregnant mares having the disease during gestation delivered normal foals after an outbreak at a breeding farm in India (Brown and Timoney, 1998). Infection and disease were produced experimentally in horses when inoculated by the intramuscular or intranasal routes (Kamada et al., 1980; Wada et al., 1982; Kamada et al., 1991a, b). The incubation period in horses is short. Horses infected experimentally by the intranasal route become symptomatic in three to four days (Kamada et al., 1991a). After intramuscular injection, the incubation period is two to six days. Kamada et al. (1991b) demonstrated that the appearance of clinical signs in equine Getah virus infection is dependent on viral inoculum size. Besides, it was assumed to be rare chance that eruptions and enlargement of the submandibular lymph node were developed simultaneously in a horse. The clinical disease persists for seven to ten days, and the horses recover fully in approximately two weeks. Subclinical infection is very common.

MORBIDITY AND MORTALITY

Although clinical disease in horses is rare, many horses are seropositive for GETV antibodies in endemic areas. In Japan, 3–50% of horses have antibodies to Getah virus; a few surveys have reported seroprevalence rates as high as 93% (Brown and Timoney, 1998; Sugiura and Shimada, 1999). Retrospective serologic studies suggest that the virus was widely distributed in Japan before the first known outbreak in 1978. The reason for the high exposure rate but paucity of clinical cases is unknown. It has been suggested that the passage of GETV through large groups of horses may result in increased virulence. During a 1978 outbreak in Japan, the virus spread slowly and irregularly over a four—to six-week period at two training centers for racehorses. The morbidity rate was 40%. During a 1990 Indian outbreak, the infection spread rapidly, and all cases appeared over a period of twelve days. In this outbreak, the morbidity rate was 37% (Brown and Timoney, 1998; Fukunaga et al., 2000). Seroprevalence of GETV has also been reported to be 17% in India and 25% in Hong Kong (Kamada et al., 1991a; Brown and Timoney, 1998; Shortbridge et al., 1994). Thus, the widespread incidence of subclinical infection of horses by Getah virus in endemic areas has been indicated.

POSTMORTEM AND MICROSCOPIC LESIONS

Deaths have not been reported in naturally infected horses. Postmortem reports of horses with disease caused by Getah virus are mostly limited to experimental studies because the disease is typically not fatal. Experimentally, horses inoculated with pathogenic GETV have shown mild changes, including atrophy of splenic and lymphoid tissue, with destruction of lymphocytes, and perivascular and diffuse infiltration of focal skin lesions by lymphocytes, histiocytes, and eosinophils. Lesions in the central nervous system (CNS) are limited to mild perivascular cuffing in the cerebrum and small hemorrhagic foci in the spinal cord (Wada et al., 1982). Generalized lymphadenopathy was reported in experimentally infected horses; the splenic and inguinal lymph nodes were particularly prominent. Some horses also had a slightly enlarged spleen and/or liver. Moderate glomerular congestion was noted in one horse, while another had congestion and slight turbidity of the piamater in the brain. In horses with a rash, the subcutaneous tissues were moderately edematous due to lymph stasis. These horses had scattered maculae in the dermis; on cut section, the maculae were thickened and circumscribed, with pale reddish foci. The histopathologic lesions consisted mainly of moderate lymphoid hyperplasia in the submandibular, axillary, splenic, renal, and inguinal lymph nodes, as well as in the spleen. The skin lesions contained perivascular or diffuse infiltrates of lymphoid cells and histiocytes, thickened blood vessel walls, and edematous smooth muscle cells. Scattered hemorrhagic foci and eosinophilic infiltrates were seen in some lesions. Perivascular cuffing with mononuclear cells was reported in the cerebrum of two horses.

Lesions have been reported after experimental inoculation in horses, mice, and chicken embryos (Scherer et al., 1962; Kumanomido et al., 1988b). The pathogenicity of GETV for swine was examined experimentally by infecting pregnant sows and piglets, and it was suggested that the virus is mildly pathogenic for swine, which may play a role as an amplifying host in nature (Izumida et al., 1988; Kumanomido et al., 1988c). Kawamura *et al.* (1987) reported a fatal case in newborn piglets with Getah virus infection. GETV has also been isolated from dead fetuses of a naturally infected sow (Shibata et al., 1991). Sentsui and Kono (1981), while examining the pathogenicity of GETV (isolated from a feverish horse) for mice, observed that the virus was transmitted horizontally among the littermates and vertically from the dam to her offspring via milk. Hiruma et al. (990) reported the virulence to skeletal muscles (produced polymyositis) in mice experimentally inoculated with GETV. Skeletal muscles of mice experimentally infected with the virus isolated from mosquitoes showed degeneration, atrophy, necrosis, and inflammatory changes of muscle fibers (Li et al., 1992).

DIAGNOSIS

Diagnosis is achieved by detection of clinical signs, virus isolation from blood of affected horses, and seroconversion to GETV (Brown and Timoney, 1998; Wekesa et al., 2001; Hinchcliff, 2007). In horses, clinical diagnosis is based on Getah virus infection suggestive of fever, hind-limb edema, and stiffness. A rash or swelling of the submandibular lymph nodes also supports the diagnosis. Hematologic abnormalities includes lymphopenia. There can be mild to moderate hyperbilirubinemia secondary to inappetence (Brown and Timoney, 1998; Wekesa et al., 2001; Hinchcliff, 2007). The differential diagnosis includes equine viral arteritis and the mild form of African horse sickness. The clinical diagnosis should always be confirmed by laboratory testing. Getah virus can be isolated in Vero, RK-13, BHK-21, and many other cell lines / cell cultures (monkey kidney cell line, mosquito cell cultures, etc.) as well as by intracerebral inoculation of suckling mice. In horses, serologic tests include serum neutralization (SN), complement fixation (CF), hemagglutination inhibition (HI), and enzyme-linked immunosorbent assay (ELISA) (Sentsui and Kono, 1980; Fukunaga et al., 2000). An ELISA has been developed for the serological survey of GETV in pigs (Hohdatsu et al., 1990). A dot-immunobinding assay for the detection of antibody to Getah virus in horses has been reported by Sugiura et al. (1989). Getah viruses can be identified and molecularly characterized by reverse transcription–polymerase chain reaction (RT-PCR) and sequencing (Wekesa et al., 2001; Wang et al., 2006; Wen et al., 2007; Zhai et al., 2007; Gur'ev et al., 2008a).

Before collecting or sending any samples from animals with a suspected foreign animal disease, the proper authorities should be contacted. Samples should only be sent under secure conditions and to authorized laboratories to prevent the spread of the disease. In horses, plasma collected at the onset of pyrexia is preferred for virus isolation; viremia appears to occur only during the first one to two days after the onset of fever. GETV has also been isolated from saliva, nasal swabs, and defribrinated blood. In addition, virus isolation may be attempted from the lungs, liver, spleen, kidneys, lymph nodes, and spinal cord at necropsy. In experimentally infected horses, the axillary and inguinal lymph nodes have the highest viral titers and seem to contain virus for the longest period.

PREVENTION AND CONTROL

Getah virus appears to be contagious to some extent. The disinfectant susceptibility of this virus has not been published; however, togaviruses are not very stable in the environment and can be inactivated by most disinfectants. Two related alphaviruses, the eastern and western equine encephalitis viruses, are susceptible to 1% sodium hypochlorite, 2% glutaraldehyde, formaldehyde, and 70% ethanol, as well as moist and dry heat. Vector-control measures may also help prevent transmission as Getah virus seems to be spread mainly by mosquitoes.

Treatment is only supportive for Getah-virus infected horses. Administration of analgesics and antipyretics is recommended; however, antimicrobials are not indicated in uncomplicated cases. Minimizing the exposure of horses to infected mosquito is prudent, although its efficacy in preventing GETV infection is unknown. During disease outbreaks, it is logical to isolate affected horses, given the potential for horse-to-horse spread of the virus.

An inactivated vaccine is available in Japan for immunization of horses against the disease caused by Getah virus (Sugiura and Shimada, 1999). In Japan, most two-year-old racehorses in training receive two doses of the vaccine, followed by a booster each year. Vaccinated horses are protected from both clinical disease and viremia. However, serological interpretation of the disease has been reported to be hindered in Japan by the widespread use of GETV vaccine that induces detectable viral antibodies in the serum (Naito et al., 1995; Sugiura and Shimada, 1999).

CONCLUSION

Getah is a mosquitoborne self-limiting viral disease of horses. Disease outbreaks have been reported from horses in Japan and India. Outbreaks of clinical disease due to Getah virus infection occur infrequently. The causative agent, Getah virus, is a member of the genus *Alphavirus* and is a small enveloped virus with a single-stranded RNA genome. It is closely related to Sagiyama virus and has similar cladistic classification as of Ross River virus. There are at least eight strains of Getah virus, which appears to mutate. A relatively high degree of conservation among Getah virus isolates has also been reported. The virus is maintained and propagated in a mosquito-pig-mosquito cycle primarily. Clinical symptoms have been reported only in horses, pigs, and experimentally infected mice. Getah viruses do not have public health implications. However, serologic studies suggest that asymptomatic Getah virus infections occur in many vertebrates/ animals including humans. Horse-to-horse contact transmission of the virus has been indicated; however, vertical transmission does not occur in horses. In horses, clinical signs of the disease are mild and occur for a short period only, characterized by pyrexia, urticarial rashes, edema of the hind legs, and stiffness. Death has not been reported, and thus the disease is not considered fatal in horses. Subclinical infection is very common. Though clinical disease in horses is rare, many horses are found seropositive for Getah virus antibodies in endemic areas.

Diagnosis is based on the detection of clinical symptoms, virus isolation from affected horses, and seroconversion status of the animal. Virus isolation can be done in various cell cultures as well as by intracerebral inoculation of suckling mice. Serological tests include SNT, CFT, HI, and ELISA. Molecular techniques of RT-PCR and sequencing are being exploited for detection and characterization of Getah viruses at genomic level. In horses, plasma collected at the onset of pyrexia is preferred for virus isolation. The virus can also been isolated from saliva, nasal swabs, and defribrinated blood. Since Getah virus seems to be spread mainly by mosquitoes, vector control measures could help prevent virus transmission. Affected horses should be isolated during disease outbreaks to check the spread of the virus to other horses. Supportive treatment can also be given to the Getah virus–infected horses accordingly. Immunization of horses against the Getah virus, by an inactivated vaccine, is practiced in Japan. Vaccination protects the horses from both clinical disease and viremia. Getah virus, first isolated in Malaysia in 1955 from mosquitoes, has now been reported from many countries. Particularly, the virus has been frequently isolated from mosquitoes from various regions. Virus has been reported from Japan, Hong Kong, Southeast Asia, the Pacific islands, Korea, and India. Recent isolation of Getah virus from various provinces in China and also in Russia and Mongolia is an indication of changes in the world distribution of this re-emerging virus.

REFERENCES

1. Asai, T., Shibata, I. and Uruno, K. 1991. Susceptibility of pregnant hamster, guinea pig, and rabbit to the transplacental infection of Getah virus. *J. Vet. Med. Sci.* 53:1109–1111.

2. Berge, T. O. 1975. Getah. In *International Catalogue of Arboviruses*, 2nd ed., 278–279. US Department of Health, Education, and Welfare.

3. Brown, C. M. and Timoney, P. J. 1998. Getah virus infection of Indian horses. *Trop. Anim. Health Prod.* 30:241–52.

4. Bryant, J. E., Crabtree, M. B., Nam, V. S., Yen, N. T., Duc, H. M. and Miller, B. R. 2005. Isolation of arboviruses from mosquitoes collected in northern Vietnam. *Am. J. Trop. Med. Hyg.* 73:470–473.

5. Calisher, C. H. and Walton, T. E. 1996. Getah virus infections. In *Virus infections of equines*, ed. M. J. Studdert, 157–168. New York, USA: Elsevier.

6. Chang, C. Y., Huang, C. C., Huang, T. S., Deng, M. C., Jong, M. H. and Wang, F. I. 2006. Isolation and characterization of a Sagiyama virus from domestic pigs. *J. Vet. Diagn. Invest.* 18:156–161.

7. Fukunaga, Y., Kumanomido, T. and Kamada, M. 2000. Getah virus as an equine pathogen. *Vet. Clin. North. Am. Equine Pract.* 16:605–17.

8. Gur'ev, E. L., Gromashevskiĭ, V. L., Prilipov, A. G. and L'vo, S. D. 2008a. Molecular genetic analysis of a diversity of Getah virus strains isolated from mosquitoes in the North-Eastern Asia. *Vopr. Virusol.* 53:9–12.

9. Gur'ev, E. L., Gromashevskiĭ, V. L., Prilipov, A. G. and L'vo, S. D. 2008b. Analysis of the genome of two Getah virus strains (LEIV 16275 Mar and LEIV 17741 MPR) isolated from mosquitoes in the North-Eastern Asia. *Vopr. Virusol.* 53:27–31.

10. Hinchcliff, K. W. 2007. Miscellaneous viral diseases: Getah and Ross rive viruses. In *Equine infectious diseases*, ed. D. C. Sellon and M. T. Long, chapter 12, 233–235. Philadelphia, USA: Saunders, Elsevier Inc.

11. Hiruma, M., Ide, S., Hohdatsu, T., Yamagishi, H., Tanaka, Y. and Fujisaki Y. 1990. Polymyositis in mice experimentally inoculated with Getah virus. *Nippon Juigaku Zasshi* 52:767–72.

12. Hohdatsu, T., Ide, S., Yamagishi, H., Eiguchi, Y., Nagano, H., Maehara, N., Tanaka, Y., Fujisaki, Y., Yago, K., Taguchi, K. et al. 1990. Enzyme-linked immunosorbent assay for the serological survey of Getah virus in pigs. *Nippon Juigaku Zasshi* 52:835–837.

13. Imagawa, H., Ando, Y., Kamada, M., Sugiura, T., Kumanomido, T., Fukunaga, Y., Wada, R., Hirasawa, K. and Akiyama Y. 1981. Sero-epizootiological survey on Getah virus infection in light horses in Japan. *Nippon Juigaku Zasshi* 43:797–802.

14. Izumida, A., Takuma, H., Inagaki, S., Kubota, M., Hirahara, T., Kodama, K. and Sasaki, N. 1988. Experimental infection of Getah virus in swine. *Nippon Juigaku Zasshi* 50:679–6784.

15. Kamada, M., Ando, Y., Fukunaga, Y., Kumanomido, T., Imagawa, H., Wada, R. and Akiyama, Y. 1980. Equine Getah virus infection: Isolation of the virus from racehorses during an enzootic in Japan. *Am. J. Trop. Med. Hyg.* 29:984–988.

16. Kamada, M., Kumanomido, T., Wada, R., Fukunaga, Y., Imagawa, H. and Sugiura, T. 1991a. Intranasal infection of Getah virus in experimental horses. *J. Vet. Med. Sci.* 53:855–858.

17. Kamada, M., Wada, R., Kumanomido, T., Imagawa, H., Sugiura, T. and Fukunaga, Y. 1991b. Effect of viral inoculum size on appearance of clinical signs in equine Getah virus infection. *J. Vet. Med. Sci.* 53:803–806.

18. Kawamura, H., Yago, K., Narita, M., Imada, T., Nishimori, T. and Haritani, M. 1987. A fatal case in newborn piglets with Getah virus infection: Pathogenicity of the isolate. *Nippon Juigaku Zasshi* 49:1003–1007.

19. Ksiazek, T. G., Trosper, J. H., Cross, J. H. and Basaca-Sevilla, V. 1981. Isolation of Getah virus from Nueva Ecija Province, Republic of the Philippines. *Trans R. Soc. Trop. Med. Hyg.* 75:312–313.

20. Kono, Y., Sentsui, H. and Ito Y. 1980. An epidemic of Getah virus infection among racehorses: Properties of the virus. *Res. Vet. Sci.* 29:162–167.

21. Kono, Y. 1988. Getah virus disease. In *The arboviruses: Epidemiology and ecology*, ed. T. P. Monath, 21–36. Boca Raton, FL: CRC Press.

22. Kumanomido, T., Fukunaga, Y., Ando, Y., Kamada, M., Imagawa, H., Wada, R., Akiyama, Y., Tanaka, Y., Kobayashi, M., Ogura, N. et al. 1986a. Getah virus isolations from mosquitoes in an enzootic area in Japan. *Nippon Juigaku Zasshi* 48:1135–1140.

23. Kumanomido, T., Fukunaga, Y., Kamada, M., Imagawa, H., Ando, Y., Wada, R., Nitta, M. and Akiyama Y. 1986b. Getah virus isolations from mosquitoes collected at two horse habitations in the western areas of Japan. *Nippon Juigaku Zasshi* 48:1191–1197.

24. Kumanomido, T., Wada, R., Kanemaru, T., Kamada, M., Akiyama, Y. and Matumoto, M. 1988a. Transplacental infection in mice inoculated with Getah virus. *Vet. Microbiol.* 16:129–136.

25. Kumanomido, T., Kamada, M., Wada, R., Kenemaru, T., Sugiura, T. and Akiyama, Y. 1988b. Pathogenicity for horses of original Sagiyama virus, a member of the Getah virus group. *Vet. Microbiol.* 17:367–373.

26. Kumanomido, T., Wada, R., Kanemaru, T., Kamada, M., Hirasawa, K., Akiyama, Y. 1988c. Clinical and virological observations on swine experimentally infected with Getah virus. *Vet. Microbiol.* 16:295–301.

27. Leake, C. J., Ussery, M. A., Nisalak, A., Hoke, C. H., Andre, R. G. and Burke, D. S. 1986. Virus isolations from mosquitoes collected during the 1982 Japanese encephalitis epidemic in northern Thailand. *Trans R. Soc. Trop. Med. Hyg.* 80:831–837.

28. Li, X. D., Qiu, F. X., Yang, H., Rao, Y. N. and Calisher, C. H. 1992. Isolation of Getah virus from mosquitos collected on Hainan Island, China, and results of a serosurvey. *Southeast Asian J. Trop. Med. Public Health* 23:730–734.

29. L'vov, S. D., Gromashevski'i, V. L., Aristova, V. A., Morozova, T. N., Skvortsova, T. M., Gushchina, E. A., Petrova, E. S. and L'vov, D. K. 2000. Isolation of Getah virus (Togaviridae, Alfavirus) strains in North-Eastern Asia. *Vopr Virusol.* 45:14–18.

30. Marchette, N. J., Rudnick, A. and Garcia, R. 1980. Alphaviruses in Peninsular Malaysia: II. Serological evidence of human infection. *Southeast Asian J. Trop. Med. Public Health* 11:14–23.

31. Morita, K., and Igarashi, A. 1984. Oligonucleotide fingerprint analysis of strains of Getah virus isolated in Japan and Malaysia. *J. Gen. Virol.* 65:1899–1908.

32. Naito, H., Murakami, S., Makabe, T. et al. 1995. Distribution of antibody titers to Japanese encephalitis, Getah, and equine influenza viruses in racehorses at the Utsonomiya racecourse. *J. Equine Sci.* 5:27–31.

33. Nakamura, T., Isahai, K., Matsumoto, M., Matsuyama, T., Oya, A. and Okuno, T. 1967. Antibody responses following natural infection of swine to group A arbovirus Getah and preliminary survey for its antibody among domestic animals. *Nihon Koshueisei Zasshi* 14:569–573.

34. Ogiso, S., Shirai, J., Tuchiya, Y. and Honda, E. 2005. Use of Getah virus for antiviral assay of human interferon. *Uirusu* 55:317–326.

35. Peiris, J. S., Amerasinghe, P. H., Amerasinghe, F. P., Calisher, C. H., Perera, L. P., Arunagiri, C. K., Munasingha, N. B. and Karunaratne, S. H. 1994. Viruses isolated from mosquitoes collected in Sri Lanka. *Am. J. Trop. Med. Hyg.* 51:154–161.

36. Scherer, W. F., Izumi, T., McCown, J. and Hardy, J. L. 1962. Sagiyama virus II. Some biologic, physical, chemical and immunologic properties. *Am. J. Trop Med. Hyg.* 11:269–282.

37. Sentsui, H. and Kono, Y. 1980. An epidemic of Getah virus infection among racehorses: Isolation of the virus. *Res. Vet. Sci.* 29:157–161.

38. Sentsui, H. and Kono, Y. 1981. Pathogenicity of Getah virus for mice. *Natl. Inst. Anim. Health Q.* (Tokyo) 21:7–13.

14. GETAH VIRUS INFECTION IN HORSES

39. Sentsui, H. and Kono Y. 1985. Reappearance of Getah virus infection among horses in Japan. *Nippon Juigaku Zasshi* 47:333–335.

40. Shibata, I., Hatano, Y., Nishimura, M., Suzuki, G., Inaba, Y. 1991. Isolation of Getah virus from dead fetuses extracted from a naturally infected sow in Japan. *Vet. Microbiol.* 27:385–391.

41. Shirako, Y. and Yamaguchi, Y. 2000. Genome structure of Sagiyama virus and its relatedness to other alphaviruses. *J Gen Virol.* 81:1353–1360.

42. Shortbridge, K. F., Mason, D. K., Watkins, K. L. and Aaskov, J. G. 1994. Serological evidence for the transmission of Getah virus in Hong Kong. *Vet. Rec.* 134:527–528.

43. Simpson, D. I., Way, H. J., Platt, G. S., Bowen, E. T., Hill, M. N., Kamath, S., Bendell, P. J. and Heathcote, O. H. 1975. Arbovirus infections in Sarawak, October 1968–February 1970: GETAH virus isolations from mosquitoes. *Trans. R. Soc. Trop. Med. Hyg.* 69:35–38.

44. Simpson, D. I., Smith, C. E., Marshall, T. F., Platt, G. S., Way, H. J., Bowen, E. T., Bright, W. F., Day, J., McMahon, D. A., Hill, M. N., Bendell, P. J. and Heathcote, O. H. 1976. Arbovirus infections in Sarawak: The role of the domestic pig. *Trans. R. Soc. Trop. Med. Hyg.* 70:66–72.

45. Srivastava, A. K. and Igarashi, A. 1986. Structural proteins of Getah virus isolates from Japan and Malaysia. *Acta Virol.* 30:126–130.

46. Strauss, J. H. and Strauss, E. G. 1994. The alphaviruses: Gene expression, replication and evolution. *Microbiol. Rev.* 58:491–562.

47. Sugiura, Y., Ohta, C. and Goto, H. 1989. A dot-immunobinding assay for the detection of antibody to Getah virus in horses. *Aust. Vet. J.* 66:340–341.

48. Sugiura, T. and Shimada, K. 1999. Seroepizootological survey of Japanese encephalitis virus and Getah virus in regional horse race tracks from 1991 to 1997 in Japan. *J. Vet. Med. Sci.* 61:877–881.

49. Takashima, I., Hashimoto, N., Arikawa, J. and Matsumoto, K. 1983. Getah virus in Aedes vexans nipponii and Culex tritaeniorhynchus: Vector susceptibility and ability to transmit. *Arch. Virol.* 76:299–305.

50. Takashima, I. and Hashimoto, N. 1985. Getah virus in several species of mosquitoes. *Trans. R. Soc. Trop. Med. Hyg.* 79:546–550.

51. Turell. M. J., O'Guinn, M. L., Wasieloski, L. P. Jr., Dohm, D. J., Lee, W. J., Cho, H. W., Kim, H. C., Burkett, D. A., Mores, C. N., Coleman, R. E. and Klein, T. A. 2003. Isolation of Japanese encephalitis and Getah viruses from mosquitoes (Diptera: Culicidae) collected near Camp Greaves, Gyonggi Province, Republic of Korea, 2000. *J. Med. Entomol.* 40:580–58.

52. Wada, R., Kamada, M., Fukunaga, Y., Ando, Y., Kumanomido, T., Imagawa, H., Akiyama, Y. and Oikawa, M. 1982. Equine Getah virus infection: Pathological study of horses experimentally infected with the MI-110 strain. *Nippon Juigaku Zasshi* 44:411–418.

53. Wang, H. Q., Liu, W. B., Yang, D. R., Liang, Y., Wang, J. W., Zhang, L. S., Liu, J. W., Tao, S. J., Lv, X. J. and Liang, G. D. 2006. Isolation and identification of arboviruses in Hebei Province. *Zhonghua Shi Yan He Lin Chuang Bing Du Xue Za Zhi* 20:52–55.

54. Weaver, S. C., Dalgarno, L., Frey, T. K. et al. 2000. Family togaviridae. In *Seventh report of the International Committee on Taxonomy of Viruses*, ed. M. H. V. van Regenmortel, C. M. Fauquet, and D. H. L. Bishop, 886–887. San Diego, CA: Academic Press.

55. Wekesa, S. N., Inoshima, Y., Murakimia and Sentsui, H. 2001. Genomic analysis of some Japanese isolates of Getah virus. *Vet. Microbiol.* 83:137–146.

56. Wen, J. S., Zhao, W. Z., Liu, J. W., Zhou, H., Tao, J. P., Yan, H. J., Liang, Y., Zhou, J. J. and Jiang, L. F. 2007. Genomic analysis of a Chinese isolate of Getah-like virus and its phylogenetic relationship with other alphaviruses. *Virus Genes* 35:597–603.

57. Yago, K., Hagiwara, S., Kawamura, H. and Narita, M. 1987. A fatal case in newborn piglets with Getah virus infection: Isolation of the virus. *Nippon Juigaku Zasshi* 49:989–994.

58. Yoshinaka, Y., Okada, S. and Shiomi, T. 1979. Hemolytic activity of a togavirus, Getah. *Microbiol. Immunol.* 23:95–103.

59. Zhai, Y. G., Wang, H. Q., Fu, S. H. and Liang, G. D. 2007. Molecular analysis on the capsid gene and 3' untranslation region of three Getah viruses isolated in China. *Bing Du Xue Bao* 23:270–5.
60. Zhai, Y. G., Wang, H. Y., Sun, X. H., Fu, S. H., Wang, H. Q., Attoui, H., Tang, Q. and Liang, G. D. 2008. Complete sequence characterization of isolates of Getah virus (genus Alphavirus, family Togaviridae) from China. *J. Gen. Virol.* 89:1446–14456.

15. Hendra Virus Infection in Horses

K. Dhama, R. V. S. Pawaiya, and S. Kapoor

Introduction

A fatal, novel respiratory disease in horses and human beings suddenly appeared in 1994 in Hendra, a suburb of Brisbane, Queensland, Australia, that affected twenty-one Thoroughbred racehorses and two persons, killing thirteen horses and a horse trainer (Murray et al., 1995a, 1995b; CDC, 1999). Another outbreak in Mackay, Queensland, claimed two horses and a second human fatality (Rogers et al., 1996; Hooper et al., 1996; Weese, 2002). The disease was characterized by severe respiratory distress, ataxia, and marked swelling of the cheeks and supraorbital fossa, aimless pacing, muscle trembling, and hemorrhagic nasal discharge over a twenty-four-hour period (Allworth et al., 1995). The disease outbreaks were attributed to a newly identified virus, which was tentatively classified as equine *Morbillivirus*, and presently referred to as Hendra virus (HeV), a new member of the new genus *Henipavirus* in the family Paramyxoviridae. These initial outbreaks were followed by further occurrences in northern Queensland of three individual sporadic deaths in horses and a suspected infection in a veterinarian, who performed postmortem examination of one of the horses, and later recovered (Field et al., 2000; Hooper et al., 2000). Repeated HeV spillover events have since occurred five times, all involving horses, with the most recent occurrence in July 2008, which also involved two human cases, one of which was lethal. Detection of antibodies in a considerable percentage of fruit bats (*Pteropus* spp.), and isolation of virus from bats suggested their role as reservoir hosts, and it is suspected that infected bat urine or reproductive fluids are involved in transmission, although the virus does not seem to be highly contagious (CDC, 1999; Williamson et al., 2000; Madić, 2001; Mackenzie et al., 2003; Mackenzie, 2005; Hance et al., 2006; Field et al., 2007b; Wong et al., 2007). Thus, bats have been mentioned as the key to the epidemiology of Hendra virus. Recently, antibodies to henipaviruses and/or Hendra virus have also been detected in bats in other regions, which indicates that distribution of henipaviruses may expand (Sendow et al., 2006; Hayman et al., 2008; Li et al., 2008).

Etiology

Previously called equine morbillivirus, Hendra virus (HeV), along with another closely related member Nipah virus (NiV), has been placed in the new genus *Henipavirus* in the family Paramyxoviridae, subfamily Paramyxovirinae, order Mononegavirales. HeV is a large pleomorphic, enveloped virus with a single-stranded, negative-sense RNA genome of 18, 234 nucleotides in length (Wang et al., 2000).

Ultrastructural features of pleiomorphism (38 to >600 nm in size), envelope with 10–18 nm of surface projections, and 18-nm-wide nucleocapsids, exhibiting a herringbone pattern with a 5-nm periodicity led to the placement of this newly identified virus in the genus *Paramyxovirus* or *Morbillivirus* of Paramyxoviridae family (Murray et al., 1995b; Hyatt and Selleck, 1996). Nonneutralization of virus by antisera from a range of paramyxoviruses, morbilliviruses, and pneumoviruses and lack of detectable hemagglutination or neuraminidase activity suggested that the virus was a morbillivirus, which was further supported by comparative sequence analyses by polymerase chain reaction (PCR) amplification of a portion of the matrix protein and phylogenetic analysis and complete nucleotide sequence of the matrix (M) and fusion (F) proteins, indicating that the virus is distantly related to other known morbilliviruses (Murray et al., 1995b; Gould, 1996; Patch et al., 2008). However, Hendra virus exhibited morphologic differences with the presence of two distinct lengths of surface projections (Hyatt and Selleck, 1996) and genetic differences demonstrated by the longer genome size of 18,234 nucleotides in comparison to that of members of the Respirovirus and Morbillivirus genera (Wang et al., 2000). These differences led to the classification of Hendra virus (HeV) as the first member (another being Nipah virus) of a new genus named aptly as Henipavirus in the family, with their designation as biosafety level 4 pathogens (ICTV, 2000; Wang et al., 2000).

EPIDEMIOLOGY
Hendra virus infections have been seen only in Australia, where this virus is endemic in fruit bats (Field et al., 2007b). Antibodies to Hendra virus (HeV) have been found in a high percentage of fruit bats (*Pteropus* spp.) in Australia, (Williamson et al., 2000). Seropositive fruit bats have been found from Darwin in north central Australia to Melbourne in southeastern Australia. A sudden outbreak of Hendra virus (HeV) infection occurred in September 1994 among Thoroughbred horses in a training complex in Brisbane, Australia, wherein thirteen horses and their trainer died (Murray et al., 1995a; 1995b). A second apparently unrelated outbreak of the HeV infection claimed two horses and their owner near Mackay, about 1000 km north of Brisbane (Rogers et al., 1996; Hooper et al., 1996 and O'Sullivan et al., 1997; Field et al., 2007b). This outbreak had actually occurred before the Hendra events and was later retrospectively identified in 1995. A single fatal equine case occurred near Cairns in North Queensland in January 1999 (Field et al., 2000; Hooper et al., 2000). Most of the cases in horses have occurred in Queensland, but one infected horse was reported from New

South Wales in 2006. HeV causes outbreaks of acute respiratory disease and high (up to 75%) mortality. In 2008 disease outbreak, infected horses had primarily neurological symptoms.

Antibodies to Hendra virus have also been detected in fruit bats in Papua New Guinea. Antibodies to henipaviruses have been found in pteropodid bats in Madagascar and Cambodia, but the circulating viruses could be distinct from Hendra or Nipah virus. Recently, Hayman et al. (2008) have detected antibodies in sera of Ghanaian fruit bats (*Eidolon helvum*) against both Nipah (39%, 95% confidence interval [CI]: 27–51%) and Hendra (22%, 95% [CI]: 11–33%) viruses using a multiplexed Luminex microsphere assay, indicating the presence of henipavirus within West Africa. Henipavirus antibodies have been found in bats (*Pteropus vampyrus*) of Indonesia (Sendow et al., 2006), various bat species in the genera Rousettus, Myotis, Miniopterus, and Hipposideros in China (Li et al., 2008) as well as in pteropid fruit bats (*Pteropus giganteus*) in northern India where Epstein et al. (2008), while testing forty-one bats for antibodies against Nipah and Hendra viruses, recorded twenty bats seropositive for Nipah virus, suggesting the circulation of virus in this species and extending the known distribution of henipaviruses in Asia westward by more than 1000 kilometers.

TRANSMISSION

Horses and humans seem to be spillover hosts for the Hendra virus. Fruit bats or flying foxes (genus *Pteropus*) appear to be the reservoir hosts. In fruit bats, Hendra virus has been isolated from blood, fetal tissues, and uterine fluids but not isolated from saliva, urine, or feces as yet. In 1996, a Hendra-like virus was isolated from the reproductive tract of a seemingly healthy pregnant, gray-headed flying fox (*Pteropus poliocephalus*). A range of tests showed the bat isolate to be indistinguishable from the Hendra virus isolated from horses (Halpin et al., 2000). However, no evidence of illness exists in flying foxes infected naturally or infected experimentally (Williamson et al., 2000) that can be attributed to infection with Hendra virus, supporting epidemiologic evidence that flying foxes are the probable hosts of Hendra virus. There has been no evidence of infection in humans even in those who have had close contact with injured bats (Selvey et al., 1995). Transmission from flying foxes to horses has not been demonstrated (Westbury, 2000); however, studies done on different species infected experimentally and flying foxes and horses infected naturally have indicated possible modes of transmission. Fogarty et al. (2008) measured the persistence of henipaviruses under various environmental conditions and thereby gained an insight into likely mechanisms of transmission. The sensitivity of henipaviruses to pH, temperature, and desiccation indicated a need for close contact between hosts for transmission to occur, although under ideal conditions henipaviruses can persist for extended periods facilitating vehicleborne transmission.

Virus has been isolated from the kidney, urine, and oral cavity of horses and from the kidney and urine of cats experimentally infected with Hendra virus. Horses have been experimentally infected by the naso-oral route, and cat-to-cat transmission and suspected cat-to-horse transmission have been reported (Westbury et al., 1995; Williamson et al., 1998). Infection and disease in reservoir and spillover hosts determine patterns of infectious agent availability and opportunities for infection, which then govern the process of transmission between susceptible species (Daniels et al., 2007). A series of further experimental inoculations of laboratory species followed, the first (Westbury et al., 1995) prompted by observations that Hendra virus was able to grow in a remarkable range of cell lines, including those derived from mammals, birds, reptiles, amphibians, and fish. Experimentally, cats and guinea pigs have been reported to develop the disease. The clinical syndrome in the cats was comparable to that seen in experimentally and naturally infected horses. Experimental infection of horses, however, did not produce the copious frothy nasal discharge that was evident in naturally occurring cases, so it cannot be ruled out that this discharge was a source of infection (Williamson et al., 1998; Hooper and Williamson, 2000). Very close contact between naturally affected horses is apparently necessary for transmission of disease.

CLINICAL SIGNS

The clinical course is very acute in horses with the time from onset of signs to death being only one to three days. Hendra virus in horses is predominantly pneumotropic and thus causes acute respiratory disease / pneumonia but may also be neurotropic resulting into encephalitis. The sick horses become anorexic, depressed, usually febrile (temperature up to 105.8°F or 41°C) with elevated respiratory rates after an incubation period of eight to eleven days (maximum sixteen days) and may show ataxia (Barclay and Paton, 2000). Signs of respiratory disease progress and copious frothy yellow nasal discharge are common terminal features. Affected animals tend not to cough. Some horses may also display neurological abnormalities. During initial outbreaks, the first human patient and equids with HeV infections died from acute respiratory disease, whereas the second human patient died from encephalitis (Mackenzie and Field, 2004). Under experimental conditions, the virus does not appear to be highly contagious between animal species, and urine is the most likely source of excretion and infection (Williamson et al., 1998).

PATHOGENESIS AND PATHOLOGY

Hendra virus in horses is predominantly pneumotropic but may also be neurotropic and, unlike morbilliviruses, has a specific tropism for vascular endothelial cells, regardless of route of challenge, generating pulmonary edema, interstitial pneumonia, or encephalitis (Hooper et al., 2001). HeV being enveloped infects cells by using membrane-anchored attachment (G) and fusion (F) glycoproteins. G possesses an N-terminal cytoplasmic tail, an external—membrane and proximal-stalk domain, and a C-terminal globular head that binds the recently identified receptors ephrinB2 and ephrinB3 (Lee et al., 2007; Negrete et al., 2007; Xu et al., 2008; Bossart and Broder, 2009). Receptor binding is presumed to induce conformational changes in G that subsequently trigger F-mediated fusion. (Bishop et al., 2008; Bossart and Broder, 2009). HeV and NiV are both able to infect cells expressing any of the ephrin-B2 and ephrin-B3 molecules (Bossart et al., 2008).

The most distinctive gross lesion in horse is a bilateral pulmonary edema characterized by gelatinous distention of subpleural lymphatics. The lungs are heavy and congested; the edema is more prominent in the ventral parts, and the lungs vary from a mottled yellowish brown to dark blue (Hooper et al., 1997). Spontaneous cases showed the airways usually filled with thick, sometimes blood-tinged foam; this lesion is not seen in the experimental cases (Murray et al., 1995a). Excess pleural and pericardial fluid, congested lymph nodes and visceral edema may also be seen. Scattered petechiae and ecchymoses may be found in the stomach, intestines, and perirenal tissues. Yellowing of the subcutaneous tissue is common.

In early infection, the microscopic vascular lesions range from edema and hemorrhage of vessel walls, fibrinoid degeneration with pyknotic nuclei in endothelial and tunica media cells, to the presence of numerous giant cells in the endothelium and sometimes the tunica media of affected both venules and arterioles. As the disease progresses, there is destruction of alveolar walls, with the appearance of alveolar and intravascular macrophages. The lesions in lungs are interstitial pneumonia, proteinaceous edema with pneumocyte and capillary degeneration (Murray et al., 1995a; Hooper and Williamson, 2000). Similar lesions were seen in the postmortem findings of the person (trainer) died of the disease (Selvey et al., 1995). Remarkably, the virus induces syncytial cells in blood vessel walls, especially in endothelium and behaves primarily as vasotropic and/or neurotropic, generating interstitial pneumonia or encephalitis (Hooper et al., 2001). Endothelial syncytium is a pathognomonic feature of henipaviral infections which is mediated by the fusion (F) and attachment (G) envelope glycoproteins of the virus (Lee et al., 2007). Nonsuppurative encephalomyelitis has been seen in some horses

(Hooper et al., 1997; Williamson et al., 1998). Virus can be located in endothelial cells by immunofluorescence, and syncytial cells may also be seen in blood vessel walls, confirming the vascular tropism of HeV (Murray et al., 1995b). Intracytoplasmic inclusion bodies may be present as characteristic nucleocapsids have been seen in the cytoplasm by electron microscopy (Hyatt and Selleck, 1996; Hooper et al., 1997). The virus becomes more widely distributed in various tissues throughout the body, presumably as a result of a leukocyte-associated viremia. In addition to its vascular tropism, HeV can also be neurotropic, causing neuronal necrosis and focal gliosis (Kahn and Line, 2008). The virus has been demonstrated in the vascular endothelium of subarachnoid and cerebral vessels and also affects the vasculature of the renal glomerulus and pelvis, lamina propria of the stomach, spleen, various lymph nodes, and myocardium.

NATURAL INFECTIONS IN HORSES AND HUMANS (ZOONOSES)

Hendra viruses are highly pathogenic in humans with case fatality rates of 40–70% (Eaton et al., 2005). The virus was the cause of fatal infections of horses and humans in Australia in 1994, 1999, and 2004 (Murray et al., 1995a, 1995b; Field et al., 2000, 2007b). During initial outbreaks in Australia, few horses died acutely showing clinical signs of fever, facial swelling, severe respiratory distress, ataxia, and copious frothy, sometimes blood-stained nasal discharge. Nonfatal cases that retained mild neurological signs and other horses found seroconverted without demonstrable clinical signs were all subsequently euthanized (Murray et al., 1995a; Baldock et al., 1996; Douglas et al., 1997). The trainer and a stable attendant fell ill with a severe influenza-like illness within a week; the trainer was hospitalized and subsequently died after respiratory and renal failure. Hendra virus infection was demonstrated in both cases (Selvey et al., 1995). In October 1995 outbreak at Mackay, two horses and a stud owner showing relapsing encephalitis died of the HeV infection (Hooper et al., 1996; Rogers et al., 1996).

Serological studies during Brisbane and Mackay incidents revealed that in-contact domestic animals (horses, cattle, goats, pigs, dogs, cats, and poultry) were not the source of infection. Hendra virus infection was not considered to be highly contagious in horses and probably required direct contact or mechanical transmission of infectious body fluids for natural transmission to occur (Baldock et al., 1996; Rogers et al., 1996).

The third focus of Hendra virus infection was reported in January 1999 in a horse near Cairns in north Queensland showing signs of inappetence, depression, and swelling of the face, lips, and neck; the case deteriorated with copious yellow frothy nasal discharge and became recumbent and had to be euthanized. A companion horse was found unaffected on clinical and serological examinations, and no human cases were involved (Field et al., 2000; 2007a). In October 2004, the death of a ten-year-old Thoroughbred gelding was reported after an acute illness (Field et al., 2007b). Hendra virus was not considered as a differential diagnosis at the time, and no samples were taken to enable a definitive retrospective diagnosis. The veterinarian who performed necropsy and his two assistants showed influenza-like symptoms after eigth days. After two weeks, the veterinarian was found positive for anti-HeV antibodies by immunofluorescent, serum-neutralization, and ELISA tests. The death of above horse was regarded as a probable case of Hendra virus infection communicated to the veterinarian (Hanna et al., 2006; Field et al., 2007b). A fifth index case occurred on December 1, 2004, in a Thoroughbred gelding. On the basis of typical gross and microscopic pathological lesions, a diagnosis of HeV virus infection was made and confirmed through viral antigen detection by immunohistochemical staining and viral RNA detection by polymerase chain reaction (PCR). Eighteen people, including the two veterinarians with possible at-risk exposure, were found negative for HeV antibodies on serial blood tests. Many epidemiological features were common on all five occasions (Field et al., 2000and Field et al., 2007b). In July 2008, the deadly Hendra virus resurfaced in Queensland, with two unrelated outbreaks at Brisbane and Proserpine. In this recent 2008 episode of He V infection in horses, one veterinarian died.

Thus, in the last fifteen years, six people have become infected with Hendra virus, and three have died as a result of the disease. In addition to the initial case in 1994, a farmer from Mackay died in 1995, and a Brisbane vet passed away in August 2008. There have also been eleven clusters of Hendra virus infection recorded in horses since the virus was first identified (CSIRO, 2008).

Flying foxes have been demonstrated to be a natural host of Hendra virus and play role in disease transmission (Halpin et al., 2000; Field et al., 2000; 2007a; 2007b). Incubation periods of eight to sixteen days (Baldock et al., 1996) and four to ten days (Murray et al., 1995b) have been reported in natural and experimental HeV infections in horses, respectively (Hall and Richards, 2000).

Though the HeV disease outbreaks have only been limited to Australia, however, recent reports of many workers have indicated that the henipavirus infections, including Nipah virus in pigs and Hendra virus in horses, are probably more widespread than at presently known, and seeing their high zoonotic potential, these viruses have been declared to be different and dangerous pathogens (Dutkiewicz, 2004; McCormack, 2005; Eaton et al., 2006; Harit et al., 2006; Epstein et al., 2008; Wild, 2009).

DIAGNOSIS

Clinical findings and gross pathological changes could be suggestive of the Hendra virus infection in the endemic areas. HeV infection can be diagnosed by virus isolation, detection of nucleic acids or antigens, or by serologic tests such as serum neutralization test (SNT), enzyme-linked immunosorbant assay (ELISA), and indirect fluorescent antibody tests (IFAT) (Studdert, 2007; Pavlin et al., 2008). HeV is classified as biosafety level 4 (BSL-4) agent as it is a dangerous human pathogen with a high case fatality rate, and for which there is no vaccination or effective antiviral treatment. Due to the high-risk consequences of human infection in the laboratory, BSL-4–containment laboratory facilities need to be highly and strictly followed.

Hendra virus can be isolated in a number of cell lines including Vero, BHK–21, MDCK, RK13, LLC-MK2, and MRC5 cells. It can also be cultured in embryonated chicken eggs, but culture in cells is preferred due to convenience. This virus can be identified in cultures by immunostaining or virus neutralization. Isolation is especially relevant in any new case or outbreak, particularly in new geographical areas or countries where HeV infection has not been previously documented. Implication of wildlife species as natural hosts of the viruses requires positive serology, polymerase chain reaction (PCR), or virus isolation from wild-caught animals (Daniels et al., 2007). In live animals, virus isolation can be attempted from the blood, nasal swabs, urine, or tissues; however, this virus is more likely to be recovered from the lung, liver, spleen, or brain at necropsy.

In serological tests including virus neutralization, cross-reactions can occur between Hendra and Nipah viruses; however, reactions to Hendra virus can be identified by comparative neutralization tests. Titers may not be detectable until ten to fourteen days after infection in horses; low-to-moderate titers can be seen in some bats, and all infected bats may not seroconvert. A virus isolate that reacts with anti-HeV and/or anti-NiV antisera in an immunofluorescence assay is considered to be serologically identical to either HeV or NiV if it displays the same sensitivity to neutralization by anti-HeV and anti-NiV antisera as HeV or NiV. Anti-HeV antiserum neutralizes HeV at an approximately fourfold-greater dilution than that which neutralizes NiV to the same extent. Conversely, anti-NiV antiserum neutralizes NiV approximately four times more efficiently than HeV (Chua et al., 2000). Crameri et al. (2002) developed a rapid immune plaque assay for the detection of HeV and NiV and antivirus antibodies.

Virus quantification procedures should be conducted at biosafety level 4 (BSL-4) facility. A new version of the differential neutralization test has been recently described, which avoids the use of infectious virus by the use of ephrin-B2–bound biospheres (Bossart et al., 2007). Although the test has yet to be formally validated, it appears to have the potential to be a screening tool for use in countries without BSL-4 facilities. Chen et al. (2006) used an antibody assay for henipaviruses using a recombinant Nipah virus nucleocapsid (N) protein. Juozapaitis et al. (2007) also successfully cloned and expressed the genes encoding HeV nucleocapsid proteins and detected the expressed protein by sera derived from fruit bats, humans, and horses infected with HeV. The use of recombinant protein as the ELISA antigen instead of inactivated virus antigens is advantageous for countries where BSL-4 facility is not available to handle this group of zoonotic viruses. Electron or immunoelectron microscopy can also be helpful for detecting HeV (Hyatt et al., 2001).

Viral antigens can be detected by immunoperoxidase or immunofluorescence assays on formalin-fixed tissues. Because HeV antigens may be cleared from the lung early in the infection, a variety of tissues should be submitted for immunohistochemistry (Daniels et al., 2001). Ideally, samples would include lung, mediastinal lymph nodes, spleen, and kidney, as well as the brain at various levels; however, all these samples should be collected only if the necropsy conditions can ensure the safety of the personnel. Whenever possible, samples of the uterus, placenta, and fetal tissues should also be collected from pregnant animals. A range of antisera to HeV and NiV may be used in immunohistochemistry, but rabbit antisera to plaque-purified HeV and NiV are particularly useful. The Nipah Virus Pathology Working Group has described a detection system for the infection (Wong et al., 2002). A biotin-streptavidin, peroxidase-linked detection system has also been used successfully (Hooper et al., 2001). Recently, Xiao et al. (2008) developed monoclonal antibodies (mAbs) with recombinant nucleocapsid protein (N) of HeV, which were able to specifically recognize HeV antigens by immunohistochemical staining of lung tissue sections of a horse experimentally infected with HeV.

The complete genomes of both HeV and NiV have been sequenced (Wang et al., 2001), and PCR-based methods, including RT-PCR, have been used on fresh and formalin-fixed tissues to detect virus and are being validated in a number of laboratories (OIE, 2008). Smith et al. (2001) reported the development of a rapid and sensitive one-tube RT-PCR assay using a fluorogenic (TaqMan) probe to improve the diagnosis of HeV infection. A particularly sensitive and useful approach to the detection of *Henipavirus* genome in specimens is real-time PCR, which has the biosafety advantage of not propagating live infectious virus (Mungall et al., 2006). These findings could be promising for the development of improved, efficient, and cost-effective HeV diagnosis system.

DIFFERENTIAL DIAGNOSIS

African horse sickness can clinically mimic Hendra virus infection and should be considered in the differential diagnosis. Other causes of sudden death that must be ruled out include anthrax, botulism, and certain other infections such as shipping fever, equine influenza, peracute equine herpesvirus 1 infection, and plant or chemical poisoning (CDC, 1999; Kahn and Line, 2008). In people, serious influenza-like signs predominate.

PREVENTION AND CONTROL

Other than supportive therapy, there is no treatment for Hendra virus infections. In some cases, surviving horses have been euthanized due to uncertainties about virus persistence. There are currently no specific antiviral drugs and neither any vaccine available for the disease caused by Nipah and Hendra viruses. Specific control program has not been considered or implemented in view of the limited transmissibility of the virus under natural conditions and the sporadic and infrequent nature of outbreaks of the disease. The disease outbreaks in Australia were handled and controlled by sacrificing all known infected horses and enforcing movement restrictions. Whenever possible, contact between horses and bat urine or uterine fluids should be avoided (Kahn and Line, 2008). Aljofan et al. (2008) have recently described a high throughput screening method using a chemiluminescent immunodetection assay for direct assessment of live henipavirus antiviral drug activity by assessing the efficacies of broad spectrum antiviral ribavirin and an experimental fusion-inhibitory peptide.

In horses, prevention is based on minimizing exposure to infected bats, their tissues and secretions. All index cases have occurred in horses, so far, stabled in open paddocks. In areas where Hendra virus infections may occur, horses should be stabled at night, and horse paddocks should not contain food or roosting trees favored by fruit bats. Feed bins and water troughs should not be placed under trees where bats might be found. Horses may also be stabled full-time or moved away from areas of high bat activity during the highest-risk months (August to January). Any dead fruit bats should be removed and destroyed by burning or burial; human exposure should be prevented while this is done. Horses that develop severe respiratory disease should be considered contagious, and standard infection control measures should be taken to avoid spreading the virus on fomites (Murray et al., 1995a; OIE, 2008). Quarantines and strict hygiene have been effective in containing past outbreaks. The low rate of horse-to-horse transmission also aids control.

Current strategies for the management of henipaviruses are directed at minimizing contact with the natural hosts, monitoring identified intermediate hosts, improving biosecurity on farms, and better disease recognition and diagnosis. Investigation of the emergence and ecology of henipaviruses warrants a broad cross-disciplinary ecosystem health approach that recognizes the critical linkages between human activity, ecological change, and livestock and human health (Field et al., 2004, 2007a).

Necropsies should be performed by trained personnel using personal protective equipment (see "Human Prevention" section). The instruments used at necropsy should be soaked in disinfectant at the site and then sealed in strong plastic clinical waste bags. Instruments should be cleaned carefully to avoid the generation of aerosols, then autoclaved. Government authorities should be consulted for the most appropriate disposal method for carcasses; deep burial has been used in the past. Contaminated areas should be cleaned and disinfected with agents such as anhydrous sodium carbonate at 40 g/L, hydrated sodium carbonate at 100 g/L, or citric acid at 2 g/L. Precaution should be taken to avoid generating aerosols or splashing material during disinfection (OIE, 2008).

In probable cases, susceptible species should not be allowed into the area until Hendra virus infection has been ruled out. If any horses are already present, they should be examined daily for signs of disease and their temperature taken if they show any signs of illness. If HeV infection is confirmed, the recommendations are that these precautions remain in place for twenty-eight days from the initial signs in the first case or twenty-two days from the death of the last case, whichever occurs later. Vaccines are not available for effective prophylaxis.

PROSPECTS FOR THE DEVELOPMENT OF ANTIVIRAL DRUGS AND VACCINE

For henipaviruses, the main research focus is on understanding virus receptors and attachment, fusion, and entry processes with the host cell, thus evolve mechanisms for targeting the very early stages of the infection process, which could make feasibility of the development of possible vaccine candidates and potential antiviral therapeutics (Bossart and Broder, 2006). Hendra viruses infect cells by a pH-independent membrane-fusion event mediated by their attachment (G) and fusion (F) glycoproteins. It has been suggested that HeV-soluble glycoprotein (sG) could offer useful receptor identification strategies and vaccine development goals for control of henipavirus infections (Bonaparte et al., 2005; Bossart et al., 2005; Lee et al., 2007). Galectin-1 (gal-1), an endogenous lectin secreted by a variety of cell types, having antiviral activity, may also augment the innate immune response against henipaviruses (Levroney et al., 2005). Recently, Xu et al. (2008) suggested the targeting of interactions between NiV glycoprotein (G) and ephrin-B2 and—B3 to disrupt viral entry. Utility of monoclonal antibodies (mAbs) are also being explored to counter HeV and NiV threats (Zhu et al., 2006a, b; Zhu et al., 2008; Prabakaran et al., 2009). Human monoclonal antibodies, m101 and m102.4, showed exceptional potency against Nipah and Hendra viruses, suggesting that these have potential for the treatment of diseases caused by henipaviruses. The monoclonal-antibody approach could be also used for prophylaxis and diagnosis and as a research reagent for these deadly pathogens. As the virus-encoded V proteins are important factors for host evasion, they represent logical targets for therapeutics directed against henipavirus epidemics (Rodriguez and Horvath, 2004). The findings of Mungall et al. (2008) demonstrating that RNA interference (RNAi) effectively inhibits henipavirus replication in vitro is also a novel approach and may provide an effective therapy for HeV and NiV too. Thus, scientific community is on the way to develop suitable antiviral and vaccine candidates for the prevention and control of HeV epidemics.

CONCLUSION

Hendra virus (HeV) is a new member of the new genus *Henipavirus* in the family Paramyxoviridae, along with a related member Nipah virus (NiV). Formerly known as equine morbillivirus, HeV has been reported to affect horses only from Australia, causing outbreaks of acute respiratory disease and high mortality; the first outbreak occurred in 1994, and the most recent one was in 2008. In horses, the clinical course is very acute with the time from onset of signs to death being only one to three days. Fruit bats act as reservoir hosts and play role in disease transmission. Very close contact between naturally affected horses is apparently necessary for transmission of disease.

There is limited information about HeV presence in other parts of the world. Recently, antibodies to henipaviruses and/or Hendra virus have also been detected in bats in few other regions outside Australia, indicating that HeV probably might expand its region, and so it is important to have an intense disease monitoring. Diagnostic tests—viz, SNT, ELISA, and FAT—are available for HeV detection, and the potent molecular tools of PCR, RT-PCR, and real-time PCR have also been developed. No vaccination or effective antiviral treatment is available for HeV infection; however, continuous studies are going on to evolve suitable candidates, which could serve as potent antiviral agent and vaccine for henipaviruses, including both HeV and NiV. Recently, utility of monoclonal antibodies, having high potency against infectious virus, have been demonstrated which could serve the purpose of developing a therapeutic agent and could be also used for prophylaxis and diagnosis and as a research reagent. The virus-encoded protein V also represents logical targets for probable therapeutics. Also, RNA-interference (RNAi) strategies could also dispense a novel therapy approach for combating the highly lethal and zoonotic pathogens like Nipah and Hendra virus.

Though, Hendra is a rare disease; however, the severity of disease and the causative virus (HeV), being a BSL-4 pathogen, warrants appropriate and high-level biosafety measures. Also, though the virus does not seem to be highly contagious, a new variant, if it appears, could behave differently, and we should be ready for that time, for which monitoring and surveillance for this virus need to be strengthened and along with rightly supported research directions need to be further advanced for developing efficient and safer diagnostics, antiviral agents, and vaccine candidates.

REFERENCES

1. Aljofan, M., Porotto, M., Moscona, A. and Mungall B. A. 2008. Development and validation of a chemiluminescent immunodetection assay amenable to high throughput screening of antiviral drugs for Nipah and Hendra virus. *J. Virological Methods* 149:12–19.
2. Allworth, A., O'Sullivan, J., Selvey, L. and Sheridan, J. 1995. Equine morbillivirus in Queensland. *Communicable Dis. Intelligence* 19:575.
3. Baldock, F. C., Douglas, I. C., Halpin, K., Field, H., Young, P. L. and Black, P. F. 1996. Epidemiological investigations into the 1994 equine morbillivirus outbreaks in Queensland, Australia. *Sing. Vet. J.* 20:57–61.
4. Barclay, A. J. and Paton, D. J. 2000. Hendra (equine morbillivirus). *Vet J.* 160:169–176.
5. Bishop, K. A., Hickey, A. C., Khetawat, D., Patch, J. R., Bossart, K. N., Zhu, Z., Wang, L. F., Dimitrov, D. S. and Broder, C. C. 2008. Residues in the stalk domain of the hendra virus g glycoprotein modulate conformational changes associated with receptor binding. *J Virol.* 82:11398–11409.
6. Bonaparte, M. I., Dimitrov, A. S., Bossart, K. N., Crameri, G., Mungall, B. A., Bishop, K. A., Choudhry, V., Dimitrov, D. S., Wang, L. F., Eaton, B. T. and Broder, C. C. 2005. Ephrin-B2 ligand is a functional receptor for Hendra virus and Nipah virus. *Proc Natl Acad Sci.* 102:10652–10657.
7. Bossart, K. N., Crameri, G., Dimitrov, A. S., Mungall, B. A., Feng, Y. R., Patch, J. R., Choudhary, A., Wang, L. F., Eaton, B. T. and Broder, C. C. 2005. Receptor binding, fusion inhibition, and induction of cross-reactive neutralizing antibodies by a soluble G glycoprotein of Hendra virus. *J Virol.* 79:6690–6702.
8. Bossart, K. N. and Broder, C. C. 2006. Developments towards effective treatments for Nipah and Hendra virus infection. *Expert Rev. Anti-infective Ther.* 4:43–55.
9. Bossart, K. N., McEachern, J. A., Hickey, A. C., Choudhry, V., Dimitrov, D. S., Eaton, B. T. and Wang, L. F. 2007. Neutralization assays for differential henipavirus serology using Bio-Plex protein array systems. *J. Virol. Methods* 142:29–40.

10. Bossart, K. N., Tachedjian, M., McEachern, J. A., Crameri, G., Zhu, Z., Dimitrov, D. S., Broder, C. C. and Wang, L. F. 2008. Functional studies of host-specific ephrin-B ligands as henipavirus receptors. *Virology* 372:*357–371.*

11. Bossart, K. N., and Broder, C. C. 2009. Paramyxovirus entry. In *Viral entry into host cells*, ed. S. Pohlmann and G. Simmons. Austin, TX: Landes Bioscience.

12. CDC-OC. 1999. Facts about Hendra Virus: CDC-OC, April 9, 1999 CDC, Division of Media Relations (404) 639–3286.

13. Chen, J., Yu, M., Morrissy, C., Zhao, Y., Meehan, G., Sun, Y., Wang, Q., Zhang, W., Wang, L. and Wang, Z. 2006. A comparative indirect ELISA for the detection of henipavirus antibodies based on a recombinant nucleocapsid protein expressed in *Escherichia coli*. *J. Virol. Methods* 136:273–276.

14. Chua, K. B., Bellini, W. J., Rota, P. A., Harcourt, B. H., Tamin, A., Lam, S. K., Ksiazek, T. G., Rollin, P. E., Zaki, S. R., Shieh, W. J., Goldsmith, C. S., Gubler, D. J., Roehrig, J. T., Eaton, B., Gould, A. R., Olson, J., Field, H., Daniels, P., Ling, A. E., Peters, C. J., Anderson, L. J. and Mahy, B. W. J. 2000. Nipah virus: A recently emergent deadly paramyxovirus. *Science* 288:1432–1435.

15. Crameri, G., Wang, L. F., Morrissy, C., White, J. and Eaton, B. T. 2002. A rapid immune plaque assay for the detection of Hendra and Nipah viruses and anti-virus antibodies. *J. Virol. Methods* 99:41–51.

16. CSIRO. 2008. *Feature article: Hendra Virus. http://www.csiro.au/science/HendraVirus.html.*

17. Daniels, P., Ksiazek, T. and Eaton, B. T. 2001. Laboratory diagnosis of Nipah and Hendra virus infections. *Microbes Infect.* 3:289–295.

18. Daniels, P., Halpin, K., Hyatt, A. and Middleton, D. 2007. Infection and disease in reservoir and spillover hosts: Determinants of pathogen emergence. *Curr. Top. Immunol. Microbiol.* 315:113–131.

19. Douglas, I. C., Baldock, F. C. and Black, P. 1997. Outbreak investigation of an emerging disease (equine morbillivirus). Epidemiol Sante Anim—Proc. of 8th ISVEE Conference, 04.081–004.008.083, Paris.

20. Dutkiewicz, J. 2004. Occupational bio hazards: Current issues. *Med. Pr.* 55:31–40.

21. Eaton, B. T., Broder, C. C. and Wang, L. F. 2005. Hendra and Nipah viruses: Pathogenesis and therapeutics. *Curr. Mol. Med.* 5:805–816.

22. Eaton, B. T., Broder, C. C., Middleton, D. and Wang, L. F. 2006. Hendra and Nipah viruses: Different and dangerous. *Nat. Rev. Microbiol.* 4:23–35.

23. Epstein, J. H., Prakash, V., Smith, C. S., Daszak, P., McLaughlin, A. B., Meehan, G., Field, H. E. and Cunningham, A. A. 2008. Henipavirus infection in fruit bats (Pteropus giganteus), India. *Emerg. Infect. Dis.* 14:1309–1311.

24. Field, H., Barratt, P., Hughes, R., Shield, J. and Sullivan, N. 2000. A fatal case of Hendra virus infection in a horse in north Queensland: Clinical and epidemiological features. *Aust. Vet. J.* 78:279–280.

25. Field, H., Mackenzie, J. and Daszak, P. 2004. Novel viral encephalitides associated with bats (Chiroptera): Host management strategies. *Arch. Virol. Suppl.* 18:113–121.

26. Field, H. E., Mackenzie, J. S. and Daszak, P. 2007a. Henipaviruses: Emerging paramyxoviruses associated with fruit bats. *Curr Top Microbiol Immunol.* 315:133–159.

27. Field, H. E., Breed, A. C., Shield, J., Hedlefs, R. M., Pittard, K., Pott, B. and Summers, P. M. 2007b. Epidemiological perspectives on Hendra virus infection in horses and flying foxes. *Aust. Vet. J.* 85:268–270.

28. Fogarty, R., Halpin, K., Hyatt, A. D., Daszak, P. and Mungall, B. A. 2008. Henipavirus susceptibility to environmental variables. *Virus Res.* 132:140–144.

29. Gould, A. R. 1996. Comparison of the deduced matrix and fusion protein sequences of equine morbillivirus with cognate genes of the Paramyxoviridae. *Virus Res.* 43:17–31.

30. Hall, L. and Richards, G. 2000. Flying foxes: Fruit and blossom bats of Australia. In *Australian natural history series*, ed. T. J. Dawson. Sydney: University of New South Wales Press Ltd.

31. Halpin, K., Young, P., Field, H. and Mackenzie, J. 2000. Isolation of Hendra virus from pteropid bats: A natural reservoir of Hendra virus. *J. Gen. Virol.* 81:1927–1932.

32. Hance, P., Garnotel, E. and Morillon, *M. 2006. Chiroptera and zoonosis: An emerging problem on all five continents. Med. Trop. (Mars)* 66:119–124.

33. Hanna, J. N., McBride, W. J., Brookes, D. L., Shield, J., Taylor, C. T., Smith, I. L., Craig, S. B. and Smith G. A. 2006. Hendra virus infection in a veterinarian. *Med. J. Aust.* 185:562–564.

34. Harit, A. K., Ichhpujani, R. L., Gupta, S., Gill, K. S., Lal, S., Ganguly, N. K. and Agarwal, S. P. 2006. Nipah/Hendra virus outbreak in Siliguri, West Bengal, India in 2001. *Indian J. Med. Res.* 123:553–560.

35. Hayman, D. T. S., Suu-Ire, R., Breed, A. C., McEachern, J. A., Wang, L., Wood, J. L. N. and Cunningham A. A. 2008. Evidence of henipavirus Infection in West African fruit bats. *PLoS ONE* 3:e2739.

36. Hooper, P. T. and Williamson, M. M. 2000. Hendra and Nipah virus infections. *Vet. Clin. North Am. Equine Pract.* 16:597–603.

37. Hooper, P. T., Gould, A. R., Russell, G. M., Kattenbelt, J. A. and Mitchell, G. 1996. The retrospective diagnosis of a second outbreak of equine morbillivirus infection. *Aust. Vet. J.* 74:244–245.

38. Hooper, P. T., Ketterer, P. J., Hyatt, A. D. and Russel, G. M. 1997. Lesions of experimental equine morbillivirus pneumonia in horses. *Vet. Pathol.* 34:312–322.

39. Hooper, P. T., Gould, A. R., Hyatt, A. D., Braun, M. A., Kattenbelt, J. A., Hengstberger, S. G. and Westbury, H. A. 2000. Identification and molecular characterization of Hendra virus in a horse in Queensland. *Aus. Vet. J.* 78:281–282.

40. Hooper, P., Zaki, S., Daniels, P. and Middleton, D. 2001. Comparative pathology of the diseases caused by Hendra and Nipah viruses. *Microbes Infect.* 3:315–322.

41. Hyatt, A. D. and Selleck, P. W. 1996. Ultrastructure of equine morbillivirus. *Virus Res.* 43:1–15.

42. Hyatt, A. D., Zaki, S. R., Goldsmith, C. S., Wise, T. G. and Hengstberger, S. G. 2001. Ultrastructure of Hendra virus and Nipah virus within cultured cells and host animals. *Microbes Infect.* 3:297–306.

43. ICTV. 2000. *Virus taxonomy classification and nomenclature of viruses: Seventh report of the International Committee on Taxonomy of Viruses.* Sydney: Academic Press.

44. Juozapaitis, M., Serva, A., Zvirbliene, A., Slibinskas, R., Staniulis, J., Sasnauskas, K., Shiell, B. J., Wang, L. F. and Michalski, W. P. 2007. Generation of henipavirus nucleocapsid proteins in yeast *Saccharómyces cerevisiae. Virus Res.* 124:95–102.

45. Kahn, C. M. and Line, S. 2008. The Merck veterinary manual [online]. Whitehouse Station, NJ: Merck and Co., Inc.; 2008. *Respiratory diseases of horses. Hendra virus infection.* http://www.merckvetmanual.com/mvm/index.jsp?cfile=htm/bc/53100.htm (accessed March 20, 2009).

46. Lee, B. 2007. Envelope-receptor interactions in Nipah virus pathobiology. *Ann. N Y. Acad. Sci.* 1102:51–65.

47. Levroney, E. L., Aguilar, H. C., Fulcher, J. A., Kohatsu, L., Pace, K. E., Pang, M., Gurney, K. B., Baum, L. G. and Lee, B. 2005. Novel innate immune functions for galectin-1: Galectin-1 inhibits cell fusion by Nipah virus envelope glycoproteins and augments dendritic cell secretion of proinflammatory cytokines. *J. Immunol.* 175:413–420.

48. Li, Y., Wang, J., Hickey, A. C., Zhang, Y., Li, Y., Wu, Y., Zhang, H., Yuan, J., Han, Z., McEachern, J., Broder, C. C., Wang, L. F. and Shi, Z. 2008. Antibodies to Nipah or Nipah-like viruses in bats, China. *Emerg. Infect. Dis.* 14:1974–1976.

49. Mackenzie, J. S. and Field, H. E. 2004. Emerging encephalitogenic viruses: Lyssaviruses and henipaviruses transmitted by frugivorous bats. *Arch. Virol. Suppl.* 18:97–111.

50. Madić, J. 2001. Zoonoses caused by new viruses in the Paramyxoviridae family. *Lijec. Vjesn.* 123:141–145.

51. Mackenzie, J. S. 2005. Emerging zoonotic encephalitis viruses: Lessons from Southeast Asia and Oceania. *J. Neurovirol.* 11:434–440.

52. Mackenzie, J. S., Field, H. E. and Guyatt, K. J. 2003. Managing emerging diseases borne by fruit bats (flying foxes), with particular reference to henipaviruses and Australian bat lyssavirus. *J. Appl. Microbiol.* 94 Suppl:59S-69S.

53. McCormack, *J. G.* 2005. Hendra and Nipah viruses: New zoonotically-acquired human pathogens. *Respir. Care Clin. N. Am.* 11:59–66.

54. Mungall, B. A., Middleton, D., Crameri, G., Bingham, J., Halpin K., Russell, G., Green, D., McEachern, J., Pritchard, L. I., Eaton, B. T., Wang, L. F., Bossart, K. N. and Broder, C. C. 2006. Feline model of acute nipah virus infection and protection with a soluble glycoprotein-based subunit vaccine. *J. Virol.* 80:12293–12302.

55. Mungall, B. A., Schopman, N. C. T., Lambeth, L. S. and Doran, T. J. 2008. Inhibition of henipavirus infection by RNA interference. *Antiviral Res.* 80:324–331.

56. Murray, K., Rogers, R., Selvey, L., Selleck, P., Hyatt, A., Gould, A., Gleeson, L., Hooper, P. and Westbury, H. 1995a. A novel morbillivirus pneumonia of horses and its transmission to humans. *Emerg. Infect. Dis.* 1:31–33.

57. Murray, K., Selleck, P., Hooper, P., Hyatt, A., Gould, A., Gleeson, L., Westbury, H., Hiley, L., Selvey, L., Rodwell, B. and Ketterer, P. 1995b. A morbillivirus that caused fatal disease in horses and humans. *Science* 268:94–97.

58. Negrete, O. A., Chu, D., Aguilar, H. C. and Lee, *B.* 2007. Single amino acid changes in the Nipah and Hendra virus attachment glycoproteins distinguish ephrinB2 from ephrinB3 usage. *J. Virol.* 81:10804–10814.

59. OIE. 2008. Hendra and Nipah Virus diseases. In *OIE Terrestrial Manual.* Ch. 2.9.6, 1227–1237.

60. O'Sullivan, J. D., Allworth, A. M., Paterson, D. L., Snow, T. M., Boots, R., Gleeson, L. J., Gould, A. R., Hyatt, A. D. and Bradfield, J. 1997. Fatal encephalitis due to novel paramyxovirus transmitted from horses. *Lancet* 349:93–95.

61. Pavlin, J. A., Hickey, A. C., Ulbrandt, N., Chan, Y. P., Endy, T. P., Boukhvalova, M. S., Chunsuttiwat, S., Nisalak, A., Libraty, D. H., Green, S., Rothman, A. L., Ennis, F. A., Jarman, R., Gibbons, R. V. and Broder, C. C. 2008. Human metapneumovirus reinfection among children in Thailand determined by an enzyme-linked immunosorbent assay using purified soluble fusion protein. *J. Infect. Dis.* 198:836–842.

62. Patch, J. R., Han, Z., McCarthy, S. E., Yan, L., Wang, L. F., Harty, R. N. and Broder, C. C. 2008. The YPLGVG sequence of the Nipah virus matrix protein is required for budding. *Virol. J.* 5:137.

63. Prabakaran, P., Zhu, Z., Xiao, X., Biragyn, A., Dimitrov, A. S., Broder, C. C. and Dimitrov, D. S. 2009. Potent human monoclonal antibodies against SARS CoV, Nipah and Hendra viruses. *Expert Opin. Biol. Ther.* 9:355–368.

64. Rodriguez, J. J. and Horvath, C. M. 2004. Host evasion by emerging paramyxoviruses: Hendra virus and Nipah virus v proteins inhibit interferon signaling. *Viral Immunol.* 17:210–219.

65. Rogers, R. J., Douglas, I. C., Baldock, F. C., Glanville, R. J., Seppanen, K. T., Gleeson, L. J., Selleck, P. N. and Dunn, K. J. 1996. Investigation of a second focus of equine morbillivirus infection in coastal Queensland. *Aust. Vet. J.* 74:243–244.

66. Selvey, L., Wells, R. M., McCormack, J. G., Ansford, A. J., Murray, P. K., Rogers, R. J., Lavercombe, P. S., Selleck, P. and Sheridan, J. W. 1995. Infection of humans and horses by a newly described morbillivirus. *Med. J. Aust.* 162:642–645.

67. Sendow, I., Field, H. E., Curran, J., Darminto, Morrissy, C., Meehan, G., Buick, T. and Daniels, P. 2006. Henipavirus in Pteropus vampyrus bats, Indonesia. *Emerg. Infect. Dis.* 12:711–712.

68. Smith, I. L., Halpin, K., Warrilow, D. and Smith, G. A. 2001. Development of a fluorogenic RT-PCR assay (TaqMan) for the detection of Hendra virus. *J. Virol. Methods* 98:33–40.

69. Studdert, M. J. 2007. Miscellaneous viral respiratory diseases. In *Equine infectious diseases,* ed. D. C. Sellon and M. T. Long, chapter 16, 171–180. Philadelphia, USA: Saunders, Elsevier Inc.

70. Wang, L. F., Yu, M., Hansson, E., Shiell, B., Michalski, W. P. and Eaton, B. T. 2000. The exceptionally large genome of Hendra virus: Support for creation of a new genus within the family Paramyxoviridae. *J. Virol.* 74:9972–9979.

71. Wang, L. F., Harcourt, B. H., Yu, M., Tamin, A., Rota, P. A., Bellini, W. J. and Eaton, B. T. 2001. Molecular biology of Hendra and Nipah viruses. *Microbes Infect.* 3:279–287.

72. Weese, J. S. 2002. A review of equine zoonotic diseases: Risks in veterinary medicine. *Proceedings of the Annual Convention of the AAEP 2002* 48:362–369.
73. Westbury, H. A. 2000. Hendra virus disease in horses. *Rev. Sci. Tech.* 19:151–159.
74. Westbury, H. A., Hooper, P. T., Selleck, P. W. and Murray, P. K. 1995. Equine morbillivirus pneumonia: Susceptibility of laboratory animals to the virus. *Aust. Vet. J.* 72:278–279.
75. Wild, T. F. 2009. Henipaviruses: A new family of emerging Paramyxoviruses. *Pathol. Biol. (Paris)* 57:188–196.
76. Williamson, M. M., Hooper, P. T., Selleck, P. W., Gleeson, L. J., Daniels, P. W., Westbury, H. A. and Murray, P. K. 1998. Transmission studies of Hendra virus (equine morbillivirus) in fruit bats, horses and cats. *Aust. Vet. J.* 76:813–818.
77. Williamson, M. M., Hooper, P. T., Selleck, P. W., Westbury, H. A. and Slocombe, R. F. 2000. Experimental hendra virus infectionin pregnant guinea-pigs and fruit Bats (Pteropus poliocephalus). *J. Comp. Pathol.* 122:201–207.
78. Wong, K. T., Shieh, W. J., Kumar, S., Norain, K., Abdullah, W., Guarner, J., Goldsmith, C. S., Chua, K. B., Lam, S. K., Tan, C. T., Goh, K. J., Chong, H. T., Jusoh, R., Rollin, P. E., Ksiazek, T. G., Zaki, S. R., and Nipah virus pathology working group. 2002. Nipah virus infection: Pathology and pathogenesis of an emerging paramyxoviral zoonosis. *Am. J. Pathol.* 161:2153–2167.
79. Wong, S., Lau, S., Woo, P. and Yuen, K. Y. 2007. Bats as a continuing source of emerging infections in humans. *Rev. Med. Virol.* 17:67–91.
80. Xiao, C., Liu, Y., Jiang, Y., Magoffin, D. E., Guo, H., Xuan, H., Wang, G., Wang, L. F. and Tu, C. 2008. Monoclonal antibodies against the nucleocapsid proteins of henipaviruses: Production, epitope mapping and application in immunohistochemistry. *Arch. Virol.* 153:273–281.
81. Xu, K., Rajashankar, K. R., Chan, Y. P., Himanen, J. P., Broder, C. C. and Nikolov, D. B. 2008. Host cell recognition by the henipaviruses: Crystal structures of the Nipah G attachment glycoprotein and its complex with ephrin-B3. *Proc Natl Acad Sci.* 105:9953–9958.
82. Zhu, Z., Dimitrov, A. S., Bossart, K. N., Crameri, G., Bishop, K. A., Choudhry, V., Mungall, B. A., Feng, Y. R., Choudhary, A., Zhang, M. Y., Feng, Y., Wang, L. F., Xiao, X., Eaton, B. T., Broder, C. C. and Dimitrov, D. S. 2006a. Potent neutralization of Hendra and Nipah viruses by human monoclonal antibodies. *J. Virol.* 80:891–899.
83. Zhu, Z., Dimitrov, A. S., Chakraborti, S., Dimitrova, D., Xiao, X., Broder, C. C. and Dimitrov, D. S. 2006b. Development of human monoclonal antibodies against diseases caused by emerging and biodefense-related viruses. *Expert Rev. Anti Infect. Ther.* 4:57–66.
84. Zhu, Z., Bossart, K. N., Bishop, K. A., Crameri, G., Dimitrov, A. S., McEachern, J. A., Feng, Y., Middleton, D., Wang, L. F., Broder, C. C. and Dimitrov, D. S. 2008. Exceptionally potent cross-reactive neutralization of Nipah and Hendra viruses by a human monoclonal antibody. *J. Infect. Dis.* 197:846–853.

16. Horse Pox

K. Dhama, P. Bhatt, R. V. S. Pawaiya, S. Kapoor, and Thankam Mathew

Introduction

Horse pox, pathologically another form of molluscum contagiosum, is a mildly contagious, self-limiting cutaneous infection in the horse caused by a poxvirus (horse pox virus, HSPV) from the genera *Molluscipoxvirus* (molluscum contagiosum virus, MCV), a virus closely related to the human molluscum contagiosum virus. The horse pox may be caused by human or cattle orthopoxviruses (Hargis and Ginn, 2007). Apparently an ancient disease of horses, horse pox is a rare dermatological viral disease characterized by usually small poxlike lesions localized to the penis, prepuce, axillary and inguinal areas, and in and around the mouth and nose. Other resembling diseases and often considered to be forms of horse pox are referred to as contagious pustular dermatitis, variola equina, grease, grease heel, viral popular dermatitis, and Uasin Gishu skin disease of the horse (McIntyre, 1949; Eby, 1958; Andrews and Pereira, 1967; Kaminjolo and Winqvist, 1975; Jayo et al., 1986; Hagen and Bruner, 1988). Horse pox has been placed in OIE list B diseases of equines.

As a family of viruses, poxviruses collectively exhibit a broad host range, and most of the individual members are capable of replicating in a wide array of cell types from various host species, at least in vitro (Werden et al., 2008). Poxviruses have been used as virus vectors to vaccination; they possess potential in cancer immunotherapy and gene therapy, and their ability to evade host-cell immune responses may provide a basis for new antipoxvirus therapies. Recombinant pox viruses expressing specific immunogenic proteins have been generated for vaccination against heterologous pathogens—viz, rabies virus, Newcastle disease virus, avian influenza, canine distemper virus, feline leukemia virus, equine influenza virus, Japanese encephalitis virus, and HIV too. Huge prospects is there in exploiting host-restricted poxvirus vectors for vaccines, gene therapy, or tissue-targeted oncolytic viral therapies for the treatment of human cancers (Paoletti, 1996; Lewis-Jones, 2004; Arlen et al., 2005; McFadden, 2005).

Numerous pathogens including viruses like West Nile virus, Chikungunya virus, Japanese encephalitis virus, hemorrhagic fever viruses like Ebola and Maburg have again entered the public arena in recent years, been reported to be causing emerging and reemerging infectious diseases, and are of much particular public health concerns. Recently, the coronavirus responsible for SARS, caused an epidemic sufficiently worrisome to challenge crisis management concepts, and presently the bird flu may be on the verge of causing a human pandemic (Bricaire and Bossi, 2006; Garavelli and Peduzzi, 2006). Pox (variola virus casing smallpox in humans) and monkeypox (miniature smallpox) are also reported to be "virtually emerging" viruses that have potential for use in bioterrorism (Georges et al., 2004; Bricaire and Bossi, 2006; Parker et al., 2007). Numerous other animal pox viruses pose potential risks for humans and animals. This risk scenario also includes recombinations between the various pox viruses, changes in hosts, and genetically engineered manipulations of pox viruses (Mayr, 2003). However, horse pox virus has not been reported to be having much public health significance.

Today the concept of globalization including global exposure to infectious diseases is becoming more apparent (Garavelli and Peduzzi, 2006). Though horse pox has been reported from Europe only, but due to an evermore connected global arena linked through international travel, politics, economics, culture, and human-human and human-animal interactions, various diseases and other poxviruses infections being reported from tropical countries worldwide, this chapter has been included in the "Tropical Viral Disease of Large Animals."

ETIOLOGY

Horse pox is caused by a poxvirus of the genera *Molluscipoxvirus* (molluscum contagiosum virus), subfamily *Chordopoxvirinae,* family Poxviridae. In 1964 Weiner et al. classified pox group of viruses into several subfamily like (1) variola vaccinia subgroup; (2) avian poxviruses; (3) Myxoma-like viruses; (4) viruses affecting ungulates including, (a) camel pox, (b) goat pox, and (c) horse pox; (5) miscellaneous group—molluscum contagiosum. Afterward, scientist working on pox group of viruses—namely, Joklik (1966), Andrews and Pereira (1972), Baxby (1975, 1984), Fenner (1976), Nakano (1979) Matthews (1979)—classified pox group of viruses. Later, Mathew (1993) reviewed the classification of the above scientists and classified pox family (Pox viridae as two families, namely, (1) Chordopox viridae (pox viruses of vertebrates) and (2) Entamopox viridae (pox viruses of insects). Included under Chordopox viridae are (a) vaccinia variola subgroup (orthopox virus), (b) orf subgroup (parapox virus), (c) fowl pox (avipox virus), (d) sheep pox (capripox virus), (e) swine pox virus, (f) Myxo subgroup (leporipox), and (g) other members of the vertebrates. In the g group is the molluscum contagiosum in which horse pox belongs (refer to bovine pox diseases in bovine section of this book). But recently horse pox is considered to be due to human or cattle orthopoxviruses (Hargis and Ginn, 2007). The disease is caused by poxvirus, a DNA epitheliotropic virus. The horse pox virus belongs to genera *Molluscipoxvirus* (molluscum contagiosum virus), a virus closely related to the human molluscum contagiosum virus. The virus is contagious in nature, 150–180 mμ in size, very much resistant to drying, and can be demonstrated under microscope through staining. It has been reported that contagious pustular dermatitis is the most common form of Jenner's horse pox (De Jong, 1917). The causative ungulate poxvirus is identical antigenically with the virus of true cowpox and is transferable to cattle and to humans (Cameron, 1908).

Poxviridae viral particles (virions) are generally enveloped. They vary in their shape depending upon the species but are generally shaped like a brick or as an oval form similar to a rounded brick. The viral genome carries a single linear, double-stranded segment of DNA. Replication of the poxvirus involves several stages like binding to a receptor on the host cell surface, entry into the cell, uncoating and then viral replication, and pathogenesis. The assembly of the virus particle occurs in the cytoskeleton of the cell and is a complex process that is poorly understood but is currently being researched. The replication of this virus is unusual for a virus with ds-*DNA* genome because it encodes its own machinery for genome replication, and therefore the replication occurs in the cytoplasm. Most viruses with a ds DNA genome replicate in the nucleus and use the host cells genome replication machinery.

Although the immune response to poxvirus infections are very similar to that seen in other viral infections, the poxviruses, unlike most other viruses (with the exception of herpesviruses), are able to defend themselves. They have been shown to carry a repertoire of proteins involved in immune evasion and immune modulation. Poxviruses encode proteins involved in blocking many of the strategies employed by the host to combat viral infections; they encode for proteins that block activity of many chemokines, cytokines, serine proteases, and even complement (Smith and Kotwal, 2002).

EPIDEMIOLOGY

Horse pox, classically known as a poxviral disease of horses, although common before the twentieth century, is rare today and is recorded in Europe with fewer occurrences as compared to the past (De Jong, 1917; Hutyra et al., 1949; Baxby, 1981; Tripathy et al., 1981; Tulman et al., 2006). Horse pox epidemic was reported in Bayan-somon of Khentei aimak Mongolia in 1976, and MNR-76 strain was isolated from sick horses, and the viral genome was studied in detail by Tulman et al. (2006). Two poxviruses antigenically similar to vaccinia were isolated from horses with natural infection in Kenya

(Kaminjolo et al., 1974a). Though in general it is a benign disease, but badly affected horses become debilitated, and occasionally young animals may die. It is spread by contact with infected grooming tools, harness, and by handling.

The study of infections of vertebrate animals by poxviruses has remained a dynamic area of research for the last century. The host range of poxviruses varies from extremely narrow to exceedingly broad, and they have been shown to enter their host by either the respiratory route or through the skin. The severity of infection varies dramatically from one specie to another, causing anywhere from a local, self-limiting infection, to a devastating systemic disease, such as smallpox (Smith Kotwal, 2002). The disease mostly affects the horses with the young ones being more susceptible. The severely affected animals may become weak with occasional mortality in young animals (Radostits et al., 2000). The disease can also be transmitted to human beings with horse attendants at high risk of getting infected.

Functionally, the known host range factors from poxviruses have been associated with manipulation of a diverse array of cellular targets, which includes cellular kinases and phosphatases, apoptosis and various antiviral pathways.

Horse pox is a benign form of pox, which produces papulovesicular eruptions, typical pox lesions either on the limbs or on the lips and buccal mucosa (Dietz and Wiesner, 1984; Fenner, 1996). The spread of horse pox occurs through direct contact from animal to animal or through attendants. Sheep pox and rabbit pox are spread by airborne infectious particles that are inhaled. Horse pox, fowl pox, and mouse pox are usually spread by skin contact. Infected grooming tools, harnesses, and handlers are potent mode of transmission of the disease (Radostits et al., 2000). Contaminated food and water may also lead to the spread of disease. Cowpox (vaccinia) and pseudocowpox (paravaccinia), localized on the udder and teats of cows, are transmissible to human beings. Inoculation of vesicular fluid, from horse pox lesions, in human and cow may also produce disease.

ZOONOTIC POTENTIAL

Poxviruses are incriminating agents of disease introduced into novel host species and among populations of the same species and have been involved with human disease associated with their zoonotic origins (Regnery, 2007). Human zoonotic poxvirus infections are rare but increasingly encountered outside their usual geographical range. Animal poxviruses occasionally produce human skin disease often associated with systemic illness. Lesions are painful blisters and crusted eschars and are usually self-limiting and rarely fatal. Treatment is generally supportive (Lewis-Jones, 2002; Essbauer et al., 2004).

Four genera of Poxviridae family are known to cause human zoonoses: *Orthopox, Parapox, Yatapox, Molluscipox*. The following are their groups:

1. *Orthopox*: variola virus, vaccinia virus, cow pox virus, monkeypox virus, smallpox (eradicated)
2. *Parapox*: orf virus, pseudocowpox, bovine papular stomatitis virus
3. *Yatapox*: tanapox virus, yaba monkey tumor virus
4. *Molluscipox*: *molluscum contagiosum virus* (MCV)

The most common are vaccinia (seen on Indian subcontinent) and molluscum contagiousum, but monkeypox infections are rising (seen in West and Central African rainforest countries).

Outbreaks of buffalo pox or poxlike infections affecting buffaloes, cows, and humans have been recorded in many parts of the world. Milkers develop poxlike lesions on the skin of the hands, forearms, and forehead accompanied by fever, axillary lymphadenopathy, and general malaise. The causative agent buffalo pox virus is a member of the orthopoxvirus, which has also been incriminated in causing horse pox and is closely related to vaccinia virus, the type species of the genus (Hargis and Ginn, 2007). Buffalo pox has been reported to be an emerging and reemerging zoonosis (Mathew 1987, 1993; Singh et al., 2006, 2007; Zafar et al., 2007). Molecular characterization using polymerase chain reaction (PCR) amplification and other methods provides accurate phylogenetic identification and suggests that a cowpoxlike virus is the probable ancestor of variola and other zoonotic poxviruses (Lewis-Jones, 2004). The discontinuation of the vaccination (with vaccinia virus) has rendered most humans vulnerable to variola virus, the etiologic agent of smallpox, if at all unfortunately this virus happens to be used in biological warfare or terrorism. Even today, we are still mostly ignorant about why most poxvirus infections of vertebrate hosts show strict species specificity or how zoonotic poxvirus infections occur when poxviruses occasionally leap into novel host species. Poxvirus tropism at the cellular level seems to be regulated by intracellular events downstream of virus binding and entry, rather than at the level of specific host receptors as is the case for many other viruses (McFadden, 2005).

There are evidences that horse pox can be directly transmitted to man (Cameron, 1908). During the smallpox epidemic in London in 1901–1902, a stableman was admitted with pain in the left arm and armpit, temperature of

100.4°F. The red spots became painful and enlarged, and others appeared as severe lymphangitis of both arms and the axillary glands on both sides; the lesions varied in size, but not in type. The local indurations and lymphangitis gradually disappeared as the lesions crusted, and the gland swelling subsided without suppuration. The patient had been engaged in treating a horse suffering from "ulcers of the mouth and throat." The patient had been successfully vaccinated in infancy and not afterward. Consideration of all the circumstances of the case led to the diagnosis of horse pox (Cameron, 1908). From time to time, other cases have been reported of the direct transmission of the disease to man from a horse suffering from "sore heels." Similarly, human cases from the horse from which the disease was contracted were "suffering from inflammation of the legs and cracked heels." The man got the infection directly from the ulcers in the horse's mouth, while experimenting on the possibility of transmitting diseases of the horse to other animals by inoculation. His horse had pustules in the mouth but no eruption elsewhere, and at first he described the condition as an aphthous stomatitis, which could be due to horse pox. Thus, human or cattle orthopoxviruses could cause horse pox.

PATHOGENESIS AND PATHOLOGY

The pathogenesis of lesion formation is more or less similar to other pox diseases. The sequence of the lesions are macule, papule, vesicle (varies in severity), umbilicated pustule, crust, and scar. It starts as multiple circular, smooth-surfaced, gray white papules 1–2 mm in diameter. Later, the lesions become umbilicated and develop a central pore from which a caseous plug is extruded, which may further turn into nodules, vesicles, and pustules. The vesicles may rupture and turn to scab, which may heal or drop off. Lesions may occur in lips, nose, oral mucosa, and genitalia. Microscopic lesions of molluscum contagiosum consist of well-demarcated foci of epidermal hyperplasia and hypertrophy, which may form invaginated lobules of the epidermis in the superficial dermis. Keratinocytes containing inclusions exfoliate though a pore that forms in the stratum corneum and enlarges into a central crater. The individual keratinocytes are markedly swollen and contain large intracytoplasmic eosinophilic inclusions, known as molluscum bodies, which can be seen histopatholocally as well as in cytoplasmic preparations. There is usually no dermal reaction (Hargis and Ginn, 2007). A solid immunity is produced after an attack of pox viral infection (Radostits et al., 2000). The large genomic-coding capacity of poxviruses enables the virus to express a unique collection of viral proteins that function as host range factors, which specifically target and manipulate host signaling pathways to establish optimal cellular conditions for viral replication (Werden et al., 2008).

CLINICAL FINDINGS

The disease generally manifests in two forms, viz, "leg form" and "buccal form." In the leg form of disease, the lesions occur mostly in back portion of pastern, and this form is characterized by moderate rise of body temperature followed by a weeping lesion, which undergoes characteristic stages like papular, vesicular, and pustular and scab formation. The pustules may rupture leading to eczematous grease condition. The lesions may cause pain leading to lameness in affected animals (Radostits et al., 2000). There may be a secondary bacterial infection leading to marked swelling of legs. The buccal form exhibits similar lesions that appear first on the insides of the lips and then spread over the whole buccal mucosa, sometimes covering the pharynx and larynx and occasionally the nostrils. The conjunctiva, the vulva, and sometimes the entire body may show lesions in very severe cases. The buccal lesions cause a painful stomatitis with salivation and anorexia as prominent signs. Most cases recuperate with lesions healing in two to four weeks (Radostits et al., 2000). In some rare cases, the lesions may spread to other parts of the body like lips, chest, forelegs, thigh, perineum, genital organs, upper respiratory tract, and then the whole body. Sometimes conjunctiva appears to be inflamed due to spread of infection via lacrimal duct.

Multiple clinical forms of horse pox include a benign, localized form with lesions in the muzzle and buccal cavity (previously known as contagious pustular stomatitis); a generalized, highly contagious form known as equine papular stomatitis; an exudative dermatitis of the pasterns described as "grease" or grease heel (a syndrome also associated with other infectious and environmental agents); equine molluscum contagiosum, which is a mild, self-limiting cutaneous disease similar to the human disease, associated with a virus similar to MCV; and Uasin Gishu disease described in nonindigenous horses of eastern Africa, associated with a poorly characterized OPV. However, generalized skin lesions are proliferative and papillomatous, and course of, the disease may be chronic (Hutyra et al., 1949; Baxby, 1981; Fenner et al., 1989; Thompson et al., 1998; Yager et al., 1993).

DIAGNOSIS

The diagnosis of the disease is based on typical clinical findings as observed in leg form, buccal form, and generalized form of the disease. Isolation of the virus from vesicular or pustular material and from blood during the viremic phase can be undertaken to confirm the disease. Presence of specific inclusion bodies in stained affected material indicates infection with poxvirus.

The leg form of horse pox may be confused with greasy heel, but no nodules, vesicles, or pustules occur in the latter disease. Vesicular stomatitis in horses has lesions that are much larger, rupture very readily, and do not undergo the typical stages of a pox lesion. Differentiation from viral papular dermatitis, which is insectborne, and Uasin Gishu, a poxlike disease of horses recorded in Kenya and assumed to be an infection contracted from wild fauna, is necessary.

Experimentally, the lesions of horse pox and papular dermatitis can be produced in horses by the injection of vaccinia virus (Studdert, 1989).

The other disease that resembles with horse pox is molluscum contagiosum (Kaminjolo et al., 1974b; Moens and Kombe, 1988), characterized by typical molluscum bodies in the skin sections (Rahaley and Mueller, 1983; Lange et al., 1991; Van Rensburg et al., 1991).

Van Rensburg et al. (1991) reported a severe papular dermatitis of especially the neck, chest, and genitalia with a marked scrotal edema in a stallion in South Africa. Histopathological examination of skin biopsies revealed the presence of numerous intracytoplasmic molluscum bodies in areas of focal epidermal hyperplasia. Electron microscopical examination showed the presence of typical pox virions in affected epidermal cells. Lange et al. (1991) also reported molluscum contagiosum in three horses in Zambia with horses found to be suffering from a slow progressive skin disease with lesions on the chest, shoulders, inner and lateral aspects of the fore—and hind limbs, the face, fetlocks, pasterns, and on the lateral surfaces of the body. The lesions varied from 4–20 mm in diameter, were hairless, but covered by soft keratin projections that, when removed, left a raw, elevated base tightly adherent to the epidermis. These lesions bled profusely when the animals were groomed. Older lesions were well circumscribed, raised above the surface, devoid of hair, and after removal of gray-white keratin flakes had a depigmented waxy appearance. Microscopically cytoplasmic inclusions containing many pox virions were found. Thompson et al. (1998) indicated that on the basis of very close homology of the viral DNA sequences (in situ hybridization studies), the causative virus of equine molluscum contagiosum is either identical with, or very closely related to, its human equivalent.

In situ detection of molluscum contagiosum virus DNA may be valuable for investigations into the cell biology of this imperfectly characterized virus and may prove useful for both retrospective and prospective epidemiological surveys. (Thompson et al., 1990). Polymerase chain reaction (PCR), a highly sensitive means of diagnosis, has also been reported to be a technique, which may also prove useful for investigations into the pathogenesis, epidemiology, and natural history of equine molluscum contagiosum infection (Thompson, 1997).

With no DNA sequence information available earlier for HSPV, only recently, Tulman et al. (2006) of USA with a group of scientist from different countries studied genome sequencing of horse pox MR-76 strain isolated from Mongolian epedimic as early as 1976 to differentiate with two other pox viral diseases of horses, namely—equine molluscum contagiosum and Uasin Gishu disease, which have been found in eastern Africa. Their studies clearly indicated that horse pox virus (HSPV) contains unique genome showing unique virulence/ host range phenotype and closely related to known vaccinia-like (VACV-like) viruses. Sequence data analysis also suggested that, while very closely related, HSPV is phylogenetically distinct from other characterized VACV-like viruses. In addition, HSPV contains potentially ancestral sequences, which is absent in other VACV-like viruses. MNR-76 may represent a naturally circulating member of the VACV lineage, as were viruses circulating among domestic animals in the era of current VACV-like viruses collected as vaccine.

Tulman et al. (2006) suggested that genomic sequence analysis of other VACV-like virus isolates may add perspective to the novel nature of HSPV relative to other viruses within the VACV lineage. It is likely that complete genomic data from uncharacterized orthopoxviruses (OPVs) isolates will aid in OPV gene identification and functional characterization while also providing information regarding the pathogenic potential of the virus, understanding the genetic basis of viral host range, and the relationships between OPVs.

Investigation of the buffalo pox disease outbreak by virus isolation in Vero cell cultures and detection of viral nucleotide sequences by polymerase chain reaction (PCR) confirmed the etiology of the disease (Singh et al., 2006). Uasin Gishu lesions are characteristically verrucose papillomas and have a poxvirus associated with it (Kaminjolo and Winqvist, 1975).

TREATMENT
The prognosis of the disease is always favorable except in cases where disease takes a prolonged course of fever. Local astringent treatment, as in the other forms of pox, may facilitate healing (Radostits et al., 2000). Tannin (10%) or potassium permanganate (1%) or hydrogen peroxide (1%) solutions may be used for the treatment of foot lesions. Mouth lesions can be treated by rinsing mouth with potassium permanganate solution. Provision of soft and palatable feeds may be offered to the affected animals.

CONTROL
Because of the contagious nature of the disease, rigid isolation and hygiene in the handling of infected horses is essential (Radostits et al., 2000). Strict

hygienic and sanitary measures should be followed in the farm premises. Effective vaccines are available for most pox diseases, though outbreaks have continued. Smallpox, a pox disease known in human beings as early as 1122 BC, was declared eradicated in 1979 by following introduction of smallpox vaccination approximately two hundred years ago. Therefore, routine smallpox vaccination was discontinued in 1980.

Vaccinia virus (VACV) is the vaccine virus used to eradicate smallpox. However, no vaccine is available for prophylaxis against this disease in horses (Radostits et al., 2000).

Conclusion

Horse pox is contagious viral infection of horses, rarely reported only from Europe. The causative agent horse pox virus belongs to genera *Molluscipoxvirus* of the family Poxviridae. Horse pox is a benign disease with typical pox lesions either on the limbs or on the lips and buccal mucosa, but severely affected horses become weak, and occasionally young animals may die. The disease generally manifests in two forms—viz, leg form and buccal form—and is spread by contact from animal to animal. The pathogenesis of lesion formation is more or less similar to other animal pox diseases. The virus can also be transmitted to human beings. Diagnosis of horse pox is based on clinical observations, presence of specific inclusion bodies in stained affected material, and isolation of the virus from affected horses. Other forms of horse pox or similar resembling diseases like grease, greasy heel, variola equina, vesicular stomatitis, viral papular dermatitis, contagious pustular dermatitis, Uasin Gishu, and molluscum contagiosum should be given due considerations. Modern diagnostic tools—viz, in situ detection and PCR tools and horse pox genome sequencing, may also be explored for laboratory confirmation of horse pox virus and for the epidemiological studies. Good management practices of isolation, hygiene, and sanitary measures need to be followed in handling of infected horses. Vaccines are available for most pox diseases, and even small pox disease of human beings have been eradicated from the world following extensive mass vaccination program; however, vaccine is not available for horse pox disease in horses. Though poxviruses (variola virus) and monkeypox posses the potential for use in bioterrorism, and buffalo pox is also of zoonotic significance, however, horse pox is not reported to be having much public health concerns. The possible use of poxviruses for biological warfare has led to renewed interest in these viruses and the antipoxviral therapies. Therefore, since literature is limited on horse pox virus, further studies are needed to be conducted on this rare viral infection of horses.

REFERENCES

1. Andrews, C. and Pereira, H. G. 1967. In *Viruses of vertebrates*. 2nd edition. London: Bailliere, Tindal and Cassell.

2. Andrews, C. and Pereira, H. G. 1972. Pox viruses. In *Viruses of vertebrates*, 3rd ed., 373–413. London: Bailliere and Tindall.

3. Arlen, P. M., Kaufman, H. L. and DiPaola, R. S. 2005. Pox viral vaccine approaches. *Semin. Oncol.* 32:549–555.

4. Baxby, D. 1975. Identification and inter relationship of variola, vaccinia subgroup of pox virus. *Prog. Med. Virol.* 19:215–246.

5. Baxby, D. 1981. *Jenner's smallpox vaccine: The riddle of vaccinia virus and its origin.* London, United Kingdom: Heinemann Educational Books Ltd.

6. Baxby, D. 1984. Pox virus. In *Topley and Wilson's principels of bacteriology, virology and immunity.* Vol. 4 *Virology*, 7th ed. New York: Arnold Publishers.

7. Bricaire, F. and Bossi, P. 2006. Emerging viral diseases. *Bull. Acad. Natl. Med.* 190:597–608.

8. Cameron, A. F. 1908. Horse-pox directly transmitted to man. *Br. Med. J.* 30:1:1293–1294.

9. De Jong, D. A. 1917. The relationship between contagious pustular stomatitis of the horse, equine variola (horse pox of Jenner) and vaccinia (cow pox of Jenner). *J. Comp. Path. Ther.* 30:242–262.

10. Eby, C. H. 1958. A note in the history of horse pox. *J. Am. Vet. Med. Assoc.* 132:420–422.

11. Essbauer, S., Pfeffer, M., Wilhelm, S. and Meyer, H. 2004. Zoonotic poxviruses. *Bundesgesundheitsblatt Gesundheitsforschung Gesundheitsschutz* 47:671–679.

12. Fenner, F. 1976. Classification and nomenclature of virus. *Intervirology* 7:1–115.

13. Fenner, F., Wittek, R. and Dumbell, K. 1989. *The orthopoxviruses*. San Diego, Calif.: Academic Press, Inc.

14. Fenner, F. 1996. Poxvirus infections. In *Virus infections of vertebrates*: *Virus infections of equines*, 6th ed. M. J. Studdert, 5. Amsterdam, USA: Elsevier.

15. Garavelli, P. L. and Peduzzi, P. 2006. Globalization and infectious diseases. *Recenti. Prog. Med.* 97:528–532.

16. Georges, A. J., Matton, T. and Courbot-Georges, M. C. 2004. Monkey-pox, a model of emergent then reemergent disease. *Med. Mal. Infect.* 34:12–19.

17. Hagan, W. A. and Bruner, D. W. 1988. Horse pox. *Hagan's and Bruner's Microbiology and Infectious Diseases of Domestic Animals*, 571.

18. Hargis, A. M. and Ginn, P. E. 2007. The integument. In *Pathologic basis of veterinary diseases*, 4th ed., M. D. McGavin and J. F. Zachary, 1173–1176. St. Louis, Missouri: Mosby Elsevier.

19. Hutyra, F., Marek, J. and Manninger, R. 1949. Pox (variola). In *Special pathology and therapeutics of the diseases of domestic animals*, vol. 1., ed. J. R. Greig, 348–393. London, United Kingdom: Bailliere, Tindall and Cox.

20. Jayo, M. J., Jensen, L. A., Leipold, H. W. and Cook, J. E. 1986. Pox virus infection in a donkey. *Vet. Pathol.* 23:635–637.

21. Joklik, W. K. 1966. The pox viuses. *Bacteriol Review* 30:33–66.

22. Kaminjolo, J. S., Nyaga, P. N. and Gicho, J. N. 1974a. Isolation, cultivation and characterization of a poxvirus from some horses in Kenya. *Zbl. Vet. Med.* B 21:592–601.

23. Kaminjolo, J. S. Jr., Johnson, L. W., Frank, H. and Gicho, J. N. 1974b. Vaccinia-like Pox virus identified in a horse with a skin disease. *Zentralbl Veterinarmed* B 21:202–206.

24. Kaminjolo, J. S. Jr. and Winqvist, G. 1975. Histopathology of skin lesions in Uasin Gishu skin disease of horses. *J. Comp. Pathol.* 85:391–395.

25. Lange, L., Marett, S., Maree, C. and Gerdes, T. 1991. Molluscum contagiosum in three horses. *J. S. Afr. Vet. Assoc.* 62:68–71.

26. Lewis-Jones, S. 2002. The zoonotic poxviruses. *Dermatol. Nurs.* 14:79–82.

16. HORSE POX

27. Lewis-Jones, S. 2004. Zoonotic poxvirus infections in humans. *Curr. Opin. Infect. Dis.* 17:81–89.
28. Mathew, T. 1987. In *Advances in medical and veterinary virology, immunology and epidemiology. Cultivation and immunological studies on pox group of viruses with special reference to buffalopx virus,* vol. 1, 4–171. N. Delhi: Thajema Publishers.
29. Mathew, T. 1993. Classification of pox group of viruses including buffalopox virus. In *Advances in medical and veterinary virology, immunology and epidemiology.* Vol. 2. *Buffalopox (Orthopox) virus and its zoonotic importance,* 11–26. N. Delhi, India: Thajema Publishers.
30. Matthews, R. E. F. 1979. Classification and nomenclature of viruses. *Intervirology* 12:3–5.
31. Mayr, A. 2003. Smallpox vaccination and bioterrorism with pox viruses. *Comp. Immunol. Microbiol. Infect. Dis.* 26:423–430.
32. McFadden, G. 2005. Poxvirus tropism. *Nat. Rev. Microbiol.* 3:201–213.
33. McIntyre, M. W. 1949. Virus popular dermatitis of the horse. *Am. J. Vet. Res.* 10:229–232.
34. Moens, Y. and Kombe, A. H. 1988. Molluscum contagiosum in a horse. *Equine Vet. J.* 20:143–145.
35. Nakano, J. H. 1979. Pox viruses. In *Diagnostic procedure for viral and rickettsial and chlamydeal infections,* 5th ed., ed. E. H. Lennette and N. Schmidt, 314–336. Philadelphia, USA: J. American Public Health Assoc. Inc. (J. B. Lippincott. Co.).
36. Paoletti, E. 1996. Applications of pox virus vectors to vaccination: An update. *Proc. Natl. Acad. Sci. USA* 93:1349–11353.
37. Parker, S., Nuara, A., Buller, R. M. and Schultz, D. A. 2007. Human monkeypox: An emerging zoonotic disease. *Future Microbiol.* 2:17–34.
38. Radostits, O. M., Gay, C. C., Blood, D. C. and Hinchcliff, K. W. 2000. Horse pox. In *Veterinary medicine,* 9th ed., 1256–1257. W. B. Saunders Co.
39. Rahaley, R. S. and Mueller, R. E. 1983. Molluscum contagiosum in a horse. *Vet. Pathol.* 20:247–250.
40. Studdert, M. J. 1989. Experimental vaccinia virus infection of horses. *Aust. Vet. J.* 66:157–159.
41. Regnery, R. L. 2007. Poxviruses and the passive quest for novel hosts. *Curr. Top. Microbiol. Immunol.* 315:345–61.
42. Singh, R. K., Hosamani, M., Balamurugan, V., Satheesh, C. C., Shingal, K. R., Tatwarti, S. B., Bambal, R. G., Ramteke, V. and Yadav, M. P. 2006. An outbreak of buffalopox in buffalo (*Bubalus bubalis*) dairy herds in Aurangabad, India. *Rev. Sci. Tech.* 25:981–987.
43. Singh, R. K., Hosamani, M., Balamurugan, V., Bhanuprakash, V., Rasool, T. J. and Yadav, M. P. 2007. Buffalopox: An emerging and re-emerging zoonosis. *Anim Health Res. Rev.* 8:105–114.
44. Smith, S. A. and Kotwal, G. J. 2002. Immune response to poxvirus infections in various animals. *Crit. Rev. Microbiol.* 28:149–185.
45. Thompson, C. H., Biggs, I. M. and de Zwart-Steffe, R. T. 1990. Detection of molluscum contagiosum virus DNA by in situ hybridization. *Pathology* 22:181–186.
46. Thompson, C. H. 1997. Identification and typing of molluscum contagiosum virus in clinical specimens by polymerase chain reaction. *J. Med. Virol.* 53:205–211.
47. Thompson, C. H., Yager, J. A. and Van Rensburg, I. B. 1998. Close relationship between equine and human molluscum contagiosum virus demonstrated by in situ hybridisation. *Res. Vet. Sci.* 64:157–161.
48. Tripathy, D. N., Hanson, L. E. and Crandell, R. A. 1981. Poxviruses of veterinary importance: Diagnosis of infections. In *Comparative diagnosis of viral diseases,* vol. 3, ed. E. Kurstak and C. Kurstak, 267–346. New York: Academic Press.
49. Tulman, E. R., Delhon, G., Afonso, C. L., Lu, Z., Zsak, L., Sandybaev, N. T., Kerembekova, U. Z., Zaitsev, V. L., Kutish, G. F. and Rock, D. L. 2006. Genome of horse pox virus. *J. Virol.* 80:9244–9258.
50. Van Rensburg, I. B., Collett, M. G., Ronen, N. and Gerdes, T. 1991. Molluscum contagiosum in a horse. *J. S. Afr. Vet. Assoc.* 62:72–74.
51. Werden, S. J., Rahman, M. M. and McFadden, G. 2008. Poxvirus host range genes. *Adv. Virus Res.* 71:135–171.

52. Weiner, L. M., Macko, I., Poulik, E. and Goodman, N. 1964. Salt requirement for precipitation of chicken antisera in agar immunoelectrophoresis. *J. Immunol.* 93:228–231.
53. Yager, J. A., Scott, D. W. and Wilcock, B. P. 1993. The skin and appendages. In *Pathology of domestic animals*, 4th ed., vol. 1., ed. K. V. F. Jubb, P. C. Kennedy, and N. Palmer, 531–738. San Diego, Calif.: Academic Press.
54. Zafar, A., Swanepoel, R., Hewson, R., Nizam, M., Ahmed, A., Husain, A., Grobbelaar, A., Bewley, K., Mioulet, V., Dowsett, B., Easterbrook, L. and Hasan, R. 2007. Nosocomial buffalopoxvirus infection, Karachi, Pakistan. *Emerg Infect Dis.* 13:902–904.

17. Japanese Encephalitis in Horses

R. V. S. Pawaiya, K. Dhama, S. Kapoor, M. Mahendran, and Thankam Mathew

Introduction

Japanese encephalitis (JE) is a mosquito-borne viral disease that affects horses, pigs, cattle, buffalo, sheep, mongoose, rodents, birds and humans. It is caused by Japanese encephalitis virus (JEV) belonging to the genus *Flavivirus* of Flaviviridae family under group B Arboviruses of *Togaviridae* (Arora et al., 1975; Mathew et al., 1976; 1977; 1979). Under B arboviruses, JE, WN, dengue, 1, 2, 3, and 4 are included and the convalescent sera cross-react with all the group B arboviruses by hemagglitination-inhibition test and modified microcomplement fixation test (Mathew and Arora, 1975). JEV is mainly transmitted by mosquito *Culex tritaeniorhynchus*, and swine play an important role as an amplifier (Buescher et al., 1959). JEV infects, in addition to humans, a number of animals such as pigs, horses, cattle, sheep, dogs, chickens, ducks, and reptiles in nature (Sugiura and Shimada, 1999; Lim et al., 2007; Zachary, 2007). Horse infected with JE may develop fatal encephalitis with anorexia, lethargy, and/or fever, etc., whereas infection in swine is generally unapparent but cause SMEDI (stillbirth, mummification, embryonic death, and infertility)—that is, stillbirths and abortions in pregnant sows and aspermia in boars (Takashima et al., 1988; Yamanaka et al., 2006; CIRAD, 2007). Swine may develop clinical signs and also amplify the virus. Cattle are often infected in endemic regions but do not become ill or develop viremia. Birds, which are infected asymptomatically, serve as important reservoir hosts. Horses and humans, recognized as manifesting the same pathological lesions from the JEV infection, are the dead-end hosts for JE. Most horses infected by JE viruses show mild clinical signs, including fever, anorexia, and depression. However, the mortality rate is high when JE infected horses show neurological symptoms (Ihara et al., 1997; Kitai et al., 2007).

In temperate regions of Asia, the Japanese encephalitis season usually begins in May or June and ends in September or October. Waterfowl are infected when mosquitoes appear in late spring, swine are infected somewhat later, and equine and human cases peak in late summer and autumn when the virus spills over into these hosts (Acha and Szyfres, 2003; Kitai et al., 2007; van den Hurk et al., 2009). In tropical regions, JEV circulates year-round in mosquitoes, birds, and swine; but there may be seasonal peaks of disease associated with irrigation, rainfall, or other factors that affect the local abundance of mosquitoes and vertebrate amplifying hosts (Mackenzie et al., 2004; Diagana et al., 2007).

Immature pigs are highly susceptible to infection, and pregnant sows often abort or give birth to stillborn and mummified fetuses. During one epidemic in Japan, 50–70% of all pigs suffered reproductive losses. Affected piglets born alive often die; however, the mortality rate is close to zero in adult pigs (Yamanaka et al., 2006; CIRAD, 2007; Arai et al., 2008). Swine are important amplifying hosts for humans and horses, and the number of swine in a region can affect the incidence of disease in other species. Wild and feral pigs may also serve as reservoir and amplifying hosts; in a recent study, 68% of wild boars in part of western Japan were seropositive (Guérin and Pozzi, 2005; Hamano et al., 2007). Where JE is seasonal, serologic surveillance in pigs can be used to predict epidemics in humans.

Viruses like West Nile virus, Chikungunya virus, JEV, Ebola, and Maburg are being reported to be causing emerging and reemerging infectious diseases possessing much public health implications. The coronavirus causing SARS epidemic earlier and presently the bird flu predicted to be on the verge of causing a human pandemic warrants the need to challenge crisis management concepts and conduct novel researches to counteract these deadly pathogens (Bricaire and Bossi, 2006; Garavelli and Peduzzi, 2006). Pox (variola virus casing smallpox in humans) and monkeypox (miniature smallpox) are also reported to be "virtually emerging" viruses having potential for use in bioterrorism (Mayor, 2003; Georges et al., 2004; Bricaire and Bossi, 2006; Garavelli and Peduzzi, 2006; Parker et al., 2007). In humans, Japanese encephalitis can be a very serious disease, although most infections are asymptomatic and clinical cases tend to manifest as severe, often-fatal encephalitis. Epidemics, which occur periodically in endemic regions, can cause significant morbidity and mortality in unvaccinated humans and animals. JEV is the most important cause of epidemic encephalitis in humans worldwide, with an estimated about fifty thousand cases and fifteen thousand deaths annually (Solomon et al., 2000; Tsai, 2000; McCormack and Allworth, 2002).

ETIOLOGY

Japanese encephalitis virus (JEV) is an arbovirus (arthropod-transmitted virus) that belongs to the genus *Flavivirus* of family Flaviviridae. JEV belongs to the Japanese encephalitis serocomplex, which is composed of ten flaviviruses, including Alfuy, Koutango, Kokobera, Kunjin, Murray Valley encephalitis, Japanese encephalitis, Stratford, Usutu, West Nile, and St. Louis encephalitis. Usutu virus has emerged recently (as of 2002), which is an African mosquito-borne flavivirus (Poidinger et al., 1996; Kuno et al., 1998; Weissenböck et al., 2002; Thiel et al., 2005; Jani and Kallen, 2009). There is only one serotype, but there are two or three subtypes of the JEV (Nakayama, Beijing-1and JaGar 01). Phylogenetic analyses of the E-protein of JaGAr 01 together with thirty-five other JE strains have revealed diversity in amino acid (AA) characteristics between the prototype strains Nakayama, JaGAr 01 and Beijing-1; Nakayama and Beijing-1 have been found to be very closely related and fall in one cluster and are different from JaGAr 01 (Mangada and Takegami, 1999; Qi et al., 2006). Comparison of AA sequences has shown a unique amino acid, arginine, for JaGAr 01 at position 123 of the E-protein, while other strains contained serine. Also, secondary structure prediction by free energy minimization revealed a unique structure for JaGAr 01, which includes an RNA segment that is conserved for all flaviviruses. Such molecular differences may play roles in the replication and antigenic characteristics of JaGAr 01 and other strains (Mangada and Takegami, 1999; Qi et al., 2006). In another study, Nakayama and Beijing-1 JE vaccines have also shown high levels of protective efficacy (Kurane and Takasaki, 2000).

The JE virus measures 40–50 nm in diameter, and structurally it is spheroidal and of cubic symmetry (Saxena, 2008). Like other flaviviruses, JEV consists of a small glycoprotein containing lipid envelope surrounding a nucleocapsid, which encloses one molecule of single-stranded, positive-sense RNA. This 11-kb molecule comprises 5'—and 3'-untranslated regions (UTRs), between which lie a single open reading frame carrying genes for three structural proteins (capsid [C], premembrane [PrM], and envelope [E]) and seven nonstructural (NS) proteins (NSI, NS2a, NS2b, NS3, NS4a, NS4b, and NS5) (Westaway et al., 1985; Sumiyoshi et al., 1987; Chambers et al., 1990; Thomas et al., 1990). The PrM protein containing hydrophobic domains presumably serves as a transmission anchor (McAda et al., 1987). E protein constitutes the major immunogen and is also expressed on the plasma membrane of infected neurons (Russell et al., 1980). It is thought to be the cell-receptor-binding protein and a mediator of membrane fusion and cell entry (Monath and Heinz, 1996). This protein is the major target of the host antiviral immune response (Heinz, 1986; Mason et al., 1991). On the basis of nucleotide sequencing of capsid/premembrane protein (C/PrM) and envelope (E) genes, five virus genotypes have been identified, including genotypes I to III (GI, GII, GIII). These have been found distributed all over southern Asia; a GIV strain was isolated from eastern Indonesia and an isolate originating in Malaysia may represent a fifth genotype (Solomon et al., 2003).

The JEV has a transmission cycle between pigs as an amplifier and mosquitoes as a vector (Buescher et al., 1959). The virus is transmitted by mosquitoes belonging to the *Culex tritaeniorhynchus, C. annulus, C. fuscocephala, C. gelidus,* and mosquitoes in the *C. vishnui* complex, which breed particularly in flooded rice fields. The virus circulates in ardeid birds (herons and egrets). Pigs are amplifying hosts in that the virus reproduces in pigs and infects mosquitoes that take blood meals but does not cause disease (CIRAD, 2007). The virus tends to spill over into human populations, and other prone animal species, when infected mosquito populations build up explosively, and the human-animal biting rate increases (these culicines are normally zoophilic; i.e., they prefer to take blood meals from animals). In temperate regions of Asia, a yearly cycle of infection is seen; mosquitoes appear in late spring, horses and swine become infected in late summer, and human cases peak during August and September. How the virus survives during the winter is unknown; however, effect of global climate change in the emergence of arbovirus diseases cannot be ruled out (Gould and Higgs, 2009). The virus may be maintained in mosquitoes, either by transovarial passage or during hibernation. Bats might also be able to carry the virus for long periods of time (CIRAD, 2007).

EPIDEMIOLOGY

JEV is distributed in temperate and tropical areas of eastern and southern Asia, occurring from the islands of the western Pacific in the east to the Pakistani border in the west and from Korea in the north to Papua New Guinea in the south (Higgins and Snyder, 2006; Lim et al., 2007; van den Hurk et al., 2009). The global importance of JE is significant, with about fifty thousand cases and fifteen thousand deaths a year worldwide (Solomon et al., 2000). Its geographic range extends from eastern Asia (China, Japan, Korea, maritime Siberia, Taiwan, the Philippines, and Vietnam), to Southeast Asia and northern Australasia (Cambodia, Indonesia, Laos, Malaysia, Papua New Guinea, Thailand, and the Torres Strait islands of northern Australia), and to southern Asia (Bangladesh, Bhutan, Myanmar, Nepal, Pakistan, and Sri Lanka) (Vaughn and Hoke, 1992; Igarashi et al., 1994; Endy and Nisalak, 2002; Parida et al., 2006a; Pant et al., 2006; Mackenzie et al., 2007; Nitatpattana et al., 2008). In India, group B arbovirus infection, including JE and WN virus in human and animals, were reported by Smithburn et al., (1954) from Maharashtra and Tamilnadu, which prompted a series of seroepidemiological and virological studies in different states of the country (Carey et al., 1968; Arora and Singh, 1974; Mathew et al., 1976, 1977, 1979, Arora and Mathew, 1977b ; Suneja et al.1977) in human as well as in animals. Outbreaks are rare in the U.S. territories of Guam and Saipan; JE develops mostly among military personnel, expatriates, and rarely in returning travelers. Because of the critical role of pigs, its presence in Muslim countries is negligible. Overall, as in other emerging pathogens, many of which are zoonotic viruses, a very complicated interplay of ecologic, climatic, environmental, and animal and human behavioral factors that have resulted in widespread distribution of JEV. Even mosquitoes pushed along by wind currents have been considered contributory to viral spread, e.g., from Papua New Guinea to the Torres Strait islands and the Australian mainland.

In horses, cases usually occur sporadically or in small clusters, but epidemics may be seen when large numbers of susceptible animals exist. Inapparent infections are common in this species (Ihara et al., 1997; Lian et al., 2002). Between 1948 and 1967, the morbidity rate in Asia was estimated to be approximately 0.045% (45 cases per 100,000 horses). Higher morbidity rates can be seen during outbreaks. During the 1948 epizootic in Japan, the morbidity rate in horses was 0.3% overall; however, in some areas, it was as high as 1.4% (Rosen, 1986; Kitai et al., 2007). The case fatality rate in horses is reported to be approximately 5.0% or less in some areas and 5.0–15.0% in others. During severe outbreaks, the case fatality rate can be as high as 30.0–40.0% (Yamanaka et al., 2006; CIRAD, 2007; Kitai et al., 2007; van den Hurk et al., 2009). In 1948 and 1949, 3679 and 1216 horses, respectively, had shown clinical illness by this disease in Japan. After utilizing an inactivated vaccine on humans and horses, incidence of the disease decreased. There has been no report of diseased horses since 1984 in Japan, while there are some reports about diseased humans and infected pigs in every year in Japan (Sugiura and Shimada, 1999). Like pigs and other animals, neonatal and young horses are particularly susceptible compared to adult animals. When one group of susceptible broodmares was introduced to an endemic area, a third of the mares died (Sugiura and Shimada, 1999; Kahn and Line, 2003). The report of JE in Korea among recently imported horses reemphasizes the serious consequences that can occur following the international movement of horses if appropriate preventive measures are not taken (Yang et al., 2008).

JE is largely a disease of rural areas, and its distribution is very significantly linked to the irrigated rice production combined with pig rearing (Arora and Singh, 1974; Mathew et al., 1979, CIRAD, 2007). In general, two epidemiological patterns of JEV have been recognized: endemic activity in tropical regions such as southern Thailand (Burke et al., 1985) and epidemic activity in temperate and subtropical regions, as first described in Japan (Kono and Kim, 1969). In endemic areas, no seasonal pattern exists, and sporadic cases of encephalitis occur throughout the year. Epidemic activity in temperate and subtropical areas occurs most commonly in summer or early autumn after the rainy season, although this may extend from spring to late autumn or even throughout the year in more southern regions. The two patterns of endemic and epidemic transmission tend to blur in subtropical regions such as northern Thailand and Vietnam, where epidemic activity may be superimposed on low-level endemic or year-round transmission. Molecular epidemiological studies on the geographic occurrence of JEV genotypes using nucleotide sequencing indicated that at least four, and possibly five, genotypes of JEV evolved from an ancestral virus in Indonesia and Malaysia and spread across Asia (Solomon et al., 2003).

TRANSMISSION

JEV is usually transmitted by mosquitoes in the genus *Culex*. The specific mosquito vectors vary with the region; however, *Culex tritaeniorhynchus* is important in spreading this virus to humans and domesticated animals across a wide geographic range. *C. tritaeniorhynchus* breeds in rice paddies and connecting canals and is active at twilight. Laboratory experiments have confirmed the vector competence of *C. tritaeniorhynchus* for JEV; this mosquito specie is susceptible to infection with titers of only 1–2 $\log_{10}$ infectious units per mosquito required to infect some strains (Takahashi, 1976; Weng, et al., 2000). Many other species of *Culex* including *C. pseudovishnui*, *C. gelidus*, *C. fuscocephala*, *C. annulirostris,* and *C. sitiens* can also transmit JEV (Muangman et al., 1972; Doi et al., 1977; van den Hurk et al., 2003). *C. tritaeniorhynchus* displays intraspecific variation in susceptibility to JEV infection, with Japanese strains generally more susceptible to infection than strains from Taiwan and Pakistan (Takahashi, 1982). It is interesting to note that in India, white cattle and buffaloes showed higher percentage of JE antibodies, but susceptibility studies carried out on buffalo calves revealed that the animals were incapable of circulating the virus adequately in the mosquito vector *Culex vishnui* group (a cattle biter), and high cattle-pig ratio in India acts as incomplete cycle of JE activity (Arora and Singh, 1974; Arora et al., 1975; Arora and Mathew, 1977a; Mathew et al., 1976; 1977; 1979). Like cattle, the dogs harboring neutralizing antibodies also fail to circulate virus, and there is no possibility of acting dog as reservoir host in India (Arora and Mathew,1977a). The genetic basis for this difference in *C. tritaeniorhynchus* susceptibility has not been established. However, the discovery of multiple cytochrome oxidase I lineages of *C. Annulirostris* may potentially explain differences in vector competence of these mosquitoes for JEV genotypes I and II in Australasia (Hemmerter et al., 2007).

Most animals are infected when they are bitten by a mosquito. Birds are the most important reservoir hosts and usually maintain the virus cycle in nature. Viremia and/or seroconversion to JEV has been observed in over ninety wild and domestic bird species belonging to a number of different avian families; however, ardeid wading birds are considered the primary enzootic hosts of JEV, who play a role in epizootic viral amplification in some areas (Buescher et al., 1959; Soman et al., 1977; Rodrigues et al., 1981). In India, many birds including egret, house crows, cattle egret, winged Jacana, mynas, and young chicken showed the presence of HI antibodies, making it difficult to point out the type of birds acting as amplifier birds (Mathew et al., 1976, 1977, 1979). However, laboratory studies indicated the involvement of young chicken in the spread of JE virus in high titer through mosquito bite; duckling can harbor the virus only for five days after infection (Arora and Mathew, 1977a). Seroepidemiological survey of Asian monkeys has also shown widespread infection of these primates with JE virus (Yuwono et al., 1984). Lizards and bats can also be infected by eating infected mosquitoes. Boars transmit the virus in semen (Guérin and Pozzi, 2005; Hamano et al., 2007). Swine are important amplifying hosts as they are bitten by the same mosquitoes that bite horses and humans. Host-preference studies indicated that cattle generally attracted more *C. tritaeniorhynchus* than pigs (Mwandawiro et al., 1999), which is suggested to be a result of physiological conditioning rather than inherent genetic factors (Mwandawiro et al., 2000). With the possible exception of bats, most other species of mammals either do not develop viremia capable of infecting mosquitoes or are unimportant in the epidemiology of the disease for other reasons. For example, although horse-to-horse transmission via mosquitoes has been demonstrated in the laboratory, too few susceptible horses are usually found in an area to maintain the virus, and the viremia in these animals may be low.

Humans are usually infected when they are bitten by a mosquito. Some cases are acquired in the laboratory or during tissue sample collection; JE virus can be transmitted through mucous membranes or broken skin, inhaled in aerosols, or acquired by needle-stick injuries. Although this virus is occasionally recovered from human blood, people are generally thought to be dead-end hosts (Tiroumourougane et al., 2002; Arai et al., 2008). JEV does not persist outside a living host. How the virus survives the winter in temperate climates is unknown. It may be maintained in mosquitoes, either by transovarial passage or during hibernation. Reptiles, amphibians, or bats might also be able to carry the virus for long periods of time when they hibernate (Doi, et al., 1983; Oya et al., 1983). Although there is some evidence for each of these hypotheses, their relative importance is unknown (van den Hurk et al., 2009).

CLINICAL SIGNS
In horses, the incubation period is usually eight to ten days. Experimentally infected horses develop clinical signs after four to fourteen days. In experimentally infected pigs, rising temperature and viremia can occur as soon as twenty-four hours after inoculation (Gould et al., 1964). The time

between exposure of pregnant swine to an infectious dose of JE virus and delivery of abnormal litters does not seem to be clearly established, although exposure early in gestation appears more likely to result in abnormal litters than later exposure. In horses, most infections are subclinical. Horses with clinical signs resemble animals with western or eastern equine encephalomyelitis (WEE, EEE), but the mortality rate is relatively low. Symptomatic cases vary in severity. Some horses have a mild illness with a transient fever, anorexia, lethargy, and congested or jaundiced mucous membranes. This syndrome usually lasts for two to three days, and the horse recovers without complications. Other horses develop encephalitis. In the milder form, the horse is lethargic and anorexic, with a fluctuating fever and neurological signs that commonly include difficulty swallowing, incoordination, transient neck rigidity, radial paralysis, or impaired vision. Jaundice or petechial hemorrhages may be found on the mucous membranes (Lian et al., 2002; Zachary, 2007). These horses often recover within a week. A more severe form, called the hyperexcitable form, is characterized by high fever, aimless wandering, violent and demented behavior, occasional blindness, profuse sweating, and muscle tremors. Although some horses recover, these symptoms are often followed by collapse and death in one to two days (Lam et al., 2005). The hyperexcitable form is uncommon and occurs in less than 5% of symptomatic horses. In some horses, neurologic defects such as ataxia may persist after recovery.

JEV cause SMEDI (stillbirth, mummification, embryonic death, and infertility) with the most common symptom being the birth of stillborn or mummified fetuses, usually at term. Piglets born alive often have tremors and convulsions and die soon after birth (Takashima et al., 1988; Yamanaka et al., 2006; CIRAD, 2007; van-den-Hurk et al., 2008). Pregnant sows may also abort. Nonpregnant animals are usually asymptomatic or experience a transient febrile illness, but symptoms of encephalitis are occasionally seen in pigs up to six months of age. A wasting syndrome was the only symptom in one group of piglets with postmortem evidence of nonsuppurative meningoencephalitis (Yamada et al., 2004). In addition, disturbances of spermatogenesis can cause infertility in boars; although this is usually temporary, it can be permanent in severely affected animals. Other domesticated animals can be infected but typically remain asymptomatic.

PATHOGENESIS
After transmission by an infected vector mosquito, JEV multiplies locally and in regional nodes (Ahmed, 1999). Two cellular characteristics are crucial to the pathogenesis: (a) the M protein, which contains hydrophobic domains that help to anchor the virus onto the host cell, and (b) the E protein, which is the

principal immunogenic feature and which is expressed on the membrane of infected cells. The E protein mediates membrane fusion of the viral envelope and the cellular membrane, promoting viral entry into the host cell (Solomon, 2003; Myint et al., 2007). On a cellular level, after attachment of virus to host cell membrane, local membrane disruption may lead to entry of virus into the cell itself. Subsequently, viremia develops, leading to inflammatory changes in the heart, lungs, liver, and reticuloendothelial system (Solomon, 2006; Jani and Kallen, 2009). Most infections are cleared before the virus can invade the CNS, leading to subclinical disease. After a phase of transient viremia, invasion of the central nervous system (CNS) occurs. JEV is thought to invade brain via vascular endothelial cells by endocytosis (Liou and Hsu, 1998). In the neurons, JEV replicates and matures in the neuronal secretory system, mainly the rough endoplasmic reticulum and Golgi apparatus, eventually destroying them (Hase et al., 1990). Experimental studies in mammalian hosts have shown JEV tropism to neurons in the CNS, indirectly indicating the presence of specific receptors with strong affinity for the virus (Oyanagi et al., 1969).

Subclinical or mild forms of Japanese encephalitis resolve in a few days if the CNS is not involved. In such cases, the infection may not produce symptoms and therefore remains undetected. However, given the neurotropic character of JEV, neurologic invasion can develop, possibly by growth of the virus across vascular endothelial cells, leading to involvement of large areas of the brain, including the thalamus, basal ganglia, brain stem, cerebellum (especially the destruction of the cerebellar Purkinje cells), hippocampus, and cerebral cortex (Myint et al., 2007). Persistent infection and congenital transmission may occur. The levels of varying immune response (intrinsic, cellular, humoral) have been characterized (Tiroumourougane et al., 2002). Higher levels of certain cytokines (interferon-alpha, interleukins 6 and 8) have been associated with an increased mortality risk (Winter et al., 2004). The types of response implicate impaired T-helper-cell immunity in patients with severe advanced disease.

JEV is believed to result in increased CNS pathology because of its direct neurotoxic effects in brain cells and its ability to prevent the development of new cells from neural stem/progenitor cells. Thus, JEV possibly represents the first mosquito-transmitted viral pathogen to affect neural stem cells, which normally serve important roles in injury recovery. This JEV-induced disruption of neural stem cell growth may be particularly important to augment morbidity and mortality (Jani and Kallen, 2009).

PATHOLOGY

In horses there are no characteristic gross lesions in the brain, and only nonspecific postmortem lesions are seen grossly; CNS lesions include mild leptomeningeal congestion and hyperemia and occasional hemorrhages within the brain and spinal cord. Mummified or stillborn fetuses can be found in litters from infected sows. Congenital neurologic defects, including hydrocephalus, cerebellar hypoplasia, and spinal hypomyelinogenesis may be seen in some litters. Experimentally infected piglets with encephalitis had swelling and edema of the brain (Yamada et al., 2004). Microscopically, neurons in the CNS are the target cells. Lesions are characterized by an early leptomeningitis and encephalitis in which neutrophils predominate followed by nonsuppurative encephalomyelitis, focal hemorrhage, and focal malacia. The virus causes neuronal degeneration, especially of Purkinje cells of the cerebellum associated with necrosis, neuronophagia, microgliosis, and axonal degeneration. Neuronal necrosis is accompanied by perivascular cuffing with lymphocytes. Inclusion bodies are not found. The lesions are distributed diffusely throughout the nervous system but affect the gray matter more than the white matter (Burns and Matumoto, 1949; Zachary, 2007).

DIAGNOSIS

1. *Clinical (field) diagnosis.* Presumptive diagnosis can be made in horses that manifest CNS disease accompanied by fever and neurological signs, particularly in an epizootic period. It has been observed that illness in horses at race tracks in Malaysia is frequently due to JE infection. The infection is manifested only by fever and a short period of lethargy (Hale and Witherington, 1953; Kheng et al., 1968). In temperate regions, this disease is most common in the late summer and early autumn. The principal sign in pigs is the birth of a litter with a large number of stillborn, mummified, or weak piglets.
2. *Collection of samples.* The samples from animals with a suspected JE disease should only be sent under secure conditions and to authorized laboratories to prevent the spread of the disease. Biosafety facilities are required for all potentially infectious material from a Japanese encephalitis case. Human encephalitis has been seen after infection through a scratch. Biosafety level 3 (BSL-3) practices are used during virus isolation.

JEV can be isolated from the corpus striatum, cortex, thalamus or spinal cord, and occasionally from the blood or cerebrospinal fluid (CSF) (Swami et al., 2008). At necropsy, samples for virus isolation should be taken from animals that have been dead for less than twelve hours or from animals killed during the acute stage of the disease. Samples for virus isolation should be kept chilled and shipped on wet ice. If shipping will be delayed for forty-eight hours or more, the samples can be frozen and sent on dry ice.

The brain should be submitted from horses that die of encephalitis; one-half of a brain should be submitted unfixed for virus isolation and the other half fixed in 10% formalin for histopathology. Alternatively, samples for virus isolation and histopathology can be collected from the cortex, midbrain, and brainstem. In live horses, whole blood should be collected into heparin. Virus isolation can also be attempted from serum and/or CSF (Tiroumourougane et al., 2002). Virus isolation is rarely successful in live horses as the viremia is usually short-lived. Paired acute and convalescent serum samples, taken two to four weeks apart, should be submitted for serology. Antibodies may also be found in CSF from acutely affected animals (Nagarkatti and Nagarkatti, 1980). In addition, a full range of tissues (including the spleen, liver, kidney, lung, and heart) should be collected for histopathology to rule out other causes of encephalitis (Lian, et al., 2002). In swine, JEV can be isolated from the brains of affected fetuses or piglets that die with encephalitis. The sow has usually cleared the virus by the time an affected litter is born. In endemic areas, serologic diagnosis is complicated by antibodies from vaccination or previous exposure. In addition, seroconversion generally occurs in the sow before reproductive symptoms are seen, and rising titers may not be observed.

3. *Laboratory diagnosis.* Confirmation of JE can be accomplished by demonstrating seroconversion in animals that survive long enough to yield properly spaced blood samples. Serologic tests include the plaque-reduction virus-neutralization test (VN), hemagglutination inhibition (HI) test, complement fixation test (CFT), enzyme-linked immunosorbent assay (ELISA), and immunofluorescence assay (IFA) (Gajanana et al., 1996; Xinglin et al., 2005; CIRAD, 2007). A latex agglutination test has been described in swine (Xinglin et al., 2002). In endemic regions, serologic diagnosis usually depends on a significant rise in titer with paired acute and convalescent samples (Mathew et al. 1976, Chang et al., 1984; Chow et al., 1996; Pant et al., 2006; Sapkal et al., 2007; Swami et al., 2008). A presumptive diagnosis may be made if a high titer is found in a single serum sample, but supportive evidence should be collected if possible. In horses, the detection of specific IgM and IgG in CSF is also good evidence of infection (Burke et al., 1985; Santhosh et al., 2007). However, demonstration of JE-specific IgM in serum of an encephalitic equine is presumptive evidence of the diagnosis. In regions where other viruses in the Japanese encephalitis serogroup are present, cross-reactions can occur in serologic tests. These reactions can be differentiated by virus-neutralization or with epitope-blocking ELISAs (Xinglin et al., 2005; Kitai et al., 2007). Reliance on seroconversion or IgM as a means of diagnosis in horses is not definitive because seroconversion may have resulted from exposure to another nonpathogenic *Flavivirus*.

Also, demonstration of antibody increase in sows bearing affected litters is probably not a reliable measure because seroconversion in such animals would probably have occurred earlier in infection.

Recently, reverse transcription–polymerase chain reaction (RT-PCR) has been used to detect flavivirus rapidly and specifically (Tanaka, 1993; Eldadah et al., 1991; Igarashi et al., 1994; Santhosh et al., 2007). Establishment of a molecular relationship among the genus *Flavivirus* with analysis of the different genomic regions has been performed (Billoir et al., 2000; Kuno et al., 1998). The application of genetic information is a useful tool in determining the correct diagnosis and evolution of pathogens. RT-PCR and RT-PCR restriction fragment length polymorphism (RFLP) analysis using a RT-PCR primer set, a nested PCR primer set, and a restriction enzyme can also detect viral nucleic acids directly in tissues or blood (Lian et al., 2002; Shirato et al., 2003). These techniques can detect and discriminate West Nile (WN) and JE viruses in infected animal brain, spleen, and serum samples and have been found to be quite useful in distinguishing WN viruses from the endemic background of JE viruses and also in discriminating the highly virulent WN strain from other WN virus strains. A one-step, single-tube accelerated quantitative reverse transcription–loop-mediated isothermal amplification (RT-LAMP) assay has been reported for rapid and real-time detection of JEV infection (Parida et al., 2006b).

Although microscopic lesions of the brain are of value, definitive confirmation is based on isolation and identification of the virus from the brain. Virus isolations are more likely to be successful from brains of animals that died after a short course of the disease. A definitive diagnosis can be made by virus isolation. The virus is isolated from blood, spinal cord samples, or portions of the corpus striatum, cortex, or thalamus of the brain. JEV can be isolated in chicken embryo, porcine or hamster kidney cells, African green monkey kidney (Vero) cells, the MDBK cell line, or mosquito cell line C3/36. Tissue samples are also inoculated into two to four-day-old mice (CIRAD, 2007). Virus isolation from sick or dead horses is often unsuccessful. The isolated virus can be identified as a flavivirus by HI or ELISA tests (Chow et al., 1996; Pant et al., 2006). It can be confirmed as JE virus by VN, RT-PCR assays or IFA for viral antigens (Lian et al., et al., 2002; Shirato et al., 2003; Zhang et al., 2005).

DIFFERENTIAL DIAGNOSIS
The disease in horses must be differentiated from other encephalitides including equine herpes myelencephalopathy, hepatic encephalopathy, bacterial or toxic encephalitis, equine protozoal myelencephalitis, rabies,

Murray Valley encephalitis, and western, eastern, and Venezuelan equine encephalomyelitis (Jani and Kallen, 2009). Various forms of toxic encephalitis must be considered in differential diagnosis. In temperate-zone Asia, the midsummer seasonal occurrence of JE in horses helps in differential diagnosis. In Asia, JE is the only recognized arboviral infection causing encephalitis in horses. Because there are many mild or subclinical infections, laboratory confirmation is essential. In pigs, other causes of SMEDI or encephalitis in newborns should be ruled out. These diseases include Menangle virus infection, porcine parvovirus infection, classical swine fever, porcine reproductive and respiratory syndrome, Aujeszky's disease (pseudorabies), blue eye (La Piedad, Michoacan) paramyxovirus disease, and porcine brucellosis, as well as common hemagglutinating DNA virus infections, which cause the same pattern of disease (Morimoto et al., 1972). There is evidence that the DNA virus infection is established in gilts in the middle or last trimester of pregnancy. Myxovirus parainfluenza 1 (Sendai) has been shown capable of producing stillbirth in swine under experimental conditions. Encephalitis in neonatal pigs is also associated with a coronavirus infection. This agent is known to cause encephalitis in piglets in at least North America and Europe (Mengeling and Cutlip, 1976).

TREATMENT AND CONTROL

For JE, there is no clearly effective antiviral agent available. However, in a recent study on anti-JE viral therapeutic efficacy of arctigenin, results from in vivo and in vitro experimentations indicated that arctigenin was capable of reducing viral load and viral replication within the brain with consequent reduction in neuronal death, secondary inflammation, and oxidative stress resulting from microglial activation, suggesting its potential for treating JE (Swarup et al., 2008).

1. *Control.* The prevention and control of JE can be achieved by three possible strategies, each targeting a specific part of the transmission cycle of JEV: (a) vaccination of the animal/human population, (b) control of amplifying hosts by either swine vaccination or changes in animal husbandry, or (c) vector control.

Options for control include elimination of the vectors, prevention of amplification of the infection cycle in birds and pigs, or immunization of horses, pigs, and people. Although some success in vector control was achieved by modification of irrigation methods to minimize breeding of *C. tritaeniorhynchus* in Southeast Asia and coincidentally by the use of agricultural pesticides, vector control has never been more than marginally successful. Reduction of the avian reservoir hosts does not appear feasible.

Stabling animals in screened barns can be partially protective, particularly during outbreaks. Peak mosquito-biting activity is usually from dusk to dawn. Barn fans are helpful as mosquitoes do not fly well in strong winds. The walls may also be sprayed with insecticides. Insect repellents can help protect individual animals. In some climates, horses may be rugged and hooded in lightweight permethrin-treated material. Environmental control of mosquitoes can reduce the number of vectors, but in many areas it is impractical. Whenever possible, pigs should be raised away from horses (CIRAD, 2007; van den Hurk et al., 2009). It would be prudent to advise those who import horses from Asian and Pacific Rim countries to outside that region to vaccinate all horses on arrival against Japanese encephalitis and avoid importation during the rainy season. Foals born to imported mares also should receive the vaccine.

JE virus does not survive well outside a living host or tissues. In the laboratory or other situations where disinfection is necessary, this virus can be inactivated with 70% ethanol, 2% glutaraldehyde, 3–8% formaldehyde, 1% sodium hypochlorite, iodine, phenol iodophors, and organic solvents/detergents. It is also sensitive to heat, ultraviolet light, and gamma irradiation (CIRAD, 2007).

2. *Vaccination.* Vaccines are protective for all genotypes. JE vaccines can prevent disease in horses and pigs. Vaccinating pigs can also decrease the amplification of the virus and help protect horses and humans. However, JEV is also amplified in birds, and some infections may still occur. An inactivated vaccine against the disease used in Japan since 1948 has significantly reduced mortality among horses over the years, and horses in Hong Kong and Singapore are routinely vaccinated against Japanese encephalitis. The only source of equine vaccine is currently from Japan, although a live, attenuated vaccine produced in hamster kidney tissue culture is in widespread use in horses in China (Han et al., 1974). This vaccine reduced disease by about 85%. An inactivated vaccine prepared in mouse brain is licensed in Japan, Korea, Taiwan, India, and Thailand for use in humans. Live, attenuated vaccines are used to immunize pigs in Japan and Taiwan (Fujisaki et al., 1975) and humans in China (Hennessy et al., 1996). Over the past few years, DNA vaccines against JEV using both structural and nonstructural genes have been developed and evaluated in animal models with different efficacies (Saxena and Dhole, 2008). Vaxfectin, used as an adjuvant, has been shown to improve the efficacy of DNA vaccine in animal model (Nukuzuma et al., 2003). A recent study promises for development of effective single-dose JE vaccine in animals using biodegradable poly(γ-glutamic acid)

nanoparticles (γ-PGA-NPs) as test adjuvant. Single dose of JE vaccine with γ-PGA-NPs enhanced the neutralizing antibody titer, and all of the immunized mice survived a normally lethal JEV infection, while only 50% of the mice that received a single dose of JE vaccine without γ-PGA-NPs survived. The results appear promising for a novel and safe γ-PGA-NPs-adjuvanted JE vaccine for animals (Okamoto, 2008).

Human vaccination is considered the most reliable method of preventing JE in humans. In human, mouse-brain-derived, formalin-inactivated vaccine developed using the prototype Nakayama strain have been used in several countries (Shlim and Solomon, 2002; Ferguson et al., 2007; Kurane, 2009), resulting into almost elimination of the incidences of JE in Japan, Korea, and Taiwan (Sohn, 2000; Igarashi, 2002), in association with other measures, viz, vector control and alternative agricultural practices (Igarashi, 2002). Inactivated cell culture vaccines prepared in primary hamster kidney (PHK) or African green monkey kidney (Vero) cells, and a live, attenuated SA14-14-2 vaccine have been used in China (Liu et al., 2006). The SA14-14-2 vaccine has also been used successfully in Nepal (Tandan et al., 2007), and most recently in India (Beasley et al., 2008). Currently, a number of vaccines are under development or in clinical trial for international use (Beasley et al., 2008; Solomon, 2008). These include the inactivated Vero cell–derived SA14-14-2 vaccines (Srivastava et al., 2001; Lyons et al., 2007) and a live, attenuated chimeric vaccine based on the ChimeriVax infectious clone of 17D yellow fever vaccine containing the *prM* and *E* genes of SA14-14-2 virus (Monath et al., 2003).

CONCLUSION

Japanese encephalitis (JE) is a disease caused by a flavivirus, a Japanese encephalitis virus (JEV) that affects membranes around the brain. The JEV is related to the St. Louis encephalitis virus, Murray Valley virus, and West Nile virus and can infect horses, pigs, humans, cattle, bats, reptiles, and various species of birds. In countries where it is endemic, the virus causes SMEDI (stillbirth, mummification, embryonic death, and infertility) in pigs and encephalitis in horses. The virus is transmitted by mosquitoes. Bats might also be able to carry the virus for long periods of time. The virus also circulates in ardeid birds (herons and egrets). Under experimental conditions, *Culex tritaeniorhynchus* mosquito can transmit the virus between horses; under natural conditions, humans and horses appear to be dead-end hosts. Cattle are often infected in endemic regions but do not become ill or develop viremia. Swine develop clinical signs and also amplify the virus. JE is a leading cause of viral encephalitis in Asia with thirty thousand to fifty thousand clinical cases of humans reported annually. JEV tends to spill over into human populations when infected mosquito populations build up explosively and human biting rate increases. The incubation period in horses is eight to ten days, and most infections are subclinical. Horses with clinical signs resemble animals with WEE or EEE, but the mortality rate is relatively low. The symptoms may include a fever, impaired locomotion, stupor, and teeth grinding. Blindness, coma, and death are possible. In some cases, the only symptoms may be a fever and short period of lethargy. The most common symptom of JE in pigs is the birth of stillborn or mummified fetuses, usually at term. There are no specific gross lesions seen in horses, similar to the signs in animals that die from EEE or WEE. Inapparent infections are common in horses; mortality in this species is approximately 5% or less. The mortality rate is high in piglets born to infected sows, but close to zero in adult pigs.

JE should be suspected in horses with fever and symptoms of a CNS disease. In horses, the different diagnosis includes toxic encephalitis and viral encephalitides such as Murray Valley encephalitis. JE can be diagnosed by virus isolation from blood, spinal cord samples, or portions of the corpus striatum, cortex, or thalamus of the brain. The virus is identified by mice inoculation, HI test, and by infection of various cell cultures. Serologic tests include the plaque reduction, VN, HI, and CFT. PCR and RFLP have also been applied for detection of JEV. In horses, virus-specific IgM and IgG antibodies can also be detected in the CSF with enzyme immunoassays and are good evidence of infection. Brains should be submitted from animals with encephalitis. Paired serum samples should be taken at least fourteen days apart for serology. Biosafety level 3 practices are recommended for investigators working with this virus.

JE vaccines can prevent disease in horses and pigs. Vaccinating pigs can also decrease the amplification of the virus. However, JEV is also amplified in birds, and some infections may still occur. For humans, an effective killed vaccine is available for Japanese encephalitis, but it is expensive and requires one primary vaccination followed by two boosters. An inexpensive live, attenuated vaccine is used in China but is not available elsewhere. Chemical vector control is not a solution as the breeding sites (irrigated rice fields) are extensive. In some rice-production systems faced with water shortages, however, certain water-management measures (alternate wetting and drying) may be applied that reduce vector populations. Personal protection (using repellents and/or mosquito nets) will be effective under certain conditions. Good management and appropriate sanitation/hygiene measures should be followed accordingly. Eliminating the pig population is often a measure taken in the wake of outbreaks. Being in the list of emerging and reemerging infectious diseases, Japanese encephalitis could cause a very serious disease; fatal encephalitis in humans can even occur in an epidemic form worldwide.

REFERENCES

1. Acha, P. N. and Szyfres, B. 2003. Zoonoses and communicable diseases common to man and animals. Volume 2. *Chlamydioses, rickettsioses, and viroses.* 3rd ed. [Pan American Health Organization (PAHO)], Washington, D.C. Scientific and Technical Publication No. 580. Japanese encephalitis, 172–179.

2. Ahmed, A. 1999. Japanese encephalitis. In *Neurology in the tropics,* 1st ed., ed. J. S. Chopra and I. M. S. Sawhney, 176–190. New Delhi: BI Churchill Livingstone.

3. Arai, S., Matsunaga, Y., Takasaki, T., Tanaka-Taya, K., Taniguchi, K., Okabe, N., Kurane, I. and Vaccine Preventable Diseases Surveillance Program of Japan. 2008. Japanese encephalitis: Surveillance and elimination effort in Japan from 1982 to 2004. *Jpn. J. Infect. Dis.* 61:333–338.

4. Arora, R. R. and Singh, N. N. 1974. Epidemiological study of an epidemic of Japanese encephalitis in Bankura Dist. of West Bengal during 1973. *J. Comm. Dis.* **6**:310.

5. Arora, R. R. Lahiri, S. K., Mathew, T., Suri, J. C., Suri, N. K. and Bhola, S. R. 1975. An outbreak of fever by group B arboviruses in Jaipur, 1973. *J. Comm. Dis.* **7**:374–376.

6. Arora, R. R. and Mathew, T. 1977a. Working paper on Japanese encephalitis. Presented to the II international seminar on zoonosis and its control in India-June 1977, 1–3. Delhi.

7. Arora, R. R. and Mathew, T. 1977b. Epidemics of Japanese encephalitis in West Bengal. Presented to the II international seminar on zoonosis and its control in India. June 1977:1–6.

8. Beasley, D. W., Lewthwaite, P. and Solomon, T. 2008. Current use and development of vaccines for Japanese encephalitis. *Expert Opin. Biol. Ther.* 8:95–106.

9. Billoir, F., De Chesse, R., Tolou, H., De Micco, P., Gould, E. A. and De Lamballerie, X. 2000. Phylogeny of the genus flavivirus using complete coding sequences of arthropod-borne viruses and viruses with no known vector. *J. Gen. Virol.* 81:781–790.

10. Bricaire, F. and Bossi, P. 2006. Emerging viral diseases. *Bull. Acad. Natl. Med.* 190:597–608.

11. Buescher, E. L., Scherer, W. F., Rosenberg, M. Z., Gresser, I., Hardy, J. L. and Bullock, H. R. 1959. Ecologic studies of Japanese encephalitis virus in Japan. II. Mosquito infection. *Am. J. Trop. Med. Hyg.* 8:651–664.

12. Burke, D. S., Nisalak, A., Ussery, N. M., Laorakpongse, T. and Chantavibul, S. 1985. Kinetics of IgM and IgG responses to Japanese encephalitis virus in human serum and cerebrospinal fluid. *J. Infec. Dis.* 151:1093–1099.

13. Burns, K. F. and Matumoto, M. 1949. Japanese equine encephalomyelitis. Review of the literature. *J. Am. Vet. Med. Assoc.* 115:112–115.

14. Carey, D. E., Myers, R. M. and Pavri, K. M. 1968. Japanese encephalitis studies in Vellore, India. Part II. Antibody response of Patients. *Indian J. Med. Res.* 56:1319–1329.

15. Chambers, T. J., Hahn, C. S., Galler, R. and Rice, C. M. 1990. Flavivirus genome organisation, expression and replication. *Annu. Rev. Microbiol.* 44:649–688.

16. Chang, H. C., Takashima, I., Arikawa, J. and Hashimoto, N. 1984. Biotin-labeled antigen sandwich enzyme-linked immunosorbent assay (BLA-S-ELISA) for the detection of Japanese encephalitis antibody in human and a variety of animal sera. *J. Immunol. Methods* 72:401–409.

17. Chow, L., Yueh, Y. Y., Hwang, Y. S., Lin, T. L., Wu, Y. C. and Horng, C. B. 1996. Detection of IgM antibody to Japanese encephalitis virus infection by enzyme-linked immunosorbent assay (ELISA). *Zhonghua Yi Xue Za Zhi* (Taipei) 58:1–6.

18. CIRAD, Centre de coopération internationale en recherche agronomique pour le développement. 2007. Japanese Encephalitis. http://pigtrop.cirad.fr/resources/encyclopedias/disease_technical_cards/japanese_encephalitis (accessed on March 1, 2009).

19. Diagana, M., Preux, P. M. and Dumas, M. 2007. Japanese encephalitis revisited. *J. Neurol. Sci.* 262:165–170.

20. Doi, R., Oya, A., Shirasaka, A., Yabe, S. and Sasa, M. 1983. Studies of Japanese encephalitis virus infection of reptiles. II. Role of lizards on hibernation of Japanese encephalitis virus. *Jpn. J. Exp. Med.* 53:125–134.

21. Doi, R., Shirasaka, A., Sasa, M., Oya, A. 1977. Studies on the susceptibility of three species of mosquitoes to Japanese encephalitis virus. *J. Med. Entomol.* 13:591–94.

22. Eldadah, Z. A., Asher, D. M., Godec, M. S., Pomeroy, K. L., Goldfarb, L. G., Feinstone, S. M., Levitan, H., Gibbs, C. J. and Gajdusek, D. C. 1991. Detection of flavivirus by reverse-transcriptase polymerase chain reaction. *J. Med. Virol.* 33:260–267.

23. Endy, T. P. and Nisalak, A. 2002. Japanese encephalitis virus: Ecology and epidemiology. *Curr. Top. Microbiol. Immunol.* 267:11–48.

24. Ferguson, M., Kurane, I., Wimalaratne, O., Shin, J. and Wood, D. 2007. WHO informal consultation on the scientific basis of specifications for production and control of inactivated Japanese encephalitis vaccines for human use, Geneva, Switzerland, 1–2 June 2006. *Vaccine* 25:5233–5243.

25. Fujisaki, Y., Sugimori, T., Morimoto, T., and Miura, Y. 1975. Development of an attenuated strain for Japanese encephalitis live virus vaccine for porcine use. *Nat. Inst. Animal Hlth. Quart.* 15:15023.

26. Gajanana, A., Samuel, P. P., Thenmozhi, V. and Rajendran, R. 1996. An appraisal of some recent diagnostic assays for Japanese encephalitis. *Southern Asian. J. Trop. Med. Public Health* 27:673–679.

27. Garavelli, P. L. and Peduzzi, P. 2006. Globalization and infectious diseases. *Recenti. Prog. Med.* 97:528–532.

28. Georges, A. J., Matton, T. and Courbot-Georges, M. C. 2004. Monkey-pox, a model of emergent then reemergent disease. *Med. Mal. Infect.* 34:12–19.

29. Gould, D. J., Byrne, R. J. and Hayes, D. E. 1964. Experimental infection of horses with Japanese encephalitis virus by mosquito bites. *Am. J. Trop. Med. Hyg.* 13:742–746.

30. Gould, E. A. and Higgs, S. 2009. Impact of climate change and other factors on emerging arbovirus diseases. *Trans. R. Soc. Trop. Med. Hyg.* 103:109–121.

31. Guérin, B. and Pozzi, N. 2005. Viruses in boar semen: Detection and clinical as well as epidemiological consequences regarding disease transmission by artificial insemination. *Theriogenol.* 63:556–572.

32. Hale, J. H. and Witherington, D. H. 1953. Encephalitis in racehorses in Malaya. *J. Comp. Pathol. Ther.* 63:195–198.

33. Hamano, M., Lim, C. K., Takagi, H., Sawabe, K., Kuwayama, M., Kishi, N., Kurane, I. and Takasaki, T. 2007. Detection of antibodies to Japanese encephalitis virus in the wild boars in Hiroshima prefecture. *Japan. Epidemiol Infect.* 135:974–977.

34. Han, G. S., Chen, B. Q., and Huang, C. H. 1974. Studies on attenuated Japanese B encephalitis virus vaccine. II. Safety, epidemiological and serological evaluation of attenuated 2–8 strain vaccine after immunization of horses. *Acta Microbiol. Sinica* 14:185–190.

35. Hase, T., Summers, P. L. and Dubois, D. R. 1990. Ultra structure changes of mouse brain neurons infected with Japanese encephalitis virus. *Int. J. Exp. Pathol.* 71:493–505.

36. Heinz, F. X. 1986. Epitope mapping of flavivirus glycoproteins. *Adv. Virus Res.* 31:103–168.

37. Hemmerter, S., Slapeta, J., van den Hurk, A. F., Cooper, R. D., Whelan, P. I., Russell, R. C., Johansen, C. A. and Beebe, N. W. 2007. A curious coincidence: Mosquito biodiversity and the limits of the Japanese encephalitis virus in Australasia. *BMC Evol. Biol.* 7:100.

38. Hennessy, S., Liu, Z., Tsai, T. F., Strom, B. L., Wan, C. M., Liu, H. L., Wu, T. X., Yu, H. J., Liu, Q. M., Karabatsos, M., Bilker, W. B., and Halstead, S. B. 1996. Effectiveness of live-attenuated Japanese encephalitis vaccine (SA14-14-2): A case-control study. *Lancet* 34:1583–1586.

39. Higgins, A. J. and Snyder, J. R. 2006. *The equine manual*, 2nd ed. 37–44. St. Louis: Elsevier Saunders.

40. Igarashi, A. 2002. Control of Japanese encephalitis in Japan: Immunization of humans and animals, and vector control. *Curr. Top. Microbiol. Immunol.* 267:139–152.

41. Igarashi, A., Tanaka, M., Morita, K., Takasu, T., Ahmed, A., Ahmed, A., Akram, D. S. and Anwar Waqar, M. 1994. Detection of West Nile and Japanese encephalitis viral genome sequences in cerebrospinal fluid from acute encephalitis cases in Karachi, Pakistan. *Microbiol. Immunol.* 38:827–830.

42. Ihara, T., Kano, R., Nakajima, Y., Sugiura, T., Imagawa, H., Izuchi, T. and Samjima, T. 1997. Detection of antibody to Japanese encephalitis virus (JEV) by enzyme-linked immunosorbent assay (ELISA). *J. Equine Sci.* 8:25–28.

43. Jani, A. A. and Kallen, A. J. 2009. Japanese Encephalitis. http://emedicine.medscape.com/article/233802-print (accessed on March 1, 2009).

44. Kahn, C. M. and Line, S. 2003. The Merck veterinary manual [online]. Whitehouse Station, NJ: Merck and Co. *Equine encephalomyelitis.* http://www.merckvetmanual.com/mvm/index.jsp?cfile=htm/bc/100900.htm (accessed March 4, 2009).

45. Kheng, C. S., Chee, T. K., Marchette, N. J., Garcia, R., Rudnick, A. and Coughlan, R. F. 1968. Japanese B encephalitis in a horse. *Aus. Vet. J.* 44:23–25.

46. Kitai, Y., Shoda, M., Kondo, T. and Konishi, E. 2007. Epitope-blocking enzyme-linked immunosorbent assay to differentiate West Nile virus from Japanese encephalitis virus infections in equine sera. *Clin. Vaccine Immunol.* 14:1024–1031.

47. Kono, R. and Kim, K. H. 1969. Comparative epidemiological features of Japanese encephalitis in the Republic of Korea, China (Taiwan) and Japan. *Bull. WHO* 40:263–277.

48. Kuno, G., Chang, G. J., Tsuchiya, K. R., Karabatsos, N. and Cropp, C. B. 1998. Phylogeny of the genus *Flavivirus. J. Virol.* 72:73–83.

49. Kurane, I. 2009. Japanese encephalitis. In *Vaccines for biodefense and emerging and neglected diseases*, ed. D. T. Alan, A. D. T. Barrett, and L. Stanberry, chapter 28, 527–535. New York: Elsevier.

50. Kurane, I. and Takasaki, T. 2000. Immunogenicity and protective efficacy of the current inactivated Japanese encephalitis vaccine against different Japanese encephalitis virus strains. *Vaccine* 18 (Suppl. 2): 33–35.

51. Lam, K. H., Ellis, T. M., Williams, D. T., Lunt, R. A., Daniels, P. W., Watkins, K. L. and Riggs, C. M. 2005. Japanese encephalitis in a racing thoroughbred gelding in Hong Kong. *Vet Rec.* 157:168–173.

52. Lian, W.-C., Liau, M.-Y. and Mao, C.-L. 2002. Diagnosis and genetic analysis of Japanese encephalitis virus infected in horses. *J. Vet. Med.* B 49:361–365.

53. Lim, S. I., Kweon, C. H., Tark, D. S., Kim, S. H. and Yang, D. K. 2007. Sero-survey on Aino, Akabane, Chuzan, bovine ephemeral fever and Japanese encephalitis virus of cattle and swine in Korea. *J. Vet. Sci.* 8:45–49.

54. Liou, M. L. and Hsu, C. Y. 1998. Japanese encephalitis virus is transported across the cerebral blood vessels by endocytosis in mouse brain. *Cell Tissue Res.* 293:389–394.

55. Liu, W., Clemens, J. D., Yang, J. Y. and Xu, Z. Y. 2006. Immunization against Japanese encephalitis in China: A policy analysis. *Vaccine* 24:5178–5182.

56. Lyons, A., Kanesa-thasan, N., Kuschner, R. A., Eckels, K. H., Putnak, R., Sun, W., Burge, R., Towle, A. C., Wilson, P., Tauber, E. and Vaughn, D. W. 2007. A phase 2 study of a purified, inactivated virus vaccine to prevent Japanese encephalitis. *Vaccine* 25:3445–3453.

57. Mackenzie, J. S., Gubler, D. J. and Petersen, L. R. 2004. Emerging flavi viruses: The spread and resurgence of Japanese encephalitis, West Nile and dengue viruses. *Nat. Med.* 10:S98–109.

58. Mackenzie, J. S., Williams, D. T. and Smith, D. W. 2007. Japanese encephalitis virus: The geographic distribution, incidence, and spread of a virus with a propensity to emerge in new areas. In *Emerging viruses in human populations*, ed. E. Tabor, 201–68. Amsterdam: Elsevier.

59. Mangada, M. N. and Takegami, T. 1999. Molecular characterization of the Japanese encephalitis virus representative immunotype strain JaGAr 01. *Virus Res.* 59:101–112.

60. Mason, P. W., Pincus, S., Fournier, M. J. et al. 1991. Japanese encephalitis virus-vaccinia recombinants produce particulate forms of structural proteins and induce high levels of protection against lethal Japanese encephalitis virus infection. *Virol.* 180:294–305.

61. Mathew, T. and Arora, R. R. 1975. Information of dengue in India-1956–74. Information given from National Institute of Communicable Disease in *Dengue News Letter* 3:3–4.

62. Mathew, T., Suri, N. K., Bhola, S. R., Suri, J. C., Arora, R. R. and Lahiri, S. K. 1976. Serological investigation of an epidemic of fever by group B arboviruses in Jaipur 1973. *Indian J. Med. Res.* 64:1136–1142.

63. Mathew, T., Srikumar, R. and George, K. 1977. Studies on human transplacental transfer of 2-Mercaptoethanol resistant and sensitive HI antibodies of Influenza and Arboviruses. *Ann. Natl. Acad. Med. Sci.* (India) 13:1–9.

64. Mathew, T., Nayar, M., Gupta, J. P., Suri, N. K., Bhola, S. R., Gosh, T. K., Suri, J. C., Talwar, V. and Pattanayak, S. 1979. Serological investigation on arbovirus activity in and around Delhi: A five year study. *Indian J. Med. Res.* 69:557–566.

65. Mayr, A. 2003. Smallpox vaccination and bioterrorism with pox viruses. *Comp. Immunol. Microbiol. Infect. Dis.* 26:423–430.

66. McAda, P. C., Manson, P. W., Schmaljohm, C. S., Dalrymple, J. M., Mason, T. L. and Fournier, M. J. 1987. Partial sequence of the Japanese encephalitis virus genome. *Virol.* 58:348–360.

67. McCormack, J. G. and Allworth, A. M. 2002. Emerging viral infections in Australia. *Med. J. AUS.* 177:45–49.

68. Mengeling, W. L. and Cutlip, R. C. 1976. Pathogenicity of field isolants of hemagglutinating encephalomyelitis virus for neonatal pigs. *J. Am. Vet. Med. Assoc.* 168:236–239.

69. Monath, T. P. and Heinz, F. X. 1996. Flaviviruses. In *Fields virology*, 3rd ed. B. N. Fields, D. M. Knipe, and M. Howley, 961–1034. Philadelphia: Lippincott-Raven.

70. Monath, T. P., Guirakhoo, F., Nichols, R., Yoksan, S., Schrader, R., Murphy, C., Blum, P., Woodward, S., McCarthy, K., Mathis, D., Johnson, C. and Bedford, P. 2003. Chimeric live, attenuated vaccine against Japanese encephalitis (ChimeriVax-JE): Phase 2 clinical trials for safety and immunogenicity, effect of vaccine dose and schedule, and memory response to challenge with inactivated Japanese encephalitis antigen. *J. Infect. Dis.* 188:1213–1230.

71. Morimoto, T., Hurogi, H., Miura., Y., Sugimori, T. and Fujisaki, Y. 1972. Isolation of Japanese encephalitis virus and a hemagglutinating DNA virus from the brain of stillborn piglets. *Nat. Inst. Anim. Hlth. Quart.* 12:127–136.

72. Muangman, D., Edelman, R., Sullivan, M. J. and Gould, D. J. 1972. Experimental transmission of Japanese encephalitis virus by *Culex fuscocephala*. *Am. J. Trop. Med. Hyg.* 21:482–486.

73. Mwandawiro, C., Boots, M., Tuno, N., Suwonkerd, W., Tsuda, Y. and Takagi, M. 2000. Heterogeneity in the host preference of Japanese encephalitis vectors in Chiang Mai, northern Thailand. *Trans. R. Soc. Trop. Med. Hyg.* 94:238–242.

74. Mwandawiro, C., Tuno, N., Suwonkerd, W., Tsuda, Y., Yanagi, T., and Takagi, M. 1999. Host preference of Japanese encephalitis vectors in Chiangmai, northern Thailand. *Med. Entomol. Zool.* 50:323–333.

75. Myint, K. S., Gibbons, R. V., Perng, G. C. and Solomon, T. 2007. Unravelling the neuropathogenesis of Japanese encephalitis. *Trans R Soc Trop Med Hyg.* 101:955–956.

76. Nagarkatti, P. S. and Nagarkatti, M. 1980. Comparison of haemagglutination inhibition (HI) and indirect fluorescent antibody (IFA) techniques for the serological diagnosis of certain flavivirus infections. *J. Trop. Med. Hyg.* 83:115–117.

77. Nitatpattana, N., Dubot-Pérès, A., Gouilh, M. A., Souris, M., Barbazan, P., Yoksan, S., de Lamballerie, X. and Gonzalez, J.-P. 2008. Change in Japanese encephalitis virus distribution, Thailand. *Emerg. Infect. Dis.* 14:1762–1765.

78. Nukuzuma, C., Ajiro, N., Wheeler, C. J. and Konishi, E. 2003. Enhancing effect of vaxfectin on the ability of a Japanese encephalitis DNA vaccine to induce neutralizing antibody in mice. *Viral Immunol.* 16:183–189.

79. Okamoto, S., Yoshii, H., Ishikawa, T., Akagi, T. Akashi, T., Takahash, M., Yamanish, K., and Mori, Y. 2008. Single dose of inactivated Japanese encephalitis vaccine with poly (-glutamic acid) nanoparticles provides effective protection from Japanese encephalitis virus. *Vaccine* 26:589–594.

80. Oya, A., Doi, R., Shirasaka, A., Yabe, S. and Sasa, M. 1983. Studies of Japanese encephalitis virus infection of reptiles. I. Experimental infection of snakes and lizards. *Jpn. J. Exp. Med.* 53:117–123.

81. Oyanagi, S., Ikuta, F. and Ross, E. R. 1969. Electron microscopic observation in mice infected with Japanese encephalitis. *Acta Neuropathol.* (Berl) 13:169–181.

82. Pant, G. R., Lunt, R. A., Rootes, C. L. and Daniels, P. W. 2006. Serological evidence for Japanese encephalitis and West Nile viruses in domestic animals of Nepal. *Comp. Immunol. Microbiol. Infect. Dis.* 29:166–175.

83. Parida, M., Dash, P. K., Tripathi, N. K., Ambuj, S., Sannarangaiah, S., Saxena, P., Agarwal, S., Sahni, A. K., Singh, S. P., Rathi, A. K., Bhargava, R., Abhyankar, A., Verma, S. K., Rao, P. V. L. and Sekhar, K. 2006a. Japanese encephalitis outbreak, India, 2005. *Emerg. Infect. Dis.* 12:1427–1430.

84. Parida, M. M., Santhosh, S. R., Dash, P. K., Tripathi, N. K., Saxena, P. Ambuj, S., Sahni, A. K., Lakshmana Rao, P. V. and Morita, K. 2006b. Development and evaluation of reverse transcription-loop-mediated isothermal amplification assay for rapid and real-time detection of Japanese encephalitis virus. *J. Clin. Microbiol.* 44:4172–4178.

85. Parker, S., Nuara, A., Buller, R. M. and Schultz, D. A. 2007. Human monkeypox: An emerging zoonotic disease. *Future Microbiol.* 2:17–34.

86. Poidinger, M., Hall, R. A. and Mackenzie, J. S. 1996. Molecular characterization of the Japanese encephalitis serocomplex of the flavivirus genus. *Virol.* 218:417–421.

87. Qi, L., Keshu, X., Huafeng, W. and Xia, Z. 2006. E sequence analysis of persistently infected mutant Japanese encephalitis virus strains. *J. Huazhong Univ. Sci. Technol.-Med. Sci.* 26:408–410.

88. Rodrigues, F. M., Guttikar, S. N. and Pinto, B. D. 1981. Prevalence of antibodies to Japanese encephalitis and West Nile viruses among wild birds in the Krishna-Godavari Delta, Andhra Pradesh, India. *Trans. R. Soc. Trop. Med. Hyg.* 75:258–262.

89. Rosen, L. 1986. The natural history of Japanese encephalitis virus. *Annu. Rev. Microbiol.* 40:395–414.

90. Russell, P. K., Brandt, W. A. and Dalrymple, J. M. 1980. Chemical and antigenic structure of flaviviruses. In *The toga viruses*, ed. R. W. Schlesinger, 503–529. New York: Academic Press.

91. Santhosh, S. R., Parida, M. M., Dash, P. K., Pateriya, A., Pattnaik, B., Pradhan, H. K., Tripathi, N. K., Ambuj, S., Gupta, N., Saxena, P. and Lakshmana Rao, P. V. 2007. Development and evaluation of SYBR green I-based one-step real-time RT-PCR assay for detection and quantitation of Japanese encephalitis virus. *J. Virol. Methods* 143:73–80.

92. Sapkal, G. N., Wairagkar, N. S., Ayachit, V. M., Bondre, V. P. and Gore, M. M. 2007. Detection and isolation of Japanese encephalitis virus from blood clots collected during the acute phase of infection. *Am. J. Trop. Med. Hyg.* 77:1139–45.

93. Saxena, S. K. 2008. Japanese encephalitis: Perspectives and new developments. *Future Neurol.* 3:515–521.

94. Saxena, V. and Dhole, T. N. 2008. Preventive strategies for frequent outbreaks of Japanese encephalitis in Northern India. *J. Biosci.* 33:505–514.

95. Shirato, K., Mizutani, T., Kariwa, H. and Takashima, I. 2003. Discrimination of West Nile virus and Japanese encephalitis virus strains using RT-PCR RFLP analysis. *Microbiol. Immunol.* 47:439–445.

96. Shlim, D. R. and Solomon, T. 2002. Japanese encephalitis vaccine for travelers: Exploring the limits of risk. *Clin. Infect. Dis.* 35:183–188.

97. Smithburn, K. C., Kerr, J. A. and Gante, P. B. 1954. Neutralizing antibodies against certain viruses in the sera of residents of India. *J. Immunol.* 72:284–257.

98. Sohn, Y. M. 2000. Japanese encephalitis immunization in South Korea: Past, present, and future. *Emerg. Infect. Dis.* 6:17–24.

99. Solomon, T. 2003. Recent advances in Japanese encephalitis. *J. Neurovirol.* 9:274–283.

100. Solomon, T. 2006. Control of Japanese encephalitis—within our grasp. *N. Engl. J. Med.* 355:869–871.

101. Solomon, T. 2008. New vaccines for Japanese encephalitis. *Lancet Neurol.* 7:116–118.

102. Solomon, T., Dung, N. M., Kneen, R., Gainsborough, M., Vaughn, D. W. and Khanh, V. T. 2000. Japanese encephalitis. *J. Neurol. Neurosurg. Psychiatry* 68:405–415.

103. Solomon, T., Ni, H., Beasley, D. W., Ekkelenkamp, M., Cardosa, M. J. and Barrett, A. D. 2003. Origin and evolution of Japanese encephalitis virus in Southeast Asia. *J. Virol.* 77:3091–3098.

104. Soman, R. S., Rodrigues, F. M., Guttikar, S. N. and Guru, P. Y. 1977. Experimental viraemia and transmission of Japanese encephalitis virus by mosquitoes in ardeid birds. *Indian J. Med. Res.* 66:709–718.

105. Srivastava, A. K., Putnak, J. R., Lee, S. H., Hong, S. P., Moon, S. B., Barvir, D. A., Zhao, B. Olson, R. A., Kim, S. O., Yoo, W. D., Towle, A. C., Vaughn, D. W., Innis, B. L. and Eckels, K. H. 2001. A purified inactivated Japanese encephalitis virus vaccine made in Vero cells. *Vaccine* 19:4557–4565.

106. Sugiura, T. and Shimada, K. 1999. Seroepizootiological survey of Japanese encephalitis virus and Getah virus in regional horse race tracks from 1991 to 1997 in Japan. *J. Vet. Med. Sci.* 61:877–881.

107. Sumiyoshi, H., Mori, C., Fuke, I., Morita, K., Kuhara, S., Kondou, J., Kikuchi, Y., Nagamtu, H. and Igarashi, A. 1987. Complete nucleotide sequence of the Japanese encephalitis virus genome RNA. *Virology* 161:497–510.

108. Suneja, R., K., Radha, S., Mathew, T., Suri, J. C., Suri, N. K. and Bhola, S. R. 1977. Clinico-laboratory study of arbovirus encephalitis in children from Delhi. Presented at II international seminar on zoonosis and its control. 16-6-1977, Delhi.

109. Swami, R., Ratho, R. K., Mishra, B. and Singh, M. P. 2008. Usefulness of RT-PCR for the diagnosis of Japanese encephalitis in clinical samples. *Scand. J. Infect. Dis.* 40:815–820.

110. Swarup, V., Ghosh, J., Mishra, M. K. and Basu, A. 2008. Novel strategy for treatment of Japanese encephalitis using arctigenin, a plant lignan. *J. Antimicrob. Chemother.* 61:679–688.

111. Takahashi, M. 1976. The effects of environmental and physiological conditions of *Culex tritaeniorhynchus* on the pattern of transmission of Japanese encephalitis virus. *J. Med. Entomol.* 13:275–284.

112. Takahashi, M. 1982. Differential transmission efficiency for Japanese encephalitis virus among colonized strains of *Culex tritaeniorhynchus*. *Jpn. J. Sanit. Zool.* 33:325–333.

113. Takashima, I., Watanabe, T., Ouchi, N. and Hashimoto, N. 1988. Ecologic studies of Japanese encephalitis virus in Hokkaido: Interepidemic outbreaks of swine abortion and evidence for the virus to overwinter locally. *Am. J. Trop. Med. Hyg.* 38:420–427.

114. Tanaka, M., 1993. Rapid identification of flavivirus using the polymerase chain reaction. *J. Virol. Methods* 41:311–322.

115. Tandan, J. B., Ohrr, H., Sohn, Y. M., Yoksan, S., Ji, M., Nam, C. M. and Halstead, S. B. 2007. Single dose of SA 14-14-2 vaccine provides long-term protection against Japanese encephalitis: A case-control study in Nepalese children 5 years after immunization. *Vaccine* 25:5041–5045.

116. Thiel, H.-J., Collett, M. S., Gould, E. A., Heinz, F. X., Houghton, M., Meyers, G., Purcell, R. H. and Rice, C. M. 2005. Flaviviridae. In *Virus taxonomy: Eighth report of the International Committee on Taxonomy of Viruses*, ed. C. M. Fauquet, M. A. Mayo, J. Maniloff, U. Desselberger, and L. A. Ball, 981–98. San Diego: Virol. Div., Int. Union Microbiol. Soc.

117. Thomas, J. C., Chang, S. H., Ricardo, G. et al. 1990. Flaviviruses genome organization, expression and replication. *Annu. Rev. Microbiol.* 44:649–688.

118. Tiroumourougane, S. V., Raghava, P. and Srinivasan, S. 2002. Japanese viral encephalitis. *Postgrad. Med. J.* 78:205–215.

119. Tsai, T. F. 2000. New initiatives for the control of Japanese encephalitis by vaccination: Minutes of a WHO/CVI meeting, Bangkok, Thailand, 13–15 October 1998. *Vaccine* 18 (Suppl. 2): 1–25.

120. van den Hurk, A. F., Nisbet, D. J., Hall, R. A., Kay, B. H., Mackenzie, J. S. and Ritchie, S. A. 2003. Vector competence of Australian mosquitoes (Diptera: Culicidae) for Japanese encephalitis virus. *J. Med. Entomol.* 40:82–90.

121. van den Hurk, A. F., Ritchie, S. A. and Mackenzie, J. S. 2009. Ecology and geographical expansion of Japanese encephalitis virus. *Annu. Rev. Entomol.* 54:17–35.

122. van den Hurk, A. F., Ritchie, S. A., Johansen, C. A., Mackenzie, J. S. and Smith, G. A. 2008. Domestic pigs and Japanese encephalitis virus infection, Australia. *Emerg. Infect. Dis.* 14:1736–1738.

123. Vaughn, D. W. and Hoke, C. H. 1992. The epidemiology of Japanese encephalitis: Prospects for prevention. *Epidemiol. Rev.* 14:197–221.

124. Weissenböck, H., Kolodziejek, J., Url, A., Lussy, H., Rebel-Bauder, B. and Nowotny, N. 2002. Emergence of usutu virus, an african mosquito-borne flavivirus of the Japanese encephalitis virus group, central Europe. *Emerg. Infect. Dis.* 8:652–656.

125. Weng, M. H., Lien, J. C., Lin, C. C. and Yao, C. W. 2000. Vector competence of *Culex pipiens molestus* (Diptera: Culicidae) from Taiwan for a sympatric strain of Japanese encephalitis virus. *J. Med. Entomol.* 37:780–783.

126. Westaway, E. G., Brinton, M. A., Gaidamovich, S. Y. A., Horzinek, M. C., Igarashi, A., Kaariainen, L., Lvov, D. K., Porterfield, J. S., Russell, P. K. and Trent, D. W. 1985. Flaviviridae. *Intervirol.* 24:183–192.

127. Winter, P. M., Dung, N. M., Loan, H. T., Kneen, R., Wills, B., Thule, T., House, D., White, N. J., Farrar, J. J., Hart, C. A. and Solomon, T. 2004. Proinflammatory cytokines and chemokines in humans with Japanese encephalitis. *J. Infect. Dis.* 190:1618–1626.

128. Xinglin, J. Huanchun, C., Qigai, H., Xiang, W., Bin, W. Dexin, Q. and Liurong, F. 2002. The development and application of the latex agglutination test to detect serum antibodies against Japanese encephalitis virus. *Vet. Res. Comm.* 26:495–503.

129. Xinglin, J., Huanchun, C., Xiang, W. and Changming, Q. 2005. Quantitative and qualitative study of enzyme-linked immunosorbent assay to detect IgG against Japanese encephalitis virus in swine sera. *Vet. Res. Comm.* 29:159–169.

130. Yamada, M., Nakamura, K., Yoshii, M. and Kaku, Y. 2004. Nonsuppurative encephalitis in piglets after experimental inoculation of Japanese encephalitis flavivirus isolated from pigs. *Vet. Pathol.* 41:62–67.

131. Yamanaka, T., Tsujimura, K., Kondo, T., Yasuda, W., Okada, A., Noda, K., Okumura, T. and Matsumura, T. 2006. Isolation and genetic analysis of Japanese encephalitis virus from a diseased horse in Japan. *J. Vet. Med. Sci.* 68:293–295.

132. Yang, D. K., Kim, B. H., Kweon, C. H., Nah, J. J., Kim, H. J., Lee, K. W., Yang, Y. J. and Mun, K. W. 2008. Serosurveillance for Japanese encephalitis, Akabane, and Aino viruses for Thoroughbred horses in Korea. *J. Vet. Sci.* 9:381–385.

133. Yuwono, J., Suharyono, W., Koiman, I., Tsuchiya, Y. and Tagaya, I. 1984 Seroepidemiological survey on dengue and Japanese encephalitis virus infections in Asian monkeys. *Southeast Asian J Trop Med Public Health* 15:194–20.

134. Zachary, J. F. 2007. Nervous system. In *Pathologic basis of veterinary diseases*, 4th ed., M. D. McGavin and J. F. Zachary, 833–971. St. Louis, Missouri: Mosby Elsevier.

135. Zhang, J. S., Zhang, P. H., Si, B. Y., Yang, H. and Cao, W. C. 2005. Comparison and discrimination of the biological characteristics between West Nile virus and Japanese encephalitis virus. [Article in Chinese.] *Zhonghua Shi Yan He Lin Chuang Bing Du Xue Za Zhi.* 19:340–343.

18. LOUPING ILL IN HORSES

R. V. S. PAWAIYA, K. DHAMA, P. BHATT, AND S. KAPOOR

INTRODUCTION

Louping ill is an acute viral disease that affects the brain and causes varying signs of incoordination, paralysis, convulsions, and death. The disease is primarily associated with sheep, but man, cattle, goats, pigs, horses, farmed red deer, llamas, dogs, wild red grouse, alpacas, and ptarmigan can also be affected (Davidson et al., 1991; Radostits et al., 2000; Simpson et al., 2002; Charrel et al., 2004; Norman et al., 2004; Macaldowie et al., 2005; Hyde et al., 2007; Cranwell et al., 2008). The term "louping ill" is ancient and was used in the eighteenth century to describe a disease of sheep, occurring in the border counties of England and Scotland, where sheep were farmed intensively on the hillsides (McFadzean, 1900). The cause is a tick-transmitted arbovirus belonging to the tickborne encephalitis (TBE) complex (Francki et al., 1991). This virus infects a number of small mammals, including shrews, wood mice, voles, and hares. Humans seem to be an accidental host. Clinical disease, including fatal outcomes, has been described for men and dogs. With regard to horses, only a limited number of case reports are available (Timoney et al., 1976; Muller et al., 2006; Hyde et al., 2007). The disease occurs regularly in certain areas throughout the British Isles where pastures are infested with the sheep tick (*Ixodes ricinus*). These are mainly hilly areas of rough upland grazing or moorland. Besides tick bites, the virus can be transmitted by contact with infected animal tissues, particularly if these are handled in a manner which generates aerosols. There is also a possibility of transmission by unpasteurized milk from viremic animals.

EPIDEMIOLOGY

The encephalomyelitic disease of sheep, louping ill has been recognized in the British Isles for at least two hundred years (McGuire et al., 1998). There are several reports describing the occurrence of louping ill in horses in Europe (Timoney, 1974; Timoney et al., 1974; Timoney, 1976; Timoney et al., 1976; Waldvogel et al., 1981; Hyde et al., 2007). Louping ill can be found throughout the upland areas of Scotland, Northern Ireland, Cornwall, and Wales (Laurenson et al., 2007). It has also been found in Norway (McGuire et al., 1998). A summary of the disease surveillance report for September 2003 from the Scottish Agricultural College Veterinary Services mentioned about the louping ill in sheep on the increase (Anonymous. 2003). A closely related disease of sheep is reported from Russia, Bulgaria,

Turkey, the Basque region in Spain, Europe, and many parts of Asia, including South Korea (Gritsun et al., 2003; Zlovin et al., 2007; Kim et al., 2008). None of the known vectors of louping ill virus are found in the United States.

In a molecular epidemiological study, phylogenetic analysis of fifty-four isolates of serologically identified louping ill virus collected from representative regions of the British Isles and Norway revealed that louping ill virus initially emerged in Ireland and that a descendant was introduced into Great Britain via Wales and was subsequently transported to the borders of Scotland, from where it was dispersed throughout Scotland, Northern England, and Norway (McGuire et al., 1998). Calculation of dates of lineage divergence in the study indicated that louping ill virus was emerged in the British Isles less than eight hundred years ago, and most louping ill virus dispersal occurred during the last three hundred years. The livestock movement was thought to be implicated in the dispersal of louping ill virus (Gao et al. 1997; McGuire et al. 1998). A disease-transmission model study describing the dynamics of louping ill virus in red grouse (the viremic host) and hares (the nonviremic host) observed that the presence of a nonviremic host allows the virus to persist more readily than it would in the presence of a host that simply amplified the tick population. More importantly, if the level of nonviremic transmission is high enough, the virus can persist in the absence of the viremic host (Norman et al. 2004). These results may have important implications for the control of louping ill and other tickborne diseases.

Etiology

Louping ill is caused by a single-stranded neurotropic RNA virus of 40–50 nm that has been classified in the Flaviviridae family, *Flavivirus* genus, and belongs to a serocomplex of fourteen related tickborne viruses that cause Russian spring-summer encephalitis, Central European encephalitis, Kyasanur Forest disease in India, Negishi encephalitis in Japan, Omsk hemorrhagic fever in Russia, Langat in Malaysia, Powassan in North America, and others (Clarke, 1964; Francki et al., 1991; McGuire et al., 1998). The strains of louping ill virus do not vary significantly in their pathogenicity. Louping ill virus differs from other members of the tickborne encephalitis (TBE) virus serocomplex by not being associated with a forest environment. For example, strains of Western European tickborne encephalitis (WTBE) virus are associated with rodent populations in Western and Central European forests. Louping ill virus, however, which is transmitted by the same vector as WTBE virus, the sheep tick (*Ixodes ricinus*), is associated with the moorland habitat of England, Wales, and Scotland. Most cases of louping ill disease seen in these countries occur in sheep and red grouse (*Lagopus lagopus scoticus*) populations, although other species of domestic animals, including horses and humans, are affected less frequently (Reid, 1984). Louping ill virus also occurs in Ireland, where a greater proportion of louping ill disease than in Great Britain is reported in domestic species other than sheep. This is attributable to the higher rainfall in Ireland, allowing *I. ricinus* to exist on better-quality pasture and therefore feed on a wider range of domestic farm animals. Several other sheep encephalomyelitis–causing flaviviruses have been isolated in Europe and are known from molecular analysis to be distinct from each other and from louping ill virus, i.e., Spanish and Turkish sheep encephalitis (Gao et al., 1993; Whitby et al., 1993; Marin et al., 1995). Although there is no evidence of any significant variation in pathogenicity between strains of louping virus from a variety of vertebrate species and from ticks (Reid, 1984), monoclonal antibody analysis has revealed antigenic heterogenicity among isolates of the virus (Hubalek, 1995). In a recent study analyzing the complete coding sequences of all recognized tickborne *Flavivirus* species—including *Gadgets Gully, Royal Farm,* and *Karshi* virus, seabird-associated *flaviviruses, Kadam* virus, and previously uncharacterized isolates of *Kyasanur Forest disease* virus and *Omsk hemorrhagic fever* virus—the authors have proposed significant taxonomic improvements, e.g., the identification of three major groups (mammalian, seabird, and Kadam tickborne flavivirus groups), the creation of a new species, (Karshi virus), and the assignment of tickborne encephalitis and louping ill viruses to a unique species (tickborne encephalitis virus), including four viral types, i.e., Western tickborne encephalitis virus, Eastern Tick-borne encephalitis virus, Turkish sheep tickborne encephalitis virus, and louping ill tickborne encephalitis virus (Grard et al., 2007). The analyses also suggested a complex relationship between viruses infecting birds and those infecting mammals.

In tissue suspensions, louping ill virus remains viable for at least eighty-two days when stored in 50% glycerol or at temperatures of—20°C or lower. It is rapidly inactivated in saline or broth, especially in dilute or acid suspensions.

TRANSMISSION
Louping ill virus can be transmitted by several species of ticks, including *Rhipicephalus appendiculatus*, *Ixodes persulcatus*, *Haemaphysalis anatolicum*, and *I. ricinus*. *I. ricinus* (Radostits et al., 2000) is thought to be the natural vector of this disease. Peak disease incidence follows seasonal

tick activity, which means louping ill is most common between April and June and in September. Louping ill virus can also be transmitted to various host species after exposure to infective aerosols and by parenteral routes. Spread on fomites has also been documented. A simple mathematical model to describe the dynamics of louping ill virus in red grouse (the viremic host) and hares (the nonviremic host) using joint threshold density curves found that the presence of a nonviremic host allows the virus to persist more readily than it would in the presence of a host that simply amplified the tick population. More importantly, if the level of nonviremic transmission is high enough, the virus can persist in the absence of the viremic host. This result has important implications for the control of tickborne diseases (Norman et al., 2004). In another study, Gilbert et al. (2004) have demonstrated experimentally a transmission route whereby red grouse (*Lagopus lagopus scoticus*) became infected with louping ill virus after eating the infected tick vector.

CLINICAL SIGNS

Louping ill is rare in horses, and most cases seem to be subclinical. The early clinical signs of louping ill are fever, depression, anorexia, and sometimes constipation. This initial phase may be mild or inapparent. A second fever spike occurs about five days after the symptoms first appear; at this time, the virus either enters the central nervous system (CNS), or the animal recovers without further signs. Horses show either a rapidly progressing nervous disease with a course of approximately two days or a transient disorder of locomotion with recovery in ten to twelve days (Timoney et al., 1976). The early symptoms of CNS involvement include muscle tremors, incoordination, ataxia, hyperesthesia, profuse salivation, protrusion of the tongue, champing of the jaw. As the disease progresses, additional symptoms appear; they may include head pressing, paraplegia, convulsions, opisthotonos, and coma. Death is not uncommon. Surviving animals may have residual CNS deficits. Experimental infection with equine strain of louping ill virus in ponies showed fever three to four days after inoculation. No gross behavioral changes were observed in any animal. Every pony was viremic for six to seven days after inoculation, with maximal titers of virus present on days 1 to 3 (Timoney, 1980a). An outbreak of louping ill infection in a group of free-range horses displayed signs of CNS disturbance, and two of these died after illnesses ranging from two to twelve days' duration. In both cases, a variable degree of viral polioencephalomyelitis was observed. A virus antigenically indistinguishable from a reference strain of louping ill virus was isolated from the brain and cervical cord of a three-year-old draft mare.

PATHOLOGY

Usually there are no major gross lesions found in the louping ill. The only gross lesion on necropsy is congestion of the meningeal vessels. Secondary pneumonia may be seen. Histopathologically, the disease is characterized by severe meningoencephalomyelitis, which is primarily a nonsuppurative although occasional neutrophils may be seen. Specific lesions include neuronal degeneration, necrosis, and neuronophagia, which are present consistently in the Purkinje cells of the cerebellar cortex; however, they may also affect neurons of the medulla oblongata, pons, and spinal cord. Lesions in Purkinje cells are considered to be responsible, though partly, for the peculiar clinical sign of louping gait showed by the affected animal. Inflammatory lesions have also been seen in sciatic nerves. The louping ill virus can consistently be revealed in nervous tissue by the use of fluorescent antibody (Doherty and Reid, 1971).

DIAGNOSIS

Louping ill should be suspected in horses with fever and signs of cerebellar and cerebral disease, particularly when the flock has recently been introduced to tick-infested pastures. The differential diagnosis in horses includes tetanus, listeriosis, rabies, pseudorabies, hypomagnesemia, hypocalcemia, acute lead poisoning, and toxic plants.

1. *Field diagnosis.* A diagnosis of louping ill must remain tentative or provisional until corroborated by confirmatory laboratory evidence. The disease should be strongly suspected, however, in horses having signs of central nervous system disturbance consistent with those seen in typical cases of louping ill virus infection and where there is a history of recent introduction onto tick-infested pastures in an endemic area. However, diagnosis of louping ill in horses cannot be based on clinical grounds alone.
2. *Specimens for laboratory.* Louping ill is a zoonotic disease; therefore, samples should be collected and handled with all appropriate precautions. For virus isolation, approximately 20 ml of uncoagulated blood should be collected during the acute stage of the disease before the neurologic signs appear. Heparinized blood should be collected during the acute viremic phase of the disease and preferably during the first three to four days after the onset of fever, which is best for virus isolation. In the majority of cases, virus isolation is attempted on the brain and spinal cord of animals that died. Although this is frequently successful in sheep, results

in horses and cattle have been variable. Unfixed portions of brain and spinal cord are best transported to the laboratory in 50% glycerol and normal saline or frozen on dry ice and dispatched in a closed, insulated container using an overnight delivery service. Paired serum samples, acute and convalescent, should be submitted for serologic examination. Half of the brain and portions of spinal cord should be submitted in 10% formalin.

3. *Laboratory tests.* Louping ill can be diagnosed by virus isolation, detection of virus antigens, or serology. Virus isolation from the blood can be successful during the acute phase of the disease but is usually unsuccessful after the neurologic signs appear. Virus may also be isolated from necropsy samples of the brain and spinal cord. Louping ill virus can be isolated in embryonated eggs, primary pig kidney or chicken embryo cell cultures, or suckling mice. The virus is identified by serum neutralization. Virus antigens can be detected by immunostaining of formalin-fixed brain or by a reverse transcriptase–polymerase chain reaction (RT-PCR) assay (Gaunt et al., 1997; van der Poel et al., 2005). A rapid and precise detection method for routine use that employs the TaqMan RT-PCR has been developed to detect louping ill virus RNA extracted from field samples (Marriott et al., 2006). This TaqMan assay is as sensitive as the cell culture infectious virus assay currently used and has the advantage of being able to detect louping ill virus in clinical specimens from which infectious virus can not be isolated possibly due to the presence of high levels of louping ill virus antibody. Recently, real-time RT-PCR assay has been used to determine the prevalence of louping ill virus in live red grouse chicks (Moseley et al., 2007). Serologic tests include hemagglutination inhibition (HI), serum neutralization (SN), and an enzyme-linked immunosorbent assay (ELISA) (Timoney, 1980b; Timoney et al., 1984). A complement fixation test (CFT) is available but rarely used; complement-fixing antibodies are transient and develop only late in the course of the disease.

The identification of louping ill virus in clinical specimens has been routinely achieved by virus isolation using susceptible pig kidney cells and subsequent serological analysis (Timoney, 1998). While this method is sensitive and detects infectious virus, it is relatively labor intensive and time consuming.

TREATMENT

There is no specific treatment for encephalitic cases of louping ill virus infection. Unlike sheep, horses and cattle affected with louping ill may respond favorably to good nursing and symptomatic treatment. An antiserum has been used and affords protection if given within forty-eight hours of exposure but is of no value once the febrile reaction has begun. It is not available commercially. Animals with clinical disease should be sedated if necessary during the acute course of the disease and should be kept in a secluded and dark area with general supportive care.

PREVENTION AND CONTROL

The limited geographical occurrence of this disease and commercial economics has restricted the availability of the vaccine. Consequently, tick control or the elimination of infection from pastures may be the required approach in the future. The intensity of tick infestation of pastures can be reduced by influencing the microclimate that they require for survival. In some areas, this can be achieved by ditching and drainage of the pastures.

1. *Vaccination.* A formalin-inactivated commercial vaccine is available that has been used successfully for many years in endemic areas (Shaw and Reid, 1981). Two doses of vaccine with an interval of two to eight weeks between injections are recommended to achieve optimal protection to natural infection. Vaccination of pregnant ewes during the last trimester is advocated to ensure that lambs receive maximal levels of passively acquired antibodies and are protected during the initial critical months of life. Vaccination of lambs after weaning when maternal immunity has waned may be advisable in areas where there is a secondary "fall rise" in tick activity (Wells and Reid, 1978). The same louping ill vaccine has been used in cattle with reasonable success based on annual revaccination against the disease.

2. *Preventive measures.* It is very doubtful whether measures aimed at reducing the tick population on infected pastures are a practical approach to controlling louping ill in areas endemic for the disease. Certainly, such measures are out of the question where rough upland or mountainous terrain is involved. Frequent acaricidal dipping or spraying of sheep and—where appropriate—cattle during the period of maximal tick activity is a valuable means of controlling the level of tick infestation and transmission of the virus.

The single most important means of controlling louping ill in areas endemic for the disease is vaccination. This should be applied initially to all stock and subsequently to all replacement animals introduced from an area in which the disease is nonendemic. Vaccination should take place at least one month before exposure to infection. Because louping ill virus is likely to be maintained in a tick-sheep cycle, systematic vaccination of a flock over a period of years may result eventually in elimination of the virus. This should not, however, prompt discontinuation of vaccination because the potential for further disease outbreaks remains as long as the tick vector is present.

3. *Quarantine and disinfection.* Prevention of infection of tick vectors is critical. Louping ill virus can also be spread in milk or contaminated tissues and by fomites. Enveloped viruses such as louping ill virus are generally susceptible to most common disinfectants.

ZOONOTIC IMPORTANCE
Louping ill virus is transmissible to humans. Humans can develop any one of four clinical syndromes: an influenza-type illness, a biphasic encephalitis, a poliomyelitis-like illness, or a hemorrhagic fever following infection with louping ill virus (Davidson et al., 1991). Transmission can take place by tick bite, exposure to aerosolized infective material, or through skin abrasions or wounds. Nonlaboratory-acquired infections most frequently result from handling infected carcasses in abattoirs. The potential for oral transmission of louping ill virus to humans also exists where milk for human consumption is obtained from goats or sheep that are in the acute phase of the infection (Reid, 1987). Humans can be infected by the louping ill virus after aerosol exposure, contamination of skin wounds, or tick bites.

CONCLUSION
Louping ill, caused by louping ill virus which is a member of *Flavivirus* genus, is an acute encephalitis of sheep but also affects other animal species, including horses. Louping ill virus variants circulate in European countries other than the UK, such as Spain (Spanish sheep encephalomyelitis virus), Turkey (Turkish sheep encephalomyelitis virus), and Greece (Greek goat encephalomyelitis virus). They are antigenically and genetically closely related to TBEV and louping ill virus and are all capable of infecting man (zoonoses). Louping ill virus is transmitted by *I. ricinus* ticks.

Louping ill is rare in horses, and most cases seem to be subclinical. The early clinical signs of louping ill are fever, depression, anorexia, and sometimes constipation. Relapse of fever occurs about five days after the symptoms first appear; at this time, the virus either enters the central nervous system (CNS), or the animal recovers without further signs. Horses show either a rapidly progressing nervous disease with a course of approximately two days or a transient disorder of locomotion with recovery in ten to twelve days. Experimental infection with equine strain of louping ill virus in ponies showed fever three to four days after inoculation. Gross lesions are not prominent, but microscopic lesions are characterized by severe nonsuppurative meningoencephalomyelitis. Diagnosis can be done by many laboratory tests, including ELISA and PCR assay. There is no treatment for louping ill; however, a formalin-inactivated commercial vaccine has been used successfully for many years in endemic areas.

REFERENCES

1. Anonymous. 2003. Problems with tickborne diseases increase in sheep flocks in northern Scotland. *Vet. Rec.* 153:611–614.
2. Charrel, R. N., Attoui, H., Butenko, A. M., Clegg, J. C., Deubel, V., Frolova, T. V., Gould, E. A., Gritsun, T. S., Heinz, F. X., Labuda, M., Lashkevich, V. A., Loktev, V., Lundkvist, A., Lvov, D. V., Mandl, C. W., Niedrig, M., Papa, A., Petrov, V. S., Plyusnin, A., Randolph, S., Süss, J., Zlobin, V. I. and de Lamballerie, X. 2004. Tick-borne virus diseases of human interest in Europe. *Clin. Microbiol. Infect.* 10:1040–1055.
3. Clarke, D. H. 1964. Further studies on antigenic relationships among the viruses of the group B tickborne complex. *Bull. WHO* 31:45–56.
4. Cranwell, M. P., Josephson, M., Willoughby, K. and Marriott, L. 2008. Louping ill in an alpaca. *Vet Rec.* 162:28.
5. Davidson, M. M., Williams, H. and Macleod, J. A. 1991. Louping-ill in man: A forgotten disease. *J. Infection* 23:241–249.
6. Doherty, P. C. and Reid, H. W. 1971. Experimental louping-ill in sheep and lambs. II. Neuropathology. *J. Comp. Pathol.* 81:331–337.
7. Francki, R. I. B., Fauquet, C. M., Knudson, D. L. and Brown, L. 1991. Classification and nomenclature of viruses: Fifth report of the International Committee on Taxonomy of Viruses. *Archives of Virol.* Supplementum 2.
8. Gao, G. F., Hussain, M. H., Reid, H. W. and Gould, E. A. 1993. Classification of a new member of the TBE flavivirus subgroup by its immunological, pathogenetic and molecular characteristics: Identification of subgroup-specific pentapeptides. *Virus Res.* 30:129–144.
9. Gao, G. F., Zanotto, P. M., Holmes, E. C., Reid, H. W. and Gould, E. A. 1997. Molecular variation, evolution and geographical distribution of louping ill virus. *Acta Virol.* 41:259–68.
10. Gaunt, M. W., Jones, L. D., Laurenson, K., Hudson, P. J., Reid, H. W. and Gould, E. A. 1997. Definitive identification of louping ill virus by RT-CPR and sequencing in field populations of *Ixodes ricinus* on the Lochindorb estate. *Arch. Virol.* 142:1181–1191.
11. Gilbert, L., Jones, L. D., Laurenson, M. K., Gould, E. A., Reid, H. W. and Hudson, P. J. 2004. Ticks need not bite their red grouse hosts to infect them with louping ill virus. *Proc. Biol. Sci.* 271 (Suppl 4): S202–205.
12. Grard, G., Moureau, G., Charrel, R. N., Lemasson, J. J., Gonzalez, J. P., Gallian, P., Gritsun, T. S., Holmes, E. C., Gould, E. A. and de Lamballerie, X. 2007. Genetic characterization of tick-borne flaviviruses: New insights into evolution, pathogenetic determinants and taxonomy. *Virol.* 361:80–92.
13. Gritsun, T. S., Lashkevich, V. A. and Gould, E. A. 2003. Tick-borne encephalitis. *Antiviral Res.* 57:129–146.
14. Hubalek, Z., Pow, I., Reid, H. W. and Hussain, M. H. 1995. Antigenic similarity of central European encephalitis and louping-ill viruses. *Acta Viol.* 39:251–256.
15. Hyde, J., Nettleton, P., Marriott, L. and Willoughby, K. 2007. Louping ill in horses. *Vet Rec.* 160:532.

16. Kim, S. Y., Yun, S. M., Han, M. G., Lee, I. Y., Lee, N. Y., Jeong, Y. E., Lee, B. C. and Ju, Y. R. 2008. Isolation of tick-borne encephalitis viruses from wild rodents, South Korea. *Vector Borne Zoonotic Dis.* 8:7–13.

17. Laurenson, M. K., McKendrick, I. J., Reid, H. W., Challenor, R. and Mathewson, G. K. 2007. Prevalence, spatial distribution and the effect of control measures on louping-ill virus in the forest of Bowland, Lancashire. *Epidemiol Infect.* 135:963–973.

18. Macaldowie, C., Patterson, I. A., Nettleton, P. F., Low, H. and Buxton, D. 2005. Louping ill in llamas (*Lama glama*) in the Hebrides. *Vet Rec.* 156:420–421.

19. Marin, M. S., McKenzie, J., Gao, G. F., Reid, H. W., Antoniadis, A. and Gould, E. A. 1995. The virus causing encephalomyelitis in sheep in Spain: A new member of the tick-borne encephalitis group. *Res. Vet. Sci.* 58:11–13.

20. Marriott, L., Willoughby, K., Chianini, F., Dagleish, M. P., Scholes, S., Robinson, A. C., Gould, E. A. and Nettleton, P. F. 2006. Detection of louping ill virus in clinical specimens from mammals and birds using TaqMan RT-PCR. *J. Virol. Methods* 137:21–28.

21. McFadzean, J. 1900. The etiology of louping ill. *J. Comp. Pathol. Ther.* 13:145–154.

22. McGuire, K., Holmes, E. C., Gao, G. F., Reid, H. W. and Gould, E. A. 1998. Tracing the origins of louping ill virus by molecular phylogenetic analysis. *J. Gen. Virol.* 79:981–988.

23. Moseley, M. H., Marriott, L., Nettleton, P., Dukes, J., Irvine, R. J. and Mougeot, F. 2007. Use of real-time RT-PCR to determine the prevalence of louping ill virus in live red grouse chicks. *Vet. Rec.* 161:660–661.

24. Müller, K., König, M. and Thiel, H. J. 2006. Tick-borne encephalitis (TBE) with special emphasis on infection in horses. *Dtsch Tierarztl Wochenschr* 113:147–151.

25. Norman, R., Ross, D., Laurenson, M. K. and Hudson, P. J. 2004. The role of non-viraemic transmission on the persistence and dynamics of a tick borne virus: Louping ill in red grouse (*Lagopus lagopus scoticus*) and mountain hares (*Lepus timidus*). *J. Math. Biol.* 48:119–134.

26. Radostits, O. M., Gay, C. C., Blood, D. C. and Hinchcliff, K. W. 2000. Louping ill. In *Veterinary medicine*, 9th ed., 1222–1225. USA: W. B. Saunders Co.

27. Reid, H. 1987. Controlling tick-borne diseases of sheep in Britain. *Practice* 9:189–191.

28. Reid, H. W. 1984. *Epidemiology of louping-ill*. In *Vector biology*, ed. M. A. Mayo and K. A. Harrap, 161–178. London: Academic Press.

29. Shaw, B. and Reid, H. W. 1981. Immune responses of sheep to louping-ill virus vaccine. *Vet. Rec.* 109:529–531.

30. Simpson, V. R. 2002. Wild animals as reservoirs of infectious diseases in the UK. *Vet. J.* 163:128–146.

31. Timoney, P. J., Donnelly, W. C., Clements, C. and Fenlon, M. 1974. Letter: Louping ill infection in the horse. *Vet. Rec.* 95:540.

32. Timoney, P. J., Donnelly, W. J., Clements, L. O. and Fenlon, M. 1976 Encephalitis caused by louping ill virus in a group of horses in Ireland. *Equine Vet. J.* 8:113–117.

33. Timoney, P. J. 1974. Serologic evidence of louping ill in the horse. *Br. Vet J.* 130:29–30.

34. Timoney, P. J. 1976. Louping ill: A serological survey of horses in Ireland. *Vet. Rec.* 41:303.

35. Timoney, P. J. 1980a. Susceptibility of the horse to experimental inoculation with louping ill virus. *J Comp Pathol.* 90:73–86.

36. Timoney, P. J. 1980b. Evaluation of the double immunodiffusion test for the diagnosis of louping ill infection. *Res. Vet. Sci.* 28:195–198.

37. Timoney, P. J. 1998. Louping ill. In *Foreign animal diseases*, 292–302. Richmond, VA: United States Animal Health Association.

38. Timoney, P. J., Geraghty, V. P., Harrington, A. M. and Dillon, P. B. 1984. Microneutralization test in PK(15) cells for assay of antibodies to louping ill virus. *J. Clin. Microbiol.* 20:128–130.

39. van der Poel, W. H., van der Heide, R., Bakker, D., De Looff, M., De Jong, J., Van Manen, N., Gaasenbeck, C. P. and Borgsteede, F. H. 2005. Attempt to detect evidence for tick-borne encephalitis virus in ticks and mammalian wildlife in the Netherlands. *Vector Borne Zoonotic Dis.* 5:58–64.

40. Waldvogel, A., Matile, H., Wegmann, C., Wyler, R. and Kunz, C. 1981. Tick-borne encephalitis in the horse. *Schweiz Arch. Tierheilkd.* 123:227–233.

41. Wells, P. W. and Reid, H. W. 1978. Antibody responses to vaccination against louping-ill virus in newborn lambs. *J. Comp. Path.* 88:425–431.

42. Whitby, J. E., Whitby, S. N., Jennings, A. D., Stephenson, J. R. and Barrett, A. D. T. 1993. Nucleotide sequence of the envelope protein of a Turkish isolate of tick-borne encephalitis (TBE) virus is distinct from other viruses of the TBE virus complex. *J. Gen. Virol.* 74:921–924.

43. Zlobin, V. I., Verkhozina, M. M., Demina, T. V., Dzhioev, I. P., Adel'shin, R. V., Kozlova, I. V., Belikov, S. I., Khasnatinov, M. A., Danchinova, G. A., Isaeva, E. I. and Grishechkin, A. E. 2007. Molecular epidemiology of tick-borne encephalitis. *Vopr. Virusol.* 52:4–13.

19. Rotavirus Diarrhea in Equines

K. Dhama, M. Mahendran, S. Kapoor, and R. V. S. Pawaiya

Introduction

Young ones of domestic animals often succumb to infectious agents at neonatal period. Among the infectious diseases of foals, neonatal diarrhea is of major concern, and multiple etiological agents like *Escherichia coli, Salmonella* species, *Clostridium perferingens, Aeromonas hydrophila, Rhodococcus equi, Strongyloides* spp., rotavirus, coronavirus, and *Cryptosporidium* have been suggested (Holland, 1990; Browning et al., 1991b; Netherwood et al., 1996; Dwyer, 2001; Steele et al., 2004; Fukai et al., 2006; Dhama et al., 2009). In equines, among these agents, equine rotaviruses (ERV), belonging to group A rotavirus, contribute significantly to enteritis and diarrhea (Hoshino et al., 1983; Murphy et al., 1999; Cullinane et al., 2006; Dwyer, 2007). In a study of foal diarrhea outbreaks in central Kentucky, rotavirus was the cause of 90% of farm outbreaks (Dwyer, 2001). The disease is usually seen in foals of two to eight weeks of age, and the susceptibility decreases as the age progresses. Besides affecting equines, rotaviruses also affect calves, piglets, lambs, kids, and young ones of pet animals and poultry; and also only recently their zoonotic potential has been documented (Studdert et al., 1978; Conner and Darlington, 1980; Holland, 1990; Cook et al., 2004; Cullinane et al., 2006; Dhama et al., 2009). The clinical signs and the outcome of the disease are similar in most of the animal species, and severity may range from a subclinical condition to severe enteritis. The virus etiology of rotaviral diarrhea in foals was first documented in the year 1975 during scours in newborn foals in England, and rotaviruses were detected in feces by electron microscopy (Flewett et al., 1975). In 1979, foal rotaviruses were reported to have an electropherotype that was distinct from those of bovine, porcine, and human rotaviruses, thus establishing the species specificity (Smith and Tzipori, 1979). By electrophoretic analysis, Legrottaglie and Agrimi (1992) also reported that equine rotavirus and bovine rotavirus strain are considerably different from each other.

Epidemiology

In equines, enteritis and diarrhea poses a great challenge for intensive horse-breeding programs, and the most commonly diagnosed etiological agent of foal diarrhea is group A rotavirus (Imagawa et al., 1994; Fukai et al., 2006). Presently, rotaviruses are well established as important etiological agents of acute gastroenteritis in various mammalian and avian species too

(Dhama et al., 2009). Rotavirus diarrhea in foals has been reported from most of the countries all over the world, and it is estimated that equine rotavirus is responsible for more than 25% of cases of foal diarrhea (Cullinane et al., 2006; Dwyer, 2007). The equine rotavirus (ERV) is ubiquitous and causes localized infection in small intestine of neonates by disrupting the efficient absorptive surfaces to produce diarrhea (Holland, 1990; Steele et al., 2004; Dhama et al., 2009). The rotaviruses, being mostly species specific and existing as geno groups, have multiple gene segments of double-stranded (ds) RNA and exhibit considerable genetic diversity as a result of genetic shift, gene rearrangements, or interchange of segments (Schroeder et al., 1982; Murphy et al., 1999; Steele et al., 2004). Also, interspecies transmission and close relationship between equine and porcine rotaviruses (PRV) have been reported (Isa and Snodgrass, 1994; Taniguchi et al., 1994). But it is suggested that rotaviruses isolated from animals, even those indistinguishable from human viruses, rarely cause natural infection in infants (Murphy et al., 1999). The ERV infection in foals has been identified in many countries—including USA (Hardy et al., 1991), UK (Netherwood et al., 1996), Argentina (Barrandeguy et al., 1998), Venezuela (Ciarlet et al., 1994), Ireland (Collins et al., 2008), Germany (Elschner et al., 2005), Japan (Watanabe et al., 1993; Imagawa et al., 1994; Takagi et al., 1993; 1994; Tsunemitsu et al., 2001; Fukai et al., 2006), Australia and New Zealand (Dwyer, 2007), and India (Gulati et al., 2007). No natural reservoir for equine rotavirus has been identified.

Etiology

Rotaviruses belong to genus *Rotavirus* within the family Reoviridae. They are icosahedral and nonenveloped (diameter of 65–70 nm), with thirty-two capsomers and eleven segments of ds RNA (16–21 kbp), well protected by an inner and outer capsid layer (Murphy et al., 1999; Desselberger et al., 2005; Dwyer, 2007; Dhama et al., 2009). The rotavirus genome encodes six structural and six nonstructural proteins (Kapikian et al., 2001). The virus has structural proteins located in the core (VP1, VP2, and VP3), inner capsid (VP6), and the outer capsid layer (VP4 and VP7). VP4 (cleaves into VP5 and VP8) and VP7 are proteins that generate neutralizing antibodies, which protect the young ones of animals from infections; VP6 is a group-specific antigen that is common to all rotaviruses. All the while, VP1, VP2 and VP3, along with other nonstructural proteins (NSPs 1–6), play an important role in viral transcription (Paul and Lyoo, 1993; Steele et al., 2004; Desselberger et al., 2005).

The functions of major structural and nonstructural proteins of rotaviruses have been identified (Murphy et al., 1999; Estes, 2001; Desselberger et al., 2005). VP1 is an RNA-dependent RNA polymerase and part of virion transcription complex with VP3; VP2 produces a protein needed for the proper functioning of the VP1 and is known to interact with VP5; VP3 (guanylyl transferase) forms complex with VP1 and have an important role in transcription; VP4, seen in outer capsid as spikes, helps the virus to attach to host cells and forms a major virulence factor and considered as P-type neutralization antigen; VP6, the group-specific antigen, have a role in transcription; and VP7 provides the protective outer capsid layer and considered as G-type neutralization antigen (Estes, 2001, 2003; Dhama et al., 2009). NSP1 is the nonstructural protein associated with cytoskeleton and have high diversity between strains; NSP2 involves in viroplasm formation along with VP5; NSP3, a nonstructural protein, have major role in translation and host shutoff; NSP4 functions as viral enterotoxin and virulence factor to increase the intracellular Ca^{2+} concentration and disturb the cellular homeostasis of the host; and NSP5 interacts with VP2, NSP2, and NSP6 (Estes et al., 1981; Prasad et al., 1988; Anthony et al., 1991; Estes, 2001, 2003).

Besides, antigenic specificities of rotaviruses have been assessed, and they are classified into groups, subgroups, and serotypes. It has been identified that the immune responses to rotavirus are essentially serotype specific (Paul and Lyoo, 1993; Steele et al., 2004; Desselberger et al., 2005; Dhama et al., 2009). The group and subgroup specificity is conferred by antigenic epitopes on VP6 protein, which differentiate the rotaviruses into seven groups (A to G) and into four subgroups (Kapikian et al., 2001; Steele et al., 2004; Desselberger et al., 2005). Group A rotaviruses comprises of important pathogens of human beings, cattle, and other animals; group B rarely affect calves, lambs, piglets, and human beings; group C may affect swine and occasionally humans; groups D, F, and G can affect poultry; and group E may affect swine. However, group A viruses are the major cause of rotaviral infections in domestic animals, including equines (Steele et al., 2004; Villarreal et al., 2006; Gulati et al., 2007; Dwyer, 2007; Dhama et al., 2009). Exploiting the RNA-PAGE technique, all the eleven segments of rotaviruses can be easily separated, and a characteristic visual pattern known as RNA electropherotype is generated (Steele et al., 2004). Based on this, group A has a 4-2-3-2 pattern; group B has 4-2-2-3 pattern; and group C viruses show a 4-3-2-2-segment migration. Rotaviruses can be classified as long or short electropherotypes (E types) based on the fast or slow electrophoretic mobility of gene segments. Human group A rotaviruses have a short RNA pattern with subgroup I specificity, while a long RNA pattern and subgroup I specificity are commonly associated with animal rotaviruses (Kapikian et al., 2001).

Similarly, there is a serotype-based classification scheme for rotaviruses based on outer capsid proteins VP7 (designated as *G* for "glycoprotein") and VP4 (designated as *P*, for "protease-sensitive protein") (Steele et al., 2004;

Desselberger et al., 2005). Based on this, rotaviruses affecting domestic animals have been reported to belong to sixteen G types and twenty-seven P types (Browning and Begg, 1996; Steele et al., 2004; Desselberger et al., 2005; Gulati et al., 2007; Dhama et al., 2009). ERV serotypes G3, G5, G10, G13, and G14 have been commonly found among isolates from different parts of the globe (Browning et al., 1991c; Imagawa et al., 1994 and 1993; Tsunemitsu et al., 2001; Gulati et al., 2007). However, majority belong to G3 or G14 with a P[12] serotype (Browning et al., 1991a; Imagawa et al., 1991 and 1993; Ciarlet et al., 1994; Browning and Begg, 1996; Tsunemitsu et al., 2001; Fukai et al., 2006). Browning et al. (1992a and 1992b) reported that serotype G3 can be further subtyped into G3A and G3B. Recently, Gulati et al. (2007) identified a G16 serotype among equine group A rotavirus.

Physical and chemical features of rotaviruses are also well-known. Rotaviruses are highly resistant and can survive up to nine months in a contaminated environment, causing a recurrent disease problem. They can survive in fecal material for long periods and remain as a source of infection to susceptible population (Chauhan and Singh, 1996; Steele et al., 2004; Chauhan et al., 2008). They are stable at low and high relative humidity and can withstand pH range of 3–9 (Murphy et al., 1999; Steele et al., 2004). Further, the rotaviruses are not inactivated in presence of ether, chloroform, quaternary ammonium disinfectants, and sodium hypochlorite (Steele et al., 2004). But it has been identified that ethanol, phenol, formalin, and chloramine-T can effectively destroy rotaviruses (Tan and Schnagl, 1981; Steele et al., 2004).

TRANSMISSION

The virus is highly contagious, and in equine facilities, the rotaviruses are spread by environmental-oral or fecal-oral transmission (Dwyer, 2001 and 2007). Also, the reduced intake of colostrum or milk, age and immune status of the foals, degree of exposure and virulence of virus, and the presence of secondary pathogens influence the disease incidence (Holland, 1990; Steele et al., 2004; Chauhan et al., 2008). Interestingly, the major stress factors that augment the infection have been found to be cold climate and marked fluctuations in the ambient temperature between day and night (Chauhan and Singh, 1996). An age-related resistance has also been observed, which is primarily due to competition between the rate of replication of rotavirus and replacement of enterocytes in older animals (Dodet et al., 1997).

CLINICAL MANIFESTATIONS

The first signs are depression and failure to suck. Other signs include inappetance, lethargy, diarrhea, mild colic, and dehydration. Pyrexia is not a major feature. Rotavirus diarrhea in neonates presents an acute disease having very short incubation period of twelve to twenty-four hours or at times ranging from eighteen to ninety-six hours evincing severe dehydrating diarrhea (Chauhan and Singh, 1996; Steele et al., 2004; Cullinane et al., 2006; Dwyer, 2007; Collins et al., 2008). Diarrhea may vary from "cow pie" to watery consistency. Watery diarrhea is of projectile nature. There is marked individual variation in the severity of the disease. Some foals remain asymptomatic while their cohorts become severely dehydrated. Foals younger than four months are most susceptible, and foals born to mares recently introduced to a stud farm are often severely affected than the foals of resident mares. The average duration of diarrhea in affected foals is three days (range, one to nine days), with fecal shedding of rotavirus particles continuing for an average of three days after return of normal feces. Electrolyte imbalances may include hypochloremia, hyponatremia, hypokalemia, and acidosis. The hemogram is often normal or reveals evidence of hemoconcentration (increased packed cell volume). Chronic diarrhea (more than fourteen days) is not typical of rotavirus infection (Cullinane et al., 2006; Dwyer, 2007).

The diarrheic feces are often devoid of blood or mucus, unless there is secondary bacterial infection (Steele et al., 2004). Repeated bouts of diarrhea may result into failure to thrive especially in young ones as the newborn calves are having less fluid reserve (Murphy et al., 1999). Older foals may not exhibit profuse watery diarrhea but show signs of abdominal pain. Outcome of infection is influenced by the strain virulence, quantity of the viral inoculum, and the age and the immune status of the foal. Virus may be shed prior to onset of diarrhea and after recovery. The infection is often nonfebrile, unless complicated by secondary pathogens. Rotavirus disease is characterized by high morbidity and low mortality. In neonates, the mortality rate due to rotavirus diarrhea may be high (50–80%) due to complicating factors but usually wavers around 5–20% (Chauhan and Singh, 1996; Dwyer, 2007). If rotavirus infection occurs in combination with *E. coli* or coronavirus, the mortality rate could be high. Several other factors like dehydration, unhygienic environment, temperature variations, and high population density in farms may also enhance disease severity (Woode and Crouch, 1978; Chauhan and Singh, 1996; Cullinane et al., 2006; Dwyer, 2007). The virus is frequently detected in feces of foals that are clinically normal, and it appears that the infective dose is an important determinant of the disease. Large quantities of the virus, up to 10^8–10^{11} particles (infective doses) per gram of feces, are shed by affected foals or diarrheic animals.

PATHOGENESIS

Rotaviruses, stable at a wide range of pH and due to buffering action of milk, survive the inclement environment of gastrointestinal tract and invade the intestinal epithelial cells (Murphy et al., 1999). The virus replicates in the cytoplasm of epithelial cells of small intestinal villi (Holland, 1990; Murphy et al., 1999). After entry through oral route, rotaviruses replicate in the mature villous epithelial cells (enterocytes). On binding to the cell surface, the virus penetrates the plasma membrane to effectively infect the cell. For infectivity, the outer capsid of the virus has to be cleaved and removed, which is facilitated by intestinal proteases like chymotrypsin (Ramig, 2004; Desselberger et al., 2005). Experimentally, it has been identified that the penetration of rotaviruses depends on trypsin treatment of the virus, which results in the specific cleavage of VP4 into polypeptides VP8 and VP5 (Steele et al., 2004; Isa et al., 2008).

The epithelial cells of the villi in duodenum are the first to become infected and release significant number of virions, which leads to more severe attack on enterocytes of mid and distal portion of small intestine (Holland, 1990; Ramig, 2004; Chauhan et al., 2008). The presence of rotavirus-specific receptors has not yet been completely elucidated, and it is assumed that the virus may gain entry into enterocytes by pinocytosis or direct penetration (Desselberger et al., 2005). However, sialic acid or galactose-based receptors, along with coreceptors like integrins, have been identified to have a role in entry of the virus into cells (Murphy et al., 1999; Desselberger et al., 2005; Dhama et al., 2009). Recently, it has been proposed that rotavirus cell entry is a multistep process, which involves virus surface proteins and several cellular molecules, including sialic acids, integrins (2 1, 4 1, v 3, and x 2), the heat shock cognate proteins, and some gangliosides. The viral capsid proteins interact sequentially with these molecules, which cause conformational changes in the virus particles to enable penetration of cell membrane (Isa et al., 2008).

The removal of outer capsid proteins result in the activation of RNA-dependent RNA polymerase (VP1), and the VP1–VP3 transcriptional complex generates positive-strand RNA molecules that act as mRNAs to get translated in the cytoplasm or serve as template for replication. Later, budding occurs through the endoplasmic reticulum and virions get released via cell lysis (Murphy et al., 1999; Desselberger et al., 2005; Chauhan et al., 2008; Dhama et al., 2009). As the multiplication progresses, the mature enterocytes are sloughed off, and immature cells from crypts take over to cover the villus surface that create a sudden change in the ratio of absorption and secretion, leading to accumulation of fluid in the lumen of intestine (Holland, 1990; Murphy et al.,

1999; Ramig, 2004; Chauhan et al., 2008). This contributes to hypermotility in intestine and generates bouts of diarrhea in young animals. There is impairment of digestion and absorption of nutrients. Mucosal damage combined with altered blood flow and a decrease in the number of goblet cells may cause ulcers (Woode and Crouch, 1978; Steele et al., 2004; Cullinane et al., 2006; Dwyer, 2007; Dhama et al., 2009). Typically, intestinal crypt cells are not affected as they are in canine parvovirus infection. Therefore, these cells continue to replicate, differentiate, and eventually replace the tip cells destroyed by the virus, resulting in a self-limiting disease.

Besides malabsorption due to destruction of mature enterocytes, activation of the enteric nervous system by vasoactive agents or secretion of a viral enterotoxin, NSP4, which alters calcium-dependent cell permeability and elevates the chloride secretion, are identified as reasons for the clinical effects contributed by rotaviruses (Estes, 2003; Desselberger et al., 2005; Chauhan et al., 2008; Dhama et al., 2009). During later stages of disease progression, enterocytes are regenerated along with recovery of the villi; hence, the rotavirus infection is considered a self-limiting one, provided the dehydration is insignificant to cause death of young ones (Holland, 1990; Steele et al., 2004).

DIAGNOSIS

Rapid and accurate detection of the etiological agent is important to further contain the spread of infection in animals. Generally, the diagnosis of rotavirus is based on isolation and identification of the virus in intestinal contents or feces (Holland, 1990; Steele et al., 2004; Cullinane et al., 2006; Dwyer, 2007; Chauhan et al., 2008; Dhama et al., 2009). One to three grams of feces should be collected from the rectum if possible. Freshly voided feces are also suitable for laboratory diagnosis. Samples should be kept cool but not frozen while they are transported to the laboratory. Rotaviruses are fastidious and difficult to isolate routinely in tissue culture. Infectivity is enhanced if samples are pretreated with trypsin, and the cell cultures are propagated in medium supplemented with trypsin. Isolation of ERV has been performed in rotavirus-specific cell line MA-104, and direct detection has been facilitated by electron microscopy (Browning et al., 1991b; Steele et al., 2004; Chauhan et al., 2008). Imagawa et al. (1981) successfully propagated ERV in MA-104 cells, while the virus from a diarrheic foal was isolated in primary African green monkey kidney cells and MA-104 cells (Hoshino et al., 1983; Browning et al., 1992a).

For diagnosis and characterization of ERV, reverse transcription—polymerase chain reaction (RT-PCR), enzyme-linked immunosorbent assay (ELISA), and polyacrylamide gel electrophoresis (PAGE) pherotyping are being used (Browning et al., 1991a; Ellis and Daniels, 1988; Tsunemitsu et al., 2001; Elschner et al., 2002, 2005; Cullinane et al., 2006; Gulati et al., 2007; Chauhan et al., 2008; Dhama et al., 2009). Serology for diagnostic purpose in foals is unreliable. Pherotyping is performed by overnight electrophoresis of segmented ds RNA in a 12.0% polyacrylamide slab gel with a 3.5% stacking gel by the discontinuous buffer system (Hardy et al., 1991). Serotyping and subgrouping by monoclonal antibody (MAb)-based enzyme-linked immunosorbent assays (ELISAs) and hybridization to VP7 and VP4 gene-specific probes has been exploited (Gouvea et al., 1990; Browning et al., 1992a). An immunochromatographic test has also been developed for the detection of group A rotavirus (de Verdier Klingenberg and Esfandiari, 1996). Commercial diagnostic assays are based on detection of VP6, the most abundant and highly conserved protein in across rotaviruses that affect many species. ELISA and latex agglutination kits designed primarily for the detection of human rotavirus provide a very useful means of rapidly diagnosing equine rotavirus (Cullinane et al., 2006). Detection of viral RNA by PAGE is the method of choice for detection of equine rotavirus, possessing maximum sensitivity and specificity. PAGE has also served as a useful tool to differentiate strains. However, some viruses that belong to different serotypes are indistinguishable by PAGE. A minimum of three negative results on samples properly obtained and stored before testing gives has been suggested to state with confirmation that a foal does not have rotaviral diarrhea (Dwyer, 2007).

Regarding the molecular detection tools, hybridization tests were developed using labeled cDNA probe (Palombo, 2002). Such probes, based on hypervariable regions of outer capsid genes of rotaviruses, could be used in hybridization assays to characterize animal rotavirus strains. Hybridization assays with specific probes have been used in P typing of equine group A rotaviruses (Imagawa et al., 1994). Nucleotide sequencing, coupled with DNA probing or RNA-RNA hybridization, has helped in characterizing the ERVs at genomic level and also to detect the interspecies relatedness (Tsunemitsu et al., 2001; Fukai et al., 2006; Gulati et al., 2007; Dwyer, 2007; Dhama et al., 2009). ERV are genetically characterized by sequence analysis of the genome segments encoding VP4 and VP7 (Takagi et al., 1994; Fukai et al., 2006). Equine rotaviruses only affect foals and are considered species specific. Though it appears that cross-infection from other species is rare, the genetic relatedness of equine rotavirus to porcine rotaviruses by molecular characterization has helped in identifying interspecies transmission from pigs to horses (Isa and Snodgrass, 1994; Taniguchi et al., 1994; Ciarlet et al., 2001; Palombo, 2002; Dhama et al., 2009). The VP4 amino acid sequence of ERV showed more than 95% homology to porcine rotavirus strains (Taniguchi et al., 1994). Similarly, the genome of serotype G10 ERV and serotype G10 calf rotavirus were found closely related to each other during molecular characterization studies (Imagawa et al., 1994). Further, regarding molecular diagnosis, rapid detection tools like PCR have caught the attention of researchers in recent years. Presently, RT-PCR, using the VP4 or VP7 gene primers, is much widely used for detection of animal rotaviruses (Buesa et al., 1996; Tsunemitsu et al., 2001; Elschner et al., 2005; Dhama et al., 2009). Also, a nested RT-PCR for the detection of group A rotaviruses was developed, which is based on a target region in gene segment 6 (Elschner et al., 2002).

PREVENTION AND CONTROL

For prevention and control of the rotavirus diarrhea in foals, commercially available inactivated vaccines have been identified to be quite effective for vaccinating dam (Barrandeguy et al., 1998; Fukai et al., 2006; Cullinane et al., 2006; Dwyer, 2007; Dhama et al., 2009). The available vaccines contain inactivated rotavirus group A and is indicated for administration to pregnant mares to enhance concentrations of colostral immunoglobulins against the virus. These vaccines, used in mares, can be considered to be reasonably safe, and pregnant mares should be vaccinated at eight, nine, ten months of gestation (Powell et al., 1997; Dwyer, 2001, 2007). For preventing infection, the local or mucosal immunity has to be enhanced as they are more crucial in providing resistance. The rotavirus antibodies transmitted through colostrums/ milk is a key factor in protecting the neonates (Saif and Fernandez, 1996; Dodet et al., 1997; Chauhan et al., 2008). Sheoran et al. (2000) have stressed the importance of prepartum equine rotavirus vaccination as it can induce strong specific IgG antibodies in mammary secretions.

Even though colostral antibodies enter the circulation, they are often considered less effective in protecting young ones when compared to those present in the intestinal lumen (Saif and Fernandez, 1996; Steele et al., 2004), but the antibody titer in serum of young ones could be considered as an indicator of protection against rotavirus diarrhea (Kohara and Tsunemitsu, 2000). To boost the maternal antibody levels, the dam has to be immunized with inactivated rotavirus vaccines a few weeks prior to parturition, which could enhance the level of protection in neonates (Holland, 1990; Saif and Fernandez, 1996; Barrandeguy et al., 1998; Steele et al., 2004; Chauhan et al., 2008; Dhama et al., 2009). In addition, it has been observed that foals given bovine colostral immunoglobulins for three to five days showed reduced morbidity due to viral diarrhea (Watanabe et al., 1993). The protection levels induced by vaccines have been extensively studied in calves when compared to foals. It has been further ascertained that the calves given pooled colostrum from vaccinated dams have been found to be devoid of diarrhea and virus shedding. Also, neonates fed for five consecutive days with colostrum obtained from vaccinated dam have been refractory to rotavirus infections (Castrucci et al., 1988). Hence, by vaccination, if serum antibodies are generated at high levels in mare, similar to bovines, the colostrum should exert sufficient protective effect in foals. Recently, it has been described that provision of one hyperimmune egg per day to newborn calves can reduce the severity of diarrhea (Bilbao et al., 2006). Also, supplementation of probiotics can prevent rotavirus-induced diarrhea in young ones (Gill and Prasad, 2008; Dhama et al., 2008a). Probiotics and natural yogurt may help to restore the normal intestinal flora. Both these strategies could also be followed in order to minimize the threat of rotavirus-induced diarrhea in foals.

Researchers are currently trying to develop new-generation vaccines that are highly efficacious and regarded as much safer during administration (Els et al., 2007; Dhama et al., 2008b). VP7 and VP4 are considered to be critical for novel vaccine development programs as they are targets for neutralizing antibodies that may provide both serotype-specific and, in some instances, cross-reactive protection (Angel et al., 2007). Investigations of the VP7 or VP4 diversity of the circulating equine viruses and the dynamics of strain replacement are important for developing novel efficacious vaccines (Collins et al., 2008). Immunization using plasmid DNA encoding the VP4 gene of rotaviruses has been found to induce humoral—and cell-mediated immune response (Garcia-Diaz et al., 2004; Herrmann, 2006). Similarly, subunit vaccines based on the VP4 protein of rotaviruses, expressed in prokaryotic system, and viruslike particles (VLPs) containing rotavirus capsid proteins that are produced in baculovirus expression system can be used as effective vaccines (Chauhan et al., 2008; Dhama et al., 2009). Also, VP5 subunits of spike protein VP4 can be exploited for outplaying the alpha-2 beta-1 integrin-based attachment of rotaviruses, and this strategy may potentially block the rotavirus infections (Graham et al., 2006). Likewise, reverse genetics, a novel methodology for generating an infectious clone of rotaviruses containing desirable gene segments, has been suggested for vaccine development (Komoto et al., 2006). Based on the current progress achieved, these novel vaccines and strategies coupled with the conventional vaccination programs are expected to make significant strides toward maintaining an equine population free of rotaviral infections.

Besides effective prophylactic strategies, management practices like strict biosecurity, quarantine, disinfection, and strict hygiene are essential for preventing the disease in foals. Overcrowding is a significant risk factor for outbreaks of foal diarrhea, which need to be avoided. Manure and bedding from stalls of affected foals should be considered a biosecurity threat to unaffected foals and therefore need to be disposed off appropriately. Good management and hygienic practices can help to reduce the incidence of rotaviral diarrhea in farm animals (Holland, 1990; Dwyer, 2001, 2007; Chauhan and Singh, 1996; Steele et al., 2004; Cullinane et al., 2006; Chauhan et al., 2008; Dhama et al., 2009). Foals suffering from rotavirus-induced diarrhea should be moved immediately with their dams to an isolation facility, and their handlers should not be in contact with other healthy horses. Appropriate antibiotics to control secondary bacterial infection and fluid and electrolyte therapy to restore the fluid reserve should be given so that the mortality rate in foals could be minimized (Murphy et al., 1999; Steele et al., 2004). Supportive care and symptomatic treatment should be followed immediately as per the nature of the case. In general, however, broad spectrum antibiotics should be avoided as they inhibit the development of the large intestine microflora. In highly compromised animal or in a danger of septicemia, broad spectrum parenteral antibiotics may be used. The administration of plasma is recommended for foals in danger of circulatory collapse. In severely affected animals, parenteral nutrition may be indicated. Assisted by a thorough understanding of the disease epidemiology as well as serotypes of the virus, prevention and control strategies have to be revised in order to protect the foals from this economically important disease.

Conclusion

Rotaviruses are being considered as the prime cause of enteritis and diarrhea in foals as it has been documented to cause 50% or more of foal diarrhea cases. Equine rotaviruses, transmitted via the fecal-oral route causes damage to the small intestinal villi resulting in cellular destruction, malabsorption, and diarrhea. These viruses have extreme genetic diversity and are resistant to many common disinfection methods. This brings additional difficulty in implementing suitable preventive measures against the infection. However, to prevent the losses, diverse approaches including good management, sanitation, and hygiene together with vaccinating the dam in order to confer protection to neonates are to be strictly followed. Awareness and implementation of strict biosecurity and disinfection procedures during the foaling season can mitigate the morbidity associated with rotavirus diarrhea. As the local or mucosal immunity in the intestinal tract is crucial for protection, the intake of rotavirus-specific antibodies via colostrum is critical for reducing the incidence of the infection in foals. As concurrent infections with other pathogens like *E. coli* can potentiate the effects of rotavirus infection, eradication of secondary pathogens from stables have to be given due importance. Further, it is important to analyze the equine rotavirus genome by serotype-specific RT-PCR or gene sequencing for assessing the interspecies transmission of these viruses between other animals and human beings also. The role of NSP4 is augmenting the severity of the diarrhea in foals, and receptor-based blocking of rotaviruses using viral protein subunits should be considered as strong points for future research.

Currently, based on the novel techniques evolved in the field of vaccinology, there is a trend for the development of new-generation vaccines against rotaviruses. DNA vaccines and subunit vaccines have been reported to develop sufficient levels of serum antibody titers in dam. Similarly, the recombinant proteins have to be utilized for developing VLP-based vaccines, which could stimulate the production of desirable quantities of specific antibodies in serum as well as colostrum. These strategies of future may provide simple and inexpensive method of immunoprophylaxis against this economically important pathogen of equines. Similarly, even when effective prophylactic products are developed, farm management practices like quarantine, disinfection, and hygiene are always of paramount importance to prevent rotavirus infection in foals.

REFERENCES

1. Angel, J., Franco, M. A. and Greenberg, H. B. 2007. Rotavirus vaccines: Recent developments and future considerations. *Nat. Rev. Microbiol.* 5:529–539.
2. Anthony, I. D., Bullivant, S., Dayal, S., Bellamy, A. R. and Berriman, J. A. 1991. Rotavirus spike structure and polypeptide composition. *J. Virol.* 65:4334–4340.
3. Barrandeguy, M., Parreno, V., Lagos, M. M., Pont Lezica, F., Rivas, C., Valle, C. and Fernandez, F. 1998. Prevention of rotavirus diarrhoea in foals by parenteral vaccination of the mares: Field trial. *Dev. Biol. Stand.* 92:253–257.
4. Bilbao, G. N., Chacana, P. A., Mendiburu, A., Rodriguez, E., Blackhall, J. O. and Terzolo, H. R. 2006. Prophylaxis of neonatal diarrhoea in dairy calves using egg yolk immunoglobulins (IgY). *Rev. Medi. Veter. Buenos Aires* 87:135–139.
5. Browning, G. F., Chalmers, R. M., Fitzgerald, T. A. and Snodgrass, D. R. 1991a. A novel group A rotavirus G serotype: Serological and genomic characterization of equine isolate FI23. *J. Clin. Microbiol.* 29:2043–2046.
6. Browning, G. F., Chalmers, R. M., Snodgrass, D. R., Batt, R. M., Hart, C. A., Ormarod, S. E., Leadon, D., Stoneham, S. J. and Rossdale, P. D. 1991b. The prevalence of enteric pathogens in diarrhoeic thoroughbred foals in Britain and Ireland. *Equine Vet. J.* 23:405–409.
7. Browning, G. F., Chalmers, R. M., Fitzgerald, T. A. and Snodgrass, D. R. 1991c. Serological and genomic characterization of L338, a novel equine group A rotavirus G serotype. *J. Gen. Virol.* 72:1059–1064.
8. Browning, G. F., Chalmers, R. M., Fitzgerald, T. A. and Snodgrass, D. R. 1992a. Evidence for two serotype G3 subtypes among equine rotaviruses. *J. Clin. Microbiol.* 30:485–491.
9. Browning, G. F., Chalmers, R. M., Fitzgerald, T. A., Corley, K. T. T., Campbell, I. and Snodgrass, D. R. 1992b. Rotavirus serotype G3 predominates in horses. *J. Clin. Microbiol.* 30:59–62.
10. Browning, G. F. and Begg, A. P. 1996. Prevalence of G and P serotypes among equine rotaviruses in the faeces of diarrhoeic foals. *Arch. Virol.* 141:1077–1089.

11. Buesa, J., Colomina, J., Raga, J., Villanueva, A. and Prat, J. 1996. Evaluation of reverse transcription and polymerase chain reaction (RT/PCR) for the detection of rotaviruses: Applications of the assay. *Res. Virol.* 147:353–361.

12. Castrucci, G., Frigeri, F., Ferrari, M., Aldrovandi, V., Tassini, F. and Gatti, R. 1988. The protection of newborn calves against experimental rotavirus infection by feeding mammary secretions from vaccinated cows. *Microbiologica* 11:379–385.

13. Chauhan, R. S. and Singh N. P. 1996. Epidemiology of rotavirus infection in calves in India. *Int. J. Anim. Sci.* 11:221–223.

14. Chauhan, R. S., Dhama, K. and Mahendran, M. 2008. Pathobiology of rotaviral diarrhea in calves and its diagnosis and control: A review. *J. Immunol. Immunopathol.* 10:1–13.

15. Ciarlet, M., Reggeti, F., Pina, C. I. and Liprandi, F. 1994. Equine rotaviruses with G14 serotype specificity circulate among Venezuelan horses. *J. Clin. Microbiol.* 32:2609–2612.

16. Ciarlet, M., Isa, P., Conner, M. E. and Liprandi, F. 2001. Antigenic and molecular analyses reveal that the equine rotavirus strain H-1 is closely related to porcine, but not equine, rotaviruses: Interspecies transmission from pigs to horses? *Virus Genes* 22:5–20.

17. Collins, P. J., Cullinane, A., Martella, V. and O'Shea, H. 2008. Molecular characterization of equine rotavirus in Ireland. *J. Clin. Microbiol.* 46:3346–3354.

18. Conner, M. E. and Darlington, R. W. 1980. Rotavirus infection in foals. *Am. J. Vet. Res.* 41:1699–1703.

19. Cook, N., Bridger, J., Kendall, K., Gomara, M. T., El-Attar, L. and Gray, J. 2004. The zoonotic potential of rotavirus. *J. Infect.* 48:289–302.

20. Cullinane, A. A., Barr, B., Bernard, W., Duncan, J. L., Mulcahy, G., Smith, M. and Timoney, J. E. 2006. Infectious diseases (Chapter 1): Rotavirus. In *The equine manual*, 2nd ed., A. J. Higgins and J. R. Snyder, 44–47. USA: Saunder, Elsevier Ltd.

21. Desselberger, U., Gray, J. and Estes, M. K. 2005. Rotaviruses. In *Topley and Wilson's microbiology and microbial infections*, ed. B. W. J. Mahy and V. T. Meulen, 946–958. USA: ASM Press.

22. de Verdier Klingenberg, K. and Esfandiari, J. 1996. Evaluation of a one-step test for rapid, in practice detection of rotavirus in farm animals. *Vet. Rec.* 138:393–395.

23. Dhama, K., Mahendran, M., Tomar, S. and Chauhan, R. S. 2008a. Beneficial effects of probiotics and prebiotics in livestock and poultry: The current perspectives. *Polivet* 9:1–13.

24. Dhama, K., Mahendran, M., Gupta, P. K. and Rai, A. 2008b. DNA vaccines of veterinary importance: Current perspectives. *Vet. Res. Commun.* 32:341–356.

25. Dhama, K., Chauhan, R. S., Mahendran, M. and Malik, S. V. S. 2009. Rotavirus diarrhea in bovines and other domestic animals. *Vet. Res. Commun.* 33:1–23.

26. Dodet, B., Heseltine, E., Mary, C. and Saliou, P. 1997. Rotaviruses in human and veterinary medicine. *Sante.* 7:195–199.

27. Dwyer, R. M. 2001. Control and prevention of foal diarrhea outbreaks. *Proc. Ann. Conven. AAEP* 47:472–475.

28. Dwyer, R. M. 2007. Equine rotavirus. In *Equine infectious diseases*, ed. D. C. Sellon and M. T. Long, chapter 17, 181–183. Philadelphia, USA: Saunders, Elsevier Inc.

29. Ellis, G. R. and Daniels, E. 1988. Comparison of direct electron microscopy and enzyme immunoassay for the detection of rotaviruses in calves, lambs, piglets and foals. *Aust. Vet. J.* 65:133–135.

30. Elschner, M., Prudlo, J., Hotzel, H., Otto, P. and Sachse, K. 2002. Nested reverse transcriptase-polymerase chain reaction for the detection of group A rotaviruses. *J. Vet. Med. B Infect. Dis.* 49:77–81.

31. Elschner, M., Schrader, C., Hotzel, H., Prudlo, J., Sachse, K., Eichhorn, W., Herbst, W. and Otto, P. 2005. Isolation and molecular characterisation of equine rotaviruses from Germany. *Vet. Microbiol.* 105:123–129.

32. Els, N. T., Walker, M. J., Peters, A., Pastoret, P. P. and Jungersen, G. 2007. Current status of veterinary vaccines. *Clin. Microbiol. Rev.* 20:489–510.

33. Estes, M. K. 2001. Rotaviruses and their replication. In *Fields virology*, ed. D. M. Knipe and P. M. Howley, 1747–1785. Philadelphia, USA: Lippincott Williams and Wilkins.

34. Estes, M. K. 2003. The rotavirus NSP4 enterotoxin: Current status and challenges. In *Viral gastroenteritis*, ed. U. Desselberger and J. Gray, 207–224. Amsterdam, Netherlands: Elsevier Science.

35. Estes, M. K., Graham, D. Y. and Mason, B. B. 1981. Proteolytic enhancement of rotavirus infectivity: Molecular mechanisms. *J. Virol.* 39:879–888.

36. Flewett, T. H., Bryden, A. S. and Davies, H. 1975. Virus diarrhoea in foals and other animals. *Vet. Rec.* 96:477.

37. Fukai, K., Saito, T., Fukuda, O., Hagiwara, A., Inoue, K. and Sato, M. 2006. Molecular characterization of equine group A rotavirus, Nasuno, isolated in Tochigi Prefecture, Japan. *Vet. J.* 172:369–373.

38. Garcia-Diaz, A., Lopez-Andujar, P., Rodriguez Diaz, J., Montava, R., Torres Barcelo, C., Ribes, J. M. and Buesa, J. 2004. Nasal immunization of mice with a rotavirus DNA vaccine that induces protective intestinal IgA antibodies. *Vaccine* 23:489–498.

39. Gill, H. and Prasad J. 2008. Probiotics, immunomodulation, and health benefits. *Adv. Experiment. Med. Biol.* 606:423–454.

40. Gouvea, V., Glass, R. I., Woods, P., Taniguchi, K., Clark, H. F., Forrester, B. and Fang, Z. Y. 1990. Polymerase chain reaction amplification and typing of rotavirus nucleic acid from stool specimens. *J. Clin. Microbiol.* 28:276–282.

41. Graham, K. L., Takada, Y. and Coulson, B. S. 2006. Rotavirus spike protein VP5* binds alpha2beta1 integrin on the cell surface and competes with virus for cell binding and infectivity. *J Gen. Virol.* 87:1275–1283.

42. Gulati, B. R., Deepa, R., Singh, B. K. and Rao, C. D. 2007. Diversity in Indian equine rotaviruses: Identification of genotype G10, P6[1] and G1 strains and a new VP7 genotype (G16) strain in specimens from diarrheic foals in India. *J. Clin. Microbiol.* 45:972–978.

43. Hardy, M. E., Woode, G. N., Xu, Z., Williams, J. D., Conner, M. E., Dwyer, R. M. and Powell, D. G. 1991. Analysis of serotypes and electropherotypes of equine rotaviruses isolated in the United States. *J. Clin. Microbiol.* 29:889–893.

44. Herrmann, J. E. 2006. DNA vaccines against enteric infections. *Vaccine* 24:3705–3708.

45. Holland, R. E. 1990. Some infectious causes of diarrhea in young farm animals. *Clin. Microbiol. Rev.* 3:345–375.

46. Hoshino, Y., Wyatt, R. G., Greenberg, H. B., Kalica, A. R., Flores, J. and Kapikian, A. Z. 1983. Isolation and characterization of an equine rotavirus. *J. Clin. Microbiol.* 18:585–591.

47. Imagawa, H., Ishida, S., Uesugi, S., Masanobu, K., Fukunaga, Y. and Nakagomi, O. 1994. Genetic analysis of equine rotavirus by RNA-RNA hybridization. *J. Clin. Microbiol.* 32:2009–2012.

48. Imagawa, H., Sekiguchi, K., Anzai, T., Fukunaga, Y., Kanemaru, T., Ohishi, H., Higuchi, T. and Kamada, M. 1991. Epidemiology of equine rotavirus infection among foals in the breeding region. *J. Vet. Med. Sci.* 53:1079–1080.

49. Imagawa, H., Tanaka, T., Sekiguchi, K., Fukunaga, Y., Anzai, T., Minamoto, N. and Kamada, M. 1993. Electropherotypes, serotypes, and subgroups of equine rotaviruses isolated in Japan. *Arch. Virol.* 131:169–176.

50. Imagawa, H., Ando, Y., Sugiura, T., Wada, R., Hirasawa, K. and Akiyama, Y. 1981. Isolation of foal rotavirus in MA-104 cells. *Bull. Equine Res. Inst.* 18:119–128.

51. Isa, P. and Snodgrass, D. R. 1994. Serological and genomic characterization of equine rotavirus VP4 proteins identifies three different P serotypes. *Virology* 201:364–372.

52. Isa, P., Gutierrez, M., Arias, C. F. and Lopez, S. 2008. Rotavirus cell entry. *Future Virol.* 3:135–146.

53. Kapikian, A. Z., Hoshino, Y. and Chanock, R. M. 2001. Rotaviruses. In *Fields virology*, 4th ed., D. M. Knipe and P. M. Howley, 1787–1833. Philadelphia: Lippincott Williams & Wilkins.

54. Kohara, J. and Tsunemitsu, H. 2000. Correlation between maternal serum antibodies and protection against bovine rotavirus diarrhea in calves. *J. Vet. Med. Sci.* 62:219–221.

55. Komoto, S., Sasaki, J. and Taniguchi, K. 2006. Reverse genetics system for introduction of site-specific mutations into the double-stranded RNA genome of infectious rotavirus. *Proc. Nat. Acad. Sci. USA* 103:4646–4651.

56. Legrottaglie, R. and Agrimi, P. 1992. Rotavirus infection in horses. Genome profile analysis of a rotavirus isolated from an infected foal. *Microbiologica* 15:209–212.

57. Murphy, F. A., Gibbs, E. P. J., Horzinek, M. C. and Studdert, M. J. 1999. Reoviridae. In *Veterinary virology*, 3rd ed., 391–404. USA: Academic Press.

58. Netherwood, T., Wood, J. L., Townsend, H. G., Mumford, J. A. and Chanter, N. 1996. Foal diarrhoea between 1991 and 1994 in the United Kingdom associated with *Clostridium perfringens*, rotavirus, *Strongyloides westeri* and *Cryptosporidium spp. Epidemiol. Infect.* 117:375–383.

59. Palombo, E. A. 2002. Genetic analysis of group A rotaviruses: Evidence for interspecies transmission of rotavirus genes. *Virus Genes* 24:11–20.

60. Paul, P. S. and Lyoo, Y. S. 1993. Immunogens of rotaviruses. *Vet. Microbiol.* 37:299–317.

61. Powell, D. G., Dwyer, R. M., Traub-Dargatz, J. L., Fulker, R. H., Whalen, J. W. Jr., Srinivasappa, J., Acree, W. M. and Chu, H. J. 1997. Field study of the safety, immunogenicity, and efficacy of an inactivated equine rotavirus vaccine. *J. Am. Vet. Med. Assoc.* 211:193–198.

62. Prasad, B. V., Wang, G. J., Clerx, J. P. and Chiu, W. 1988. Three-dimensional structure of rotavirus. *J. Mol. Biol.* 199:269–275.

63. Ramig, R. F. 2004. Pathogenesis of intestinal and systemic rotavirus infection. *J. Virol.* 78:10213–10220.

64. Saif, L. J. and Fernandez, F. M. 1996. Group A rotavirus veterinary vaccines. *J. Infect. Dis.* 174:98–106.

65. Schroeder, B. A., Street, J. E., Kalmakoff, J. and Bellamy, A. R. 1982. Sequence relationships between the genome segments of human and animal rotavirus strains. *J. Virol.* 43:379–385.

66. Sheoran, A. S., Karzenski, S. S., Whalen, J. W., Crisman, M. V., Powell, D. G. and Timoney, J. F. 2000. Prepartum equine rotavirus vaccination inducing strong specific IgG in mammary secretions. *Vet. Rec.* 146:672–673.

67. Smith, M. and Tzipori, S. 1979. Gel electrophoresis of rotavirus RNA derived from six different animal species. *Aust. J. Exp. Biol. Med. Sci.* 57:583–585.

68. Steele, A. D., Geyer, A. and Gerdes, G. H. 2004. Rotavirus infections. In *Infectious diseases of livestock*, 2nd ed., J. A. W. Coetzer and R. C. Tustin, 1256–1264. Southern Africa: Oxford.

69. Studdert, M. J., Mason, R. W. and Patten, P. E. 1978. Rotavirus diarrhea of foals. *Aust. Vet. J.* 54:363–364.

70. Takagi, M., Hoshi, A., Ohta, C., Shirahata, T., Goto, H., Urasawa, T., Taniguchi, K. and Urasawa, S. 1993. A minor prevalent strain in a severe outbreak of foal diarrhea associated with serotype 3 rotavirus. *J. Vet. Med. Sci.* 55:661–663.

71. Takagi, M., Taniguchi, K., Urasawa, T., Urasawa, S., Shirahata, T. and Goto, H. 1994. Characterization of a G14 equine rotavirus (strain CH3) isolated in Japan. *Arch. Virol.* 139:209–215.

72. Tan, J. A. and Schnagl, R. 1981. Inactivation of a rotavirus by disinfectants. *Med. J. Aust.* 1:19–32.

73. Taniguchi, K., Urasawa, T. and Urasawa, S. 1994. Species specificity and interspecies relatedness in VP4 genotypes demonstrated by VP4 sequence analysis of equine, feline, and canine rotavirus strains. *Virology* 200:390–400.

74. Tsunemitsu, H., Imagawa, H., Togo, M., Shouji, T., Kawashima, K., Horino, R., Imai, K., Nishimori, T., Takagi, M. and Higuchi, T. 2001. Predominance of G3B and G14 equine group A rotaviruses of a single VP4 serotype in Japan. *Arch. Virol.* 146:1949–1962.

75. Villarreal, L. Y. B., Uliana, G., Valenzuela, C., Chacon, J. L. V., Saidenberg, A. B. S., Sanches, A. A., Brandao, P. E., Jerez, J. A. and Ferreira, A. J. P. 2006. Rotavirus detection and isolation from chickens with or without symptoms. *Rev. Bras. Cien. Avicola* 8:187–191.

76. Watanabe, T., Ohta, C., Shirahata, T., Goto, H., Tsunoda, N., Tagami, M. and Akita, H. 1993. Preventive administration of bovine colostral immunoglobulins for foal diarrhea with rotavirus. *J. Vet. Med. Sci.* 55:1039–1040.
77. Woode, G. N. and Crouch, C. F. 1978. Naturally occurring and experimentally induced rotavirus infection of domestic and laboratory animals. *J. Am. Vet. Med. Assoc.* 173:522–526.

20. West Nile Virus Infection of Horses

K. Dhama, R. V. S. Pawaiya, S. Kapoor, and Thankam Mathew

Introduction

The West Nile Virus (WNV), which is a flavivirus, belongs to the family Flaviviridae; it is a mosquito-borne virus that can result in fatal encephalitis in human beings, equines, and avian species (Hubalek and Halouzka, 1999; Rappole et al., 2000; Rappole and Hubalek, 2000; Komar, 2000; Castillo-Olivares and Wood, 2004; Kramer et al., 2008). The virus is closely related to Japanese encephalitis and St. Louis encephalitis viruses that are primarily maintained in nature by transmission cycles between mosquitoes and birds. Occasionally, WNV infects and causes disease in other vertebrates, including humans and horses.

In the recent past, the coronavirus caused severe acute respiratory syndrome (SARS) in humans; and presently, the threat of few emerging and reemerging infectious viruses like the West Nile, Chikungunya, Japanese encephalitis, Ebola, and Maburg are posing much public health implications, with avian influenza (bird flu) virus predicted to be on the verge of causing a human pandemic. This situation warrants the need of conducting novel researches, proper monitoring at global level, and focusing on crisis management concepts to encounter these deadly pathogens. Variola virus that caused smallpox in humans and the monkeypox (miniature smallpox) are also being reported to be "virtually emerging" viruses having high potential for use in bioterrorism (Mayr, 2003; Georges et al., 2004; Bricaire and Bossi, 2006; Garavelli and Peduzzi, 2006). In recent times, West Nile virus has reemerged as an important pathogen worldwide.

The West Nile virus (WNV) was first isolated in 1937 from a human being who had fever. He resided in the West Nile province of Uganda and hence named as WN virus (Smithburn et al., 1940; Guharov, 2004). Since then, sporadic and major outbreaks, mainly in humans but also in horses, have been reported in Africa, the Middle East, and Europe (Murgue et al., 2002). In the last decade, WNV has reemerged as an important pathogen for humans and horses as frequent outbreaks with increased proportion and severity of neurological disease cases and high bird mortality have been reported (Hubalek and Halouzka, 1999; Cantile et al., 2000; Chowers et al., 2001; Murgue et al., 2001a Weinberger et al., 2001; Weiss et al., 2001; Blitvich et al., 2003b; Dupuis et al., 2003). During the last few years, WNV-related disease in humans and horses have been reported on higher side and in a wider way (Mailles et al., 2003). Since 1999, it has been reported from USA, and more than 23,500 human cases have been reported till 2006. Out of that cases, 9,800 patients showed neuroinvasive disease, and 943 died because of WN infection (Sejvar, 2007).

ETIOLOGY

The West Nile virus belongs to genus *Flavivirus* of the family Flaviviridae, whereas earlier it was classified in Togaviridae, and is an arbovirus (Monath and Heinz, 1996). Flaviviruses are further classified into twelve serogroups based on cross-reactivity in virus-neutralization assays. WNV, together with Japanese encephalitis (JE), St. Louis encephalitis (SLE), Murray Valley encephalitis (MVE), Kunjin (KUN), Usutu (USU), Koutango (KOU), Cacipacore (CPC), Alfuy (ALF), and Yaounde (YAO) viruses belongs to the Japanese encephalitis sero-complex group (Heinz et al., 1999).

The genome of WNV is a positive-sense, single-stranded RNA without any polyadenylation at the 3'end. The icosahedral core is composed of multiple copies of a highly basic capsid protein (C) (12 kDa) surrounded by a host-cell envelope modified by the insertion of two virus-encoded proteins, the major envelope protein E (53 kDa), and the membrane protein M (8 kDa) (Deubel et al., 2001; Brinton, 2002). The viral genome contains a 5' and a 3' noncoding region of 96 and 631 nucleotides, respectively, which flanks one single open reading frame of 10,302 nucleotides encoding a polyprotein, which gets processed by viral and cellular proteases into three structural proteins (namely, C, E, and M or pr-M) and five nonstructural proteins (namely, NS1, NS2a/NS2b, NS3, NS4a/NS4b, and NS5). Tertiary structures at genomic end play important regulatory role in replication and assembly. NS1 and NS4A take part in virus replication; NS2A in assembly and virion release; NS3 and NS2B possess proteolytic activities; and NS5 acts as a RNA-dependent RNA polymerase and methyltransferase playing role in methylation of the 5'-cap structure (Brinton, 2002).

The E protein contains the neutralizing epitopes and cell-binding receptors and is associated with biological activities of virulence, tropism, antigenicity, and hemagglutination (Monath and Heinz, 1996; Beasley and Barrett, 2002; Brinton, 2002; Castillo-Olivares and Wood, 2004; Beasley, 2005; Long, 2007). Antigenic relationships between flaviviruses show the existence of flavivirus group, subgroup, sero-complex, type-specific, and strain-specific antigenic determinants (Heinz et al., 1999) based on virus neutralization and indirect immunofluorescence tests and nucleotide sequences analysis. There are two distinct lineages of WNVs (Berthet et al., 1997; Savage et al., 1999; Porter et al., 2003). Lineage 1 comprise viruses isolated from animals in African continent (Central and North Africa, Europe, Israel, and North America), which have been associated with epidemics of increased severity in humans and horses, whereas lineage 2 comprises of viruses that have only been found to circulate in enzootic cycles in birds in Central and

South Africa. Proteins prM, NS1, NS3, and NS5 of flaviviruses also have been reported to be antigenic (Kaufman et al., 1989; Tan et al., 1990; Falconar and Young, 1991; Davis et al., 2001; Jozan et al., 2003; Wong et al., 2003).

TISSUE CULTURE SUSCEPTIBILITY

West Nile virus grows in a wide variety of primary cells and continuous cell lines from mammalian (Vero cells, BHK-21, RK-13, SW-13) and mosquito species (C6/36, *Aedes albopictus, A. Aegypti* cells) (Monath and Heinz, 1996). Depending on the host species, the virus can grow in vivo in a variety of cells from different tissues such as neurons, glial cells, and cells from spleen, liver, heart, lymph nodes, and lung (Cantile et al., 2001). Virus replicates in the perinuclear region of the rough endoplasmic reticulum and the virions are finally released by exocytosis or by budding. Cytopathic effects of the virus include cell lysis, syncytia formation, and virus persistence may occur (Pogodina et al., 1983; Despres et al., 1993; Westaway et al., 1997; Deubel et al., 2001; Xiao et al., 2001; Monath and Heinz, 1996).

ROLE OF BIRDS AND MOSQUITOES IN WNV TRANSMISSION

Birds act as the major amplifying host in the natural cycle of all members of the JE antigenic complex of flaviviruses, with several species of mosquitoes playing as vectors; and *Culex* species have special role in case of WNV life cycle. The lesser-discriminant species *Cx. pipiens, Cx. Nigripalpus,* and *Cx. tarsalis* may function as important bridge vectors that spread infection to horses and man from birds (Bernard and Kramer, 2001). Primary vectors and vertebrate host species dependent on the geographic area and the levels of virus that are circulating among both the avian and mosquito species that are infected by WNV plays a significant role in virus transmission. (Komar, 2000; Bernard and Kramer, 2001; Blitvich et al., 2003a). WNV is carried by the infectious mosquitoes in their salivary glands, and susceptible vertebrate hosts get infected at the time of feeding of these mosquitoes; viremia occurs in vertebrate hosts for up to five days. Other insect vectors then must feed on these hosts during viremia to become infected, and thus further transmission occurs (Cornel et al., 1993; Bernard and Kramer, 2001). The reproduction activity of mosquitoes and viral replication in insect vectors being temperature dependence accounts for the highly seasonal variation in WNV transmission and disease outbreaks. This is the reason that most encephalitis cases in temperate regions such as Europe, Canada, and the northern states of USA occur during late summer or autumn when insect numbers and temperatures are elevated.

Transmission from vertebrate host to mosquito is highly dependent on the state of viremia in the vertebrate. However, development of titers sufficient to infect mosquito species is a rare event reflected in both horse and man, although they are typically referred to as dead-end hosts (McIntosh et al., 1969; Hubalek and Halouzka, 1999; Komar, 2000; Bunning et al., 2002; Ng et al., 2003; Cullinane et al., 2006; Long, 2007). It is likely that out of various species of mosquito reported to be virologically competent vectors of WNV (Komar, 2000), only fewer are likely to be considered important.

WNV is maintained in an epizootic transmission cycle between mosquitoes and birds with humans and horses as incidental hosts (Work et al., 1955; Nasci et al., 2001; Komar, 2000; Komar et al., 2000). The migrating or wild birds may also transmit WNV to susceptible animal species and play role in repeated reintroduction of WNV (Rappole and Hubalek, 2000; Rappole et al., 2000; 2003; Dhama et al., 2008a). Such examples are in some areas like the temperate area of Camargue in Southern France, where transmission has been reported to occur sporadically and where irregular epidemics in horses have been reported, and also in Africa, where there are large populations of migratory birds with WNV endemic activity, introducing the infection to the Middle East (Bernard and Kramer, 2001, Murgue et al., 2001a; 2002; Malkinson et al., 2002; Buckley et al., 2003; Dhama et al., 2008a). The speed and pattern of spread make the role of migratory birds less likely than that from dispersal movements from nonmigratory birds such as the house sparrow. Transovarian transmission of WNV has been identified in one species of mosquito and also been demonstrated experimentally in a range of *Culex* and *Aedes* species mosquitoes and the *Cx. pipiens* (Baqar et al., 1993; Miller et al., 2000; Turrell et al., 2001); however, this mode of transmission of WNV is probably unimportant, though could help viral persistence (Bernard and Kramer, 2001).

The similarity of the viruses involved in the North American mortality of birds in 1999, the crow deaths in the USA, and the Israeli outbreaks with mortality in geese in 1998 and 1999 strongly suggests a unique feature of the virus strain involved since they also involved avian mortality in all these outbreaks. There was also a similarity in appearance and spread of WNV during these outbreaks in both equine and human cases of disease (Lanciotti et al., 1999; OIE, 1999; Bernard et al., 2001; Eidson et al., 2001; Komar et al., 2002).

EPIDEMIOLOGY
WNV has been reported in different countries like, Romania, Morocco, Tunisia, Italy, Russia, Israel, France, Canada, Mexico, North America, other parts of Africa, the Middle East, and the Caribbean region (Blitvich et al., 2003b; Dupuis et al., 2003, Schuler et al., 2004). Serological investigations in birds in Britain suggest that a WN-like virus has been circulating among bird populations (Buckley et al., 2003). During the twentieth century, sporadic and major WNV outbreaks, mainly in humans, but also in horses, have

been reported in Africa, the Middle East, and Europe (Murgue et al., 2002). However, during the past few years, mostly in the twenty-first century, frequent disease outbreaks have been recorded worldwide both in humans and horses with increased proportion and severity of neurological disease cases or high mortality in birds, confirming the reemergence of WNV as an important pathogen (Hubalek and Halouzka, 1999; Roehrig et al., 2002; Castillo-Olivares and Wood, 2004; Durand et al., 2004; L'vov et al., 2004; Mackenzie et al., 2004; Schuler et al., 2004; Ward, 2006; Sejvar, 2007; Takasaki, 2007; Blitvich, 2008; CDC, 2008; Klinkhamer and Lipman, 2008; Kramer et al., 2008; Long, 2007; Ndiva et al., 2008; Rudolf et al., 2008; Alonso-Padilla et al., 2009).

Taylor et al. (1956) first demonstrated the viral activity in birds from Egypt. Later, the serological survey conducted by Schmidt and Elmansoury (1963) in the same Nile region of Egypt revealed a 54% seropositivity rate in equines but with only one death among the equine population. Before 1994, WNV did not seem to be having much public health implications till the virus was isolated from different parts of world (Europe [Spain, Portugal, Russia, the former Czechoslovakia, Romania, France], Africa (South Africa, Senegal, Kenya), and Asia (Israel, Iran, India). Till this time, WNV was regarded as a mosquito-borne infection of birds, which was rarely associated with clinical disease in either horse or man, except the epidemic in France in 1962–1963, where eighty horses were affected with ataxia and weakness and 25–30% died (Joubert et al., 1970), and the outbreak in South Africa in 1974, where eighteen thousand humans got affected too although with no deaths recorded, and no information reported about disease in equines (McIntosh et al., 1969; Jupp, 2001). The number of disease outbreaks and their severity has been reported to increase since the mid-1990s with deaths in humans also documented in Algeria, Romania, Morocco, Tunisia, Congo, Russia, and Israel (Le Guenno et al., 1996; Tber-Aldelhaq, 1996; Tsai et al., 1998; Nur et al., 1999; Platonov et al., 2001; Triki et al., 2001; Murgue et al., 2001b; Malkinson et al., 2002). Morbidity and mortality was also reported among horses in the outbreaks of Morocco and Israel but not in Romanian and Russian epidemics. The outbreak in Israel was very unusual as extensive mortality in birds was noted, and the virus was isolated from the brain of a stork. And in 1999, WN virus was identified in commercial geese from Israel (Murgue et al., 2001b; Steinman et al., 2002; Banet-Noach et al., 2003). Besides these outbreaks, there were limited outbreaks restricted only to horses from Northern Italy and France in 1998 (Cantile et al., 2000; Murgue et al., 2001b; Autorino et al., 2002). The serological survey showed 38% of horses were affected in a 700-km² area of Tuscany, Italy. There was no difference in age-specific prevalence noted as the horses were not exposed for WN virus earlier. WNV human cases were not reported from the WNV outbreaks of Italy in 1998 despite the fourteen equine cases (Mugue et al., 2001b).

Subsequent serological studies revealed a 58% seroprevalence in equines in the area of the outbreak, a far higher frequency than that for those with clinical signs (Autorino et al., 2002). Subsequently, many WNV cases of human, equine, birds, and other mammals were reported in the Western Hemisphere from New York, Florida, and from other American states, Mexico, Canada, and the Caribbean areas (Anonymous, 1999, 2003 ; Anderson et al., 1999; Asnis et al., 2000; Petersen and Roehrig, 2001; Trock et al., 2001; Weese et al., 2003; Sejvar, 2007). Seropositive to WNV (approximately 20%) was also reported in contact animals. As in Israel, there was substantial avian mortality, in particular in crows, that preceded the human and horse disease reports (Anderson et al., 1999).

WNV infection in human and horses in United States were recorded as follows: The 2002 epidemic of North Dakota spread to forty-three states of USA (Schuler et al., 2004; Ndiva et al., 2008), and the 2002 Texas WN epidemic was in the high plains of North Texas and north central Texas among the equids, (Ward, 2006). The other states that recorded WNV was in Northern Indiana during the 2002 outbreak (Ward et al., 2004), in Nebraska and Colorado (Salazar et al., 2004), and in Northern California from 2003 onward (Nielsen et al., 2008). WN virus epidemic was also recorded from Canada in 2001 onward, from Saskatchewan in 2002 and from Ontario in 2002 (Epp et al., 2007; Weese et al., 2003, Takasaki, 2007). In Mexico and the Caribbean region, WNV was recorded by Blitvich et al., 2003b; Dupuis et al., 2003, Blitvich et al., 2003c and in Japan from 2005 by Takasaki (2007). For the first time in Cuba, the WNV was detected from four asymptomatic horses and three human encephalitic cases by serologic methods in 2003 and 2004, respectively (Pupo et al. 2006).

In 2003, WNV cases were again diagnosed in equines and humans in France (Mailles et al., 2003). Durand et al. (2002) reported WN virus outbreaks in horses in Southern France in 2000, and out of the seventy-six equine cases, twenty-one horses died. The serological survey of 5,107 samples showed 42% of the IgG-positive animals were positive for IgM, indicating a recent infection. Furthermore, recent serological investigations in birds in Britain suggest that a WN-like virus has been circulating among resident bird populations (Buckley et al., 2003).

CLINICAL SIGNS

WNV infection in horses generally does not result in clinical illness. However, of late, WNV was reported to be associated with an increased proportion of neurological disease in both infected humans (1%) and horses (10%) (Petersen and Roehrig, 2001; Bunning et al., 2002). Except for pyrexia, clinical signs of WNV in horses are almost exclusively of neurological nature reflecting the pathology in the central nervous system (CNS), which occurs predominantly in the spinal cord (Cantile et al., 2000; 2001). A transitory febrile period might occur after infection, although this is not always observed. The spinal cord injury causes ataxia, paresis, or paralysis of the limbs, affecting either the hind limbs or all four limbs, the latter resulting in recumbency. Skin fasciculations, muscle tremors, and muscle rigidity also often accompany these signs. In an outbreak in the United States, some of the horses displayed symptoms of ataxia, dysmetria, phases of somnolence to hyperexcitability or even aggression, hyperesthesia, facial nerve paralysis, paresis of the tongue, and dysphagia, primarily due to damage of the medulla oblongata, thalamus, the reticular formation, cerebellum, and brain cortex and also from deficits in cranial nerves (Ostlund et al., 2000, 2001; Castillo-Olivares and Wood, 2004; Ward, 2006; Long, 2007). Mortality rates of around 38% in USA, 57% in France, and 42% in Italy among the clinically affected horses during different disease outbreaks have been recorded (Cantile et al., 2001; Murgue et al., 2001a; Ostlund et al., 2001). Few horses that suffered from WNV infection may have been required to be euthanized on humane grounds, and 71.2% of the horses were euthanized in Texas outbreak in 2002. The most important symptoms noticed were ataxia (69%), abnormal gait (52%), muscle fasciculations (49%), depression (32%), and recumbency (28%) (Ward et al., 2006). Severe neurological disease in horses does not appear to occur preferentially in old animals as has been the cases with human disease.

PATHOGENESIS AND PATHOLOGY

Following arthropod (mosquito or tick) bite, the virus replicates in local tissues and in regional lymph nodes and reaches the bloodstream via lymphatic vessels. In mice, Langerhans cells of the skin have been shown to play a role for WNV transport to the lymph nodes (Johnston et al., 2000). This virus replication and viremia may result in infection of extraneural tissues, increasing the virus titers in blood and perhaps preceding the invasion of the CNS. Many different mechanisms of neuroinvasion by WNV have been put forward: (1) passive diffusion across the capillary endothelium, (2) virus replication in endothelial cells and budding of virus into the CNS parenchyma, or (3) retroaxonal virus transport of infected neurons of the olfactory epithelium. Because of the low titer and short duration of viremia in horses as opposed to birds and failure to detect WNV antigen in vascular endothelial cells, the first two neuroinvasion pathways are not likely expected (Cantile et al., 2001; Bunning et al., 2002). Many degenerating neurons in WNV-infected hamsters underwent apoptosis, but this was not associated with inflammatory cells. Neurological damage in natural WNV infection of horses has been suggested due to an immunopathological component (Cantile et al., 2001)

Virus strain and the host factors probably decide the outcome of WNV infection. The virus isolated from brain tissue of the 2000 WN virus outbreak in Southern France was closely related to the Morocco 1996 and Italy 1988 isolates from horses, from mosquitoes of the Senegal 1993 and Kenya 1998, and to the human isolate of Volgogard 1999 epidemic. But the isolate from the Southern France in 2000 was different from Israel 1998, New York 1999, and Tunisia 1997 isolates (Murgue et al., 2001b).

WNV pathogenicity is dependent on innate immune responses (Lobigs et al., 2003). The E protein and, to a lesser extent, NS1 and NS2b influence the neurovirulence and neuroinvasiveness of flaviviruses (McMinn, 1997). The WNV outbreaks of increased virulence are caused by lineage 1 strains rather than lineage 2 and are dependent on nucleotide sequences of the genome region encoding the E protein (Lanciotti et al., 1999). Like many other flaviviruses, WNV have been reported to cause persistent infections both in vitro and in vivo, associated with the generation of defective interfering particles, temperature-sensitive mutants, and nonplaquing mutants (Brinton, 1981, 1982, 1983; Brinton et al., 1985; Pogodina et al., 1983; Chen et al., 1996; Lancaster et al., 1998; Xiao et al., 2001; Vlaycheva and Chambers, 2002). Whether persistent infections occur in vivo during WNV infection of horses or these genetic variations represent immune-evasion strategies employed by the virus is not known (Castillo-Olivares and Wood, 2004).

Lesions of WNV infection in the horse are predominantly limited to the CNS, and lesions affecting extraneural tissues are rarely described, which is in contrast with widespread lesions observed in many internal organs of WNV-infected birds (Cantile et al., 2000, 2001; Steele et al., 2000; Cullinane et al., 2006; Long, 2007). WNV causes polioencephalomyelitis in horses, particularly in the lower brain stem and ventral horns of the spinal cord. Lesions include perivascular cuffs of lymphocytes and macrophages with frequent hemorrhages but generally in the absence of viral infection of vessel walls, scattered foci of microgliosis, and in the most severe cases, neuronal degeneration with cytoplasmic swelling and chromatolysis. These lesions are less commonly observed in the cortex of cerebellum and cerebrum.

DIAGNOSIS

Due to the subclinical nature of many WNV infections and the similarity of encephalomyelitis to other equine neurological syndromes, laboratory confirmation directly by identification of the virus or indirectly by testing for antibodies in clinical specimens (postmortem tissues, cerebrospinal fluid, whole blood, or serum) is necessary for the presence of WNV infection.

Diagnosis of WNV in field cases in horses is hampered by the typically short duration and low level of the viremia in horses. Therefore, negative virus detection test results should never be regarded as evidence of absence of WNV. Virus isolation can be attempted from cerebrospinal fluid (CSF), blood or tissues in Vero, RK-13 cells, or mosquito cell lines (Ostlund et al., 2001). The cytopathic effect is not always evident, especially in mosquito cells, and therefore, indirect immunofluorescence using a monoclonal antibody (MAb) of well-defined specificity or detecting viral nucleic acid is necessary to confirm the presence of and/or to identify virus isolates. As diagnostic tools, reverse transcription and nested polymerase chain reaction method have been reported to be sensitive and quite successful in differentiating clinical samples from the suspected cases of WNV encephalitis (Johnson et al., 2001; Ostlund et al., 2001). This method could detect WNV nucleic acid in brain tissues of serologically confirmed cases of WNV encephalitis. Sample for virus isolation should be collected during viremia in early stages.

Routinely used non-nested PCR techniques for diagnosis of infection in man and birds are unsuitable for use in horses due to their relative insensitivity at detecting low titers of virus. Immunocytochemistry on CNS tissues (including cortex, cerebellum, brain stem, and spinal cord) using WN-specific Mab can also be used (Cantile et al., 2001). Antigen-capture ELISA tests have been used to confirm the presence of WNV in avian tissues and mosquito pools (Hunt et al., 2002) but are unsuitable for use in horses due to the low level of viremia.

For flaviviruses, hemagglutination inhibition (HI) and complement fixation tests (CFT) have been widely used for the diagnosis, including JE in horses, and these are available for WNV also; but being laborious, time consuming, slow, and cross-reactive with other flaviviruses, they are not widely used for diagnosis of WNV infection in the horse (Monath and Heinz, 1996; Autorino et al., 2002; Omilabu et al., 1990; OIE, 2000; Ostlund et al., 2000). HI test and CFT were done to diagnose arboviral encephalitis infections in children from Delhi, India. Out of the twelve paired sera tested, eleven pairs were positive. Among the positive, eight showed conversion or fourfold rise in titer for one or more than one group B arboviruses. Out of the eight sera, five cases showed conversion for both with JE and WN antibodies, one case showed conversion only for WN alone, another one case showed conversion for JE alone, and another case for all group B arboviral antigens, indicating that encephalomyelitis due to single infection with JE alone or by WN alone occurred in Delhi, India. Both the HI-positive single sera were also positive for CFT for one or more group of arboviruses suggesting recent infection. Thus, proved WN infection was also there in Delhi during 1973–1974 in children (Suneja et al., 1977). Mathew et al. (1976) also did HI and CFT using the paired sera of patients from group B arbovirus epidemic in Jaipur, India, (1973) and indicated that pyrexia of unknown origin (PUO) was caused by one or more of types of dengue or West Nile viruses.

Even though, the HI and CFT can be valuable in areas free of circulating WNV-related flaviviruses and also have the advantage of being species independent, instead, WNV-specific IgM and IgG-capture ELISA tests and the plaque reduction neutralization test (PRNT) have been preferred for serological diagnosis and surveillance. This test has relevant diagnostic value since WNV-specific IgM appear in the circulation by day 6–7 postinfection and are believed to last less than three months (Bunning et al., 2002; Ostlund et al., 2000). Since IgM cannot cross the hematoencephalic barrier, the presence of IgM in CSF is highly indicative of a recent WNV infection.

Being very sensitive, the ELISA test is particularly valuable for serosurveillance of WNV infection, and virus-specific IgG lasts for at least fifteen months after infection (Murgue et al., 2001; Ostlund et al., 2001; Autorino et al., 2002). A recent infection can be demonstrated by a fourfold increase in antibody titer on paired serum samples collected two weeks apart. IgG—and IgM-based ELISA tests appear sensitive but can cross-react with antibodies against other flaviviruses. An epitope-blocking ELISA test has been developed, which can be used to detect WNV-specific antibodies in serum samples from birds and various mammalian species, including horses (Blitvich et al., 2003b, c). The NS1 protein of WNV has also been used as a diagnostic reagent in antibody-capture ELISA procedures (Jozan et al., 2003). The more specific PRNT has been used successfully as a diagnostic tool for WNV infection in horses (Bunning et al., 2002; Ostlund et al., 2001).

Recently, new tests are used to detect WN virus as well as to differentiate WN virus from JE. Some of them are (1) TaqMan RT-PCR assay for detection and quantification of both lineages of West Nile virus RNA (Tang et al., 2006), (2) the rE MIA (recombinant non structural proteins fluorescent microsphere immunoassay) (Balasuriya et al., 2006), (3) epitope-blocking, enzyme-linked immunoabsorbent assay (Kitai et al., 2007), and (4) polyvalent ELISA and (5) plaque-reduction neutralization test (PRNT) (Magnarelli et al., 2008) to measure serum antibodies to WN virus in horses that were naturally exposed as well as vaccinated against flavivirus in Connecticut and New York, USA. Dauphin and Zientara (2007) have described the recently developed tests for serological survey and virological detection of WN virus in horses, humans, and birds and also the new vaccines developed for WN virus prevention.

DIFFERENTIAL DIAGNOSIS
To have a correct diagnosis, it is helpful to make a careful interpretation of the history, clinical, and laboratory data. WNV infection needs to be differentially diagnosed from JE, alphavirus encephalitides (VEE, WEE, EEE), protozoal meningoencephalitis, EHV-1 myelitis, rabies, and

Borna disease (Castillo-Olivares and Wood, 2004; Cullinane et al., 2006; Long, 2007). Botulism, hypocalcaemia, leukoencephalomalacia, and hepatoencephalopathy may also need to be included in differential diagnosis at some times.

THERAPY

Treatment guidelines for horses with WNV encephalomyelitis can be found in recent publications (Long et al., 2002; Porter et al., 2003). Treatment is aimed at reducing CNS inflammation, preventing self-inflicted injuries, supportive measures, symptomatic therapy, and nutritional care.

PREVENTION AND CONTROL

Strategies for prevention of West Nile encephalitis in endemic areas include vaccination, reduction of virus circulation through measures influencing mosquito populations, and reduction of contact with infected mosquito vectors through altered behavior or management. Vaccination is considered to be effective in preventing development of disease and has been demonstrated to decrease mortality in horses with West Nile encephalitis by approximately two to three times (Steinman et al., 2002; Porter et al., 2003; Salazar et al., et al., 2004; Schuler et al., 2004). Vaccination also prevents viremia in most horses following exposure to WNV-infected horses (Siger et al., 2004). Both whole virus-killed vaccine and recombinant canary pox WNV vaccine are available in North America (Ng et al., 2003; Geiser et al., 2003).

There is a long history of environmental insecticide use in the management of arbovirus outbreaks, particularly in North America, and undoubtedly their use is beneficial during periods of intense challenge. Other effective methods of reducing the local populations of some mosquito species include control of standing water and removal of larval breeding sites. An important area in West Nile prevention is management of horses to prevent exposure to infected mosquitoes. Stabling, particularly at dawn and dusk, in insect-proof stabling may form an inexpensive, safe, and effective means of preventing infection. Normal stabling could be enhanced by the use of insecticides within stables and topical insect repellents, but the efficacy of such measures has not been fully evaluated.

VACCINATION

Protective immunity against various flavivirus infections is associated with both humoral and cellular immune responses and comprise effector mechanisms, namely, cytotoxic T lymphocytes, virus-neutralizing antibody and possibly nonneutralizing antibody responses, and antibody-dependent cell-mediated cytotoxicity (ADCC) ; anti-NS1 antibodies have protective efficacy (Monath and Heinz, 1996). For the prevention of WNV infection in horses, various immunization strategies employing inactivated vaccines, live, attenuated vaccines, genetically modified live vaccines, and DNA vaccines have been devised (Monath, 2001; Ng et al., 2003; Dhama et al., 2008b). Traditionally, inactivated vaccines against flaviviruses have been prepared in mouse brain or tissue culture followed by inactivation with formalin or betapropiolactone.

Most inactivated vaccines do not elicit cellular immunity and rely on the stimulation of strong antibody responses for protection. DNA and live vaccines have the capacity to stimulate adaptive cellular immunity. The potential of DNA vaccination for WNV has been demonstrated in mouse and horse infection models (Chang et al., 2000; Davis et al., 2001).

The strategy of chimeric yellow fever (YF) viruses (YF-17D vaccine strain) expressing WNV antigens has also been used (Monath, 2001; Monath et al., 2001) as has been used for JE and dengue, offering advantages of live vaccines: stimulation of humoral as well as cellular immunity (M and E are targeted by neutralizing antibodies and by CTLs) with a single dose and long-lasting immunological memory, with the added advantage of increased safety. A prototype YF/WNV vaccine has been constructed and shown to be protective against WNV challenge of hamsters (Tesh et al., 2002). This vaccination approach is currently being explored in horses and humans.

Since then, various vaccines were prepared and studied for their efficiency to protect WN virus infection in horses. Minke et al. (2004) prepared an ALVAC (canary pox virus–based recombinant-vCP2017) expressing the prM and E genes derived from a 1999 New York isolate of WNV and assessed its protective efficacy in horses by two experiments. The first study was to evaluate both serum-neutralizing antibody response to WN and duration of immunity. In the second experiment, the onset on protection of the horses was studied. They found that two doses of vCP207 provided both antibody response and an early immunity in horse against WNV viremia. Singer et al. (2004) conducted experiments to determine the onset immunity after IM administration of a single dose of recombinant canary pox virus vaccine against WN virus in horses in a blind challenge trial. They found that the recombinant canary pox virus vaccine provided early protection against viremia after challenge with WNV-infected mosquitoes despite the absence of measurable antibody titers in horses. Later, Long et al. (2007) developed an improved vaccine to get immunogenicity with a single dose of live flavivirus chimera (WN-FV) vaccine, which generates a protective immune response to WNV infection in horse within ten days after a single dose. The immunity lasts for one year. This is an USDA-licensed vaccine for the equine WNV vaccine. ElGarch et al. (2008) also studied whether WN virus recombinant canary pox virus vaccine can produce WNV-specific neutralizing antibodies and cell-mediated immune responses in the horse and showed that the recombinant ALVAC-WNV vaccine produced neutralizing antibodies and prM/E insert-specific IFN-gamma(+)-producing cells against WNV in vaccinated horses. They also showed that both WNV-specific IFN-gamma-producing cells and anti-WVN neutralizing antibody responses are not inhibited by subsequent vaccinations with the same vector vaccine. Very recently, Bonafe et al. (2009) demonstrated that baculovirus-produced WNV envelope protein antigen (rWNV-E) could produce a stable and safe vaccine to protect against WNV infection.

CONCLUSION

West Nile virus (WNV) is a flavivirus responsible for a life-threatening neurological disease (WN encephalitis) in man and horses. The virus has recently reemerged as an important zoonosis, has leaped geographical barriers, and has demonstrated a capacity to spread over an entire continent like the America in a few years, causing illness and deaths in humans and horses. Recent scientific advances have contributed to a better understanding of WNV and the disease it causes, but many aspects about immunity, pathogenesis, and molecular basis of virulence, especially in the horse, are still to be understood properly. Also, revealing the host's feeding preferences of vector species (mosquitoes) involved in the transmission of WNV is critical to the understanding of WNV ecology, which is vital to evolve effective control strategies. The effective means to determine an infection are detection of viral nucleic acid and/or viral-specific immunoglobulin, IgM and/or IgG, and viral culture of CSF and/or serum. The latest improvements in laboratory diagnosis will reveal important epidemiological features of WNV. Preventive and control measures include an effective surveillance system, good management practices, vector control, and vaccination. Effective vaccines are available for horses including inactivated vaccine, DNA vaccine, a chimeric live, attenuated vaccine, and recombinant vaccines. Currently, there is no vaccine for treating WNV infection in humans. Being a mosquito-borne virus, WNV can spread to and colonize new areas. Also, considering the movement and migration of reservoir birds, there is concern that WNV may be introduced into wider arenas. Added to these, globalization and global warming can also have impact on WNV expansion. Coordinated research and networking surveillance program are the need of the hour for this zoonotic pathogen, which has acquired marked attention of the scientific community world over.

REFERENCES

1. Alonso-Padilla, J., Loza-Rubio, E., Escribano-Romero, *E.*, *Córdoba, L., Cuevas,* S., Mejía, F., Calderón, R., Milián, F., Travassos, *D. A., Rosa, A., Weaver, S. C.*, Estrada-Franco, J. G. and Saiz, J. C. 2009. The continuous spread of West Nile virus (WNV): Seroprevalence in asymptomatic horses. *Epidemiol. Infect.* 2009 17:1–6 [Epub ahead of print].

2. Anderson, J. F., Andreadis, T. G., Vossbrinck, C. R., Tirrell S., Wakem, E. M., French, R. A., Garmendia, A. E. and Van Kruiningen, H. J. 1999. Isolation of West Nile virus from mosquitoes, crows, and a Cooper's hawk in Connecticut. *Science* 286:2331–2333.

3. Anonymous. 1999. Outbreak of West Nile-like viral encephalitis–New York. *MMWR Morb. Mortal. Wkly Rep.* 48:845–849.

4. Anonymous. 2003. Provisional surveillance summary of the West Nile virus epidemic–United States, January–November 2002, CDC. *MMWR Morb. Mortal. Wkly Rep.* 52:1160–1160.

5. Asnis, D. S., Conetta, R., Teixeira, A. A., Waldman, G. and Sampson, B. A. 2000. The West Nile virus outbreak of 1999 in New York: The Flushing Hospital experience. *Clin. Infect. Dis.* 30:413–418.

6. Autorino, G. L., Battisti, A., Deubel, V., Ferrari, G., Forletta, R., Giovannini, A., Lelli, R., Murri, S. and Scicluna, M. T. 2002. West Nile virus epidemic in horses, Tuscany region, Italy. *Emerg. Infect. Dis.* 8:1372–1378.

7. Balasurya, U. B., Shi, P. Y., Wong, S. J., Demarest, V. L., Gardner, I. A., Hullinger, P. J., Ferraro, G. L., Boone, J. D., De Cino, C. L., Glaser, A. L. Renshaw, R. W., Ledizet, M., Koski, R. A. and MacLachlan, N. J. 2006. Detection of antibodies to West Nile virus in equine sera using microsphere immunoassay. *J. Vet Diagn Invest.* 18:392–5.

8. Banet-Noach, C., Malkinson, M., Brill, A., Samina, I., Yadin, H., Weisman, Y., Pokamunski, S., King, R., Deubel, V. and Stram, Y. 2003. Phylogenetic relationships of West Nile viruses isolated from birds and horses in Israel from 1997 to 2001. *Virus Genes* 26:135–141.

9. Baqar, S., Hayes, C. G., Murphy, J. R. and Watts, D. M. 1993. Vertical transmission of West Nile virus by *Culex* and *Aedes* mosquitoes. *Am. J. Trop. Med. Hyg.* 48:757–762.

10. Beasley, D. W. and Barrett, A. D. 2002. Identification of neutralizing epitopes within structural domain III of the West Nile virus envelope protein. *J. Virol.* 76:13097–13100.

11. Bernard, K. A. and Kramer, L. D. 2001. West Nile virus activity in the United States, 2001. *Viral Immunol.* 14:319–338.

12. Bernard, K. A., Maffei, J. G., Jones, S. A., Kaufman, E. M., Ebel, G. D., Dupuis, A. P. 2nd, Ngo, K. A., Nicholas, D. C., Young, D. M., Shi, P. Y., Kulasekera, V. L., Eidson, M., White, D. J., Stone, W. B. and Kramer, L. D. 2001. West Nile virus infection in birds and mosquitoes, New York State, 2000. *Emerg. Infect. Dis.* 7:679–685.

13. Berthet, F. X., Zeller, H. G., Drouet, M. T., Rauzier, J., Digoutte, J. P. and Deubel V. 1997. Extensive nucleotide changes and deletions within the envelope glycoprotein gene of Euro-African West Nile viruses. *J. Gen. Virol.* 78:2293–2297.

14. Bonafé, N., Rininger, J. A., Chubet, R. G., Foellmer, H. G., Fader, S., Anderson, J. F., Bushmich, S. L., Anthony, K., Ledizet, M., Fikrig, E., Koski, R. A. and Kaplan, P. 2009. A recombinant West Nile virus envelope protein vaccine candidate produced in Spodoptera frugiperda expresSF+ cells. *Vaccine* 27:213–222.

15. Bricaire, F. and Bossi, P. 2006. Emerging viral diseases. *Bull. Acad. Natl. Med.* 190:597–608.

16. Blitvich, B. J., Marlenee, N. L., Hall, R. A., Calisher, C. H., Bowen, R. A., Roehrig, J. T., Komar, N., Langevin, S. A. and Beaty, B. J. 2003a. Epitope-blocking enzyme-linked immunosorbent assays for the detection of serum antibodies to West Nile virus in multiple avian species. *J. Clin. Microbiol.* 41:1041–1047.

20. WEST NILE VIRUS INFECTION OF HORSES

17. Blitvich, B. J., Bowen, R. A., Marlenee, N. L., Hall, R. A., Bunning, M. L. and Beaty, B. J. 2003b. Epitope blocking enzyme-linked immunosorbent assays for detection of West Nile virus antibodies in domestic mammals. *J. Clin. Microbiol.* 41:2676–2679.

18. Blitvich, B. J., Fernandez-Salas, I., Contreras-Cordero, J. F., Marlenee, N. L., Gonzalez-Rojas, J. I., Komar, N., Gubler, D. J., Calisher, C. H. and Beaty, B. J. 2003c. Serologic evidence of West Nile virus infection in horses, Coahuila State, Mexico. *Emerg. Infect. Dis.* 9;853–856.

19. Blitvich, B. J. 2008. Transmission dynamics and changing epidemiology of West Nile virus. *Anim. Health Res. Rev.* 9:71–86.

20. Brinton, M. A. 1981. Isolation of a replication-efficient mutant of West Nile virus from a persistently infected genetically resistant mouse cell culture. *J. Virol.* 39:413–421.

21. Brinton, M. A. 1982. Characterization of West Nile virus persistent infections in genetically resistant and susceptible mouse cells. I. Generation of defective nonplaquing virus particles. *Virology* 116:84–98.

22. Brinton, M. A. 1983. Analysis of extracellular West Nile virus particles produced by cell cultures from genetically resistant and susceptible mice indicates enhanced amplification of defective interfering particles by resistant cultures. *J. Virol.* 46:860–870.

23. Brinton, M. A. 2002. The molecular biology of West Nile virus: A new invader of the Western Hemisphere. *Annu. Rev. Microbiol.* 56:371–402.

24. Brinton, M. A., Davis, J. and Schaefer, D. 1985. Characterization of West Nile virus persistent infections in genetically resistant and susceptible mouse cells. II. Generation of temperature sensitive mutants. *Virology* 140:152–158.

25. Buckley, A., Dawson, A., Moss, S. R., Hinsley, S. A., Bellamy, P. E. and Gould, E. A. 2003. Serological evidence of West Nile virus, Usutu virus and Sindbis virus infection of birds in the UK. *J. Gen. Virol.* 84:2807–2817.

26. Bunning, M. L., Bowen, R. A., Cropp, C. B., Sullivan, K. G., Davis, B. S., Komar, N., Godsey, M. S., Baker, D., Hettler, D. L., Holmes, D. A., Biggerstaff, B. J. and Mitchell, C. J. 2002 Experimental infection of horses with West Nile virus. *Emerg. Infect. Dis.* 8:380–386.

27. Cantile, C., Di Guardo, G., Eleni, C. and Arispici, M. 2000. Clinical and neuropathological features of West Nile virus equine encephalomyelitis in Italy. *Equine Vet. J.* 32:31–35.

28. Cantile C., Del Piero F. and Di Guardo G. 2001. Arispici M., Pathologic and immunohistochemical findings in naturally occuring West Nile virus infection in horses. *Vet. Pathol.* 38:414–421.

29. Castillo-Olivares J. and Wood, J. 2004. West Nile virus infection of horses. *Vet. Res.* 35:467–483.

30. Chang, G. J., Hunt, A. R. and Davis, B. 2000. A single intramuscular injection of recombinant plasmid DNA induces protective immunity and prevents Japanese encephalitis in mice. *J. Virol.* 74:4244–4252.

31. Chen, L. K., Liao, C. L., Lin, C. G., Lai, S. C., Liu, C. I., Ma, S. H., Huang, Y. Y. and Lin, Y. L. 1996. Persistence of Japanese encephalitis virus is associated with abnormal expression of the nonstructural protein NS1 in host cells. *Virology* 217:220–229.

32. Chowers, M. Y., Lang, R., Nassar, F., Ben-David, D., Giladi, M., Rubinshtein, E., Itzhaki, A., Mishal, J., Siegman-Igra, Y., Kitzes, R., Pick, N., Landau, Z., Wolf, D., Bin, H., Mendelson, E., Pitlik, S. D. and Weinberger, M. 2001. Clinical characteristics of the West Nile fever outbreak, Israel, 2000. *Emerg. Infect. Dis.* 7:675–678.

33. Cornel, A. J., Jupp, P. G. and Blackburn, N. K. 1993. Environmental temperature on the vector competence of *Culex univittatus* (Diptera: culicidae) for West Nile virus. *J. Med. Entomol.* 30:449–456.

34. Cullinane, A. A., Barr, B., Bernard, W., Duncan, J. L., Mulcahy, G., Smith, M. and Timoney, J. E. 2006. Infectious diseases (Chapter 1): Togaviral and flaviviral encephalitides. In *The equine manual*, 2nd ed., A. J. Higgins and J. R. Snyder, 37–44. USA: Saunder, Elsevier Ltd.

35. Davis, B. S., Chang, G. J., Cropp, B., Roehrig, J. T., Martin, D. A., Mitchell, C. J., Bowen, R. and Bunning, M. L. 2001. West Nile virus recombinant DNA vaccine protects mouse and horse from virus challenge and expresses in vitro a noninfectious recombinant antigen that can be used in enzyme-linked immunosorbent assays. *J. Virol.* 75:4040–4047.

36. Dauphin, G. and Zientara, S. 2007. West Nile virus: Recent trends in diagnosis and vaccine development. *Vaccine* 25:5563–76.

37. Centers for Disease Control and Prevention (CDC). 2008. West Nile virus activity—United States, 2007. *MMWR Morb. Mortal. Wkly Rep.* **57**:720–723.

38. Despres, P., Frenkiel, M. P. and Deubel, V., 1993. Differences between cell membrane fusion activities of two dengue type-1 isolates reflect modifications of viral structure. *Virology* 196:209–219.

39. Deubel, V., Fiette, L., Gounon, P., Drouet, M. T., Khun, H., Huerre, M., Banet, C., Malkinson, M. and Despres, P. 2001. Variations in biological features of West Nile viruses. *Ann. N.Y. Acad. Sci.* 951:195–206.

40. Dhama, K., Mahendran, M. and Tomar, S. 2008a. Pathogens transmitted by migratory birds: Threat perceptions to poultry health and production. *Int. J. Poult. Sci.* 7:516–525.

41. Dhama, K., Mahendran, M., Gupta, P. K. and Rai, A. 2008b. DNA vaccines and their applications in veterinary practice: Current perspectives. *Vet. Res. Commun.* 32:341–356.

42. Dupuis, A. P. 2nd, Marra, P. P. and Kramer, L. D. 2003. Serologic evidence of West Nile virus transmission, Jamaica, West Indies. *Emerg. Infect. Dis.* 9:860–863.

43. Durand, B., Chevalier, V., Pouillot, R., Labie, J., Marendat, I. Murgue, B., Zeller, H. and Zientara, S. 2002. West Nile virus outbreak in horses, Southern France, 2000: Result of a serosurvey. *Emerg Infect Dis.* 8:777–82.

44. Durand, J. P., Simon, F. and Tolou, H. 2004. West Nile virus: In France again, in humans and horses. *Rev. Prat.* 54:703–710.

45. Eidson, M., Komar, N., Sorhage, F., Nelson, R., Talbot, T., Mostashari, F. and McLean, R. 2001. Crow deaths as a sentinel surveillance system for West Nile virus in the Northeastern United States, 1999. *Emerg. Infect. Dis.* 7:615–620.

46. El Garch, H., Minke, J. M., Rehder, J., Richard, S., Edlund Toulenmonde, C., Dinic, S., Andreoni, C., Audonnet, J. C., Nordgren, R. and Juillard, V. 2008. *Vet Immunol. Immunopathol* 123:230–239.

47. Epp, T., Waldner, C., Corrigan, R. and Curry, P. 2007. Public health use of surveillance for West Nile virus in horses, Saskatchewan, 2003–2005. *Vet Res.* 38:109–116.

48. Falconar, A. K. and Young, P. R. 1991. Production of dimer-specific and dengue virus group crossreactive mouse monoclonal antibodies to the dengue 2 virus non-structural glycoprotein NS1. *J. Gen. Virol.* 72:961–965.

49. Garavelli, P. L. and Peduzzi, P. 2006. Globalization and infectious diseases. *Recenti. Prog. Med.* 97:528–532.

50. Geiser, S., Seitzinger, A., Salazar, P., Traub-Dargatz, J., Morley, P., Salman, M., Wilmont, D., Steffen, D. and Cunningham, W. 2003. Economic impact of West Nile virus on the Colorado and Nebraska equine industries: 2002, United States Department of Agriculture. *Animal and Plant Health Inspection Services: Veterinary Services Info Sheet* N394.0403, 2003.

51. Georges, A. J., Matton, T. and Courbot-Georges, M. C. 2004. Monkey-pox, a model of emergent then reemergent disease. *Med. Mal. Infect.* 34:12–19.

52. Heinz, F. X., Purcell, R. H., Gould, E. A., Howard, C. R., Houghton, M., Moormann, R. J. M., Rice, C. M. and Thiel, H. J. 1999. Family: Flaviviridae. In *Virus taxonomy: 7th report of the International Committee on Taxonomy of Viruses*, ed. M. H. V. Van Regenmortel, D. H. L. Bishop, E. B. Carstens, M. K. Estes, S. M. Lemon, J. Maniloff, M. A. Mayo, D. J. McGeoch, C. R. Pringle, and R. B. Wickner, 859–878. San Diego: Academic Press.

53. Hubalek, Z. and Halouzka, J. 1999. West Nile fever: A reemerging mosquito-borne viral disease in Europe. *Emerg. Infect. Dis.* 5:643–650.

54. Hunt, A. R., Hall, R. A., Kerst, A. J., Nasci, R. S., Savage, H. M., Panella, N. A., Gottfried, K. L., Burkhalter, K. L. and Roehrig, J. T. 2002. Detection of West Nile virus antigen in mosquitoes and avian tissues by a monoclonal antibody-based capture enzyme immunoassay. *J. Clin. Microbiol.* 40:2023–2030.

55. Johnston, L. J., Halliday, G. M. and King, N. J. 2000. Langerhans cells migrate to local lymph nodes following cutaneous infection with an arbovirus. *J. Invest. Dermatol.* 114:560–568.

56. Johnson, D. J., Ostlund, E. N., Pedersen, D. D. and Schmitt, B. J. 2001. Detection of North American West Nile virus in animal tissue by a reverse transcription-nested polymerase chain reaction assay. *Emerg. Infect. Dis.* 7:739–741.

57. Joubert, L., Oudar, J., Hannoun, C., Beytout, D., Corniou, B., Guillon, J. C. and Panthier, R. 1970. Epidemiology of the West Nile virus: Study of a focus in Camargue. IV. Meningo-encephalomyelitis of the horse. *Ann. Inst. Pasteur* (Paris) 118:239–247.

58. Jozan, M., Evans, R., McLean, R., Hall, R., Tangredi, B., Reed, L. and Scott, J. 2003. Detection of West Nile virus infection in birds in the United States by blocking ELISA and immunohistochemistry. *Vector Borne Zoonotic Dis.* 3:99–110.

59. Jupp, P. G. 2001. The ecology of West Nile virus in South Africa and the occurrence of outbreaks in humans. *Ann. N.Y. Acad. Sci.* 951:143–152.

60. Kaufman, B. M., Summers, P. L., Dubois, D. R., Cohen, W. H., Gentry, M. K., Timchak, R. L., Burke, D. S. and Eckels, K. H. 1989. Monoclonal antibodies for dengue virus prM glycoprotein protect mice against lethal dengue infection. *Am. J. Trop. Med. Hyg.* 41:576–580.

61. Kitai, Y., Shoda, M., Kondo, T. and Konishi, E. 2007. Epitope-blocking enzyme-linked immunosorbent assay to differentiate West Nile virus from Japanese encephalitis virus infection in equine sera. *Clin Vaccine Immunol.* 8:1024–31.

62. Klinkhamer, K. and Lipman, L. J. 2008. Introduction of West Nile virus in the Netherlands. *Tijdschr Diergeneeskd.* 133:106–107.

63. Komar, N. 2000. West Nile viral encephalitis. *Rev. Sci. Tech.* 19:166–176.

64. Komar, N., Davis, B., Bunning, M. L. and Hettler, D. L. 2000. Experimental infection of wild birds with West Nile virus (New York 1999 strain). *Am. J. Trop. Med. Hyg.* 62:229–230.

65. Komar, N., Lanciotti, R. S., Bowen, R., Langevin, S. and Bunning, M. L. 2002. Detection of West Nile virus in oral and cloacal swabs collected from bird carcasses. *Emerg. Infect. Dis.* 8:741–742.

66. Kramer, L. D., Styer, L. M. and Ebel, G. D. 2008. A global perspective on the epidemiology of West Nile virus. *Annu. Rev. Entomol.* 53:61–81.

67. Lancaster, M. U., Hodgetts, S. I., Mackenzie, J. S. and Urosevic, N. 1998. Characterization of defective viral RNA produced during persistent infection of Vero cells with Murray Valley encephalitis virus. *J. Virol.* 72:2474–2482.

68. Lanciotti, R. S., Roehrig, J. T., Deubel, V., Smith, J., Parker, M., Steele, K., Crise B., Volpe, K. E., Crabtree, M. B., Scherret, J. H., Hall, R. A., Mac-Kenzie, J. S., Cropp, C. B., Panigrahy, B., Ostlund, E., Schmitt, B., Malkinson, M., Banet, C., Weissman, J., Komar, N., Savage, H. M., Stone, W., McNamara, T. and Gubler, D. J. 1999. Origin of the West Nile virus responsible for an outbreak of encephalitis in the northeastern United States. *Science* 286:2333–2337.

69. Le Guenno, B., Bougermouh, A., Azzam, T. and Bouakaz, R. 1996. West Nile: A deadly virus? *Lancet* 348:1315.

70. Lobigs, M., Mullbacher, A., Wang, Y., Pavy, M. and Lee, E. 2003. Role of type I and type II interferon responses in recovery from infection with an encephalitic flavivirus. *J. Gen. Virol.* 84:567–572.

71. Long, M. T. 2007. Flavivirus infections. In *Equine infectious diseases*, ed. D. C. Sellon and M. T. Long, chapter 21, 198–206. Philadelphia, USA: Saunders, Elsevier Inc.

72. Long, M. T., Ostlund, E. N., Porter, M. B. and Crom, R. L. 2002. Equine West Nile encephalitis: Epidemiological and clinical review for practitioners. *AAEP Proceedings* 48:1–6.

73. Long, M. T., Gibbs, E. P., Mellencamp, M. W., Bowen, R. A., Seino, K. K., Zhang, S., Beachboard, S. E. and Humphrey, P. P. 2007. Efficacy, duration and onset of immunogenecity of a West Nile virus vaccine, live flavivirus chimera, in horses with a clinical disease challenge model. *Equine Vet J.* 39:491–497.

74. Lvov, D. K., Butenko, A. M., Gromashevsky, V. L., Kovtunov, A. I., Prilipov, A. G., Kinney, R., Aristova, V. A., Dzharkenov, A. F., Samokhvalov, E. I., Savage, H. M., Shchelkanov, M. Y., Galkina, I. V., Deryabin,

P. G., Gubler, D. J., Kulikova, L. N., Alkhovsky, S. K., Moskvina, T. M., Zlobina, L. V., Sadykova, G. K., Shatalov, A. G., Lvov, D. N., Usachev, V. E., Voronina, A. G. 2004. West Nile virus and other zoonotic viruses in Russia: Examples of emerging-reemerging situations. *Arch Virol Suppl.* 18:85–96.

75. Lustig, S., Olshevsky, U., Ben-Nathan, D., Lachmi, B. E., Malkinson, M., Kobiler, D. and Halevy, M. 2000. A live attenuated West Nile virus strain as a potential veterinary vaccine. *Viral Immunol.* 13:401–410.

76. Mackenzie, J. S., Gubler, D. J. and Petersen, L. R. 2004. Emerging flaviviruses: The spread and resurgence of Japanese encephalitis, West Nile and dengue viruses. *Nat. Med.* 10:S98–109.

77. Mailles, A., Zeller, H., Durand, J. P., Zientara, S., Goffette, R., Gloaguen, C., Armengaud, A., Schaffner, F., Hars, J., Chodorge, E. and Barbat, J. 2003. Human and equine West Nile virus infections in France, August–September 2003. *Eurosurveillance Weekly Archives 43 (October 23, 2003):* 7.

78. Malkinson, M., Banet, C., Weisman, Y., Pokamunski, S., King, R., Drouet, M. T. and Deubel, V. 2002. Introduction of West Nile virus in the Middle East by migrating white storks. *Emerg. Infect. Dis.* 8:392–397.

79. Magnarelli, L. A., Busmich, S. L., Anderson, J. E., Ledizet, M. and Koski, R. A. 2008. Serum antibodies to West Nile virus in naturally exposed and vaccinated horses. *J. Med Microbiol.* 57:1087–93.

80. Mathew, T., Suri, N. K., Bhola, S. R., Suri, J. C., Arora, R. R. and Lahiri, S. K. 1976. Serological investigation of an epidemic of fever by group B arboviruses in Jaipur 1973. *Indian J. Med. Res.* 64:1136–1142.

81. Mayr, A. 2003. Smallpox vaccination and bioterrorism with pox viruses. *Comp. Immunol. Microbiol. Infect. Dis.* 26:423–430.

82. McIntosh, B. M., Dickinson, D. B. and McGillivray, G. M. 1969. Ecological studies on Sindbis and West Nile viruses in South Africa. V. The response of birds to inoculation of virus. *S. Afr. J. Med. Sci.* 34:77–82.

83. McMinn, P. C. 1997. The molecular basis of virulence of the encephalitogenic flaviviruses. *J. Gen. Virol.* 78:2711–2722.

84. Miller, B. R., Nasci, R. S., Godsey, M. S., Savage, H. M., Lutwama, J. J., Lanciotti, R. S. and Peters, C. J. 2000. First field evidence for natural vertical transmission of West Nile virus in *Culex univittatus* complex mosquitoes from Rift Valley Province, Kenya. *Am. J. Trop. Med. Hyg.* 62:240–246.

85. Minke, J. M., Sige, L., Karaca, K., Austgen, L., Gordy, P., Bowen, R., Renshaw, R. W., Loosmore, S., Audonnet, J. C. and Nordgren, B. 2004. Recombinant canary poxvirus vaccine carrying the prM/E genes of West Nile virus protects horses against a West Nile virus-mosquito challenge. *Arch Virol Suppl.* 18:221–30.

86. Monath, T. P. 2001. Prospects for development of a vaccine against the West Nile virus. *Ann. N.Y. Acad. Sci.* 951:1–12.

87. Monath, T. P. and Heinz, F. X. 1996. Flaviviruses. In *Fields virology*, vol. 1, ed. B. N. Fields and P. M. Howley, 961–1034. Philadelphia: Lippincott-Raven Publishers.

88. Monath, T. P., Arroyo, J., Miller, C. and Guirakhoo, F. 2001. West Nile virus vaccine. *Current Drug Targets: Infectious Disorders1* 1 (May 2001): 37–50.

89. Murgue, B., Murri, S., Zientara, S., Durand, B., Durand, J. P. and Zeller, H. 2001a. West Nile outbreak in horses in southern France, 2000: The return after 35 years. *Emerg. Infect. Dis.* 7:692–696.

90. Muruge, B., Murris, S., Trki, H., Deubel, V. and Zeller, H. G. 2001b. West Nile in the Mediterranean basin: 1950–2000. *Ann NY Acad Sci.* 951:117–26.

91. Murgue, B., Zeller, H. and Deubel, V. 2002. The ecology and epidemiology of West Nile virus in Africa, Europe and Asia. *Curr. Top. Microbiol. Immunol.* 267:195–221.

92. Nasci, R. S., Savage, H. M., White, D. J., Miller, J. R., Cropp, B. C., Godsey, M. S., Kerst, A. J., Bennett, P., Gottfried, K. L. and Lanciotti, R. S. 2001. West Nile virus in overwintering *Culex* mosquitoes, New York City, 2000. *Emerg. Infect. Dis.* 7:1–3.

93. Ndiva, M. M., Hearne, R., Dyer, N. W. and Khaitsa, M. L. 2008. The economic impact of West Nile virus infection in horses in the North Dakota equine industry in 2002. *Trop Anim. Health Prod.* 40:69–76.

94. Nielsen, C. F., Reisen, W. K., Armijos, M. V., Maclachan, N. J. and Scott, T. W. 2008. High sub-clinical West Nile virus incidence among nonvaccinated horses in northern California associated with low vector abundance and infection. *Am. J. Trop. Med. Hyg.* 78:45–52.

95. Ng, T., Hathaway, D., Jennings, N., Champ, D., Chiang, Y. W. and Chu, H. J. 2003. Equine vaccine for West Nile virus. *Dev. Biol.* (Basel) 114:221–227.

96. Nur, Y. A., Groen, J., Heuvelmans, H., Tuynman, W., Copra, C. and Osterhaus, A. D. 1999. An outbreak of West Nile fever among migrants in Kisangani, Democratic Republic of Congo. *Am. J. Trop. Med. Hyg.* 61:885–888.

97. OIE (Office International des Epizooties). 1999. West Nile fever in Israel in geese. *OIE Dis. Info.* 12:166.

98. OIE (Office International des Epizooties). 2000 In Manual 2000.

99. Omilabu, S. A., Olaleye, O. D., Aina, Y. and Fagbami, A. H. 1990. West Nile complement fixing antibodies in Nigerian domestic animals and humans. *J. Hyg. Epidemiol. Microbiol. Immunol.* 34:357–363.

100. Ostlund, E. N., Andresen, J. E. and Andresen, M. 2000. West Nile encephalitis. *Vet. Clin. North Am. Equine Pract.* 16:427–441.

101. Ostlund, E. N., Crom, R. L., Pedersen, D. D., Johnson, D. J., Williams, W. O. and Schmitt, B. J. 2001. Equine West Nile encephalitis, United States. *Emerg. Infect. Dis.* 7:665–669.

102. Petersen, L. R. and Roehrig, J. T. 2001. West Nile virus: A reemerging global pathogen. *Emerg. Infect. Dis.* 7:611–614.

103. Platonov, A. E., Shipulin, G. A., Shipulina, O. Y., Tyutyunnik, E. N., Frolochkina, T. I., Lanciotti, R. S., Yazyshina, S., Platonova, O. V., Obukhov, I. L., Zhukov, A. N., Vengerov, Y. Y. and Pokrovskii, V. I. 2001. Outbreak of West Nile virus infection, Volgograd Region, Russia, 1999. *Emerg Infect. Dis.* 7:128–132.

104. Pogodina, V. V., Frolova, M. P., Malenko, G. V., Fokina, G. I., Koreshkova, G. V., Kiseleva, L. L., Bochkova, N. G. and Ralph, N. M. 1983. Study on West Nile virus persistence in monkeys. *Arch. Virol.* 75:71–86.

105. Porter, M. B., Long, M. T., Getman, L. M., Giguere, S., MacKay, R. J., Lester, G. D., Alleman, A. R., Wamsley, H. L., Franklin, R. P., Jacks, S., Buergelt, C. D. and Detrisac, C. J. 2003. West Nile virus encephalomyelitis in horses: 46 cases. *J. Am. Vet. Med. Assoc.* 222:1241–1247.

106. Pupo, M., Guzman, M. G., Fernandez, R., Llop, A., Dickinson, F. O., Perez, D., Cruz, R., Gonzalez, T., Estevez, G., Gonzalez, H., Santos, P., Kouri, G., Andonova, M., Lindsay, R., Artsob, H. and Drebot, M. 2006. West Nile virus infection in humans and horses, Cuba. *Emerg Infect Dis.* 12:1022–1024.

107. Rappole, J. H. and Hubalek, Z. 2000. Migratory birds and West Nile virus. *J. Appl. Microbiol.* 94:47–58.

108. Rappole, J. H., Derrickson, S. R. and Hubalek, Z. 2000. Migratory birds and spread of West Nile virus in the Western Hemisphere. *Emerg. Infect Dis.* 6:319–328.

109. Rappole, J. H., Reed, K. D., Meece, J. K., Henkel, J. S. and Shukla, S. K. 2003. Birds, migration and emerging zoonoses: West Nile fever, lyme disease, influenza A and enteropathogens. *Clin. Med. Res.* 1:5–12.

110. Roehring, J. T., Layton, M., Smith, P., Cambell, G. L., Nasci, R. and Lanciotti, R. S. 2002. The emergence of West Nile virus in North America: Ecology, epidemiology and survelliance. *Curr. Top. Microbiol. Immunol.* 267:223–240.

111. Rudolf, I., Hubálek, Z., Sikutová, S. and Svec, P. 2008. Neglected arthropod-borne viral infections in the Czech Republic. *Epidemiol. Mikrobiol. Imunol.* 57:80–89.

112. Salazar, P. J. Traub-Dargatz, L., Morley, P. S., Wilmont, D. D., Steffen, D. J., Cunningham, W. E. and Salman, M. D. 2004. Outcome of equids with clinical signs of West Nile virus infection and factors associated with death. *J. Am Vet. Med. Assoc.* 225:267–74.

113. Savage, H. M., Ceianu, C., Nicolescu, G., Karabatsos, N., Lanciotti, R., Vladimirescu, A., Laiv, L., Ungureanu, A., Romanca, C. and Tsai, T. F. 1999. Entomologic and avian investigations of an epidemic of West Nile fever in Romania in 1996, with serologic and molecular characterization of a virus isolate from mosquitoes. *Am. J. Trop. Med. Hyg.* 61:600–611.

114. Schmidt, J. R. and Elmansoury, H. K., 1963 Natural and experimental infection of Egyptian equines with West Nile virus. *Ann. Trop. Med. Parasitol.* 57:415–427.

115. Schuler, L. A., Khaitsa, M. L., Dyer, N. W. and Stoltenow, C. L. 2004. Evaluation of an outbreak of West Nile virus infection in horses: 569 cases, 2002. *J. Am Vet Med. Assoc.* 225:1084–89.

116. Sejvar, J. J. 2007. The long term outcomes of human West Nile virus infection. *Clin Infect Dis.* 44:1617.

117. Siger, L., Bowen, R. A., Karaca, K. Murray, M. J., Gordy, P. W., Losmore, S. M., Audonnet, J. C., Nordgren, R. M. and Minke, J. M. 2004. Assessment of the efficacy of a single dose of a recombinant vaccine against West Nile virus in response to natural challenge with West Nile virus-infected mosquitoes in horses. *Am J Vet. Res.* 65:1459–62.

118. Smithburn, K. C., Hughes, T. P., Burke, A. W. and Paul, J. H. 1940. A neurotropic virus isolated from the blood of a native of Uganda. *Am. J. Trop. Med.* 20:471–492.

119. Steele, K. E., Linn, M. J., Schoepp, R. J., Komar, N., Geisbert, T. W., Manduca, R. M., Calle, P. P., Raphael, B. L., Clippinger, T. L., Larsen, T., Smith, J., Lanciotti, R. S., Panella, N. A. and McNamara, T. S. 2000. Pathology of fatal West Nile virus infections in native and exotic birds during the 1999 outbreak in New York City, New York. *Vet. Pathol.* 37:208–224.

120. Steinman, A., Banet, C., Sutton, G. A., Yadin, H., Hadar, S. and Brill, A. 2002. Clinical signs of West Nile virus encephalomyelitis in horses during the outbreak in Israel in 2000. *Vet. Rec.* 151:47–49.

121. Suneja, R. K., Radha, S., Mathew, T., Suri, J. C., Suri, N. K. and Bhola, S. R. 1977. Clinico-laboratory study of arbovirus encephalitis in children from Delhi, India. Presented the II international seminar on zoonosis and its control. 16-6-77, Delhi.

122. Tan, C. H., Yap, E. H., Singh, M., Deubel, V. and Chan, Y. C. 1990. Passive protection studies in mice with monoclonal antibodies directed against the non-structural protein NS3 of dengue 1 virus. *J. Gen. Virol.* 71:745–749.

123. Tang, Y., Annie Hapip, C., Liu B. and Fang, C. T. 2006. Highly sensitive TaqMan RT-PCR assay for detection and quantification of both lineages of West Nile virus RNA. *J Clin Virol.* 200636177–82.

124. Takasaki, T. 2007. West Nile fever/encephalitis. *Uirusu.* 57:199–205.

125. Taylor, R. M., Work, T. H., Hurlbut, H. S. and Rizk, F. 1956. A study of the ecology of West Nile virus in Egypt. *Am. J. Trop. Med. Hyg.* 5:579–620.

126. Tber-Aldelhaq, A. 1996. West Nile fever in horses in Morocco. *Bull. OIE* 11:867–869.

127. Tesh, R. B., Arroyo, J., Travassos Da Rosa, A. P., Guzman, H., Xiao, S. Y. and Monath, T. P. 2002. Efficacy of killed virus vaccine, live attenuated chimeric virus vaccine, and passive immunization for prevention of West Nile virus encephalitis in hamster model. *Emerg. Infect. Dis.* 8:1392–1397.

128. Triki, H., Murri, S., Le Guenno, B., Bahri, O., Hili, K., Sidhom, M. and Dellagi, K. 2001. West Nile viral meningo-encephalitis in Tunisia. *Med. Trop.* (Madr.) 61:487–490.

129. Trock, S. C., Meade, B. J., Glaser, A. L., Ostlund, E. N., Lanciotti, R. S., Cropp, B. C., Kulasekera, V., Kramer, L. D. and Komar, N. 2001. West Nile virus outbreak among horses in New York State, 1999 and 2000. *Emerg. Infect. Dis.* 7:745–747.

130. Tsai, T. F., Popovici, F., Cernescu, C., Campbell, G. L. and Nedelcu, N. I. 1998. West Nile encephalitis epidemic in southeastern Romania. *Lancet* 352:767–771.

131. Turrell, M. J., O'Guinn, M., Dohm, D. J. and Jones, J. W. 2001. Vector competence of North American mosquitoes (Diptera: Culicidae) for West Nile virus. *J. Med. Entomol.* 38:130–134.

132. Vlaycheva, L. A. and Chambers, T. J. 2002. Neuroblastoma cell-adapted yellow fever 17D virus: Characterization of a viral variant associated with persistent infection and decreased virus spread. *J. Virol.* 76:6172–6184.

133. Ward, M. P., Levy, M., Thacker, H. L. Ash, M., Norman, S. K., Moore, G. E. and Web, P. W. 2004. Investigation of an outbreak of encephalomyelitis caused by West Nile virus in 136 horses. *J. Am. Vet. Med Assoc.* 225:84–89.

134. Ward, M. P. 2006. Spread of equine West Nile virus encephalomyelitis during the 2002 Texas epidemic. *Am J. Trop. Med. Hyg.* 74:1090–95.

135. Ward, M. P., Schuermann, J. A., HighField, L. D. and Murray, K. O. 2006. Characteristics of an outbreak of West Nile virus encephalomyelitis in a previously uninfected population of horses. *Vet Microbiol.* 118:255–9.

136. Weese, J. S., Baird, J. D., DeLay, J., Kenney, D. G., Staempfli, H. R., Viel, L., Parent, J., Smith-Maxie, L. and Poma, R. 2003. West Nile virus encephalomyelitis in horses in Ontario: 28 cases. *Can. Vet. J.* 44:469–473.

137. Weinberger, M., Pitlik, S. D., Gandacu, D., Lang, R., Nassar, F., Ben David, D., Rubinstein, E., Izthaki, A., Mishal, J., Kitzes, R., Siegman-Igra, Y., Giladi, M., Pick, N., Mendelson, E., Bin, H. and Shohat, T. 2001. West Nile fever outbreak, Israel, 2000: Epidemiologic aspects. *Emerg. Infect. Dis.* 7:686–691.

138. Weiss, D., Carr, D., Kellachan, J., Tan, C., Phillips, M., Bresnitz, E. and Layton, M. 2001. Clinical findings of West Nile virus infection in hospitalized patients, New York and New Jersey, 2000. *Emerg. Infect. Dis.* 7:654–658.

139. Westaway, E. G., Mackenzie, J. M., Kenney, M. T., Jones, M. K. and Khromykh, A. A. 1997. Ultrastructure of Kunjin virus-infected cells: Colocalization of NS1 and NS3 with double-stranded RNA, and of NS2B with NS3, in virus induced membrane structures. *J. Virol.* 71:6650–6661.

140. Wong, S. J., Boyle, R. H., Demarest, V. L., Woodmansee, A. N., Kramer, L. D., Li, H., Drebot, M., Koski, R. A., Fikrig, E., Martin, D. A. and Shi, P. Y. 2003. Immunoassay targeting nonstructural protein 5 to differentiate West Nile virus infection from dengue and St. Louis encephalitis virus infections and from flavivirus vaccination. *J. Clin. Microbiol.* 41:4217–4223.

141. Work, T. H., Hurlbut, H. S. and Taylor, R. M. 1955. Indigenous wild birds of the Nile Delta as potential West Nile virus circulating reservoirs. *Am. J. Trop. Med. Hyg.* 4:872–888.

142. Xiao, S. Y., Guzman, H., Zhang, H., Travassos da Rosa, A. P. and Tesh, R. B. 2001. West Nile virus infection in the golden hamster (*Mesocricetus auratus*): A model for West Nile encephalitis. *Emerg. Infect. Dis.* 7:714–721.

SECTION B

LIST OF BOVINE AND OVINE TROPICAL VIRAL DISEASES

1. BLUE TONGUE
(Sore Mouth, Sore Muzzle, Ovine Catarrhal Fever, Pseudofoot-and-Mouth Disease)

M. R. SASEENDRANATH, M. KRISHNAN NAIR, Z. MATHEW, AND THANKAM MATHEW

INTRODUCTION

Bluetongue (BT) is an arthropod-borne virus disease of ruminants, primarily of sheep and less frequently of cattle, goats, buffalo, deer, dromedaries, and antelope, transmitted by the *Culicoides* midges, characterized by fever; edema of face, ears, and nose; erosion of buccal mucous membrane; hyperemia of coronary band; sensitivity of the lamina of the hoof; respiratory distress; and marked cachexia.

ETIOLOGY

Bluetongue virus (BTV) is an *orbivirus* in the family Reoviridae. So far twenty-five serotypes of BTV have been isolated worldwide (Radostits et al., 2000), which are designated as BLU 1–BLU 25.

Bluetongue virus is complex nonenveloped virus with seven structural proteins and an RNA genome with an icosahedral-shaped particle consisting of ten double-stranded(ds) RNA segments of different sizes, encapsulated in a double-layered protein coat. Removal of the outer protein layer activates a viral-associated RNA polymerase that transcribes the ten genome segments into ten mRNAs, which are in turn translated into at least seven structural (VP1–VP7) and three nonstructural (NS1–NS3) proteins (Huismans and Dijk, 1990). The three nonstructural (NS) proteins, namely, NS-1, NS-2, NS-3 and the related NS3 A are produced in the bluetongue-infected cells. NS-1 and NS-2 are synthesized in the cytoplasm and are involved in virus replication, assembly, and morphogenesis (Roy, 2008). The virions have a diameter of 68–70 nm, comprising an outer capsid around a 54-nm core. VP2 and VP5 form the outer capsid, and the other five structural proteins are in the core. VP2 is primarily responsible for the induction of type-specific neutralizing antibodies (Verwoerd and Erasmus, 1994). Genetically and structurally, BTV is well characterized (Roy, 2008).

BTV is comparatively a resistant virus and withstands decomposition and is stable in decaying organic matter. But the virus is sensitive to acid, and the infectivity is lost easily in mild acidic condition and inactivated by 3.0% formalin and 70.0% alcohol. It resists 20.0% diethyl ether, chloroform, and

0.1% per cent sodium deoxycholate, indicating lack of essential lipids in the virus particles. The virion is stable at 4°C and—70°C but loses its infectivity when rapidly frozen at—20°C. It survives drying in air and retains its infectivity in serum, defibrinated blood, and in a glycerol-oxalate-phenol mixture for twenty-five years at room temperature. The virus survives at pH 5.6 to 8.0. BTV cross-reacts with many other antigenically related viruses like those causing epizootic hemorrhagic disease of deer and African horse sickness. BTV multiplies in both arthropod and mammalian host cells. The virulence of BTV varies markedly; even strains with matching serotypes vary in virulence. The world reference center for serotyping BTV is in South Africa.

EPIDEMIOLOGY

DISTRIBUTION
Even though bluetongue was first described in South Africa after Merino sheep were imported from Europe during the late eighteenth century, there was an early report of an acute febrile disease of sheep resembling bluetongue as early as 1652 in Merino and other European breeds (Verwoerd and Erasmus, 1994). The disease was confined to South Africa for many years, and the studies on the viral nature of the disease, its insect spread, and the various serotypes of the virus were mainly done in that country, mostly at the Onderstepoort Institute (Howell, 1960, 1970). BT has been reported from Africa, Asia, South America, North America, Australia, and some islands of tropics and subtropics (Buxton and Fraser, 1977). BTV was also found in Netherland, Germany, and Luxembourg. Belgium had an outbreak of BT in 2006 (Toursaint et al., 2007a). In UK, the first out break of BTV was reported in Highland cow on a rare breeds farm in Suffplk (BBC News, 2007). In the same year, BTV spread in Scandinavia, Switzerland, and Denmark (International Society for Infectious Diseases, 2007). Norway had its first epidemic of bluetongue in February 2009 (Right health.com, 2009). In 2009, cattle imported to UK were found to be carrying of BTV inspite of having been tested before shipping. May be because the animals can develop low-level viremia when bitten by an infective midge even after vaccination, and the PCR test showed positive. But the animals will not have enough viruses to infect the midges and also have severe disease (Internet news, 2009).

The prevalence of BT is determined by the climatic conditions, geography, and altitude, which facilitate the survival of the vectors.

The Office International Des Epizooties has placed BT in list A category considering its importance.

SOURCE OF INFECTION

Infected animals act as a source of infection for vectors. Cattle and other wild ruminants are reservoirs and amplifying hosts while suffering mildly. Transplacental transfer of BTV infection is noted in the ruminant calves, and it would be the possible way for BTV to overwinter, and midges can then spread the diseases from the calves to other animals during the start of new season. Outbreaks of the disease typically occur either when susceptible sheep are introduced to endemic areas or when infected midges carry the virus from endemic regions to adjacent areas containing susceptible population.

TRANSMISSION

BTV is transmitted biologically by certain species of culicoids. Though there are more than 1,400 species of culicoids, nearly 20 species of them have been found to be involved in the transmission of BT (OIE, 1998). *Culicoides veriipennis, C. insignis, C. fulvus, C. wadai, C. actoni, C. brevitarsis, C. imicola, C. oxystoma, and C. orientalis* are some among them (Ventor et al., 2006; Patel et al., 2007). The insect vectors of BTV breed in moist conditions in a variety of habitats, particular damp and muddy areas, and in decaying organic matter.

There is evidence that infected midges are carried by the wind for long distances up to 100 km (Sellers, 1981; Gloster et al., 2007). Competent midges are infected when biting viremic vertebrates. The chance of infection depends on the genotype of the midge, the strain of the virus, the level of viremia and environmental factors (Mellor et al., 2000). The extrinsic incubation period (the period between feeding on infected blood and the appearance of the virus in the saliva of the midge) is one to two weeks (Erasmus, 1990). The vectors that carry the virus prefer to feed on large animals. The main transmission cycle is between the culicoid midge and cattle. Sheep are infected when cattle are not present or the midge population is high.

Although BTV can be found in the semen of some rams and bulls, it has been isolated only at the time of peak viremia, and this occurrence could be due to the presence of blood cells in the semen as these viruses are closely associated with them. Virus also can be transferred from viremic dams (sheep and cattle) to the developing fetus (Stott, 1998). Transmissibility depends on the stage of development, viral strain, and the immune status of the dam. Sheep are most affected in the first trimester whereas cattle are highly susceptible between 60 and 140 days of gestation, with a transmission rate of 15–20%. The virus does not spread through meat, milk, or dairy products. The potential for BTV transmission also exists due to poor management practices, such as using the same needle for injections or infected surgical equipments.

HOSTS

BT is primarily a disease of sheep. In cattle and goats, the disease is rare, and they suffer mildly. BTV affects domestic and wild ruminants and some other herbivores such as elephants, antelope deer, and buffaloes (Righthealth. com, 2009). Dogs are also found to be affected by BTV, leading to abortion. Even though BTV affects most of the domestic animals, it is not a threat to humans but can mislead the bluetongue with some type of heart disease.

PATHOGENESIS

The extrinsic incubation period is one to two weeks. After introduction by the bite of an infected midge, bluetongue virus first replicates in the local lymph nodes and subsequently induces a primary viremia, which seeds other lymph nodes, spleen, lung, and vascular endothelium (Gibbs and Greiner, 1988). Circulating virus associates with blood cells, mostly with erythrocytes and platelets, though virus associated with mononuclear cell is critical for dissemination of virus throughout the animal. Later in viremia, the virus is exclusively associated with erythrocytes. Virus particles appear to be sequestered in invaginations of the erythrocyte membrane, allowing prolonged viremia even in the presence of neutralizing antibodies (OIE, 1998). Vascular endothelial damage causes changes in capillary permeability and fragility and subsequent disseminated intravascular coagulation and necrosis of tissues supplied by the damaged capillaries. These changes result in edema, congestion, hemorrhage, inflammation, and necrosis.

In animals dying acutely, the oral mucosa is hyperemic and shows petechiae or ecchymoses. Excoriations may be in areas subject to mechanical abrasion, the edges of lips, dental pad, tongue, and cheeks opposite the molar teeth. There is no vesiculation in BT. There is hyperemia in the fore stomachs. The lungs are hyperemic with severe alveolar and interstitial edema, and there is froth in the bronchi and fluid in the thoracic cavity. There is severe hydropericardium. A variable-sized hemorrhage in the tunica media near the base of the pulmonary artery is almost pathognomonic. Subepicardial and subendocardial hemorrhages, particularly involving the left ventricle, are common. Animals that die later than fourteen days after infection often show dramatic degeneration and necrosis of the skeletal musculature. Muscles lose pigmentation, and the intermuscular fascia are infiltrated with a clear gelatinous fluid (Erasmus, 1990). In sheep, death occurs mostly as a result of secondary pneumonia.

Microscopic examination of mucosal lesions shows mononuclear cell infiltration and degeneration and necrosis of epithelial cells in which large acidophilic intracytoplasmic masses accumulate. Affected muscles have edema, hemorrhage, hyaline degeneration, and necrosis. Infiltration by neutrophils, macrophages, and lymphocytes is present in acute cases.

CLINICAL FINDINGS

After an incubation period of less than a week, severe febrile reaction leading to body temperature of 40–41°C is observed, for four to twelve days.

After two days of febrile reaction, congestion of oral and nasal mucosa along with serous nasal discharge and profuse salivation is noticed. The nasal discharge subsequently becomes mucopurulent, and the saliva becomes frothy. Congestion of conjunctiva, skin, and coronary bands is also observed. The congestion of the nose and nasal cavity produces a sore muzzle effect.

Other common clinical signs include edema of lips, gums, dental pad, nose, face, submandibulum, eyelids, and sometimes ears. The edema of lips and nose can give the sheep a monkey-face appearance.

Affected sheep occasionally have swollen, congested, cyanotic tongue. Ulcers and necrotic lesions are noticed by three days, and by a week excoriation of buccal mucosa leads to bloodstained frothy salivation. Lenticular necrotic ulcers develop on the lateral aspect of tongue. Swallowing often becomes difficult. Stertorous type of respiration is observed. Diarrhea and dysentery may also occur in some cases.

Dark red to purple band in the skin just above the coronet due to coronitis is an important sign that leads to knee walking. Constant changing of position of the feet gives bluetongue the nickname the dancing disease (BBC NEWS, UK, 2008-10-24). Coronitis and laminitis are manifested by lameness and recumbency. Torticollis and wryneck (opisthotonos) with twisting of head and neck to one side are observed in some cases. This is due to the direct viral action on skeletal muscles. Muscle stiffness and weakness often prevent the animals in lowering their head and in turn from eating. This leads to marked loss of condition.

The other clinical signs soon follow with death occurring during the second week following infection. Many of these deaths are the result of pulmonary edema and/or cardiac insufficiency. Further, sheep may die from chronic disease three to five weeks after infection with bacterial complications, especially pasteurellosis (OIE, 1998).

Though the severe form of BT is occurring in sheep, cattle population is also suffering mildly, and their importance is in epidemiology of this disease by helping the pathogen to survive in nature. The frequency of infection of cattle with bluetongue virus is generally higher than in sheep, even though the severe form of the disease in cattle is rare. Clinical infection in cattle is mild and manifested by fever, stiffness or lameness, and increased respiratory rate. There may be lacrimation and increased salivation. The skin of the muzzle is often inflamed and may crack and peel. The lips and tongue may be swollen, with ulcers on the oral mucosa. Similarly, the skin of the neck, flanks, perineum, and teats may be affected (Erasmus, 1990).

Hydroencephaly, microcephaly, curvature of the limbs, blindness, and deformity of the jaw are the common congenital deformities recorded in bovine and sheep fetuses in bluetongue virus–infected dams. The severity of lesions depends on the stage of gestation. Fetuses seem to be most susceptible during the period of active brain development (Erasmus, 1990). Fetal death leading to abortion or resorption and birth with debilitated and weak lambs are observed in ewes affected in the first trimester of pregnancy.

Morbidity rate reaches up to 100%, while mortality is about 50%. Mild or inapparent form of the disease is also noticed with slight pyrexia, off feed, and change in the white cell count.

Pregnant bitches abort or give birth to stillborn pups and die within a week (Wilbur et al., 1994).

Immune Response
Because of the plurality of viral strains and variation in the susceptibility among various breeds of sheep, the duration of immunity after an infection has not been well defined.

Animals typically seroconvert between seven and fourteen days after infection. Generally, sheep challenged with homologous strain are immune for a period of twelve months after vaccination. Newborn lambs that ingest colostrum from immune dams have immunity for a period of sixty-eight days.

Diagnosis
This disease is diagnosed from the clinical signs, by the isolation and identification of the virus, and by the demonstration of antigen and antibody. Isolation and identification is done in laboratory animals, embryonated chicken eggs, and in tissue culture.

Antibody against BTV is demonstrated by using serological tests like complement fixation, agar gel immunodiffusion (Wilson, 1999), counter immunoelectrophoresis, monoclonal-based competitive enzyme linked immunosorbent assay, and virus neutralization. Agar gel immunodiffusion is relatively simple, rapid, and economical to carry out and generally applied to screen animals involved in international trade, though it is less sensitive. The demonstration of antibody has diagnostic value if the antibody titer is found increased in the subsequent sampling after a fortnight which indicates current infection. Demonstration of IgM antibody is also suggestive of current infection.

Detection of antigen or nucleic acid using immunohistochemical tests, immunoperoxidase, and immunoelectron microscopic techniques using monoclonal antibody are very rapid, sensitive, and specific. Molecular techniques like reverse transcriptase–polymerase chain reaction (PCR) can be used for the detection of the virus and have the advantage of speed and accuracy over other methods (Antony et al., 2007; Toursaint et al., 2007b). Nested PCR is serotype-specific for BTV. The best clinical materials to be collected for the above tests are blood in heparin during viremia, spleen, liver, bone marrow, and lymph nodes. Molecular techniques like detecting viral nucleic acid are more reliable as the various serological tests vary in their results. Isolation and identification of the BTV is time-consuming.

DIFFERENTIAL DIAGNOSIS
Contagious caprine pleuropneumonia, (CCPP) contagious ecthyma, foot-and-mouth disease, *peste des petits* ruminants, coenurosis, and plant poisoning are the conditions to be differentiated from BT.

In CCPP and BT, fever and respiratory distress are common, but there is no digestive system involvement in CCPP, and clinical signs are restricted to respiratory system and pericardium.

In contagious ecthyma, the orf virus causes proliferative, not necrotic lesions, that involve the lips rather than the whole oral cavity. Absence of nasal discharge and diarrhea also distinguishes it from BT.

Foot-and-mouth disease occurs mildly in small ruminants. In FMD, respiratory distress and diarrhea are absent. But BT differs from PPR in the presence of edema of head region, the coronary band of the hooves, and the less hairy parts of the body. There is lameness in BT.

In coenurosis, sheep shows nervous signs without any diarrhea, respiratory involvement, and coronitits. In plant or mineral poisoning, case history and absence of fever distinguishes poisoning from PPR.

TREATMENT

There is no specific treatment for bluetongue disease. Antibiotics to prevent secondary bacterial complications are recommended along with supportive therapy as the animal can not ingest anything orally. Anti-inflammatory and pain relief medications can be used to alleviate the symptoms.

PREVENTION AND CONTROL

Bluetongue-free areas are established by border animal movement control, quarantine of imported animals, control of vectors (especially in transportation), and by routine serologic surveys of susceptible population.

Prevention of bluetongue in endemic area has done by the immunization of vertebrate hosts, especially sheep and cattle, and removal of vectors or prevention of vector attack.

Farmers generally do not accept the concept of vaccination if the possibility of severe infection is limited. So farmer education is important in such situations. The control of midges by the application of insecticides and larvicides to insect resting and breeding sites or systemically to cattle has not been fully investigated but is likely to have local success only. Protecting sheep from exposure to midges is a more practical approach and can be achieved by moving sheep from insect resting and breeding sites, stabling animals overnight, or the use of insect repellents.

Limiting vector exposure number and habitat can help control virus transmission. Keeping the animals indoors during peak vector times and conditions is recommended (from dusk to dawn). Vectors may be active during daytime when overcast and in shady areas. Changing water levels and removing organic matter (manure) frequently help to limit vector habitats. Vector repellents like diethyltoluamide (DET) can be used. Application of larvicides in breeding sites can be done, though this may pollute the environment. Bluetongue disease does not cause infection in humans; therefore, there are no public health issues to be considered.

VACCINATION

Prophylactic immunization of sheep is the most practical and effective control measure, requiring polyvalent vaccines. Both live and inactivated vaccines (Ramakrishnan et al., 2006) are available globally and are made as per the need of the region, depending on the geographical distribution of the serotypes. A modified live vaccine (serial passage through eggs or cell culture) is available and is used in endemic areas.

The live vaccine carries some risks for pregnant animals causing teratogenicity and early embryonic death. It is hypothesized that the virus may be transmissible to the vector from a vaccinated animal and may reassort in the vector, so it is advisable that the vaccine is administered outside the peak *Culicoides* season. Live, attenuated bluetongue vaccines have wide use. Teratogenicity of attenuated virus for the developing fetus and the propensity for vaccine virus to be excreted in the semen of bulls and rams have to be studied thoroughly. Colostral immunity in young sheep, which usually persists for more than two months, can interfere with the development of active immunity to vaccination. Young lambs can be effectively vaccinated at the age of three months. Breeding ewes and rams should be vaccinated before mating. Ewes should not be vaccinated within three weeks of mating. The vaccination has to be repeated annually in all the cases, one month before the expected occurrence of the disease in endemic areas. Serotype 8, serotype 4, and serotype 1 vaccines are produced for large animals and sheep by various vaccine companies namely Fort Dodge Animal Health (Wyeth), Merial, and Intervet. Recombinant canary poxvirus vaccine coexpressing genes encoding VP2 and VP5 outer capsid proteins of blue tongue virus induces high-level protection in sheep (Boone et al., 2006).

REFERENCES

1. Antony, S., Jones, H., Darpel, K. E., Elliot, H., Maan, S., Samuel, A., Mellor, P. S. and Marten, P. P. C. 2007. A duplex Rt-PCR assay for detection of genome segment 7(VP7 gene) from 24 BTV serotypes. *J. Virological Methods* 41:188–197.

2. BBC NEWS UK 2008. "Dancing disease set for long run." News.bbc.co.uk.hhtp://news.bbc.co.uk/1/hi/uk/7019511.stm (retrived on 2008-10-24).

3. "Bluetongue—Europe (50)." International Society for Infectious Diseases. 2007-10-30. www.promedmail.org/pls/promed/f?

4. Bluetongue outbreak detected in Denmark-EU. *http://www.reuters.com/*article/latest Crisis/idUSL13660817.

5. Blue Tonguevirus and vaccination UK. 2009. http://www.warmwell.com/about fmd08.html.

6. Boone, J. D., Balasurya, U. B., Karaca, K., Audonnet, J. C., Yao Jiansheng, He Ling, Nordgren, R., Monaco, F., Savini, G., Gardner, I. A. and MacLachlan, N. J. 2006. Recombinant canary pox virus vaccine co-expressing genes encoding VP2 and VP5 outer capsid proteins of blue tongue virus induces high level protection in sheep. *Vaccine* 5:672–678.

7. Buxton, A. and Fraser, G. 1977. In *Animal microbiology*, 629–632. Oxford: Blackwell Scientific Publications.

8. Erasmus, B. J. 1990. Bluetongue virus. *Virus infections of ruminants* 31:227–237.

9. Howell, P. G. 1960. A preliminary antigenic classification of strains of bluetongue virus. *Onderstepoort J. Vet. Res.* 28:357–363.

10. Howell, P. G. 1970. The antigenic classification and distribution of naturally occurring strains of bluetongue virus. *J. South Afr. Vet. Med. Assoc.* 41:215–223.
11. Huismans, H. and Dijk A. Avan. 1990. Bluetongue virus structural components. *Current Topics in Microbiology and Immunology* 162:21–41.
12. Gloster, J., Mellor, P. S., Manning, A. J., Webster, H. N. and Host, M. C. 2007. Assessing the risk of windborne spread of blue tongue in 2006 outbreak of disease in northern Europe. *Vet. Rec.* 160:45–56.
13. Internet Blue tongue–RightHealth. http://www.righthealth.com/topic/Blue_tongue overview /wiki _ detailed? modp=bluetongue.
14. Mellor, P. S., Boorman, J. and Baylis, M. 2000. Culicoides biting midges: Their role as arbovirus vectors. *Annual Review of Entomology* 45:307–340.
15. Office International des Epizooties. 1998. Supporting document for the OIE International Animal Health Code chapter 2.1.9 on bluetongue. OIE Ad hoc working group on bluetongue, September 1998.
16. Patel, R., Chandel, B. S., Chauwan, H. C., Pawar, D. W., Bulbule, N. R., Bhalodia, S. D. and Khan, H. N. 2007. Prevlence of potentioal vector of blue tonguevirus in Gujarat. *Royal Vet. J. India* 3:33–36.
17. Radostits, O. M., Gay, C. C., Blood, D. C. and Hinchcliff, K. W. 2003. In *Veterinary medicine*, 9th ed., 1128–1134. China: Book Power.
18. Ramakrishnan, M. A., Pandey, A. B., Singh, K. P., Singh, R., Nandi, S. and Mehrothra, M. L. 2006. Immune response and protective efficacy of binary ethyleneimine (BEI) inactivated blue tongue vius vaccine in sheep. *Vet. Res. Commun.* 30:873–880.
19. Righthealth.com. 2009. http://www.righthealth.com/topic/Blue_tongue/ overview/ wiki_ detailed?modp=blue tongue (retrived on 2/24/2009).
20. Roy, P. 2008. Molecular dissection of Bluetongue virus. In *Animal viruses: Molecular biology*, 305–354. Caister Academic Press.
21. Sellers, R. F. 1981. Bluetongue and related diseases. In *Virus diseases of food animals*, ed. E. P. J. Gibbs, 567–584. London, UK: Academic Press.
22. Stott, J. L. 1998. Bluetongue and epizootic hemorrhagic disease. In *US Animal Health Association, Committee on Foreign Animal Disease. Foreign animal diseases: The gray book.* 6th ed, part IV, 24. Richmond, VA: US Animal Health.
23. Toursaint, J. F., Sailleau, C., Mast, J., Houdart, P., Czaplicki, G., Demeestere, L., Vanden Bursche, F., Dessel, W. Van, Goris, N., Breard, E., Bounaadja, L., Thiry, E., Zienbara, S. and Clercq, K. De. 2007a. Blue tongue in Belgium, 2006. *Emerging infectious diseases* 1:614–616.
24. Toursaint, J. F., Sailleau, C., Breard, E., Zientara, S. and Clercq, K. De. 2007. Blue tongue virus detection by 2 real time RT-PCR targeting 2 different genomic segments. *J. Virol. Methods* 140:115–123.
25. Ventor, G. J., Mellor, P. S. and Pawesk, J. T. 2006. Oral susceptibility of South African stock associated Culicoides species to blue tongue virus. *J. Medical Veterinary Entomology* 20:329–334.
26. Verwoerd, D. W. and Erasmus, B. J. 1994. Bluetongue. In *Infectious diseases of livestock with special reference to Southern Africa. Cape Town, South Africa*, ed. J. A. W. Coetzer, G. R. Thomson, and R. C. Tustin, 443–459. Oxford University Press.
27. Wilbur, L. A., Evermann, J. F. and Mertens, P. P. 1994. Abortion and death in pregnant bitches associated with a canine vaccine contaminated with bluetongue virus. *J. Am. Vet. Med. Assoc.* 204:1762–65.

2. Bovine Coronaviral Infection
(Nebraska Calf Diarrhea, Winter Dysentery)

M. R. Saseendranath, and M. Krishnan Nair

Introduction
Bovine coronavirus (BCV) is an important cause of enteric and respiratory disease in young calves and winter dysentery (WD) in adult cows.

Etiology
Bovine coronavirus (BCV) is group 2 member of the genus *Coronavirus,* belonging to the family Coronaviridae (Loa, 2006). Coronaviruses are enveloped viruses with single-stranded RNA genome. The name "coronavirus" is derived from the Latin *corona,* meaning "crown," as the virus envelope appears to be crowned by a characteristic ring of small bulbous structures. BCV is a medium-sized virus (75–160nm) with club-shaped peplomers projecting from envelope.

Proteins that contribute to the overall structure of all coronaviruses are the spike (S), envelope (E), membrane (M), and nucleocapsid (N). Bovine coronavirus (BCV) was first isolated in 1971. BCV can be isolated in BEK and Vero cells (Benfield and Saif, 1990). The virus is stable at pH 3. BCV survives well at low temperatures and at low levels of ultraviolet light. BCV hemagglutinate RBCs of hamster, mouse, and rat.

Epidemiology

Distribution
BCV infection is an important causative agent of neonatal diarrhea and respiratory illness in calves in beef and dairy cattle worldwide (Mebus et al., 1972; Acres et al., 1975; Woode et al., 1978; Tsunemitsu, et al., 1991; Hasoksuz et al., 2005). The virus may be detected in both diarrheic and healthy calves. Winter dysentery (WD) in adult cattle caused by BCV is a clinically and economically important disease in many countries (Loa et al., 2006). Disease is more common during winter months mainly due to the enhanced capacity of the virus to survive in cool, moist condition. It is characterized by high morbidity (50–100%), but low mortality (1–2%). Bovine coronavirus infection is more observed in calves older than three months (Gumusova et al., 2007).

SOURCE OF INFECTION

Diseased calves and carrier and infected cows are the source of the infection in a herd. BCV has been detected in the dung of a high proportion of clinically normal adult cows despite the presence of specific antibodies in the serum (Crouch and Acres, 1984; Crouch et al., 1985). The virus excretion is found to be more during cold season and around parturition; hence, calves born to carrier animals are more prone to develop diarrhea (Collins et al., 1987). Recovered calves that are apparently immune to disease can still shed BCV in their nasal secretions or feces.

TRANSMISSION

Infection is established by ingestion or inhalation of BCV. The respiratory tract infection allows virus transmission by the aerosol-nasal route in addition to the fecal-oral route.

HOSTS

The calves from cows with low serum antibody titers and low antibody titers in their colostrum and milk are susceptible to infection. Calves born to primiparous cows are particularly vulnerable. Adult cows suffer from winter dysentery and respiratory tract infection as a result of BCV infection. Coronavirus infection was reported in another species of animals like camel calves of sixty-five weeks of ages.

PATHOGENESIS

The virus infection starts in the proximal small intestine and spreads throughout the small and large intestines. BCV replicates in "rapidly dividing" cells such as those that line intestinal villi. Virus replication occurs in the surface epithelial cells, particularly in those on the distal half of the villi. Infected cells die, slough off, and are replaced by immature cells. In the small intestine, these changes result in stunting and fusion of adjacent villi, and in the large intestine they lead to atrophy of the colonic ridges.

Histologically, it is observed that the tall columnar epithelial cells, which usually line the small intestinal villi and colonic ridges, are replaced by cuboidal and squamous epithelial cells, and in severe infections, there may be areas of complete desquamation, resulting in the decreasing the number of goblet cells. These changes lead to the reduced absorptive capacity of the gut due to the reduction in the surface area as well as by the presence of immature cells. These cells retain some of their secretory capacity, which leads to the increase in the volume of the fluid in the gut lumen. At the same time, the immature cells are unable to secrete the digestive enzymes, resulting in the impaired digestion. Undigested lactose accumulate in the gut, leading to an increased osmolarity and further drawing fluid into the gut. The decrease in the digestive and absorptive capacity leads to diarrhea, with loss of water and electrolytes leading to dehydration, acidosis, and hypoglycemia. Death may occur due to acute shock and heart failure. As the virus is not attacking the crypt of the intestinal villi, the disease is self-limiting.

BCV can also cause a respiratory syndrome that is usually quite mild or even subclinical. Clinical signs are usually seen in calves two to sixteen weeks old and include sneezing (from rhinitis) and coughing (from tracheitis). Because BCV can infect respiratory epithelium, it can predispose calves to opportunistic bacterial infections. Calves with respiratory BCV infection can shed high numbers of virus in their nasal discharge, and this virus can cause enteric and/or respiratory disease in other cattle.

Microscopic lesions of winter dysentery (WD) are most evident in the spiral colon where crypt epithelium exhibits varying degrees of degeneration and necrosis. Grossly, hemorrhage (including petechiae) can be found in the mucosa of both the small and large intestine. Villous atrophy in small intestinal mucosa leads to severe shortening of the villi and leading to malabsorption and loss of enzymatic activity.

CLINICAL SIGNS
The incubation period is twenty hours. The clinical severity of BCV enteritis varies with age, immunological status of the calf, infective dose, and strain of virus. Diarrhea is more common in very young colostrum-deprived calves. Coronaviral diarrhea in young calves is characterized by yellow diarrhea and can last three to six days. Listlessness, anorexia, pyrexia, and dehydration are the other important signs. In some, calves feces contain flecks of blood. Calves with bloody diarrhea can die of hypovolemia within a few hours of the onset of clinical signs. Majority of the calves recover, but a few die if diarrhea is severe (Mebus et al., 1973; Bridger et al., 1978; Saif et al., 1986).

Winter dysentery (WD) in adult cows is characterized by severe watery diarrhea (sometimes with blood and mucus), decreased milk production, listlessness, depression, anorexia, weight loss, and sometimes cough and/or nasolacrimal discharge. Excess salivation, lethargy, weakness, dehydration and shock. Diarrhea persists for five to six days.

Inadequate colostrum intake, immunodeficiency, and secondary viral, bacterial, and parasitic infections contribute to the severity of the clinical signs.

Postmortem finding reveals distended bowl and small intestine with liquid feces. No gross lesions are found.

BCV can also cause respiratory tract infections in calves of different ages. Infection is generally subclinical and is seen in calves between two and sixteen weeks of age (Thomas et al., 1982; Tsunemitsu et al., 1991).

IMMUNE RESPONSE

Following natural infection, calves develop active immunity to the virus and its IgA antibodies at the mucosal surface, which protect against reinfection (Saif, 1987; Heckert et al., 1991). Cows that recover from WD are apparently immune for one to five years. IgM is the predominant copro antibody to BCV infection followed by IgG (Zakaria et al., 1996).

DIAGNOSIS

IDENTIFICATION OF THE AGENT

Virus isolation is the conventional methods of diagnosis, but difficult and time-consuming. Hemagglutination test (HA) and hemagglutination inhibition (HI) test can be used for the identification and confirmation of the agent (Sharpee et al., 1976; Muniapa et al., 1985). Enteric BCV infections are diagnosed by examination of fecal samples for the presence of virus. Electron microscopy can detect coronavirus particles in feces or intestinal contents (Saif et al, 1991). Immunofluorescent microscopy can detect coronavirus antigens in infected tissues (e.g., small intestine and spiral colon of calves, spiral colon of cows, or trachea and lungs of calves with respiratory syndrome). In calves with BCV enteric infection, viral particles can be detected by electron microscopy in the feces one to two days before the onset of diarrhea and for several days after the diarrhea has resolved (Durham et al., 1979). Viral antigen can also be demonstrated by the use of specific antibodies and gold conjugated probes (Langpap et al., 1979; Saif et al., 1986; Heckert et al., 1989). Enzyme linked immunosorbent assay (ELISA) are the most widely used diagnostic test for BCV (Crouch and Acres, 1984). Indirect antigen capture ELISA was especially useful for diagnosing BCV feces and nasal secretions of calves (Hasoksuz et al., 2005).

A dot blot hybridization test using a cDNA probe labeled with either p32 or biotin to detect BCV RNA is also in use (Shockley et al., 1987). Multiplex polymerase chain reaction is found to be very effective in differentiating turkey coronavirus, infectious bronchitis virus, and bovine coronavirus (Loa et al., 2006).

Serology can detect seroconversion or a fourfold increase in serum immunoglobulin levels. Virus neutralization assay of serum (detecting a fourfold increase in antibody liters) is valuable for diagnosing WD and BCV-associated respiratory disease.

DIFFERENTIAL DIAGNOSIS
BCV has to be differentiated from other bacterial, viral, parasitic, and protozoan infections of calves. Bacterial and viral antigen identification by various serological and molecular methods are useful for differentiation of coronaviral infection. The presence of characteristic ova or oocysts in the feces helps to differentiate various parasitic and protozoan diseases.

TREATMENT
There is no specific therapy for bovine coronaviral enteritis. The aim of the treatment is to replace the loss of fluids and electrolytes parenterally. Oral administration of astringent can be adopted to reduce the severity of diarrhea, which can otherwise lead to dehydration and acidosis. Warm bedding and surrounding will help to early recovery.

PREVENTION AND CONTROL
Identification and segregation of carrier cows and calves decrease the incidence of BCV infection, though practically a difficult procedure. Because mucosal immunity is important in preventing or recovering from BCV infection, calves that do not receive colostrum are especially susceptible to BCV enteritis. Hence, colostrum feeding immediately after birth helps to prevent the infection.

VACCINATION
Vaccination of herds can provide protection. BCV diarrhea can be prevented either by increasing their levels of specific immunity. The immune status of the susceptible calves can be raised by vaccination of pregnant cows or by oral immunization of neonatal calves to stimulate active immunity. Vaccination prevents the increase in the BCV shedding which usually occurs from carrier cows at parturition (Collins et al., 1987). Live, attenuated vaccine is effective if given to newborn calves after birth.

Active immunization of calves by oral inoculation with live, attenuated BCV vaccines has been found to protect colostrum-deprived calves (Thurber et al., 1977). Aerosol route of vaccine administration has also been tried as an alternate method to prevent the neutralization of the vaccine virus by gut immunoglobulins. In utero vaccination of bovine fetuses resulted in protective levels of immunity in six days old calves, but incidence of abortions and premature births limit this method of vaccination (Mullaney et al., 1988). Combined rota and corona vaccine is also available, which can be given to calves as well as to adult cows during pregnancy.

ERADICATION

Eradication of bovine coronaviral infection is practically very difficult.

REFERENCES

1. Acres, S. D., Laing, C. J., Saunders, J. R. and Radostitis, O. M. 1975. Acute undifferentiated neonatal diarrhea in beef calves. 1. Occurrence and distribution of infectious agents. *Can. J. Comp. Med.* 39:116–132.

2. Benfield, D. A. and Saif, L. J. 1990. Cell culture propagation of a coronavirus isolated from cows with winter dysentery. *J. Clin. Microbiol.* 28:1454–1457.

3. Bridger, J. C., Woode, G. N. and Meyling, A. 1978. Isolation of corona viruses from neonatal calf diarrhea in Great Britain and Denmark. *Vet. Microbiol.* 3:101–113.

4. Collins, J. K., Reigel, C. A., Olson, J. D. and Fountain, A. 1987. Shedding of enteric corona virus in adult cattle. *Am. J. Vet. Res.* 48:361–365.

5. Crouch, C. F. and Acres, S. D. 1984. Prevalence of rota virus and corona virus antigen in the feces of normal cows. *Can. J. Comp. Med.* 48:340–342.

6. Crouch, C. F., Ohmann, H. B., Watts, T. C. and Babiuk, L. A. 1985. Chronic shedding of bovine corona virus antigen-antibody complexes by clinically normal cows. *J. Gen. Virol.* 66:1489–1500.

7. Durham, P. J. K., Stevenson, B. J. and Farquharson, B. C. 1979. Rotavirus and corona virus associated diarrhea in domestic animals. *New Zealand Vet. J.* 27:30–32.

8. Gumusova, S. O., Yaziro, Z., Albayarak, H. and Meral, Y. 2007. Rota virus and Corona virus prevalence in healthy calves and calves with diarrhea. *Medyiyna Weterynaryjna* 63:62–64.

9. Heckert, R. A., Saif, L. J. and Myers, G. W. 1989. Developmemnt of protein A–gold immuno electronmicroscopy for detection of bovine coronavirus in calves: Comparison with ELISA and direct immunofluorescence of nasal epithelial cells. *Vet. Microbiol.* 19:217–231.

10. Heckert, R. A., Saif, L. J., Mengel, J. P. and Myers, G. W. 1991. Isotype specific antibody responses to bovine corona virus structural protein in the serum, feces and mucosal secretion from experimentally challenged-exposed colostrum deprived calves. *Am. J. Vet. Res.* 52:692–699.

11. Hasoksuz, M., Kayar, A., Dodurka, T. and Ilgazit, T. 2005. Detection of respiratory and enteric shedding of bovine corona virus in cattle in Northwestern Turkey. *Acta Veterinaria Hungarica* 53:1367–146.

12. Langpap, T. J., Bergel, M. E. and Reed, D. E. 1979. Corona viral enteritis of young calves: Virologic and pathologic findings in naturally occurring infections. *Am. J. Vet. Res.* 40:1476–1478.

13. Loa, C. C., Lin, T. C., Wu, C. C., Bryan, T. A., Hooper, T. A. and Schrader, D. L. 2006. Differential detection of Turkey corona virus, infectious bronchitis virus and Bovine corona virus by a multiplex polymerase chain reaction. *J. Virol. Methods* 131:86–91.

14. Mebus, C. A., White, R. G., Stair, E. I., Rhodes, M. B. and Twiehaus, M. J. 1972. Neonatal calf diarrhea: Results of a field trial using a reo like virus vaccine. *Vet. Med/Small Anim. Clin.* 67:173–178.

15. Mebus, C. A., Stair, E. L., Rhodes, M. B. and Twiehaus, M. J. 1973. Pathology of neonatal calf diarrhea induced by a corona virus like agent. *Vet. Pathol.* 10:45–64.

16. Mullaney, T. P., Newman, L. E. and Whitehair, C. K. 1988. Humoral immune response of the bovine fetus to *in utero* vaccination with attenuated bovine corona virus. *Am. J. Vet. Res.* 49:156–159.

17. Mullanay, T. P., Newman, L. E. and Whitehair, C. K. 1988. Humoral immune response of the bovine fetus to *in utero* vaccination with attenuated bovine corona virus. *Am. J. Vet. Res.* 49:156–159.

18. Muniappa, L., Mitov, B. K. and Kharalambiev, Kh. T. 1985. Demonstration of corona virus infection in buffalos. *Vet. Med. Nauki.* 22:27–32.

19. Saif, L. J. 1987. Development of nasal, fecal and serum isotype specific antibodies in calves challenged with bovine corona virus and rota virus. *Vet. Immunol. Immunopathol.* 17:425–439.

20. Saif, L. J., Redman, D. R., Moorehead, P. D. and Theil, K. W. 1986. Expeimentally induced corona virus infections in calves: Viral replication in the respiratory and intestinal tracts. *Am. J. Vet. Res.* 47:1426–1432.

21. Saif, L. J., Brock, K. V., Redman, D. R. and Kohler, E. M. 1991. Winter dysentery in dairy herds: Electron microscopic and serological evidence for an association with corona virus. *Vet. Rec.* 128:447–449.

22. Sharpee, R. L., Mebus, C. A. and Bass, E. P. 1976. Characterization of calf diarrhoeal corona virus. *Am. J. Vet. Res.* 37:1031–1041.

23. Shockley, L. J., Kapke, P. A., Lapps, W., Brian, D. A., Potgiete, L. N. D. and Woods, R. 1987. Diagnosis of porcine and bovine enteric corona virus infections using cloned cDNA probes. *J. Clin. Microbiol.* 25:1591–1596.

24. Thomas, L. H., Gourlay, R. N., Stott, E. J., Howard, C. J. and Bridger, J. C. 1982. A search for new microorganism in calf pneumonia by inoculation of gnotobiotic calves. *Res. Vet. Sci.* 33:170–182.

25. Thurber, E. T., Bass, E. P. and Beckenhauer, W. H. 1977. Field trial evaluation of a reo corona virus calf diarrhea vaccine. *Can. J. Comp. Med.* 41:131–136.

26. Tsunemitsu, H., Yonemichi, H. and Hirai, T. 1991. Isolation of bovine corona virus from feces and nasal swabs of calves with diarrrhoea. *J. Vet. Med. Sci.* 53:433–437.

27. Woode, G. N., Bridger, J. C. and Meyling, A. 1978. Significance of bovine corona virus infection. *Vet. Rec.* 102:15–16.

28. Zakaria, R., Kanwati, E. L., Tsenemitsu, H., Smith, D. R. and Saif, L. J. 1996. Infection and cross protection studies of winter diarrhea, bovine corona virus strains in colostrum deprived and gnotobiotic calves. *Am. J. Vet Res.* 57:48–53.

3. Bovine Ephemeral Fever
(*Three-Day Sickness, Bovine Epizootic Fever, Stiff Sickness Dragon, Boat Disease*)

M. R. Saseendranath, and M. Krishnan Nair

Introduction
Bovine ephemeral fever (BEF) is an acute, noncontagious, epizootic arthropod transmitted disease of cattle and buffaloes, characterized by sudden onset of high fever, stiffness, lameness, and uneventful recovery in few days with high morbidity and low mortality.

Etiology
BEF is caused by an ss RNA virus belonging to the genus *Ephemerovirus* in the family Rhabdoviridae having a size of 80 × 120–140 nm. The virus isolated from South Africa was cone shaped while the strain studied in Japan and Australia were bullet shaped (Lecatsas, 1970). The virus is enveloped and has five structural proteins and ether sensitive. The pH lower than 2.5 and higher than 12.0 destroys the virus in ten minutes. Inactivation takes place within 10 minutes at 56°C, 18 hours at 37°C, and 120 hours at 25°C. The virus is antigenically related to at least three other viruses which are nonpathogenic to cattle—viz., Kimberly virus, Berrimah virus, and Adelide River virus. Kotonkan and Puchong viruses in Africa and Malaysia respectively produce a disease in cattle similar to ephemeral fever (Chandra et al., 2004).

Epidemiology

Distribution
This disease was first reported from Central Africa in 1867. It is now enzootic in many parts of tropical and subtropical countries. There has been no report of BEF from Europe and North or South America (Sharma and Adlaka, 1994) and Egypt (Madbouly et al., 2006a).

Wild ruminants appear to act as reservoirs of bovine ephemeral fever virus (BEFV). The disease tends to disappear for long periods and return in an epizootic form when the resistance of the population is reduced.

Source of Infection
The diseased animals and biological vectors are the sources of infection.

The virus never exists in recovered animals, and it is suggested that some fauna may be carrying the virus from season to season. Wild ruminants appear to act as reservoirs or amplifying hosts and are implicated in the interepizootic maintenance of the infection.

Hosts

Cattle and buffaloes are mainly affected. Sheep and goat do not suffer generally. All breeds of cattle are susceptible, but younger-age groups ranging from six months to two years are more vulnerable. BEF has also been recorded in some wild ruminants.

Transmission

BEF is transmitted by the bite of insects, mosquitoes, and culicoids. The vectors pick up the infective agent from the blood of diseased animal. The vectors become infective within a week of feeding on a diseased animal. The biologically transmitted arbovirus multiplies in the vectors and are inoculated with saliva when a blood meal is obtained, whereas mechanically transmitted agents are transported directly from host to host. Even 0.002 ml of blood has been found to produce the disease in susceptible animals, experimentally. The virus does not spread through semen or meat. Transmission never occurs through close contact with infected animals or saliva or ocular discharge.

Pathogenesis

After entry of the virus, the organism multiplies in blood and leads to viremia. The virus is closely associated with leucocytes and platelets. The virus localizes in the mesodermal tissues like joints, muscle, and lymph nodes and causes severe inflammation leading to the various clinical signs. There is vasculitis and thrombosis. Serofibrinous inflammation in serous and synovial cavities is seen, along with and increased endothelial permeability. No evidence of tissue destruction is observed.

Clinical Signs

The incubation period ranges from two to ten days, with an average of three days. Considerable individual variations in clinical signs are observed depending upon the dose and strain of the virus and resistance of the host.

The characteristic finding of BEF is its sudden onset and spontaneous recovery even in the absence of any treatment. The main symptoms are biphasic fever (104–108°F) with peaks twelve to twenty-four hours apart. Increased heart and respiratory rates, anorexia, ruminal atopy, depression, serous nasal and ocular discharge, salivation, muscle twitching, and shivering are observed. The affected animals show shifting lameness, from the second day of fever, in one or more limbs. The lameness may be similar to that in acute laminitis. The suffering animals will be depressed, stiff, and stand with drooping head. Majority of the animals will be reluctant to lie down and prefer to stand. Some may be recumbent for one or two days. Animals in early lactation or heavy yielders may become downer resulting in permanent paresis in some. The muscles of the affected limb become stiff, hard, and painful. Sudden drop in milk production is also observed in lactating animals. The animals do not return to their full production even after the recovery, if it is in lactation. Pneumonia, mastitis, locomotor dysfunction, abortion, and infertility are the other complications noticed in affected animals. In uncomplicated cases, the temperature returns to normal in three to four days' time, and the animal becomes normal (Davies et al., 1984; Lino et al., 1998; Rehman et al., 2002). Morbidity is about 50–100%. Mortality is very low, unless it is complicated by secondary infections.

IMMUNE RESPONSE
After experimental infection, two-year immunity against homologous strains of BEF was recorded. Generally after an attack, there is solid immunity for a period of two to three years.

DIAGNOSIS
Clinical signs are pathognomonic. Virus isolation and identification by culture, and various serological (Ali et al., 2001), molecular, and biotechnological (Eto et al., 1991) laboratory methods are employed for diagnostic confirmation. Paired serum samples for the assessment of antibody by any of the serological methods are effective in diagnosis. Early leukocytosis with neutrophilia with shift to left, increased plasma fibrinogen, marked rise in creatinine kinase, and decreased calcium levels are also characteristic in BEF (Uren and Murphy, 1985). Significant reduction was noticed in total erythrocyte count, hemoglobin concentration, and lymphocyte count. Serum biochemistry in BEF revealed a decrease in total protein, albumin, globulin, calcium, phosphorous, and zinc and an increase in copper, creatinine, blood urea nitrogen, aspartate aminotransferase, and alanine aminotransferase (Hamoda et al., 2002). Necropsy findings are not pathognomonic. Serofibrinous polyserositis involving synovial, pericardial, and peritoneal cavities are characteristic. Pulmonary emphysema and edematous and enlarged lymph nodes are noted in BEF (Sayed et al., 2001).

DIFFERENTIAL DIAGNOSIS

BEF has to be differentiated from Rift Valley fever, bluetongue, babesiosis, blackleg, and foot-and-mouth disease.

Rift Valley fever leads to high mortality in lambs and calves and much lower incidence in adult animals. Hepatic lesion on necropsy is also noticed, whereas in BEF, mortality is very negligible and seen in all age groups without any lesions in liver.

Bluetongue in sheep leads to severe lesions on muzzle, eye, and face and severe laminitis with lameness. These lesions are not present in BEF.

In babesiosis along with pyrexia, coffee-colored urine due to hemoglobinuria is observed without any lameness. Intraerythrocytic demonstration of the organism confirms the diagnosis.

Blackleg can be differentiated by severe localized inflammatory lesions of the affected muscle with crepitating sound. The lameness will not be shifting from one leg to another. Moreover in blackleg, there is low morbidity and high fatality.

In foot-and-mouth disease pyrexia is followed by vesicular development and ulceration on the tongue, gum, nostril, interdigital area, teat and udder, which are absent in BEF.

TREATMENT

Symptomatic treatment is done to alleviate pain, fever, lameness and to restore the appetite. Broad-spectrum antibiotics to prevent the secondary bacterial complications and nonsteroidal anti-inflammatory agents like phenylbutazone, diclofenac, ketoprofen, ibuprofen, and salicylates are being used widely to alleviate the other clinical signs. Cows in lactation, and in recumbency must be supported with parenteral calcium, vitamins, and dextrose. The ailing animals should be nursed carefully. They should not be drenched as far as possible. In uncomplicated cases, the recovery occurs in three to four days.

PREVENTION AND CONTROL

Isolation of diseased animals in fly-proof shed will reduce the chance of transmission from the ailing animal to other susceptible population. Livestock can be protected from vectors by proper housing in fly-proof sheds in endemic areas, especially during an outbreak. Keeping the premises free of decaying organic matter, avoiding stagnation of water by providing proper drainage, and periodic disinfection will reduce the vector population considerably and thereby the arthropod-borne diseases like BEF.

VACCINATION

Vaccines against BEF have been developed in Australia, Japan, Egypt, and South Africa. There are two types of commercially available vaccines. The live vaccine provides immunity for twelve months with a single injection, which has to be repeated every year. The inactivated vaccine gives immunity for only six months, if given two doses of vaccine at an interval of four weeks (Bai et al., 1992; Madbouly et al., 2006b). Park et al. (1994) studied the effect of binary ethylenimine–inactivated tissue culture vaccine in cattle and observed virus-neutralizing antibody one week after vaccination, which was persistent up to thirty-two weeks in cattle. Cattle vaccinated with recombinant vaccinia virus expressing G protein produced neutralizing antibodies and were protected against experimental BEFV infection.

REFERENCES

1. Ali, N. M., Ahmed, L. A. and Shahein, M. A. 2001. Isolation and identification of three day sickness virus in Egypt. *Vet. Med. J. Giza.* 49:425–434.
2. Bai, W. B., Yan, J. D., Chang, I. J., Jiang, C. L. and Lin, X. Y. 1992. Studies on vaccine against ephemeral fever. In Bovine ephemeral fever and related rhabdoviruses. Proceedingss of the 1st International Symposium-Beijing, August 1992.
3. Chandra, R., Kumar, R. and Pradhan, V. K. 2004. Bovine ephemeral fever: An update. *Intas Polyvet.* 5:9–15.
4. Davies, S. S., Gibson, D. S. and Clark, R. 1984. The effect of Bovine ephemeral fever on milk production (Dairy cattle). *Aus. Vet. J.* 1:128–130.
5. Eto, N., Yamada, K., Koga, A., Shirahata, S. and Murakami, H. 1991. Establishment and characterization of monoclonal antibodies against bovine ephemeral fever virus. *Agricultural and Biological Chemisty* 55:167–172.
6. Hamoda, F. K., Khalaf, S. S. and Khoder, M. H. 2002. Some clinical, epidemiological and laboratory studies on bovine ephemeral fever (Three day sickness). *Vet. Med. J. Giza.* 50:203–220.
7. Lecatsas, G. 1970. Further observations on the ultrastructure of ephemeral fever virus. *Onderstpoort J. Vet. Res.* 37:145–146.
8. Lino, Y. K., Inaba, Y., Li, N. J., Chain, C. Y., Luu, S. L. and Liou, P. P. 1998. Epidemiology of Bovine ephemeral fever virus infection in Taiwan. *Microbiol. Research* 53:289–295.
9. Madbouly, H. M., Hegazi, A. G., El-Shabrawy, M., Tamam, S. M. and Gamil, G. S. 2006a. Isolation and identification of ephemeral fever virus from cattle in Middle Egypt. *Vet. Med. J. Giza.* 54:877–886.
10. Madbouly, H. M., Hegazi, A. G., El-Shabrawy, M., Tamam, S. M. and Gamil, G. S. 2006b. Preparation of inactivated bovine ephemeral fever virus vaccine (BEF) from locally isolated strain using different adjuvants. *Vet. Med. J. Giza.* 54:955–970.
11. Park, B. K., Chang, C. H., Lee, P. S., Rhee, J. C., Son, D. and Lee, K. W. 1993. Bovine ephemeral fever virus vaccine inactivated with binary ethyleneimine. *J. Agri. Sci.* 35:6850–6890.

12. Rehman, A. A. A., Sayed, A. S., Sadiek, A. H. and Mohamed, N. A. 2002. Bovine ephemeral fever: Isolation of the causative virus and the associating bacterial respiratory complications. *Assint Veterinary Medical Journal* 6:196–212.

13. Sayed, A. S., Sadiek, A. H. and Ali, A. A. 2001. Bovine ephemeral fever in Assint governorate: Clinical laboratory and therapeutic studies. *Assint Veterinary Medical Journal* 4:157–175.

14. Sharma, J. N. and Adlakha, S. C. 1994. In *Virus diseases of animals in India*. 1st ed., 104. New Delhi: ICAR.

15. Uren, M. F. and Murphy, G. M. 1985. Studies on the pathogenesis of bovine ephemeral fever in sentinel cattle. II. Hematological and biochemical data. *Vet. Microbiol.* 10:505–515.

4. BOVINE LEUKOSIS
(Lymphosarcoma, Enzootic Bovine Leucosis, Malignant Lymphoma)

M. R. SASEENDRANATH, AND M. KRISHNAN NAIR

INTRODUCTION

Bovine leukosis is a lymphoproliferative disease of cattle caused by bovine leukemia virus (BLV) and is characterized by various manifestations in different age groups and lymphosarcoma in a minor percentage of infected adult cattle.

ETIOLOGY

Bovine leukosis virus (BLV) is an exogenous C type oncovirus belonging to the family Retroviridae, subfamily Orthoretrovirinae, and the genus *Deltaretrovirus.*

Virion consist of an envelop, a nucleocapsid, and a nucleoid and is spherical to pleomorphic.

BLV genome is positive-sense, single-stranded RNA virus measuring 80–100 nm in diameter. The virus is cell associated, and its genome is inserted into the genome of host lymphocytes and monocytes. The virus possesses a nucleoprotein and surface glycoprotein. It is genetically and antigenically related to ovine leukemia virus, and immunological cross-reaction has been demonstrated between these two viruses.

The infectivity of the BLV is abolished by lipid solvents, phenol, trypsin, and formaldehyde. Infectivity is rapidly destroyed at 56°C. Pasteurization destroys the infectivity of this virus.

EPIDEMIOLOGY

DISTRIBUTION

Bovine leukemia is worldwide in distribution. The initial description of bovine leukosis in cattle appeared in German medical literature in 1871. Europe is considered to be the homeland of enzootic bovine leukosis. Later, BLV has been reported from United States (Burridge et al., 1981), Israel (Brenner et al., 1986), Taiwan (Wang et al., 1986); Egypt (Zaghawa et al., 2002), Brazil (Carneiro et al., 2003), and later from many other countries. BLV infection is pandemic, and the prevalence of infection in cattle herds can reach 60–90%. It is not the disease actually, but the seropositivity that restricted the trade, which resulted in severe economic loss.

SOURCE OF INFECTION

Seropositive cattle with lymphocytosis is a major source of BLV for susceptible cattle (Itohara et al., 1985). Blood, saliva, nasal secretions, broncheoalveolar washings, colostrum, milk, urine, feces, uterine discharge, and embryos are the main sources through which the virus transmission mainly occurs.

BLV can be transmitted through colostrum or milk if the dams are infected (Meas et al., 2002). In countries where beef and dairy industries make up a large part of the economy, majority of the herds are infected. Eighty-four percent of herds of Argentina and seventy percent herds of Canada are found to harbor BLV (Sargeant, 1997; VanLeeuwen, 2001; Trono, 2001).

TRANSMISSION

The virus is cell associated, and transmission between animals is by blood or tissue containing lymphocytes. Main mode of transmission is by contact with infected animals. Since the virus is transmitted to the newborn through colostrum or milk, infection mainly takes place early in the life of a calf.

The spread of infection in cattle occurs as a result of the manageable practices in the cattle industry such as feeding blood from slaughtered cows and feeding pooled colostrum to calves, the use of syringes, tattooing and dehorning instruments on multiple animals without proper sterilization between uses (Gonda, 1992). Rectal palpation of infected and healthy cows using a common gloves resulted in transmission of bovine leukemia (Kohara et al., 2006).

The infection can also occur through the wounds on skin. Bloodsucking flies can also transmit the disease. Very small amount of infected blood can transmit the disease. In utero transmission has also been documented. The virus remains within the lymphocytes and not inactivated by the antibody. The presence of antibody indicates the infection. It is usually difficult to predict which infected animal will develop the disease, which depends on the genetic makeup of the individual animals.

BLV is found in the marketed milk and meat of dairy and beef cattle. Consumption of unpasteurised dairy products or undercooked beef could possibly allow transmission to humans (McClure et al., 1974).

Host

BLV mainly affects cattle and can infect other species, including sheep and goats, naturally and several species experimentally, including nonhuman primates. BLV can also infect the cells of many species cultured in flasks including cells from human, simian, canine, caprine, equine, and nonhuman primates (Graves and Ferrer, 1976).

Under natural conditions, the oncogenic potential of BLV appears to be expressed only in cattle and sheep. An increased incidence of leukemia has been found among dairy farmers (Donham, 1980).

Pathogenesis

Most of the BLV infections are asymptomatic. There is a brief viremia soon after infection, followed by a long incubation period, when the virus remains quiescent as provirus that is randomly integrated into the genome of the infected cells.

Whether or not the animal becomes infected or develop any of the other form of the disease depends on the recipient's genetic constitution. The outcome may also depend on the animal's immune status and the size of the dose of the virus. The lesions develop at varying rates in different animals. Only 2–5% of the cattle that becomes infected develop malignant lymphoma and persistent lymphocytosis, a benign proliferation of lymphoid cells (Johnson and Kaneene, 1992). Some develop only transient viremia without seroconversion. Some develop persistent lymphocytosis within months or years. Neoplasms in cattle with enzootic bovine leukosis involve a combination of internal and superficial lymph nodes, heart, abomasum, intestine, kidney, uterus, liver, spleen and epidural space of lumbar spinal cord. Both T and B lymphocytes are infected, but the tumors are composed of B lymphocytes.

Immune Response

Antibodies against bovine leukosis virus appear as early as three weeks postexposure (Merion et al., 1985). Most of the BLV-infected cattle develop antibodies to BLV structural proteins. A greater response is usually noted to the glycosylated proteins of the envelope, gp51 and gp30, than the internal proteins, gp24, gp15, gp12 and gp10. Antibodies and BLV are also detected in the milk and colostrum and are partially protective against infection of calves. The initial appearance of antibodies depends upon the dose of the virus received by the host as well as by the other unique differences of the immune system of the individual cattle. Antibody to gp51 is having neutralizing capacity. About 80% of the adult form of the disease has a marked depression of IgM globulin.

CLINICAL SYMPTOMS

Bovine leukemia is reported in four different forms—namely, (1) adult or enzootic form, (2) skin, (3) thymic, and (4) calf forms. The first two are in adults and the latter two in younger animals.

The adult form is seen in cattle over three years of age. The incubation period appears to be three to five years. Most cattle infected with BLV do not exhibit clinical signs. BLV infection is lifelong in cattle, and so demonstration of serum antibodies indicates persistent lymphocytosis. Lymphoma or lymphosarcoma develops in minor percentage of BLV-infected cattle, but it is a fatal disease characterized by lymphomatous involvement of multiple organs. These include lymph nodes, heart, gastrointestinal tract (especially abomasum), liver, spleen, uterus, and kidneys. Clinical signs reflect the organ involvement. Peripheral lymph nodes may be visually or palpably enlarged. Cardiac involvement usually includes the right atrium and can result in congestive heart failure with dependent edema. Poor reproductive performance and palpable enlargement of the uterine wall or intrapelvic lymph nodes are also observed in malignant lymphoma. The clinical signs depend on the location of the tumors.

Loss of weight, decreased milk yield, external and internal lymphadenopathy, decreased appetite, posterior paresis, fever, respiratory involvement, exophthalmous, diarrhea, constipation, and cardio vascular involvement are the common signs observed in adults. Occasionally, peracute death is also observed due to the infiltration of cardiac muscle with lymphocytes.

Skin form usually appears in cattle in the age group of eighteen to thirteen months. Grayish white raised circular nodules are formed and widely distributed over the entire body. There is generalized enlargement of superficial and visceral lymph node. Skin form regresses and reappear.

The thymic form usually appears in cattle one to two years of age. This form is characterized by massive lymphocytic infiltration in the thymus and regional lymph nodes. There is massive enlargement of thymus with clinical signs related to compression in this area leading to neck and brisket edema and dysphagia.

The calf form or juvenile form is most often recognized in calves under six months of age. In this form, there is generalized enlargement of lymph nodes and lymphocytic infiltration in bone marrow and internal organs. There is gradual loss of weight, weakness, and other associated signs depending on location of the lesions.

DIAGNOSIS

Bovine leukemia (BL) can be diagnosed from the clinical signs, and the confirmation can be made by either antigen or antibody detection.

BL can be diagnosed on routine reproductive palpations as the tumors often develop in the uterus. BL should always be suspected in older cows with enlarged internal lymph nodes. Antemortem diagnosis of BL can be established by aspiration cytology of enlarged lymph nodes. Hematological finding reveals persistent lymphocytosis. Often the lymphocyte count approaches 100 000/ μL. Neoplastic tumors are identified by histological examinations.

BLV infection can be assumed when postmortem examination of adult cattle reveals lymphomatous tumor in multiple sites. Grossly these tumors are soft, gray-white, and can include friable areas of necrosis.

Microscopically, lymphoid cells are observed in abundance in affected organs. BLV causes a persistent infection and demonstration of antibodies can be used to identify infected animals. Seroconversion occurs from three weeks to three months.

The first serological test developed for the diagnosis of bovine leukemia virus infection was the agar gel immunodiffusion test using an internal protein gp24 polypeptide (Miller and Olson, 1972). Later, the gp51 protein was found to give higher sensitivity to this test, and this antigen was either mixed with or used to replace gp24 antigen.

Radioimmunoassay(RIA) employing both gp24 and gp51 antigens (Davare et al., 1976; Box et al., 1979; Choi et al., 2002) is being used in the epidemiological studies.

Enzyme-linked immunosorbent assay (ELISA) using serum samples and milk samples was developed and found to have higher sensitivity and specificity (Memmerickx et al., 1984; Memmerickx et al., 1985; Ridge and Galvin, 2005). The Herdchek anti-BLV test is an enzyme immunoassay for the detection and verification of antibody to highly immunogenic envelope glycoprotein gp51 of the bovine leukemia virus, which can be applied on serum or milk. The Chekit leukotest screening milk test kit is an enzyme immunoassay for the detection of antibody to bovine leukemia virus.

Polymerase chain reaction (PCR) has been effectively used in the diagnosis of BLV (Gutierrez et al., 2001; Lew et al., 2004; Felmer et al., 2006; Kohara et al., 2006).

Specific tumors-associated antigens (TAA) had been detected on bovine leucosis tumor cells and lymphocytes of cattle infected with BLV without any evidence of lymphosarcoma (Onuma and Olson, 1977).

DIFFERENTIAL DIAGNOSIS
Wide range of clinical signs at various age groups makes the definitive diagnosis of BL often difficult. Tuberculosis, Johne's disease, traumatic pericarditis, and theileriosis are some of the diseases to be differentiated. Tuberculosis and Johne's diseases can be differentiated using specific allergic tests and molecular tests, whereas traumatic pericarditis by the characteristic hematological changes, clinical signs, and absence of weakness. Theileriosis can be diagnosed by identification of the organisms and their response to therapy.

TREATMENT
There is no specific therapy for bovine leukemia.

PREVENTION AND CONTROL
All new cows entering the herd should be screened for BLV before adding to the herd. Simultaneously, the calves should be prevented from picking up the infection from the dam by separating them from the mother before they suck. Transmission to the newborn calves are also reduced by avoiding exposure to maternal blood at the time of parturition. Colostrum should be heated or frozen to inactivate the virus. No bloody milk is fed to the calves. Only disposable needles should be used for injections, and all instruments such as dehorners, taggers, tatooers, or surgical equipments should be disinfected between uses. Hand gloves can be cleaned or changed between cows in high-risk areas.

Prevention of entry of infection into a herd can be achieved by ensuring that all the imports into the herd have been tested at least days prior to arrival and are seronegative. Control of insect vectors is another point to be born in mind. Blood transfusions and vaccines containing blood such as those used against babesiosis and anaplasmosis must be carefully screened to ensure that they are free of the infection.

VACCINATION
So far no effective vaccine is developed and in use against bovine leucosis.

ERADICATION
BLV has been eradicated from many countries using a test and slaughter policy. In 1996 after thirty years of effort, Finland completely eradicated the infection from its cattle (Nutio et al., 2003).

REFERENCES

1. Box, F., Bruck, C., Mammerickx, M., Portetelle, D., Ghysdael, J., Cleuter, X., Leclercq, M., Dekegel, D. and Burny, A. 1979. Humoral immune response to bovine leukemia virus infection in cattle and sheep. *Cancer. Res.* 39:1118–1123.

2. Brenner, J., Meriom, R., Avraham, R., Trainin, Z. and Sevir, D. 1986. Prevalence of Bovine leukemia virus (BLV) infectivity in some Israeli dairy herds. *Israel Journal of Veterinary Medicin* 42:11–15.

3. Burridge, M. J. Puhr, D. M. and Hennemann, J. M. 1981. Prevalence of Bovine leukemia virus infection in Florida. *J. Am. Vet. Med. Assoc.* 7:704–707.

4. Carneiro, P. A. M., Ascujo, W. P., Bergel, E. H. and Souza, K. W. 2003. Prevalence of infection with bovine leucosis virus in dairy cattle raised in Amazon state, Brazil. *Acta Amazonica* 33:111–125.

5. Choi, K. Y., Liu, R. B. and Buehring, G. C. 2002. Relative sensitivity and specificity of AGID, EIA and immunoblotting for detection of anti bovine leukemia virus antibodies in cattle. *J. Virol. Methods* 104:33–39.

6. Davare, S. G., Stephenson, J. R., Sarma, P. S., Aaronson, S. A. and Chander, S. 1976. Bovine lymphosarcoma: Development of a radioimmunologic technique for detection of the etiologic agent. *Science USA* 194:1428–1430.

7. Donham, K. J. 1980. Epidemiologic relation of bovine population and human leukemia in Iowa. *Am. J. Epidemiol.* 112:80–92.

8. Felmer, R., Zuniga, I., Recabel, M. and Charez, R. 2006. Diagnosis and typing of bovine leukemia virus using a PCR-RFLP test on DNA extracted from somatic cells in milk. *Archieves de Medicina Vetrianria* 38:252–257.

9. Gonda, M. 1992. Bovine immunodeficiency virus. *AIDS* 6:759–776.

10. Graves, D. C. and Ferrer, J. F. 1976. *In vitro* transmission and propagation of the bovine leukemia virus in monolayer cell cultures. *Cancer Res.* 36:4152–4159.

11. Gutierrez, S. E., Dokini, G. L., Arroyo, G. H., Rodriguez-Dubra, C., Ferrer, J. F. and Esteban, E. N. 2001. Development and evaluation of an highly sensitive and specific blocking ELISA and PCR assay for diagnosis of leukemia virus infection in cattle. *Am. J. Vet. Res.* 62:1571–1577.

12. Itohara, S., Oikawa Terui, S., and Mizuno, Y. 1985. Infectivities of bovine leukemia virus in peripheral blood lymphocytes from naturally infected cattle and their relation to persistent lymphocytosis and antibody titres. *Japanese Journal of Veterinary Science* 47:807–810.

13. Johnson, R. and Kaneene, J. B. 1992. Bovine leukemia virus and enzootic bovine leucosis. *Vet. Bull.* 62:287–312.

14. Kohara, J., Konnai, S. and Ohema, M. 2006. Experimental transmission of bovine leukemia virus in cattle *via* rectal palpation. *Japaneses J. Vet. Res.* 54:25–30.

15. Lew, A. E., Bock, R. E., Molloy, J. B., Minchin, C. M., Robinson, S. J. and Steer, P. 2004. Sensitive and specific detection of proviral bovine leukemia virus by 5'Taq nucleases PCR using a 3'mirror groove binder fluorgenic probe. *J. Virol. Methods* 115:167–175.

16. McClure, H. M., Keeling, M. E., Custer, R. P., Marshak, R. R., Abt, D. A. and Ferrer, J. F. 1974. Erythroleukemia in two infant chimpanzees fed milk from cows naturally infected with the bovine C-type virus. *Cancer Res.* 34:2745–2757.

17. Mammerickx, M., Portetelle, D. and Bruck, C. 1984. Diagnosis of enzootic bovine leucosis with an enzyme linked immunosorbent assay test (ELISA) utilizing monoclonal antibody. *Anneles de Medicine Veterinaire.* 128:55–63.

18. Mammerickx, M., Portetelle, D. and Burny, A. 1985. Application of an immunosorbent assay (ELISA) involving monoclonal antibody for detection of BLV antibodies in individual or pooled bovine milk samples. *Zentralblattfurr Veterimedicine* B 32:526–533.

19. Meas, S., Usui, T., Ohashi K., Sugimold, S. and Onuma, M. 2002. Vertical transmission of bovine leukemia virus and bovine immunodeficiency virus in dairy cattle herds. *Vet. Microbiol.* 84:275–282.

20. Merion, R., Brenner, J., Gluckman, A., Avraham, R. and Trainin, Z. 1985. Humoral and cellular responses in calves experimentally infected with bovine leukemia virus (BLV). *Vet. Immunol. Immunopathol.* 9:105–114.

21. Miller, J. M. and Olson, C. 1972. Precipitating antibody to an internal antigen of the C-type virus associated with bovine lymphosarcoma. *J. National Cancer Institut* 49:1459–1462.

22. Nutio, L., Rusanen, H., Sihvonen, L. and Neuvonen, E. 2003. Eradication of enzootic bovine leukosis from Finland. *Prev. Vet. Med.* 30:43–49.

23. Onuma, M. and Olson, C. 1977. Tumour associated antigen in bovine and ovine lymphosarcoma. *Cancer. Res.* 37:3249–3256.

24. Ridge, S. E. and Galvin, J. W. 2005. A comparison of two ELISAs for the detection of antibodies to bovine leucosis virus in bulk milk. *Aust. Vet. J.* 83:431–434.

25. Sargeant, J. M. 1997. Associations between farm management practices, productivity and bovine leukemia virus infection in Ontario dairy herds. *Prev. Vet. Med.* 31:211–221.

26. Trono, K. G. 2001. Seroprevalence of bovine leukemia virus in dairy cattle in Argentina: Comparision of sensitivity and specificity of different detection methiods. *Vet. Microbiol.* 83:23–248.

27. VanLeeuwen, J. A. 2001. Seroprevalence of infection with *Mycobacterium avium subspecies paratuberculosis,* bovine leukemia virus and bovine viral diarrhoea virus in martime Canada dairy cattle. *Can. Vet. J.* 42:193–198.

28. Wang, C. T., Chang, C. H. and Lin, P. C. 1986. Serological survey on bovine leukemia virus infection in Taiwan. *J. Chinese Soc. Vet. Sci.* 12:7–14.

29. Zaghawa, A., Beier, D., El-Rahim, I. H. A. A., El-Ballal, S., Karim, J., Conraths, J. J. and Marquardt, O. 2002. An outbreak of enzootic bovine leucosis in upper Egypt: Clinical, laboratory and molecular-epidemiological studies. *J. Vet. Med* B 49:123–129.

5. BOVINE POX: COWPOX AND BUFFALO POX
(Variola, Vaccinia)

COWPOX: THANKAM MATHEW, M. R. SASEENDRANATH, AND M. KRISHNAN NAIR

BUFFALO POX: THANKAM MATHEW

INTRODUCTION

Under bovine pox, there are two pox diseases affecting cattle, namely, (a) cowpox and (b) buffalo pox. Since antiquity, pock diseases were affecting human and animals. The earliest pock diseases as epidemic noted was in China 1122 BC (Smadel, 1948). Hutyra et al. (1946) reported that the pock disease was known in ancient India. In the blacks of Central Africa, the pock disease occurred long before Christian era. But in Europe, pock disease first appeared in the sixteenth century. In Western Hemisphere, after the first voyage of Columbus, pock disease was introduced with a rapid spread all over the Central and South Africa.

Goodpasture (1933) was the first to place the poxviruses in genus *Borreleota* in memory of Borrel, who was the first to describe the elementary bodies of fowl pox. Fenner and Burnet (1957) classified poxviruses according to the morphology, antigenic relationship, presence of DNA in the virus as pox group as (1) the pox variola (smallpox), (2) pox officinale (vaccinia), (3) pox bovis (cowpox), (4) pox muris (ectromelia), (5) pox avium (fowl pox), and (6) pox myxomatosis. Weiner et al. (1964) classified pox group of viruses into several subgroups as follows:

1. *Variola vaccinia subgroup.* (a) variola major, (b) variola minor, (c) vaccinia, (d) cowpox, (e) ectromelia, (f) monkey pox, and (g) rabbit pox.
2. *Avian poxviruses.* (a) fowl pox, (b) canary pox, (c) pigeon pox, and (g) turkey pox.
3. *Myxoma-like viruses.* (a) rabbit myxoma and (b) rabbit fibroma,
4. *Viruses affecting ungulates.* (a) camel pox, (b) goat pox, and (c) horse pox.
5. *Miscellaneous group.* (a) molluscum contagiosum.

Later (Joklik, 1966); Andrews and Pereira (1972); Baxby (1975, 1984b); Fenner (1976); Nakano (1979); Matthews (1979) classified pox group of viruses, including buffalo poxvirus, which is given in detail by Mathew

(1993). In 1993, Mathew reviewed the previous scientist classification and classified the pox group of viruses as follows:

FAMILY POXVIRUS (POX VIRIDAE)

Subfamily

I. **Chordopox Viridae** (poxviruses of vertebrates)
II. **Entamopox Viridae** (poxvirus of insects)

1. **Chordopox Viridae**

Generae

A. **Vaccinia Variola Subgroup (Orthopoxvirus)**

1. Vaccinia virus (vaccine strain)
2. Buffalo poxvirus (buffaloes)
3. Camel poxvirus (camel)
4. Cowpox (bovines, man, and unknown reservoir host, probably rat and cat)
5. Ectromelia virus (mice)
6. Monkey pox (monkey, man, and unknown reservoir hosts)
7. Rabbit poxvirus (rabbit)
8. Lenny virus (probably buffalo pox, hybrid of variola and vaccinia)
9. Variola virus (man) a. Variola major b. Variola intermedia c. Variola minor

B. **Orf Subgroup (Parapoxvirus)**

1. Orf
2. Bovine pustular stomatitis virus
3. Contageous ecthyma virus
4. Milker's nodule virus

C. **Fowl Pox (Avipox Virus)**

1. Fowl pox
2. Canary pox
3. Junco poxvirus
4. Pigeon poxvirus
5. Quail poxvirus
6. Sparrow poxvirus

7. Starling virus
8. Turkey poxvirus
9. Peacock poxvirus

D. Sheep Pox (Capripoxvirus)

1. Sheep poxvirus
2. Goat poxvirus
3. Lumpy skin virus (white cattle)

E. Swine Poxvirus

1. Swine poxvirus

F. Myxo Subgroup Leporipox

1. Hare fiboma virus
2. Rabbit (Shope fibroma virus)
3. Squirrel fibroma virus

G. Other Members of the Vertebrates

1. Carnivore pox (cat, cheetah, okapi, and anteaters)
2. Elephant poxvirus (elephant)
3. Molluscum contagiosum
4. Racoon poxvirus (raccoon)
5. Tana poxvirus
6. Yaba monkey pox (from Yaba, Nigeria)
7. White pox (variant of monkey pox) in monkeys
8. Gerbil poxvirus (in gerbil)
9. Auzduk (camel pox, contagious ecthyma of camel)
10. Seal poxvirus (seal)
11. Cotiapox (from sentinel mice in Cotia Colony, Brazil)
12. Fish poxvirus (fish)

Cowpox

Thankam Mathew, M. R. Saseendranath, and M. Krishnan Nair

Cowpox is a contagious viral disease of cows characterized by development of vesicles, pustules, and scabs on teat and udder.

Etiology

Cowpox is caused by a virus belonging to the family Poxviridae and the genus *Orthopoxvirus*. It is a double-stranded (ds) DNA virus. The virus particles are brick shaped having a diameter of 250–300 nm in diameter. Cowpox virus is very closely related to vaccinia and buffalo poxviruses (Mathew, 1987). There is complete cross-protection between buffalo pox and cowpox. This virus grows well on the chorioallantoic membrane of seven to thirteen-day-old embryonated eggs with hemorrhagic spots at the center without perforation and with embryo mortality of 30%, which can be differentiated from vaccinia and buffalo pox (Mathew, 1987). Hemagglutinin of cowpox virus agglutinates turkey and fowl erythrocytes. The virus can also be grown on chicken, human, bovine, rabbit, (RK) kidney, and Vero cell lines. Mathew (1987) reported a detailed study of cowpox in comparison with buffalo pox, vaccinia on RK, monkey kidney (MK), hamster kidney (HK), and human amnion (HuA) cell culture with the production of CPE. Hemadsorption studies in tissue culture was reported by Mathew (1967a, b) as sunflower-like hemadsorption with fowl, human "O", rabbit, guinea pig, and dog red cells with cowpox, in comparison with other mammalian poxvirus—namely, buffalo pox, vaccinia, and sheep pox.

Epidemiology

Cowpox is sporadic in occurrence. There is loss of milk production as a result of improper letting down of milk due to pain because of soreness of teat and rarely mastitis. It was the observation of Jenner in 1798 that milkmaids who had been infected with cowpox virus were resistant to smallpox that led to the science of vaccinology (Willis, 1997).

Distribution

Sporadic cases of cowpox occur in UK, European, and Asian countries.

Source of Infection

This virus is endemic in small rodents such as wild ground squirrels, gerbils, voles (*Microtus* sp.), and wood mice in Europe and Asia. Marennikova and Sheluhina (1976) also reported that in Russia, cowpox virus produced panzootic infection among Felidae animals like lion, cheetah, etc., in Moscow. Marennikova et al. (1978) and Marennikova (1979) pointed out that rodents acted as reservoir for cowpox and became a source of infection in okapi and elephants. Wild and domestic felids are usually affected by hunting rodents. Cheetah, panther, lion, puma, jaguar, ocelot, lynx, anteater, elephant, and rhinoceros also act as sources of infection (Chantrey et al., 1999; Hazel et al., 2000). Cowpox virus infection can occur in a number of different mammalian species, one of which is cattle. Hence, cattle is acting as an incidental host.

TRANSMISION
Cows can be infected from farm cats or human beings. Cow-to-cow transmission is mainly from through milker's hand or teat cup of milking machine. According to Baxby (1977), cowpox can bring about severe, infection in human beings. Although cowpox infections in cows were usually very mild, it becomes more virulent when it affected an unusual host. Marennikova and Sheluhina (1976) proved that white rats used as food were a source of infection, which in turn contracted infection from wild rodents. Introduction of infected animal facilitates transmission from herd to herd. Cowpox can also be transmitted by biting insects.

HOSTS
Endemic in certain rodents in Europe and East Asia, cattle are a rare and incidental host. Young calves are more susceptible than old cows. Incidence is more in female because of contact with milker's hand. Incidence has been recorded more in temperate zones during winter. In an area where the disease is endemic, only heifers and newly introduced animals are likely to develop the clinical signs. Cowpox virus has got a wide range of hosts like rabbit, guinea pig, mouse, monkey, and human being. The disease mainly occurs in cows and is transmissible to human beings. But in human beings, the infection is likely to occur from infected cats rather than from cows. Baxby et al. (1982) studied an outbreak of pox in captive cheetahs at Whipnande park of UK in 1977. Their investigation proved that virologically, the virus resembled cowpox in pock appearance on CAM and ceiling temperature. Cow pox infection in cows were usually very mild, but it becomes more virulent when it affected an unusual host. Rodents can also act as reservoir host of cowpox virus, which can also infect another carnivorous host. Baxby et al. (1979 and 1982) reported pox outbreak in two out of three cheetahs in another English zoo in November 1978. Thomasett et al. (1978) were the first to show that domestic cats could be infected by poxvirus, and they could isolate the virus resembled that of cowpox. Later, Horne et al. (1984) reported seven cases of cat pox in UK. Gaskell et al. (1983) reproduced pock infection by intravenous injection in cats and on cultivation on CAM

produced hemorrhagic pock, and the morphology of the particles was identified as orthopoxvirus. The virus isolated neutralized the cow pox antiserum. Thomsett et al. (1978), Gaskell et al. (1983), and Horne et al. (1984) identified cat pox as cowpox because of the above findings. Baxby (1984a) also identified seventeen isolates of cat pox as cowpox. Bennet et al. (1986, 1990) reviewed feline cowpox virus infection in domestic cats, and they also concluded that cowpox virus infection was an increasingly recognized condition of cats in UK. Schonabauer et al. (1982) studied pox infection in domestic cats and suggested the possible pathogenicity of the poxvirus in man.

Pether et al. (1986) reported the occurrence of cowpox virus infection in a man and in his six-year-old daughter, who got the infection from their ten-year-old cat. Mathew (1990) also reported poxlike infection of her pet cat in Delhi, India, and her fourteen-year-old daughter also got infection from the cat, showing rise in temperature with small pinpoint scabs with itching all over the body. According to Ganiev and Farzaliev (1964), cows get infected on the teats of following vaccination of the workers on a farm in North Ossetian, Byelorussia, USSR, and Tatar in USSR. The skin lesion appeared after nine to thirteen days after vaccination of the workers. Korzenko (1964) reported the disease spread through udder cloths, from one farm to another, and also by milk cans and streams. Baxby and Bennet (1994) reviewed cowpox infection in fifty-four cases of human cases.

Dogs are relatively resistant (Smith et al., 1999), but a case of cowpox in human being had been reported to be transmitted from a dog (Baxby et al., 1982).

PATHOGENESIS
Virus access to tissues is through injuries of teat and udder. Papules appear on the second or third day. Vesicles are seen in one to two days. Central umbulication, rupture and secondary complication, suppuration drying into crusts and scabs occur.

CLINICAL SIGNS
The clinical pox syndrome in cows can be brought about by the virus of vaccinia, cowpox, and paravaccinia. The true cowpox is identical with Downie cowpox, produced only by the cowpox that is different from vaccinia and paravaccinia.

The incubation period is three to seven days. The cattle may show slight fever, anorexia, and cessation of rumination followed by appearance of lesions on teat and udder, which pass through all stages of pox infection. Typical pox lesions are on the teats and udder. Erythema, papules with a zone of hyperemia around the base, vesiculation, pustular stage, and scab formation are noticed in that order. True cowpox scabs are 1–2 cm in diameter and are thick, tenacious, and yellow brown to red in color. Secondary mastitis is seen in some cases. Udder becomes hyperemic, swollen, and painful. In bulls, the lesions are seen on the scrotum.

Generally, the lesions heal in two weeks' time, but in some animals, fresh crops of lesions may develop and may cause the disease to persist for a month or more. Lesions are confined to teats and lower parts of udder. In severe cases, the lesions may spread to inside the thighs and rarely to perineum, vulva, and mouth. Lesions heal in two weeks' time. Sometimes fresh crops of lesions may cause the disease to persist for a month or more. Sucking calves develop pock lesions around mouth.

Immune Response

Recovery results in solid immunity. Calves acquire passive immunity from colostrum of immunized dam. Hence, following an outbreak, subsequent immunity protects the cows for several years.

Diagnosis

Cow pox can be diagnosed from clinical signs. Firm dark red circular lesions with raised edges and depressed centers on teat and udder are characteristic.

Isolation and identification of the virus in tissue cultures and embryonic egg inoculation is a routinely adopted method for the isolation and identification of the virus. Hemorrhagic pock lesions on the chorioallantoic membrane (CAM) of embryonated egg is of diagnostic value to differentiate from other poxlike vaccinia and buffalo pox (Mathew, 1987). Inoculation on cornea and scarified skin rabbit is another method of diagnosis. Demonstration of the virus by electron microscopy is a confirmatory method.

Serological tests like immunofluorescence and enzyme-linked immunosorbent assay (Hazel et al., 2000; Jana and Mehrothra, 2000) are also being used widely. Individual strains of cowpox virus can be identified by using restriction endonucleases digestion pattern (Loperev et al., 2001).

Differential Diagnosis

Cowpox has to be differentiated from pseudocowpox, foot-and-mouth disease (FMD), vesicular stomatitis, vesicular exanthema ulcerative mammillitis.

Pseudocowpox is caused by a parapoxvirus. Pseudocowpox primarily affects cows in early lactation, slow spreading, and long healing time. Disease lasts for eighteen months in a herd.

Vesicles of FMD, vesicular exanthema, and vesicular stomatitis are larger, which do not develop from papules as in the case of pox. There will not be any vesicular lesions in oral and nasal mucous membrane and at interdigital space in cowpox.

Bovine ulcerative mammilitis is caused by a bovine herpes virus 2 (BHV-2) and rarely BHV-4, which occurs usually two weeks after calving, followed by persistent infection in the herd. There is vesicle leading to sloughing of skin, which leads to severe ulceration. Clinical course is prolonged.

TREATMENT
Palliative therapy like cleaning the pock lesions with antiseptic lotions and application of mild antiseptic to prevent secondary bacterial infection is the line of treatment.

PREVENTION AND CONTROL
Quarantine of new addition, segregation of the affected animals from healthy ones, separate attendants for the affected and diseased, milking the affected last and the healthy first in order to reduce the transmission through the hands of the milker or through the milking machine are some important control measures to be adopted. Udder, cloths, milking machines, and hands should be disinfected after contact with infected animals. Quaternary ammonium compounds are the best disinfectants.

As the flies are also playing a role in the transmission of the infection, measures to reduce fly population have to be undertaken by avoiding breeding places for flies and by spraying insecticides.

VACCINATION
No specific vaccine is available at present, though vaccinia virus can be used prophylactically.

ERADICATION
Measure to reduce the rodent population, fly population, avoidance of contact with rodents and cats are some measures to achieve eradication of this disease.

REFERENCES

1. Andrewes, C. and Pereira, H. G. 1972. Pox viruses. In *Viruses of vertebrates* ED. III, 373–413. London: Bailliere and Tindall.
2. Baxby, D. 1975. Identification and interrelationship of variola, vaccinia subgroup of pox virus. *Prog. Med. Virol.* 19:215–246.
3. Baxby, D. 1977. Is cow pox misnamed? A review of 10 human cases. *Brit. Med. Journal* 1:137–1381.
4. Baxby, D., Shackletor, W. B., Wheeler, J. and Turner, A. 1979. A comparison of cow pox like virus isolated from European zoos. *Arch. Virol.* 61:337–340.
5. Baxby, D. 1984a. Cow pox infection of cats. *Vet. Record* 115:91.
6. Baxby, D. 1984b. Pox virus. In *Topley and Wilson's principales of bacteriology, virology, and immunity.* Vol. 4 *Virology*, 7th ed. New York: Arnold Publishers.
7. Baxby, D., Ashton, D. G., Jones, D. M. and Thomsett, L. R. 1982. An outbreak of cowpox in captive cheetahs: Virological and epidemiological studies. *J. Hyg.* (London) 89:365–372.
8. Baxby, D. and Bennett, M. 1994. Human cowpox 1969–1993. A review based on 54 cases. *Brit. J. Dermatology* 131:598–607.
9. Bennett, M., Gaskell, C. J., Gaskell, R. M., Baxby, D. and Gruffydd Jones, T. J. 1986. Pox virus infection in domestic cat. *Vet. Record* 118:387–390.
10. Bennett, M., Gaskell, C. J., Baxby, D., Gaskell, R. M., Kelly, D. F. and Naidoo, J. 1990. Feline cowpox virus infection. *J. Small Anim. Pract.* 31:167–173.
11. Chantrey, J., Meyer, H., Baxby, D., Begon, M., Bown, K. J., Hazel, S. M., Jones, T., Montgomery, W. I. and Bennett, M. 1999. Cowpox reservoir hosts and geographic range. *Epidemiol. Infect.* 122:455–460.
12. Fenner, F. 1976. Classification and Nomenclature of virus. *Intervirology* 7:1–115.
13. Fenner, F. and Burnet. F. M. 1957. A short description of the pox virus group (vaccinia and related virus group). *Virology* 4:305–314.
14. Ganiev, M. K. and Farzaliev, I. A. 1964. Pox in buffaloes from contact with vaccinated human beings. *Veterinariya Moscow* 41:31–34.
15. Gaskell, R. M., Gaskell, C. J., Evans, R. J., Dennis, P. E., Bennett, R. M., Udall, N. D., Voyle, E. and Hill, T. J. 1983. Natural and experimental pox virus infection in the domestic cat. *Vet. Record* 112:164.
16. Goodpasture, E. W. 1933. Boreliotoses, fowlpox, molluscum contagiosum, variola, vaccinia. *Science* 77:119–121.
17. Hazel, S. M., Bennet, M., Cantrey, J., Bown, K., Cavanagh, R., Jones, T. R., Baxby, D. and Begon, M. 2000. A longitudinal study of an endemic disease in its wildlife reservoir: Cowpox and wild rodents. *Epidemiology and Infection* 124:551–562.
18. Horne, C. M., Gruffydd-Jone, J. J., Bennett, M., Gaskell, R. M. and Baxby, D. 1984. Cow pox in Cats. *Vet Record* 11:22–22.
19. Hutyra, F., Marek, J. and Manninger, R. 1946. In *Special pathology and therapeutics of the disease of domestic animals.* Vol. 1, 4th ed., 367–403. London: Tindall and Cox.
20. Jana, D. and Mehrothra, M. L. 2000. Standardization of a dot enzyme linked immunosorbent assay for the sero diagnosis of experimental cow pox virus infection and humoral immunity in rabbits. *Indian Vet. J.* 77:281–284.
21. Joklik, W. K. 1966. The pox viruses. *Bacterial Review* 30:33–66.
22. Korzenko, V. N. 1964. Pox in cows during vaccination of the human population. *Veterinarya. Moscow* 41:31–34.

23. Loperev, V. M., Messing, R. F., Esposito, J. J. and Meyer, H. 2001. Detection and differentiation of old world Orthopox viruses. Restriction fragment length polymorphism of the crm B gene region. *J. Clinical. Microbiol.* 39:94–100.

24. Marennikova, S. S. 1979. Field and experimental studies of pox viruses infection in rodents. *Bull. WHO* 57:467–464.

25. Marennikova, S. S. and Sheluhina, E. M. 1976. White rats as a source of pox infection in carnevores of the family felidae. *Acta. Virol.* 20:442.

26. Marennekova, S. S., ladnyi, I. D., Ogorodnikova, Z. I., Shelukhina, E. M. and Maltseva, M. M. 1978. Identification and study of pox virus isolated from wild rodents in Turkmenia. *Arch. Virol.* 56:7–14.

27. Mathew, T. 1967a. Virus study of pock disease among buffaloes. *Indian. J. Path. Bact.* 10:101–102.

28. Mathew, T. 1967b. Cultivation and immunological studies on pox group of viruses. PhD thesis, Madras University–Haffkine Institute Bombay.

29. Mathew, T. 1987. In *Advances in medical, and veterinary virology, immunology and epidemiology. Cultivation and immunological studies on pox group of viruses with special reference to buffalo pox virus.* Vol. 1, 4–171. New Delhi: Thajema Publishers.

30. Mathew, T. 1990. Clinical picture of pox like infection of cats in India. *Indian Vet. J.* 67:61–62.

31. Mathew, T. 1993. Classification of pox group of viruses including buffalopox virus. In *"Advances in medical and veterinary virology, immunology and epidemiology. Vol. 2. Buffalopox(ortho pox) virus and it's zoonotic importance.",* 11-26. New Delhi: Thajema publishers.

32. Matthews, R. E. F. 1979. Classification and nomenclature of viruses. *Intervirology* 12:3–5.

33. Nakano, J. H. 1979. Pox viruses. In *Diagnostic procedure for viral and rickettsial and chlamydeal infections,* 5th ed., ed. E. H. Lennette and N. Schmidt, 257–308.

34. Pether, J. V. S., Trevains, P. H., Harrison, S. R. B., Baxby, D. Bennet, M. and Gibbs, E. P. J. 1986. Cow pox from cat to man. *Lancet* 1:38–39.

35. Smadel, J. E. 1948. Viral and rickettesial infection of man. T. M. Rivers and F. L. Horsfall Jr. 1st ed. 314–336. Philadelphia: J. B. Lippincott Co.

36. Schonabauer, M. Schonbauer, A., Langle, A. and Kolbl, S. 1982. Pox infection in a domestic cat. *Zentral blatt fur veterinary medizin* 29:434–440.

37. Smith, K. C., Bennett, M. and Garett, D. C. 1999. Skin lesions caused by *Orthopox* virus infection in a dog. *J. Small Anim. Pract.* 44:495–497.

38. Thomasett, L. R., Baxby, D. and Denham, E. M. 1978. Cow pox in the domestic cat. *Vet. Record* 108:567.

39. Weiner, L. M., Macko, I., Poulik, E. and Goodman, N. 1964. Salt requirement for precipitation of chicken antisera in agar immunoelectrophoresis. *J. immunol.* 93:228–231.

40. Willis, J. N. 1997. Edward Jenner and the eradication of small pox. *Scottish Med. J.* 42:118–121.

Buffalo Pox

Thankam Mathew

Introduction

Buffalo poxvirus, an important zoonotic diseases, affects buffaloes with high morbidity and productivity losses, and it is closely related to vaccinia virus than cowpox (Mathew, 1967). Buffalo pox (BP) was reported from the countries where buffaloes are reared, mainly in India, Pakisthan, Indonesia, and Egypt. For the first time, BP infection was reported from India by Sharma from Lahore in 1934 (at that time Lahore was in India).

History

Coming to the history of pox infection, due to poxviruses, it was present in antiquity. The first evidence of smallpox was found in Egyptian mummies of the Eighteenth Dynasty (1580–1350 BC). In India, variola became endemic in the first millennium BC and spread to Asia and, ultimately, to Europe in the eighteenth century. In the fifteenth and sixteenth centuries, the introduction of smallpox to the New World destroyed the Native American populations. During the French-Indian Wars, the British used smallpox as a biological weapon. Smallpox continued to be a major worldwide problem well into the twentieth century and produced half-million deaths per year in Europe. In the twentieth century, naturally occurring smallpox was eradicated through an intense program of vaccination. The smallpox was reduced through the origin of vaccination. By applying the dried material of smallpox to the skin, it caused a milder infection in human and produced permanent immunity, which led to the practice of variolization. In the nineteenth century, inoculation with cowpox virus, a close relative of smallpox, led to smallpox immunity by Jenner, and this established the practice of vaccination, although variolization continued into the twentieth century.

The Chronological Occurrence of Buffalo Pox

As early as 1934, Sharma named buffalo pox as an interesting outbreak of variola vaccinia from Lahore. Bhatia (1936), from Hissar, reported as variola on the eyes and around the ears of buffaloes; Mukundu, in 1936, reported from Bangalore, Ramapratab, (1937) as an acute mastitis as a sequel of variola in buffaloes; Warrier (1937) reported as variola in buffaloes from Vadakachery, Kerala; Maqsuid (1944) reported as generalized vaccinia in buffaloes in Punjab; Mohan (1948) reported pox infection in buffaloes followed by *Corynebacterium* infection in

Utterpradesh; Haddow and Idnani (1949) reported buffalo pox in Punjab; Ramkrishnan and Anandapadmanabhan (1957) reported protection against buffalo pox by vaccinia from Andra Pradhesh; Maqsood (1958) again reported buffalo pox infection in Pakisthan; Paranaik et al. (1963) reported as cowpox in buffaloes in Bombay; Mathew (1963–64) reported buffalo pox from Arey Milk Colony, Goregaon, Bombay, and took up a detailed study during 1963 to 1967 on buffalo poxvirus by collecting buffalo pox scabs from dairy farms at Jogeswari and Goregaon in Bombay as follows: (1) cultivation of buffalo poxvirus in different tissue cultures on (a) primary monkey kidney, (b) rabbit kidney, (c) hamster kidney, and (d) human amnion tissue cultures by primary passages as qualitative and quantitative studies; (2) serial passages as qualitative and quantitative in tissue cultures; (3) studies on CAM in comparison with other poxviruses (namely, vaccinia, cowpox, goat pox, sheep pox, swine pox, and fowl pox); (4) hemadsoption study with various species RBC on tissue culture-passaged poxviruses; (5) immunological studies of buffalo poxvirus to find out the antigenic components and cross-reaction with other members of poxviruses by using gel diffusion test and hemagglutination inhibition test; and (6) interference of buffalo pox and other poxviruses by the Ranikhet disease virus (Lasota strain) chick interferon for the PhD research. Again, Mathew et al. (1978) reported buffalo pox from Dhulia Dt. Maharashtra during 1975–76; Arnold et al. (1976) also reported buffalo pox epidemic from Egypt; Mallik and Dwivedi (1982) reported clinical outbreak of buffalo pox in Barely, UP; Sulochana et al. (1983) reported buffalo pox outbreak in Mannarghat of Kerala State, India.; Chandra et al. (1986) reported pox infection of buffaloes from India. Kolhapure et al. (1997) investigated buffalo pox outbreaks in Maharastra State during 1992–1996 and isolated twenty-two virus from the skin scabs of humans infected and milch cattles. They also noted that a few children showed clinical manifestations on the face, arm, and buttocks, who have no contact with the infected animals but contact with parents or other members of the family who had infection, which clearly indicated the possibility of man-to-man transmission of buffalo pox infection. Nedunchellivan et al. (1992) also reported buffalo pox infection in man from Namakkal Tamilnadu (Madras State). WHO (1996) reported five pediatric cases of buffalo poxvirus infection from two villages of Maharashtra where cattle were also infected. According to Ligda (1998) during buffalo pox outbreaks in India, 33.3% buffaloes were infected, while 25% cattle were infected with B. pox, and 20% milkers were affected, and the lesions by B. poxvirus was larger, and the duration of the diseases was shorter compared to cowpox virus infection. Also, sporadic infection in children were noted with B. poxvirus, which resembled more to human smallpox. Anand Kumar and Butchaiah have done the partial antigenic characterization of buffalo poxvirus in 2004. Singh et al. (2006 a) studied in detailed way on the outbreak of buffalo pox in dairy herds of Aurangabad and isolated the virus in Vero cells and detected the viral nucleotide sequence by polymerase chain reaction (PCR), serum neutralization, and nucleic acid sequencing. Singh et al. (2006b) again gave details of various tests to identify the BP isolates in tissue culture. During outbreaks of BP in buffaloes, human beings who have contact with the infected animals were also affected.

As per Shanley et al. (2006), infections due to the members of the Poxviridae family occur in humans and animals, and the Orthopoxviruses include smallpox (variola), monkey pox, vaccinia, cowpox, buffalo pox, cantagalo, and aracatuba viruses. Parapoxviruses contain orf virus, bovine papular stomatitis virus, pseudocowpox virus, deer poxvirus, and seal poxvirus. Yata poxviruses consist of tana poxvirus and Yaba poxviruses, which are found primarily in Africa, include the human poxvirus. Molluscum contagiosum virus is in Molluscipoxviruses. In humans, smallpox and molluscum are specific. In humans, vaccinia virus also produce generalized infection, which has been used for vaccination.

Afia Zafar et al. (2007) reported the buffalo pox infection in human beings in Pakisthan who were admitted in the burns unit. The lesions noted were very near the burn wounds of their body. The human beings were not having the contact with infected buffaloes. According to Afia Zafir et al. (2007), the infection they got through the application of butter on the wound that was made from buffalo milk fat, which is the usual practice in Karachi, Pakistan. In the same year, Ramanan et al. (2007) notified two human cases of BP infection in Bhilai, MP, India, in a twenty-two-year-old milker and a twenty-year-old man working in the same dairy. Three other milkers also had the same skin lesions history and subsided within two weeks. The patient had high fever (40°C) with bilateral axillary lymphadenitis and tender lymph nodes. In the second case, blackish lesions on both hands for twelve days in palm side of the fingers, on both hands. In the second case, neither fever nor lymphadenopathy were noticed. The virus was isolated in primary chick embryo's fibroblast tissue culture as well as on the CAM. The second patient was comfortable and had no fever and lymphadenopathy. Eight out of twenty buffaloes in the diary showed multiple ulcerative lesions on the teats with reduction of milk yield almost nil. Singh et al. (2007) reviewed buffalo poxvirus diseases affected throughout the world, and they are of the opinion that buffalo pox infection is an emerging and reemerging zoonoses. According to them, generalized buffalo poxvirus infection are now rare than before.

Instead severe local infections on the udder, teat producing, mastititis and reduces the milk yield of the animals, and BP virus is phylogenetically closely related to vaccinia.

Even though buffaloes are reared in different nations, buffalo pox infection was recorded mainly from India as buffaloes are mainly used as milking cattle in India, and the infection get to buffaloes through milking man who vaccinated with calf lymph earlier as buffalo pox is more related to vaccinia than cowpox or variola.

ETIOLOGY
Buffalo pox infection is caused by a virus belonging to the family Pox Viridae and the genus *Orthopoxvirus*. It is a double-stranded DNA virus of 130 kbp. Virion is of brick shaped or oval virus with a diameter of 200–400nm.

EPIDEMIOLOGY
Buffalo pox infection was mainly reported from different countries of the world where buffaloes are reared, namely, India, Indonesia, Egypt, Pakistan, and Italy. In India, Sharma (1934) reported BP for the first time, and thereafter, it was reported from different states of India as shown in the history of BP infection.

DISTRIBUTION
Pox infection in buffaloes were noted as early as 1917 by Mr. P. P. Devassy, educated father of the author Thankam Mathew, in Trichur District, Kerala, India, and was called as *vasuri* in buffaloes as it occurred simultaneously with smallpox (*vasuri*, named from Malayalam language) in human being in Kerala, India. Sporadic cases were reported from Egypt (Arnold et al., 1976) and Asian countries where buffaloes are reared for milk production or for field work. Thus, buffalo pox was reported from India, Bangladesh, Pakistan, Russia, Indonesia, and Egypt. Mansjoer in 1951 reported outbreak as variola in buffaloes in Indonesia. Mammerickx (1960) reported buffalo pox infection as vaccinia infection from Italy.

TRANSMISSION
Buffaloes are infected through milker's hand or teat cup of milking machine as in cowpox. Nosocomal infection of buffalo pox in human was recorded in Pakisthan (2007) by Afia Zafar through buffalo milk butterfat applied on burn wounds. Usually human being recovered within three to four weeks. Man-to-man infection of BP was recorded by Kolhapure et al. (1997) in children through contact with infected person or by inhalation of infected air.

HOSTS

According to Kataria (1969), Srinivasppa and Garg (1976), and Chandra (1986), BP can be produced in rabbits and guinea pigs, but sheep, goats, adult mice, and zebu cows are not infected by BP virus. Dhogra et al. (1978) could infect Swiss infant mice with BP virus. Sulochana et al. (1983) reported that applied pox scab suspension collected from the ear lesions of buffaloes on the comb of chicken by scarification did not produce any lesions. But when they applied the same material on rabbit skin by scarification, it produced small vesicles. However, when it was applied on the skin of buffalo abdomens by scarification, it produced good vesicles with tendency to generalize and create scab formation. But in white cattle, skin scarification produced mild lesions, and in goats still milder inflammatory reactions were noticed at the site of scarification.

In humans, it can be transmitted from buffaloes who are having contact with infected buffaloes. In humans it produces localized pox lesions on the skin of the hands and forehead with fever usually for three days with lymphadenopathy and general malaise.

PATHOGENESIS AND LESIONS

Pox lesions appear on the udder, teats, and hind quarters of the infected animals. Characteristic ulcerated pox lesions with raised edges, accompanied by pain on palpitation were noted. About 50% of the infected buffaloes produce mastitis and reduced milk yield also. In addition, it reduces the working capacity of infected animals. Pockmarks with otorrhea in and around the ears were also noted by Mullick et al. (1990) in buffaloes affected near Bareilly Village. No mortality was noted in any of the buffalo pox outbreaks in Arey Milk Colony, Bombay, Dhulea, Aurangabad, epidemics or any of the epidemics reported (Mathew, 1967; Mathew and Mathew, 1986; Singh, 2006; Ramanan et al., 2007). Adult females are more prone to the buffalo poxvirus infection. Usually the incubation period is six to ten days (Mullick et al., 1990).

EFFECT OF PHYSICOCHEMICAL AGENT

Mohanty and Rai (1988) studied the effect of various physicochemical agents on buffalo poxvirus and reported that the virus grown in Vero cell culture was found to be sensitive to heat at 56°C for sixty minutes, pH 3, and chloroform. But it is ether resistant. Formalin 1:4000 inactivated completely the BP virus in eight hours, 0.05% acetyl ethyleneimine in six hours, and 0.05% beta-propiolactone in fifteen minutes.

IMMUNE RESPONSE

As in cow pox, once infected, recovered animals from BP get solid immunity. Mohanty and Rai (1989) reported immune response induced by Vero cell culture adapted BP virus in rabbit and buffaloes.

DIAGNOSIS

As in other diseases, BP can be diagnosed from clinical signs by seeing the pock lesions on the udder and teat of the buffaloes, isolation, and identification of the virus on tissue culture as well on CAM of chick embryo. The characteristic pock lesions on the CAM of chick embryo distinguish it from cowpox and vaccinia (Mathew, 1967a). In the tissue culture, by noting the CPE as well as characteristic sunflower-like hemadsoption noted with fowl RBC are of diagnostic method (Mathew, 1967b). Serum neutralization test like hemagglutination inhibition test (HI) Mathew (1967a), polymerize chain reaction (Singh et al., 2006a), counterimmunoelectroporesis (Singh et al, 2006b) are the reliable methods for identification of BP virus from other poxviruses.

DIFFERENTIAL DIAGNOSIS

BP should be differentiated from pseudocowpox caused by parapoxvirus, foot-and-mouth diseases (FMD), vesicular stomatitis, vesicular exanthema, which are larger, and there will not be any vesicular lesions in the oral and nasal mucous membrane and at interdigital space; ulcerative mammilitis caused by bovine herpes virus occurs two weeks after calving and cowpox infections by isolating the virus on the CAM and noting the hemorrhagic spots at the center of the pox lesions on CAM (Mathew, 1967a).

TREATMENT

Earlier there was no treatment for BP as in cowpox. But recently Bhanuprakash et al. (2007) succeeded by in vitro studies that the extract of leaves of the plant *Eugenia jambolana* inhibit BP virus (98.52%) without any toxic effect by conducting different cytopathic effect assays inhibition tests.

Vaccinia-specific immunoglobulin (VIG), which is an isotonic sterile solution of the immunoglobulin fraction of plasma from persons vaccinated with vaccinia vaccine, can be used to humans infected with BP. But Food and Drug Administration (FDA) has not approved yet the use of antiviral compound. Another antiviral drug ST246 have been reported to be 100% active against vaccinia and other orthopoxvirus infection, and FDA is also under study to give permission for treatment (Wikipedia the Free Encyclopedia, 2007).

PREVENTION AND TREATMENT

More or less same prevention and control for cow pox can be followed for BP prevention and treatment. Segregation of the affected animals from healthy ones is the best method. Separate milkers for the infected and healthy buffaloes to prevent transmission through milker's hand. After contact with infected buffaloes, milking machine and hands should be disinfected.

VACCINATION

No vaccination available except vaccinia virus vaccine even for buffaloes.

ERADICATION

As in cowpox, reduce fly population and avoid contact of buffaloes with the human infected with BP.

REFERENCES

1. Afia Zafar, Swanepoel, R., Hewson, R., Nizam, M., Ahmed, A., Hussain, A., Grobbelaar, A., Bewley, K., Mioulet, V., Dowsett, B., Easterbrook, L. and Hasan, R. 2007. *Emerg. Infect. Dis. (serial on the Internet)* 13:1–4.

2. Anand Kumar, P. and Butchaiah, G. 2004. Partial antigenic characterization of buffalopox virus. *Veterinary research communications* 28:543–552.

3. Arnold, D. H. L., Odom, R. B. and Jasmes, W. B. 1976. In *Viral diseases, diseases of the skin* by Andrews 8th ed. Philadelphia. From *J. Egyptian Vet. Med. Assoc.* 36:151–159.

4. Bhanuprakash, V., Hosamani, M., Balamurugan, V., Singh, R. K. and Swarup, D. 2007. *Invitro* antiviral activity of *Eugenia jambolana* plant extract on buffalopox virus: Convention and qPCR methods. *International J. Tropical Med.* 2:3–9.

5. Bhatia, S. N. 1936. Variola in the ears and around the eyes of buffaloes. *Indian Vet. J.* 12:236–2137.

6. Chandra, R., Singh, I. P., Garg, S. K. and Varshney, K. C. 1986a. Clinico pathological studies of buffalopox virus in rabbits. *Acta Virol.* 30:390–396.

7. Chandra, R., Garg, S. K., Rana, U. V. S. and Rao, V. D. P. 1986b. Pox infection of Buffaloes. *Farm Animals* 2:57–69.

8. Dhogra, S. C., Sharma, V. K. and Pandey, R. 1978. Susceptiblity of infant Swiss mice to buffalopox virus. *Vet. Rec.* 102:382–383.

9. Haddow, J. R. and Idnani, J. A. 1949. Outline of Veterinary Science Manager of Publication Karachi, Ist ed., 61–65.

10. Kataria, R. S. and Singh, I. P. 1969. A research note on the antigenic analysis of the buffalo pox virus and its comparison with vaccinia and cow pox virus. *PunjabVeterinarian* 8:25–26.

11. Kolhapure, R. M., Deolankar, R. P., Tupe, C. D., Raut, C. G., Basu, A., Dama, B. M., Pawar, S. D., Joshi, M. V., Padbiri, V. S., Goverdhan, M. K. and Banerjee, K. 1997. Investigation of buffalopox outbreak in Maharastra state during 1992–1996. *Indian. J. Med. Res.* 106:441–446.

12. Ligda, D. J. 1998. Diseases of water buffaloes. *Internet* Feb. 16, 1998.

13. Mallik, K. P. and Dwivedi, S. K. 1982. Clinical observations in an outbreak of buffalopox. *Indian Vet. J.* 59:397–398.

14. Mansjoer, M. 1951. Variola in buffaloes in Indonesia. *Hamera Zoa* 58:547–556.

15. Mammerickx, M. 1960. Le buffle, monographie du genere bubalus. *Bull. agric. congobelge.* 51:171–211.

16. Mathew, T. 1966. Cultivation and immunological studies on pox group of viruses. Propagation of vaccinia virus in hamster kidney cell culture. *Indian J. Path. Bact.* 10:101–102.

17. Mathew, T. 1967a. Virus study of pock disease among buffaloes. *Indian. J. Path. Bact.* 10:101–102.

18. Mathew, T. 1967b. Cultivation and immunological studies on pox group of viruses. PhD thesies, University of Madras–Haffkine Institute Bombay.

19. Mathew, T. 1987. In *Advances in medical, and veterinary virology, immunology and epidemiology. Cultivation and immunological studies on pox group of viruses with special reference to buffalo pox virus.* Vol. 1, 1st ed., 4–171. New Delhi: Thajema Publishers.

20. Mathew, T. 1990. Clinical picture of pox like infection of cats in India. *Indian Vet. J.* 67:61–62.

21. Mathew, T. 1993. Classification of pox group of viruses including buffalo pox virus. In *Advances in medical, and veterinary virology, immunology and epidemiology. Buffalopox (Ortho pox) virus and its zoonotic importance.* Vol. 2, 1st ed., 11–26. New Delhi: Thajema Publishers.

22. Mathew, T. and Mathew, Z. 1986. Isolation, cultivation and haemadsoption of buffalo pox virus in BHK-21 cell line from Dhule epidemic (Western India). *Int. J. Zoonoses* 13:45–48.

23. Mathew, Z., Mathew, T., Choudhary, P. G., Naik, B. I. and Menon, M. N. 1978. Buffalopox outbreak in Maharashtra (India). *Livestock Adviser* 3:17–21.

24. Maqsood, M. 1944. Generalized vaccinia in buffaloes. *Indian J. Vet. Sci. Anim. Husbandry* 14:213–215.

25. Maqsood, M. 1958. Generalized buffalo pox. *Vet. Record* 70:321–322.

26. Mohan, R. N. 1968. Diseases and parasites of buffaloes. Part 1. Viral mycoplasmal, rickettsial diseases. *Vet. Bull.* 38:567–576.

27. Mohanty, P. K. and Rai, A. 1988. Immunogenicity of cell culture vaccines against buffalopox. Proceeding of 2nd World Buffalo Congress, New Delhi, 1988.

28. Mohanty, P. K. and Rai, A. 1988. Effect of various physico-chemical agents on buffalopox virus. *Indian J. Comp. Microbiol. Immunol. Infect. Dis.* 9:112–117.

29. Mohanty, P. K. and Rai, A. 1989. Immune response induced by Vero cell culture adapted BP virus in rabbit and buffaloes. *Indian J. Exp. Biol.* 27:350–355.

30. Mukundu, P. A. 1936. Cow pox and its seaquale. *Indian Vet. J.* 13:50–51.

31. Mullick, S. G., Rama Rao, D., Mallick, K. P. and Sastry, M. S. 1990. Some epidemiological aspects of an outbreak of buffalo pox. *Indian J. Comp. Microbiol. Immunol. Infect. Dis.* 11:135–140.

32. Nedunchelliyan, S., Reddy, D. S. and Venkataraman K. S. 1992. Buffalopox infection in man. *Indian J. Public Health* 36:57.

33. Paranaik, D. I., Gorhe, D. S., Khoth, J. B. and Hattangady, S. R. 1963. A note of two cases of cow pox in buffaloes. *Bombay Vet College Mag.* 10:42–44.

34. Rama Pratab, L. V. P. 1937. Acute mastitis: A sequele to variola in buffaloes. *Indian Vet. J.* 13:367–370.

35. Ramkrishnan, M. and Ananthapadmanabhan, K. 1957. An experimental study on the virus of buffalopox. *Indian Vet J.* 34:23–30.

36. Shanley, J. D., Lwlwick, L. I., Talavera, F., Sanders, C. V., Mylonakis, F. H. and Cunha, B. A. 2006. Pox viruses, Wiley Interscience.

37. Sharma, G. K. 1934. An interesting outbreak of variola vaccinia in Lahore. *Miscellaneous Bulletin of Imperial Council of Agriculture Research. Selected Clinical Articles* 8:1–4.

38. Singh, R. K., Hosamani, M., Balamurugan, V., Satheesh, C. C., Singal, R. K., Tatwarti, S. B., Bambal, R. G., Ramteke, V. and Yadav, M. P. 2006a. An outbreak of buffalopox in buffalo (*Bubalus bubalis*) dairy herds in Aurangabad, India. *Rev. Sci. Tech. Off. Int. Epiz.* 25:981–987.

39. Singh, R. K., Hosamani, M., Balamurugan, V., Satheesh, C. C., Rasool, T. J. and Yadav P. 2006b. Comparative sequence analysis of envelope protein genes of Indian buffalopox virus isolates. *Arach. Virol* 151:1995–2005.

40. Singh, R. K., Hosamani, M., Balamurugan, V., Bhanuprakash, V., Rasool, T. J. and Yadhav, M. P. 2007. Buffalopox: An emerging and re-emerging zoonoses. *Animal Research Reviews* 8:105–114.

41. Srinivasppa, J. and Garg, S. K. 1976. A study of buffalopox virus in the internal organs of the artificially infected rabbit. *Current Res. University Agricultural Sci.* (Bangalore) 5:85–86.

42. Sulochana, S., Pillai, M., Jayaprakashan, V., Nair, G. K., Murugan, M. R. and Abdulla, P. K. 1983. An outbreak of pox in buffaloes in Kerala. *Kerala. J. Vet. Sci.*14:145–151.

43. Wariyar, K. C. 1937. Variola in buffaloes. *Indian Vet. J.* 14:169–170.

44. Wikipedia. 2007. *Orthopoxvirus.* In Wikipedia, the free encyclopedia.

6. Bovine Rotaviral Enteritis

M. R. Saseendranath, and M. Krishnan Nair

Introduction

Rotaviral enteritis is characterized by severe diarrhea and is seen in neonatal calves, lambs, kids, piglets, foals, and human infants. Mebus et al. (1969) reported the association of rotavirus with diarrhea in calves.

Etiology

Rotavirus belongs to the family Reoviridae. Currently seven serogroups A to G are recognized. Rotavirus is comprised of a number of structural and nonstructural proteins. The major structural proteins include VP4, VP7, and VP6. Rotavirus serogroups are classified into serotypes based on the specificity of the outer capsid protein VP7 (G types) and VP4 (P types). VP4 protein has hemagglutinating property. At least fourteen G and twelve P serotypes of group A rotavirus are recognized. Group A rotavirus is the most frequently detected one causing diarrhea in the farm animals and man, whereas group B has been isolated from adult cows. All the rotaviruses from different species share a common group A antigen located on the major inner capsid protein, VP6. The outer capsid is composed of two proteins, the VP7 and VP4. Both of these proteins have been shown to independently induce neutralizing antibodies (Ester and Cohen, 1989).

The virus measures 65–75 nm in diameter and has a wheel-like structure and hence the name. Rotaviruses differ in their virulence. They are trilayered, and only the complete trilayered virions are infective.

The virus is relatively stable in feces and resistant to commonly used disinfectants such as iodophores and hypochlorites. The survival of rotaviruses in air and on surface is directly influenced by relative humidity. The virus is stable between pH 3 and 9 and is capable of surviving for thirty minutes at 60°C and seven to nine months at 18–20°C.

Epidemiology

Distribution

Rotaviral infection is reported worldwide in different species. Grover et al. (1998) reported rotaviral enteritis in calves from India. Rotavirus from one species can rarely infect members of other species. Experimental infection of pigs, calves, and lambs with human rotavirus has been demonstrated. The calf rotavirus can infect piglets. Morbidity ranges from 5–80% and case fatality from 5–60%. High morbidity and mortality are recorded in first calf heifer, where there is low colostrum antibody. Rotavirus infection is more related to meteorological changes than to age as more cases are found during spring months (Wani et al., 2004). Gumusova et al., (2007) reported widespread rotaviral infection in zero-to three-month-old animals.

SOURCE OF INFECTION
The adult animals are the source of infection to neonates. As the intestinal tract is the main site of multiplication, viruses are excreted only in the feces. The virus is excreted before the onset of clinical signs, during the disease, and during convalescent period for several weeks by the infected calves as well as by adult cows. Pregnant cows excrete the virus intermittently throughout pregnancy.

The virus has also been absorbed into soil, which become a source of contamination of feed and water.

TRANSMISSION
The main mode of transmission is fecal-oral. Feed and water contamination with dung and licking the soiled body and udder by the calves are the other modes of transmission.

HOSTS
Each species of animals has its specific rotavirus, though broad similarities exist in pathogenesis in general viruses are not cross-infective among species. Neonates of various species of animals, which are lacking maternal antibody, are the main victims of the rotaviral infection. Host susceptibility mainly depends on the presence of maternal antibody in the lumen of intestine of the newborn. The protective effect of the maternal antibody depends on the titer of the antibody, which in turn depends on the quantum of colostrum intake. Newly born calves up to three weeks of age are commonly affected. Though the adult animals are also affected, they suffer mildly or subclinically.

Immune status of the dam, colostrum intake, viral exposure, and the presence of the other enteropathogens are the factors involved in the outcome of severity of the clinical signs. Mortality is also more in young animals that have received insufficient colostrum and are subjected to severe environmental stress.

Erdogan et al. (2003) observed mean age of rotavirus-positive cases as 6.5 days with a range of 1.0-19.0 days. As the calves grow, rotavirus positivity also decreases. Calves born in larger herds or grouped in large numbers are more likely to be positive for the virus.

PATHOGENESIS

After ingestion of the virus, being resistant to the proteolytic enzymes, it reaches the small intestines and infects the epithelial cells lining the villi of small intestine. In the intestinal tract, the virus is activated to infectious form by the enzymes such as lactase and trypsin. VP4 protein of the virus is cleaved by trypsin into VP5 and VP8 polypeptides, and the cleavage of protein by trypsin is essential for the infectivity and penetration of the virus into the susceptible cells.

Rotavirus infects mature brush border villous epithelial cells in small intestine and to a lesser extent in large intestine. The infected cells are sloughed leading to partial villous atrophy, and the atrophic villi are rapidly replaced in four to six days of diarrhea. The activity of galactosidase (lactase) in the brush border of the villous epithelium is reduced, which results in decreased utilization of lactose. Reduction in enzymes is associated with immature enterocytes in the villi during rotavirus infection.

Viral multiplication in the cells causes malfunctions of the absorptive epithelium and result in profuse diarrhea. There is dehydration, loss of electrolytes, acidosis, and death.

The presence of other enteropathogens like *E. coli.*, parasites, and viral infections like corona increases the severity of clinical outcome. No gross pathognomonic lesions are noted. The stomach may be filled with casein curd or milk. The small intestine appears thin walled and translucent, flaccid, and may contain more fluid than usual. The colon and cecum are distended, voluminous, and may contain yellow fluid or dark gray fluid.

Histologicaly, lesion areas are mostly confined to the mucosal layer of small intestine. The villi are either desquamated or the lining columnar epithelial cells transformed into cuboidal epithelial cells. The lamina propria shows varying degree of infiltration with lymphocytes and macrophages.

CLINICAL SIGNS

Disease occurs in five to seven days of age. Calves are most susceptible to rotavirus infection between one to three weeks of age, more at five to seven days. This is correlated with the rapid decline in the maternal antibody titer. Incubation period is eighteen to twenty-four hours.

There is mild to severe diarrhea, depression, dehydration, and occasionally death. Feces may be light colored, semiliquid, or pasty in nature.

Immune Response

Neonates are protected from rotavirus during first few days after birth when colostral antibody is active in the gut, which declines after third day of age. Recovered animals are solidly immune to further rotavirus infection.

Diagnosis

Diarrhea during first three weeks of life has to be suspected for rotaviral infection. Rectal swabs, dung or intestinal contents, smears from intestinal mucosa, or section of intestine are the best clinical materials to be collected from suspected cases. The virus being cytolytic, often the diarrheic feces is negative for viral antigen as the virus-laden cells have been shed previously in the feces.

Electron microscopy, reverse transcriptase–polymerase chain reaction (RT-PCR) (Gouvea et al., 1994a and Gouvea et al., 1994b; Chinsangasam et al., 1995; Minakshi, 2002), nested multiplex PCR (Saravnanan et al., 2006), ELISA (Sunilchandra and Mahalingam, 1994 ; Minakshi et al., 2001; Ekik and Oztur, 2002; Polanco et al., 2004; Wani et al., 2004; Wani et al., 2007), RNA-PAGE (Burgue et al., 1999; Jindal et al., 2000; Dighe et al., 2003; Wani et al., 2007), lateral flow immunoassay (Al-yousif et al., 2002), and dot hybridization technique by using DNA probes are the tests employed for the identification of the rotaviral antigen. Specificity and sensitivity of immunochromatography test are found to be 97.3% and 82.1% respectively (Reschova et al., 2000).

Antibody detection test like serum-neutralization test and ELISA are also being used effectively (Wassel et al., 1999).

Differential Diagnosis

Rotaviral infection has to be differentiated from diseases like coronaviral enteritis, colibacillosis, coccidiosis, parasitic enteritis, and indigestion either by demonstration of the antigens or concerned antibody. Parasitism can be ruled out by detecting the specific ova.

Treatment

Aim of the treatment comprises mainly maintenance of hydration and electrolyte balance of the calves by isotonic fluid therapy and to prevent secondary bacterial infection by antibiotic therapy.

Prevention and Control

Enhancement of the immune status of the dam during pregnancy to increase the maternal antibody to calves helps to prevent the disease. Administration of bovine colostral immunoglobulin has a preventive effect on rotavirus diarrhea in beef calves when it was given soon after calving (Osame et al., 1991).

VACCINATION

Vaccination of the dam against rotavirus and colostrum feeding of calves reduces the incidences dramatically (Rousie et al., 2000). Combined vaccination against rotavirus, coronavirus, and *E. coli* induced high levels of antibodies in the colostrum and milk for twenty-eight days (Wassel et al., 1999; Moro et al., 2000; Crouch et al., 2001). Hence, vaccination of the dam during the last trimester of pregnancy enhances the colostral antibody.

The CBRV epitope expressed in plants has been found to be effective in inducing an antirotavirus response in adult female mice when administered either intraperitoneal or orally. Suckling mice born from immunized female are seen protected against oral challenge with virulent rotavirus. These findings demonstrate the feasibility of inducing lactogenic immunity against enteric pathogens like rotavirus (Wigdorovitz et al., 2004).

ERADICATION

Eradication of rotaviral infection is practically impossible.

REFERENCES

1. Al-Yousif, Y., Anderson, J., Chard-Bergstom, C. and Kapil, S. 2002. Development evaluation and application of lateral flow immunoassay (Immunochromatography) for detection of rota virus in bovine fecal samples. *Clinc. Diagnostic. Immunol.* 9:723–724.

2. Burgue, D., Ozkul, A., Karoglu, T., Yesilbag, K., Oguzoglu, T. C., Bilage-dagalp, S., Akca, Y., Alkan, F. and Tan, M. T. 1999. The investigation of rota virus infections in diarrheic and non-diarrheic sheep using PAGE and ELISA. *Veteriner Fakultesi Dergisis, Ankara Universitesi* 46:243–247.

3. Chinsangasam, J., Schore, C. E., Guterbock, W., Weaver, L. D. and Osburn, B. I. 1995. Prevalence of group A and group-B rota viruses in the feces of neonatal dairy calves from California. *Comp. Immunol. Microbiol. Infect. Dis.* 18:93–103.

4. Crouch, C. F., Oliver, S. and Francis, M. J. 2001. Serological and milk responses of cows vaccinated with a single dose of a combined vaccine against rota virus, corona virus and *E. coli* F5(K99). *Vet. Rec.* 149:105–108.

5. Dighe, V. D., Grover, V. P. and Pandey, R. 2003. Epidemiological studies on bovine rota virus in neonatal diarrheic calves at organized dairy farms in Haryana and adjoining areas using RNA-PAGE. *Indian. J. Anim. Sci.* 73:623–626.

6. Ekik, M. and Oztur, K. F. 2002. Detection of rota virus antigens in newborn calves with diarrhea by ELISA and detection of Rota virus antibodies from their dams in Konya region. *Veterinarian* 13:1–10.

7. Erdogan, H. M., Unver, A., Gunes, V. and Citil, M. 2003. Frequency of rota virus and corona virus in neonatal calves in Kars district. *Kafkas universitesi Veteriner Fakultesi Dergisi. Kars Turkey* 9:65–68.

8. Ester, M. K. and Cohen, J. 1989. Rota virus gene structure and function. *Microbiol. Rev.* 53:410–449.

9. Gouvea, V., Santoes, N., Timenetsky, C. and Do, M. 1994a. Identification of bovine and porcine rota virus G types by PCR. *J. Clin. Microbiol.* 32:1338–1340.

10. Gouvea, V., Santoes, N., Timenetsky, C. and Do, M. 1994b. VP4 typing of bovine and porcine group A rotavirus by PCR. *J. Clin. Microbiol.* 32:1333–1337.

11. Grover, Y. P., Minakshi, Patanayak, D. P. and Pandey, R. 1998. Epidemiological studies on bovine rota virus in diarrhoeic calves at organized dairy farms in Haryana and adjoining areas during 1996–1997. *Indian J. Comp. Microbiol. Immunol. Infect. Dis.* 19:121–123.

12. Gumusova, S. O., Yaziro, Z., Albayarak, H. and Meral, Y. 2007. Rota virus and Corona virus prevalence in healthy calves and calves with diarrhea. *Medyiyna Weterynaryjna* 63:62–64.

13. Jindal, S. R., Maiti, N. K. and Oberoi, M. S. 2000. Genomic diversity and prevalence of rota virus in cow and buffalo calves in northern India. *Revue scientifique technique-Office International des Epizooties* 19:871–876.

14. Mebus, C. A., Underdahi, N. R., Rhodes, M. B. and Teeihaus, M. J. 1969. *University Nebraska Agri. Exp. Stn. Res. Bull.* 233:1.

15. Minakshi, Malik, V., Prasad, G. and Pandey, R. 2001. VP4 gene specific RT-PCR for detection of bovine group A rota virus. *Indian. J. Anim. Sci.* 71:611–613.

16. Minakshi and Pandey, R. 2002. VP7 gene based RT-PCR assay for detection of bovine group A rota virus. *Indian. J. Microbiol.* 42:73–76.

17. Moro, E. and Umehara, O. 2000. Control of neonatal diarrhoea in calves by vaccination of pregnant cows with Scourguard 3K/C and antibodies transfer through colostrum. *A. Hora Veterinaria* 20:39–43.

18. Osame, S., Ichijo, S., Ohta, C., Watanabe, T., Benkele, W. and Goto, H. 1991. Preventive administration of bovine Colostral immunoglobulin for bovine diarrhoea. *J. Vet. Med. Sci.* 53:87–96.

19. Saravanan, M., Parthiben, M. and Ramdoss, P. 2006. Genotyping rota virus of neonatal calves by nested multiplex PCR in India. *Veterinarski Arhiv* 76:497–505.

20. Sunilchandra, N. P. and Mahalingam, S. 1994. Application of ELISA in the diagnosis of rotavirus infections in buffalo calves. *Buffalo J.* 10:237–248.

21. Polanco, G., Gonzalez, M., Mansano, L., Camara, J. and Puerto, M. 2004. Rotavirus in asymptomatic animals: Detection and antigenic classification. *Archives de Medicina Veterinaria* 36:65–70.

22. Reschova, S., Frenz, J., Stepanek, J. and Rozkos, N. A. 2000. Immunochromatographic detection of bovine rota virus using egg yolk antibodies. *Veterinaria Medicina* 45:33–37.

23. Rousie, S. Le., Klein, N., Houghton, S. and Charleston, B. 2000. Use of colostrum from rotavirus-immunized cows as a single feed to prevent rotavirus-induced diarrhoea in calves. *Vet. Rec.* 147:160–161.

24. Wani, S. A., Bhat, M. A., Samanta, D., Ishaq, S. M., Ashrafi, M. A. and Buch, A. S. 2004. Epidemiology of diarrhea caused by rota virus and *E. coli* in lambs in Kashmir valley, India. *Small Ruminant Research* 52:145–153.

25. Wani, S. A., Bhat, M. A. and Ishaq, S. M. 2007. Molecular epidemiology of rota virus in calves and lambs with diarrhea in Kashmir valley. *Indian J. Virol* 18:17–19.

26. Wassel, M. S., Shafey, S. M. and Saleh, M. S. 1999. Preparation and evaluation of an inactivated combined vaccine of bovine rota, corona virus and K99 enterotoxigenic *E. coli. Egyptian. J. Agri Res.* 77:957–969.

27. Wigdorovitz, A., Mozgovoj, M., Santoes, M. J., Parreno, V., Gomez, C., Figueira, D. M., Trono, K. G., Rios, R. D., Franzone, P. M., Fernandez, F., Carrillo, C., Babiuk, L. A., Escribano, J. M. and Borca, M. V. 2004. Protective lactogenic immunity conferred by an edible peptide vaccines to bovine rota virus produced in transgenic plants. *J. Gen. Virol.* 85:1825–1832.

7. Bovine Viral Diarrhea (BVD) and Mucosal Disease Complex (MDC)
(Bovine Pestivirus Disease Complex, Mucosal Disease Complex)

M. R. Saseendranath, M. Krishnan Nair, Thankam Mathew, and Z. Mathew

Introduction

Bovine viral diarrhea (BVD) is usually a benign infection resulting in minimal clinical changes but also occurs as mucosal disease complex (MDC) with severe clinical manifestation and heavy mortality. The BVD virus may also cause congenital defects in calves, reproductive failure, and severe immunosuppression contributing to the severity of other infectious diseases or disease complex depending on the stage of infection and immune status of the host.

Etiology

Bovine viral diarrhea virus (BVDV) is a small enveloped, single-stranded RNA virus. BVDV belongs to the genus *Pestivirus* of the family Flaviviridae. Hog cholera virus and border disease virus in sheep are also members of the *Pestivirus* genus and have close antigenic relationship with BVDV. There are two biotypes of BVDV, designated as cytopathic and noncytopathic, depending upon the ability to cause cytopathic effect in cell culture. The noncytopathic BVDV only causes persistent infection (PI) by crossing the placenta and invading the fetus, whereas the superinfection with cytopathic biotype causes mucosal disease in animals already persistently infected with noncytopathic biotype. Both the cytopathic and noncytopathic types can be isolated from animals dying of mucosal disease.

The BVDV genome encodes both structural and nonstructural proteins. The structural proteins include the capsid protein C (p14) and three glycoproteins—gp48, gp25, and gp53. The capsid protein functions to package the genomic RNA and to provide structure for the formation of the virion envelope. The three glycoproteins are associated with the lipid envelope. The major glycoprotein E2 (gp53 protein) has been shown to possess virus-neutralizing activity (Donis et al., 1988).

The virus particles are sensitive to low pH, ether, chloroform, and other lipid solvents. The virus is readily inactivated at 56°C in thirty minutes.

EPIDEMIOLOGY

DISTRIBUTION

The virus causing bovine viral diarrhea (BVD) and mucosal disease (MDC) is distributed worldwide. Olafson et al. (1946) reported BVD for the first time. BVD has been recorded in most cattle-rearing countries of the world. In 1965, Milles et al. doubted that the original Oregon C24V cytopathogenic virus is that of BVD or of MDC. Two strains of virus namely, Nantwich noncytopathic pathogenic and FS virus cytopathic nonpathogenic were isolated by Darbyshire (1963). Six serotypes of viruses i.e. M62, M63, M80, M153, F2 66A, and T11 were isolated by Huck and Cart Wright (1964) from MDC having different properties. The Nantwich and Oregon C24V strains produced similar antibodies. Similarly, the M6 serotype of Huck and Cartwright (1964) resembled to the FS strain of Darbyshire (1963). In 1956, Pandey and Murthy, for the first time, reported the occurrence of MDC from UP, India, (Pandey and Murthy, 1961) and later by Sapre (1962 and 1964). Parnaik et al. (1964) reported MDC from Maharashtra and Chandrashekaran and Balasubramanyam (1962) from Madras, Tamil, Nadu. They could isolate the virus by propagating in the same host or rabbit. But Mathew et al. (1968) could isolate the MDC virus in chick embryo as well as tissue culture from the lesions of young buffalo calves aged fifteen days to three months suffering from MDC in the young stock farm of Arey Milk Colony, Bombay.

BVD infections are seen in all ages of cattle and have major economic impact due to productive and reproductive losses. Poor reproductive performance due to infertility and embryonic death, abortion, prenatal growth retardation, stillbirth, congenital defects, and death from mucosal disease result in severe economic loss to the dairy farmers. Clinical MDC is usually sporadic and only a small percentage, less than 5%, of the herd is affected.

SOURCE OF INFECTION

Cattle acutely or chronically infected with BVDV are the primary source of virus. Discharge from the reproductive tract of an infected cow or PI cow or aborted fetus can also be the source of infection. Persistently infected white-tailed deer (*Odocoileus virginianus*) also pose a threat to BVD control programs (Passler et al., 2006). Infected animals shed virus in all secretions or excretions including nasal discharge, saliva, semen (Coria and McClurkin, 1978), feces, urine, tears, and milk. Carrier cows can remain clinically normal for years, during which time they breed successfully. Their progeny may be apparently normal but are invariably persistently viremic carriers, resulting in a maternal viremic family (Little Johns and Walker, 1985).

TRANSMISSION

Transmission is usually by direct contact with a carrier (Roeder and Drew, 1984). Nose-to-nose contact is an effective method of transmitting the virus from infected to healthy animal. The primary route of viral entry is probably oro-nasal. Introduction of a PI bull into a susceptible herd is a potent source of infection through semen. The fetus can be infected by transplacental transmission of the virus from the infected dam, whether the dam is transiently or persistently infected (Uttenthal et al., 2007). Epidemics of abortion and congenital defects have been attributed to the transplacental virus infection of the fetuses of the cows in the first trimester of pregnancy. Other less important routes of entry may be by biting insects and contaminated instruments. Infection has also been introduced into herds through the use of vaccines for other diseases, which were contaminated with the BVDV (Lohr et al., 1983).

HOSTS

BVD occurs in all classes of cattle. Most cases occur between six to twenty-four months of age. Rarely calves as young as four months of age or cattle older than two years of age are affected. Serological surveys in sheep and goats revealed that 11% of sheep and 16% of goats as seropositive (Lamontagne and Roy, 1984), though the clinical form of the disease is rare in small ruminants.

PATHOGENESIS

Following entry of the virus and contact with the mucosal lining of the mouth or nose, initial replication occurs in epithelial cells with a predilection site for the tonsils. From here, the virus is able to spread systemically through the bloodstream. Spread can occur either as free virus in the serum or as virus-infected leucocytes, particularly lymphocytes and monocytes. Isolation of virus from serum or leucocytes is generally possible between three and ten days postinfection. During systemic spread, the virus is able to gain entry to most tissues with a preference for lymphoid tissues. However, the tissues infected may vary between different virus strains.

Mucosal disease in nature is probably a rare event because of the special circumstances that are required for it to occur. The first factor that must be present for mucosal disease to occur is that an animal must be persistently exposed to BVDV. The persistent infection occurs when a fetus becomes infected in utero between one to four months of gestation with noncytopathic BVDV. If BVDV virus is present during this time, it too is recognized as self and allowed to survive and replicate in the fetus and the postnatal animal. In most cases, persistently infected fetus do not perform well, often dying in utero or soon after birth. However, calves that do survive remain infected for life. Virus is allowed to replicate unchallenged and is continuously shed into the environment. The host mounts no immune response against the original virus. However, if the host becomes infected with another BVD virus, which is antigenically different from the persistent virus, an immune response can occur to the second virus. The second factor needed for mucosal disease to occur is the superinfection of the persistently infected animal with an antigenically similar cytopathic BVDV. This may be in several ways. The most common occurrence is by a mutation at specific sites in the noncytopathic virus genome. This mutation may occur in several different ways, including insertion of RNA into or deletion of RNA from the noncytopathic BVDV genome. The end result of the mutation is that a new protein, termed "p80," is produced during translation of the cytopathic BVDV RNA genome. This protein is present in noncytopathic BVDV as part of a larger protein termed "p125." The role that "p80" plays in causing cytopathology is not understood. It should be noted that the mutation does not change the antigenic makeup of the virus, and therefore the cytopathic virus is not recognized by the host's immune system and is allowed to replicate without challenge. Other sources of cytopathic viruses would include modified live vaccines or experimental challenge. Antigenic homology between the cytopathic and noncytopathic virus must be maintained for mucosal disease to occur.

PATHOLOGY

The lesions of the buccal mucosa consist of discrete, shallow erosions that become confluent, resulting in large areas of necrotic epithelium which become separated from the underlying tissue. These erosions occur inside the lips and on the gums, and dental pad, on the posterior part of the hard palate, at the commissures of the mouth and on the tongue. The entire oral cavity may have a cooked appearance with the gray necrotic epithelium covering the deep pink raw base. Similar lesions occur on the muzzle, which become confluent and covered with scabs and debris.

Although the mechanisms of cellular damage are unclear, the replicating cytopathic BVDV results in rapid depletion of the gut-associated lymphoid tissue (Peyer's patches) with subsequent necrosis of the gastrointestinal mucosa. Severe diarrhea ensues, which eventually leads to the animal's death.

CLINICAL SIGNS

The clinical signs associated with BVD virus infection vary widely depending on the individual and the strain of virus involved and stage of infection. BVD is an in apparent or subclinical infection with high morbidity and low fatality characterized by fever, leucopenia, inappetency, and mild diarrhea followed by rapid recovery in a few days and the production of viral-neutralizing antibodies. Similar infection, with no long-term consequences other than the development of antibody, occurs in fetuses over about 150–180 days of gestation.

Only persistently infected (PI) animals will be developing MDC and die of this disease, usually between six months and two years of age. Mucosal disease, however, can be seen affecting calves as young as only a few weeks of age, and some PI animals may survive and in apparently good health for many years.

Acute mucosal disease complex is characterized by the sudden onset of clinical disease in animals of six to twenty-four months of age that were infected before 125 days of gestation and acting as persistently infected animals and later superinfected with cytopathic form of the BVDV. The morbidity is low, but fatality is high, reaching 100%. The affected animals are depressed, anorectic, and with slobber saliva and wetting hair around the mouth. Their body temperature is elevated to 40–41°C. Tachycardia and polypnea are common. Ruminal movements are usually absent. Profuse watery diarrhea occurs two to four days after the onset of clinical illness. Their feces are foul smelling and may contain mucus and variable quantities of blood. Occasionally, small fibrinous intestinal casts are present. Straining at defecation is common, and the perineum is usually stained and smeared with feces. There is mucopurulent nasal discharge associated with some minor erosions on the external nares, and similar lesions are seen in the pharynx. Lacrimation and corneal edema are sometimes observed. Lameness occurs in some animals and appears to be due to laminitis, coronitis, and erosive lesions of the skin of the interdigital space. Usually dehydration and weakness are progressive, and death occurs in five to seven days after the onset of the signs.

Some animals with acute mucosal disease complex may not die and become chronic cases. There may be intermittent bouts of diarrhea, inappetency, progressive emaciation, rough and dry hair coat, chronic bloat, hoof deformities, and chronic erosions in the oral cavity and skin. Shallow, erosive lesions covered with scabs can be found on the perineum, around the scrotum, preputial orifice, vulva, between the legs and at the skin horn junction around the dew claws, in the interdigital clefts, and at the heels. The failure of these skin lesions to heal is an important clinical findings suggestive of chronic mucosal disease. Chronic cases sometime survive for several weeks or months during which time they are unthrifty and ultimately die from chronic debility.

If the infected animal is a pregnant female, in addition to the effects of infection on the adult, those on the fetus have to be considered. The clinical signs vary dependant on the strain of virus involved and on the age of the fetus. At almost any stage of the pregnancy, and particularly during the first and second trimesters, infection of the fetus can result in fetal death. This may manifest as conception failure, early embryonic death with delayed returns to estrous, the production of mummified calves, or later abortions. If the BVD infection does not result in the death of the fetus, it may be responsible for causing various fetal abnormalities, which classically affect the CNS, especially the cerebellum and the eyes. The stage of fetal development determines the type of defect that occurs. The most common defect is cerebellar hypoplasia. Other defects that have been described include cataract, retinal degeneration and hypoplasia, optic neuritis, skeletal malformations, hypotrichosis, and general growth retardation. Possible explanations include direct cell damage by the replicating virus or indirect cell damage by the immune response to the virus. The result of this will be the delivery of a calf that has difficulty in standing and balancing or which has ocular lens cataract (or both). If fetal infection occurs during the first trimester of pregnancy, prior to the development of the fetal immune system, a further possibility is the production, at term, of a persistently infected (PI) calf. Calves that are born to be persistently viremic carriers may be smaller than their contemporaries and may fail to grow normally. They may survive and appear unthrifty for several months or more until they develop fatal MD or some other infectious conditions.

IMMUNE RESPONSE

Postnatal BVDV infection cause severe immunosuppression leading to the outbreak of other diseases like pneumonia and enteritis. BVDV interferes with lymphocyte and macrophage function. Impaired neutrophil functions and immunoglobulin secretion by plasma cells are also observed in BVDV infection. Recovery from mild form of BVD causes solid immunity to the particular type of BVDV. The E2 surface glycoprotein of BVDV is an immunodominat epitope inducing protective neutralizing antibodies in infected as well as vaccinated animals (Donofrio et al., 2006).

DIAGNOSIS

In addition to the clinical and postmortem signs of BVD infection, a variety of laboratory methods exists to assist in the diagnosis of this disease. These include virus isolation, demonstration of antigen in various body secretions, and excretions or specific antibody in blood or milk. Confirmation of a diagnosis of BVD in acute cases depends upon demonstration of either antigen or seroconversion in paired serum samples. The definitive etiological diagnosis of MDC by virus isolation is time-consuming and expensive. Virus isolation can be attempted by inoculation of nasopharyngeal swabs, ocular swabs, intestinal tissues, spleen, most other tissues, or any fraction of blood into cell culture. Virus isolation using microtiter immunoperoxidase detection method is the most common method used for testing large numbers of samples. Presence of virus or viral antigen is recognized by cytopathic effects and in case of noncytopathic strains by various serological methods.

The serological methods used to detect noncytopathic virus or antigen in cell culture or tissues, such as intestine, kidney, or spleen from affected animals or aborted fetal tissues, include direct or indirect immunofluorescent antibody staining (FAT), immunoperoxidase staining (Ward and Kaeberle, 1984; Katz et al., 1987), gel diffusion technique (Mathew et al., 1968; Hopkinson et al., 1979). Nasal epithelial cells collected on cotton swabs can be used to conduct FAT for the diagnosis of field cases of BVD in calves (Silim and Masy, 1983). RT-PCR is being applied for testing semen (Amen et al., 2003) and milk for the detection of BVDV. Positive identification of BVDV can be done by preliminary PCR screening from bulk milk sample would give good justification for further herd testing by virus isolation.

Serological techniques like complement fixation test, immunofluorescent staining, enzyme-linked immunosorbent assay (ELISA) (Krametter-Frotscher et al., 2007) are also used for the detection of antibody. The infection status of a herd may be established by additional methods such as testing bulk milk for anti-BVDV antibody. Commercial ELISA kits are available for detection of BVD virus in serum and skin biopsy (Hill et al., 2007).

Most BVDV-associated congenital defects occur following infection after the onset of immunological competence, and therefore, calves with these defects have BVDV antibody. The diagnosis of BVDV-induced congenital defects in calves should include both virus isolation and serology to detect BVDV-specific antibody prior to uptake of colostrum. The identification of persistently infected animals is most routinely done by virus isolation. The level of viremia in persistently infected animals is generally quite high (10^6 $CCID_{50}$/ml of serum) but may vary from 10^2–10^7 $CCID_{50}$/ml. In addition, the level of viremia may decline in individual animals over time. In most cases, for routine identification of persistently infected animals, serum is adequate for virus isolation. In young calves, maternal antibody causes a decrease in the level of free virus in serum, and so virus isolation may be false negative.

Due to colostral antibody in young calves less than three months of age, the best sample remains to be whole blood in which the mononuclear cells are separated for virus isolation. Persistent infections should only be determined by identification of BVDV by virus isolation in sequential samples collected thirty days apart. By testing the animal thirty days apart, it is possible to assess for a fourfold increase in antibody titer.

The most common approach to herd screening would be to obtain serum samples from all the animals in the herd over three months of age. In addition, whole blood samples should be collected from calves less than three months of age. Basically, all animals in the herd should be tested. A pregnant animal must be considered as to represent two animals. Using this method, results from two serial passages are generally available within five to nine days. In addition, calves born during the next nine months must be tested to ensure that no additional persistently infected animals are born that were in utero at the time of testing. Pregnant animals may be in a convalescent period from an acute infection and may be negative for virus isolation, while a persistently infected fetus remains in utero. Due to the interference of maternal antibody, it is recommended that calves be retested at three to four months of age prior to vaccination to ensure that no persistently infected animals would be advanced and placed in the replacement heifer-breeding groups.

DIFFERENTIAL DIAGNOSIS
BVD/MD complex has to be differentiated from other diseases of cattle with or without diarrhea and with or without oral lesions. Erosive stomatitis and gastroenteritis are characteristics of BVD, rinderpest, and bovine malignant catarrh. The identification of the antigen or the agent or antibody is the only method by which we can differentiate these diseases. The presence of vesicles in vesicular diseases and the highly contagious nature help to identify diseases like foot-and-mouth disease and vesicular stomatitis. Salmonellosis and Johne's disease can be diagnosed by demonstration of the agent or antigen. Parasitism can be differentiated by demonstration of the characteristic ova and by absence of erosive lesions. Poisoning of molybdenum and copper are the other diseases, which can be differentiated by the history and other epidemiological findings.

TREATMENT
No specific treatment is available for BVD. Symptomatic therapy is advised. Animals with chronic BVD should be culled and destroyed.

CONTROL AND PREVENTION

The successful control and prevention of the BVD-MD complex in a herd depends on the prevention of introduction of infection into the herd, the identification and eradication of carriers, and immunization of the breeding stock before their first breeding. It is important to emphasize that vaccination be done at least three weeks before breeding so that breeding females become seropositive to the virus before conception.

The main objective of eradication of the disease is the identification and culling of all PI animals. The eradication of BVD from a herd by identifying and removing PI animals will, however, take a considerable and variable period of time and dependent on the size of the herd because of the slow recirculation of acute infection between susceptible individuals within the herd. This recirculation can, however, be halted by vaccination, and so the gold standard in BVD control and eradication is to combine the identification and removal of all PI animals with whole herd vaccination. Following the eradication of BVD from a herd, careful consideration should be given to biosecurity precautions aimed at preventing the reintroduction of the virus and the need for continued vaccination before future management strategies are defined.

VACCINATION

Due to the high prevalence of BVDV in the cattle population, it is mandatory that BVDV vaccination be done. The use of killed or modified live vaccines can provide protection by decreasing the consequences of acute infections. The unprotected animals are at very high risk while vaccinated animals are at low risk from BVD virus.

In recent years, the development of effective and safe vaccines, which provide fetal as well as maternal protection, allowed the option of controlling BVD by vaccination. This usually involves giving unvaccinated animals two doses of initial course of the vaccine. Previously vaccinated animals should receive a single booster dose of vaccine each year. In the ideal situation, a whole-herd vaccination policy should be implemented although strategic vaccination of all replacement breeding animals before they enter the herd can be useful in certain situations.

Commercially available inactivated and modified live BVDV (MDV, modified live virus vaccine) vaccines have been extensively used for more than thirty years, but since their introduction the problems of BVDV-related infections appear to have become worse instead of better (Bolin, 1995). It is important to understand that vaccination against BVD virus only protects against the clinical effects of the disease in the animal but does not protect against infection. MLV is a potential source of in utero infection and/or immunosuppression (Liess et al., 1984; Roth and Kaeberle, 1983). BVD vaccination programs have not always been 100% successful. Live vaccines induce reasonably good immunity against field infections, preventing clinical manifestation of BVD as well as giving fetal protection. However, there is always a concern about the risk associated with the use of live vaccines in pregnant animals and also the possibility of spread of vaccine virus from vaccinated animals to susceptible ones. Inactivated vaccines are generally safe, but the immunity they offer does not offer reliable fetal protection against virulent field strains.

E2 subunit vaccine has been reported to induce protection in immunized animals (Bolin and Ridpath, 1996; Bruschke et al., 1997). The use of cloned viral genes holds great promise for the development of new vaccines to control BVDV. DNA vaccine can serve as an alternative to conventional immunization with MLV or inactivated vaccines to induce protection (Robinson et al., 1993; Sedgah et al., 1994). Direct injection of plasmid DNA into animals offers several advantages over classical vaccine preparations and virus vectors for vaccinations. Simple, rapid, and inexpensive production of plasmid DNA, thermal stability of the plasmid product, and the potential for a long shelf life of stabilized plasmid DNA are characteristics that make genetic vaccination very attractive for the next generation of vaccines against BVDV (Siegrist and Lambert, 1997). Harpin et al. (1999) demonstrated that vaccination of cattle using a DNA construct encoding only E2 protein of BVDV was able to induce both neutralizing antibody production and lymphocyte proliferation. It appeared that both humoral and cell-mediated responses are involved in the development of protective response in cattle, and so this vaccine offers great promise for the control of BVD.

REFERENCES

1. Amen, A. S., Abid-Elmonem, M. F. I., and Ali, N. M. 2003. Application of nested RT-PCR for detection of BVDV in semen. *Vet. Med. J. Giza* 51:497–500.
2. Bolin, S. R. 1995. Control of bovine viral diarrhea infection by use of vaccination. *Veterinary Clinics of North American Food Animal Practice* 11:615–625.
3. Bolin, S. R. and Ridpatah, J. F. 1996. Glycoprotein E2 of bovine viral diarrhea virus expressed in insect cells provides calves with limited protection from systemic infection and disease. *Arach. Virol.* 141:1463–1477.
4. Bruschke, C. J., Mooremann, R. J., van Oirschot, J. T. and van Rijn, P. A. 1997. A subunit based on glycoprotein E2 of bovine virus diarrhea induces fetal protection in sheep against homologous challenge. *Vaccine* 15:1940–1945.

5. Chandrasekharan, K. P. and Bala Subramaniam, G. 1962. A preliminary report on a disease resembling mucosal disease complex in buffalo calves. *Indian Vet. J.* 39:141–147.

6. Coria, M. F. and McClurkin, A. W. 1978. Specific immune tolerance in an apparently healthy bull persistently infected with bovine viral diarrhea virus. *J. Am. Vet. Med. Assoc.* 172:449–451.

7. Darbyshire, J. H. 1963. The isolation, separation and identification of 2 viruses from a case of bovine mucosal disease. *J. Comp. Path.* 73:309–318.

8. Donis, R. O., Corapi, W. and Dubovi, E. J. 1988. Neutralizing monoclonal antibodies to bovine viral diarrhea virus bind to the 56k to58 K glycoprotein. *J. Gen. Virol.* 69:77–86.

9. Donofrio, G., Bottarelli, E., Sando, C. and Flammini, C. F. 2006. Expression of bovine viral diarrhea glycoprotein E2 as a soluble secreted from mammalian cell line. *Clinic. Vaccine Immunol.* 13:698–701.

10. Harpin, S., Hurley, D. J., Mbikay, M., Talbot, B. and Elazhary, Y. 1999. Vaccination of cattle with a DNA plasmid encoding the bovine viral diarrhea virus major glycoprotein E2. *J. Gen. Virol.* 80:3137–3144.

11. Hill, F. I., Reichel, M. P., McCoy, R. J. and Tisdall, D. J. 2007. Evaluation of two commercial enzyme linked immunosorbent assays for detection of bovine viral diarrhea virus in serum and skin biopsy of cattle. *New Zealand Vet. J.* 55:45–48.

12. Hopkinson, M. F., Hart, L. T., Segar, C. L., Larson, A. D. and Fulton, R. W. 1979. An immunodiffusion test for the detection of bovine virus diarrhea virus antibodies in bovine serum. *Am. J. Vet. Res.* 40:1189–1191.

13. Huck, R. A. and Cartwright, S. F. 1964. Isolation and classification of viruses from cattle during outbreaks of mucosal or respiratory disease and from herds of reproductive disorders. *J. Comp. Path.* 74:346–365.

14. Katz, J. B., Ludemann, L. Pemberton, J. and Schmerr, M. J. 1987. Detection of bovine virus diarrhea virus in cell cultures using an immunoperoxidase technique. *Vet. Microbiol.* 13:153–157.

15. Krametter-Frotscher, R., Loitsch, A., Kohler, H. Schleiner, A., Schiefer, P., Mosti, K., Goija, F. and Baum Gartner, W. 2007. Serological survey for antibodies against pestiviruses in sheep in Australia. *Vet. Rec.* 160:726–730.

16. Lamontagne, L. and Roy, R. 1984. Presence of antibodies to bovine viral diarrhea-mucosal disease virus (Border disease) in sheep and goat flocks in Quebec. *Can. J. Comp. Med.* 48:225–227.

17. Liess, B., Orban, S., Frey, H. R., Trautwien, G., Wiefel, W. and Lindow, H. 1984. Studies on transplacentaly transmissibility of a bovine virus diarrhea (BVD) vaccine virus in cattle. *Zentralblatt fur Veterimedizin Reihe* B 31:669–681.

18. Littlejohns, I. and Walker, K. H. 1985. Etiology and pathogenesis of mucosal disease of cattle, current concepts, observations and speculations. *Aust. Vet. J.* 62:101–103.

19. Lohr, C. H., Evermann, J. F. and Ward, A. C. 1983. Investigations of dams and their offspring inoculated with a vaccine contaminated by bovine virus diarrhea virus. *Vet. Med. Small Anim. Clin.* 78:1263–1266.

20. Mathew, T., Mathew, Z., Manjrekar, L. and Vangurlkekar, K. G. 1968. Isolation of virus from buffalo calves with mucosal disease complex syndrome. *Indian J. Microbiol.* 8:11–17.

21. Mills, J. H. L., Neilson, S. W. and Lugenbuhl, R. E. 1965. Current status of mucosal disease. *J. Amer. Vet. Med. Assn.* 146:691–696.

22. Olafson, P., Mac Callum, A. D. and Fox, F. H. 1946. An apparently new transmissible disease of cattle. *Cornell Vet.* 36:205–213.

23. Pandey, P. G. and Murthy, K. 1961. Incidence and pathology of some recently recognized mucosal disease like syndrome amongst cattle and buffaloes in India. *Bull. International Epizootics.* 55:706–714.

24. Parnaik, D. T., Gorhe, D. S. and Khot, J. B. 1964. Observations on outbreak of a disease similar to the British mucosal disease in a diary farm in Bombay. *Indian J. Vet. Sc.* 34:171–176.

25. Passler, T., Walz, P. H., Ditchkoff, S. S., Givens, M., Maxwell, H. S. and Brock, K. V. 2006. Experimental persisitent infection with bovine viral diarhoea virus in white tailed deer. *Vet. Microbiol.* 122:50–356.

26. Robinson, H. L., Hunt, L. A. and Webster, R. G. 1993. Protection against lethal influenza virus challenge by immunization with a hemagglutinin expressing plasmid DNA. *Vaccine* 11:957–960.

27. Roeder, P. L. and Drew, T. W. 1984. Mucosal disease of cattle: A late sequel to fetal infection. *Vet. Rec.* 114:309–313.

28. Roth, J. A. and Kaeberie, M. L. 1983. Suppression of neutrophil and lymphocyte functaion induced by a vaccinal strain of bovine diarrhea virus with or without administration of ACTH. *Am. J. Vet. Res.* 44:2366–2372.

29. Sapre, S. N. 1962. A preliminary note on field observations in an epidemic of Ajanta disease commonly known as mucosal disease. *Indian Vet. J.* 39:1–10.

30. Sapre, S. N. 1964. A note on further observations on mucosal disease complex in Maharashtra. *Indian Vet J.* 41:255–258.

31. Sedgah, M., Hedstrome, R., Hobart, and Offman, S. L. 1994. Protection against malaria by immunization with plasmid DNA encoding circumsporozoite protein. *Prooced. Nat. Acaemy Sci.*, USA 9:9866–9870.

32. Sharma, S. N. and Adlakha, S. C. 1994. In *Virus diseases of Animals in India*, 1st ed.1994, 91. New Delhi: Indian Council of Agricultural Research.

33. Siegrist, C. A. and Lambert, P. H. 1997. Immunization with DNA vaccines in early life:advantages and limitations as compared to conventional vaccines. *Springer seminars in Immunopathology* 19:233–243.

34. Silim, A. and Massy, E. 1983. Detection of infectious bovine rhinotracheitis and bovine viral diarrhea virus in the nasal epithelial cells by the direct Immunofluorescence technique. *Can. J. Comp. Med.* 47:18–22.

35. Uttenthal, A., Hoye, M. J., Grondahl, C., Houe, H., Maanen, C., van Rasmussen, T. B. and Larsen, L. E. 2007. Vertical transmissionof bovine virus diarrhea virus (BVDV) in mouse deer (*Tragulus javanicus*) and spread to domestic cattle. *Arach. Virol.* 151:2379–2380.

36. Ward, A. C. S. and Kaeberle, M. L. 1984. Use of an immunoperoxidase stain for the demonstration of bovine viral diarrhea virus by light and electron microsopies. *Am. J. Vet. Res.* 45:165–170.

8. Foot-and-Mouth Disease

(Aphthous Fever, Panzootic Aphtha, Vesicular Aphtha, Eczema Contagiosa)

M. R. Saseendranath, M. Krishnan Nair, and Thankam Mathew

Introduction

Foot-and-mouth disease (FMD) is an acute contagious viral disease of cloven-footed animals characterized by fever and formation of vesicles on the tongue, gum, nasal mucous membrane, interdigital space, and on the teat and udder.

Etiology

The causative agent of foot-and-mouth disease (FMD) as a filterable agent was first discovered by Loeffler and Frosch in 1897 (Merchant and Barner 1973). The viral agent belongs to the genus *Aphthovirus* of the family Picornaviridae. There are seven main serotypes of FMD virus, namely O, A, C, SAT-1, SAT-2, SAT-3, and Asia-1 (Pereira, 1977). The serotypes O, A, and C were recorded from various part of the globe, whereas the serotypes SAT-1, SAT-2, SAT-3 were reported from South African territories in 1948. Asia-1 was reported from Pakistan in 1957. Thereafter more than sixty subtypes were recorded under various serotypes. Each of these serotypes is immunologically independent and never gives any cross-protection to others. Hence, animals after suffering from infection with one serotype are susceptible to infection with other serotypes.

FMD virus has an icosahedral shape with a diameter of 25 nm, comprising single-stranded RNA enclosed in a protein capsid consisting of thirty-two capsomers. It has got four main viral proteins namely, VP1 to VP4 of which VP1 stimulates the production of serum-neutralizing antibody and is associated with the adsorption of the virus to the host cell. VP1, VP2, and VP3 are seen on the capsid surface while VP4 is associated with the viral genome. The virus is very sensitive to pH and temperature changes, and this has clear implications for the shelf life of vaccines where cold chains are not efficient. Sunlight destroys the virus quickly. The virus is relatively sensitive to heat but insensitive to cold. Hence, survival of the virus outside the body of host in tropical countries is practically nil.

The thermal stability of different serotypes of virus varies. The A and Asia-1 are the most stable, and the Southern African strains are least stable, and O and C have intermediate stability (Carillo et al., 1997). Sodium carbonate (4%), sodium hydroxide (2%), and formaldehyde (2%) are the best disinfectants to be used during an outbreak. The virus may persist nearly for a year in infected premises in temperate zones.

EPIDEMIOLOGY

DISTRIBUTION
The first FMD outbreak in Europe was described by Fracastorius in 1546 (Merchant and Barner, 1973).

This disease is widespread globally except in North and Central America, Caribbean Islands, Australia, New Zealand, Japan, and UK, although UK had a severe outbreak during 2001 after a long gap since 1969. This disease is endemic in most of the Asian (Chandranaik et al., 2007) and African countries except some island nations. In 2007 summer, there was an outbreak in UK and Cyprus due to the leakage from the laboratory, and the laboratory in UK was closed and planned to rebuild (Internet news). Another FMD outbreak occurred in Isingiro, Uganda, in January 2008. In the same year, foot-and-mouth outbreak reached in Ngami, Botswana. In Vietnam, FMD was confirmed in two cows and twenty-four buffaloes in Hoa Binh Province in Cun Pheo commune, Mai Chau District, and laboratory tests were also positive. In three other districts namely, Kon Tum, SonLa, and Hoa Binh of Vietnam, foot-and-mouth outbreak also occurred in 2009 (Internet news, February 2009). In USA since 1929, no outbreak was noted and was eradicated.

SOURCE OF INFECTION
The main source of infection is from infected or diseased or convalescent animals or reservoir animals. The infected animals start excretion of the virus twenty-four hours before the onset of clinical signs. The excretion continues during the course of the disease and even during the convalescent period. The period of excretion after recovery varies between species. Cattle can excrete the virus for up to nine months to three years after recovery, sheep for nine months, and goats for three months, whereas pigs never act as carriers though they act as amplifier hosts. A minor percentage of FMD-vaccinated animals, when they become infected with field strains of the virus, turns to become carriers. The virus localize at the esophagopharyngeal area; because of this, some of the FMD-free countries want to maintain their FMD-free status by stamping out policy

rather than going for vaccination programs. But it has been observed that these animals never become a source of virus for an outbreak to occur unless such animals are slaughtered and meat scrapes are fed to pigs (Toma et al., 2002). The African buffalo *Syncerus caffer* acts as lifetime carrier for FMD virus (Vosloo et al., 2007). Significant reduction in duration of excretion of FMD virus has been observed following vaccination in lambs under experimental condition (Orsel et al., 2007).

TRANSMISSION

The most common route of transmission of FMD virus is by inhalation. Close contact with diseased animals, animals in incubation, and convalescent animals lead to transmission in tropical environment. The disease can spread over considerable distances by aerosol transmission and by wind (Gleeson et al., 1995). This mode of transmission is quite common in temperate zones where the atmospheric temperature is low with high humidity.

The second most important route is ingestion of contaminated feed, fodder, water, milk from suffering animals, and meat from diseased animals. Pigs can become infected when fed with meat scrapes and blood meals from diseased animals. Transmission can also occur indirectly by means of contaminated utensils, vehicles through attendants, milkers, and veterinarians. FMD virus crosses the placenta and causes death in fetal lambs (Ryan et al., 2007).

HOSTS

Cattle are the most susceptible species. Buffaloes, pigs, sheep, goats, camels, and wild animals such as deer, bison, antelope, llamas, wild pigs, alpacas, giraffes, elephants, elk, moles, rats, and hedgehogs are also susceptible to this disease. Birds also get infected. Rarely, man can also develop vesicles in the mouth or hands. Horses, donkeys, mules, and zebras are resistant to this disease.

Young animals are affected more severely and may die of the infection without showing premonitory signs. Native breeds are more resistant comparing pure breeds. Weak and debilitated animals are more likely to succumb to secondary infection.

PATHOGENESIS

The incubation period of FMD varies from one to twenty-one days with an average of two to seven days. The virus after entering the hosts multiplies in the cells at entry site to cause destruction of the cells and release of virions.

The released virions infect neighboring cells as well as mononuclear cells leading to viremia. They get localized in epithelial tissues in the oral cavity, in the interdigital space, and teat.

The initial lesion is a localized balloon degeneration of the cells in the middle of the stratum spinosum of the epithelium. Edema, with bits of fibrin, accumulates and cause separation of cells. Liquification necrosis and accumulation of serum and leucocytes cause production of vesicles, which results to form bullae. The virus also causes lesions in myocardium especially in young animals with hyaline degeneration and necrosis. Secondary bacterial infection generally complicates the lesion.

CLINICAL SIGNS
The clinical signs vary with the strain of the virus, exposure dose, the host species, the age and breed of the animal, and the level of immunity.

After an incubation period of two to seven days, the animal becomes dull, anorectic with cessation of rumination, and pyretic (105–107°F). The oral as well as the nasal mucous membranes become highly hyperemic. There is serous salivation and nasal discharge and is soon followed by development of vesicles on the tongue, gum, muzzle, snout, nasal mucous membrane, interdigital space, teats, and rarely on the vulva. The vesicles rupture, and ulcers develop. In a day or two, the serous nature of saliva changes over to frothy, ropy, and stringy type. The affected animals show uneasiness, discomfort, and may become lame and even recumbent. Pregnant animals may abort. Lactating animals may develop mastitis.

The course of the disease may take two to three weeks. Young animals may die due to multifocal myocarditis. Now, it is known that strains like O cause myocarditis in adult animals also. Though FMD is not a killer disease; sequela to FMD are very important, often leading to infertility, abortion, stillbirth, retention of placenta, mastitis, and improper response to subsequent vaccination by poor immune response. Diabetes mellitus in bovines is also observed as complication. The condition *panter* with raised hair and low heat tolerance is very characteristic in animals, which have recovered from FMD. The milk production falls drastically. The work efficiency of draft animals suffers markedly.

IMMUNE RESPONSE
Serum immunoglobulin M (IgM) may be detected three to five days after infection, reaching a peak between five to ten days. Serum IgG1 and IgG2 appears from the fourth day onward and reach maximum level between

fifteen to twenty days. Virus-neutralizing antibodies may be present for years, whereas IgM does not generally persist (Abu Elzein and Crowther 1981; Carillo et al., 1997). Mucosal immune responses have also been studied following infection in cattle. A peak of neutralizing activity attributed to IgM and IgA was observed in the pharyngeal fluids seven days after the virus exposure. Between twenty to sixty days postinfection, the neutralizing activity of the pharyngeal fluid was attributed exclusively to IgA produced at mucosal surfaces rather than by serum transudation (Francis et al., 1983).

DIAGNOSIS

Diagnosis is often done based on clinical signs, demonstration of viral antigens, and demonstration antibody to viral proteins. Demonstration of the viral antigen is being done usually by complement fixation test (CFT) and enzyme-linked immunosorbent assay (ELISA) and polymerase chain reaction (RT-PCR) (Reid et al., 1998; El-Kohly et al., 2007).

A liquid phase blocking ELISA was developed to quantify FMD antibodies (Gruia et al., 1995; Chen et al., 2007) and is being used internationally. Demonstration of specific antibody in unvaccinated animal is also being used for diagnosis.

The latex agglutination test is simple, rapid, and sensitive for the detection of antibody of FMD virus in the surveillance of FMD (Sugimura et al., 2000). The clinical materials to be collected for the diagnosis are vesicular fluid, epithelial covering from unruptured as well as freshly ruptured vesicles, blood at the height of pyrexia, esophageal/pharyngeal fluid using a probang cup in ruminants, throat swabs in pigs, and myocardial tissues and blood from fatal cases. The clinical materials can be collected in viral transport medium consisting of equal amounts of glycerol and 0.04M phosphate buffer (pH 7.2–7.6) with antibiotics (penicillin 1000 IU, neomycin 100 IU, polymixin bisulphate 50 IU, and Mycostatin 100 IU per ml of the medium). The detection of FMD virus persistent carriers among convalescent ruminants is of paramount importance in the aftermath of a field outbreak, and it is possible to demonstrate the mucosal rather than serum antibody. Infected animals regularly mount antibody response in oropharyngeal fluids, in contrast to vaccinated cattle, which can be demonstrated by neutralization assay and/or immunoglobulin–specific (IgA-specific) kinetic ELISA (Archetti et al., 1998). Vaccinated cattle seldom show mucosal antibody response (Berinstein et al., 1993). An epitope-blocking, enzyme-linked immunosorbent assay has been used for the detection of antibodies to nonstructured proteins (NSPs) to differentiate

FMD-infected and FMD-vaccinated animals (Perkins et al., 2006; Oem Jaeku et al., 2007).

TREATMENT

There is no specific treatment for FMD. Supportive therapy with fluids and vitamins along with broad spectrum antibiotics to prevent secondary bacterial complications can be employed. Cleaning and dressing of the wounds and ulcers with antibiotic and antiseptics lotions and ointments have to be done to heal the oral, foot, and udder lesions.

PREVENTION AND CONTROL

Different strategies are employed to control FMD in different parts of the world.

For FMD-free zones, prevention of contact with infection, strict quarantine of livestock and their products, stamping out (by slaughter) of all suspected or infected animals, and proper disposal of contaminated products and surveillance are recommended. Vaccination is not advocated since a minor proportion of vaccinated animals may become carriers.

For FMD-semifree zones control program mainly depends on the combination of strict quarantine, zoo sanitary measures, slaughter of infected animals, and wherever necessary a compulsory regular vaccination and surveillance.

For FMD endemic zones, epidemiological studies are conducted, and a major percentage of the susceptible population is covered under compulsory vaccination at regular intervals with strict surveillance. The vaccination program must be coupled with supportive zoo sanitary measures and legislative support. In the event of an outbreak, immediate ban must be enforced on the movement of livestock, animal products (milk, meat, semen, etc.), fodder, feed, vehicle, etc., from the foci of infection. The diseased animals should not be let loose for grazing. Ban on visitors in organized farms must be implemented during an outbreak. No assembling of animals in vaccination and health camps should be allowed during an outbreak. Immediate containment/ring vaccination at a radius of 10 km has to be carried out starting from the periphery. In most of the endemic zones, stamping-out policy cannot be implemented due socioeconomic reasons.

VACCINATION

Depending on the epidemiological studies and according to the requirement of each region, the different combinations of polyvalent and monovalent-inactivated FMD vaccines are recommended. There are a number critical elements in the production of FMD vaccines, such as the selection of appropriate strains, which have direct bearing on the quality of the immune response and proper and timely application of good-quality vaccine.

The efficient control of FMD by immunization depends not only on the appropriate choice of the vaccine in terms of infectivity, potency, and strain composition but also on a series of interrelated zoo sanitary factors, which are also equally important. These include national centralized planning (including contingency planning) and control, vaccination and revaccination policy, the availability of epizootiological intelligence based on adequate diagnostic capability and ongoing immunological surveillance, the logistics of supply with its components of storage, transport and distribution, proper vaccine application, cleaning and disinfection of premises, vehicle and belongings of personnel, control of animal movements, recording, ongoing economic outcome and benefit analysis, training and retraining of technical staff, public relations, and commitment of agricultural community. In most of the tropical countries where vaccinations is practiced, inactivated quadrivalent FMD (O, A, C, Asia-1) vaccine is being used.

There are two types; the difference is only in the adjuvants used. They are aluminum hydroxide gel and oil adjuvanted vaccines. Aluminum hydroxide gel vaccine is mainly used for the ruminants, whereas oil adjuvanted vaccine is used for ruminants as well as for pigs. In India where this disease is endemic, aluminum hydroxide gel vaccines was being used, but during the last few years, the oil adjuvant vaccine has started replacing the aluminum gel vaccine. Now in India, trivalent oil adjuvanted vaccine is being produced excluding the serotype C as the outbreak due to C had never occurred for the last several years. Arlacal A, Mannide Monoleate, Bayfol F, Drakeol 6VR, Marcol 52 are some of the common oils used in the production of FMD vaccines.

Three FMD vaccine formulations viz, aluminum hydroxide saponin, Marcol oil emulsion and paraffin oil emulsion were tried, and it is seen that Marcol oil emulsion vaccine provides better immune response than the other two vaccines. Booster vaccination carried out after 21 days of primary did not have any significant effect on antibody titer. The titer also remained protective for 270 days. The maternal antibodies also had no effect of immune response with oil adjuvant vaccines (Anand Rao et al., 1993).

The duration of immunity, protection, stimulation of immunocompetent cells producing long-lasting secondary response and IgG response by oil adjuvanted vaccines had been reported (Berinstein et al., 1993).

The structural protein G-H loop of VP1 of FMD virus has been expressed and shown to induce virus-neutralizing antibodies and protection in more than 40% experimental and natural hosts (Taboga et al., 1997). By transplanting the gene-encoding VP1, transformed plants (*Arabidopsis thaliana*) expressing VP1 elicited specific antibody responses to synthetic peptides representing amino acid residue 135 to 160 of VP1 and protected against challenge with FMDV in immunized mice (Carillo et al., 1997).

FMD antigen harvests used to prepare vaccine contain a high proportion of irrelevant proteins and small quantities of structural proteins of FMDV. The structural proteins include whole virus particles (146S particles) and various subunits, including natural empty particles (75S) and pentameric clusters (12S) of virus proteins, VP1, VP2, and VP3. The immunogenicity of 146S particles exceed that of 75S particles, and the 12S particles by about ten and one hundred times respectively (Doel and Chong, 1982). The integrity of 146S particles is thus crucial to the efficacy of vaccine, and poor thermal stability probably accounts for some FMD vaccines (Doel and Baccarini, 1981). Another aspect of antigenic integrity is the VP1 proteins within the 146S particles. Many enzymes, including trypsin, cleave important antigenic determinant on VP1 and while not affecting the stability of the capsid, seriously reduce the immunogenicity of the virus and hence the vaccine (Doel and Collen, 1982). The 146S particles of different serotypes vary considerably in their immunogenicity of the virus; hence, it is a common practice to use five to tenfold of O virus than the other serotypes per dose of vaccine.

Inactivation with acetylethyleneimine (AEI) and binary ethyleneimine (BEI) reduces the thermal stability of all serotypes (Gomez and Doel, 1984) particularly with serotype O, whereas the inactivation by aldehydes are reported to enhance the thermal stability. The main drawback with formaldehyde treatment is its residual infectivity leading to vaccine-induced outbreak.

FMD remains the most important disease of livestock and one of the most difficult to control, nationally and internationally, because of the rapidity and ease with which it can spread. Thus, a serious outbreak in any one country should never be taken lightly. It represents not only a threat to neighboring countries but also a dangerous source of disease, which could be transferred to a distant trading partner. So it is in the interest of all concerned to do everything possible to control this disease by strict measures. Some countries are planning to develop support a system for managing FMD epidemic by using variety of computer technologies, including data-based management system and geographic information system.

REFERENCES

1. Abu Elzein, E. M. E. and Crowther, J. R. 1981. Detection and quantification of IgM, IgA, IgG1 and IgG2 antibodies against foot and mouth disease virus from bovine sera using and enzyme linked immunosorbant assay. *J. Hyg. Camb.* 86:79–85.

2. Ananda Rao, K., Palanisamy, R., Kalanidhi, A. P., Azad, H. M. and Srinivasan, V. A. 1993. Use of oil adjuvant vaccine in cattle. *Indian Vet. J.* 70:490–497.

3. Archetti, I. L., Amadori, M., Donn, A., Salt, J. and Lodetti, E. 1998. Detection of foot and mouth disease virus-infected cattle by assessment of antibody response in oropharyngeal. *J. Virol.* 72:1688–1690.

4. Berinstein, A., Perez Filgueira, M., Schudel, A., Zamorano, P., Borca, M. and Sadir, A. 1993. Avridine and LPS from *Brucella ovis*: Effect on the memory induced by foot and mouth disease virus vaccination in mice. *Vaccine* 11:1295–1301.

5. Carillo, C., Wigdorovitz, A., Oliveros, J. C., Zamorano, P. I. Szadir, A. M., Gomez, N., Salinas, J., Escribano, J. M. and Borca, M. V. 1997. Protective immune response to foot and mouth disease virus with VP1 expressed in transgenic plants. *J. Virol* 71:2606–2614.

6. Chandranaik, B. M., Girsh, V. R., Harish, B. R., Ravindra Hedge, Mamta, G. S., Renukaprasad, C. and Krishnappa, G. 2007. Isolation of Asia-1 FMD virus from an outbreak in Karnataka. *Indian Vet. J.* 84:434–435.

7. Chen, S. P., Lee, M. C., Sun, Y. F., Cheng, I. C., Yang, P. C., Lin, Y. I., Jing, M. H., Robetson, I. D., Edward, J. R. and Ellis, T. M. 2007. Immune response of pigs to commercialized emulsion FMD vaccines and live virus challenge. *Vaccine* 25:4464–4469.

8. Doel, T. R. and Baccarini, P. J. 1981. Thermal stability of foot and mouth disease virus. *Arch. Virol.* 70:21–32.

9. Doel, T. R. and Chong, W. K. T. 1982. Comparative immunogenicity of 146S, 75S and 12S particles of foot and mouth disease virus. *Arch. Virol.* 73:185–191.

10. Doel, T. R. and Collen, T. 1982. Qualitative assessment of 146S particles of foot and mouth disease virus in preparation destined for vaccine. *J. Biol. Standard* 10:69–81.

11. El-Kohly, A. A., Soliman, H. M. T. and Rehman, A. O. A. 2007. Molecular typing of a new foot and mouth disease virus in Egypt. *Vet. Rec.*160:695–697.

12. Francis, M. J., Ouldridge, E. J., and Black, L. 1983. Antibody response in bovine pharyngeal fluid following foot and mouth disease vaccination and or exposure to live virus. *Res. Vet. Sc.* 35:206–210.

13. Gleeson, L. J., Chamnanpood, P., Cheunprasert, S., Srimasartitkol, N. and Trisasarom, A. 1995. Investigation of an outbreak of foot and mouth disease in vaccinated dairy cattle in Thailand. *Aust. Vet.* 72:21–24.

14. Gomez, G. J. and Doel, T. R. 1984. Effect of temperature and inactivating agents on Colombian strains of apthovirus. *Revta lat. amer. Microbiol.* 26:21–26.

15. Gruia, M., Danes, M. and Borca, M. 1995. Liquid phase blocking ELISA in (foot and mouth disease) FMD antibody detection. *J. Pasteur Institute of Romania* 3:22–25.

16. Intenet News. 2008. *http://www.earlywarninginc.com/*outbreaks.php?m=1&y=2008.

17. Internet News. 2009. http://www.thecattlesite.com/footandmouth/26133/disease-spreads-in-viet-nam.

18. Merchant, I. A. and Barner, R. D. 1973. *An outline of infectious diseases of domestic animals.* 3rd ed., 199. New Delhi: Oxford & IBH Publishing Company.

19. Oem Jaeku, Chang Byung Sik, Joo too Don, Yang Mi Young, Kim G. Wang Jae, Park Jee Young, Ko Young Joon, Kim yong Jn, Park Jong Hyeon and Joo Yi Seok. 2007. Development of an epitope-blocking-enzyme linked immunosorbent assay to differentiate between animals infected with and vaccinated aginst foot and mouth disease virus. *J. Virol. Meth.* 142:174–181.

20. Orsel, K., Dekker, A., Bouma, A., Stageman, J. A., and Jong, M. C. M. 2007. Quantification of foot and mouth disease virus excretion and transmission within groups of lambs with and without vaccination. *Vaccine* 25:2673–2679.

21. Pereira, H. G. 1977. Subtyping of foot and mouth disease virus. *Developments in Biological Standardization* 35:165–174.

22. Perkins, J., Clavijo, A., Hindson, B. J., Lenhoff, R J. and McBride, M. T. 2006. Multiplexed detection of antibodies to non structured proteins of foot and mouth diseased virus. *Analytical Chemistry* 78:5462–5468.

23. Ryan, E., Zhang, Z., Brooks, H. W., Horisington, J. and Brownlie, J. 2007. Foot and mouth disease viruss crosses the placenta and causes death in fetal lambs. *J. Comp. Path.* 136:256–265.

24. Sugimura, T., Suzuki, T., Chatchawanchonteera, A., Sinuwonkwat, P., Tsuda, T. and Murakami, Y. 2000. Application of Latex beads agglutination tests for the detection of antibody against virus infection associated (VIA) antigen of foot and mouth disease virus. *Vaccine* 17:1767–1771.

25. Taboga, O., Tami, C., Carrillo, E., Nunez, J. I., Radrigues, A., Saiz, J. C., Blanco, E., Valero, M. L. and Roig, X. 1997. A large scale evaluation of peptide vaccines against foot and mouth disease; lack of solid protection in cattle and isolation of escape mutants. *J. Virol.* 71:2606–2614.

26. Toma, B., Moutou, F., Dufour, B. and Durand, B. 2002. Ring vaccination against foot and mouth disease. *Comp. Immune. Microbiol. Infect. Dis.* 25:365–372.

27. Reid, S. M., Frosyth, M. A., Hutchings, G. H. and Ferris, N. P. 1998. Comparison of RtPCR ELISA and virus isolation for the routine diagnosis of FMD. *J. Virol. Meth.* 70:213–214.

28. Vosloo, W., Klerk, L. M. De., Boshoff. C. I., Botha, B., Dwaraka, R. M., Keet, D. and Haydon, D. N. 2007. Characterisation of a SAT-1 outbreak of foot and mouth disease in captive African buffalo (*Syncerus caffer*): Clinical symptoms, genetic characterization and phylogenetic comparison of outbreak isolates. *Vet. Microbiol.* 120:226–240.

9. Infectious Bovine Rhinotracheitis (IBR)

(Red Nose, Infectious Pustular Vulvovaginitis, Infectious Balanoposthitis, Summer Pink Eye, Bovine Herpesvirus)

M. R. Saseendranath, and M. Krishnan Nair

Introduction

Infectious bovine rhinotracheitis (IBR) is a highly contagious disease caused by bovine herpesvirus 1 (BHV-1) showing different clinical forms as rhinotracheitis, pustular vulvovaginitis, pustular balanoposthitis, abortions, conjunctivitis, encephalitis, and enteritis. The infection is seen both in cattle and buffaloes. Generalized systemic infection is seen in calves.

IBR is placed in list B disease in the Office International Des Epizooties (OIE) classification.

Etiology

IBR is caused by BHV-1 virus. The viral etiology of the disease was confirmed by Madin et al. (1956). The different subtypes of BHV-1 are capable of attacking various tissues in the body leading to a variety of clinical signs. Bovine herpes virus 1(BHV-1) is a ssDNA virus belonging to the family Herpesviridae.

Genetic analysis of various clinical isolates has found different BHV-1 subtypes, designated as BHV-1.1; BHV-1.2a; BHV-1.2b; and BHV-1.3. Afterward, BHV-1.3 has been renamed as BHV-5. BHV1.1 causes mainly the respiratory form of the disease while BHV1.2a and BHV-1.2b cause genital infection. BHV-1.3 (BHV-5) is responsible for the encephalitic form. Viruses belonging to subtypes 1.1 and 1.2a are more virulent than those belonging of subtype 1.2b.

The virus is stable between pH 6–9. BHV is extremely susceptible to lipid solvents such as ether, acetone, ethyl alcohol, and chloroform. The virus is inactivated within twenty-one minutes at 56°C within ten days at 37°C and stable for up to one month at 4°C and for nine months at -60°C (Snowden, 1964). The virus may survive for up to one year in frozen semen at -196°C.

Distribution

IBR was first recorded as a specific disease syndrome in Colorado feedlot cattle in the early1950s, and the first clinical description of the disease was published in 1955 (Miller, 1955). IBR was originally recognized as a respiratory disease of cattle in the Western United States. Later, IBR became recognized as a complex of disease syndromes occurring throughout the world wherever intensive cattle rearing was going on, except in several European countries that had eradicated the infection. IBR is known to exist in India since 1976 (Mehrotra, 1977). Since then various reports have come from different parts of the country (Sulochana et al., 1982; Renukaradhya et al., 1996 and Suresh et al., 1999). Morbidity can go up to 100%, and mortality is about 10%.

SOURCE OF INFECTION

Main sources of infection are the nasal exudates and coughed-up droplets, genital secretions, semen, fetal fluids and tissues from infected, diseased, and recovered animals. One peculiarity of IBR infection is its latency, and when there is immunosuppression or any other kind of stress, reactivation can occur, and the virus is shed in secretions from the eyes, nose, and reproductive organs (Miller, 1991). Such animals become source of BHV-1 infection for other animals. IBR virus can persist in clinically recovered animals for years.

TRANSMISSION

IBR transmission is by airborne-infected materials, or by contact (Noordegraaf et al., 1998). Other methods of spread are coital (Collings et al., 1972), by artificial insemination (Suresh et al., 1991; Renukaradhya et al., 1996), in utero, and congenital during passage of the newborn through the infected vagina at calving.

HOSTS

IBR is a highly infectious disease of cattle. Holstein Friesian showed higher incidence of BHV-1 seropositivity than Jersey cattle (Masolla et al., 1981). The virus naturally infects cattle, water buffaloes, goats, pigs, mule deer, and some wild ruminants. All ages and breeds of cattle are susceptible but is most commonly found in aged cattle (McDermott et al., 1997).

PATHOGENESIS

The virus can cause different clinical syndromes depending upon the route of infection and also the subtype that causes the infection. The primary infection is restricted to the respiratory tract, eyes, and the reproductive tract.

The virus invades the epithelial cells of the upper respiratory tract, conjunctiva, nostril, digestive and genital tracts, resulting in hyperemia, edema, and necrosis of epithelial cells and eventually resulting in various clinical manifestations.

The systemic form of the infection in calves is characterized by severe inflammation and necrosis of the respiratory and alimentary tract, including the pharynx, esophagus, lungs, larynx, lymph nodes, liver, kidney, and brain.

The virus spreads from the nasal mucosa via the trigeminal nerve to the trigeminal ganglion and to the brain resulting in a nonsuppurative encephalitis.

CLINICAL SIGNS

Clinical symptoms depend on the tissue infected, the strain of the virus, environmental conditions, managemental practices, and the resistance of the animal. The incubation period is usually four to six days, and the infection lasts for ten to fourteen days.

In general, the IBR virus produces different clinical forms of disease in cattle respiratory, ocular (Timoney et al., 1971), abortion (Kennedy and Richards, 1964), infectious pustular vulvovaginitis (Kendrick et al., 1958; Cook, 1998), infectious pustular balanoposthitis, encephalitis (Barenfus et al., 1964), and generalized infections of newborn calves (Miller, 1955; Gibbs and Rweyemamu, 1977). The outcome of BHV-1 infection can vary from subclinical to a systemic infection in neonatal calves that is often highly fatal.

Respiratory form of IBR was the first to be reported in association with the disease. Depression, fever (104–108°F), and decreased appetite accompany the respiratory signs. Dyspnea, hyperemia of nasal mucous membrane, and profuse watery nasal discharge are the initial signs. The nasal discharge becomes thicker and darker as the disease progresses. The animal stands with its head and neck extended. Later, small necrotic foci appear on the nasal mucous membrane and becomes crusted.

The upper respiratory tract is involved affecting the nasal turbinates, sinuses, pharynx, larynx, and trachea. Dry, nonproductive cough is noted. Death is uncommon unless the disease is complicated with secondary bacterial infection. Ulcers are common in the nose and mouth.

Reproductive form of the disease causes infectious pustular vulvovaginitis in cows and infectious pustular balanoposthitis in bulls (Studdert et al., 1964).

Infectious pustular vulvovaginitis (IPV) is characterized by a thick yellow to brown vulvar discharge that attaches to the vulvar tufts of hairs. The vulva is swollen, and the vulvar and vaginal lining is reddened, and small whitish necrotic foci are seen. The irritation at the vulvar and vaginal mucous membrane leads to frequent tail-switching and urination. Upon spreading vulval lips, red spots and discrete pustules may be noted. The course of IPV is usually two to three weeks. Sometimes infertility also accompanies the infection. Lesions similar to the IPV may appear on the penis and prepuce of the bulls. Symptoms include fever, depression, loss of appetite, and painful urination. Usually the lesions both in cows and bulls resolve in two to three weeks' time.

Abortion occurs two to seven days after death of the fetus. Usually an incubation period of eighteen days to three months is observed, and abortion may occur at any stage of the gestation period but is usually noticed in the second half of the gestation. Often this abortion is preceded by a mild respiratory and/or eye infection (pink eye). The aborted fetus has no consistent gross characteristic lesions, and in utero infection can occur at any stage of gestation. The dam looks apparently healthy, and there are no signs of impending abortion. Abortion occurs as a result of fetal death, and the fetus is usually partially decomposed. Such animals usually breed back without any problem.

Abortion may also be produced by vaccination of pregnant animals with some modified live vaccines. Calves may be born with the IBR virus. The calves may be weak and may have enteritis or respiratory symptoms. Keratoconjunctivitis is another form of IBR infection characterized by reddened, swollen mucous membrane. There is clear watery lacrimation in the beginning, which becomes purulent in the subsequent days due to secondary complication. The secretion causes the hair to mat and closure of the eyelids.

Encephalitic form of IBR results in depression, ataxia, and other nervous signs. BHV-1 also causes generalized disease in newborn calves, characterized by generalized infection, bronchopneumonia, enteritis, and death.

Systemic infection of IBR in calves under ten days of age is severe and highly fatal. Anorexia, fever, salivation, and rhinitis, accompanied by unilateral or bilateral conjunctivitis are common in calves. The oral mucous membrane becomes hyperemic, and erosions on the soft palate covered with tenacious mucopurulent exudate are characteristic.

All clinical signs may subside within a fortnight, but the infected animals remain as a lifelong carrier. These convalescent carriers may spread the virus when reactivated either by stress or by infection by other agents like BVDV or subsequent immunosuppression.

IMMUNE RESPONSE

A natural infection or vaccination with modified live vaccine induces both cell-mediated and humoral immunity. The level of neutralizing antibody is not a reliable indicator of resistance to clinical disease. Nine to thirteen days after infection, the serum-neutralizing antibody IgM appears in the serum, and nasal and ocular secretions and are detectable up to a month. The IgA antibodies appear few days later than the IgM antibodies. In the serum IgA antibodies are no longer detectable after three weeks but persist for prolonged periods in mucosal secretions. No antibody responses are detectable in genital secretions.

The intranasal vaccine has the ability to induce local or mucosal immunity. The vaccine has also been reported to induce interferon production, which can provide early protection against the viral infection. The interferon appears in three days and persists for ten days. Use of these vaccines in combination should be considered for immunization of young calves. Primary vaccination with intranasal vaccine provides early resistance to the virus. Secondary vaccination with inactivated virus markedly enhances circulating antibody titer, which may result in giving further resistance to infection. Maternal antibody in the calf may interfere with the successful vaccination of calves before six months of age.

DIAGNOSIS

Although the clinical findings of respiratory disease, abortion, or IPV may be highly suggestive of IBR, laboratory confirmation is necessary for the diagnosis.

The isolation of the organism from the affected tissues and secretions, demonstration of the virus, viral antigens, and antibodies by a battery of serological and molecular test are applied to confirm the diagnosis. The virus is also detected by electron microscopy. The most widely applied antigen detection test is immunofluorescence.

Rapid diagnosis of IBR antigen in the tissues such as liver, brain, and fetal spleen using immunofluorescence is found to be very effective (Reed et al., 1971).

Immunoprecipitation test (Aruna and Suribabu, 1982), neutralization tests, passive hemagglutination test (Suresh et al., 1992), and ELISA are also employed for detection of BHV-1 antibodies.

Antibody detection by ELISA is one among the best and is a rapid, inexpensive, and simple method for screening sera samples (Sharma et al., 2006). Avidin-biotin ELISA is found to be very sensitive and specific (Suersh et al., 1999).

Herd screening is commonly based on serological tests such as ELISA and virus-neutralization test.

Confirmation of exposure to BHV-1 infection is also facilitated by measurement of antibody in serum, plasma, or milk. Paired serum samples should show an increase in the titer. From the live animal, nasal or ocular swabs may be taken for virus isolation or antigen detection test using molecular tests like PCR (Salomskas et al., 2006).

DIFFERENTIAL DIAGNOSIS

IBR has to be differentiated from pasteurellosis, which shows all the pneumonic signs. Pasteurellosis can be diagnosed by blood smear examination and from the treatment response with antibiotics. The erosive lesions are absent in pasteurellosis.

Bovine viral diarrhea is another important disease to be differentiated, which is characterized by depression, fever, anorexia, oral lesions and ulcers, persistent diarrhea, dehydration, and death in few days, whereas the mortality is less in IBR and diarrhea is not always present. Calf diphtheria and viral pneumonia are the other diseases to be differentiated from neonatal form of IBR, which can be done by serological and molecular tests.

TREATMENT

As in the case of other viral infections, there is no specific therapy. Antibiotics to prevent secondary bacterial infection may be necessary.

PREVENTION AND CONTROL

Biosecurity measures and vaccination are the tools for control of IBR. Control of IBR infection can be done by sero-monitoring of herds at regular intervals and by elimination of the reactors.

All new additions should be examined and must be free of infection. Isolate all new additions for at least thirty days and reexamine them before adding to the herd.

Isolate all diseased animals immediately upon detection. Eliminate the reactors by slaughter or by incineration. Assure hygienic standards to prevent the spread of the virus. Rodent control, fly control, disinfection, optimized housing, and good management conditions would help to prevent the occurrence of the disease. Always purchase animals from BHV-negative herds.

VACCINATION

Vaccination using modified live and inactivated vaccines is used for the prevention of IBR. Fast-acting intranasal vaccine, which confers shorter immunity, is very useful. Live vaccines stimulate serum-neutralizing antibody response, but inactivated vaccines do not elicit any serological response (Frerichs et al., 1982). Vaccinate young calves intranasally with live vaccine, revaccinate after a month, and with booster dose as per manufacturer's direction every year. Nasal vaccines and killed vaccines can be used in pregnant animals. Two doses at four weeks' interval are recommended and then repeated annually. The main types of vaccines stimulate the production of local interferon, local secretory immunoglobulin, cell-mediated antibody, and humoral antibody.

The major surface glycoproteins of the BHV-1 are the antigen responsible for the induction of protective immunity. The major glycoproteins of BHV-1 are gI, gIII, and gIV are now renamed as gB, gC, and gD.

ERADICATION

As a first step, the disease has to be made notifiable. Annual screening and elimination of the reactors, testing of animals before addition to the herd, and vaccination of the susceptible populations are the key points of eradication.

Countries that have IBR control programs require IBR-free certification prior to shipping cattle to their regions. ELISA is the test preferred by many European countries. The reactors are culled, slaughtered, and disposed of either by deep burial or by burning. Vaccination of all susceptible population is mandatory in IBR-eradicated countries.

REFERENCES

1. Aruna, D. and Suribabau, T. 1982. Immunoprecipitation tests for detection of IBR virus. *Indian J. Anim. Sci.* 62:414–415.
2. Barenfus, M., Delliqiuadri, C. A., Mc Intyre, R. W. and Schroeder, R. J. 1964. Isolation of infectious bovine rhinotracheitis virus from calves with meningoencephlitis. *Am. Vet. Med. Ass.* 143:725–728.
3. Collings, D. F., Gibbs, E. P. J. and Stafford, L. P. 1972. Concurrent respiratory and genital disease associated with infectious bovine rhinotracheitis/infectious pustular vulvovaginitis (IBR/IPV) virus in a dairy herd in the United Kingdom. *Vet. Rec.* 91:214–219.
4. Cook, N. 1998. Bovine herpes virus-1. Clinical manifestations and an outbreak of infectious pustular vulvo vaginitis in a UK dairy herd. *Cattle Practice* 6:341–344.

9. INFECTIOUS BOVINE RHINOTRACHEITIS (IBR)

5. Frerichs, G. N., Woods, S. B., Lucas, M. H. and Sands, J. J. 1982. Safety and efficiency live and inactivated infectious bovine rhionotrachietis vaccines. *Vet. Rec.* 111.116–122.

6. Gibbs, E. P. J. and Rweyemamu, M. M. 1977. Bovine herpes viruses. Part I. *Vet. Bulletin* 47:317–343.

7. Kendrick, J. W., Gillepie, J. H. and McEntee, K. 1958. Infectious pustular vulvovaginitis of cattle. *Cornell Vet.* 48:458–495.

8. Kennedy, P. C. and Richards, W. P. C. 1964. The pathology of abortion caused by the virus of infectious bovine rhinotracheitis. *Path. Vet.* 1:7–17.

9. Madin, S. H., York, C. J. and Mc Kercher, D. G. 1956. Isolation of infectious bovine rhinotracheitis virus. *Science* 124:721–722.

10. Massola, D. M., Welsman, A. and Soleman, I. E. 1981. The prevalence of serum neutralizing antibodies to infectious bovine rhinotracheitis virus in Scotland. *J. Hygeine* 86:209–215.

11. Mc Dermott, J. J., Kadohira, M., O'Callaghan, C. J. and Shoukri, M. M. 1997. A comparison of different models for assessing variations in the seroprevalence of infectious bovine rhinotracheitis by farm, area, and district in Kenya. *Preventive Vet. Med.* 32:219–234.

12. Mehrotra, M. L.1977. Isolation of respiratory viruses from cattle and their possible role in genital disorders. PhD thesis, Agra University.

13. Miller, N. J. 1955. Infectious bovine rhinotracheitis of cattle. *J. Am. Vet. Med. Ass.* 126:463–467.

14. Miller, J. M. 1991. The effects of IBR virus infection on reproductive function of cattle. *Vet. Med.* 1:95–98.

15. Noordegraaf, A. V., Buijtels, J. A. A. M., Dijkhuizen, A. A., Franken, P., Stegman, J. A. and Verhoeff, J. 1998. An epidemiological and economic simulation model to evaluate the spread and control of infectious bovine rhinotracheitis in the Netherlands. *Preventive Vet. Med.* 36:219–238.

16. Reed, D. E., Bicknell, E. J. and Bury, R. J. 1973. Systemic form of infectious bovine rhinotrachieits in young calves. *J. Am. Vet. Med. Assoc.* 163:753–755.

17. Renukaradhya, G. J., Rajasekhar, M. and Raghavan, R. 1996. Prevalence of infectious bovine rhinotracheitis in southern India. *Rev. Sci. Tech. off. Int. Epiz.* 15:1021–1028.

18. Salomskas, A., Mokeeliuniene, V., Jacevicius, E., Lelesius, R., Mockeliunas, R., Kliucinskas, R. and Petkevicius, S. 2006. Diagoisis and prevention of infectious bovine rhinotracheitis and bovine viral diarrhoea in Lithuania. *Veterinariarija ir zootechnika* 33:55.

19. Sharma, M., Katoch, R. C. and Charanjeet Dhar, P. 2006. Seroprevalence of IBR among cattle in Himachal Pradesh. *Indian Vet. J.* 83:1–3.

20. Snowden, W. A. 1964. Infectious tracheitis and infectious pustular vulvovaginitis in Australian cattle. *Aust. Vet. J.* 40:277–288.

21. Studdert, M. J., Barker, C. A. V. and Savan, M. 1964. Infectious pustular vulvo vaginitis virus infection in bulls. *Am. J. Vet. Res.* 25:303–314.

22. Sulochana, S., Pillai, R., Nair, G. K. and Abdulla, P. K. 1982. Serological survey on the occurrence of infectious bovine rhinotracheitis in Kerala. *Indian J. Comp. Micro. Imm. Inf. Dis.* 3:7–11.

23. Suresh, S., Gunaseelan, L., Kumanan, K. and Manorama Dhinakaran 1992. A modified passive haemagglutination test for the detection of Bovine herpes virus1 antibodies in bovines. *Cheiron* 21:137–140.

24. Suresh, K. B., Sudharsana, K. J. and Jasekhar, M. 1999. Seroprevalence of infectious bovine rhinotracheitis in cattle. *Indian Vet. J.* 76:5–9.

25. Timoney, P. J. and O'Connor, P. J. 1971. An outbreak of conjunctival form of infectious bovine rhinotracheitis virus infection. *Vet. Res.* 89:370.

10. LUMPY SKIN DISEASE

(Dermatosis Nodularis, Exanthema Nodularis Bovis, Lumpy Disease, Knowpvelsiekte Neethling Virus Disease, Pseudourticaria)

M. R. SASEENDRANATH, M. KRISHNAN NAIR, Z. MATHEW, AND THANKAM MATHEW

INTRODUCTION

Lumpy skin disease (LSD) is an economically important viral disease of cattle and rarely of buffaloes, characterized by eruption of variably sized skin nodules, edema of the limbs, and swelling of the superficial lymph nodes. It causes damage to hides, loss of milk and beef production, abortions in females, and sterility in males (Green, 1959), while lesions in the mouth, pharynx, and respiratory tract cause a rapid deterioration in condition and sometimes severe emaciation persisting for months. An epizootic in South Africa, which lasted until 1949, affected eight million cattle and consequently incurred enormous economic losses (Thomas and Mare, 1945; von Backstrom, 1945; Diesel, 1949). Office International Des Epizooties (OIE) has classified LSD under list A disease.

ETIOLOGY

LSD is caused by lumpy skin disease virus belonging to the genus *Capripoxvirus* under the family Poxviridae (Fenner, 1976).

Poxviridae viruses are large-sized, double-stranded DNA organisms. LSD viruses are brick or oval shaped; over one hundred polypeptides exist within the virions, which are arranged in a core, two lateral bodies, a membrane, and an envelope. The envelope contains two layers of cellular lipids and several virus-specific polypeptides. Mature virions that are released from the cell without disruption are enveloped, most are released by the rupture of the host cell, and therefore are nonenveloped. Both enveloped and nonenveloped virions are infectious.

The average size of *Capripoxvirus* is 260–320 nm. LSD virus is closely related to sheep and goat poxvirus, with cross immunity between the three viruses. LSD has only one serotype. LSD virus is susceptible to 55°C for two hours, 65°C for thirty minutes, and susceptible to high alkaline or acid pH. The virus is inactivated by direct sunlight but survives well at cold temperatures.

Sodium hypochlorite 2%, sodium hydroxide 2%, gluteraldehyde 2%, formalin 1%, and phenol 2% are found to be very effective in disinfection of the premises during an outbreak of LSD.

LSD virus can survive up to six months in a suitable environment and can persist for up to thirty-three days in dried skin lesions.

EPIDEMIOLOGY

LSD has a morbidity of 5–85% and mortality ranging from 2–40%. Death rate is more among calves.

Incidence of LSD is highest in summer, but it may occur in winter also. It is more prevalent along water courses and on low ground. African buffaloes (*Syncerus caffer*) are suspected of being carriers of LSD virus in Kenya.

DISTRIBUTION

LSD is a disease of cattle, primarily in Africa and Madagascar and rarely in the Middle East. LSD has occurred in a wide range of ecotypes in Africa, where it appears to have spread to virtually all countries on the continent.

The clinical syndrome of LSD was first described in Zambia (formerly Northern Rhodesia) in 1929, in Botswana (Bechuanaland) in 1943, the Republic of South Africa in 1944, Zimbabwe (Southern Rhodesia) in 1945, Mozambique in 1946, Swaziland in 1946, Basutoland in 1947, Madagascar in 1954, and Belgian Congo in 1955 (Burdin and Prydie, 1959). LSD was first identified in East Africa in Kenya in 1957 and the Sudan in 1972. It was first time reported in West Africa in 1974, and also reported in Nigeria for the first time in 1974 by Nawathe et al. (1978). Then it was spreading into Somalia in 1983. Sporadic outbreaks occurred in Nigeria between 1974–1978. In 1979, there was an epidemic of LSD in Nigeria when the third author was working as principal scientific officer of Veterinary Public Health Laboratory of the federal govt. of Nigeria, Kaduna State, and have observed the cases. During the epidemic, the virus strain was more virulent than the previous epidemic of 1974. In the 1979 epidemic in Nigeria, there was high morbidity, and mortality was as low as 2%. Also in the 1979 epidemic, the disease was in association with the anaplasmosis, babesiosis, and listeriosis (Asagba and Nawathe, 1982). In Nigeria, lumpy skin–attenuated vaccine was tried for to control of the disease. Attenuated lumpy skin virus vaccine had tried to control the disease in South Africa also (Weiss, 1963). From 1929 to 1986, the disease was restricted to countries in sub-Saharan Africa, although its potential to extend beyond this range had been suggested (Davies, 1981). It has recently extended its range to include Egypt and Israel. In 1989, a focus of LSD was identified in Israel and subsequently eliminated by the slaughter of all infected cattle as well as contacts. Ring vaccination with a sheep pox strain was carried out around the focus area, and no further clinical cases have occurred. LSD was reported from Egypt in 1988. In 2001, lumpy skin disease was recorded in Mauritius and Senegal.

CULTIVATION

Tissue culture, Most of the ovine and bovine primary cell culture are good for lumpy skin diseases virus growth. But lamb testes tissue culture gives good yield of the virus (Plowright and Witcomb, 1959).

Embryonated egg. The virus grows on fertile embryonated five to seven days old egg at 33.5°C to 35.0°C. After four to six days' incubation, small white discrete plaques were seen on the CAM with out hemorrhage or necrosis.

SOURCE OF INFECTION

Capripoxviruses are very resistant to inactivation and remain viable for long periods on or off the animal host. Fomites, such as clothing and equipment, readily transport the virus where it may persist for six months. Skin lesions contain infective LSD virus when shed. Virus is also present in blood, nasal and lachrymal secretions, semen, milk, and saliva, which may be sources for transmission. Virus has been detected in semen up to twenty-two days after infection. Virus can be transmitted through milk.

There is no carrier state for LSD in recovered animals. Movement of infected animals is the main means of transmission to new areas.

TRANSMISSION

The virus of LSD does not spread readily among animals held in insect-proof pens. While infection by contact can occur, this is thought to occur only at a low rate and is not considered a major component of transmission during epizootics. Most infection is thought to be the result of insect transmission of the virus (von Backstrom, 1945; Thomas and Mare, 1945; Diesel, 1949; MacOwan, 1959; Weiss, 1968). Mechanical transmission occurs primarily by biting insects, particularly mosquitoes and flies. In Nigeria, it has been noted that the spread of LSD was more during rainy season when vectors are more and with the combined effect of wind and movement of host and vector. But in some states of Nigeria during 1979, the spread of LSD was more in dry season from March onward (Nawathe et al., 1982).

LSD virus has been isolated from *Stomoxys* spp., commonly associated with cattle and from the *Biomyia fasciata* mosquito species found in large numbers and associated with LSD-infected cattle. *Tabanidae*, *Glossina*, and *Culicoides* spp. have all been found in situations where there has been ongoing LSD transmission and have been suspected to be involved. Transmission is thought to be mechanical rather than biological.

Aedes aegypti female mosquitoes are capable of the mechanical transmission of lumpy skin disease virus (LSDV) from infected to susceptible cattle. Mosquitoes that had fed upon lesions of LSDV-infected cattle were able to transmit virus to susceptible cattle over a period of two to six days postinfective feeding (Chihota et al., 2001).

Ingestion and direct contact transmission are minor sources of infection, even though the virus is present in nasal and lachrymal secretions.

HOST

LSD only affects cattle, although European (*Bos taurus*) cattle are more susceptible than zebu (*Bos indicus*) cattle. Dairy breeds such as Jersey, Guernsey, and Ayrshires are recognized as particularly susceptible. LSD is an acute infectious disease of cattle of all ages.

Sheep and goats do not become infected during outbreaks of LSD even when held in close contact with infected cattle. But LSD virus replicates in sheep and goats following inoculation. African buffaloes (*Syncerus caffer*) do not show lesions in the field during epizootics of LSD and nor did the majority of Asian water buffaloes, *Bubalus bubalis*, exposed during the Egyptian LSD epizootic, although five cases have been seen in Asian water buffalo (All et al., 1990). Oryx (*Oryx beisa*), giraffe (*Giraffe camelopardalis*), and impala (*Aepyceros melampus*) are susceptible to experimental infection.

PATHOGENESIS

The length of the viremic period does not correlate with the severity of clinical disease. Viremia can be detected from one to twelve days using virus isolation and from four to eleven days using the PCR (Tuppurainen et al., 2005). There is pyrexia at the time of viremia, and subsequently the virus gets localized in skin and subcutis, producing typical nodules. On postmortem, nodules are found in the subcutaneous tissues, muscle fascia, and muscles. They are gray-pink with necrotic cores. Nodules may also be found through the nasopharynx, trachea, bronchi, lungs, rumen, abomasum, renal cortex, testicles, and uterus. Bronchopneumonia may be present. Hemorrhages may occur in the spleen or the liver and rumen. Raised nodules may occur on the mucous membrane of the stomachs. Ulcers form in the abomasum, as well as inflammation and hemorrhages in the intestines.

Histopathological sections of the skin lesions show vasculitis and perivascular infiltration with leukocytes with resultant thrombosis of the vessels in the dermis and subcutis. The cells infiltrating the lesion are of a predominantly epithelioid type, known as the *"celles claveleuses"*, which was described by Borrel in 1903 in sheep pox. There are also eosinophilic intracytoplasmic inclusions in the epidermal elements of the lesion and the inflammatory cells (Burdin, 1959). The lesions gradually become necrotic as a result of the thrombosis.

CLINICAL SIGNS

The incubation period of lumpy skin disease is four to fourteen days. LSD symptoms range from inapparent to severe disease.

Fever is the first clinical sign accompanied by depression, salivation, nasal, and eye discharge. Fluctuating fever of 40.0–41.5°C either transitory or lasting up to two weeks are observed. Swollen limbs of the animals with difficulty in walking were noted in LSD-affected animals in Nigeria (Nawathe et al., 1982). Ten days after the temperature rise, nodules or lumps appear on the skin, initially circular, flat, and firm. Nodules up to 0.5–7.0 cm in diameter appear throughout the full depth of the skin. These are raised about 3 mm above the skin and can occur all over the body. Painful nodules develops especially in the skin of the head, neck, muzzle, nares, back, limbs, penis, prepuce, vagina, perineum, eyelids, lower ear, nasal mucosa, and under the tail. The skin nodules contain a firm, creamy gray, or yellow mass of tissue. These nodules may become necrotic, and deep scabs may form ("sitfast"). Removal or shedding of sitfast leaves a deep ulcer, which slowly fills with granulation tissue. In severe cases, nodules can also develop inside the mouth, nose, and many other internal organs, which may result in excessive salivation, respiratory distress, and abortion. Yellowish gray lesions occur on the tongue, on the cheeks, on the hard palate and gums, and in the nostrils. Most nodules heal over several weeks but leave a disfiguring scar, which damages the hide. Some nodules may become permanent, hard lumps and some may disappear completely. Mild lesions heal in a few weeks, whereas severe lesions usually take several months.

The regional lymph nodes become enlarged, and edema develops in the udder, brisket, and legs. Superficial lymph nodes draining areas of the infected skin may become enlarged to four to ten times their normal size.

Often LSD leads to complications like secondary bacterial infection of teat lesions, which may lead to severe mastitis and loss of the quarter. Secondary bacterial infection of tendon and joint may result in permanent lameness. Abortion, intrauterine infection, and temporary sterility may occur.

Very few animals die of lumpy skin disease. Up to 10% of calves affected with LSD die. Systemic signs may be absent in mild cases. The greatest loss from the disease is the decrease in milk yield, the loss in condition, and the rejection or reduced value of the hide.

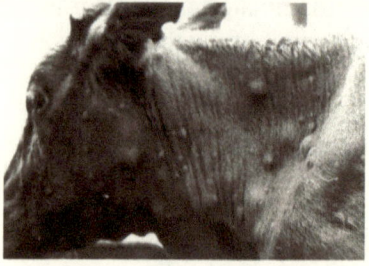 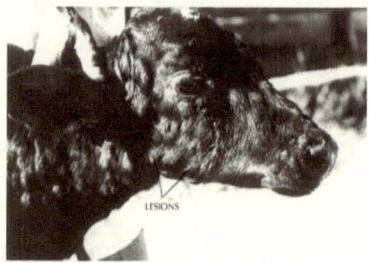

Photo of the lesions of LSD from Dr. Nawathe
(Courtesy from Dr. D. R. Nawathe).

IMMUNE RESPONSE
The recovered animals are solidly immune for life.

DIAGNOSIS
A tentative diagnosis can be made from the clinical signs. Laboratory confirmation is desirable. To confirm the diagnosis, samples should be collected from the live animals. Serum from both acute and convalescent animals, nodular fluid, scabs, and skin biopsies are the best clinical materials. Both fresh and fixed samples should be taken from skin lesions and lesions in the visceral organs.

Electron microscopy, agar gel immunodiffusion, inoculation of primary cell culture of lamb or calf testis and kidney, hematoxylin and eosin staining for intracytoplasmic inclusion bodies, direct immunofluorescent staining, virus neutralization, enzyme-linked immunosorbent assay (ELISA), and polymerase chain reaction (PCR) are used for the identification of the antigen.

Serological tests like indirect fluorescent antibody test, virus neutralization, ELISA, and PCR are employed for the detection of antibody.

PCR is found to be superior in detecting LSD virus from blood and skin samples to transmission electron microscopy. However, virus isolation is still required when the infectivity of the LSD virus is to be determined (Tuppurainen et al., 2005; Bagla et al., 2006).

The early skin lesions contain large numbers of virus particles, which can be readily seen with an electron microscope. Simple negative staining of a few small skin fragments taken from the lesions with phosphotungstic acid will show large numbers of the roughly brick-shaped poxvirus particles.

Virus isolation is best carried out in primary or secondary prepubertal lamb testis cell cultures. They are more sensitive than kidney, muscle, lung, skin, thymus, or endothelial cells, although can be used. Cultures are infected with suspensions of the early skin lesions, preferably in tubes or wells with cover slips. These can then be stained at forty-eight to fifty-six hours to show the eosinophilic intracytoplasmic inclusions, or the viral antigen may be identified by immunological methods with fluorescent or peroxidase conjugated antibodies. This is possible as early as twenty-four hours after inoculation of the cultures (Davies et al., 1971).

DIFFERENTIAL DIAGNOSIS

Lumpy skin disease has to be differentiated from pseudo-lumpy skin disease, which is a milder form of disease caused by bovine herpesvirus 2. This diseases can be similar clinically, although the herpesvirus lesions seem confined mainly to the teats and udder of cows, and the disease is called herpes mammillitis. Lumpy skin disease could also be confused with other diseases such as skin tuberculosis, onchocercosis, *dermatophilus congolensis* infection, besnoitiosis, rinderpest, hypoderma bovis infection, bovine lymphangitis, cowpox, mycotic dermatitis, uticaria, photo sensitization, severe infestations with demodectic mange and insect, or tick bite allergy. These diseases have to be differentiated by identifying the causative organisms.

TREATMENT

No specific treatment is available for LSD. Strong antibiotic therapy may avoid secondary infections. There is no specific antiviral treatment available for LSD-infected cattle. Sick animals may be removed from the herd and given supportive treatment consisting of local wound dressing to discourage fly worry and prevent secondary infections. Systemic antibiotics may be given for skin infections, cellulitis, or pneumonia, and food and water should be made readily available. Local applications of insecticides to infected cattle have been made in an attempt to reduce further transmission, but no apparent benefit has been noticed.

PREVENTION AND CONTROL

Vaccination is the most effective method to control the disease.

LSD-free countries should monitor the disease while importing livestock, hides, skins, and semen from endemic areas. In endemic areas, strict quarantine should be enforced to avoid introduction of infected animals into safe herds. In cases of outbreaks, isolation and ban of animal movements, slaughtering of all sick and infected animals, scientific disposal of dead animals by incineration or deep burial, disinfection of premises and implements, vector control in premises and on animals should be observed. Vector control in ships and aircraft is also highly recommended.

A vaccination cover with a 25–50-km radius may then be established around the focus and all cattle movements stopped within that zone.

VACCINATION

In Africa, vaccination against LSD were effectively done using Neethling strain of LSD virus and Kenya sheep and goat poxvirus. The Neethling strain of LSD virus was passaged fifty times in tissue cultures of lamb kidney cells and then twenty times in embryonated eggs and used as vaccine. The strain proved to be immunogenic for cattle, although local reactions do occur in a high proportion of animals at the vaccination site. No generalization of infection has ever followed its use (Weiss, 1968). Neethling strain immunity has been confirmed to last up to three years. Sheep and goat pox vaccines may cause severe local reactions. An attenuated vaccine made from a capripoxvirus that affected both sheep and goats in Kenya has been produced. Immunity lasts at least for two years and probably for life (Capstick and Coackley, 1961). It is not advised in countries free from sheep and goat pox. Studies with both the Neethling and the Kenya SGPV strains show that an immunizing dose of $10^{3.5}$ TCID$_{50}$ is desirable for field vaccination campaigns. Good protection has been obtained with 10^2 in the face of an epizootic.

Osuagwuh et al. (2006) observed the ability of LSD vaccination to prevent the excretion of LSD virus in semen of vaccinated bulls.

Two other strains of sheep pox vaccine have recently been used as a prophylaxis against LSD. The Romanian strain, prepared in the skin of lambs for use against sheep pox, was used in several million cattle in Egypt and appeared to be immunogenic. Another sheep pox strain, the RM 65 prepared in tissue culture, was used in Israel. No complications have followed the use of these strains in cattle.

Caprirab is a live recombinant lumpy skin disease virus (Neethling vaccine strain) expressing the glycoprotein of rabies virus. Caprirab is aimed at cattle and will confer dual immunity to both lumpy skin disease LSD and rabies. It is envisaged with more widespread testing that Caprirab may be used as a rabies vaccine for a wide variety of animals. It has the potential of being given orally in bait form because of its stability. The LSDV vaccine, used as the base of Caprirab, confers lifelong immunity against lumpy skin disease after a single vaccination. Furthermore, due to its stability, the maintenance of a cold chain is unnecessary. This is the most important advantage for vaccines aimed at the developing world (Aspaden, 2007).

Cattle have been protected against challenge with rinderpest and lumpy skin disease viruses by vaccination with a recombinant capripoxvirus containing the fusion protein (F) gene of rinderpest virus. The minimum protective immunizing doses for rinderpest and lumpy skin disease were found to be 5.5×10^4 plaque forming units (pfu) and 1.5×10^3 pfu, respectively (Romero et al., 1994).

ERADICATION
In the event of an outbreak, the sick animals should be kept in fly-free places and all the in-contact animals vaccinated. Affected animals would have to be slaughtered, and a 3-km protection zone and 10-km surveillance zone set up around the infected premises. After cleansing and disinfection, the restrictions should remain in force for at least twenty-eight days, this being the assumed maximum incubation period of this disease.

LSD is not transmissible to humans.

REFERENCES

1. Asagba, M. C. and Nawathe, D. R. 1982. Lumpy skin disease: The present status in Nigeria. Proceedingof XII World congress on diseases of cattle, the Netherlands. Sept. 7–10,1982.
2. All, A. A., Esmet, M., Attia, H., Selim, A. and Abdel Hamid, Y. M. 1990. Clinical and pathological studies on lumpy skin disease in Egypt. *Vet. Rec.* 127:549–550.
3. Aspaden, K. 2007. Caprirab: A novel dual vaccine developed for use against rabies and lumpy skin diseases in the developing world. *Science in Africa online* 19:34:40.
4. Bagla, V. P., Osuagwuh, V. I., Annandalf, C. U. and Irons, P. C. 2006. Elimination of toxicity and enhanced detection of lumpy skin disease virus on cell culture from experimentally infected bovine semen samples. *Onderstepoort J. Vet. Res.* 73:263–268.
5. Burdin, M. L. 1959. The use of histopathological examination of skin material for the diagnosis of lumpy skin disease in Kenya. *Bull. Epizootic Dis. Africa.* 7:21–36.
6. Burdin, M. L. and Prydie, J. 1959. Lumpy skin disease of cattle in Kenya. *Nature* 183:949–950.
7. Capstick, P. B. and Coackley, W. 1961. Protection of cattle against lumpy skin disease. 1. Trials with a vaccine against Neethling type infection. *Res. Vet. Sci.* 2:362–368.
8. Chihota, C. M., Rennie, L. F., Kitching, R. P. and Mellor, P. S. 2001. Mechanical transmission of lumpy skin disease virus by *Aedes aegypti* (Diptera: *Culicidae*). *Epidemiol. Infecion* 126:317–321.
9. Davies, F. G. 1981. Lumpy skin disease. In *Virus diseases of food animals*, vol. 2, ed. E. P. J. Gibbs. 751–764. London: Academic Press.
10. Davies, F. G., Kraus, H., Lund, L. J. and Taylor, M. 1971. The laboratory diagnosis of lumpy skin disease. *Res. Vet. Sci.* 12:123–127.

10. LUMPY SKIN DISEASE

11. Diesel, A. M. 1949. The epizootiology of lumpy skin disease in South Africa. *Proc. 14th Int. Vet. Cong.* London, 2:492–500.
12. Fenner, F. 1976. Classification and nomenclature of viruses. *Intervirolog y* 6:112.
13. Green, H. F. 1959. Lumpy skin disease: Its effect on hides and leather and a comparison in this respect with some other skin diseases. *Bull. Epizootic Dis. Africa* 7:63–79.
14. MacOwan, K. D. S. 1959. Observations on the epizootiology of lumpy skin disease during the first year of its occurrence in Kenya. *Bull. Epizootic Dis. Africa* 7:7–20.
15. Nawathe, D. R., Gibbs, E. P. J., Asagba, M. O. and Lawman, M. J. P. 1978. Lumpy skin disease in Nigeria. *Trop. Anim. Hlth. Prod.* 10:49–54.
16. Nawathe, D. R., Asagba, M. O., Abegunde, A., Ajayi, S. A. and Durkwa, L. 1982. Some observations on the occurrence of lumpy skin disease in Nigeria. *Zbl. Vet. Med.* B 29:31–36.
17. Osuagwuh, U. I., Bagla, V., Venter, E. H., Annandale, C. H. and Irons, P. C. 2006. Absence of lumpy skin disease virus in semen of vaccinated bulls following vaccination and subsequent experimental infection. *Vaccine* 10:1016.
18. Plowright, W. and Witcomb, H. A. 1959. The growth in tissue culture of a virus derived from lumpy skin disease of cattle. *J. Path. Bacteriology* 78:397–407.
19. Romero, C H., Barrett, T., Kitching, R. P., Carn, V. M. and Black, D. N. 1994. Protection of cattle against rinderpest and lumpy skin disease with a recombinant capripoxvirus expressing the fusion protein gene of rinderpest virus. *Vet. Rec.* 135:152–154.
20. Thomas, A. D. and Mare, C. V. E. 1945. Knopvelsiekte. *J. S. Afr. Vet. Med. Assoc.* 16:36–43.
21. Tuppurainen, E. S., Venter, E. H. and Coetzer, J. A. 2005. The detection of lumpy skin disease virus in samples of experimentally infected cattle using different techniques. *Onderstepoort J. Vet. Res.* 72:153–164.
22. Von Backstrom, U. 1945. Ngamil and cattle disease. Preliminary report on a new disease, the aetiologica l agent probably being of an infectious nature. *J. S. Afr. Vet. Med. Assoc.* 16:29–35.
23. Weiss, K. E. 1963. In *Emerging diseases of animals*, FAO, Rome, 179–201.
24. Weiss, K. E. 1968. Lumpy skin disease. In *Virology monographs*, vol. 3, 111–131. Vienna-New York: Springer Verlag.

11. MALIGNANT CATARRHAL FEVER (MCF)

(Malignant Head Catarrh, Catarrhal Fever, Gangrenous Coryza, Bovine Malignant Catarrh, Snotziekte)

M. R. SASEENDRANATH, AND M. KRISHNAN NAIR

INTRODUCTION

Malignant catarrhal fever (MCF) is a generalized and fatal disease of ruminants, especially cattle, buffalo, and deer, caused by either alcelaphine herpesvirus 1(AHV-1) or ovine herpesvirus 2 (OvHV-2), characterized by high fever, profuse nasal discharge, bilateral corneal opacity, lymphadenopathy, and inflammation and ulceration of digestive and respiratory organs.

ETIOLOGY

MCF is caused by a highly cell associated lymphotrophic herpesvirus of the family Herpesviridae, subfamily Gammaherpesvirinae, and the genus *Rhadinovirus.* The causative virus exists in nature in some hosts where they are well adopted without producing visible clinical symptoms. MCF is caused by two gamma herpesviruses. Alcelaphine herpesvirus 1(AHV-1) and ovine herpes virus 2 (OvHV-2). MCF caused by these two viruses are clinically and pathologically indistinguishable and produces a wide spectrum of clinical entities.

This virus is relatively unstable in environment, losing its infectivity within three hours in hot dry weather (Rossiter et al., 1983). This virus is quickly inactivated by sunlight. The AHV-1 can be propagated in vitro, which readily induces experimental infections and can be reisolated from tissues and secretions of clinically susceptible hosts, whereas the in vitro isolation of OvHV-2 virus is very difficult. SA-MFC virus was isolated from domestic cattle in Minnesota in 1977 and from domestic cattle in Austria in 1990. Plowright isolated wildebeest strain MCF virus from a blue wildebeest (*Connochaetes taurinus taurinus*) in 1960.

EPIDEMIOLOGY

MCF is predominantly a disease of domestic cattle (*Bos taurus* and *B. indicus*), water buffalo (*Bubalus bubalis*) (Martucciello et al., 2006), Bali cattle (banteng) (*Bos javanicus*), American bison (*Bison bison*), and deer (cervid species). Both strains of MCF virus, the ovine and the wildebeest strains, are capable of causing indistinguishable disease in any of these species. In Africa, MCF is responsible for very significant losses in domestic cattle and wild ruminants (Plowright et al., 1975).

DISTRIBUTION

MCF has been recognized as a disease for over two hundred years, and the disease was first recorded in late 1700. The association between wildebeest and MCF in domestic cattle was recognized early on by Maasai pastoralists and by South African farmers, who referred the disease as *snotziekte* (snotting disease) (Plowright, 1965).

MCF is present throughout the world where the two principal natural hosts, wildebeest and sheep, are present. Wildebeest, hartebeest, and topi are carriers of AHV-1. All wildebeest in the wild and most wildebeest in the zoo appear to be infected with the virus. Several other wild ruminants in Africa as *Oryx* and *Addax* may also act as reservoirs, although MCF virus has not been isolated from these species.

SA-MCF has been reported from Europe (Martucciello et al., 2006), Asia, and Africa. Morbidity ranges from 28–45% and mortality 90–100%.

SOURCE OF INFECTION

The causative virus exists in nature in carriers like wildebeest and sheep to which they are well adapted. MCF affected animals never or rarely transmit the infection, and it is only the natural hosts that can act as a source of infection. Wildebeest appears to be efficient transmitters of the virus to other ruminants.

The WA-MCF virus is harbored in all species of wildebeest as a lifelong, asymptomatic infection. Viral shedding by adults is at relatively low levels, except during periods of stress or parturition, at which time virus titers in oropharyngeal and ocular secretions rise significantly (Plowright, 1986). Most of the clinical MCF originates from young wildebeest calves, up to the age of about four months. The virus transmission between wildebeest species involves both horizontal and vertical methods. Neutralizing antibodies develop around three months of age, after which the viral shedding declines dramatically (Mushi et al., 1981). WA-MCF occurs most frequently in Africa during the wildebeest calving season and in zoological parks sporadic cases occur throughout the year.

Intense viral shedding from the wildebeest occurs during the first ninety days of life, whereas lambs do not begin to shed significantly until after five months of age. Sheep and goats (both domestic and wild species) are the carriers of OvHV-2 (Plowright et al., 1960).

Both strains of MCF viruses are shed into the environment via oral, nasal, and ocular secretions from their respective well-adapted reservoir hosts.

TRANSMISSION

AHV-1 is cell associated in wildebeest, hartebeest, and topi. The cell-associated form is rarely transmitted to other animals. But under stress conditions, cell-free viruses are isolated from nasal secretions. Wildebeest calves can also be infected in utero and shed the virus in nasal and ocular secretions and in the dung.

Efficient transmission via infected secretions of the well-adapted hosts is favored by close contact and in cool and moist environment. It has also been observed that there is a possibility of remote transmission by shared water sources and mechanical vectors. Transmission over considerable distances up to couple of miles has been observed. Susceptible hosts acquire the virus through inhalation and ingestion of virus-laden secretions or through ingestion of contaminated foodstuff or water.

WA-MCF is not transmitted by natural means from one clinically susceptible to another. Affected animals are dead-end hosts. OvHV-2 transmission is relatively difficult from one cow to another. Transmission of clinical SA-MCF occurs both from adolescent lambs and from adults. The mode of transmission of OHV-2 is still not clear. It seems that close contact between susceptible animals and sheep, especially lambing ewes, is thought to be necessary (Brenner and David, 2005). The role of goats in transmission is also not known. Transmission of diseases in the absence of any carriers has also been recorded, leading to a suspicion of alternate transmission modes ranging from insect vectors to horizontal transmission between the susceptible animals (Barnard and Pypekamp, 1983; Huck et al., 1961; Piercy, 1954).

HOSTS

The natural hosts for the MCF viruses are found in the artiodactyl families Bovidae, Cervidae, and Giraffidae (Bridgen et al., 1989). Two types of hosts exist, well-adapted asymptomatic carriers and poorly adapted hosts, in which both clinical disease and latent, subclinical infection occur. The well-adapted hosts are shedding the virus in environment, whereas the poorly adapted viruses generally do not shed viruses and therefore considered as dead-end hosts.

Clinical disease has been recorded over thirty species of ruminants. The susceptibility to OvHV-2 varies. *Bos taurus* and *Bos indicus* are relatively resistant to this infection whereas water buffalo (Hill et al., 1993; Martucciello et al., 2006) and many species of deer are more susceptible. Bison, Bali cattle, and Pere Davids deer are extremely susceptible.

In cattle and all susceptible wild ruminants, MCF affects all ages, breeds, and sexes. The disease has been described in pigs, giraffe, and species of antelopes.

The domestic rabbit (*Oryctolagus cuniculus*) is readily infected with wildebeest and ovine MCF viruses and develop significant lymphoproliferative disease. Other laboratory animals that have been successfully infected include the rat and hamster.

PATHOGENESIS

The virus mainly induces a vasculitis and consequent degeneration and necrosis of tissues. Lesions may be seen in the upper gastrointestinal and respiratory tract and characterized by erythema, hemorrhage, inflammation, and erosions. Erosions are mainly seen in the mouth, nasal septum, turbinates, esophagus, and trachea. Lungs are not generally involved.

The mucosa of the fore stomach may exhibit erythema, sparse hemorrhages, or erosions. Catarrhal enteritis and ulcerations of Peyer's patches may be noticed. The lymph nodes are swollen, edematous, and hemorrhagic with inflammatory changes. Congestion and petechial hemorrhages may be visible in brain and meninges. Synovitis is noticed especially in the tibiotarsal joints.

Histologically, there is necrotizing vasculitis and is characterized by fibrinoid necrosis of the media with infiltration of lymphoid cells in the walls. Perivascular lymphoid accumulation has been seen. In severe cases, endothelial damages can occur. A very characteristic feature is the infiltration of lymphocytes and mononuclear cells in most of the organs (Amano et al., 1998). The epithelial tissue show degeneration accompanied by inflammatory changes.

CLINICAL SIGNS

Incubation period under field condition is unknown, and it varies as numerous complicating factors influence the disease expression. Recrudescence of existing infection can occur at any time, giving a prolonged incubation period of several months. Experimental studies showed that the incubation period varies from nine to sixty days (Plowright et al., 1960; Huck et al., 1961; Plowright, 1968). It is considered that it may extend up to two hundred days. Some animals appear to be subclinically infected and develop clinical signs after a period of severe stress.

A wide variety of clinical symptoms are seen in MCF. Four forms of MCF have been described.

1. Peracute Form

Fever, severe inflammation of the oral and the nasal mucosa, and hemorrhagic gastroenteritis are seen with a course of one to three days.

2. Intestinal Form

There is fever, diarrhea, hyperemia of oral and nasal mucosa with accompanying discharges, and lymphadenopathy with a course of four to nine days.

3. Head and Eye Form

This is the typical form of MCF. There is sudden onset of symptoms. Dullness, anorexia, agalactiae, pyrexia (106-107°F), profuse serous nasal and ocular discharges which later become mucopurulent, severe dyspnea due to the obstruction of the nasal cavity with exudates, and open-mouthed breathing and salivation may be seen (Nielson et al., 1988; Martucciello et al., 2006).

Blepherospasms and bilateral corneal opacity that begins at the corneoscleral junction and progresses inward is a common finding. The oral mucosa may contain multifocal or diffuse areas of necrosis. Erosions may be found at the tip of the oral papilla.

Superficial necrosis is evident in the anterior nasal mucosa and on the buccal mucosa. Discrete local area of necrosis appears in the hard palate and gums. Animal moves its jaws carefully because of pain. Dung becomes dry in the beginning, and but there is fetid diarrhea later on.

Sometimes skin becomes ulcerated; vulva, vagina, and teats may show swelling and ulceration; and hardened scabs may be seen on the udder, perineum, and teats. In some animals, the horn and hoof covering may become loosened and get sloughed. Skin lesions are common in cattle and deer with ovine strain of MCF virus but less so with the wildebeest strain.

The joints become swollen, milk production may drop, and the superficial lymph nodes may be enlarged. Constipation is common, but diarrhea and hemorrhagic gastroenteritis can also be seen.

Nervous signs such as muscular twitching, convulsions, hyperesthesia, nystagmus, staggering gait, paresis, and head-pressing syndrome against walls or objects may be present.

Pregnant animals may abort. Animal becomes highly dehydrated, temperature falls below normal, pulse becomes faster and weaker, and death may occur in twenty-four hours. The course of the disease varies from four to fourteen days.

4. Mild Form

Mild form more commonly occurs in experimental animals. There is transient fever, and mild erosions appear on the nasal and oral mucosa. Mild disease may be followed by complete recovery, recovery with recrudescence, or chronic MCF.

Highly susceptible animals, such as bison, banteng, generally suffer shorter, more acute courses than do somewhat less susceptible species such as domestic cattle. Many deer die within forty-eight hours of the first sign of MCF, but this time frame is highly variable. Bison usually die within two to five days of initial signs.

IMMUNE RESPONSE
Cattle and experimentally infected rabbits recovered from MCF have a solid immunity against all strains of MCF virus.

DIAGNOSIS
MCF should be suspected in animals having clinical signs such as sudden death or fever with nasal and lachrymal discharge; lymphadenopathy; corneal edema; erosive; and inflammatory changes in the GI tract, skin, and bladder; and bilateral corneal opacity. The history of contact with sheep, goat, antelopes, or wildebeest is also taken into account.

Histopathological demonstration of multisystem lymphoid infiltration, disseminated vasculitis, and degenerative epithelial lesions are characteristic.

Virus isolation (Mushi et al., 1980) is a method of diagnosis, though it is difficult in OvHV-2 infections. A volume of 10–20 ml of blood in EDTA, pieces of spleen, lung, lymph nodes, adrenal gland and thyroid should be collected for the virus isolation.

Serological tests like virus neutralization, complement fixation test (CFT) (Sentsui et al., 1996), immunoblotting, a monoclonal-based competitive inhibition enzyme-linked immunosorbent assay (CI-ELISA) (Li et al., 1995; Li et al., 2001), indirect fluorescence antibody test (IFAT), and immunohistochemistry are being used for demonstration of antibody. Paired serum samples, three weeks apart, should be collected for the confirmation of the diagnosis. Polymerase chain reaction is being used as the diagnostic method of choice (Crawford et al., 1999; Martucciello et al., 2006). Bremer et al. (2005) developed a single-tube duplex nested PCR for differentiation of OvHV-2 and AHV-1.

DIFFERENTIAL DIAGNOSIS
MCF has to be differentiated from bovine viral diarrhea–mucosal disease (BVD-MD), bluetongue, rinderpest, infectious bovine rhinotracheitis, foot-and-mouth disease, vesicular stomatitis, and the conditions caused by the ingestion of caustic materials or some poisonous plants or mycotoxins.

An erosive stomatitis and gastroenteritis are characteristic of rinderpest, BVD, and MCF. As the signs are more or less similar, antigen detection is the main mode of differentiation. The stomatitis and hyperemia are severe in MCF along with a corneoscleral opacity, lymph node enlargement, and terminal encephalitis. Rinderpest is characterized by high morbidity and mortality. The vesicular diseases like foot-and-mouth disease and vesicular stomatitis are characterized by the presence of the vesicles on the tongue and buccal mucosa, teats and, coronets and can be distinguished from erosions. Bluetongue is a fatal clinical disease of sheep, whereas sheep never suffer clinically from MCF.

TREATMENT

There is no specific treatment. Antibiotics, corticosteroids, antiviral drugs, vitamins, and other supportive therapy have been tried. Occasional recovery of animals following corticosteroid therapy has been reported (Milne and Reid, 1990), but the role of the treatment remains unknown since significant numbers of cattle also recovered without treatment (Hamilton, 1990; Kalunda et al., 1981; O'Toole, et al., 1997).

PREVENTION AND CONTROL

Preventing contact between carriers and clinically susceptible species remains the primary control method. Reduction of stress is also beneficial in reducing the number of cases, particularly with the more susceptible species. General preventive measures include separation of known carrier and susceptible species and separation of keeper staff and equipments between these species. Most commonly used disinfectants are effective. Containment of an outbreak usually means the immediate separation of cattle or the susceptible host from sheep and goats in the case of the SA-MCF and the susceptible host from alcelaphine or wild ruminants in the case of WA-MCF. There is no evidence that OvHV-2 or AHV-1 infection in humans.

VACCINATION

No vaccine has been developed for the disease so far. Some viral strains have undergone limited attenuation after serial passage in cell cultures and offer hope for a future modified live virus vaccine. Killed virus vaccines have been inconsistent in inducing protection against virulent virus challenge, although some have induced significant titers of serum virus-neutralizing antibodies.

ERADICATION

Cattle should be kept separated from potential reservoir hosts such as sheep, goats, and wildebeest, especially during lambing, kidding, or calving seasons, respectively. The stocking of cattle ranches with alcelaphine antelopes, wild sheep, or goats should be discouraged or should require a negative MCF serologic test, preferably by the serum virus-neutralization methods or a negative PCR test for any wild ruminants destined for such a facility. Similar testing of such wild ruminants before being placed in or transferred between zoos is also recommended as a means to prevent the introduction of potential carriers of MCF virus.

REFERENCES

1. Amano, H., Kajio, N., Sujioka, T., Mizoguchi, T., Ohmura, K., Katai, N. and Nakajima, Y. 1988. MCF in Japanese deer. *J. Jap. Vet. Med. Assoc.* 41:188–191.

2. Barnard, B. J. H. and Pypekamp, H. E. 1983. Wildebeest derived malignant catarrhal fever: Unusual epidemiology in South Africa. *Ondeerstepoort J. Vet. Res.* 55:69–71.

3. Bremer, C. W., Swarat, H., Doboro, F. A., Dungu, B., Romito, M. and Viljoen, G. 2005. Discrimination between sheep associated and wildebeest associated MCF virus by means of a single-tube duplex nested PCR. *Onderstepoort J. Vet. Res.* 72:285–291.

4. Brenner, J. and David, D. 2005. Sheep associated malignant catarrhal fever in cattle (SA-MCF): Recent clinical and epidemiological aspects in Israel. *Israel J. Vet. Med.* 60:19–22.

5. Bridgen, A., Herring, A. I., Inglis, N. F. and Reid, H. W. 1989. Preliminary characterization of the Alcelaphine herpesvirus1 genome. *J. Gen. Virology* 70:1141–1150.

6. Crawford, T. B., Li, H. and O'Toole, D. T. 1999. Diagnosis of malignant catarrhal fever by PCR using PCR using formalin fixed paraffin embedded tissue. *J. Vet Diagn. Invest.* 11:111–116.

7. Hamilton, A. F. 1990. Account of three outbreaks of malignant catarrhal fever incattle in Republic of Ireland. *Vet. Rec.*127:231–232.

8. Hill, F. D., Arthrur, D. G. and Thompson, J. 1993. Malignant catarrhal fever in a swamp buffalocalf in Newzeland. *Newzeland Vet. J.* 41:35–38.

9. Huck, R. A., Shand, A., Allsop, P. J. and Peterson, A. B. 1961. Malignanat catarrh of deer. *Vet. Rec.*73:457–465.

10. Kalunda, M. D., Ardiri, A. H. and Lee, K. M. 1981. Malignanat catarrhal fever. Response of American cattle to malignant catarrhal virus isolated in Kenya. *Can. J. Com. Med.* 45:70–76.

11. Li, H., Shen, D. T., O'Toole, D., Knowles, D. P., Gorhan, J. R. and Crawford, T. B. 1995. Investiation of sheep associated malignant fever virus infection in ruminants by PCR and competitive ELISA. *J. Clin. Microbiol.* 33:2048–2053.

12. Li, H., Snowder, G., O'Toole, D. T. and Crawford, T. B. 1998. Transmission of Ovine herpesvirus-2 in lambs. *J. Clin. Microbiol.* 36:223–226.

13. Martucciello, A., Marianelli, C., Capuano, M., Astarita, S., Alfano, D. and Galiero, G. 2006. An outbreak of malignant catarrhal fever in Mediterranean water buffalo (*Bubalus bubalis*). *Large Animal Review* 12:21–24.

14. Milne, E. M. and Reid, H. W. 1990. Recovery of a cow from malignant catarrhal fever. *Vet. Rec.*126:640–641.

15. Mushi, E. Z., Karstad, L. and Jessett, D. M. 1980. Isolation of Bovine malignant catarrhal fever virus from ocular and nasal secretions of wildebeest calves. *Res. Vet. Sci.* 29:168–171.

16. Mushi, E. Z., Rurangirwa, F. R. and Karstad, L. 1981. Shedding of malignant catarrhal fever virus by wildebeest calves. *Vet. Microbiol.* 6:281–286.

17. Nielson, N. O., Oosterhuis, J., Janssen, D., McColl, K., Anderson, M. P. and Heuschele, W. P. 1988. Fatal respiratory disease in Nilgai Tahr. *CanadianJ. Vet. Res.* 52:216–221.

18. O'Toole, D. T., Li, H., Miller, D., Williams, W. R. and Crawford, T. B. 1997. Chronica and recovered cases of Sheep associated malignant catarrhal fever in cattle. *Vet. Rec.*140:519–524.

19. Piercy, S. E. 1954. Studies in bovine malignant catarrh. V. The role of sheep in the transmission of the disease. *Brit. Vet. J.* 110:508–516.

20. Plowright, W. 1965. Malignant catarrhal fever in East Africa. *Res. Vet. Sci.* 6:57–83.

21. Plowright, W. 1968. Malignant catarrhal fever. *J. Am. Vet. Med. Assoc.* 152:795–796.

22. Plowright, W. 1986. Malignant catarrhal fever. *Revue Scientifique et Technique, Office International des Epizooties* 5:897–958.

23. Plowright, W., Ferris, R. D. and Scott, G. R. 1960. Bluewildebeest and the etiological agent of Bovine malignant catarrhal fever virus. *Nature* 188:1167–1169.

24. Plowright, W., Herniman, A. J., Jessent, D. M., Kalunda, M. and Pampton, C. S. 1975. Immunization of cattle against herpes virus causing malignant catarrhal fever. *Res. Vet. Sci.* 13:37–45.
25. Rossiter, P. B., Jessent, D. M. and Karstad, L. 1983. Role of the wildebeest fetal membranes and fluids in the transmission of malignant catarrhal fever virus. *Vet. Rec.* 113:150–152.
26. Sentsui, H., Nishimori, T., Nagai, T. and Nishioka, N. 1996. Detection of sheep associated malignant catarrhal fever virus antibodies by CFT. *J. Vet. Med. Sci.* 58:1–5.

12. PESTE DES PETITS RUMINANTS
(Goat Plague, Kata)

M. R. SASEENDRANATH, M. KRISHNAN NAIR, THANKAM MATHEW, AND Z. MATHEW

INTRODUCTION

Peste des petits ruminants (PPR) is a highly contagious acute viral disease of goats and sheep and small wild ruminants characterized by fever, oculo-nasal discharge, necrotizing and erosive stomatitis, enteritis, and pneumonia caused by a RNA virus. Infected animals present clinical signs similar to rinderpest disease in cattle. Office Des Internatioanl Epizootes (OIE) has classified PPR under list A diseases.

ETIOLOGY

PPR virus belongs to the family Paramyxoviridae and the genus *Moribillivirus*. This virus is antigenically related to rinderpest virus of cattle and other large ruminants, human measles virus, and canine distemper virus (Gibbs, et al., 1979; Barrett, 1996). Four lineage of PPR virus has been reported so far, three from the African continent and one from Asia (Dhar et al., 2002). One African strain was also isolated from an outbreak in South India. This virus has six structural proteins, the nucleoprotein (Np), which encapsulate the DNA; the phosphoprotein (P) associated with polymerase; the large (L) protein; the matrix (M) protein; the fusion (F) protein, helping in attachment and viral penetration; and the hemagglutinin (H) protein. The matrix protein which is intimately associated with the internal face of the viral envelope and makes a link between the nucleocapsid and the virus external glycoproteins, H and F. The half-life of the virus has been estimated to be 2.2 minutes at 56°C and 3.3 hours at 37°C, is stable between pH 4–10, and susceptible to alcohol, ether, detergents, and disinfectants like iodophore and chlorine. It survives long in chilled and frozen tissue.

EPIDEMIOLOGY

DISTRIBUTION

PPR was first reported from Cote d'Ivoire, West Africa, in 1942. PPR was reported in 1981 in the dwarf goats of Oyo, Ogun, and Ondo states of Nigeria. Since it was initially suspected to be a rinderpest disease outbreak in goats, the Epidemiology Unit, Federal Livestock Dept. (FLD), conducted a three-day international conference at FLD Kaduna, with the experts from

UK on rinderpest, experts on PPR from France, and scientists from NVRI, Vom, Nigeria. After reviewing the field reports on clinical symptoms in goats and the epidemiology of the outbreak, a detailed discussion was conducted, and it was concluded that those were outbreaks of PPR. The conference requested FLD and National Veterinary Research Institute (NVRI) Vom to conduct further laboratory tests to confirm diagnosis (Mathew, 1981). Later, Nawathe (1984) described control measures for PPR in Nigeria as it is of great economic importance on the basis of mortality, morbidity, loss of meat, milk and milk products, and poor feed efficiency. In 2003, Ogunsanmi et al. reported PPR virus antibodies in 10.5% sera of African gray Duiker (*Sylvicapra grimmia*) in Nigeria, and 0% was positive for RP virus. Recently Sailu et al. (2008) conducted a comparative study for the prevention of the PPR by PPR vaccine and ethanoveterinary herbs. They found approximately 60% protection among the PPR exposed sheep and goats with ethonoveterinary herbs in Kogi State, Nigeria. In India, PPR was recorded for the first time in 1987 and has been reported regularly from different states (Saravanan et al., 2007). PPR has also been reported from many countries in Africa, Middle East, and Asia. PPR was reported from China in 2008 by OIE and in Tibet in July 2007 (OIE, 2007). The spread of PPR in Kenya and Uganda was reported by Amanfu (2008), regional manager of FAO Unit in Nairobi, Kenya. The animals affected are goat and sheep, cattle, and domestic buffaloes. Serological evidence were also detected in the following animals, namely, gazelles and ibex, gray duiker, waterbuck, bush buck, cape buffalo, and roan antelope. The disease PPR is endemic in Sudan, Ethiopia, Kenya, Uganda, Somalia, and Tanzania (OIE, 2007).

The first report of PPR in Morocco was in 2008 in sheep and goats. The outbreak was mainly in sheep with 133 outbreaks. It affected twenty-nine provinces with a mortality rate of 80%. The outbreak of PPR in Morocco was brought about by livestock crossing the national barrier of the Sahara producing risk in North Africa. It also produced great economic loss. FAO is preventing the outbreak by ring vaccination around field outbreaks in high-risk areas, control of animal movement, and quarantine measures (FAO report9th September2008).

SOURCE OF INFECTION

An infected animal is always the source of infection. Tears, nasal discharge, coughed-up secretion, and excretion of incubating sick animals contain the virus that transmits the infection (Couacy-Hymann et al., 2007). The virus is present in the nasal secretion three days after infection. No carrier status has been reported in recovered animals.

TRANSMISSION

Close, direct contact is necessary for this labile virus to spread that occurs mainly by aerosol transmission. Livestock trade markets, livestock shows, vaccination camps, and places where goats and sheep gather facilitate transmission of infection by close contact or by droplet inhalation.

It was observed that pastoral cattle in Nigeria grazing along with the PPR-infected goats did not show the symptoms of PPR/rinderpest since the cattle are not susceptible to PPR infection (Mathew, 1981).

The virus can also be transmitted through contaminated feed and water. Introduction of recently purchased animals from endemic areas often happens to be the source of infection. Subclinical infection and viral shedding before the onset of overt clinical signs facilitate spread of infection. More frequent outbreaks are observed during rainy season or dry cold season.

HOSTS

It is mainly a disease of goats and sheep. Wild small ruminants, cattle, buffalo, camel, and pigs develop inapparent infections. Mortality rate is more in goats of the age groups from four to eighteen to twenty-four months. Effective control of this disease is of economic importance in Africa, Asia, and Middle East. PPR virus has also been isolated from buffaloes (*Bubalus bubalis*) from District Livestock Farm, Tanjaore, Tamil Nadu. During that epidemic, fifty buffaloes were affected out of 385 buffaloes (Govindarajan et al., 1997). Roeder et al. (1994) reported PPR in camel.

Haroum et al. (2002) reported detection of antibodies against PPR virus in sera of cattle camels, sheep, and goat in Sudan. There is no public health risk of transmission.

PATHOGENESIS

The portal of entry of PPRV is the epithelium of upper respiratory tract and tonsil. PPRV replicates in the local lymph nodes and causes viremia. The virus spreads via blood to other lymph nodes and different parts of body and localizes in the alimentary, respiratory, and lymphoid system causing necrosis of cells leading to erosive lesions.

There is conjunctivitis and erosive lesions inside the lower lips, on the gums, tongue, the hard palate, pharynx, and upper esophagus. Streaks of hemorrhage and erosions are seen in duodenum and ileum. Necrosis and severe ulcerations in Peyer's patches and congestion on the ileo-cecal and ceco-colic junctions are characteristics. Linear hemorrhages or zebra stripes in the large intestine in colon and rectum are the prominent lesions observed.

Erosion and petichiae of nasal mucosa and turbinates, larynx, and trachea are common findings in PPR. Epithelial cells in affected parts show cytoplasmic and intranuclear eosinophilic inclusions. Bronchial epithelium shows squamous metaplasia. In lung, there is giant cell pneumonia and intranuclear and intracytoplasmic inclusions. There will be necrosis in spleen, lymph nodes, and tonsils. Lymphocytes and the cells show inclusions. Ikede (1983) and Uzuokwu (1983) described gross and microscopic lesions in the natural and experimental domestic small ruminants and in wild white-tailed deer (*Odocoileus virginianus*) in Nigeria.

CLINICAL SIGNS

Incubation period is four to six days but may range from three to ten days. The disease is manifested with pyrexia of 104–106°F, which may last for three to five days. The animal becomes depressed and anorectic with suspended rumination and has a dry muzzle. The serous nasal discharge becomes mucopurulent and occludes the nasal cavity. There is respiratory distress, and the animal may sneeze. The serous ocular discharge becomes mucopurulent, which mats the eyelids.

Within four days of onset of fever, the gums, tongue, lips, dental pad, and buccal mucosa become hyperemic, and erosive lesions develop in seven to eight days. A profuse watery diarrhea develops at the time the oral lesions appear. A watery, bloodstained diarrhea is common in the later stage of the disease. Pneumonia with coughing, pleural rales, and abdominal breathing are also seen. The animal becomes dehydrated and emaciated, and death usually occurs in about five to ten days after the onset of clinical signs.

IMMUNE RESPONSE

Sheep and goats that recover from PPR develop an active immunity against the disease. Antibodies have been demonstrated even four years after infection.

DIAGNOSIS

Diagnosis can be done mainly from clinical signs, isolation and identification of the agent, and demonstration of antigen and antibody by various methods.

Specimens for the diagnosis has to be collected from several animals in the acute phase of the disease. Swabs of conjunctival discharge and scrapings from nasal, buccal and rectal mucosa, and whole blood at the peak of pyrexia during the early stage of the disease are the clinical materials to be collected. If blood is used for PCR technique, heparin should not be used as the anticoagulants because it seems to inhibit the reaction. At necropsy, mesenteric and bronchial lymph nodes, spleen, lung, and large intestine should be collected aseptically, chilled on ice, and transported under refrigeration. Pieces of organs for histopathology are collected in 10% formalin.

Identification of PPRV has been carried out by virus isolation in primary lamb kidney cells or in African green monkey kidney (Vero cell cultures), virus neutralization, and electron microscopy (Nanda et al., 1996). The cytopathic effects produced by PPRV develop in five days and consist of rounding and aggregation, culminating in syncytia formation in lamb kidney cells. Antigen detection is done by hemagglutination inhibition (Brindha et al., 2007), agar gel immunoprecipitation, counterimmunoelectrophoresis, immunocapture enzyme-linked immunosorbent assay (Libeau et al., 1994; Nanda et al., 1996), and immunohistopathology.

PPR diagnosis is made by detecting viral ribonucleic acid using PPR-specific cDNA clones (Roeder et al., 1994). A polymerase chain reaction (PCR) based on the amplification of the Np and F protein genes has been developed for the specific diagnosis of PPR (Shaila et al., 1996; Nanda et al., 1996; Couacy-Hyman et al., 2002). This technique is very sensitive, and the result can be obtained in a few hours.

Anderson et al. (1991) developed a test, namely, monoclonal antibody based on competitive enzyme-linked immunosorbent assay (cELISA) to differentiate rapidly the infections with PPRV from those of RPV. Seroconversion occurs in ten to fourteen days, and the antibody can be demonstrated by virus neutralization, competitive ELISA (Libeau et al., 1995), CIE, and AGID. Detection of antibodies requires paired sera samples taken three weeks apart if one sample is taken late in the course of the disease. A simple, rapid, and easy to perform field dot-ELISA has been developed for the diagnosis of PPR (Saravanan et al., 2006).

DIFFERENTIAL DIAGNOSIS
Rinderpest (RP), contagious caprine pleuropneumonia, bluetongue, hemorrhagic septicemia, foot-and-mouth disease, coccidiosis, and heart water disease are the diseases to be differentiated from PPR.

Clinical signs of RP and PPR are quite similar, but RP should be the prime suspect if both cattle and small ruminants are involved.

Hemorrhagic septicemia is characterized by respiratory signs and diarrhea. Fatality rate never exceeds 10%.

In CCPP and PPR, fever and respiratory distress are common, but there is no digestive system involvement in CCPP.

Bluetongue differs from PPR in the presence of edema of head region, the coronary band of the hooves, and in the less hairy parts of the body. There is lameness in bluetongue.

In heart water disease, there is often central nervous system involvement, including convulsions, and no diarrhea as in PPR.

Contagious ecthyma can be distinguished from the PPR by the absence of nasal discharge and diarrhea. The orf virus causes proliferative, not necrotic, lesions involving the lips rather than the whole oral cavity.

Foot-and-mouth disease occurs mildly in small ruminants. In FMD, respiratory distress and diarrhea are absent. FMD lesions are more pronounced among sheep than in goat.

In coccidiosis, there is absence of fever and no involvement of upper digestive tract and respiratory tract organs.

Case history and absence of fever distinguishes plant or mineral poisoning from PPR.

TREATMENT
There is no specific therapy. Antibiotic therapy is recommended to prevent secondary bacterial complications along with fluid administration to combat dehydration.

PREVENTION AND CONTROL

VACCINATION
Tissue culture rinderpest vaccine was being used to prevent PPR (Taylor, 1979). The use of rinderpest vaccine to protect small ruminants against PPR is now contraindicated because it produces antibodies to rinderpest, which interfere with serosurveillance for rinderpest and the Global Rinderpest

Eradication Program. Homologous PPR vaccine is preferred over RP vaccine to avoid confusion when retrospective serological survey is done.

OIE, Paris, has to issue special guidelines on PPR vaccination of sheep and goats in the countries like India, which are declared free from rinderpest but are endemic to PPR infection in sheep and goats.

A homologous PPR vaccine is available now. Live, attenuated tissue culture vaccine is being used internationally. Genetically engineered vaccinia and capripox recombinant vaccines are also under trial. It has been found that goats, when vaccinated with a recombinant capripox vaccine containing either fusion (F) gene or the hemagglutinin (H) gene of rinderpest virus, survived when challenged with a lethal dose of PPR virus (Jones et al., 1993; Romero et al., 1995).

The genes of the PPRV immune-protective proteins and the fusion and the hemagglutinin proteins have been introduced into the genome of capripox vaccine strain. Viruses have proved to be effective as a dual vaccine to protect against the two major diseases of small ruminants (Sinnathampy et al., 2001). The live, attenuated PPR vaccine could also protect goats against rinderpest challenge (Couacy-Hymann et al., 1995).

ERADICATION

Quarantine, slaughter, and disposal of infected animals and disinfection of affected premises should be effectively practiced. PPR-free countries should ensure that only vaccinated animals are allowed to enter in endemic areas. The unrestricted movement of PPR-susceptible animals from areas infected with PPR should be prohibited. If the disease is introduced, it can be eradicated by quarantine and slaughter and disposal of infected animals and decontamination of the affected premises.

High-risk countries or countries trading with or geographically close to infected countries can protect themselves by having all susceptible animals vaccinated before they enter the country and/or vaccinating the national herd. Since Tissue culture RP vaccine is now contraindicated in rinderpest-free countries to protect against PPR, OIE/FAO has to give necessary guidelines to use the safest vaccine and make it available for the PPR-endemic countries to avoid reappearance of rinderpest with the use of TCRP vaccine. If an outbreak occurs in an area, the animals should be quarantined and ring vaccination adopted. In endemic areas, all the susceptible animals should be vaccinated.

REFERENCES

1. Amanfu, W. 2008. *PPR Spread in Kenya/Uganda: Threat to the rest of Eastern Africa.* FAO Animal Health ServiceAGAH.
2. Anderson, J., Mckay, L. A. and Butcher, R. N. 1991. IAEA Technical document 623, Proceedings of a final research coordination meeting of the FAO/IAEAJSIDA/OAU Coordinted research Programme. Bingerville, Cote d'Ivoire. November 19–23, 1990, 4.
3. Barrett, T. 1996. Geographic distribution and epidemiology of *peste des petits ruminants* virus. *Virus Res.* 43:149–153.
4. Brindha, K., Govindarajan, R., Ravikumar, G., Chandran, N. D. J. and Kotteeswaran, A. 2007. Seromonitoring of *Peste des des petits ruminants* virus in bovines. *Indian Vet. J.* 84:238–40.
5. Couacy-Hymann, E., Bodjeh, K., Angba, A., Domenech, J. and Diallo, A. 1995. Protection of goats against rinderpest by vaccination with attenuated *peste des petits ruminanats* virus. *Res. Vet. Sci.* 59:106–109.
6. Couacy-Hyman, E., Roger, F., Hurard, C., Gillou, J. P., Libeau, G. and Diallo, A. 2002. Rapid and sensitive detection of *peste des petits ruminanats* virus by a polymerase chain reaction assay. *J. Virol Methods* 100:17–25.
7. Couacy-Hymann, E., Bodjo, S. C., Donho, T., Koffi, M. Y., Libean, G. and Diallo, A. 2007. Early detection of viral excretion from experimentally infected goats with PPR virus. *Preventive Vet. Med.* 78:85–88.
8. Dhar, P., Sreenivasa, B. P., Barrett, T., Corteyn, M., Singh, R. P. and Bandhopadhyay, S. K. 2002. Recent epidemiology of *peste des petitis ruminants* virus (PPRV). *Vet. Microbiol.* 88:153–159.
9. FAO. 2008. FAO report September 9, 2008. First ever outbreak of Peste des petits ruminants in Morocco. Internet Morocco Newslines.
10. Gibbs, E. P., Taylor, W. P., Lawman, M. J. and Bryant, J. 1979. Classification of *peste des petitis ruminanats* virus as the fourth member of the genus *morbillivirus. Intervirology* 11:5, 268–274.
11. Govindarajan, R., Koteeswaran, A., Venugopalan, A. T., Shyam, G., Shaouna, S., Shaila, M. S. and Ramachandran, S. 1997. Isolation of *peste des petits ruminants* virus from an Indian buffalo (*Bubalus bubalis*). *Vet. Rec.* 14:573–574.
12. Haroum, M., Hajer, I., Mukhtar, M. and Ali, B. B. 2002. Antibodies against peste des petitisruminants virus in sera of cattle, camels, sheep and goats in Sudan. *Vet. Res. Commun.* 26:537–541.
13. Ikede, B. O. 1983. Histopathologyof natural cases of PPR characteristic lesions and changes occurring during the disease peste des petits ruminants (PPR) in sheep and goats In *Proceedingsof the international work shop held at IITA Ibadan, Nigeria.* 24–26 September., ed. D. H. Hill. Addis Ababa, Ethiopia: ILCA.
14. Jones, L., Giavedoni, L., Slaiki, J. T., Brown, C., Mebus, C. and Yilma, T. 1993. Protection of goats against *peste des petits ruminants* with a vaccinia virus double recombinant expressing the F and H genes of Rinderpest virus. *Vaccine* 11:961–964.
15. Libeau, G., Diallo, A., Colas, F. and Guerre, L. 1994. Rapid differential diagnosis of rinderpest and *peste des petits ruminanats* using an immunocapture ELISA. *Vet. Rec.*134:12, 300–304.
16. Libeau, G., Prehaud, C., Lancelot, R., Colas, F., Guerre, L., Bishop, D. H. and Diallo, A. 1995. Development of a competitive ELISA for detecting antibodies to the *peste des petits ruminants* virus using a recombinant nucleoprotein. *Res. Vet. Sci.* 58:50–55.
17. Mathew, Z. 1981. Personal communication as he had organized the PPR conference at Epidemiology Unit, FLD Kaduna, Nigeria.
18. Nanda, Y. P., Chatterjee, A., Purohit, A. K., Diallo, A., Innui, K., Sharma, R. N., Libeau, G., Thevasagayam, J. A., Bruning, A., Kitching, R. P., Anderson, J., Barrett, T. and Taylor, W. P. 1996. The isolation of *peste des petits ruminanats* virus from northern India. *Vet. Microbiol.* 51:207–216.
19. Nawathe, D. D. 1984. The control of peste des petits ruminants in Nigeria. *Prev. Vet. Med.* 2:147–155.
20. OIE. 2007. Peste des petits ruminants, PPR in China (Peoples Rep. of) OIE Alert Message CHN-27-07-07. Internet News.

12. PESTE DES PETITS RUMINANTS

21. OIE. 2008. Peste des petits ruminants in China (Peoples Rep. of) OIE Alert Message CHN 11-07-08. Internet news.
22. Ogunsanmi, A. O., Awe, E. O., Obi, T. U. and Taiwo, V. O. 2003. Peste des petits ruminants (PPR) virus antibodies in African Grey Duiker (*Sylvicapra grimmia*). *African J. Biomed. Research* 6:59–61.
23. Roeder, P. L., Abraham, G., Kenef, G. and Barrett, T. 1994. *Peste des petisis ruminants* in Ethiopian goats. *Trop. Anim. health Pro.* 26:69–73.
24. Romero, C. H., Barret, T., Kitching, R. P., Bostock, C. and Black, D. N. 1995. Protection of goats against *peste des petits ruminanats* with a recombinant Capri poxviruses expressing the fusion and hemagglutinin protein gene of rinderpest virus. *Vaccine* 13:1, 36–40.
25. Saravanan, P., Balamurugan, V., Sen, A., Sahay, B., and Singh, R. K. 2006. Development of Dot-Elisa for diagnosis of PPR in small ruminanats. *J. Applied Animal Research* 30:121–124.
26. Saravanan, P., Balamurugan, V., Sen, A., Sarkar, J., Sahay, B., Rajak, K. K., Hosmani, M., Yadav, M. P. and Singh, R. K. 2007. Mixed infection of PPR and Orf in a goat farm in Shahjahanpur, India. *Vet. Rec.* 160:410–412.
27. Sailu, O. J., Audu, S. I., Sanda, M. E., Aribido, S. O. and Olaou, M. 2008. Adoption of vaccination and etnoveterinary treatment for peste des petits ruminants (PPR) among sheep and goat in Ijumu local government area of Kogi State, Nigeria. *Agricultural Journal* 3:404–408. Medwell online journal, 2008.
28. Shaila, M. S., Shamaki, D., Forsyth, M. A., Diallo, A., Goatley, L., Kitchin, R. P., Couacy-Hymann, E., Bidjeh, K., Angba, A., Domenech, J. and Diallo, A. 1996. Protection of goats against rinderpest by vaccination with attenuated *peste des petits ruminants* virus. *Res. Vet. Sci.* 59:106–109.
29. Sinnathampy, G., Renukaradhya, G. J., Rajasekhar, M., Nayak, R. and Shaila, M. S. 2001. Immune responses in goats to recombinant hemagglutinin-neuraminidase glycoprotein of *peste des petits ruminants* virus; identification of a T cell determinanat. *Vaccine* 19:4826–23.
30. Taylor, W. P. 1979. Protection of goats against *peste des petits ruminants* with attenuated Rinderpest virus. *Res. Vet. Sci.* 27:321–324.
31. Uzuokwu, M. 1983. The pathology of peste de petits ruminants (PPR caprine pneumoenterits) in sheep and goats. In *Proceedings of the international workshop* held at IITA Ibadan, Nigeria, 24–26 September 1980, ed. D. H. Hill. Addis Ababa, Ethiopia: ILCA.

13. Rabies in Bovines and Ovines
(*Hydrophobia, Lyssa*)

M. R. Saseendranath, M. Krishnan Nair, Thankam Mathew, and Z. Mathew

Introduction
Rabies is a viral encephalitis affecting all warm-blooded animals, including human being, usually transmitted by the bite of an infected animal.

Etiology
Rabies is caused by a RNA virus belonging to the genus *Lyssavirus* and family Rhabdoviridae (King and Turner, 1993). The genus *Lyssavirus* includes six serotypes. Sereotype 1 causes classical rabies. Other rabies-related viruses are European bat lyssavirus I and II and the recently isolated Australian bat lyssavirus.

Crick (1981) reported other rabies-related viruses namely, Lagos virus (isolated from bats in Nigeria), Mokola virus (isolated from man and shrews in Nigeria), Duvenhage (isolated from man in South Africa), Kotonkan (*Culicoides* in Nigeria), Obodhiang (mosquitoes in Sudan).

Rabies viruses are approximately 180 nm × 75 nm in size. This bullet-shaped virus contains a lipid envelope and negative-stranded RNA. The rabies genome encodes five proteins classified as nucleoprotein (N), phosphoprotein (P), matrix protein (M), glycoprotein, (G) and polymerase (L). The virus has a phospholipids envelop, which has glycoprotein spikelike structures measuring 5–8 μm (microns) in length with a knob on the tip of the spike

Rabies virus is stable between pH 3 and 11 and may survive for many years at-70°C or when freeze dried and kept at 0-4 °C. Desiccation, UV and x-ray exposure, sunlight, beta-propiolactone, ether, chloroform, acetone, iodine preparations, quarternary compounds, and detergents rapidly inactivate the virus. The virus is also inactivated at 60°C for thirty seconds.

Culture of Rabies Virus
Kanazawa (1936) and Webster and Clow (1937) cultivated rabies virus in mouse embryo tissue culture. The Flury strain was originally isolated from the nervous tissue of a girl named Flury, who got infected through vaginal mucosa (Leach and Johnson, 1940). Later, the LEP (low egg passage) variant of Flury strain was developed by passaging through 136 intracerebral passage in

day-old chicks (Koprowaski and Cox, 1948). Then Kissling (1958) cultivated fixed and street virus in hamster kidney tissue culture, which provided new system for the study of rabies virus, and Fenge (1960) produced the first tissue culture vaccine by cultivating the rabies virus in hamster kidney tissue culture. Ver et al. (1964) studied the factor affecting the yield of rabies virus in tissue culture. Hronovsky et al. (1966) adapted the street virus to the dog kidney primary tissue culture, with specific reproducible cytopathic effect.

EPIDEMIOLOGY

The ancient physicians described a disease resembling rabies in dogs and humans around 3000 BC. Rabies in animals was described in detail by Democritus in 500 BC and by Celcus in the first century. Zinke (1804) reported the first experimental transmission of rabies by the inoculation of saliva from a rabid dog to a normal dog. Pasteur et al. (1881) reported the isolation of the infective agent from the brain of the animal that died of rabies. Later, Pastuer et al. (1884) passaged the street virus hundred times in rabbits and obtained fixed virus, and later in 1885, Pastuer carried out the successful vaccination against rabies in a peasant boy bitten by rabid dog. Rabies is worldwide in distribution. Indian subcontinent, Africa, parts of Central and South America are highly endemic zones for rabies. Spain, UK, Sweden, Finland, Norway, Greece, Portugal, New Zealand, Japan, Caribbean islands, Ireland, Lakshadweep and Andaman and Nicobar islands in India, parts of Indonesia, and Singapore are currently free of rabies. Season had no influence on incidence of rabies among domestic animals (Praveena et al., 2006).

SOURCE OF INFECTION

In most of the cases, rabid animal is the source of infection. Infected animals excrete the virus three to four days before the onset of symptoms. Hence, unprovoked bite from an otherwise normal animal has to be viewed seriously, and necessary treatment has to be started immediately. In most countries of Africa and Asia, dogs continue to be the main hosts and are responsible for most of the human rabies cases. It has been recorded that 96.2% of the human rabies cases are occurring due to dogbite in India. Dog rabies virus variants are the major circulating rabies viruses that transmit the disease to other domestic animals and man in India (Nagarajan et al., 2006). The virus is also maintained by wild animals like jackal, foxes, raccoons, arctic fox, skunks, mongoose, wolves, and hyenas. Nair et al. (1978) reported the role of bandicoots in the transmission of rabies in India. Bat rabies has emerged as an important agent in transmission of rabies in Latin American countries.

TRANSMISSION

Bite of an infected animal is considered as the primary mode of transmission. The bite wound is likely to be contaminated with virus-laden saliva.

The most common mode of transmission is by the bite of diseased dogs and cats. Wild carnivores like foxes, raccoons, skunks, jackals, wolves, and insectivores and vampire bats also transmit the disease in sylvatic rabies. Cattle, horses, sheep, goat, deer, and other domestic animals can become infected with rabies and but rarely transmit the disease. Rodents, monkeys, and mongoose also play a minor role in transmission.

Ingestion of meat from animals that died of rabies is one important method of transmission in the wild. Milk consumption from rabid animals may also to be a source of infection. Lambs develop rabies by sucking milk from rabid dam. Intrauterine transmission has also been recorded in animals. Aerosol transmission has been recorded in people who entered the vampire bat dwelling caves without mask and protective clothing. The bloodsucking vampire bat found in South and Central America and also the fruit bats act as carrier of rabies virus. Very few reports of dogs acting as carrier was reported by Veeraraghavan et al. (1966) and Bell (1966). In India, the disease is prevalent throughout the year in an epidemic form. According to Horsefall and Tamm (1965) during summer season, rabies is more as the dogs are free moving, and contact among them are more. In contrast during winter season, spread of rabies is less due to lack of contact among the animals. Inhalation of rabies virus may also cause the infection (Atanasiu, 1965; Constatine, 1962; and Winkler, 1968). Transmission from person to person is rare and can happen through transplant surgery. A case of transmission via organ transplant happened when organs from a man infected with rabies caused the death of three recipients. Unknowingly, eyes collected from a rabies patient had led to the transmission of rabies in man. Rabies diseases exists in two epizotic forms: (1) urban type, which spread mainly through dogs; and (2) sylvatic type, which is prevalent in wild animals and bats (WHO, 966).

Hosts

All warm-blooded animals, including human beings, are susceptible to infection. Foxes, coyotes, jackals, wolves, and certain rodents are among the most susceptible animal groups. Skunks, raccoons (Rosatte et al., 2007), bats (Hester et al., 2007), rabbits, and cattle have high susceptibility. Animal species with only moderate susceptibility include dogs, sheep, goats, horses, man, and nonhuman primates. Mongoose in India are known to suffer from rabies, and the possibility of transmission of the disease from infected mongoose to other rodents and human beings cannot be ruled out. Therefore, cases of bites by rodents, which show a tendency to be unusually aggressive, must be viewed with suspicion and treated. All birds and primitive mammals such as opossum have low susceptibility. Cats are more resistant than dogs to the experimental infection with some canine rabies isolates form wild life. Gopal (1984), Wimalaratne and Kodikara (1999), and Aravind et al. (2006) reported rabies in elephants.

PATHOGENESIS

The incubation period of rabies is variable and depends upon the site of bite, the quantity of virus deposited at the site of bite (if the bite is nearer to the brain, the onset of rabies will be quicker than the bite on hand and leg), the strain and the virulence of the virus, species of animals involved (foxes can carry up to 10 × 6 infectious units of virus per milliliter of saliva), and innervation at the site of bite. Usually, the incubation period varies from few days to weeks, months, and to years depending on the above mentioned biological factors. But a case of rabies with a long incubation period of nineteen and a half years was there in record. Long incubation period may be due to latent infection, becomes active, due to some stress factor on the host (Horsefall and Tamm, 1965). According to Veeraraghavan (1954), in human being only 43% of the people bitten by rabid dogs and have not undergone any treatment suffer from rabies.

The virus has a phase of local replication in myocytes before entering the nervous system through the neuromuscular junctions and neuromuscular spindles. The virus specifically attaches to the receptors for the neurotransmitter, nicotinic acetylcholine receptors at the neuromuscular junctions, facilitating the entry of the virus into nerves. The virus spreads by retrograde (centripetal) passive intraaxonal flow in peripheral nerves. Neuronal infection and intraaxonal flow deliver the virus to the central nervous system via the spinal cord. Although uncommon, infection by other routes is possible. Following intranasal exposure, virus enters the trigeminal nerves and ganglia in its course to the central nervous system (CNS).

Once the virus reaches the CNS, it spreads in the brain within forty-eight hours. Following the replication in the CNS, the virus spreads centrifugally to salivary glands and other organs by means of peripheral nerves. Virus spreads via cranial nerves to salivary glands, and higher titers of virus have been found in salivary glands than in the brain, and high titers have also been found in lungs, indicating that the agent may replicate outside the CNS. The virus has been isolated from different organs and tissues such as the adrenal glands, subcutaneous fat of bats, kidneys, bladder, ovaries, testicles, sebaceous glands, germinal cells of hair follicles, cornea, tongue, papillae, intestinal wall, and pancreas. The rabies virus excretion begins three to four days before the onset of clinical signs, and the victims die in three to five days of onset of clinical signs.

CLINICAL FINDINGS

Rabies virus infection has been classically divided into three major stages: prodromal, furious, and paralytic. All the animals may not pass through these three clinical stages. Behavioral changes are mainly observed in prodromal stage. Dogs behave abnormally, hide in dark corners, friendly dogs become aggressive, and aggressive dogs behave in a friendly manner and become restless. During the furious stage, there is aggressiveness, tendency to attack and bite whatever comes on the way. This is the stage of transmission of the disease. Often the dog leaves the home at this stage and never returns. This stage is followed by paralytic stage and finally death due to respiratory failure. In dumb form of rabies, the furious stage is missing. The animal passes from the prodromal stage to the paralytic stage.

In cats, the incubation period is two to six weeks, and the disease is usually of furious type. Among farm animals, cattle are the highly susceptible group. Usually, the incubation period is three weeks and may range up to months. The disease starts with excitation and off feed. Yawning a few hours before the start of bellowing is a pathognomonic sign in cattle. The yawning movements are described as voiceless attempt to bellow. Drooling of saliva is a consistent finding. Other important signs are bellowing, tenesmus with paralysis of anus, resulting in the sucking in and blowing out air, frequent urination, increased sexual excitement, tendency to mount on other animals and to charge.

Animal bellows till the animal reaches paralytic stage. The sound is characteristically hoarse, and actions are exaggerated. The animals at this stage are hypersensitive to sounds. Unlike in human beings, animals drink water till the paralytic stage. Bulls at this stage often have paralysis of penis. Death usually ensues forty-eight hours after the animal becomes recumbent. The course of the disease usually extends six to seven days in cattle, and death is due to respiratory failure. In sheep and goats, the clinical signs are similar to those in cattle.

IMMUNE RESPONSE
The glycoprotein (G) and nucleoprotein (N) are dominant antigens in antirabies virus immune response. G protein induces virus-neutralizing antibodies while N protein has dominant T helper epitopes. Incorporation of N protein in the vaccine preparation offers added advantage as there is extensive cross-reactivity among N protein as compared with G protein of various *Lyssaviruses*. Mice immunized with rabies nucleoprotein (RNP) are also protected from peripheral challenge of rabies virus in the absence of neutralizing antibody. Protection of RNP-immune mice from peripheral challenge has been ascribed to the role of gamma interferon secreted by T helper cells.

Mathew (1971) took up a detailed study of interference phenomenon of rabies virus using different viral and nonviral inducers of interferon and found that the interferon inhibit the multiplication of rabies virus by way of the interference phenomenon.

DIAGNOSIS

Diagnosis is based on history of rabid animal bite, clinical signs, and by different laboratory tests for the detection of inclusion bodies, antigen and antibody.

Several techniques can be used for the detection of rabies antigen. The biological test by inoculating brain suspension intracerebrally into one-day-old Swiss albino mice is the most confirmative test and takes ten to twenty-one days, but it is most reliable (Lennette and Schimidt, 1964). Demonstration of Negri bodies by Seller's staining (Praveena et al., 2006), fluorescent antibody test (FAT) (Goldwasser and Kissling, 1958), rabies rapid enzyme immunodiagnosis (RREID), agar gel diffusion test, counterimmunoelectrophoresis test, latex agglutination test, virus isolation in newborn mice, virus isolation in cell culture, immunoperoxidase test, (IPT), peroxidase antiperoxidase test (PAP), avidin-biotin test, dipstick dot-ELISA test, reverse transcriptase–polymerase chain reaction (RT-PCR) (Kimura et al., 2006), and electron microscopy are some among them. Recently monoclonal antibodies are used in several laboratories to detect the strain variations. Detection of viral RNA by dot and slot hybridization, in situ hybridization, and different types of polymerase chain reactions are recent advanced techniques.

Many serological procedures have been described for measuring rabies antibody. These include the following: (1) hemagglutination test (HA) and hemagglutination inhibition test (HI) (Mathew, 1971), (2) complement fixation test (CFT), (3) plaque reduction test, (4) gel diffusion test, (5) counterimmunoelectrophoresis test, (6) mouse neutralization test, (7) radioimmunoassay, and (8) rapid fluorescent focus inhibition test (RFFIT).

The hemagglutination (HA) for the virus was first reported by Halonen et al. (1968) and Kuwart et al. (1968) for the rabies virus of tissue culture origin. Later, Murphy et al. (1968) also reported a detailed study of hemagglutination of rabies virus. Hemadsorption also was demonstrated by street rabies virus adapted to tissue culture by Selimov et al. (1965). (Mathew, 1971) showed that different strains of rabies virus, namely, CVS, street virus, Paris fixed virus, Flury, LEP, and HEP strains, showed HA with fowl, goose, and frog red cells at pH range of 6.2–6.4 and also done the HI test with horse hyperimmune antirabies serum and dog antirabies serum to prove the specific rabies antigen and antibody reaction.

Mathew (1971) standardized a new test PCA (passive cutaneous anaphylaxis) reaction. It was found to be specific test for rabies diagnosis and is a quick and easy test to conduct in guinea pig for the diagnosis of rabies infection.

In the PCA test, rabies hyperimmunized antiserum (0.1 ml) is intradermally injected on one side of the back into the shaved skin of adult white guinea pig (Hartley strain). As a control, normal sheep serum is also injected on the opposite side of the back of guinea pig. Rabies antigen was prepared mixing 1.0 ml of 10% brain suspension from mouse injected with street virus, showing symptoms of paralysis, with 1.0 ml of 10% Evans blue (vital dye). After three hours of injecting rabies antiserum (time given to fix the antibodies in the skin), 1.0 ml of rabies brain suspension antigen mixed with Evans blue is injected slowly by intracardial route into the above guinea pig. If the antigen (brain suspension) is positive for rabies infection, there will be intense bluing of the skin around the site of rabies antiserum injection. This is caused by passive cutaneous anaphylaxis (PCA) reaction with the extravasations of blood containing colored rabies antigen when reacted with rabies antibody at the site where rabies antiserum is injected. The control skin injection site where normal serum is injected will not show any significant bluing, indicating that no antigen antibody reaction has taken place as normal serum did not contain any antibodies to the rabies antigen injected by i/c route. So the PCA test can be considered specific for the diagnosis of rabies.

DIFFERENTIAL DIAGNOSIS

The following diseases with nervous disorders are often confused with rabies: lead poisoning, lactation tetany, vitamin A deficiency, polioencphalomalacia, listeriosis, enterotoxemia, and ketosis.

Acute and subacute lead poisoning are characterized by blindness, convulsion, champing of jaws, twitching of eye lids and ears, and pressing of head against a wall. In rabies, there is no blindness, convulsion, and facial muscle paralysis; but bellowing, yawning, and tendency to attack are very characteristic.

Lactation tetany is common in milking animals showing hyperesthesia, tremor, convulsion, and recumbency followed by death.

Avitaminosis is common in young animals up to two years, where blindness, tremors, and convulsion are common. Polioencephalomalacia is characterized by blindness, nystagmus, opisthotonos, convulsion, and bellowing.

In listeriosis, circling and head-pressing syndrome are common. Animals with enterotoxemia show diarrhea and nervous signs. Nervous form of ketosis is seen in lactating animals and also characterized by presence of ketone bodies in urine and milk, with a history of reduction in milk yield.

TREATMENT

The case fatality is cent percent; hence, treatment after the onset of clinical signs is not rewarding. Immediately after the bite, application of first aid by washing the bite wound with clean water and soap for fifteen minutes, followed by application of antiseptics like spirit, tincture iodine, dettol, savlon, etc., are indicated. It is important to start antirabies vaccine treatment immediately in the case of deep wounds near the brain. Being a viral disease, specific treatment is lacking. Postexposure antirabies therapy is indicated in animals wherever euthanasia is not possible. The Essen schedule (zero-, three-, seven-, fourteen-, eighteen-, and ninety-day optional of vaccination) of postexposure antirabies therapy is done in animals also. Any inactivated tissue culture antirabies vaccine can be used which contains an antigenic titer of at least 2.5 IU/dose. In severe cases of third class of exposure, rabies immunoglobulins are also administered. Equine rabies immunoglobulins (at the dose rate of) 40.0 IU/kg can be administered in small animals. So far, no such studies were undertaken in cattle.

PREVENTION AND CONTROL

VACCINATION

The best way of prevention is the prophylaxis of the vectors mainly dogs. The primary immunization of dogs is done at two months of age and give booster dose four weeks later followed by then annual vaccination. In endemic areas, other susceptible population like cattle, sheep, and goats are also immunized at three months of age, and then annual vaccination is done. The control of rabies in India has been reported by Menon et al. (1976) during the OIE meeting in Paris.

Mathew et al., (1978) prepared and studied the BPL-inactivated (beta propiolactone–inactivated) suckling mouse brain antirabies vaccine to protect animals and humans and found better than sheep brain BPL-inactivated vaccine during that period.

Inactivated tissue culture antirabies vaccine containing 2.5 IU/ml/dose is used for the prophylactic immunization and postexposure therapy. DNA vaccines can be produced at low cost, which can be stored at room temperature. They are ideally suited for prophylactic immunization against rabies in developing countries. Studies have shown that DNA rabies vaccine (DRV) comprising plasmid DNA encoding rabies virus surface glycoprotein protects mice, dogs, and nonhuman primates against rabies virus infection (Xiang et al., 1994, 1995; Ray et al., 1977; Bahloul et al., 1998; Biswas et al., 1999; Jallet et al., 1999; Perrin et al., 1999).

Several strategies are being examined for improving the potency of DRV so that they can be used for both prophylactic and postexposure therapy in man and animals (Xiao Yue Qiang et al., 2007). Coinoculation of a plasmid expressing granulocyte-macrophage colony stimulating factor was shown to enhance the potency of DRV (Xiang and Ertl, 1995). Adjuvants such as monophosphoryl lipid A, when administered together with DRV, enhanced rabies virus–neutralizing antibody (RVNA) titers after an initial intradermal vaccination in nonprimed animals but not in animals that have been immunologically primed (Lodmell et al., 1999). Biswas et al. (2001) demonstrated that mice immunized with combination rabies vaccine containing a low dose of cell-culture-derived inactivated rabies virus vaccine and DNA rabies vaccine induced higher levels of rabies virus–neutralizing antibodies than those immunized with DRV alone and are completely protected against peripheral as well as intracerebral rabies virus challenge. The quantity of inactivated rabies virus vaccine for enhancing the potency of DRV can be 625-fold lower than that of a standard dose of inactivated rabies virus vaccine. DNA combined tissue culture antirabies vaccine in different postexposure immunization schedules provided protection in rabies exposed goats (Raji and Saseendranath, 2006).

An effective and economical tool to combat the threat of stray and community dogs is by immunizing them with oral vaccines. Live oral vaccines have already been in use for decades for foxes in Europe and for raccoons in USA to control wild life rabies. Mebatsion et al. (2004) reported an improved live oral vaccine based on the modification of original Alabama-Dufferin (SAD) strain. An SAD mutant has been derived wherein arginine residue of glycoprotein G at position 333 is replaced with aspartic acid to obtain strain ORA-D. ORA-D. These all are various strains made in that particular study out of SAD by genetic manipulations, for oral vaccination of stray dogs and wild animals. It is nonpathogenic to adult mice but retain residual pathogenicity for baby mouse. A further deletion was introduced to the P protein. This removes the LC8 binding site, thereby preventing axonal transport of the virion core along a neural tract. This steps lead to the development of a stable ORA-DP vaccine virus, which is safe for even suckling mice. Further, to enhance the immunogenicity of the vaccine, the ORA-DPC strain has been developed in which the insertion is realized on addition glycoprotein G derived from CVS strain. ORA-DPC is the best candidate rabies vaccine strain for oral immunization of dogs. Oral bait vaccine, Rabidog SAG2, has been safe and highly immunogenic in Indian stray dogs under captivity without any adverse reaction, salivary excretion and absence of replication of the vaccine strain in brain and salivary glands (Cliquet et al., 2007).

The control of rabies should aim at reduction of rabies in wildlife by wild life immunization, immunization of main vectors like dogs and cats, reduction of the population of stray dogs by animal birth control (ABC) program, and finally through the public education.

RABIES CONTROL MEASURES IN NIGERIA

Epidemiology Unit, Federal Livestock Dept., Nigeria, awarded consultancy projects to the veterinary professors in the Nigerian university to conduct a survey and suggest method of control of various livestock diseases, including rabies. The project report on rabies concluded that there is a great need to create awareness about rabies in Nigeria to get the public cooperation for the control of rabies in humans and dogs. There are some misgivings in Nigeria attributed to rabies. In Nigeria, the people suffering from rabies symptoms are always attributed to the practice of juju (sending evil spirit) by their enemy. So the people who are infected by rabid dogbite and showing symptoms of rabies are always taken to local village doctor (juju practitioner) to get rid of the evil spirit, without giving any rabies treatment vaccination. On the basis of this finding in 1981, Epidemiology Unit, Federal Livestock Dept. (FLD), Kaduna, Nigeria, conducted First National Rabies Awareness Campaign to create awareness among villagers about the horror of rabies and remove the myth of rabies infection, the necessity to control it by vaccinating all the pet dogs and stray dogs, and giving immediate treatment vaccination for those exposed the dogbite.

The preparation for the two-week campaign started one year in advance. The campaign was given great publicity through mass media like local newspapers, pictorial wall papers (displayed in the schools and local govt. offices), distribution of rabies education leaflets, veterinarians and veterinary students giving talks to high school / college students, five-minute TV film on *Horror of Rabies* by showing the tragic suffering and death of a person who had not undergone any treatment vaccination after a rabid dogbite. The National Rabies Awareness Campaign was launched in each state by the governor or his representative and in the capital by the president of Nigeria/his representative with wide TV coverage. It created such a great impact among the public, encouraging the priests in the church mentioning the importance of rabies vaccination in their sermon. Throughout Nigeria, dog vaccination camps were arranged during the fifteen days of the National Rabies Campaign. Large number of pet dogs were given rabies vaccine with three-year immunity against rabies. Large doses of human rabies treatment and prevention vaccine were imported. The veterinarians and veterinary students were given preventive vaccination against rabies. It was a great success in creating great awareness, removing the myth on rabies, the necessity to protect dogs against rabies, and providing urgent treatment to people exposed to the bite of a rabid dog.

REFERENCES

1. Atanasiu, P. 1965. Transmission of rabies by respiratory route to laboratory animals. *C. R. Acad. Sci.* 261. 277–279.
2. Aravind, B., Anilkumar, M., Raju, S. and Saseendranath, M. R. 2006. A case of rabies in an Indian elephant *Elephas maximus. Zoos Print J.* 21:2172.
3. Bahloul, C., Jacob, Y., Tordo, N. and Perrin, P. 1998. DNA based immunization for exploring the enlargement of immunological corss-reactivity against Lyssa viruses. *Vaccine* 16:417–425.
4. Bell, J. F. 1966. In *Proc. Nat. Rabies Symposium,* 117. National Communicable Disease Centre, Atlanta, USA.
5. Biswas, S., Ashok, M. S., Reddy, G. S., Srinivasan, V. A. and Rangarajan, P. N. 1999. Evaluation of protective efficacy of rabies DNA vaccine in mice using an intracerebral challenge model. *Curr. Sci.* 76:1012–1016.
6. Biswas, S., Reddy, G. S., Srinivasan, V. A. and Rangarajan, P. N. 2001. Pre-exposure efficacy of a novel combination DNA and inactivated Rabies virus vaccine. *Human Gene Therapy* 12:1917–1922.
7. Cliquet, F., Gurbaxani, J. P., Pradhan, H. K., Pattnaik, K. B., Patil, S. S., Regnault, A., Begouen, H., Guiot, A. L., Sood, R., Mahi, P., Singh, R., Meslin, F. X., Picard, C., Subert, M. F. A. and Barrat, J. 2007. The safety and efficacy of oral bait vaccine SAG2 in Indian stray dogs. *Vaccine* 25:3409–3418.
8. Constatine, D. G. 1962. Rabies transmission by nonbite route. *Publ. health Resp.* (Wasb) 77:287–289.
9. Crick, J. 1981. Rabies. In *Virus diseases of food animals,* vol. 2, ed. E. P. J. Gibbs, 469–508. London: Academic Press.
10. Gopal, T. 1984. Rabies in an Indian elephant calf. *Indian Vet. J.* 61:82–83.
11. Goldwasser, R. A. and Kissling, R. E. 1958. Fluorescent antibody staining of street and fixed rabies virus antigen. *Proc. Soc. Exp. Biol. Med.* 98:219–223.
12. Halonen, P. E., Murphy, F. A., Fields, B. N. and Reese, D. R. 1968. Haemagglutinin of rabies and other bullet shasped viruses. *Proc. Soc. Exp. Biol. Med.* 127:1037–42.
13. Hester, L. C., Best, T. L. and Hudson, M. K. 2007. Rabies in bats from Alabama. *J. wild life Diseases* 43:291–299.
14. Horsfall, F. L. Jr. and Tamm, I. 1965. In *Viral and rickettsial infectionsof man,* 4th ed. London: Pitman Medical Publishing Co. Ltd.
15. Hronovsky, V., Benda, R. and Cinatl, J. 1966. In *Viral and rickettsial infections of man,* 4th ed. London: Pitman Medical Publishing Co. Ltd.
16. Jallet, C., Jacob, Y., Bahloul, C., Drings, A., Desmezieres, E., Tordo, N. and Perrin, P. 1999. Chimeric Lyssa virus glycoproteins with incressed immunological potential. *J. Virol.* 73:225–233.
17. Kanazawa, K. 1936. Study of fixed rabies virus propagated in the brain. *Jap. J. Exp. Med.*14:519.
18. Kimura, L. M. S., Dautar Junior, J. V., Monta, W. C., Kotcut, I., Marens, V. A. and Brandas, P. E. 2006. PCR technique for rabies diagnosis. *Revista Baasiterta de Medicine Veterinaria* 28:104–109.
19. King, A. A. and Turner, G. S. 1993. Rabies: A review. *J. Comp. pathol.* 108:1–3.
20. Kissling, R. E. 1958. Fluorescent antibody study of street and fixed rabies virus antigen. *Proc. Soc. Exp. Biol.* (NY) 98:223.
21. Koprowaski, H. and Cox, H. N. 1948. Studies on chick embryo adapted rabies virus culture characteristics and pathogenesis. *J. Immunol.* 60:533.–554.
22. Kuwert, R., Wiktor, T. J., Sokol, F. and Koprowaski, H. 1968. Haemagglutin by rabies virus. *J. Virol.* 2:1381–1392.
23. Leach, C. N. and Johnson, H. N. 1940. Human rabies with special reference to virus distribution and titer. *Amer. J. Trop. Med.* 20:335–340.
24. Lennette, E. H. and Schimidt, N. J. 1964. In *Diagnostic procedures for viral and Rickettasial Diseases,* 3rd. ed. American Public Health Assn. Inc. 1970 Brodway New York.

25. Lodmell, D. L., Ray, N. B., Ulrich, J. T., and Ewalt, L. C. 1999. DNA vaccination of mice against rabies virus: Effects of the routes of vaccination and the adjuvant monophophoryl lipid A. *Vaccine* 18:1059–1066.

26. Mathew, Z. 1971. Haemagglutination and haemadsoption by rabies virus. PhD thesis, Haffkine Institute, University of Bombay.

27. Mathew, Z. 1971. Diagnosis of rabies infection by passive cutaneous anaphylaxis reaction. PhD thesis, Haffkine Institute, University of Bombay, 53–95.

28. Mathew, Z. 1971. Interferon studies on rabies virus. PhD thesis, Haffkine Institute, University of Bombay, 97–124.

29. Mathew, T., Rai Chowdhuri, A. N., Bhola, S. R. and P. K. Topa. 1978. Studies on BPL inactivated suckling mouse brain antirabies vaccine. *Indian J. Med. Res.* 68:197–203.

30. Mathew, Z. 1981. Personal communication. Zachariah Mathew, Chief Veterinary Officer and Head of Epidemiology Unit, Federal Livestock Dept. Kaduna.

31. Mebatsion, T., Van Braber, M., Visser, N., Kilari, S. and Singh, S. N. 2004. Development of an oral rabies vaccine with improved safety and efficacy to control canine rabies in stray dogs. Proceedings of 6th National conference, APCRI. 2004.

32. Menon, M. N., Mathew, Z., Mathew, T. and S. C. Adlakha. 1976. Control of rabies in India. *Bull. Off. Int. Epiz.* 86:341–349.

33. Murphy, F. A., Halonen, P. E., Gary, Jun, G. W. and Reese, D. R. 1968. Physical characterization of rabies haemagglutinin. *J. Gen. Virol.* 3:289.

34. Nagarajan, T., Mohansubramanain, B., Seshagiri, E. V., Nagendrakumar, S. B., Saseendranth, M. R., Satyanarayana, M. L., Thiagarajan, D., Rangarajan, P. N. and Sreenivasan, P. A. 2006. Molecular epidemiology and rabies virus isolates in India. *J. Clin. Microbiol.* 44:3218–3224.

35. Nair, S., Dighe, P. Y. and Nanavati, A. N. D. 1978. Role of bandicoots in rabies transmission. *Indian J. Med. Research.* 67:347–353.

36. Pasteur, L., Chamberland Roux and Thuillier. 1881. *Sur Larage, C. R. Acad. Sc.* 92:1259. Cited by Horsfall, F. L. and Tamm, I. 1965.

37. Pasteur, L. Chamberland Roux. 1884. Nouvelle Communication Sur. In *Rage C. R. Acad. Sc.* 98:457. Cited by Horsfall, F. L. and Tamm, I. 1965.

38. Pasteur, L. 1885. *C. R. Acad. Sc.* 101:765. Cited by Horsfall, F. L. and Tamm, I. 1965.

39. Perrin, P., Jacob, Y., Aguilar-Setien, A., Loza-Rubio, E., Jallet, C., Desmezieres, E., Aubert, M., Cliquet, F. and Tordo, N. 1999. Immunization of a dog with a DNA vaccine induces protection against rbies virus. *Vaccine* 18:479–485.

40. Praveena, P. E., Manohar, B. M., Balachandran, C. and Rao, V. N. A. 2006. A study on the occurrence of rabies. *Indian Vet. J.* 83:1251–1252.

41. Raji James and Saseendranath, M. R. 2006. Efficacy of DNA combined tissue culture antirabies vaccine in different post exposure immunization schedule in rabies exposed goats. *Indian J Vet. Med.* 26:93–95.

42. Ray, N. B., Ewalt, L. C. and Lodmell. 1997. Nanogram quantities of plasmid DNA encoding the rabies virus glycoprotein protect mice against lethal virus infection. *Vaccine* 15:892–895.

43. Rosatte, R., Donovan, D., Allen, M., Bruce, L., Buchanan, T., Sobey, K., Davies, C., Wandeler, A. and Muldoon, F. 2007. Rabies in vaccinated raccoons from Ontario, Canada. *J. Wildlife Disease* 43:300–301.

44. Selimov, M. A. and Lliasova, R. S. H. 1968. Vop. Virus 13:76 (cited in Index Medicus,.10, Part. II. 1969), 510.

45. Sreenivasan, P. A. 2006. Molecular epidemiology and rabies virus isolates in India. *J. Cln. Microbiol.* 44:3218–3224.

46. Veeraraghavan, N. 1954. Phenolised vaccine treatment of peopleexposed to rabies in South India. Annual Report (1954), Pasteur Institute of South India, Coonor.

47. Veeraragavann, N., Gajnana, A. R., Rangasami, R., Saraswathi, K. C., Devaraj, R. and Hallan, K. M. 1966. In *The Scientific and Annual Report (1968)*, Pasteur Institute of South India, Coonor.

48. Webster, L. T. and Clow, A. D. 1937. Propagation of rabies virus in tissue culture. *J. Exp. Med.* 66:125–131.

49. WHO. World Health Org. Tech. Rep. Ser. No. 321. 1966. (Expert committee on Rabies 5th Report).

50. Wimalaratne, O. and Kodikara, D. S. 1999. First reported case of elephant rabies in Srilanka. *The Vet. Rec.* 144:98.

51. Winkler, W. G. 1968. Airborne rabies virus isolation. *Wild Life Disease* 4:37–40.

52. Xiang, Z. Q. and Ertl, H. C. J. 1995. Manipulaton of immune response to a plasmid encoded viral antigen by co inoculation with plasmid expressing cytokines. *Immunity* 2:129–135.

53. Xiang, Z. Q., Spitalink, S., Tran, M., Cheng, J. and Ertl, H. C. J. 1994. Vaccination with a plasmid vector carrying the rabies virus glucoprotein gene induces protective immunity against rabies virus. *Virology* 199:132–140.

54. Xiang, Z. Q., Spitalink, S., Tran, M., Cheng, J., Erikson, J., Wojczyk, B. and Ertl, H. C. J. 1995. Immune response to nucleic acid vaccines to rabies virus. *Virology* 209:569–579.

55. Xiao Yue Qiang, Li Hai Tao, Lui Lan, Zhang Shou Feng, and Hu Rong Liang. 2007. Field immunoassay of RV glycoprotein and nucleoprotein "bivalent" DNA vaccine in dogs. *J. Vet. Sci.* 27:195–199.

56. Zinke. 1804. Cited by Johnson, H. In *Viral and Rickettsial infections of Man*. By Rivers and Horsfall, F. L. 1959. 3rd Ed.

14. Rift Valley Fever

M. R. Saseendranath, and M. Krishnan Nair

Introduction
Rift valley fever (RVF) is a peracute or acute insectborne viral disease of man and animals, characterized by hepatitis and high mortality in lambs and calves, abortion in livestock especially in sheep and influenza-like disease or hemorrhagic fever in human beings. The disease can cause very serious economic loss in livestock, particularly in sheep, goats, cattle, camels, Asian water buffaloes, and wild antelopes.

Etiology
The RVF virus belongs to the family Bunyaviridae and genus *Phlebovirus*. The RVF virus is an RNA lipid-enveloped spherical structure, 80 nm–120 nm in diameter and contains 5–10 nm surface spikes (G1 and G2). These spikes mediate the attachment of the virus to the host cell receptors, serve as hemagglutinin, and are the targets for the host's neutralizing antibodies. The virus has a helical nucleocapsid and three single-stranded negative sense (L, M, S) RNAs. The virus lipid envelope contains 20–30% lipids totally derived from the host cell membrane.

The virus survives for several months at 4°C and gets inactivated at 56°C in two hours. It is resistant to alkaline pH but inactivated by pH <6.8. Lipid solvents like ether and chloroform inactivate the virus. Areas contaminated with blood spillage can be decontaminated with 2% acetic acid or 5% sodium hypochlorite. Blood, even dried blood, may remain infective for humans for some months at ambient temperature. Pasteurization renders milk safe. Hides and skins, bones, and manure are rendered safe if sun dried.

Epidemiology
Outbreaks of RVF occur generally when particularly heavy, prolonged, and, often, unseasonal rainfall favors the breeding of mosquito vectors. Epidemics in most of Eastern and Southern Africa occur in five to twenty-year cycles, but in the dry semiarid zones of Eastern Africa, the periodicity is fifteen to thirty years.

Mechanical transmission of infection by mosquitoes, midges, phlebotomids, stomoxids, simulids, and other biting flies appears to play a significant role in epidemics. It has been suggested that *Hyalomma* species of cattle ticks might have spread RVF infection to West Africa and Egypt.

Approximately 1% of human sufferers die of the disease. Among livestock, the fatality level is significantly higher. In pregnant livestock infected with RVF, there is the *abortion* of virtually 100% of fetuses, and the fatality rate for newborn lambs is 90%.

Livestock epizootics can occur after heavy rainfall and flooding that result in hatching of *Aedes* mosquitoes and other vectors that feed on nearby mammals (CDC, 1997–98). An epizootic of RVF is generally observed during years in which unusually heavy rainfall and localized flooding occur. The excessive rainfall allows mosquito eggs, usually of the genus *Aedes*, to hatch. The mosquito eggs are naturally infected with the RVF virus, and the resulting mosquitoes transfer the virus to the livestock on which they feed. Once the livestock is infected, other species of mosquitoes can become infected from the animals and can spread the disease. In addition, it is possible that the virus can be transmitted by other biting insects. *Aedes vexans*, *A. ochraceus*, and *A. dalzieli* mosquitoes, as well as other mosquitoes and bloodsucking insects, such as the sand fly *Phlebotomus duboscqui*, are known vectors for RVF. Because mosquitoes are easily carried long distances by wind, RVF has the potential to spread rapidly to new countries and even to new continents.

DISTRIBUTION
RVF was first reported among livestock in Kenya in the Rift Valley of Kenya around 1915, but the virus was not isolated until 1931. The virus was first isolated in 1930 from humans in Kenya (Daubney, 1931). The disease was first observed in Southern Africa in 1950. The most notable epizootic occurred in Kenya in 1950–1951 and resulted in the death of an estimated one hundred thousand sheep. Imported European animals were found especially susceptible to RVF.

Most epidemics have occurred in Eastern and Southern Africa, and until 1977, the farthest north that the disease was known to have occurred was the Sudan. During 1977 and 1978, a major epidemic occurred in the Nile Delta and Valley in Egypt. A severe epidemic affected the Senegal River basin in Mauritania and Senegal in 1987 and again in Egypt in 1993. In September 2000, an outbreak was confirmed in Saudi Arabia and Yemen.

SOURCE OF INFECTION
Wild fauna, viremic people, diseased animals, and infected mosquitoes are the important sources of infection leading to outbreak in most of the countries.

The virus is maintained through a cycle involving mosquito vectors and domestic livestock. *Aedes* mosquito transmit the virus transovarially, which lay drought-resistant eggs and survives for several years without hatching. Ruminants act as amplifying hosts. Human beings pick up infection from nasal discharge, blood, vaginal secretions after abortion in animals and from infected meat, in addition to mosquito bites.

TRANSMISSION

Transcutaneous transmission by mosquito and fly bite constitutes the major mode of transmission of RVF. Studies have shown that sleeping outdoors at night in geographical regions where outbreaks occur could be a risk factor for exposure to mosquito and other insect vectors.

International travelers increase their chances of getting the disease when they visit RVF-endemic locations during periods when sporadic cases or epidemics are occurring.

Unlike in humans, nonvector transmission of RVF virus is not considered to be important in livestock.

Humans acquire RVF more frequently through exposure to the blood, body fluids, or tissues of diseased animals with abraded skin, wounds, or mucous membranes. The virus is transmitted via contact with the blood, secretions, or excretions of infected animals. Because the virus affects livestock, contact with diseased animals can be via slaughtering or handling of infected animals. Direct exposure to infected animals can occur during slaughter or through veterinary and obstetric procedures. Many of the cases were in persons who had recently been involved in the dissection, slaughter, or care of sick animals (Joubert et al., 1951; Van Veldman et al., 1977). A high attack rate has been demonstrated for abattoir workers (Abu-Elyazeed et al., 1996 *http://www.cdc.gov/ncidod/EID/vol8no2/01-0023.htm—21*), herdsmen (Zaki et al., 1995), and veterinary personnel (Mundel and Gear, 1951), all of whom have extensive contact with animal blood or other body fluids in the course of their work (Wilson et al., 1994 *http://www.cdc.gov/ncidod/EID/vol8no2/01-0023.htm—21*). The risk of human-to-human infection through direct contact appears also to be very low.

Aerosol transmission of the disease via contact with laboratory specimens has also been documented.

Low concentrations of RVF virus are found in the milk of infected animals and may lead to transmission of RVF by the consumption of raw milk (Alexander, 1951; Jouan et al., 1989).

The infection can be transferred between animals when they are vaccinated or blood-sampled using the same needle without proper sterilization during an epidemic.

HOST
Clinical disease has been observed in sheep, goats, cattle, domesticated Asian buffaloes, camels, and humans, of which the most susceptible has been sheep. The susceptibility of wild antelopes to disease has not been established fully, but it is believed that at least some species suffer mortality and abortion. Some breeds of sheep and goats appear to be relatively resistant to the disease.

African monkeys and domestic carnivores present a transitory viremia.

PATHOGENESIS
RVF virus spreads from the site of introduction in the body, and initial replication occurs in spleen, liver, and brain. These are either directly damaged by the effects of the virus or by immunopathologiocal mechanisms.

Hepatocytes are the primary site of viral replication in lambs and calves. Hepatic lesions progress from degeneration and necrosis of individual hepatocyte to extensive necrosis throughout the liver leading to hepatic insufficiency.

Even in benign infections of livestock, there is a marked leukopenia during the first three to four days of infection, corresponding with the peak fever and viremia. At the same time, there are marked increases in the serum concentrations of some enzymes indicative of liver cell damage.

The most severe lesions are found in aborted sheep fetuses and newborn lambs. The liver is usually enlarged, soft, friable, and yellowish brown to dark reddish brown in color. Irregular congested patches and hemorrhages of varying size are often present in the substance of the liver together with pale foci. Jaundice is seen in only a relatively small proportion of lambs because of the short time to death. In older sheep, the hepatic lesions are generally not so severe, but jaundice may be more marked. Pale areas of cell necrosis combined with large hemorrhages give a mottled appearance to the liver. Hemorrhages and edema of the gall bladder are common, and the bile may contain blood. Elsewhere, in newborn lambs, peticheal and echymotic hemorrhages are found in the abomasal mucosa, and the contents are often dark brown from the presence of partly digested blood. The contents of the small intestine may be similar. Most mature sheep have hemorrhages and edema in the abomasal folds and sometimes free blood in the intestinal lumen.

Aborted cattle fetuses, calves, and older cattle show lesions essentially similar to those in sheep fetuses, lambs, and older sheep.

In all animals, the peripheral and visceral lymph nodes are enlarged, edematous, and may contain peticheal hemorrhages. The spleen is enlarged with hemorrhages in the capsule.

Hepatic necrosis of varying degree is the most striking microscopic lesion in all animals. Many animals have congestion, edema, hemorrhage, and emphysema in the lungs.

IMMUNE RESPONSE

As animals mature, their susceptibility to RVF disease decreases. Innate immunity varies between breeds, and some breeds of sheep and goat appear to be relatively resistant. Herd immunity levels are high after epidemics, the immunity appears to be lifelong. Immune dams transfer immunity to their offspring via colostrum, and this affords some protection for up to five months in lambs.

After natural infection, domestic animals lose a detectable amount of IgM antibody within six months of infection (Morven et al., 1992).

In a large percentage of humans, experimental inoculation with a killed vaccine results in an early IgM response that wanes and is undetectable by four to six weeks, but this is not a model for natural infection (Niklasson et al., 1984).

Of the few clinical infections that have been followed closely for serologic conversion, IgM antibody appears around day 5, is absent in 50% by day 45, and is undetectable four months later (VanVelden et al., 1977), whereas IgG appears about day 4 and may persist indefinitely at high titer.

CLINICAL SYMPTOMS

Incubation period varies from one to six days. In animals, the first sign of an epidemic of RVF is normally numerous abortions in infected pregnant sheep, goats, cattle, Asian buffaloes, and camels. Abortion can occur at any stage of gestation, with autolysis of fetus. The most severe reactions occur in newborn lambs and kids, which die within hours of infection, rarely surviving more than thirty-six hours. Onset is marked by high fever, which subsides sharply before death. Affected animals are listless, disinclined to move or feed, and respiration is rapid. Mortality reaches 90% or more in animals less than one week of age. Fatality is attributed to hepatic damage (Erasmus and Coetzer, 1981; Yedloutsching et al., 1981).

Older lambs and kids and mature sheep and goats may develop inapparent, peracute, or acute disease. In peracute disease, death occurs before the development of notable signs. Acute disease is characterized by high fever for one to three days, anorexia, weakness, listlessness, and rapid respiration. Some animals regurgitate ruminal contents and exhibit bloodstained nasal discharge, fetid diarrhea, and dysentery. Jaundice may be evident. Death occurs after about three days of illness. The mortality rate is lower than in week-old lambs but can still reach 50% or more. Eighty percent of pregnant ewes abort after infection (Mundel and Gear, 1951).

Inapparent infections are quite frequent in other species than sheep. Adult cattle exhibit clinical signs of disease infrequently, but some may develop acute disease with fever for two to three days, with anorexia, lacrimation, hyper salivation, nasal discharge, dysgalactia, and diarrhea, which may be bloodstained. The mortality rate does not usually exceed 10% but can be higher. A prolonged course of ten to twenty days with marked jaundice has been described in the Sudan.

RVF in man characteristically manifests as an acute influenza-like illness with transient fever, headache, severe muscle and joint pain, photophobia, and anorexia and sometimes with a peticheal rash, nausea, vomiting, and epistaxis. The course is four to seven days leading to full recovery in two weeks. The most frequent complication is retinitis, usually bilateral, occurring one to three weeks after the primary febrile illness. Permanent loss of central vision occurs in about 50% of those affected. There may be permanent unilateral or bilateral blindness. In a proportion of RVF cases, a biphasic fever is seen with encephalitis developing during the second febrile phase. Patients suffer confusion, hallucinations, vertigo, and choreiform movements, which is sometimes leading to coma. The case mortality rate is generally low, but full recovery may be protracted and long-term neurological complications have been reported. Hemorrhagic diathesis with hepatitis is a relatively new form of the disease. There is an acute febrile illness of two to four days' duration, followed by jaundice, and widespread hemorrhages in mucosa and subcutaneously. Bleeding occurs at needle puncture sites, from the gums, and nose, and there may be hematemesis and diarrhea with melena. Death usually occurs within another three to six days, and a few patients recover after a long slow convalescence. Approximately 1% of infected people die of the disease.

DIAGNOSIS
RVF has to be suspected when there is simultaneous occurrence of numerous cases of abortion and disease in ruminants, together with disease of humans, following heavy and prolonged rainfall. The clinical diagnosis can be

confirmed by a number of tests for the demonstration of the antigen and antibody. Specimens required include heparinized and clotted peripheral blood, heart blood, tissue samples (liver, spleen, kidney, and lymph nodes), and serum. Samples from aborted fetuses should include brain. Where delay is anticipated in samples reaching a laboratory or where samples have to be transported at ambient temperature, tissue samples can be preserved in glycerol-saline solution (50:50).

Virus isolation is by cell culture (BHK21, Vero, mosquito cell line, primary calf, lamb, or goat kidney cell line) or by intraperitoneal or intracerebral inoculation of weanling mice or hamsters. Confirmation can be made by immunofluorescent or immunoperoxidase staining and inoculation of one-to two-days old lambs and of embryonated chicken egg.

Detection of viral antigen is made by immunofluorescent or immunoperoxidase staining of frozen sections, immunodiffusion, complement fixation, and ELISA.

Detection of viral RNA can be made by reverse transcriptase polymerase–chain reaction (RT-PCR).

Virus neutralization and ELISA helps to detect antibodies. Paired samples collected during the acute phase and again two to three weeks later provide evidence of recent infection. IgM-capture ELISA allows diagnosis of recent infection to be made on a single serum sample.

DIFFERENTIAL DIAGNOSIS

Wesselsbron disease tends to occur under the same climatic conditions as RVF. Both cause mortality in lambs, kids, and calves and abortion in ewes, but RVF is associated with much higher mortality and abortion rates. Wesselsbron disease is usually inapparent in adult animals and is limited to southern Africa.

RVF could also be confused with Nairobi sheep disease (transmitted by *Rhipicephalus* and *Amblyomma* species ticks) of sheep and goats because of abortion, mortality, and jaundice and can be identified by serological tests.

Intoxication by poisonous plants can cause mortality associated with hepatic lesions, hemorrhages, and jaundice superficially resembling RVF.

Conditions of high rainfall and humidity favor the occurrence of leptospirosis, which can mimic many of the clinical signs of RVF. Leptospirosis can be differentiated by various bacteriological, serological, and molecular tests.

TREATMENT

There is no specific therapy for RVF. Various antiviral agents had been tried with little effect. Other treatment with interferon, immune modulators, and convalescent plasma are found useful.

CONTROL

Control of disease involves protection from mosquito vectors. Personal protection is important and effective. Using appropriate protective clothing and insect repellents and avoiding outdoor activity at peak biting times of the vector species. Measures to control mosquitoes during outbreaks, like use of insecticides, are effective if conditions allow access to mosquito-breeding sites.

Treatment of livestock with a systemic insecticide (e.g., an avermectin) or a topical insecticide (e.g., a synthetic pyrethroid) over a wide area could assist in reducing the populations of potential vectors. Biological control systems using *Bacillus thuringiensis* or hormones suppressing larval development are more acceptable alternatives.

Animals may be moved from low-lying areas to well-drained and windswept pastures at higher altitudes and confine livestock in mosquito-proof stables. There should be control of livestock movements. All infected livestock should be slaughtered and disposed. However, such measures are usually impractical, instituted too late, and at best palliative in the face of a RVF epidemic. Public awareness programs are essential to keep the public fully and accurately informed, not only to reduce concern but also to assist in diagnosis of disease and to take appropriate control measures.

Avoiding exposure to blood or tissues of animals that may potentially be infected is an important protective measure for persons working with animals in RVF-endemic areas.

New systems that monitor variations in climatic conditions are being applied to give advance warning of impending outbreaks by signaling events, which may lead to increases in mosquito numbers. Such warnings allow authorities to implement measures to avert an impending epidemic. Remote sensing satellite technology, which can predict rainfall patterns likely to result in disease emergence, has been suggested as a means to monitor RVFV activity (Linthicum et al., 1987, 1999).

VACCINATION

Immunization remains the only effective means of protecting livestock. RVF can be prevented by animal vaccination. Both live, attenuated and killed vaccines have been developed for veterinary use. All ruminants in herds within the infected area should be vaccinated immediately with an inactivated RVF vaccine and revaccinated after two to four weeks and annually.

The live vaccine requires only one dose and produces long-lived immunity. But the presently available vaccine may cause abortion if given to pregnant animals. The mouse-adapted Smithburn strain of RVF virus is used to produce live vaccines. They are highly immunogenic and induce durable, probably lifelong immunity within seven days after a single inoculation, although cattle may not be fully protected. However, the virus is only partially attenuated and can cause abortion or fetal damage and prolonged gestation in a proportion of pregnant animals. It is also conceivable that the virus could be transmitted between animals by mosquitoes and revert to full virulence. The use of such vaccines is therefore inadvisable in countries where the presence of the virus has not been proven. This vaccine is pathogenic to human beings. The killed vaccines do not cause any of the untoward reactions, but multiple doses must be given to produce protective immunity. This may prove problematic in endemic areas. Vaccines prepared by the inactivation of wild strains of RVF virus with formalin or beta-propiolactone give low antibody responses. Repeated inoculation after an initial double vaccination with an interval of two to four weeks is required to maintain immunity, which is short-lived. They are safe in pregnant animals but are expensive to produce. Sheep are protected better than cattle while colostral immunity is inadequate.

A human live, attenuated vaccine, MP-12, is currently undergoing trials but is not approved for human use. Other attenuated strains have been developed as potential live vaccines. Formalin-inactivated vaccines have been used to protect laboratory workers. A viral glycoprotein vaccine has also been developed.

An inactivated vaccine has been developed for human use. This vaccine is not licensed and is not commercially available but has been used experimentally to protect veterinary and laboratory personnel at high risk of exposure to RVF. Other candidate vaccines are under investigation.

The risk of transmission from infected blood or tissues exists for people working with infected animals or people during an outbreak. Gloves and other appropriate protective clothing should be worn and care taken when handling sick animals or their tissues. Healthcare workers looking after patients with suspected or confirmed RVF should employ universal precautions when taking and processing specimens from patients. Hospitalized patients should be nursed using barrier techniques. As noted above, laboratory workers are at risk, so samples taken for diagnosis from suspected human and animal cases of RVF should be handled by trained staff and processed in suitably equipped laboratories.

ERADICATION

Activities undertaken should attempt to contain the virus at the site of introduction (by movement controls) and then eliminate it (destruction of infected and potentially infected livestock). It is very important that the timing and sequence of operations give the greatest chance of eliminating the virus before it becomes widespread in an insect vector or animal populations, including wildlife.

Immediately on suspicion of the disease, an infected area should be designated extending at least 10 km from the foci of infection, and movements in and out of the area are prohibited. The area at risk is also determined with respect to geographical features, prevailing winds, the presence of possible vectors, and the density of prospective hosts. Infected humans can play an important role in the transmission of RVF, and it will be necessary to trace both animal and human movements. Close collaboration between human and medical staff is called for to trace both the source of infection and possible secondary cases. Surveillance involves clinical examination of livestock at risk and serological monitoring of a statistically significant sample at short intervals to determine if virus transmission is occurring.

Clinical cases should be slaughtered first (by shooting preferably), followed by animals in direct contact and then the remaining susceptible animals. It is not necessary to slaughter healthy animals outside the affected herd. Care must be taken not to generate aerosols and expose animals and people to infection. Disposal by burial is preferable (*http://www.fao.org/ag/aga/agah/ empres/Info/rvf/RVF198.htm—Contents*).

Climatic forecasting in conjunction with satellite imaging of flooded areas has been suggested as a method for predicting where and when RVF outbreaks might occur, potentially enabling earlier interventions (Linthicum et al., 1999) (*http://www.fao.org/ag/aga/agah/empres/Info/rvf/RVF198. htm—Contents*).

REFERENCES

1. Abu-Elyazeed, R., El-Sharkawy, S., Olson, J., Botros, B., Soliman, A. and Salib, A. 1996. Prevalence of anti-Rift Valley fever IgM antibody in abattoir workers in the Nile Delta during the 1993 outbreak in Egypt. *Bull World Health Organ.* 74:155–158.

14. RIFT VALLEY FEVER

2. Alexander, R. A. 1951. Rift Valley fever in the Union. *J. S. Africa Vet. Med. Association* 22:105–109.

3. CDC. Rift Valley fever-East Africa, 1997–1998. 1998. *MMWR.* 47:261–264.

4. Daubney, R., Hudson, J. R. and Garnham, P. C. 1931. Enzootic hepatitis or Rift Valley fever: An undescribed virus disease of sheep, cattle and man from East Africa. *J. Pathol. Bacteriol.* 34:545–579.

5. Erasmus, B. J. and Coetzer, J. A. W. 1981. The symptomology and pathology of Rift Valley fever in domestic animals. *Contr. Epidem. Biostatist.* 3:77–82.

6. Jouan, A., Coulibaly, I., Adam, F., Philippe, B., Riou, O. and Leguenno, B. 1989. Analytical study of a Rift Valley fever epidemic. *Res. Virol.* 140:175–86.

7. Joubert, J. D. S., Ferguson, A. L. and Gear, J. H. S. 1951. Rift Valley fever in South Africa. 2. The occurrence of human cases in the Orange Free State, the North-Western Cape Province, the Western and Southern Transvaal. A. Epidemiological and clinical findings. *S. Afr. Med. J.* 1951:25:890–891.

8. Linthicum, K. J., Bailey, C. L., Davies, F. G. and Tucker, C. J. 1987. Detection of Rift Valley fever viral activity in Kenya by satellite remote sensing imagery. *Science* 27:1656–1659.

9. Linthicum, K. J., Anyamba, A., Tucker, C. J., Kelley, P. W., Myers, P. F., Peters, C. J. 1999. Climate and satellite indicators to forecast Rift Valley fever epidemics in Kenya. *Science* 285:397–400.

10. Morven, J., Rollin, P. E., Lanventure, S. and Roux, J. 1992. Duration of immunoglobulin M antibodies against Rift Valley fever virus in cattle after natural infection. *Trans. R. Soc. Trop. Med. Hyg.* 86:675–680.

11. Mundel, B. and Gear, J. 1951. Rift Valley fever. I. The occurrence of human cases in Johannesburg. *S Afr Med J.* 25:926–930.

12. Niklasson, B., Peters, C. J., Grandien, M. and Wood, O. 1984. Detection of human immunoglobulins G and M antibodies to Rift Valley fever virus by enzyme-linked immunosorbent assay. *J Clin Microbiol.* 19:225–229.

13. Van Velden, D. J. J., Meyer, J. D., Olivier, J., Gear, J. H. S. and McIntosh, B. 1977. Rift Valley fever affecting humans in South Africa: A clinicopathological study. *S. Afr. Med. J.* 51:867–871.

14. Wilson, M. L., Chapman, L. E., Hall, D. B., Dykstra, E. A., Ba, K. and Zeller, H. G. 1994. Rift Valley fever in rural northern Senegal: Human risk factors and potential vectors. *Am. J. Trop. Med. Hyg.* 50:663–675.

15. Yedloutschnig, R. J., Dardiri, A. H. and Walker, J. S. 1981. Persistence of Rift Valley fever virus in the spleen, liver, and brain of sheep after experimental infection. *Contr. Epidem. Biostatist.* 3:72–76.

16. Zaki, S. R., Greer, P. W., Coffield, L. M., Goldsmith, C. S., Nolte, K. B., and Foucar, K. 1995. Hantavirus pulmonary syndrome: Pathogenesis of an emerging infectious disease. *Am. J. Pathol.* 146:552–579.

15. RINDERPEST
(Cattle Plague, Peste Bovine, Pestis Bovina)

M. R. SASEENDRANATH, M. KRISHNAN NAIR, THANKAM MATHEW, AND Z. MATHEW

INTRODUCTION
Rinderpest is a highly contagious viral disease of ruminants especially of cattle, manifested as peracute, subacute, or in subclinical forms, characterized by inflammation, necrosis, and erosion of the mucous membranes particularly of respiratory and digestive tract.

ETIOLOGY
Rinderpest (RP) virus is a single-stranded RNA virus belonging to the family Paramyxoviridae under the genus *Morbillivirus*. The RP virus has many strains with considerable variation in virulence, but all are immunologically identical. Immunity, which develops as a result of infection or vaccination with one strain, protects all other strains. RP virus is antigenically related to the viruses, which causes canine distemper, peste des petits ruminants of goats and sheep, measles in humans, porcine distemper in seals, and equine influenza.

The virus particle is spherical or ovoid in morphology and measures 90–250 nm in diameter. Some filamentous and elongated forms vary up to 500–1000nm. The RP virus is having six major proteins, viz, H, F, N, L, P, and M proteins. The virus is covered with spiked envelope, which contains H protein that binds to the cell receptor, and the fusion F protein that induces formation of syncytia. The H and F proteins of the envelope confer protective immunity against RP virus in cattle. The RNA is protected by N nucleoprotein. Transcription in infected cell is mediated by polymerase L protein and polymerase-associated P protein. The M protein forms the matrix and is lying within the virus.

The RP virus is not shown to be having any hemagglutinating property. The virus is sensitive to ether, chloroform, and trypsin and is highly fragile and easily destroyed by heat, drying, and disinfectants. Strong alkalies like sodium hydroxide (2.5%) and sodium carbonate (4%), phenol (5%), cresol (3.5%), and formalin (4%) are found to be the best disinfectants.

In manure, this virus remains infective for about forty-eight hours. The optimum stability of the virus is between pH 7.2–8.0 and is rapidly inactivated by putrefaction within twenty-four hours in cadavers. It loses its infectivity on exposure to sunlight or when dried under natural conditions.

EPIDEMIOLOGY

DISTRIBUTION

Rinderpest is one of the oldest diseases of cattle recorded from the fifth century. It is believed that this disease is originated from Asia, and epizootics of this disease swept over Europe until about the end of nineteenth century, reducing the cattle population considerably. It is this disease that was responsible for the establishment of first veterinary school of Europe at Lyons, France, in 1762, for giving training to veterinarians to control this dreadful malady, which used to wipe out the entire cattle population.

Rinderpest is one of the major economic problems in Asia and Africa (Yilma, 1989). The last disastrous outbreak of RP had occurred in Great Britain in 1865. Europe is free from the disease since 1880. The disease is now mainly reported from Asian and African countries. In 1983, a severe epidemic of rinderpest disease occurred in Nigeria with the import of trade cattle from the neighboring countries like Chad. This has happened due to the lack of quarantine stations in the trade cattle route. A large number of Fulani white cattle died. An outbreak of rinderpest in the wild buffaloes in the Yankari Wildlife Sanctuary, Nigeria, was also reported. As some Fulani owners lost their entire herd of cattle wealth, they committed suicide, resulting in political repercussions at national level. This led the federal govt. of Nigeria to implement urgently strict rinderpest control measures and vaccinations. To overcome the shortage of vaccine, the federal govt. imported one million doses of TCRP vaccine from BAIF, India. (Mathew, 1983; Mathew et al., 1984; Mathew et al., 1989). Iran is free of rinderpest since1982 (WHO, 1989).

During the fifteen-year period (1974–1988) of National Project on Rinderpest Eradication (NPRE) program in India, it was found that the average incidence of RP to be between 0.0020 and 0.0009% (Dutta et al., 1991). Since 2006, India is free from rinderpest disease. Bhutan is free from RP, but as it is prevalent in neighboring countries, the threat of reintroduction is constant (Rai, 1991).

SOURCE OF INFECTION

The main source of infection is always an infected animal, during incubation, clinical manifestation, and convalescent period. Mild or in apparent form of infection also acts as a source. The virus occurs in the excretion and secretion of affected animals, like urine, milk, dung, and nasal and lacrimal discharges.

TRANSMISSION

Close contact with infected and susceptible animal is usually necessary for the spread of the disease through inhalation of viral droplets as this virus is not in a position to survive outside for long.

Ingestion of contaminated feed, water, and fodder with excretion or secretion from diseased animal is the next important mode of transmission. Pigs pick up infection by ingesting infected meat scraps. Though insects carry this virus on their body mechanically, they are not likely to transmit infection.

HOSTS

The cloven-hoofed animals are the natural hosts of RP. In addition to cattle, the infection was recorded in water buffalo, sheep and goat, pig, yak, free living wild animals like water buck, wart hog, African buffalo, eland, wildebeest, bush buck, giraffe, kudu, gazelle, and impala. Rinderpest outbreak was reported in Indian wild goats, Nilgiri Tahr, and in European wild sheep during 1991 at Vandallur Zoo, Chennai (Madras), India (Chandran et al., 1991). Cattle and buffalos of all ages are susceptible. European breeds of cattle are more susceptible than zebu cattle. RP virus is not communicable to human beings.

PATHOGENESIS

The incubation period ranges from two to six days depending on the virulence of the virus, quantum of the virus entered, and resistance of the host. The RP virus after entry into the system penetrates through the epithelium of upper respiratory tract and multiplies in tonsils and regional lymph nodes, from where it is released into the blood leading to viremia. The virus is attached to mononuclear cells and is disseminated throughout the body.

The virus has got high affinity to the lymphoid tissue and epithelial cells of alimentary and respiratory tracts. The initial changes are noted in the deep layers of stratum malphigii just above the basal layer. The epithelial cells undergo necrosis but do not form vesicles. As the lesions increase in size and extend toward the surface, the cornified layer becomes raised, and the necrotic area are seen grossly as tiny slightly elevated grayish white foci (1 mm in diameter). These lesions then coalesce, and the detachment of overlying necrosed tissue from the underlying basal layer results in formation of shallow erosions. In these sites, there is extensive cellular necrosis as well as development of multinucleated giant cells or syncytia, which contain intranuclear and intracytoplasmic inclusions. The infection causes necrosis of lymphocytes in lymph nodes, spleen, and Peyer's patches. The mucosal changes are characterized by necrosis of stratified squamous epithelium of the upper alimentary tract and necrosis of crypts in the intestine, resulting in erosion. Inflammatory cells are minimal, but multinucleated syncytia are characteristic.

There is abomasitis and ulcerative lesions in the pyloric region. The Peyer's patches are frequently dark in color and friable. The cecum and colon zones of hemorrhage and erythema running transversally across the colonic mucosa produce a characteristic striped appearance of *zebra striping*. Hemorrhage in caeco-colic junction and bands of congestion in rectum are also noticed (Rautmare et al., 1992). Erosions in the upper respiratory tract are uncommon. But there may be hemorrhage and discoloration. The virus replicates in monocytes, lymphocytes, and epithelial cells. Because of destruction of lymphocytes in tissues, there is marked leucopenia. The focal necrotic stomatitis and enteritis, which are characteristic of this disease, are the direct result of viral infection and replication in epithelial cells in the alimentary tract. Death usually results from dehydration and due to secondary bacterial and parasitic infestation as a result of immunosuppression.

CLINICAL FINDINGS

The intensity of clinical signs varies depending on the strain of virus, dose of the virus, route entry, concurrent infections, and resistance of the host. In a newly infected area, the mortality may reach 90% and morbidity 100%. The peracute form is characterized by fever (105–107°F), congested mucous membranes, respiratory distress, and death in one to two days; whereas in acute form, the course of the disease may last four to seven days; and in subacute case, the animal may live up to three weeks or longer. Plowright (1968) divided the pathogenesis of the disease into four stages as incubation, prodromal, mucosal, and convalescent and presented a very comprehensive description of the host-virus interaction and the sequence of events, which result in the development of clinical signs and lesions. Scott (1981) added a diarrheic phase in between the mucosal and convalescent phase.

In the acute form, the initial symptoms noticed are fever (105–107°F) (without mucosal lesions phase of prodromal fever), restlessness, loss of appetite, cessation of rumination, reduction of milk yield, dryness of muzzle, and constipation. This is followed in day or two by nasal and ocular discharges, photophobia, thirst, anorexia, and excessive salivation.

This stage is followed by mucosal phase characterized by inflammation of buccal, nasal, and conjunctival mucosa and in some cases hyperemia and swelling of vaginal and vulval mucosa. The lacrimation becomes more profuse and purulent, and there is blepherospasm. Bubbly salivation of clear bloodstained saliva is followed by purulent saliva and halitosis (fowl smell). Serous nasal discharge becomes purulent. Discrete grayish necrotic lesions (1–5 mm in diameter) develop inside lower lip, gum, cheek, lower surface of tongue mucosa, and the dorsum of tongue, and these may become extensive and coalesce. Similar lesions are common on nasal, vulval, and vaginal mucosa. The necrosis on the tongue mucosa may slough off, leaving raw red areas with sharp edges. Vesicles are not found in rinderpest.

The temperature reaches a high level on the peak of viremia on the third or fifth day since onset of symptoms, and then drops as diarrhea starts. The onset of diarrhea is correlated with the intestinal lesions in the mucosal phase. The animal arches its back, and severe tenesmus and grinding of teeth are noticed. As the abdominal pain increases, restlessness becomes more pronounced. The shooting diarrhea converts into fetid dysentery. Abortion may occur in pregnant animals, discharging infective viruses in the fetal and vaginal secretions for up to twenty-four hours.

The skin at certain parts of body becomes hyperemic, and vesicles may develop, which subsequently cause thickening of skin and scab formation. The animal loses condition and become dehydrated, emaciated, and exhausted. In the terminal stage, there is prostration and subnormal temperature, and death occurs within six to twelve days.

A few animals recover and pass on to a convalescent phase during which mucosal lesions heal rapidly, and diarrhea stops. Body condition recovers after several weeks. Subacute and skin form occur with lower morbidity and mortality. The inflammation of mucosa is catarrhal, and there is no dysentery. In the skin form, there is no systemic involvement. Small pustules develop on the neck, over the withers, inside the thigh, and on the scrotum. Pigs with fatal cases of RP develops fever, nasal and lacrimal discharge, congestion of nasal mucosa, and acute gastroenteritis followed by death in a day or two.

IMMUNE RESPONSE

Immunity after recovery from disease or by vaccination is long and durable. The protection is provided by secretory immunoglobulins. IgM and IgG appear in that order. Local immunoglobulin IgA is also playing an important role in the control of the severity of the clinical symptoms. As the virus causes severe leucopenia and lymphopenia, there is immunosuppression, and so secondary disease flare up is also common, which is an important factor for high mortality.

DIAGNOSIS

RP is diagnosed from the clinical signs and by various serological tests for the demonstration of viral antigen and antibody. Lymph nodes, tonsils, alimentary tract, fresh spleen, and blood are the best clinical materials for the antigen detection, whereas the serum is collected for the antibody assessment.

RP antigen can also be detected by counterimmunoelectrophoresis (CIEP) in the lymph node and spleen of affected animals shortly after death (Chandran et al., 1991; Chandran et al., 1993). Das and Sarkar (1993) had employed ELISA, reverse passive hemagglutination, CIEP, and fluorescent antibody test (FAT) for the demonstration of RP antigen in the clinical materials.

Chauhan et al. (1993) reported that serum samples from convalescent and in-contact buffaloes were positive for RP antibodies in gel precipitation and CIEP tests. Reddy and Giridhar (1992) observed avidin-biotin ELISA and SNT could detect RP antibodies in the sera of vaccinated cattle, whereas none of the samples were positive by either AGPT or CIEP. Ramdass et al. (1993) demonstrated the use of dip-stick ELISA for the demonstration of RP antibodies. Renukaradhya et al. (2003) developed competitive-ELISA for the demonstration of antibodies to RP virus.

Pandey et al. (1992) had developed a modified hybridization technique for the detection of RP virus using biotinylated DNA probes prepared from clones D-74 (RPVC N gene).

A reverse transcription–PCR (RT-PCR) test was extensively used by Forsyth and Barret (1995) for the diagnosis of rinderpest. A rapid chromatographic strip test for the pen-side diagnosis of RP virus from the lacrimal fluid was developed by Bruning et al. (1999) using the clear view TM chromatographic strip test technology.

TREATMENT

There is no specific therapy for RP. Broad-spectrum antibiotic therapy to prevent secondary bacterial complications and supportive fluid and vitamins therapy to avoid dehydration are adopted as part of symptomatic treatment. But in areas where the eradication program is going on, therapy is not indicated. The affected and all in-contact animals are slaughtered and disposed of properly, followed by disinfection of the area.

PREVENTION AND CONTROL

Control measures include slaughter of infected and in-contact animals, strict quarantine, and countrywide vaccination of cattle, calves, and buffaloes (WHO, 1989).

Rinderpest can be easily controlled by slaughter of infected animals and rigid quarantine of in-contact animals. Introduction of new animals from diseased areas only after quarantine and, if seronegative, vaccination three weeks before mixing with the existing stock are advised. An immune belt has to be built along the border with endemic areas. All livestock and livestock product movement should be banned during outbreaks. All susceptible and in-contact animals must be slaughtered and properly disposed of or burned. Infected premises should be cleaned and disinfected. Rinderpest is amenable to eradication provided there is a professional determination and firm will to carry it out. In 1998, India declared herself provisionally free from rinderpest disease for the entire country. But the rules and regulations of World Trade Organization (WTO) require that the country should be free from RP outbreak for more than ten years before declaring it free from rinderpest. Hence, international declaration of freedom from RP has been done following three stages of disease surveillance for freedom from RP. The first stage of provisional freedom from RP for entire India was declared on March 1, 1998.

The second stage of freedom from RP disease for various zones was approved by OIE (Office of International Epi. Des Zootes) on May 27, 2004. The third final stage was approved by OIE in 2006, and the final certificate from OIE was awarded to the joint secretary and animal disease commissioner, Govt. of India, in the Seventy-fourth Annual General Session of OIE, Paris, held in May 2006.

Pan African Rinderpest Campaign (PARC), South Asia Rinderpest Eradication Campaign (SAREC), West Asia Rinderpest Eradication Campaign (WAREC), and NPRE are some of the important projects launched to eradicate RP in various countries. The Joint Project 15 (JP15) for the control of rinderpest in Nigeria was implemented by the Epidemiology Unit of Federal Livestock Department (FLD), Kaduna, and conducted RP vaccinations using the TCRP virus vaccine manufactured by National Veterinary Research Institute Vom, Nigeria. The TCRP vaccine was also imported from India to increase the coverage of livestock vaccinated. Under the supervision of Epidemiology Unit, Fulani cattle owners were educated to get their cooperation by sending publicity film units and vaccination teams to each village (Mathew, 1983).

Mathur (1995) opined that the maintenance of freedom from rinderpest in the Middle East will depend on the freedom from the disease in South Asia and Africa. Nearly seventeen thousand animals died due to RP in 1985 in Iraq, and the disease was controlled by culling, vaccination, and movement restrictions. Eighty to ninety percent of the bovine population in Iraq was vaccinated in 1990 and 1991 (Anbari and Jassim, 1992).

In Turkey, RP outbreak was reported in1992, killing 2,700 cattle and the outbreak was controlled by slaughtering 12,000 and vaccinating 12 million animals (Sahal, 1992). The Joint FAO/IAEA (International Atomic Energy

Agency) started sero-monitoring of RP as part of PARC (Pan African Rinderpest Campaign) using ELISA-based system.

"The goal of complete freedom from rinderpest from the world is within our grasp, and this would mark only the second example of a disease to be eradicated worldwide, after smallpox" (Internet: Global Eradication of Rinderpest Animal Production and Health (APH) Joint FAO/ IAEA. 2009).

VACCINATION

RP can be prevented by immunization. Effective live tissue culture vaccine is being used, which provides long and durable immunity for three years. An effective vaccinia virus recombinant vaccine for RP is developed that protects cattle against challenge by more than one thousand times the lethal dose of the virus, which can be easily propagated and administered by scarification. This vaccine is thermostable and does not require any cold chain, which is a distinct advantage in the hot arid regions of Africa and Asia (Yilma, 1989; Yamanouchi et al., 1993). Romero et al. (1994) and Ngichabe et al. (2002) protected cattle against RP and lumpy skin disease by vaccination with a recombinant capripox containing F gene of RP virus. The minimum protective immunizing dose for RP and LSD were 5.5×10 pfu and $1.5 \times 10 3$ pfu respectively. Verardi et al. (2002) had constructed a recombinant vaccinia virus vaccine that expresses both fusion (F) hemagglutinin and (H) gene of RP virus. It was observed that calves born from vaccinated dam and fed colostrum were protected for 105 days against RP by maternal antibodies. Therefore, the first vaccination to these calves could be done by 3–3.5 months (Erturk and Burgu, 2002). Sinnathamby et al. (2001) had constructed a recombinant RP virus vaccine expressed in baculovirus.

REFERENCES

1. Anbari, A. and Jassim, F. A. 1992. Country report rinderpest eradication, 1991. Republic of Iraq. *Operation Rinderpest* 1992,10–11:13–15.

2. Bruning, A., Bellamy, K., Talbot, D. and Anderson, J. 1999. A rapid chromatographic strip test for the pen side diagnosis of rinderpest virus. *J. Virological Methods* 81:143–154.

3. Chandran, N. D. J., Albert, A., Jayaprakash, R. and Venketesan, R. A. 1991. Occurrence of rinderpest in small wild ruminants. *Indian J. Anim. Sci.* 61:1176–1177.

4. Chandran, N. D. J., Albert, A. and Venketesan, R. A. 1993. A rapid method for diagnosing RP in live animals. *Indian J. Comp. Microbiol. Immunol.* 14:36.

5. Chauhan, R. S., Mahajan, N. K. and Kaushik, R. K. 1993. Emergence of rinderpest epidemics in buffaloes in Haryana (India). *Indian. Vet. J.* 70:695–698.

6. Das, A. K. and Sarkar, P. 1993. Comparative efficiency of ELISA and FAT for the detection of RP antigen in clinical materials from experimentally infected calves. *Indian J. Anim. Sci.* 63:5485–487.

7. Das, A. K. and Sardar, P. 1993. Detection of RP antigen in clinical materials of experimentally infected calves using CIE and Reverse Passive Haemagglutination (RPHA) test. *Indian Vet. J.* 70:889–892.

8. Dutta, J., Rathore, B. S. and Mallick, S. G. 1991. Status of rinderpest in India—an epidemiological study. *Indian Vet. J.* 68:99–103.

9. Erturk, A. and Burgu, I. 2002. The determination of the first vaccination time and the control of the maternal antibodies using competitive ELISA of the calves born from mothers that have been vaccinated against rinderpest disease. *Etlik-Veteriner–Mikrobiyoloji-Dergisi.* 13:1–14.

10. Forsyth, M. A. and Barrett, T. 1995. Evaluation of PCR for detection and characterization of RP and PPR viruses for epidemiological studies. *Virus Research* 39:151–163.

11. FAO/ IAEA. 2009. Global Eradication of Rinderpest Animal Production and Health (APH) Internet. 2009. Internet. 2005. http://www-naweb.iaea.org/nafa/stories/2005-rinderpest-eradication.html (accessed Feb. 2009).

12. Mathew, Z. 1983. Personal Communication.

13. Mathew, T., Adeola, C. O. and Olukun, S. B. 1984. Clinico epidemiological and laboratory studies of rinderpest malady during 1983 epidemic in Nigeria. Poster presentation, 6th International Congress of Virology Japan.

14. Mathew, T., Mathew, Z., Adeola, C. O., and Olukun, S. B. 1989. Rinderpest outbreak in Nigeria. *Indian J. Virol.* 5:30.

15. Mathur, S. C. 1993. Rinderpest: Surveillance and control in the Middle East. *Operation Rinderpest, 1993* 14–15:1–10.

16. Ngichabe, C. K., Wamwayi, H. M., Ndungu, E. K., Mirangi, P. K., Bostock, C. J., Black, D. N. and Barrett, T. 2002. Long-term immunity in African cattle vaccinated with recombinant capripox rinderpest virus vaccine. *Epidemiol. Infection* 128:343–349.

17. OIE. 2006. 74th Annual General Session of OIE, Paris, May 2006.

18. Pandey, K. D., Baron, M. D. and Barrett, T. 1992. Differential diagnosis of RP and PPR using biotynylated cDNA probes. *Vet. Rec.* 131:199–200.

19. Plowright, W. 1968. Rinderpest virus. In *Monographs in virology*, ed. J. Parker and R. Pstape, 3:25–110. Vienna and New York: Springer-Verlag.

20. Rai, M. K. 1991. Rinderpest in Bhutan. An appraisal of the current status. *Bhutan J. Anim. Hus.* 12:19–22.

21. Ramdass, P., Meerarani, S. and Padmanabhan, V. D. 1993. Dipstick enzyme immunoassay for RP antibody in cattle. *Vet. Micbiol.* 36:385–388.

22. Rautmare, S. S., Kamatii, G. R., Kulkarni, S. G., Kulkarni, S. V. and Pathak, S. V. 1992. Occurrence of mixed infection of rinderpest and foot and mouth disease at an organized farm. *Indian J. Anim. Sci.* 62:1137–1138.

23. Reddy, G. K. and Giridhar, P. 1992. A comparative evaluation of A-B ELISA, SNT, AGPT and CIE for the detection of RP antibodies in cattle sera. *Indian J. Anim. Health* 31:35–38.

24. Renukaradhya, G. J., Suresh, K. B., Rajasekhar, M. and Shaila, M. S. 2003. Competetive enzyme linked immunosorbent assay based on monoclonal antibody and recombinant hemagglutinin for sero-surveillance of rinderpest virus. *J. Clin. Microbiol.* 41:943–947.

25. Romero, C. H., Barrett, K., Itching, R. P., Carn, V. M. and Black, D. N. 1994. Protection of cattle against RP and lumpy skin disease with a recombinant capripox virus expressing the fusion protein gene of RP virus. *Vet. Rec.* 135:152–154.

26. Sahal, M. 1992. Brief report on rinderpest in Turkey in 1991/92. *Deutsch-Tierarztliche-Wochenschrift. 1992* 99:349–350.

27. Scott, G. R. 1981. Rinderpest and peste des petits ruminants. In *Virus diseases of food animals. A world geography of epidemiology and control. Disease Monographs*, vol. 2, ed. E. P. J. Gibbs, 401–32. New York: Academic Press.

28. Sinnathamby, G., Sangeetha, N., Renukaradhaya, G. J., Rajasekhar, M., Nayak, R., Shaila, M. S. and Naik, S. 2001. Recombinant hemagglutinin protein of rinderpest virus expressed in insect cells induces humoral and cell mediated immune responses in cattle. *Vaccine* 19:28–29.

29. Verardi, P. H., Aziz, F. H., Ahmad, S., Jones, L. A., Beyene, B., Ngotho, R. N., Wamwayi, H. M., Yesus, M. G., Egziabher, B. G. and Yilma, T. D. 2002. Long-term sterilizing immunity to rinderpest in cattle vaccinated with a recombinant vaccinia virus expressing high levels of the fusion and haemagglutinin glycoproteins. *J. Virology* 76:484–491.

30. Yamanouchi, K., Inui, K., Sugimoto, M., Asano, K., Nishinaki, F., Kitching, R. P., Takamatsu, H. and Barrett, T. 1993. Immunization of cattle with a recombinant vaccinia vaccine expressing the haemagglutinin gene of RP virus. *Vet. Rec.* 132:152–156.

31. Yilma, T. D. 1989. Prospects for the total eradication of rinderpest. *Vaccine* 7:484–485.

32. WHO. 1989. New outbreaks of rinderpest in Islamic Republic of Iran and their control. *WHO Report, 1989*, 5 (pt. 1): 317–318.

16. Vesicular Stomatitis
(Pseudo–Foot-and Mouth Disease, Sporadic Apthae, Mouth Rash)

M. R. Saseendranath, and M. Krishnan Nair

Introduction
Vesicular stomatitis (VS) is a viral disease of cattle, horse, and swine characterized by vesicular lesions on the tongue, oral mucosa, teats, and coronary bands.

Apart from its economic impact, VS is significant because its outward signs are similar to those of foot-and-mouth disease. The only way to diagnose and differentiate these diseases is by laboratory tests.

Etiology
The viral etiology of VS was first confirmed in 1926 by Cotton. The causative agent, vesicular stomatitis virus (VSV), is a member of genus *Vesiculovirus* in the family Rhabdoviridae. It is a large bullet-shaped RNA virus measuring 150nm × 180nm ×50nm. Two strains of VSV are New Jersey and Indiana. The three subtypes of Indiana found in South America are cocal, Alagoas, and Piry.

The genome of the virus is a single molecule of negative-sense RNA that encodes five major proteins: glycoprotein (G), matrix protein (M), nucleoprotein (N), large protein (L), and phosphoprotein (P). The G protein enables viral entry into the cell by mediating both virus attachment to host cell and fusion of the viral envelop with the endosomal membrane following endocytosis.

The viral envelop is covered by short spikes of about 10 nm long. The virus agglutinates goose RBC at 0–4°C. The virus is inactivated at 56°C in thirty minutes. VSV is susceptible to various disinfectants including 1% sodium hypochlorite, 70% ethanol, 2% gluteraldehyde, 2% iodophore, 4% sodium carbonate, 2% sodium hydroxide, 2% formaldehyde and is sensitive to ether and other lipid solvents. VSV is stable between pH 4–10.

Epidemiology

Distribution
Vesicular stomatitis (VS) was first described in Africa in 1884 and in France in 1915. VS is more common in the United States. The most recent outbreak

of vesicular stomatitis occurred in the Southwestern United States in 1995. Morbidity rate may vary from 5–90%, and the rate of mortality is usually low.

VS is endemic in some of the warmer regions of North, Central, and South America, including parts of United States (Rodriguez et al., 1990). Outbreaks also occur in the more temperate regions of the Western Hemisphere. The disease is more common during rainy season but occasionally occurs during dry season also.

SOURCE OF INFECTION
Infected animals are the main source of infection. Saliva, exudates, and tissues from open vesicles are the common source of infection.

TRANSMISSION
VSV is transmitted by insect vectors, especially sand flies and blackflies. Transovarian transmission has been demonstrated in both sand flies (Nunamaker et al., 2001) and blackflies. Black flies (*Simulium vittatum*) (Mare et al., 1991; Mead et al., 2004) transmit the infection biologically, whereas *Culicoides* sp. (Nunamaker et al., 2001) and flies and eye gnats transmit by mechanical means. VSV has also been isolated from mosquitoes. Ingestion of infected grasshoppers is also likely to transmit the infection. Once VSV is introduced into a herd, it can spread rapidly within the herd through direct contact between animals, through feed, insects, inanimate objects that can harbor the virus (fomites), feeding equipment, and bedding. Humans are infected by contact with vesicular fluid or saliva from infected animals. Aerosol transmission occurs in laboratories. Insect vectors, mechanical transmission, and movement of animals are responsible for the spread of the infection from one area to another.

HOSTS
Members of the Equidae, Bovidae, and Suidae are the domestic hosts. Horses, donkeys, mules, cattle, swine, camels, and humans are the common susceptible hosts. Calves are more resistant than the adult.

Feral pigs are acting as reservoir and amplifier hosts. Sheep and goats are relatively resistant and rarely show clinical signs. Most cases occur in adult and young cattle and horses under a year of age. Many species of wild animals, including white-tailed deer (Fletcher et al., 1991), bobcats, raccoons, and monkeys, are also susceptible. People who handle infected animals also can become infected with VS. Laboratory animals like guinea pig, mice, ferrets, hamsters, and chinchillas are susceptible to this infection. Chicken embryo is commonly used for the isolation of this virus.

PATHOGENESIS

The VSV, after entering the body, localizes in the regional lymphnodes and multiplies leading to viremia. The virus localizes to the mucous membrane of the oral mucosa, the skin around the mouth, on the teat, and udder and coronets. Viral antigens localized in keratinocytes at coronary band suggesting these cells as one of the primary sites of viral replication (Scherer et al., 2007). Subsequently, there is vesicular development and ulcerations.

Postmortem lesions include vesicles, ulcers, erosions and crusting on the lips, nostrils, hooves or teats, and in the mouth. Heart and rumen lesions as in foot-and-mouth disease are not seen in VS.

CLINICAL SIGNS

The incubation period for VS ranges from two to eight days. Symptomatology is more or less similar to that of foot-and-mouth disease. Excessive salivation and frothing at mouth is often the first symptom. Fever can occur immediately before or at the same time lesions first appear but is of short duration and thus is rarely detected. Examination reveals the characteristic lesions like blanched, raised vesicles (blisters) on the lips, dental pad, hard palate, muzzles, tongue, nostrils, hooves, teats, and in the mouth (Kim et al., 2000). The vesicles vary in size while some are as small as a pea; others cover the entire surface of the tongue. Eventually, the vesicles swell and break resulting in painful ulcers and erosions, which can cause anorexia and refusal to drink. Foot lesions cause lameness in less than 5% of infected cattle. Cows with painful teat lesions may refuse to permit milking and resulting in reduction in yield, often leading to mastitis. Infected animals usually experience severe weight loss.

The number of infected cattle in a herd varies. Five to ten percent of animals within an infected herd may show clinical signs, and up to eighty percent of the animals in a herd may become infected. If there are no complications, such as secondary infections, infected animals recover in about two weeks. However, the ulcers may take up to two months to heal, and healing animals may still spread the disease.

IMMUNE RESPONSE

Immunity after an attack is transient and never lasts for more than six months.

DIAGNOSIS

Clinical findings are the important indications for diagnosis. However, laboratory confirmation is needed as vesicular stomatitis cannot be reliably distinguished from other vesicular diseases including foot-and-mouth disease, vesicular exanthema, and swine vesicular disease. However, presence of symptoms in horses suggests vesicular stomatitis.

Materials to be collected for the identification of the agent include epithelial tissue covering, the vesicles, or vesicular fluid in buffered glycerol saline, whereas for the identification of the antibody, paired serum samples have to be collected one to two weeks apart. If epithelial tissue is not available, samples of esophageal/pharyngeal fluid can be collected from cattle.

IDENTIFICATION OF AGENTS
Virus isolation is done by inoculating embryonated chicken eggs or unweaned mice and tissue culture systems (chick fibroblasts, pig kidney, BHK-21, Vero); VSV can also be isolated after intracerebral inoculation of three-week-old mice, inoculation of footpad of guinea pigs, interdigital space of horses and cattle, and snout of pigs. Viral identification in cultures is by immunofluorescence, complement fixation test (CFT), and enzyme-linked immunosorbent assay (ELISA) (Alonsa et al., 1991; Enmin et al., 2001; Alyarado et al., 2002). In tissues, the viral identification can be done by ELISA, CFT, virus-neutralization test (VNT), and polymerase chain reaction assay (RT-PCR). Antibody assessment can also be done using various types of ELISA (Herhandez et al., 1992; Afshar et al., 1993a, 1993b).

DIFFERENTIAL DIAGNOSIS
VS closely resembles foot-and-mouth disease, foot rot, rinderpest, infectious bovine rhinotracheitis, bovine viral diarrhea, and malignant catarrhal fever. Vesicular diseases can be differentiated from VS by laboratory methods only. Animals do not suffer from foot lesions in rinderpest. The diarrhea is not manifested in any of the vesicular diseases, which is common in rinderpest, mucosal disease, bovine viral diarrhea, and malignant catarrhal fever. Infectious bovine rhinotracheitis is manifested by respiratory as well as by genital symptoms, which is not a sign in VS.

TREATMENT
There is no specific treatment. Antibiotics may be used to avoid secondary bacterial infection. Supportive therapy helps to heal the lesions inside oral cavity and on feet and teat.

PREVENTION AND CONTROL
Isolate infected animals and maintain them in an area physically away from other cattle as soon as signs appear. Minimize interpen movement of all animals.

Spray on the carcasses around the mouth, teats, and feet with disinfectant and treat them with insecticide. Avoid putting cattle into contact with other animals, such as dogs, cats, rodents, birds, and insects. The goal is to minimize or prevent the entrance of any potential biological or mechanical vector of VSV into the herd.

Clean and sanitize manger and water sources daily. Use different boots or disinfectant footbaths when moving between clean and infected areas. Phenolic, and halogen-based disinfectants are found to be the best. Sunlight and heat also destroy the virus quickly. Clean and sanitize feeding and cleaning equipment before using for healthy animals. All animal movements must be banned till thirty days after healing of all lesions in affected animals.

Cattle that are already infected with VS or that have been in contact with infected animals can introduce the disease into healthy beef herds. New cattle should be permitted only from sources that have not had animals with clinical signs of VS during the past three months. Isolate newly arrived cattle and calves from the rest of the herd for at least twenty-one days.

Farm vehicles that are used for transporting cattle to slaughter or that are driven to places where other cattle-hauling trucks congregate should be cleaned and disinfected. Drivers of these vehicles should change contaminated clothing.

Implement a vector-control program for animals.

VACCINATION

Inactivated and attenuated virus vaccines have been experimentally tested (House et al., 2003) but are not yet available commercially. Studies using DNA vaccine that expresses G gene of the vesicular stomatitis (New Jersey virus) shows encouraging results, which may be a useful tool in future to control this disease (Cantlon et al., 2000).

ERADICATION

People who handle an infected animal can contract vesicular stomatitis if they fail to follow proper biosafety methods. In humans, vesicular stomatitis causes an acute influenza-like illness with symptoms of fever, muscleache, headache, and malaise. Vesicular lesions are rare in humans. Prevalence in humans may be under reported because the disease often goes undetected or is misdiagnosed. People who handle potentially infected cattle should wear gloves to protect their hands and should not allow saliva and blister fluids to come in contact with open wounds or with their mucous membranes, such as the membranes in their eyes or mouth.

References

1. Afshar, A., Dulac, G. C., Wright, P. F. and Martin, D. 1993a. Application of indirect ELISA for detection of bovine antibody against vesicular stomatitis virus. *J. Vet. Diagnostic Investigation* 5:26–32.

2. Afshar, A., Shkarchi, N. H. and Dulac, G. C. 1993b. Development of a competitive ELISA for detection of bovine, porcine and equine antibody to VSV. *J. Clin. Microbiol.* 31:1860–1865.

3. Alonsa, A., Martin, M. A., Gomes, P. D., Allende, R. and Sondahl, M. S. 1991. Development and evaluations of an enzyme linked immunosorbent assay for detection—typing and subtyping of VSV. *J. Vet. Diagnostic Investigation* 3:287–292.

4. Alyarado, J. F., Dolz, G., Herrero, M. V., McCluskey, B. and Salman, M. 2002. Comparision of the serum neutralization test and competitive enzyme linked immunosorbent assay for the detection of antibodies to vesicular stomatitis and New Jersey virus. *J. Vet. Diagnostic Investigation* 14:290–292.

5. Cantlon, J. D., Gordy, P. W. and Bowen, R. A. 2000. Immune response in mice, cattle and horses to a DNA vaccine for vesicular stomatitis. *Vaccine* 18:2368–2374.

6. Enmin, Z., Riva, J. and Clavijo, A. 2001. Development of an immunoglobulin (IgM) capture enzyme linked immunosorbent assay for detection of equine and swine IgM antibodies to vesicular stomatitis virus. *Clinical diagnostic Lab. Immunol.* 8:475–481.

7. Fletcher, W. O., Stallknecht, D. E., Kearney, M. T. and Eernisse, K. A. 1991. Antibodies to vesicular stomatitis New Jersey type virus in white tailed deer in Ossoban Island, Georgia. *J. Wild Life Dis.* 27:675–680.

8. Herhandez, D. J., Salman, M. D., Webb, P. A., Keefa, T. J., Arevalo, A. A. and Mason, J. 1992. Evaluataion of an ELISA for detection of antibody to VSV in cattle in enzootic region of Mexico. *Am. J. Vet. Res.* 53:440–443.

9. House, J. A., House, C., Dubouget, P. and Lombard, M. 2003. Protective immunity in cattle vaccinated with a commercial scale, inactivated, bivalent vesicular stomatitis vaccine. *Vaccine* 21:1932–1937.

10. Kim, L. M., Morley, P. S., McCluskey, B. J., Mumford, E. L., Swenson, S. L. and Salman, M. D. 2000. Oral vesicular lesions in horses without evidence of vesicular stomatitis virus infecetion. *J. Am. Vet. Med. Assoc.* 216:1399–1404.

11. Mare, C., Cupp, E. V. and Cupp, M. M. 1991. Vesicular stomatitis virus (New Jersey) infection and replication in black flies (*Simulium vittatun*). *Proceedings-annual meeting of the United States Animal Health Association* 95:179–188.

12. Mead, D. G., Gray, E. W., Noblet, R., Murphy, M. D., Howerth, E. W. and Stallknecht, D. E. 2004. Biological transmission of vesicular stomatitis virus (New Jersey serotype) by *Simulium vittatum* (Diptera: Simulidae) to domestic swine. *J. Med. Entamology* 41:78–82.

13. Nunamaker, R. A., Perez de Leon, A. A., Campbell, C. L., and Lonning, S. M. 2001. Oral infection of *Culicoides sonorensis* (Diptera: Ceratopogonidae) by vesicular stomatitis virus. *J. Medical Entomology* 37:784–786.

14. Rodriguez, L. L. Vernon, S., Morales, A. I. and Letchworth, U. J. 1990. Serological monitoring of vesicular stomatitis New Jersey virus in enzootic regions of Costa Rica. *Am. J. Trop. Med. Hyg.* 42:272–281.

15. Scherer, C. F. C., O'Donneli, V., Golde, W. T., Gregg, D., Estes, D. M. and Rodriguez, L. L. 2007. Vesicular stomatitis New Jersey virus (VSNJV) infects keratinocytes and is restricted to lesion sites and local lymph nodes in the bovines a natural host. *Vet. Res.* 38:75–390.

SECTION C

LIST OF SWINE TROPICAL VIRAL DISEASES

1. African Swine Fever

D. Nandi, and S. Nandi

Introduction

African swine fever (ASF) is an acute to chronic febrile viral disease of swine characterized by pyrexia, hyperemia of the skin, abortions, edema, and hemorrhages in internal organs particularly in lymph nodes. Pigs are the only mammal naturally susceptible to the disease in which acute hemorrhagic disease is produced with high mortality and morbidity (Penrith et al., 2004). In Africa, warthogs (*Phacochoerus aethiopicus* and *P. africanus*) and to a lesser extent bush pigs (*Potamochoerus porcus*) serve as reservoirs of the virus. *Ornithodoros* ticks also serve as vector cum reservoir of the virus (Radostits et al., 2007). ASF is an economically significant disease of domestic pigs in the Southern African subregion, where outbreaks regularly occur (Boshoff et al., 2007).

Etiology

Causative virus

ASF virus (ASFV) is a double-stranded DNA (dsDNA) containing enveloped virus with icosahedral symmetry. The virus shares structural features with both Poxviridae and Iridoviridae family viruses, and thus it has been earlier classified under both of them. Subsequently, it has been removed from both the families. Recently, it is the sole member of the newly created family Asfaviridae (African swine fever and related viruses) within the genus *Asfavirus* (Fauquet and Mayo, 2001). ASF is placed in list A of diseases by Office International des Epizooties due to virulence, economic significance, and importance in international security and trade (OIE, 2004). ASFV is the only known DNA containing arbovirus (arthropod borne) (Poterfield, 1975; Kleiboeker and Scoles, 2001). ASF virion has an average diameter of 200–220 nm and is comprised of five concentric layers of varying electron densities. They comprise of a central electron dense nucleoprotein core consisting of a DNA containing nucleoid, which is surrounded by a thick protein coat (Carrascosa et al., 1984; Andres et al., 1997). Within the envelope, there is an icosahedral capsid containing 1,892 to 2,172 capsomers, each 13 nm in diameter resembling hexagonal prism with a central hole (Carrascosa et al., 1984). The capsid in turn encloses a second lipoprotein membrane that surrounds the DNA containing core. The genome is a single molecule of dsDNA, 95–105 kbp in size and has covalently closed ends and terminal repetitions. Sequence analysis of the most variable fragment, within the B602L gene, from eighty-one different isolates from different countries has distinguished thirty-one subgroups of virus isolates, which varied in sequence and number of a tandem repeat encoding four amino acids (Nix et al., 2006). This provided information about strains of viruses circulating in different countries and can be used in future to study the molecular epidemiology and evolution of virus isolates and to trace the sources of disease outbreaks (Nix et al., 2006).

PHYSICAL AND SEROLOGICAL PROPERTIES OF THE VIRUS

ASF virus has remarkable pH stability and remains viable for two hours in a pH range of 1.9–13.4, but it is inactivated in twenty minutes at 60°C and by most lipid solvents (Coggins, 1966). All the secretions, excretions, blood, tissue fluids, and internal organs are rich sources of the virus. The virus is exceptionally stable and can survive in the blood stored in cold dark room for six years. ASF virus has been recovered from processed hams after five months and from bone marrow after six months of storage. Infected premises have been found to remain infective for pigs even three months after depopulation (Sanchez Botiza, 1961).

Serotypes of ASF virus have not yet been recognized and differences in antigenicity, and hemadsorption patterns among different ASF virus isolates have been reported (Penrith et al., 2004). It has been reported that the most pathogenic strains exist in nature in Africa where soft ticks, warthogs, and domestic pigs coexist in the same ecologic environment. In Spain and Portugal, where wild hogs are not a factor and ticks serve as a vector and reservoir of ASF virus, the virus strains are less virulent. Generally, when ASF enters a new country or area, disease is acute in nature with high morbidity and mortality, but after several months of circulation, it becomes less virulent and mild in nature with low mortality and morbidity (Penrith et al., 2004). The survivors are likely to act as carriers and shed the virus into the environment.

HOST RANGE

Domestic and wild pigs are the only animals naturally susceptible to the disease (Chakrabarti, 2007). They may harbor the virus without showing any symptoms and thereby act as carriers for prolonged periods (Mare, 1976). Warthogs serve as a better source of ASFV for *Ornithodoros* ticks than for domestic swine as contact with the latter is less likely. Domestic swine of all breeds and ages appear to be fully susceptible. Cattle, sheep, goat, horse, mouse, guinea pigs, and rabbit are not susceptible to the disease.

TISSUE CULTURE

ASFV replicates in the cytoplasm of histiocytes, reticuloendothelial (RE) cells, and lymphocytes of infected pigs (Petisca and Goncalves, 1977) and certain *Ornithodoros* ticks (Greig, 1972). Swine leukocytes and bone marrow cell cultures are used for primary isolation of the virus (Malmquist and Hay, 1960). After adaptation, the virus can be grown in PK-15, MVPK, BHK-21, Vero, and MS cells (Malmquist, 1962).

EPIZOOTIOLOGY

HISTORY AND PREVALENCE

Montgomery (1921) first reported ASF from East Africa, which showed close resemblance to classical swine fever (CSF) in its clinical manifestation. Studies conducted during early 1900s revealed that the causative virus produce higher mortality in domestic pigs, and the disease differed epidemiologically and immunopathologically from CSF (Montgomery, 1921). Unlike CSF, neutralizing antibody was not produced in the recovered pigs, and antisera to CSF failed to protect pigs from the disease. Steyn (1928) reported ASF from South Africa. In 1957, ASF spread to Portugal (Ribeiro et al., 1958), in 1960 to Spain, in 1971 to Cuba, and subsequently to Brazil, Malta, Dominican Republic, Haiti, and Sardinia. In 1982, ASF entered Cameroon in West Africa. In Malta, the disease caused death or slaughter of eighty thousand pigs within twelve months of diagnosis, which is rare example where a country opted for extermination of a species for ensuring particular disease freeness. Outside Europe, Cuba was first infected in 1971, and the disease was only eradicated after the loss of forty thousand pigs. The consistent difference between the manifestation of ASF in Africa and outside Africa was the occurrence of relatively less virulence and chronic disease in the latter. The degree to which the decline in pathogenicity in non-African outbreaks of ASF that may be attributed to the large-scale release of vaccine strains attenuated by passage in cell cultures in early 1960s is debatable (Hess, 1981). The disease attracted international attention and become a concern to pig raisers when it reached Portugal and created havoc by establishing in Iberian Peninsula. ASF was also reported from Angola and northern Mozambique due to contact of domestic pigs with free-ranging pigs, which acted as reservoir (Mendes, 1961, 1971). The arrival of the disease in Europe evoked considerable attention, and concerted research has been directed toward containing the infection with the use of a suitable vaccine. However, attempts made to vaccinate pigs with an attenuated vaccine in order to confer strong and durable immunity have largely remained unsuccessful. Rather, it produced a relatively less virulent form of the virus with resultant mild infection and high proportion of survivors (Penrith et al., 2004). ASF has never been reported on the North American continent, Asia, or Australia.

Two distinct epizootiological patterns, namely, (1) a sylvatic cycle in warthogs in Africa and (2) an enzootic cycle in domestic swine are thought to exist. However, a maintenance cycle of the virus in domestic pig population independent of the agency of wild suids or ticks also persist.

SYLVATIC CYCLE

In Southern and Eastern Africa, ASFV is maintained in a sylvatic cycles causing asymptomatic infection in wild pigs (warthogs, *Phacochoerus aethiopicus*) and to a lesser extent in bush pigs (*Potamochoerus porcus*) and argasid ticks (soft ticks) belonging to the genus *Ornithodoros*. The ticks remain in burrows used by these wild hogs and act as a biological vector of the virus. After ingestion during feeding on viremic swine, the virus replicates in the midgut of the tick and infects its reproductive system (Kleiboeker et al., 1999). The transovarian and venereal transmission of the virus between the ticks has been reported. The virus is also transmitted between developmental stages of the ticks, i.e., transtadial transmission resulting in excretion of virus through tick saliva and coxal gland and Malpighian excrement. Infected ticks may live several years and transmit the disease at each feeding. After primary infection, young warthogs develop viremia but older warthogs are persistently infected and seldom exhibit viremia. Thus, the virus is maintained in a cyclical manner between young warthogs and ticks.

Domestic Cycle

Primary outbreaks of ASF in domestic swine in Africa occurred due to bite of infected ticks or ingestion of carcasses of acutely infected warthogs. Once infected, the domestic swine become the important source of virus for remaining susceptible swine population. In west-central Malawi, a cycle involving domestic pigs and *Ornithodoros* sp. ticks that live in pig houses (Kholas) has been described (Penrith et al., 2004).

TRANSMISSION

The disease is transmitted through contact with wild pigs (warthogs, *Phacochoerus* sp.) and bush pigs (*Potomochoerus* sp.), which act as reservoir of infection. The virus is abundantly present in all the secretions and excretions from nasopharynx, conjunctiva, and urogenital tract. ASF has been recovered from swine louse (*Haematopinus suis*) and soft ticks

(*Ornothodoros moubata*) in Africa and *O. erraticus* (now *O. macrocanus*) in Spain and Portugal (Sanchez Botiza, 1963). Transovarian and transtadial transmission of the virus in ticks has been reported in experimental study (Plowright et al., 1970; Ayoade and Adeyemi, 2003). The disease may be transmitted through indirect contact with infected pens and ingestion of uncooked contaminated garbage material. Semen from viremic boar also contains ASFV and may transmit the same during insemination (Guerin and Pozzi, 2005). *Ornithodoros sonrai*, a soft tick from Senegal, was also found to carry ASFV DNA and thus act as a vector cum reservoir of the virus (Vial et al., 2007). The infection is maintained in ticks for up to four months after last blood meal and is able to transmit the virus to pigs during feeding. Hard-shield ticks (*Rhipicephalus* spp.) are not infected with ASFV. Female ticks have higher infection rate than males and the later can transmit the virus to females during copulation, but the reverse direction of transmission from female to male is not reported. ASFV do not have any adverse effects on the survival of the ticks that suggest a mechanism of viral replication in ticks, which is compatible with host survival. The mechanical transmission of the virus by people and inanimate objects is also possible because of the stability of the virus in blood, feces, and tissue. The international spread of ASF virus has been linked to feeding of swine with food containing scraps of uncooked meat from infected swine as it happened in Portugal in 1957, Brazil in 1978, and Caribbean and Mediterranean Islands in 1978.

PATHOGENESIS AND IMMUNOPATHOLOGY

The incubation period of the disease is five to nine days in natural infection and two to five days in experimental infection in pigs. ASFV enters cell by receptor-mediated endocytosis (Valdeira and Geraldes, 1985). Two proteins p^{12} and p^{54} have been implicated in viral attachment and p^{30} in virus internalization (Gomez-Puertas et al., 1998). Viral and cell membrane cholesterol was found to have profound effects on ASFV infection in host cell, and thymidine kinase (TK) gene is required for efficient replication of the virus in swine macrophages and for virulence (Bernardes et al., 1998; Moore et al., 1998). On uncoating replication of the virus occurs primarily in the cytoplasm; however, an early nuclear replicative phase that precedes this is characterized by synthesis of small DNA fragments of 2000nt length (Garcia-Beato et al., 1992; Rojo et al., 1999). Replication of viral DNA reaches peak at eight hours postinfection, during which dimeric head-to-head concatameric forms of DNA are observed (Rojo et al., 1999). DNA replication regulates virus gene expression in the host cell and divides transcription and translation into an early and late phase. Approximately thirty-five early proteins and seventy-one late proteins appear during viral replications that undergo posttranslational modification like proteolytic cleavage, phophorylation, and myristylation. By around ten hours postinfection, virions are released from the infected cells by budding through plasmalemma or by rupturing the cell membrane (Penrith et al., 2004). Viral morphogenesis is colocalized with viral DNA replication and occurs in discrete cytoplasmic regions designated as "viral factories" located close to the nucleus (Rojo et al., 1999). This area is rich in fibrillar and membranous organelles and surrounded by enlarged Golgi apparatus, huge number of ribosomes, and mitochondria (Rojo et al., 1998).

The virus on entry usually invades the tonsils and lymph nodes of the gastrointestinal tract and respiratory tracts followed by dissemination throughout the body by a primary viremia in which virions are predominantly associated with red blood cells (RBCs) in 90% cases and to some extent with white blood cells (WBCs) (Wardley and Wilkinson, 1977). When the infection is through tonsil, large number of virus may be detected in mandibular lymph nodes (Greig, 1972). A generalized infection follows with titers up to 109 ID50/ml of blood or per gram of tissue. Consequently, all secretions and excretions contain infectious virus. Experimental studies have shown that ASF virus replicates in several cell types within the RE system and causes a severe leucopenia. ASFV shows a predilection for antigen presenting cells of macrophage-mononuclear system (Rodriguez et al., 1996). The virus attaches to the cell surface protein membrane receptors and in the viral factories within the cytoplasm (Gomez-Villamandos et al., 1997). Virus replication may also take place in other cell types like endothelial cells, pericytes, glomerular mesangial cells, renal collecting duct epithelial cells, hepatocytes, neutrophils, and megakariocytes (Gomez-Villamandos et al., 1995a, b, c). However, replication in these sites does not contribute significantly to the outcome of the disease. Although marked lymphopenia is a characteristic feature of ASF, replication rarely takes place within lymphocytes (Oura et al., 1998a). However, there is widespread destruction of T and B lymphocytes due to apoptosis (programmed cell death) precipitated by the release of cytokines such as tumor necrosis factor (TNK-) from infected macrophages (Ramiro-Ibanez et al., 1996; Oura et al., 1998b). An early increase in TNF- , IL-1 , IL-1 , and IL-6 expression were detected in lymphoid organs from ASF infected animals, together with an increase in the serum concentrations of TNF- and IL-1 . These changes were accompanied by increased apoptosis of lymphocytes and the presence of infected and uninfected macrophages showing changes indicative of secretory and phagocytic activation (Salguero et al., 2005). Interestingly, ASFV genome contains at least one conserved gene p21 that is reported to inhibit apoptosis of infected macrophages and sustains their survival, which, in turn, allows productive viral replication and persistence of the virus in cells (Revilla et al., 1997). This was proved by detection of viral DNA in macrophages by PCR technique for more than five hundred days postinfection. Virus recovery from the lymph nodes of pigs infected with ASF was achieved forty-five days after infection (Oura et al., 1998a).

Hemorrhage in multiple organs, which is a characteristic finding in this viral infection, may be caused due to severe thrombocytopenia or as a result of disturbed homeostasis subsequent to massive macrophage destruction and release of active molecules like enzymes, cytokines, complement factors, and arachidonic acid metabolites, including prostaglandin E_2 and prostacyclins (Rodriguez et al., 1996). There is also increased vascular permeability and disseminated intravascular coagulation; death is due to excessive fluid exudation in lungs with resultant respiratory failure (Villeda et al., 1993). Thrombocytopenia may also be due to immune mediated process involving antigen-antibody complex that causes platelet aggregation and consumption due to coagulopathy (Villeda et al., 1993). Pathological changes in liver are particularly due to release of inflammatory mediators like TNF- , thomboxane A_2 and decreased prostacyclins (Grau and Lou, 1993; Gomez-Villamandos et al., 1995c). Hemorrhages in kidney are due to phagocyte activation and endothelial destruction in renal interstitial capillaries accompanied by disseminated intravascular coagulation (Gomez-Villamandos et al., 1995b). Changes in lungs particularly alveolar edema are ascribed to activation of pulmonary macrophages with release of IL-1, TNF- , LTB4, and oxygen-free radicals (Carrasco et al., 1996; Carrasco et al., 2002). Apoptosis of lymphocytes in both spleen and lymph nodes is assumed to occur as a result of the release of cytokines from infected macrophages. In general, apoptosis of T cell occur prior to and to a greater extent than that of B cells, which are again earlier to that observed in spleen and lymph glands (Oura et al., 1998b). A close relation has been demonstrated between viral replication and number of mononuclear cells undergoing apoptosis (Oura et al., 1998b). Immune suppression in infected pigs may also be attributed to release of viral protein p^{36} by macrophages and resultant reduction in expression of class I and II major histocompatibility (MHC) antigens (Gonzalez-Juarrero et al., 1992; Childerstone et al., 1998). However, immune suppression in naturally infected pigs is not generally apparent due to rapid course of infection and quick death. The pigs that recover generally develop solid immunity to challenge with the same virus but not the heterologous virus. Repeated infection with one strain of the virus appears to broaden the spectrum of resistance to heterologous viruses (Plowright, 1986). Antibody to ASFV is effective in neutralizing the virus; however, in vitro extensively passaged virus loses phophatidylinositol residues from viral envelope and thereby becomes refractory to neutralization by homologous antibody (Gomez-Puertas et al., 1997). Viral proteins p^{73}, p^{54} and p^{30} are primarily thought to be associated with neutralization process (Gomez-Puertas et al., 1996). Except macrophages, though other lymphocytes do not support replication of ASFV inside cells, due to indirect effects of cytokines released by the former, these surviving cells (CD4+, CD8+ T cells, and B cells) show reduced proliferative response to in vitro stimuli with mitogens (Childerstone et al., 1998).

Current evidence suggests that ASFV modulate signaling pathways in infected macrophages, thus interfering with the expression of a large number of immunomodulatory genes like A238L, which inhibits both activation of the host NF kappa B transcription factor and inhibits calcineurin phosphatase activity (Dixon et al., 2004). Another ASFV-encoded protein CD2v, which resembles host CD2 protein, causes the adsorption of red blood cells around virus-infected cells and extracellular virus particles, thereby helps in virus dissemination in pig's body and has a role in impairing lymphocyte function (Dixon et al., 2004). Two ASFV proteins, an IAP and a Bcl2 homologue, inhibit apoptosis in infected cells and thus facilitate production of progeny virions. Half to two-thirds of the approximately 150 genes encoded by ASFV are not essential for replication in cells but have an important role for virus survival and transmission in its hosts. However, manipulation of these genes may provide means for discovery of novel immunomodulatory drugs (Dixon et al., 2004). Serum concentrations of C-reactive protein, serum amyloid A, and haptoglobin were found to increase in pigs inoculated with African swine fever virus (Sánchez-Cordón et al., 2007).

CLINICAL SIGNS

Generally ASF is manifested as acute or hyperacute disease in Africa; however, outbreaks recently documented from this country as well from other areas revealed a relatively less acute but rather chronic from of the disease (Penrith et al., 2004). Swine infected with ASF virus develop fever (105–108°F), which occurs five to fifteen days after exposure and persists for about four days. Other clinical signs observed one to two days after the onset of fever are inappetance, incoordination, huddling and disinclination to move, muscle tremor, convulsion, and recumbency. There is increasing congestion and cyanosis of the skin of tail, limbs, ears, snout, and abdomen that can be easily visualized on naked eyes (Radostits et al., 2007). Hyperemia and hemorrhages of the skin is usually marked over the snout, ears, under the belly, over the hindquarters, and around the fetlocks (Maurer, 1975; Carnero et al., 1977). Pregnant sows often abort at any stage of pregnancy. There is extreme weakness of the hindquarters and extreme difficulty in walking. Respiratory rates are increased as soon as body temperature rises, and after two to four days of fever, breathing becomes painful. Slight mucopurulent ocular and nasal discharges are often present, followed by a profuse, watery, or frothy, bloodstained nasal discharge (Chakrabarti, 2007). The pulse is extremely rapid; cough and accelerated respiration appear in one-third of cases. With some strains of virus, bloody diarrhea and vomiting may occur. Death usually occurs by the seventh day after onset of fever. In East and South Africa, mortality is often 100%, but in Spain and Portugal, where the disease occurs as subacute or chronic form, mortality is about 30%. In subacute from, disease lingers up to few weeks with development of intermittent fever, anorexia, loss of condition, cough, and pneumonia. Some animals may develop cardiac insufficiency due to extensive serofibrinous pericarditis and adhesions. Painful swelling of the joints of the limbs as a result of joint and tendon sheath effusions may also appear, with edema of periarticular tissues. The survivors are persistently infected and constitute a source of infection (Penrith et al., 2004).

PATHOLOGY

In general, lesions are in proportion to the amount of damage to the circulatory and reticuloendothelial system. In acute ASF due to highly virulent virus, marked lesions are observed, whereas in subclinical, mild, and in chronic form, minimal or no lesions are observed. The circulatory system is mostly severely affected as evidenced by congestion, edema, ascites, hydrothorax, hydropericardium, hemorrhage, infarctions, and necrosis in many visceral organs (Chakrabarti, 2007; Radostits et al., 2007). Like in hog cholera, there is around 40–50% fall in leukocyte count. The pericardial sac may become thickened and opaque. Petechial hemorrhages are present over all serous surfaces, lymph nodes under pericardium and endocardium. There is accumulation of excessive fluid in all the body cavities. The visceral lymph nodes are hemorrhagic and edematous, and the gastric, periorbial, and renal mesenteric lymph nodes are also affected and attain more than normal size

(Radostits et al., 2007). Severely hemorrhagic lymph nodes often look like hematoma.

The majority of the spleen from animals with ASF is grossly normal. Severe engorgement is commonly noted in African cases of ASF. When enlarged spleen is incised, the pulp appears deep purplish black and bulges from the cut surface. There is often a marked depletion of lymphocytes in lymphoid tissue and infiltrations of lymphocytes and macrophages in liver, brain, and other tissues. In acute ASF, total leukocyte count may be reduced or normal, but the differential counts reveal lymphopenia and neutrophilia with left shift (Gomez-Villamandos et al., 1997). The mucous and serous membranes of the respiratory system appear congested, and blood vessels are virtually engorged. Petechial and ecchymotic hemorrhages are often found on the pleural surfaces of the lungs. A straw color or blood-tinged fluid is present in the thoracic cavity. Scattered petechial and ecchymoses are also found on the serous surfaces and in the parenchyma of the lungs. When affected lungs are incised, the cut surface appears uniformly congested, and frothy fluid exudes from the cut air passages and alveoli. In chronic cases, circumscribed, caseous, or pneumonic areas are found in the lungs.

The liver is usually congested and slightly enlarged. Mottling with dark areas of congestion is the commonest abnormality. Engorgement of superficial blood vessels in the wall of the gall bladder is commonly seen. Petechiae and ecchymoses may be scattered over the serous mucosal surfaces. The gall bladder is usually distended with bile and blood. Kidneys are congested and often hemorrhagic. Usually petechiae are most numerous on the cortical surfaces and in the pelvis of kidneys. In some cases, kidneys appear as big hematomas as clotted blood appears to encircle the kidney. Some of the clotted blood may be outside the renal capsule and some between renal capsule and kidney. The renal hemorrhages are considered almost pathognomonic and are consistent feature following inoculation of pigs with virulent or moderately virulent virus (Radostits et al., 2007). The urinary bladder appears as normal in less virulent forms of ASF, but in more virulent forms petechiae may be found on the mucosa.

Congestion, edema, and hemorrhages are found in the gastrointestinal tract. The stomach is filled with ingesta. The gastritis may be marked with mucosal surface appearing red. Rarely free blood may be found in the stomach. Ulcers often covered with necrotic debris appear in the pyloric and fundic regions in about one-fourth of the cases. The petechial and ecchymotic hemorrhages are found on the mucosa of small and large intestines. The region of the ileocecal valve normally contains mucus-filled crypts and numerous lymphoid nodules. Mild reddening to severe hemorrhages with ulceration of the mucosa of cecum is found in 50% of the cases. Lesions similar to button ulcer of hog cholera are unusual and occur in the cecum or colon only. The ulcers are small, deep, and covered with necrotic debris. Inflammation of the colon occurs in 50% of the cases. In 10–20% of the cases, the colon contains large quantity of blood mixed with ingesta. These pigs have a bloody diarrhea before death. Congestion of the meninges is frequent but usually mild and small perivascular hemorrhages may be present. Generalized acute neuronal degeneration was observed in all parts of the brain. Sometimes neuronal degeneration is associated with neuronophagia and focal glial proliferation (Radostits et al., 2007). Histopathological lesions of acute ASF include fibrinoid vasculitis particularly in lymphoid organs and severe karyorrhexis of macrophages in lymphoid tissues (Radostits et al., 2007). In the spleen, the Schweiger-Seidel (SS) sheaths are often obliterated due to destruction of macrophages. Infiltration of monocyte, macrophages into periovascular spaces have been described in many organs, including tonsils, periocular tissues, splenic red pulp, lymph nodes, gastrointestinal tracts, liver, lung, brain, kidneys, and adrenal glands (Moulton and Coggins, 1968). The pericardium and epicardium may be thickened with granulation tissue covered by fibrinous exudates and infiltrated by mononuclear cells. Lung septa are thickened with discrete foci of high mineralization, necrosis, and fibrosis. Articular swellings are characterized by granulation tissue infiltrated by mononuclear cells (Moulton and Coggins, 1968). Cutaneous lesions, as observed by immunohistochemical and ultrastructural study, revealed vascular changes ranging from hyperemia, mild edema, scarce fibrin microthrombi, microhemorrhages, and secondary pustules and superficial folliculitis (Mozos et al., 2003).

DIAGNOSIS

The diagnosis can be made on the basis of clinical signs and pathological lesions. The clinical signs and necropsy lesions resemble hog cholera, salmonellosis, and other diseases. So laboratory confirmation is imperative to diagnose and differentiate ASF from most similar hog cholera.

DIFFERENTIAL DIAGNOSIS

The clinical features and gross lesions of ASF are similar to hog cholera. ASF should be suspected when the disease is cholera-like, highly contagious, 100% fatal, and gross lesions are similar to but more severe than those of hog cholera. The most significant gross lesions are cyanosis and hemorrhages of the lymph nodes, hemorrhages of the heart and kidneys, pulmonary interlobular edema, and congestion and edema of the gall bladder and found in animals only immunized to hog cholera. Inoculation of uninfected pigs with 10 ml of a 10% suspension of spleen, lymph nodes, or whole blood from suspected cases of ASF is one of the most sensitive and reliable methods available for detecting ASF virus. The test pigs can be given prophylactic doses of hog cholera antiserum simultaneously with the test inoculum. If the inoculum contains ASF virus, the inoculated pigs should be sick by five days postinoculation. Direct fluorescent antibody test (FAT) of spleen, lymph nodes, and blood collected during early febrile stage readily gives positive result. Bacterial septicemias as observed in cases of salmonellosis, erysipelas, or pasteurellosis are important differential diagnosis for acute ASF. However, high mortality across the age spectrum, failure to respond to antimicrobial agents, and failure to isolate bacterial pathogens will suggest possible ASF when CSF is ruled out. Neitz (1963) identified certain protozoal and rickettsial diseases of pigs for differentiation with ASF like *Babesia* sp., *Trypanosoma* sp., and *Eperythrozoon* spp., which produce overlapping clinical signs. Sudden death due to poisoning by coumarin rodenticides, mycotoxins should also be contemplated for differentiation with ASF.

CONFIRMATORY DIAGNOSIS

Hemadsorption test developed by Malmquist and Hay (1960), Tubiash (1963), and Coggins (1968) is a reliable and practical test for detection of ASF virus. But some low virulent strains of ASFV may not produce any hemadsorption and may require two to three serial passages in swine leukocyte cultures before hemadsorption test is conclusive (Pini and Waghaar, 1974; Mebus et al., 1978). The ability of ASF virus to produce hemadsorption in leukocyte cultures is still regarded as mostly reliable test. However, confirmatory diagnosis may be accomplished by means of modified direct complement fixation test (CFT) (Boulanger et al., 1967a), agar gel precipitation test (AGPT) (Coggins and Heuschele, 1966; Boulanger et al., 1967b), immunodiffusion test, radioimmnuoassay, radio immunoprecipitation and immunoblotting, dot immunobinding assay, immunofluorescence, or Giemsa stained cytoplasmic inclusion bodies in circulating leukocytes of infected pigs (Colgrove, 1968, 1969). The use of an enzyme-linked immunosorbent assay (ELISA) based on p^{30} and a Western blot based on p^{54} protein was found to be highly sensitive and specific (Oviedo et al., 1997). ASF antibodies are usually present in detectable amounts before fever subsides when the disease runs a protracted period. They continue to increase twenty-eight days postinfection and persist for life (Hess and Pan, 1977). The indirect FA test is most widely used for detecting antibodies to ASF virus. Immunoelectrophoresis, AGPT (Coggins and Heuschele, 1966), and radial immunodiffusion (RID) (Pan et al., 1974) are useful in screening serum samples. At present, ELISA test is the most useful method for large-scale ASF serological studies, although false positives have been detected, mainly on poorly preserved sera. Recently with some modifications in this technique, diagnosis of ASF virus has become more rapid and specific. Gallardo et al. (2006) used recombinant ASF virus polyprotein pp62 expressed in the baculovirus expression system as antigens in ASF serological tests and studied its suitability for use in a novel ELISA. Results indicated that the use of these recombinant proteins as antigens in the ELISAs improves the sensitivity and specificity of the test making pp62 protein as one of the most interesting viral proteins to be used for serological ASF diagnosis. Recombinant viral proteins p32 and p54 expressed in insect cells may be used for the detection of African swine fever virus-specific antibodies using Western blot analysis and indirect ELISA (Sakamoto et al., 2006). Similarly, recombinant protein p^{30} expressed in insect larvae has been exploited for serodiagnosis of ASFV (Barderas et al., 2000). Hutchings and Ferris (2006) used both polyclonal and monoclonal antibodies–based indirect sandwich ELISA for antigen detection of African swine fever virus where the former was found to be more sensitive.

Impression smears or cryosections of lymph nodes or spleen may be stained with fluorescein-isothicyanate-conjugated anti-ASF immunoglobulin and examined microscopically under ultraviolet light for characteristic granular immunofluorescence, using positive and negative controls for detection of viral antigen; however, doubtful cases may be confirmed by hemadsorption (Bech-Nielsen et al., 1990). Viral antigen and DNA can be detected in preserved and paraffin-embedded tissues by immunocytochemical methods and in situ hybridization (Oura et al., 1998c). Due to acute nature of the disease in most outbreaks, production of antibody do not occur; therefore, antibody-detection tests are of limited value. However, they are valuable for studying endemic ASF in pigs or for serosurveillance in certain African and other nations where the disease is believed to be persistent in order to support eradication and restocking operations (Wensvoort et al., 1988). Hernaez et al. (2006) visualized ASFV infection in living cells by incorporation into the virus particle of enhanced green fluorescent protein-p54 (EGFP) membrane protein chimera and analyzed virus progression along the infection cycle and infected cell death as time-lapse animations.

Recently polymerase chain reaction (PCR) has been contemplated as the method of choice for rapid, sensitive, and most specific detection of ASF. Molecular beacon assays are one type of real-time PCR technology capable of fast, specific, sensitive, and reliable detection of ASF virus (McKillen et al., 2007). Genomic DNA of ASFV has been detected by PCR from spleen, lymph node, liver, and lung tissues of a red river hog (*Potamochoerus porcus*) in Nigeria (Luther et al., 2007). A nested PCR assay, with an internal control system, was developed to detect DNA of ASFV in *Ornithodoros erraticus*, and the assay revealed a better analytical sensitivity than conventional PCR protocol (Basto et al., 2006). A fluorogenic probe hydrolysis (TaqMan) PCR assay for ASFV was developed and evaluated for application in preclinical diagnosis of the disease and surveillance and/or emergency management of an outbreak (Zsak et al., 2005). Aguero et al. (2004) developed and standardized a highly sensitive and specific gel-based multiplex RT-PCR assay for the simultaneous detection and differential diagnosis of ASF and CSF in clinical samples. A novel, highly sensitive, hot-start PCR method for rapid and specific detection of ASFV that can be used as a routine diagnostic test in surveillance, control, and eradication programs have been developed (Aguero et al., 2003). A plaque assay has been developed for African swine fever virus on swine macrophages, which can be used for virus titration and isolation/purification of recombinant viruses (Bustos et al., 2002). Cell culture, ELISA, and PCR are the most accurate and widely used methods for detection of virus from semen of infected boar (Guerin and Pozzi, 2005).

TREATMENT AND PREVENTION

No effective treatment is available. In an attempt ribavirin, an antiviral drug, has been tried in case of ASF infection and was found that a concentration 15 μg/ml that is not toxic for the host cells can inhibit ASFV infection (Valdeira, 2001) However, good husbandry and supportive therapy may enhance clinical recovery in some pigs depending on the virulence of the virus.

Control of ASF will entirely depend on preventing contact between domestic pigs and the sources of the virus. In the event of a confirmed outbreak, the entry of ASF virus must be prevented by preventing movement of infected pigs and their products and stamping out of all infected and in-contact pigs, with proper disposal of carcasses by burial or incineration. The infected premises should be disinfected, and it should remain empty for at least forty days as recommended by OIE (IAHC, 2001). It is generally advised that sentinel pigs (which are healthy, fully susceptible to infection, and seronegative) at the rate of 10% of stock (minimum 2 in number) must be allowed to roam freely in the disinfected premises after thirty days, with careful observation. If after six weeks they remain healthy and seronegative, the farm may be allowed for full stocking, perceiving that the area is virus free (Penrith et al., 2004). All inanimate objects should be properly disinfected using standard disinfectants. The practice of feeding garbage, which contain table scraps, and trimmings of pork carrying ASF virus must be discouraged. Cured pork and pork sausages are especially hazardous since the curing process is not likely to inactivate ASF virus. Proper disposal of garbage from international airport and seaports to prevent consumption by swine inhibit the international spread of ASF virus. Strict quarantine and slaughter should be adopted to prevent further spread of the disease. Serological surveillance should be conducted in all sows and boars in every herd. Hygiene and sanitation (overall biosecurity) should be improved. All livestock transaction must be brought to the knowledge and inspection by veterinary health professionals. Health certificate may be issued to every tested herd (Radostits et al., 2007). Usually control of ASF is complicated by ticks (tampans), which can thrive in the environment for years together in cracks and crevices. Due to wild life reservoir of the disease, lack of an effective vaccine, transmission of the virus through meat and meat products, persistent infection in survivors, and biological transmission by ticks, complete eradication is a difficult task to achieve. Stamping-out policy has some socioeconomic constraints, which is compounded by lack of political support with respect to emergency financing and paying of indemnities to swine raisers.

No effective vaccine is available till date. Numerous attempts to develop a useful vaccine against ASF have failed. Heat, Lugol's solution, formalin, toluol, crystal violet, BPL, AEI, and glyceraldehydes inactivation and attenuation of the virus in cell culture system have been tried with varied results (Walker, 1933; De Kock et al., 1940; Stone and Hess, 1967). Both recovered and animals vaccinated with attenuated virus vaccine following exposure to wild virus remain as carriers. As ASF is a notifiable disease, every outbreak should be brought to the knowledge of concerned authority for adopting early necessary action to contain further spread of the disease nationally and internationally (Bulletin of OIE, 2000).

Conclusion

ASFV is a double-stranded DNA virus, which shares structural features with both Poxviridae and Iridoviridae families. The disease has gained considerable attention due to its clinical similarity with CSF and difficulties in managing an outbreak. Control of ASF has been complicated due to presence of wildlife reservoir and role of ticks in disease transmission. Efforts should be made to minimize contact of domestic pigs with warthogs or biting by an infected tick along with strict imposition of farm biosecurity to prevent entry of the virus into a naive farm. A prompt confirmatory diagnosis after taking into consideration similar conditions will help adopt an early control measure. All international organizations should remain alert and instrumental in preventing spread of the disease to other countries from Africa, where it is originally present.

References

1. Aguero, M., Fernandez, J., Romero, L., Sanchez-Mascaraque, C., Arias, M. and Sanchez-Vizcaino, J. M. 2003. Highly sensitive PCR assay for routine diagnosis of African swine fever virus in clinical samples. *J. Clin. Microbiol.* 41:4431–4434.

2. Aguero, M., Fernandez, J., Romero, L. J., Zamora, M. J., Sanchez, C., Belak, S., Arias, M. and Sanchez-Vizcaino, J. M. 2004. A highly sensitive and specific gel-based multiplex RT-PCR assay for the simultaneous and differential diagnosis of African swine fever and classical swine fever in clinical samples. *Vet. Res.* 35:551–563.

3. Andres, G., Simon-Mateo, C. and Vinuela, E. 1997. Assembly of African swine fever virus: Role of polyprotein p2020. *J. Virol.* 71:2331–2341.

4. Ayoade, G. O. and Adeyemi, I. G. 2003. African swine fever: An overview. *Revue-d'-Elevage-et-de-Medecine-Veterinaire-des-Pays-Tropicaux.* 56:129–134.

5. Barderas, M. G., Wigdorovitz, A., Merelo, F., Beitia, F., Alonso, C., Borca, M. V. and Escribano, J. M. 2000. Serodiagnosis of African swine fever using the recombinant protein p30 expressed in insect larvae. *J. Virol. Methods* 89:129–136.

6. Basto, A. P., Portugal, R. S., Nix, R. J., Cartaxeiro, C., Boinas, F., Dixon, L. K., Leitao, A. and Martins, C. 2006. Development of a nested PCR and its internal control for the detection of African swine fever virus (ASFV) in Ornithodoros erraticus. *Archiv. Virol.* 151:819–826.

7. Bech-Nielsen, B., Arias, M. L., Panadero, J., Escribano, J. M., Gomez-Tejedor, C., Bonilla, Q. P. And Sanchez-Vizcaino, J. M. 1990. Laboratory diagnosis and disease occurrence in the current African swine fever eradication program in Spain. *Prev. Vet. Med.* 17:225–234.

8. Bernardes, C., Antonio, A., Pedroso-de-Lima, M. C. and Valdeira, M. L. 1998. Cholesterol affects African swine fever virus infection. *Biochimica-et-Biophysica-Acta,-Lipids-and-Lipid-Metabolism* 1393:19–25.

9. Boshoff, C. I., Bastos, A. D. S., Gerber, L. J. and Vosloo, W. 2007. Genetic characterisation of African swine fever viruses from outbreaks in southern Africa (1973–1999). *Vet. Microbiol.* 121:45–55.

10. Boulanger, P., Bannister, G. L., Gray, D. P., Ruckerbauer, G. M. and Willis, N. S. 1967a. African swine fever. II. Detection of the virus in swine tissues by means of the modified direct complement fixation test. *Can. J. Comp. Med. Vet. Sci.* 31:7–9.

11. Boulanger, P., Bannister, G. L., Gray, D. P., Ruckerbauer, G. M. and Willis, N. S. 1967b. African swine fever. III. The use of the agar double diffusion precipitation test for the detection of the virus in swine

tissue. Detection of the virus in swine tissues by means of the modified direct complement fixation test. *Can. J. Comp. Med. Vet. Sci.* 31:12–14.

12. Bulletin-Office-International-des-Epizooties. 2000. Notifiable diseases reported to the OIE. 112:673.

13. Bustos, M. J., Nogal, M. L., Revilla, Y. and Carrascosa, A. L. 2002. Plaque assay for African swine fever virus on swine macrophages. *Archiv. Virol.* 147:1453–1459.

14. Carnero, R., Costes, C. and Pichard, M. 1977. African swine fever: A contribution to the pathogenesis and immunology. Agric. Res. Semin. on hog cholera/classical swine fever and African swine fever, Hannover, Germany, 1976, EUR 5094, 591–601.

15. Carrasco, L., Chacon, M. L., Gomez, V. J. C. And Bautista, M. J. 1996. The pathogenic role of pulmonary intravascular macrophages in acute African swine fever. *Res. Vet. Sci.* 61:193–198.

16. Carrasco, L., Nunez, A., Salguero, F. J., Diaz-San-Segundo, F., Sanchez-Cordon, P., Gomez-Villamandos, J. C. and Sierra, M. A. 2002. African swine fever: Expression of interleukin 1—alpha and tumour necrosis factor—alpha by pulmonary intravascular macrophages. *J. Comp. Pathol.* 126:194–201.

17. Carrascosa, J. L., Carazo, J. M., Carrascosa, A. L., Garcia, N., Santisteban., A. and Vinuela, E. 1984. General morphology and capsid fine structire of African swine fever virus particles. *Virology* 132:160–172.

18. Chakrabarti, A. 2007. African swine fever. In *A textbook of preventive veterinary medicine*, 4th ed., 128–131. Ludhiana, India: Kalyani Publishers.

19. Childerstone, A., Talamatsu, H., Yang, H., Denver, M. and Parkhouse, R. M. E. 1998. Modulation of T cell and monocyte function in the spleen following infection of pigs with African swine fever virus. *Vet. Immunol. Immunopathol.* 52:281–295.

20. Coggins, G. S. 1968. Immunofluorescence and inclusion bodies in circulating leukocytes of pigs infected with African swine fever virus. *Bull. Epiz. Dis. Afr.* 16:341–343.

21. Coggins, L. 1966. Growth and certain stability characteristics of African swine fever virus. *Am. J. Vet. Res.* 27:1351.

22. Coggins, L., and Heuschele, W. P. 1966. Use of agar diffusion precipitation test in the diagnosis of African swine fever. *Am. J. Vet. Res.* 27:485–487.

23. Colgrove, G. S. 1968. Immunofluorescence and inclusion bodies in circulating leukocytes of pigs infected with African swine fever virus. *Bull. Epiz. Dis. Afr.* 16:341–343.

24. Colgrove, G. S. 1969. Diagnosis of African swine fever by fluorescent antibody staining of blood films and buffy coat smears. *Bull. Epiz. Dis. Afr.* 17:39–44.

25. De Kock, G., Robinson, E. M. and Keppel, J. J. G. 1940. Swine fever in South Africa. *Onderstepoort J. Vet. Sci.* 14:31–33.

26. Dixon, L. K., Abrams, C. C., Bowick, G., Goatley, L. C., Kay-Jackson, P. C., Chapman, D., Liverani, E., Nix, R., Silk, R. and Zhang-Fu, Q. 2004. African swine fever virus proteins involved in evading host defence systems. *Vet. Immunol. Immunopathol.* 100 (3/4): 117–134.

27. Fauquet, C. M. and Mayo, M. A. 2001. The 7th ICVT report. *Archiv. Virol.* 146:189–194.

28. Gallardo, C., Blanco, E., Rodriguez, J. M., Carrascosa, A. L. and Sanchez-Vizcaino, J. M. 2006. Antigenic properties and diagnostic potential of African swine fever virus protein pp62 expressed in insect cells. *J. Clin. Microbiol.* 44: 950–956.

29. Garcia-Beato, R., Salas, M., Vinuela, E. and Sala, J. 1992. Role of the host cell nucleus in the replication of African swine fever virus DNA. *Virology* 188:637–649.

30. Gomez-Puertas, P., Rodriguez, F., Oviedo, J. M., Ramiro-Ibanez, F., Ruiz, G. F., Alonso, C. and Escribano, J. M. 1996. Neutralizing antibody to different proteins of African swine fever inhibits both viral attachment and internalization. *J. Virol.* 70:5689–5694.

31. Gomez-Puertas, P., Oviedo, J. M., Rodriguez, F., Coll, J. and Escribano, J. M. 1997. Neutralization susceptibility of African swine fever virus is dependent on the phopholipid composition of viral particles. *Virology* 228:180–189.

32. Gomez-Puertas, P., Rodriguez, F., Oviedo, J. M., Brun, A., Alonso, C. and Escribano, J. M. 1998. The African swine fever virus proteins p54 and p30 are involved in two distinct steps of virus attachment and both contribute to the antibody-mediated protective immune response. *Virology* 243:451–471.

33. Gomez-Villamandos, J. C., Hervas, J., Mendez, A., Carrasco, L., Villeda, C. J., Wilkinson, P. J. and Sierra, M. A. 1995a. Ultrastructural study of the renal tubular system in acute experimental African swine fever: Virus replication in glomerular mesangial cells and in the collecting ducts. *Archiv. Virol.* 140:581–589.

34. Gomez-Villamandos, J. C., Hervas, J., Mendez, A., Carrasco, L., Villeda, C. J., Wilkinson, P. J. and Sierra, M. A. 1995b. Pathological in the renal interstitial capillaries of pigs inoculated with the two different strains of African swine fever virus. *J. Comp. Pathol.* 112:283–298.

35. Gomez-Villamandos, J. C., Hervas, J., Mendez, A., Carrasco, L., Villeda, C. J., Wilkinson, P. J. and Sierra, M. A. 1995c. A pathological study of the perisinucidal unit of the liver in acute African swine fever. *Res. Vet Sci.* 59:146–151.

36. Gomez-Villamandos, J. C., Bautista, M. J., Carrasco, L., Caballero, M. J., Hervas, J., Villeda, C. J., Wilkinson, P. J. and Sierra, M. A. 1997. African swine fever virus of bone marrow: Lesions and pathogenesis. *Vet. Pathol.* 34:97–107.

37. Gonzalez-Juarrero, M., Lunney, J. K., Sanchez, V. J. M. and Mebus, C. 1992. Modulation of splenic macrophages and swine leucocyte antigen (SLA) and viral antigen expression following African swine fever virus (ASFV) inoculation. *Archiv. Virol.* 123:145–156.

38. Grau, G. E. and Lou, J. 1993. TNF in vascular pathology: The importance of platelet-endothelium interactions. *Res. Immunol.* 144:355–363.

39. Greig, A. 1972. Pathogenesis of African swine fever in pigs naturally exposed to the disease. *J. Comp. Pathol.* 82:73–79.

40. Guerin, B. and Pozzi, N. 2005. Viruses in boar semen: Detection and clinical as well as epidemiological consequences regarding disease transmission by artificial insemination. *Theriogenology* 63:556–572.

41. Hernaez, B., Escribano, J. M. and Alonso, C. 2006. Visualization of the African swine fever virus infection in living cells by incorporation into the virus particle of green fluorescent protein-p54 membrane protein chimera. *Virology* 350:1–14.

42. Hess, W. R. and Pan, I. C. 1977. The immune response in African swine fever. Agric. Res. Semin. on hog cholera/classical swine fever and African swine fever. Hannover, Germany, EUR 5904, 602–611.

43. Hess, W. R. 1981. African swine fever: A reassessment. *Adv. Vet. Sci. Comp. Med.* 25:39–69.

44. Hutchings, G. H. and Ferris, N. P. 2006. Indirect sandwich ELISA for antigen detection of African swine fever virus: Comparison of polyclonal and monoclonal antibodies. *J. Virol. Methods* :213–217.

45. IAHC. 2001. *International Animal Health Code*—mammals, birds and bees, 10th ed., OIE, Paris.

46. Kleiboeker, S. B. and Scoles, G. A. 2001. Pathogenesis of African swine fever virus in *Ornithodoros* ticks. *Anim. Hlth. Res. Rev.* 2:121–128.

47. Kleiboeker, S. B., Scoles, G. A., Burrage, T. G. and Sur, J. H. 1999 African swine fever virus replication in the midgut epithelium is required for infection of *Ornithodoros* ticks. *J. Virol.* 73(10): 8587–8598.

48. Luther, N. J., Majiyagbe, K. A., Shamaki, D., Lombin, L. H., Antiagbong, J. F., Bitrus, Y. and Owolodun, O. 2007. Detection of African swine fever virus genomic DNA in a Nigerian red river hog (*Potamochoerus porcus*). *Vet. Rec.* 160:58–59.

49. Malmquist, W. A. 1962. Propagation, modification and haemadsorption of African swine fever in cell culture. *Am. J. Vet. Res.* 23:241.

50. Malmquist, W. A. and Hay, D. 1960. Haemadsorption and cytopathic effect produced by African swine fever virus in swine bone marrow and buffy coat cultures. *Am. J. Vet. Res.* 21:104–106.

51. Mare, C. J. 1976. The role of wild pigs in the epidemiology of African swine fever. In *Wildlife diseases*, 3rd ed., ed. L. A. Page, 227–234. New York.

52. Maurer, F. D. 1975. African swine fever. In *Diseases of swine*, 4th ed., ed. H. W. Dunne and A. D. Leman, 256–272. Ames: Iowa State Univ. Press.

53. McKillen, J., Hjertner, B., Millar, A., McNeilly, F., Belak, S., Adair, B. and Allan, G. 2007. Molecular beacon real-time PCR detection of swine viruses. *J. Virol. Methods* 140:155–165.

54. Mebus, C. A., Dardiri, A. H., Hamdy, F. M., Ferris, D. H., Hess, W. R. and Callis, J. J. 1978. Some characteristics of African swine fever virus isolated from Brazil and the Dominican Republic. Proc. 82nd Annual Meet US Anim. Health Assoc, 232–236.

55. Medes, A. M. 1961. Considerations sur la diagnostique et la prophylaxie de la porcine africaine. *Bulletin de OIE* 57:591–600.

56. Mendes, A. M. 1971. Algumas doencas dos animais em Angola e Mozambique e sua importancia na hygiene das carnes. *Rev Portuguesa das Ciencias Veterinarias* 66:271–286.

57. Montgomery, R. E. 1921. On a form of swine fever occurring in British East Africa (Kenya Colony). *J. Comp. Pathol.* 34:242–244.

58. Moore, D. M., Zsak, L., Neilan, J. G., Lu, Z. and Rock, D. L. 1998. The African swine fever virus thymidine kinase gene is required for efficient replication in swine macrophages and for virulence in swine. *J. Virol.* 72:10310–10315.

59. Moulton, J. and Coggins, I. 1968. Comparison of lesions in acute and chronic African swine fever. *Cornell Vet.* 58:364–388.

60. Mozos, E., Herráez, P., Pérez, J., Fernández, A., Blanco, A., Martín, M. P. and Jover A. 2003. Cutaneous lesions in experimental acute and subacute African swine fever: An immunohistopathological and ultrastructural study. *Dtsch Tierarztl Wochenschr* 110:150–154.

61. Neitz, W. O. 1963. African swine fever. In *Emerging diseases of animals*. FAO agricultural studies no. 61, Food and Agricultural Organization of United Nations, Rome, Italy.

62. Nix, R. J., Gallardo, C., Hutchings, G., Blanco, E. and Dixon, L. K. 2006. Molecular epidemiology of African swine fever virus studied by analysis of four variable genome regions. *Arch. Virol.* 151:2475–2494.

63. OIE. 2004. *Manual of diagnostic tests and vaccines for terrestrial animals*. Office-International-des-Epizooties. 5th ed., vol. 1, Paris, France, 233.

64. Oura, C. A. I., Powel, P. P., Anderson, E. and Parkhouse, R. M. E. 1998a. The pathogenesis of African swine fever in the resistant bush pigs. *J. Gen. Virol.* 79:1439–1443.

65. Oura, C. A. I., Powel, P. P. and Parkhouse, R. M. E. 1998b. African swine fever: A disease characterized by apoptosis. *J. Gen. Virol.* 79:1427–1438.

66. Oura, C. A. I., Powel, P. P. and Parkhouse, R. M. E. 1998c. Detection of African swine fever virus in infected pig tissues by immunocutochemistry and in situ hybridization. *J. Virol. Methods* 72:205–217.

67. Oviedo, J. M., Rodriguez, F., Gomes-Puertas, P., Brun, A., Gomez, N., Alonso, C., and Escribano, J. M. 1997. High level expression of the major antigenic African swine fever virus proteins p54 and p30 in baculovirus and their potential use as diagnostic reagents. *J. Virol. Methods* 64:27–35.

68. Pan, I. C., Trautaman, R., Hess, W. R., De Boer, C. J. and Tessler, J. 1974. African swine fever: Detection of antibody by reverse single radial immunodiffusion. *Am. J. Vet. Res.* 35:351–3654.

69. Penrith, M. L., Thomson, G. R. and Bastos, A. D. S. 2004. African swine fever. In *Infectious diseases of livestock*, 2nd ed., vol. 2, ed. J. A. W. Coetzer and R. C. Tustin, 1088–1119. Oxford, UK: Oxford University Press.

70. Petisca, J. L. N. and Goncalves, J. M. M. 1977. The evolution of the histopathological picture on pigs experimentally infected with acute African swine fever virus (lymph nodes, spleen, thymus and bone marrow). Agric. Res. Semin. on hog cholera/classical swine fever and African swine fever. Hannover, Germany, 1976, EUR 5904, 612–627.

71. Pini, A. and Wagehaar, G. 1974. Isolation of a non-haemadsorbing strain of African swine fever (ASF) virus from a natural outbreak of the disease. *Vet. Rec.* 94:12–14.

72. Plowright, W. 1986. African swine fever: A retrospective view. *Rev. Sci. Tech. Off. Int Epiz.* 5:455–468.

73. Plowright, W., Perry, C. T. and Peirce, M. A. 1970. Transovarial infection with African swine fever virus in the argasid tick (*Ornithodoros moubata porcinus*). *Vet. Rec.* 2:582–584.

74. Porterfield, J. S. 1975. The basis of arbo virus classification. *Med. Biol.* 53:400–405.

75. Radostits, O. M., Gay, C. C., Hinchcliff, K. W. and Constable, P. D. 2007. *Veterinmary medicine: A textbook of the diseases of cattle, sheep, pigs, goats and horses*, 10th ed. Philadelphia: WB Saunders. 1027–1032.

76. Ramiro-Ibanez, F., Ortega, A., Brun, A., Escribano, J. M. and Alonso, C. 1996. Apoptosis: A mechanism of cell killing and lymphoid organ impairment during acute African swine fever virus infection. *J Gen Virol.* 77:2209–2219.

77. Revilla, Y., Cebrian, A., Baixeras, E., Martinez, A., Vinuela, E. and Salas, M. L. 1997. Inhibition of apoptosis by African swine fever virus Bcl-2 homologue: Role of the BH1 domain. *Virology* 228:400–404.

78. Ribeiro, J. M., Azevedo, R. J., Teixero, M. J. O., Braco Forte, M. C., Rodrigues, R., Ribeiro, A. M., Oliveiro, E., Noronha, F., Grave Pereira, C. and Dias Vigario, J. 1958. Peste porcine provoquee par une souche differente (SL) de la souche classique. *Bull OIE* 50:516.

79. Rodriguez, F., Fernandez, A., Perez, J., Martin, D. L. A. J., Sierra, M. A. and Jover, A. 1996. African swine fever: Morphology of a viral hemorrhagic disease. *Vet Rec.* 139:249–154.

80. Rojo, G., Chamoro, M., Salas, M. L., Vinuela, E., Cuezva, J. M. and Salas, J. 1998. Migration of mitochondria to viral assembly sites in African swine fever virus-infected cells. *J. Virol.* 72:7583–7588.

81. Rojo, G., Garcia-Beato, R., Vinuela, E., Salas, M. L. and Salas, J. 1999. Replication of African swine fever virus DNA in infected cells. *J. Virol.* 257:524–536.

82. Sakamoto, K., Yamakawa, M., Tsuda, T. and Murakami, Y. 2006. Detection of African swine fever virus-specific antibodies using the recombinant viral proteins p32 and p54 expressed in insect cells. *Japan Agric. Res. Quart.* 40:271–276.

83. Salguero, F. J., Sanchez-Cordon, P. J., Nunez, A., Fernandez-de-Marco, M. and Gomez-Villamandos, J. C. 2005. Proinflammatory cytokines induce lymphocyte apoptosis in acute African swine fever infection. *J. Comp. Pathol.* 132:289–302.

84. Sanchez Botiza, C. 1961. Comptes rendus des séances de la conference exceptionelle OIE-FAO sur la peste porcine aricaine et al peste equie africaine. *Bull. OIE* 55:371–372.

85. Sanchez Botiza, C. 1963. Reservorios del virus de la peste procina africana. *Bull. OIE* 60:895.

86. Sánchez-Cordón, P. J., Cerón, J. J., Núñez, A., Martínez-Subiela, S., Pedrera, M., Romero-Trevejo, J. L., Garrido, M. R. and Gómez-Villamandos, J. C. 2007. Serum concentrations of C-reactive protein, serum amyloid A, and haptoglobin in pigs inoculated with African swine fever or classical swine fever viruses. *Am. J. Vet. Res.* 68:772–777.

87. Steyn, D. G. 1928. Preliminary report on a South African virus disease amongst pigs. 13th and 14th Rep. Dir. Vet. Educ. Res. Onderstepoort, S. Africa, 415.

88. Stone, S. S. and Hess, W. R. 1967. Antibody response to inactivated preparations of African swine fever virus in pigs. *Am. J. Vet. Res.* 28:475.

89. Tubiash, H. S. 1963. Quantity production of leukocyte cultures for use in haemadsorption tests with African swine fever virus. *Am. J. Vet. Res.* 24:381–384.

90. Valdeira, M. L., and Geraldes, A. 1985. Morphological study on the entry of African swine fever virus into cells. *Biol. Cell.* 55:35–40.

91. Valdeira, M. L. 2001. Effect of ribavirin on the African swine fever virus replication. *Revista-Portuguesa-de-Ciencias-Veterinarias* 96:183–189.

92. Vial, L., Wieland, B., Jori, F., Etter, E., Dixon, L. and Roger, F. 2007. African swine fever Virus DNA in Soft Ticks, Senegal. *Emerg. Infect. Dis.* 13:1928–1931.

93. Villeda, C. J., Williams, S. M., Wilkinson, P. J. and Vinuela, E. 1993. Consumption coagulopathy associated with shock in acute African swine fever. *Archiv. Virol.* 133:467–475.

94. Walker, J. 1933. East African swine fever. Thesis, Univ. Zurich, Balliere, Tindall and Cox, London, 1.

95. Wardley, R. C. and Wilkinson, P. J. 1977. The association of African swine fever virus with blood components of infected pigs. *Archiv. Virol.* 55:327–334.

96. Wensvoort, G., Terpstra, C. and Blemraad, M. 1988. Detection of antibodies against African swine fever virus using infected monolayers and monoclonal antibodies. *Vet. Rec.* 122:536–539.

97. Zsak, L., Borca, M. V., Risatti, G. R., Zsak, A., French, R. A., Lu, Z., Kutish, G. F., Neilan, J. G., Callahan, J. D., Nelson, W. M. and Rock, D. L. 2005. Preclinical diagnosis of African swine fever in contact-exposed swine by a real-time PCR assay. *J. Clin. Microbiol.* 43:112–119.

2. Classical Swine Fever

G. Saikumar

Introduction

Classical swine fever (CSF; synonyms: hog cholera, swine fever, and swine plague) is probably economically the most important viral infectious disease of domestic pigs (Moennig, 2000). In India, according to 1999–2000 annual report of the Project Directorate on Animal Disease Monitoring and Surveillance (PD-ADMAS), CSF was present in twenty of thirty-two states/union territories, and based on outbreak rate per ten thousand villages, it was ranked the topmost among the seven OIE list A diseases reported in India. As per the reports of the World Organization for Animal Health, fifty-nine outbreaks of CSF were recorded in India during 2004. The exact number of CSF outbreaks and prevalence of CSFV infections in India could be much higher than that is apparent from occasional reports that have appeared from time to time.

Etiology

The CSF virus (CSFV) is a member of the genus *Pestivirus*. Pestiviruses are a small group of ssRNA viruses comprising CSFV, BVDV of cattle, and BDV of sheep. Based on their morphology, type of nucleic acid, genome organization, and replication strategy, pestiviruses are classified in the family Flaviviridae. CSFV is an enveloped, positive-sensed, single-stranded RNA virus, which is spherical in shape and 40–60 nm in size with a genome of approximately 12.3 kb. The pestivirus genomic RNA contains a single long open reading frame (ORF) that is flanked by a 5' and 3' nontranslated region (NTR). The resulting polyprotein of about 3,900 amino acids is processed (Co and post translationally) by viral as well as cellular proteases to yield four structural and seven to eight nonstructural viral proteins. The proteins are arranged in the order No: Npro/C/Erns/E1/E2/P7/NS2-3/NS4A/NS4B/NS5A/NS5B; and NS2-3 can be processed to yield NS2 and NS3.

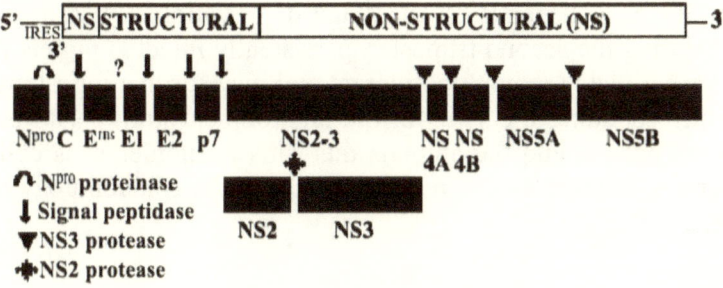

Genomic organization of CSFV

The envelope glycoproteins E1 (55 kDa) and E2 (46 kDa) are located at the surface and nonglycosylated protein C of 36 kDa in the core of the virion. Also, the envelope protein E1 of CSFV contains major antigenic determinants, which are conserved and involved in neutralization. "Erns" protein has Rn ase activity and is secreted in considerable amounts from infected cells and has pathological significance.

CSFV strains can be classified into (1) high virulent, (2) moderate virulent, and (3) avirulent types. High virulent strains kill nearly all pigs irrespective of age, moderate virulent strains generally lead to subacute illness in postnatally infected piglets but may cause abnormalities in porcine fetuses, and avirulent strains are attenuated and pathogenic for fetuses only.

PATHOGENESIS

The most important mode of CSFV transmission is via the oronasal route. The superficial epithelial cells, as well as those that cover the tonsillar crypts, are the principal sites of viral multiplication. Viremia occurs between 16 and 24 hpi (hr.post infection), and the virus reaches the spleen, peripheral lymph nodes, bone marrow, and Peyer's patches of the intestinal mucosa by hematogenous spread.

The infection can run an acute, subacute, chronic, atypical, or inapparent course. Virulent virus causes acute CSF, where as infections with low virulent virus may cause inapparent disease. The virus readily crosses the placenta in pregnant sows and may cause persistent infection or various fetal malformations (Dewulf et al., 2001). The degree of pathogenicity varies from one pig to another, and the low virulent CSFV strains may cause high mortality in young pigs and recovery in older pigs. Moreover, possibly due to the practice of vaccination, a gradual shift in the trend of virulence of viral strains from high to low is being noticed, and pigs infected with such strains do not manifest characteristic lesions. Low virulent strains may be propagated unnoticed by carrier sows. The outcome of transplacental passage of CSFV depends on the stage of gestation. When a sow gets infected during the second trimester, persistently infected piglets may be born. These piglets are immunotolerant and may survive for a long time, persistently shedding the virus in the environment until a late onset of the disease occurs, and the animals die. This phenomenon is called the carrier-sow syndrome and is very important in the epidemiology of CSF (Bouma, 2001).

CSFV grows readily in vitro and is able to cause a persistent, noncytopathic infection of cell cultures. This indicates that the virus can avoid the antiviral effects of type I interferon (IFN) and prevents apoptosis. The first protein encoded by the genome Npro is an autoprotease that cleaves itself from the nascent viral polyprotein and whose function has been enigmatic. Recently, it has been shown that CSFV lacking Npro induces rather than inhibits an interferon response in infected monocytes (Ruggli et al., 2002).

Since the virus is so innocuous in vitro, it has long been suspected that the serious lesions found in vivo must have an immunopathological origin. During infection, there are profound changes in the bone marrow and in the circulating white cell population, and such changes may precede widespread infection of these cell types (Summerfield et al., 2001). This suggests an indirect cytopathic effect induced in mainly uninfected cells, damaged by a soluble viral factor or by some other disturbance of cellular homeostasis. There is evidence for both of these mechanisms. First, there is a soluble viral protein "Erns" that at high concentrations is able to induce apoptosis in lymphocytes in vitro (Bruschke et al., 1997). Second, virus replication in monocytes and macrophages induces the release of proinflammatory cytokines, including prostaglandin-E2 and interleukin-1, which have a probable role in fever and hemorrhages (Knoetig et al., 1999).

Leucopenia (in particular, lymphopenia) is a characteristic early event during CSF. The leucopoenia involved leukocyte subpopulations in a disparate manner, with B lymphocytes, helper T cells and cytotoxic T cells being the most affected. Depletion of lymphocyte subpopulations occurs one to four days before virus is detectable in the serum.

CSFV infects and efficiently replicates in monocyte, and bone marrow-derived dendritic cells (DCs) also. The T cell stimulatory capacity of CSFV-infected DCs is maintained both in a polyclonal T cell stimulation and in specific-antigen-presentation assays, requiring antigen uptake and processing (Dewulf et al., 2001). Recent studies to elucidate the mechanism of hemorrhagic pathology of the disease suggests that infection of the vascular endothelial cells has central role in the pathogenesis of the disease as various proinflammatory cytokines (interleukins 1, 6, and 8) and coagulation factor, tissue factor, and vascular endothelial cell growth factor involved in endothelial cell permeability are increased, and this may disrupt the hemostatic balance and leads to the coagulation and thrombosis seen in acute disease (Bensaude et al., 2004).

CLINICAL DISEASE

CSF is manifested in four different forms: (1) the peracute form resulting in a high morbidity and death within five days postinfection, (2) the acute form terminating in death between ten and twenty days postinfection, (3) the subacute form terminating in death between twenty and twenty-nine days postinfection, and (4) the chronic disease, having a duration of thirty or more days.

In the peracute form, sudden death may occur in young piglets without any sign of illness. Typical acute CSF cases are characterized by dullness, anorexia, and pyrexia (up to 40–41°C) within two to six days with usual peak between fourth and eighth day of illness, followed by exudative conjunctivitis and huddling of animals in a corner of the pen. The other clinical symptoms usually observed include constipation followed by diarrhea, incoordination of movements manifested as weaving and staggering gait, and convulsions. Skin of white pigs may reveal hyperemic rashes, followed by petechial hemorrhages as well as purple discoloration of ears.

Chronic or persistent CSF may occur both after prenatal or postnatal infection of pigs. Based on the clinical signs, chronic CSF can be divided into three clinical phases: an early acute reaction characterized by anorexia, depression, and fever; a period of general clinical improvement; and a period of relapse and death. Chronically, sick pigs often suffer from a partial alopecia characterized by thinning of bristles. There is evidence of general depression and unthriftiness, emaciation with or without diarrhea, persistent mild fever, and terminal deep purple coloration of the abdominal skin. Chronic, persistent infection leads to development of runted pigs.

The clinical picture of CSF is not always characterized by a febrile disease with typical clinical signs and high morbidity and mortality. Atypical cases of CSF may go unnoticed in affected farm. Some recent CSFV isolates from across the world have been observed not to produce overt clinical signs and hence believed to be of low or moderate virulence (Sandvik et al., 2000; Terpstra and deSmit, 2000). In newborn pigs with congenital CSFV infection of low virulence, muscular tremors of whole body, neck tremors causing the affected piglets to nod their heads in a vertical direction, inability to stand, and loss of equilibrium have been observed. The late-onset disease is a sequel of congenital CSFV infection.

Infection in the early stage of gestation up to seventy days leads to still born or aborted fetuses with typical lesions like hydrops and subcutaneous edema (jelly piglets). Persistent infections of the litters occur when sows are infected between seventy and ninety days of gestation. In chronic or persistent CSF, usually single-organ system (such as respiratory system, GI system, and CNS) is affected. A high incidence of myoclonia congenita (congenital trembles) associated with cerebellar hypoplasia is observed (Trautwein, 1988). Persistently infected piglets constantly shed large amounts of virus and are a dangerous virus reservoir, spreading the disease and maintaining the infection within the pig population. Persistently infected piglets may be born if the fetus's own immune system is not yet capable of recognizing the virus (phase of immunotolerance) (Kaden et al., 2005). Persistently infected piglets may appear clinically normal at birth, but they invariably die from CSF after survival periods of eleven months (late-onset CSF). Leucopenia is a consistent manifestation of persistent CSF, but in the terminal stages of disease, leucocytosis may develop. Body temperature of such piglets remains normal. Growth retardation is the most common finding.

PATHOLOGY

GROSS LESIONS

In acute CSF, the gross lesions include erythema and petechial or ecchymotic hemorrhages in the skin; enlarged edematous, swollen, and hemorrhagic lymph nodes; necrotic tonsillitis; petechial hemorrhages in epiglottis and larynx; petechial subcapsular hemorrhages in the kidneys; and infarcts in the spleen.

In chronic CSF, the carcasses are often emaciated, the spleen is smaller than normal, and button ulcers are present in the large intestine. Lesions of pneumonia, atrophy of the thymus, and exostoses at the costochondral junctions of the ribs of young pigs are the commonest lesions in chronic or inapparent or late-onset infections. A single-organ system (lungs, gastrointestinal tract, and central nervous system) may predominantly be affected, and secondary bacterial infections are frequently observed. Button ulcers or diffuse diphtheroid necrotizing enteritis may be present. In lymph nodes, the pathological signs may only consist of hyperplasia instead of typical hemorrhages as described in acute course of the disease (Terpstra, 1991). Pathological changes are less typical, especially the lack of hemorrhages on organs and serosa. In animals displaying chronic diarrhea and necrotic and ulcerative lesions on the ileum, the ileocecal valve, and the rectum are common. The clinical signs and lesions of chronic CSF are of nonspecific type (Moennig et al., 2003).

Congenital CSFV infections can result in mummification, stillbirth, and malformations. Abnormalities include residual septa in the gallbladder, edema and petechial hemorrhages in the mesocolon, fissures in the renal cortex, excessive fluid in abdominal and thoracic cavities, extensive hypoplasia of the lungs, hydrocephalus, cerebellar hypoplasia, small cerebral gyri, malformation of pulmonary artery, and congestion of tissues. The pathological picture varies from edema in prenatal deaths to hemorrhages in piglets that died after birth. Hemorrhages are mainly observed in skin, lymph nodes, and kidneys. Postnatal death is highest in litters from sows infected at sixty-five days of pregnancy. Growth retardation is a common feature, and diarrhea, lymphadenopathy, and locomotor disturbances are also seen in the persistently infected pigs.

MICROSCOPIC LESIONS
In acute CSF, there is marked hemorrhage and necrosis. The lesions in the lymph nodes include severe peripheral hemorrhage and also in the cell-poor substance, causing typical marbled gross appearance. Primarily, CSFV attacks the reticuloendothelial system. Microscopic kidney lesions follow a pattern of hemorrhage, edema, and lymphocyte infiltration, with tubular epithelium showing varying retrogressive changes.

In the spleen, there is swelling and hyalinization of blood vessel walls, obstruction with thrombotic material, and resulting infarction (Terpstra, 1991). Hemorrhages of tonsil, skin, heart, and intestinal mucosa are seen. Lungs show hemorrhages, catarrhal to fibrinous bronchopneumonia, and pleuritis. The heart shows myocardial congestion, swelling, and dissociation of the perinuclear sarcoplasm. Stomach may be markedly congested and hemorrhagic. Catarrhal to necrotic enteritis is found in the intestines. Mesenteric blood vessels are usually markedly engorged. Occasionally, subserous ecchymotic and suffusive hemorrhages occur in the small and large intestines. Brain shows congestion, hemorrhage, encephalitis, perivascular cuffing, microgliosis, and focal necrosis (Van Oirschot, 1999).

In chronic CSF, general depletion of lymphoid tissue is the most prominent histopathological lesion. Other important lesions are lymphocytic interstitial nephritis, glomerulonephritis, nonsuppurative diffuse meningoencephalitis, diphtheroid necrotizing enteritis, and hyperplastic lymphadenitis.

The most outstanding lesions in pigs with persistent CSF are thymic atrophy and severe depletion of lymphocytes and germinal follicles in peripheral lymphoid organs. Histiocytic hyperplasia with phagocytosis of lymphocytic debris is also frequently seen. Persistent CSFV infections induce adrenal cortical hyperplasia characterized by an increased width of the zona fasciculata and atrophy of the zona glomerulosa and zona reticulate. In fetuses infected with low virulent congenital CSFV infection, the changes include endothelial swelling, hydropic degeneration, pyknotic nuclei, and infiltrating mononuclear cells in the tunica media of blood vessels. Areas normally myelinated in the cerebrum, pons, medulla oblongata, cerebellum, and spinal cord have a lacy appearance and stain faintly by the H&E method.

DIAGNOSIS

CSF is suspected when characteristic postmortem lesions are seen, but often no pathognomonic lesions are seen at necropsy (Van Oirschot, 1999). Symptoms vary considerably depending on the age and breed of the affected animal and virulence of the infecting virus. In acute cases, fever and leucopenia in ailing animals and hemorrhagic lesions in lymph nodes, kidneys, and infarction of the spleen are highly suggestive for CSF but may be confused with African swine fever, septicemic salmonellosis, pasteurellosis, erysipelas, and others. It is therefore mandatory that suspected cases are thoroughly investigated by laboratory tests. The subacute, chronic, or late-onset CSF is generally manifested with a wide variety of clinical signs and pathological lesions.

Isolation of virus in cell culture is considered to be the gold standard, but it takes at least three days and is labor intensive. CSFV can be isolated from buffy coat cells or organ suspensions from tonsil, spleen, lymph nodes, and kidneys by inoculating cell lines of porcine origin such as PK-15 and SK-6. The virus does not produce cytopathic effect, and hence, inoculated cultures need to be tested by immunohistochemical methods using specific antibodies.

Detection of viral antigen in the tonsil, lymph nodes, and kidney samples by immunohistochemical methods—i.e., the direct immunofluorescence antibody technique (FAT) on cryostat tissue sections—is preferred when quick diagnosis is required as it takes less than twenty-four hours. In formalin-fixed, paraffin wax–embedded tissues, CSFV antigen can be demonstrated by using a monoclonal antibody based avidin-biotin-complex

(ABC) immunoperoxidase method. The advantage of this method is the good preservation of histological details, but the test takes a long time to complete.

For screening of large number of samples, antigen-capture enzyme-linked immunosorbent assays may be used. Detection of CSF antibody is useful for surveys, and the virus-neutralization test is the most specific and sensitive method for CSF-antibody detection. Porcine serum samples are incubated with a CSF reference virus to check for presence of neutralizing antibodies. The limitation with this test is that cross-neutralizing antibodies specific to ruminant pestivirus (BVDV) infections of pigs also give a positive result, and it takes about three days to complete the test. Large numbers of serum samples are preferably processed by ELISA tests.

Immunoassays have low sensitivity, especially if infected animals are to be detected during the incubation phase or in a chronic state of the disease when viremia is low or intermittent. Serology or immunohistochemical methods are not efficient for the detection of clinically inapparent viral state in which a particular viral marker is synthesized at below-threshold level (Kaden et al., 1999). CSFV-infected cells may express no or very little viral antigen on the cellular surface, especially in low-virulent CSFV-infected tissues (Van Oirschot, 1999).

Detection of CSFV nucleic acids by reverse transcription (RT) and then PCR (RT-PCR) is a rapid and highly sensitive diagnostic tool. RT-PCR seems promising when compared with other established assays, such as virus isolation or an antigen-capture assay (Lowings, et al., 1996). Additionally, the RT-PCR amplicons can be sequenced and directly used for the typing of the isolated virus (Greiser Wilke et al., 1998). Because an internationally standardized method is not yet available and is yet to be recognized by the OIE (WOAH) as a recommended test for CSF diagnosis, the test has not gained the desired level of adoption in the diagnostic laboratories. Handel et al. (2004) noted that RT-PCR could reliably detect infected pigs beginning at 3 dpi (3 days post infection) regardless of whether animals were inoculated with a low, moderate, or high virulent strain of CSFV. Of the three assays for detecting pigs infected with low-, moderate-, and high-virulent CSFV strains-e.g., RT-PCR, virus isolation, and immunoperoxidase assays, RT-PCR gave the most consistent results. For clinical samples, nested RT-PCR was more sensitive than RT-PCR, and RT-PCR was more sensitive than virus isolation.

Real-time (fluorogenic) RT-PCR methods are rapid (one day or less, including RNA extraction), are not influenced by neutralizing antibody, have very large dynamic range, and allow precise quantitation of as little as twofold differences in viral RNA amounts (Uttenthal et al., 2003). A flurogenic-probe hydrolysis (TaqMan) reverse transcriptase (RT) PCR assay for CSFV developed by Risatti et al. (2003) detected the presence of the virus before the appearance of the disease. Van Rijn et al. (2004) developed a multiplex assay for detection of five economically important viruses, including CSFV in swine semen. Evaluation of the diagnostic sensitivity and specificity of a TaqMan probe–based RT-PCR for CSFV using nasal swab samples taken from both symptomatic and asymptomatic animals clearly showed the superior diagnostic sensitivity of real-time RT-PCR over virus isolation (100% versus 72.4%, respectively) with little loss of specificity (98.9% versus 100%, respectively) (Risatti et al., 2005). The assay can be used to analyze virus genetic load in tissues. In experimentally infected pigs, virus infection appeared first in tonsil (day 1), then submandibular lymph node, spleen, ileum, and mesenteric lymph node (by day 3).

At this institute, nucleic acid–based techniques like RT-PCR are routinely used for and have been employed for diagnosis of CSFV infections in fresh and archival formalin-fixed, paraffin-embedded tissues (Singh et al., 2005a). Other nucleic acid–based tests that are used as, and when required, are phylogenetic analysis of CSFV isolates (Singh et al., 2005b). In situ hybridization (ISH) using DNA and RNA probes for localization of CSFV and real-time PCR assays (SYBR green and TaqMan assays) for detection of virus genetic load in a wide variety of tissue samples originating from experimentally and naturally infected pigs (Nagarajan et al., 2006, 2007). It is anticipated that nucleic acid–based tests will soon replace many of the conventional tests used for CSF diagnosis because of their increased sensitivity and specificity. It's only a matter of time that more and more laboratories in India will increasingly adopt these techniques as is happening in most laboratories in the European Union. For control of this deadly disease, detailed epidemiological information needs to be gathered. This cannot be accomplished without a proper established system for laboratory confirmation of every suspected case/outbreak of CSF. Infrastructural facilities and trained manpower would be required for virus isolation, characterization of the isolates with respect to its virulence, and genotyping of all virus strains circulating in different regions of the country, both in endemic regions and in areas where sporadic outbreaks occur with serious consequences. The prevalence of this deadly disease can be drastically reduced by active surveillance disease and strategic vaccination campaigns.

2. CLASSICAL SWINE FEVER

REFERENCES

1. Bensaude, E., Turner, J. L., Wakeley, P. R., Sweetman, D. A., Pardieu, C., Drew, T. W., Wileman, T. and Powell, P. P. 2004. Classical swine fever virus induces proinflammatory cytokines and tissue factor expression and inhibits apoptosis and interferon synthesis during the establishment of long-term infection of porcine vascular endothelial cells. *J. Gen. Virol.* 85:1029–37.

2. Bouma, A., Stegeman, J. A., Engel, B., de Kluijver, P., Elbers, A. R. W. and de Jong, M. C. M. 2001. Evaluation of diagnostic tests for the detection of classical swine fever in the field without a golden standard. *J. Vet. Diagn. Invest.* 13:383–388.

3. Bruschke, C. J. M., Hulst, M. M., Moormann, R. L. M., van Rijn, P. A. and van Oirschot, J. T. 1997. Glycoprotein erns of pestivirus induces apoptosis in lymphocytes of several species. *J. Virol.* 71:6692–6696.

4. Callens, M. and de Clercq, K. 1999. Highly sensitive detection of swine vesicular disease virus based on a single tube RT-PCR system and DIG-ELISA detection. *J. Virol. Meth.* 77: 87–99.

5. Dewulf, J., Laevens, H., Koenen, F., Mintiens, K. and de Kruif, A. 2001. An experimental infection with classical swine fever virus in pregnant sows: Transmission of the virus, course of the disease, antibody response and effect on gestation. *J. Vet. Med.* B 48:583–591.

6. Greiser-Wilke, I., Depner, K., Fritzemeier, J., Haas, L. and Moennig, V. 1998. Application of a computer program for genetic typing of classical swine fever virus isolates from Germany. *J. Virol. Meth.* 75:141–150.

7. Handel, K., Kehler, H., Hills, K. and Pasick J. 2004. Comparison of reverse transcriptase-polymerase chain reaction, virus isolation and immunoperoxidase assays for detecting pigs infected with low, moderate, and high virulent strains of classical swine fever virus. *J. Vet. Diagn. Invest.* 16:132–8.

8. Kaden, V., Steyer, H., Strebelow, G., Lange, E., Hubert, P. and Steinhagen, P. 1999. Detection of low virulent classical swine fever virus in blood of experimentally infected animals: Comparison of different methods. *Acta Virol.* 43:373–80.

9. Kaden, V., Steyer, H., Schnabel, J. and Bruer, W. 2005. Classical swine fever (CSF) in wild boar: The role of the transplacental infection in the perpetuation of CSF. *J. Vet. Med. B. Infect. Dis. Vet. Pub. Hlth.* 52:161–4.

10. Knoetig, S. M., Summerfield, A., Spagnuolo-Weaver, M. and Mccollough, K. C. 1999. Immunopathogenesis of classical swine fever: Role of monocytic cells. *Immunol.* 97:359–366.

11. Lowings, J. P., Ibata, G., Needham, J. and Paton, D. J. 1996. Classical swine fever diversity and evolution. *J. Gen. Virol.* 77:1311–1371.

12. Moennig, V. 2000. Introduction to classical swine fever: Virus, disease and control policy. *Vet. Microbiol.* 73:93–102.

13. Moennig, V., Floegel-Niesmann, G. and Greiser-Wilke, I. 2003. Clinical signs and epidemiology of classical swine fever: A review of new knowledge. *Vet. J.* 165:11–18.

14. Nagarajan, K., Saikumar, G., Dandapat, S. and Paliwal, O. P. 2006. Classical swine fever: Clinicopathological studies in piglets infected with CSFV (INB/03) isolate. *Indian J. Anim. Sci.* 76:199–203.

15. Nagarajan, K., Saikumar, G., Singh, V. K. and Paliwal, O. P. 2007. Clinico-pathological changes and tissue distribution of viral nucleic acids following experimental infection of piglets with a north Indian isolate (INB/03) of classical swine fever virus. *Indian J. Anim. Sci.* 77:281–287.

16. Risatti, G., Holinka, L., Lu, Z., Kutish, G., Callahan, J. D., Nelson, W. M., BreaTio, E., and Borca, M. V. 2005. Diagnostic evaluation of a real-time reverse transcriptase PCR assay for detection of classical swine fever virus. *J. Clin. Microbiol.* 43:468–71.

17. Risatti, G. R., Callahan, J. D., Nelson, W. M. and Borca, M. V. 2003. Rapid detection of classical swine fever virus by a portable real-time reverse transcriptase PCR assay. *J. Clin. Microbiol.* 41:500–5.

18. Ruggli, N., Tratschin, J. D., Schweizer, M., Hofmann, M. A. and Summerfield, A. 2002. Interaction of classical swine fever virus with innate antiviral defense mechanisms: The viral protein Npro is required for

prevention of double-stranded RNA-induced cell death and type 1 interferon synthesis. In 5th Pestivirus Symposium, St. John's College, Cambridge, UK, 26–29th August, 24 (*http://www.ploufragan.afssa.fr/esvv/Programmes/absbookp.doc*).

19. Sandvik, T., Drew, T. W. and Paton, D. J. 2000. CSF virus in East Anglia: Where from? *Vet. Rec.* 147:251.

20. Singh, V. K., Saikumar, G. and Paliwal. O. P. 2005a. Detection of classical swine fever in archival formalin-fixed tissues by reverse transcription-polymerase chain reaction. *Res. Vet. Sci.* 79:81–84.

21. Singh, V. K., Saikumar, G. and Paliwal. O. P. 2005b. Phylogenetic analysis of classical swine fever (CSFV) by cloning and sequencing of partial 5' non-translated genomic region. *Indian J. Anim. Sci.* 74:1093–1097.

22. Summerfield, A., Zingle, K., Inumaru, S. and Mccullough, K. C. 2001. Induction of apoptosis in bone marrow neutrophil-lineage cells by classical swine fever virus. *J. Gen. Virol.* 82:1309–1318.

23. Terpstra, C., and de Smit, A. J. 2000. The 1997/1998 epizootic of swine fever in the Netherlands: Control strategies under a non-vaccination regimen. *Vet. Microbiol.* 77:3–15.

24. Terpstra, C. 1991. Hog cholera: An update of present knowledge. *British Vet. J.* 147:397–406.

25. Trautwein, G. 1988. Pathology and pathogenesis of the disease. In *Classical swine fever and related infections*, ed. B. Liess, 24–27. Boston, USA: Martinus Nijhoff Publishing.

26. Uttenthal, A., Storgaard, T., Oleksiewicz, M. B. and de Stricker, K. 2003. Experimental infection with the Paderborn isolate of classical swine fever virus in 10-week-old pigs: Determination of viral replication kinetics by quantitative RT-PCR, virus isolation and antigen ELISA. *Vet. Microbiol.* 92:197–212.

27. Van Oirschot, J. T. 1999. Classical swine fever (Hog cholera). In *Diseases of swine*, 8th ed., 159–72. Ames, Iowa, USA: Iowa State University Press.

28. Van Rijn, P. A., Wellenberg, G. J., Hakze-van der Honing, R., Jacobs, L., Moonen, P. L. and Feitsma, H. 2004. Detection of economically important viruses in boar semen by quantitative RealTime PCR technology. *J. Virol. Meth.* 120:151–60.

3. Nipah Virus Infections in Humans and Pig

S. Nandi, and P. K. Dash

Introduction

Nipah virus infection is an emerging zoonotic disease first described in 1999, and the virus is under the genus *Henipavirus* and family Paramyxoviridae. The disease is similar to another emerging zoonotic disease caused by Hendra virus and can spread from its wildlife reservoir to pigs and humans where it causes an often-fatal disease (Wang et al., 2001). It is a notifiable disease in most countries and to be handled under highest biological security level 4 (BSL-4). In Malayasia, an outbreak of viral encephalitis occurred over a thirty-five-week period from September 29, 1998, to May 31, 1999, among pig farmers, creating considerable anxiety and fear. Of the 265 cases reported to the Ministry of Health in Malaysia, 105 were fatal, and the case fatality rate was 39.6% (Chua et al., 1999; Chong et al., 2000). The outbreak also spread to neighboring Singapore, where 11 workers of an abattoir developed the disease with one fatality. Ninety-three percent of the reported cases involved those directly in the pig-farming industries—namely, pig farmworkers, pig farm proprietors, housewives, and family members assisting in the farms. The majority of the cases occurred in those aged twenty and above (92.4%) and actively engaged in pig industry followed by the age group ten to nineteen years (6.4%). About 82.6% of the cases are male (Lam, 2003; Chong et al., 2000; Chua, 2003).

Etiology

Henipavirus is a genus of the family Paramyxoviridae and order Mononegavirales containing two members, Hendravirus and Nipah virus. The henipaviruses are naturally harbored by pteropid fruit bats (flying foxes) and are characterized by a large genome (18.2 kb), wide host range, and their recent emergence as zoonotic pathogens capable of causing illness and death in domestic animals and humans (Wang et al., 2001; Chua et al., 2000).

The viruses are pleomorphic ranging in size from 40–600 nm in diameter. They possess a lipid membrane overlying a shell of viral matrix protein. At the core is a single helical strand of genomic RNA tightly bound to N (nucleocapsid) protein and associated with the L (large) and P (phospoprotein) proteins, which provide the RNA polymerase activity. F (fusion) protein trimers and G (attachment) protein tetramers are embedded within the lipid membrane. The genome of the Nipah virus consists of a nonsegmented, single-stranded, negative-sense RNA. In common with other members of the

Paramyxovirinae subfamily, the number of nucleotides in the *Henipavirus* genome is a multiple of six, known as the rule of six. The Nipah virus has been classified by the CDC as a category C agent (Wang et al., 2001; Chan et al., 2001; Harcourt et al., 2000).

OUTBREAKS

After initial outbreak of the disease in Malaysia, seven more outbreaks of Nipah virus have occurred since 1998 all within Bangladesh and neighboring parts of India, where *Pteropus* species (*P. giganteus*) are available (Bellini et al., 2005; Chadha et al., 2006).

DIFFERENT OUTBREAKS OF NIPHA VIRUS ARRANGED

Year	Months	Place	Total	Mortality
2001	January 31–February 23	Siliguri, India	66	74%
2001	April–May	Meherpur District, Bangladesh	13	69%
2003	January	Naogaon District, Bangladesh	12	67%
2004	January–February	Manikganj and Rajbari provinces, Bangladesh	42	33%
2004	February–April	Faridpur District, Bangladesh	36	75%
2005	January	Tangail District, Bangladesh	12	92%
2007	February–May	Nadia District, India	50	12%

TRANSMISSION

The symptoms of Nipah virus infection in Malayasia were primarily encephalitic in humans and respiratory in pigs. Later, respiratory illness in humans has been reported, and likelihood human-to-human transmission indicates the presence of more dangerous strain of the virus. Based on the seroprevalence data and virus isolations, the primary reservoir for Nipah virus was identified as pteropid fruit bats including *Pteropus vampyrus* (Malayan flying fox) and *Pteropus hypomelanus* (island flying fox), both available in Malaysia. The transmission of Nipah virus from flying foxes to pigs is thought to be due to an overlap of bat habitats and piggeries in Peninsular Malaysia. The fruit orchards were in close proximity to the piggery, allowing the spillage of urine, feces, and partially eaten fruits onto the pigs. Certain species of fruit bats are the natural hosts of Nipah virus and distributed across an area encompassing northern, eastern, and southeastern areas of Australia, Indonesia, Malaysia, the Philippines and some of the Pacific Islands. The bats appear to be susceptible to infection with these viruses without showing any symptoms. Serologically positive dogs, cats, bats, horses, and goats were found in the infected areas (Yob et al., 2001; Eason et al., 2006; Chua et al., 2002).

BAT INFECTION WITH NIPHA VIRUS IN DIFFERENT COUNTRIES

Bat types	Scientific name	Country
Fruit bat	*Pteropus vampyrus* and *P. hypomelanus*	Malaysia
Fruit bat	*Pteropus lylei*	Cambodia
Fruit bat	*Pteropus lylei* and *Hipposider oslarvartus*	Thailand
Fruit bat	*Pteropus rufus* and *Eidolon dupreanum*	Madagascar

However, no infection of human or other species have been observed in Cambodia, Thailand, or Madagascar. The apparent source of infection for humans is direct contact with pigs. Transmission of virus is thought to be from body fluids of infected pigs. Human-to-human transmission has not been documented.

EPIDEMIOLOGY

Fruit-eating bats (*Pteropus* sp.) are the natural reservoir for the *Henipaviruses*. Humans are usually infected via the intermediate hosts. In case of Nipah virus, pigs are the usual intermediate hosts. But exposure to infected fruit bats or materials contaminated by infected bats or direct human-to-human transmission is also possible. Bats are classified under the order Chiroptera, family Pteropodidae, and genus *Pteropus*, commonly referred to as flying foxes. Sixty-five *Pteropus* species are distributed from Madagascar through the Indian subcontinent to southeastern Asia and Australia and far east as the Cook Islands. Some *Pteropus* species are among the largest of all bats weighing as much as 1.2 kg and displaying a wingspan of up to 1.7 m. *Pteropus* species are unique because they lack the complex neural and behavioral mechanisms required for echolocation that characterize the vast majority of bat species. Instead, they have large eyes, navigate visually and feed mainly on fruits and flowers, which they locate by smell. Nipah virus and Hendra virus, having close genomic similarity, were difficult to differentiate serologically earlier. The word "Nipah" originated from the name of a village Sungai Nipah in the Malaysian Peninsula, one of the first villages where pig farmers developed an encephalitic disease (Johara et al., 2001; Olivae and Daszak, 2005).

The first known human infection with Nipah virus was detected during an outbreak of severe febrile encephalitis in Peninsular Malaysia and Singapore in 1998–1999. Direct contact with pigs was the primary source of human infection. Most of the victims were adult males involved in pig farming or pork production. The spread of virus within the pig farms and between states of Malaysia was due to movement of pigs. Transmission between pigs in the same farm was attributed to direct contact with excretions and secretions such as urine, saliva, and laryngeal and pharyngeal secretions. Iatrogenic transmission by use of same needles was also implicated. The spillage of virus from its natural reservoir into the pigs remains a subject of speculation. Species jumping of viruses can be due to evolutionary or ecological reasons. Nipah virus is an old virus and has not undergone any evolutionary change. Most authorities believe that ecological factors led to their emergence. This can be due to a change in the number density and management of pigs. The deforestation and drought prompted migration of bats from their natural habitat in the coastal forest on to the villages where piggeries were located (Wong, 2000; Mohd Nor et al., 2000).

Unlike the Malaysia outbreak, bat-to-pig-to-human transmission was unlikely to have occurred in Bangladesh. For religious reason, pig farming is not practiced in Bangladesh, and pig population is low. Hence, direct bat-to-human transmission and then human-to-human transmission seemed most likely. The route might be through contaminated date palm juice, which humans consume. The palm juice collected in earthen pots hung atop date palm trees is a common practice in rural areas of Eastern India and Bangladesh during winter months. The bats feed on the juice, thus contaminating the juice with their saliva, which is subsequently drunk by humans. The Siliguri epidemic clearly resembled the Bangladesh epidemic (Eason et al., 2006).

Symptoms in Pigs

The clinical disease in pigs can be very subtle, and a large proportion of pigs in a farm may not exhibit any clinical signs. The incubation period varies from seven to fourteen days. In suckling pigs, mortality is high, and infected piglets showed symptoms of open-mouth breathing.

In weaners (older than four weeks) and growers, clinical signs include fever (>39°C) with respiratory signs ranging from rapid and labored breathing to harsh nonproductive coughing. Blood-tinged mucous discharge from the nostrils appeared in severe cases. Neurological signs included trembling, twitching, muscular spasms, rear leg weakness, and varying degree of lameness or spastic paresis.

In sows and boars, clinical signs included sudden death or acute febrile illness with labored breathing, increased salivation, and serous or mucopurulent nasal discharge. Neurological signs observed included agitation, head pressing, tetanus-like spasms and seizures, champing of mouth, and apparent pharyngeal muscle paralysis. Abortions occur in first trimester of pregnancy in affected sows. In animals, especially in pigs, the virus causes porcine respiratory and neurologic syndrome also known as barking pig syndrome or one-mile cough (Mohd Nor et al., 2000; WHO, 2001; FAO/APHCA, 2002).

Clinical Signs in Human

The incubation period in humans varies from several days to two months with four to eighteen days in most of the cases. The symptoms include fever, headache, drowsiness, cough, abdominal pain, nausea, vomiting, weakness, problems with swallowing, and blurred vision. A majority of patients had impaired level of consciousness (55%) with brain stem dysfunction, abnormal doll's eye reflex, pinpoint pupils, hypertension, and tachycardia. Neurological signs include seizures and ataxia. The salient clinical features of Nipah virus encephalitis that distinguish it from JE include early brain stem signs, early ataxia, segmental myoclonus, and terminal autonomic dysfunction (Goh et al., 2000; Lee et al., 1999).

Laboratory Findings

Thrombocypenia with platelet counts of <140 000 mm^{-3} and leucopenia with WBC count of <4000 mm^{-3} have been reported. Blood urea, creatinine, and electrolyte levels were normal in all patients. Elevated levels of alanine aminotransferase and aspartate aminotransferase have been reported.

Cerebrospinal fluid examination showed elevated level of protein and WBC counts (Tan et al., 2000).

TREATMENT

Ribavirin is the drug of choice against Nipah virus infection as it has broad spectrum activity against both RNA and DNA viruses. The drug has been shown to cross the blood-brain barrier following oral administration, making it useful for the treatment of viral encephalitis. The preliminary study showed that ribavirin treatment in acute Nipah encephalitis was associated with 36% reduction in mortality and increased survival without neurological deficits. The ribavirin and 6 azauridine were able to delay but not prevent Nipah virus–induced mortality. Poly I:C, an interferon inducer, was found to be effective.

Monoclonal antibodies against F and G glycoproteins can be used in prophylaxis and treatment (Chong et al., 2001).

POSTMORTEM LESIONS

In pigs, the postmortem lesions are relatively nonspecific. The lungs present mild to severe lesions with varying degree of consolidation, emphysema, and petechial to ecchymotic hemorrhages and blood-tinged exudates in the airways. The meninges show generalized congestion and edema. Kidneys showed congestion both on surface and in the cortex. Histologically, interstitial pneumonia with widespread hemorrhages and syncytial cell formations in the endothelial cells of the blood vessels of the lungs has been noticed. Generalized vasculitis, hemorrhages, and infiltration of mononuclear cells were observed in the lungs, kidneys and brain tissue. Immunohistology showed a high concentration of the viral antigens in the endothelium of the blood vessels of lungs. It indicates that respiratory secretions from infected pigs were likely to be a rich source of infectious virus (Chua et al., 2000).

In human beings, the virus after entry causes a systemic multiorgan vasculitis. CNS is most commonly affected. However, endothelial affection is observed in the heart, lung, kidney, and spleen. Immunohistochemistry showed intense staining of endothelial and parenchyma cells and multinucleate giant cells characteristic of paramyxovirus infections. Nipah virus has been isolated from CSF, tracheal secretions, throat swabs, nasal swabs, and urine (Chua et al., 1999; Chua et al., 2000a).

ECONOMIC ASPECTS

The Nipah outbreak in pigs in Malaysia causes considerable loss of revenue to the pig farmers, animal feed suppliers, lorry transport companies, abattoir workers, food vendors, etc. The economic losses were also significant when neighboring countries stopped importing the live pigs.

In Malaysia, during the outbreak, many humans died. And about 8,500 workers directly involved in the pig-breeding activities; 9,400 workers engaged in supporting industries; and 3 lakhs workers in related industries nationwide were affected. Although the outbreak is over and the pig farms declared free of Nipah virus, many still remain unemployed (Lam, 2003).

Diagnosis

1. **Virus isolation.** Nipah virus grows well in Vero cells. The tissues collected from the animals during postmortem examination could be used after processing for inoculation in cell cultures. Virus isolates are then identified using immunostaining, neutralization, PCR, electron microscopy, and immune electron microscopy. A cytopathic effect develops within three days, but two 5 days passages are recommended before declaring it as negative (Daniel et al., 2001).
2. **RT—PCR.** RT-PCR can be used for M gene or N gene–specific amplification and has allowed for phylogenetic-based study and comparison of the strains responsible for the various outbreaks (Daniel et al., 2001; WHO, 2001).

Prevention

In the absence of any widely accepted treatment modality, the importance of the prevention of the spread should be emphasized. Singapore controlled the outbreak in 1998 by stopping pig export from Malaysia. The Malaysia outbreak was contained by mass culling of over one million pigs. Very strict hygienic measures by way of wearing gloves and masks seem mandatory. Pig farms should be located at a distance from human habitat, and periodic serological checkup may be conducted (Halder and Chakravarty, 2006).

Control and Eradication

With the discovery of the Nipah virus causing the disease, monitoring the pig farms and the abattoirs to detect the antibodies to Nipah virus should be initiated. A Nipah IgG ELISA is already available. All the farms outside the previously designated high-risk areas were screened by taking statistically valid random samples of sows for Nipah virus antibodies. Farms with two consecutive negative tests performed within an interval of three weeks were accorded as free status. Farms found positive during first or second blood tests should be depopulated. Besides, proper zoosanitary measures should be adopted, including good animal husbandry practices (Mohd Nor et al., 2000).

Conclusion

The emergence of henipavirus parallels the emergence of other zoonotic viruses in recent decades. SARS coronavirus, Australian bat *Lyssavirus*, Menangle virus, and probably Ebola virus and Marburg virus are also harbored by bats and are capable of infecting a variety of other species. The emergence of each of these viruses has been linked to an increase in contact between bats and humans, sometimes involving an intermediate domestic animal host. The increase contact is driven both by human encroachment into bats' territory (in case of Nipah, specifically piggery in the said territory) and movement of bats toward human populations due to changes in food distribution and loss of habitat particularly in South Asia and Australia, thus creating the overlap of human and flying fox distributions.

Nipah virus is an emerging and deadly zoonotic disease caused by *Henipavirus* under the family Paramyxoviridae. There were considerable social disruptions and tremendous economic loss to pig-rearing industry. This highly virulent virus, believed to be introduced into pig farms by fruit bats, spread easily among pigs and was transmitted to humans who came into close contact with infected animals. As there is no vaccine available for Nipah virus and handling of virus needs a BSL-4 laboratory, only a handful of laboratories have access to the virus. Because of the high virulence of henipaviruses, the absence of therapeutic intervention strategies and vaccines, and their classification as BSL-4 pathogens, a plan for emergency response to Nipah virus outbreak should always consider the diagnostic and laboratories preparedness and eradication and surveillance program. As the Nipah virus outbreaks in pigs cause enormous economic losses and widespread panic and fear because of its zoonotic importance, high mortality, and absence of suitable therapeutic interventions, people are going to be frightened in case of its outbreak. The handling of the outbreak is a delicate and sensitive problem and could easily be turned into a serious political, religious, and racial issue. So proper planning in seromonitoring of the disease and culling of the positive and infected pigs must be adopted, which may lead to the control of the disease to a great extent.

References

1. Bellini, W. J., Horcourt, B. M., Bowden, N. and Rota, P. A. 2005. Nipah virus: An emergent paramyxovirus causing severe encephalitis in humans. *J. Neurovirol.* 11:481–487.
2. Chadha, M. S., Comer, J. A., Lowe, L., Rota, P. A., Rollin, P. E. and Bellini, W. J. 2006. Nipah virus associated encephalitis outbreak, Siliguri, India. *Emerging Infectious Diseases* 12:235–240.
3. Chan, Y. P., Chua, K. B., Koh, C. L., Lim, M. E. and Lam, S. K. 2001. Complete nucleotide sequences of Nipah virus isolates from Malaysia. *J. Gen. Virol.* 82:2151–2155.

4. Chong, H. T., Kamarulzaman, A., Tan, C. T., Goh, K. J., Thayaparan, T., Kunjapan, S. R., Chew, N. K., Chua, K. B. and Lam, S. K. 2001. Treatment of acute Nipah encephalitis with ribavirin. *Ann. Neurol.* 49:810–813.

5. Chong, H. T., Kunjapan, S. R., Thayaparan, T. and Tong, J. M. G. 2000. Nipah encephalitis outbreak in Malaysia, clinical features in patients from Seremban. Neurol. *J. Southeast Asia* 5:61–67.

6. Chua, K. B. 2003. Nipah virus outbreak in Malaysia. *J. Clin. Virol.* 26:265–275.

7. Chua, K. B., Bellini, W. J., Rota, P. A. and Harcourt, B. H. 2000. Nipah virus: A recently emergent deadly paramyxovirus. *Science* 288:1432–1435.

8. Chua, K. B., Goh, K. J., Wong, K. T., Kamarulzaman, A. and Tan, P. S. K. 1999. Fatal encephalitis due to Nipah virus among pig-farmers in Malaysia. *Lancet* 354:1257–1259.

9. Chua, K. B., Koh, C. L., Hooi, P. S., Wee, K. F., Khong, J. H., Chua, B. H., Chan, Y. P., Lim, M. E. and Lam, S. K. 2002. Isolation of Nipah virus from Malaysian Island flying foxes. *Microbes and Infection* 4:145–151.

10. Chua, K. B., Lam, S. K., Tan, C. T., Hooi, P. S., Goh, K. J., Chew, N. K., Tan, K. S., Kamarulzaman, A. and Wong, K. T. 2000a. High mortality in NIpah encephalitis is associated with presence of virus in cerebrospinal fluid. *Ann. Neurol.* 48:803–805.

11. Daniel, P., Ksiazek, T. and Eaton, B. T. 2001. Laboratory diagnosis of Nipah and Hendra virus infection. *Microbes and Infectio* 3:289–295.

12. Eason, B. T., Broder, C. C., Middleton, D. and Wang, L. F. 2006. Hendra and Nipah viruses: Different and dangerous. *Nat. Rev. Microbiol.* 4:23–35.

13. FAO/APHCA. 2002. Manual on the diagnosis of Nipah virus infection in animals, RAP publication 2002/01, Thailand, 90P.

14. Field, H., Young, P., Yob, J. M., Mills, J., Hall, L. and Mackenzie, J. 2001. The natural history of Hendra and Nipah viruses. *Microbes and Infectio.* 3:307–314.

15. Goh, K. J., Tan, C. T., Chew, N. K., Tan, P. S. K., Kamarulzaman, A. and Sarji, S. A. 2000. Clinical features of Nipah virus encephalitis among pig farmers in Malaysia. *New Engl. J. Med.* 342:1229–1235.

16. Halder, A. and Chakravarty, A. 2006. Nipah virus encephalitis: A cause for concern for Indian neurologists? *Ann. Indian Acad. Neurol.* 9:137–144.

17. Harcourt, B. H., Tamin, A., Ksiazek, T. G. and Rota, P. A. 2000. Molecular characterization of Nipah virus, a newly emergent paramyxovirus. *Virolog* 271:334–349.

18. Johara, M. Y., Field, H., Rashdi, A. M. and Jamaluddin, A. 2001. Nipah virus infection in bats (order Chiroptera) in Peninsular Malaysia. *Emerg. Infect. Dis.* 7, 439–441.

19. Lam, S. K. 2003. Nipah virus—a potential agent of bio-terrorism. *Antiviral Research* 57:113–119.

20. Lee, K. E., Umapathi, T., Tan, C. B., Tjia, H. T. L. and Lee, W. L. 1999. The neurological manifestations of Nipah virus encephalitis, a novel paramyxovirus. *Ann. Neurol.* 46:428–432.

21. Mohd Nor, M. N., Gan, C. H. and Ong, B. L. 2000. Nipah virus infection of pigs in peninsular Malaysia. *Rev. Sci. Tech. Off. Int. Epiz.* 19:160–165.

22. Olivae, K. J. and Daszak, P. 2005. The ecology of emerging neurotropic viruses. *J. Neurovirol.* 11:441–446.

23. Tan, K. S., Sarji, S. A., Tan, C. T., Abdullah, B. J. J., Chong, H. T., Thayaparan, T. and Koh, C. N. 2000. Patients with asymptomatic Nipah virus infection may have abnormal cerebral MRI. *Neurology J. Southeast Asia* 5:69–73.

24. Wang, L., Harcourt, B. H. and Yu, M. 2001. Molecular biology of Hendra and Nipah viruses. *Microbes and Infection* 3:279–287.

25. WHO. 2001. Nipah virus fact sheet no. 262.

26. Wong, K. T. 2000. Emerging and re-emerging epidemic encephalitis: A tale of two viruses. *Neuropathol. Appl. Neurobiol.* 26:313–318.

27. Yob, J. M., Field, H., Rashdi, A. M. and Morrissy, C. 2001. Nipah virus infection in bats (order Chiroptera) in Peninsular Malaysia. *Emerg. Infect. Dis.* 7:439–441.

4. Porcine Circovirus 2–Associated Diseases

G. Saikumar

Introduction

Porcine circovirus 2 (PCV2) has been associated with a number of disease syndromes in pigs. Postweaning multisystemic wasting syndrome (PMWS) first identified in Western Canada is now a global pig disease. PCV2 has also been associated with porcine dermatitis and nephropathy syndrome (PDNS), with proliferating and necrotizing pneumonia (PNP), and reproductive disorders in pigs. Some recent reports from the USA have identified PCV2 as an important agent in porcine respiratory disease complex (PRDC) (Allan and Ellis, 2000). Porcine circovirus 2–associated diseases (PCVAD) are worldwide in distribution, with outbreaks being observed in North and South America, Europe, and Asia.

Etiology

Porcine circovirus (PCV), a member of the newly recognized Circoviridae family, was first detected as a contaminant of the pig kidney cell line PK-15 (Tischer et al., 1974). Circoviruses are the smallest viruses identified so far with a diameter of 17 nm having a single-stranded circular DNA genome of about 1.76 kb (Tischer et al., 1982; Mankertz et al., 2004). The genome consists of two potentially functional open reading frames (ORFs): ORF1 (930 bp) encodes the Rep protein involved in viral replication, and ORF2 (690 bp) encodes the immunogenic capsid protein (Fenaux et al., 2000; Cheung, 2003). Nucleotide sequence analysis of the PCV associated with PMWS is different from PCV derived from PK-15 cells. The cell-culture derived virus is nonpathogenic for swine and is referred as PCV type 1 (PCV1), and the virus associated with the new disease is referred as PCV2 (Allan et al., 1999a). The two viruses share 76% nucleotide homology with each other (Roca et al., 2004). Both viruses are nonenveloped with icosahedral symmetry. The two other animal circoviruses included in this family are chicken anemia virus (CAV) and psittacine beak and feather disease virus. These three circoviruses-i.e., PCV, CAV, PBFDV, do not share nucleotide sequence homology or antigenic determinants with one another (Todd et al., 1991).

Occurrence

Serological studies indicated that the prevalence and incidence of PCV2 infection is high, affecting up to 100% of pig herds in parts of Canada, the USA, and Europe (Cottrell et al., 1999; Allan and Ellis, 2000). PCV2 has also been isolated from pigs in North America, many parts of Europe, and Southeast Asia. More recently, the presence of this virus among Indian pigs associated with reproductive failure was also demonstrated by Sharma and Kumar (2008). Apparently, PCV2 is widely distributed in pig populations throughout the world.

A retrospective serological survey conducted in Canada to determine the presence of antibodies to PCV1 and PCV2 in serum samples collected from sows at slaughterhouses in Canada in 1985, 1989, and 1997 indicated that PCV2 had been circulating in the Canadian pig population at least ten years before the PMWS was reported (Magar et. al., 2000). In another study conducted in the UK, archival tissues tested for presence of PCV2 DNA/antigen by PCR and IHC were found positive in 32.0–41.0% of the samples collected between 1970 to 1990 (Grierson et al., 2004). In Spain, testing of archived tissues and sera samples collected from pigs between 1985 to 1997 revealed 41.3% of the tissues and 72.7% of the sera positive for PCV2 nucleic acids and antibodies, indicating enzootic infection since 1985 (Rodriguez-Arrioja et al., 2003). In Belgium, the presence of PCV2 could be traced back to 1969 (Sanchez et al., 2001).

PATHOGENESIS

PCV2 can be transmitted through direct contact via oronasal, fecal, and urinary routes (Bolin et al., 2001, Magar et al., 2000). Experimental studies revealed that PCV2 is excreted through respiratory and oral secretions besides urine and feces of both PCVAD-affected and clinically healthy pigs, with higher viral loads in the PCVAD-affected pigs (Segales et al., 2005). Vertical transmission can result in birth of viremic or persistently infected piglets. PCV2 can also be transmitted through semen (Larochelle et al., 2000).

Disease attributed to PCV2 has been studied at the field level (Madec et al., 2000; Quintana et al., 2001; Rodriguez-Arrioja et al., 2002) and under experimental conditions (Rosel et al., 1999). The primary etiological role of PCV2 has been established, but experimental infection in conventionally reared pigs often induces low-grade lesions without manifestation of clinical signs of disease. Probably, additional factors, mainly concurrent viral infections, are necessary for manifestation of clinical disease (Balasch et al., 1999). Under experimental conditions, clinical signs and lesions of PMWS could be induced in conventional young piglets coinfected with PCV2 and PRRSV, PPV, or other pathogens (Allan et al., 1999 b; Kennedy et al., 2000; Madec et al., 2000; Quintana et al., 2001; Segales et al., 2002). In gnotobiotic pigs, the synergistic effect of PCV2 and PPV has been demonstrated by reproducing clinical disease and lesions typical of PMWS in coinfected pigs (Krakovka et al., 2000).

Investigations into possible differences in virulence among some field isolates of Midwestern United States indicated that marked difference in virulence can occur with minimal changes in the nucleic acid sequence of ORF2 (Opriessnig et al., 2006a). Recent increase in the incidence and severity of PCV2-associated diseases in Canada and United States was attributed to new emerging genotypes of PCV2 (Cheung et al., 2007, DeLay et al., 2005). At this stage, it is not clear what makes the new PCV2b genotype more virulent. The association of another unidentified etiological agent responsible for the increased severity of disease in recent times cannot be ruled out. Host genetics may also have a role in susceptibility. While most purebred and crossbred pigs are susceptible to PCVAD, purebred Landrace pigs appear to be more susceptible to PCVAD (Opriessnig et al., 2006b).

Circoviruses probably depend on host DNA synthesis for their replication and, therefore, replicate most efficiently in rapidly dividing cells. Since PCV2 preferentially targets lymphoid cells, the replication of PCV2 may be enhanced by lymphoid stimulation caused by another coinfecting virus, e.g., PRRSV, PPV, or immune stimulation, following vaccination. Pigs vaccinated with commercial *Actinobacillus pleuropneumonia* and *M. hyopneumoniae* vaccines and inoculated with PCV2 showed significantly longer length of viremia, a higher copy number of the PCV2 genome in serum, a wider range of tissue distribution of PCV2 antigen, and an increased severity of lymphoid depletion (Opriessnig et al., 2003). In pigs, general immunostimulation (injections of keyhole limpet hemocyanin emulsified in incomplete Freunds adjuvant and of thioglycollate medium) could enhance the severity of PMWS in specific-pathogen-free six-week-old piglets (Grasland et al., 2005).

Following infection, viral antigen is detectable in the cytoplasm and nuclei of a wide range of lymphoid and nonlymphoid tissues, including smooth muscle cells and fibroblasts. Lymphoid depletion and presence of large amounts of PCV2 antigen or nucleic acids in the cytoplasm of macrophages and dendritic cells in the depleted follicles is a consistent finding. However, there is no evidence that PCV2 replicates in these cells (Vincent et al., 2003). Probably these cells only help transport of the virus to different organs of the body. It is still not clear whether lymphopenia is due to decreased production in the bone marrow or increased loss due to necrosis or apoptosis.

Pigs suffering from PMWS show severe alterations of hematological parameters (anemia, lymphopenia with decrease of CD8+ and IgM+ cells, monocytosis, and neutrophilia) and extensive lymphocyte depletion in all lymphoid organs (Segales et al., 2001; Darwich et. al., 2002). Changes in the cytokine expression profiles include an overexpression of IL-10 in thymus and general decrease of cytokines IL-2, IL-4, IL-10, IL-12, and IFN-gamma in other lymphoid organs. Thymic IL-10 mRNA overexpression in PMWS pigs is associated with depletion and atrophy of the organ. These changes lead to severe T-cell immunosuppression.

CLINICAL SIGNS
PMWS-affected pigs show poor weight gain, hairy coat, and emaciation. Some pigs may show high fever (40–42°C), dyspnea, anemia, jaundice, mild diarrhea, and respond poorly to antibiotic therapy. Superficial inguinal lymph nodes become enlarged and palpable, and some of them may appear pale and yellow in color. Mortality rates vary between 10–25%, and duration of illness may be two to three weeks.

Porcine respiratory disease complex (PRDC) caused by PCV2 in association with other respiratory pathogens such as PRRSV, SIV, and *M. hyopneumoniae* is clinically manifested as decreased growth rate, decreased feed efficiency, anorexia, fever, cough, and dyspnea.

In pigs affected with PDNS, there may be anorexia, depression, stiff gait, and reluctance to move. The prominent sign is the presence of irregular red or purple patches (macules and papules) in the skin that may coalesce with time, especially around the hind legs and perineal area. Affected animals generally die within a few days after showing clinical signs, and the mortality rate may reach 100% in older pigs.

In gilts, reproductive problems are characterized by late-term abortions and increased numbers of mummified fetuses, stillbirth, and weak piglets. Congenital tremor, characterized by tremor of the head and limbs of the newborn pigs possibly associated with PCV2, has also been observed (Hines and Lukert, 1994).

PATHOLOGY
POSTWEANING MULTISYSTEMIC WASTING SYNDROME (PMWS)
In subclinical infection, necrotizing lymphadenitis, mainly follicular necrosis, limited to one or two lymph nodes may be seen. Grossly, enlargement of lymph nodes is observed. Lungs are noncollapsible and show tan-colored mottling. Kidneys are generally enlarged and may have grayish white streaks or spots. Gastric ulceration may be seen in some cases. Histopathological

changes include lymphohistiocytic to granulomatous inflammatory lesions in lymphoid tissues and organs. Severe depletion of lymphocytes, particularly in follicles and paracortical zones of the lymph nodes and in the periarteriolar lymphoid sheaths of the spleen is seen. The depletion is prominent in lymph nodes that are enlarged. It is accompanied by infiltrations of histiocytes, particularly in the cortical sinuses, which often contain single large or multiple small basophilic, cytoplasmic inclusion bodies. Multinucleate syncytia are frequently seen in lymphoid tissues, particularly in lymph nodes, spleen, and gut-associated center of follicles depopulated of lymphocytes. In affected lungs, there is commonly a lymphohistiocytic interstitial pneumonia, with destruction of bronchial and bronchiolar epithelium and inflammatory cells in the alveoli. Lymphohistiocytic infiltrations are also found in the liver, kidney, and pancreas. Extensive necrosis of hepatocytes, often with parenchymal collapse, is a feature of liver lesions. In the kidney, there may be multifocal interstitial nephritis with vasculitis. In the stomach, colon, cecum, and duodenum, there can be marked gland and crypt necrosis, with mononuclear cell infiltrations.

In cases of PRDC, granulomatous bronchointerstitial pneumonia with mild to severe necrotizing and ulcerative bronchiolitis and bronchiolar fibrosis and abundant PCV2 antigen associated with the lesions is noticed. In PCV2-associated enteritis, the intestinal mucosa is thickened, and mesenteric lymph nodes are enlarged (Jensen et al., 2006). Microscopically, granulomatous enteritis with lesions in Peyer's patches is characteristic.

In pigs showing PDNS, there are necrotizing skin lesions (mainly on rear legs and perineal region) and/or swollen and pale kidneys with generalized cortical petechiae. The other prominent lesions are systemic necrotizing vasculitis and necrotizing and fibrinous glomerulonephritis. Currently, PDNS is considered as type III hypersensitivity reaction, although the antigen associated with this immunecomplex disease is not definitively known.

In stillborn and weak neonatal piglets, chronic passive congestion, cardiac hypertrophy, and diffuse nonsuppurative to necrotizing or fibrosing myocarditis associated with abundant PCV2 antigen is observed. Heart is the target organ in the fetuses. The affected piglets show hepatic chronic venous congestion, cardiac hypertrophy, and severe diffuse myocarditis (O'Connor et al., 2001). When experimentally inoculated into pregnant sows at different stages of gestation, PCV2 resulted in variable gross pathology. Fetuses when inoculated at fifty-seven days of gestation were pale, edematous with distended abdomens. Hemorrhages, congestion, edema, and enlarged liver were observed in the fetuses. However, no gross abnormality was observed in fetuses of sows inoculated at seventy-five and ninety-two days of gestation (Sanchez et al., 2001). PCV2 infection resulted in abortion, premature farrowing, and stillbirths in six pregnant sows inoculated intranasally at three weeks before expected farrowing date. Microscopic lesions limited to the lungs of stillborn and live-born piglets were mild pneumonic changes characterized by infiltration of mononuclear cells in the alveolar spaces (Park et al., 2005).

Congenital tremor subtype AII resulting from myelin deficiency has been associated with PCV2. No gross or microscopic lesions were recorded from four different farms experiencing outbreaks of CT. However, PCV2 nucleic acid was detected in neural tissues and liver of both CT-affected and normal pigs (Stevenson et al., 2001). On the other hand, recent work conducted in Europe (Kennedy et al., 2003) on cases of CT AII did not show any association with PCV2. Therefore, the association between PCV2 and CT needs further confirmation.

Immunolabeling of tissue sections from pigs with clinical PMWS, using PCV2 specific antibodies, often reveals large concentrations of virus antigen in lymphoid tissues, particularly lymph nodes. Viral antigen is most frequent in the cytoplasm of cells, but labeling in the nucleus is also observed. Labeled cells appear to be principally mononuclear phagocytes and dendritic cells; epithelial cells and lymphocytes can also contain virus antigen (Sanchez Jr., et al., 2004).

Retrospective and prospective studies have indicated that while virtually all PMWS cases are associated with the presence of PCV2 nucleic acid and antigen in lesions, a proportion of cases also contain porcine parvovirus, porcine respiratory and reproductive syndrome virus (PRRSV), or other agents. The mechanisms involved in the potentiation of PCV2 replication in PCV2/PRRSV and PCV2/porcine parvovirus (PPV) dually infected pigs may relate to the fact that monocyte/macrophage cell types are common targets of these three viruses (Allan et al., 2000). In cases of respiratory disease, PCV2 is usually found together with PRRSV, swine influenza (SIV), or other recognized pneumonic pathogens (Pallares et al., 2002). PCV2 has also been identified in, and isolated from, cases of abortion and fetal death (Pensaert et al., 2004). In these cases, severe myocarditis was often found associated with viral antigen in myocardiocytes, thus directly associating the virus with fatal myocardial failure. The virus has also been demonstrated in kidneys and lymphoid tissue from pigs affected with porcine dermatitis and nephropathy syndrome (PDNS). In PDNS, pronounced lymphoid depletion and renal and cutaneous lesions were seen (Rosell et al., 2000). PCV2 nucleic acid can be detected in macrophages, histiocytes, and dendritic cells of several tissues and organs, including lymph nodes, gut-associated lymphoid tissue, tonsil, lung, spleen, liver, kidney, and skin.

DIAGNOSIS

Clinical signs and lesions can be suggestive of PCV2 infection. A definitive diagnosis can only be made by laboratory testing for demonstration of virus in affected tissues. Diagnosis of PCVAD is based on the combination of clinical signs, gross and microscopic lesions, and demonstration of PCV2 antigen or nucleic acid in lesions.

Porcine circoviruses can be isolated from the tissues of pigs affected by PMWS and other disease syndromes in specially treated tissue cultures. Virus isolation is carried out by inoculation of PCV1-free PK15 cell lines with clarified organ suspension or plasma or serum. Since the virus grows in the cells without producing cytopathic changes, infection is confirmed by PCR detection of viral nucleic acids or by staining the cultures using an immunofluorescent or immunoperoxidase technique with polyclonal antiserum.

Isolation in cell culture is tedious; hence, diagnostic methods that rely on the direct detection of viral antigens or DNA are more popular. PCV2 antigen in the PMWS-affected pigs is usually found in the cytoplasm of histiocytes, multinucleate giant cells, and other monocyte/macrophage lineage cells such as alveolar macrophages, Kupffer cells, and follicular dendritic cells of lymphoid tissues (Rosell et al., 1999; Allan and Ellis, 2000).

Viral antigen can be detected using indirect immunofluorescence on acetone-fixed cryostat sections. PCV2 antigen can be detected in tissues using monoclonal antibodies. In affected animals, PCV2 antigen is easily demonstrated in the cytoplasm of infected macrophages (Sanchez Jr. et al., 2001; Kim and Chae, 2004). In the tissues of stillborn and neonatal piglets, the antigen can be detected in the germinal centers of lymph nodes in the cells resembling macrophages. In spleen, PCV2-positive cells may be found scattered in the red pulp in macrophage-like cells. Lung, thymus, liver, and tonsil may also reveal the presence of PCV2 antigen (Park et al., 2005).

PCR, although sensitive and specific when used by itself, can be problematic in routine diagnosis because many pigs can be viremic without developing disease. Amplification of the specific sequence of PCV2 by PCR followed by RFLP (Hamel et al., 1998), PCR using type specific primers (Allan et al., 1999), and multiplex PCR (Larochelle et al., 1999) have been used to detect and differentiate PCV1 from PCV2 in infected cells. Several PCR and nested PCR reactions have been reported for the diagnosis of PCV2 infections from tissues of PMWS-affected pigs and sera of stillborn piglets (Kim and Chae, 2003).

Nucleotide sequencing and phylogenetic analysis helps to determine the extent of genetic similarity among the PCV2 isolates. The value of diagnosing PCV2 infections and studying the pathogenesis of PCV2 by PCR and other molecular approaches will depend on knowledge of the extent of genetic variation among PCV2 isolates from different geographic regions.

Nonradioisotopically labeled DNA probes have been used to detect the PCV2 nucleic acid sequences in the lesions (Choi and Chae, 1999). Digoxigenin-labeled DNA probes that can differentiate PCV1 from PCV2 in formalin-fixed, paraffin-wax-embedded tissues of field cases of PMWS revealed that in some cases, both PCV1 and PCV2 were detected mainly in the macrophages of lymph nodes and spleen (Kim and Chae, 2001). In PCV2-ssociated cases of congenital tremor, the virus could be demonstrated by ISH in large and small neurons, Purkinje cells, and a few oligodendrocytes in the CNS (Stevenson et al., 2001).

There are varieties of serological tests that can detect antibodies against PCVs. A new specific test for PCV2 antibodies has been developed (Blanchard et al., 2003). Since subclinical infections with PCV2 are known to be widespread in pigs, the use of serology in the diagnosis of PCV2-related diseases is limited. Serology can be used as a management tool in breeding herds.

CONTROL STRATEGIES

PCVAD can be controlled by ensuring good management practices that include good hygiene, good nutrition, minimum stress, and elimination of concurrent infections and potential factors that induce immune stimulation. Vaccines have been developed for use in growing pigs and breeding animals. The inactivated, oil-adjuvanted PCV2-vaccine (CIRCO-VAC) used in Europe is said to be efficacious in breeding-age animals. Suvaxyn PCV2 One Doseis a commercial vaccine available in the United States. This is a killed version of the live chimeric PCV1-2 virus (Fenaux et al., 2003, Fenaux et al., 2004). A baculovirus expressed PCV2 vaccine Ingelvac CIRCOFLEX has shown promising results in Canada. Autogenous vaccines prepared from lung or lymphoid tissue homogenates obtained from PCVAD pigs and inactivated with 2% formaldehyde was found to reduce mortality from 20–3%.

REFERENCES

1. Allan, G. M. and Ellis, J. A. 2000. Porcine circoviruses: A review. *J. Vet. Diagn. Invest.* 12:3–14.

2. Allan, G. M., McNeilly, F., Mechan, B. M., Kennedy, S., Mackie, D. P., Ellis, J. A., Clark, E. G., Espuna, E., Saubi, N., Riera, P., Botner, A. and Charreyre, C. E. 1999a. Isolation and characterization of circoviruses from pigs with wasting syndromes in Spain, Denmark and Northern Ireland. *Vet. Microbiol.* 66:115–123.

3. Allan, G. M., Kennedy, S., McNeilly, F., Foster, J. C., Ellis, J. E., Krakowa, S. J., Meehan, B. M. and Adair, B. M. 1999b. Experimental reproduction of severe wasting disease by co-infection of pigs with PCV and PPV. *J. Comp. Pathol.* 121:1–11.

4. Allan, G. M., McNeilly, F., Meehan, B. M., Ellis, J. A., Connor, T. J., McNair, I., Krakowka, S. and Kennedy, S. 2000. A sequential study of experimental infection of pigs with porcine circovirus and porcine parvovirus: Immunostaining of cryostat sections and virus isolation. *J. Vet. Med, Series B.* 47:81–94.

5. Balasch, M., Segales, J., Rosell, C., Domingo, M., Mankertz, A., Urniza, A. and Plana-Duran, J. 1999. Experimental inoculation of conventional pigs with tissue homogenates from pigs with postweaning multisystemic wasting syndrome. *J. Comp. Pathol.* 121:139–48.

6. Blanchard, P., Mahe, D., Cariolet, R., Truong, C., Le Dimna, M., Arnauld, C., Rose, N., Eveno, E., Albina, E., Madec, F. and Jestin, A. 2003. An ORF2 protein-based ELISA for porcine circovirus type 2 antibodies in postweaning multisystemic wasting syndrome. *Vet. Microbiol.* 17:183–94.

7. Bolin, S. R., Stoffregen, W. C., Nayar, G. P. and Hamel, A. L. 2001. Postweaning multisystemic wasting syndrome induced after experimental inoculation of cesarean-derived, colostrums-deprived piglets with type 2 porcine circovirus. *J. Vet Diagn Invest.* 13:185–194.

8. Cheung, A. K. 2003. The essential and non-essential transcription units of viral protein synthesis and DNA replication of porcine circovirus type2. *Virology* 313:452–9.

9. Cheung, A. K., Lager, K., M., Kohutyuk O. I., Vincent, A. L., Henry, S. C., Baker, R. B., Rowland, R. and Dunham A. G. 2007. Detection of two porcine circovirus type 2 genotypic groups in United States swine herds. *Arch. Virol.* 152:1035–1044.

10. Choi, C. and Chae, C. 1999. *In situ* hybridization for detection of PCV in pigs with PMWS. *J. Comp. Pathol.* 121:265–270.

11. Cottrell, T. S., Friendship, R. M. and Dewey, C. E. 1999. A study investigating epidemiological risk factors for PCV2 in Ontario. *The Pig. J.* 44:10–17.

12. Darwich, L., Segales, J., Domingo, M. and Mateu, E. 2002. Changes in the CD4+, CD8+, CD4+CD8+ and immunoglobulin M-positive peripheral blood mononuclear cells of postweaning multisystemic wasting syndrome affected pigs and age matched in infected wasted and healthy pigs correlate with lesions and porcine circovirus type2 in lymphoid tissues. *Clin. Diagn. Lab. Immunol.* 9:236–242.

13. DeLay, J., McEwen, B., Carman, S., Fairles, J. and van Dreumel, T. 2005. Porcine circovirus type 2-associated disease is increasing. *AHL Newsletter* 9:22.

14. Fenaux., M., Halbur, P. G., Gill, M., Toth, T. E. and Meng, X. J. 2000. Genetic characterization of PCV2 from pigs with PMWS in different geographic regions of North America and development of a differential PCR-RFLP assay to detect and differentiate between infections with PCV1 and PCV2. *J. Clin. Microbiol.* 38:2494–2503.

15. Fenaux, M., Opriessnig, T., Halbur, P. G. and Meng, X. J. 2003 Immunogenecity and pathogenecity of chimeric infectious DNA clones of pathogenic porcine circovirus type 2 (PCV2) and nonpathogenic PCV1 in weanling pigs. *J. Virol.* 77:11232–11243.

16. Fenaux, M., Opriessnig, T., Halbur, P. G., Elvinger, F. and Meng, X. J. 2004. A chimeric porcine circovirus (PCV) with the immunogenic capsid gene of the pathogenic PCV type 2 (PCV2) cloned into the genomic backbone of the non-pathogenic PCV1 induces protective immunity against PCV2 infection in pigs. *J. Virol.* 78:6297–6303.

17. Grasland, B., Loizel, C., Blanchard, P., Oger, A., Niguol, A. C., Bigarre, L., Morvan, H., Cariolet, R. and Jestin, A. 2005. Reproduction of PMWS in immunostimulated SPF piglets transfected with infectious cloned DNA of type 2 porcine circovirus. *Vet. Res.* 36:685–97.

18. Grierson, S. S., King, D. P., Sandvik, T., Hicks, D., Spencer, Y., Drew, T. W. and Banks, M. 2004. Detection and genetic typing of type 2 porcine circoviruses in archived pig tissues from the U.K. *Arch. Virol.* 149:1171–1183.

19. Hamel, A. L., Lin, L. L. and Nayar, G. P. S. 1998. Nucleotide sequence of PCV associated with PMWS in pigs. *J. Virol.* 72:5262–5267.

20. Hines, R. K. and Lukert, P. D. 1994. PCV as a cause of congenital tremors in newborn pigs. *Proc. Am. Assoc. Swine Pract.* 344–345.

21. Jensen, T. K., Vigre, H., Svensmark, B. and Bille-Hansen, V. 2006. Distinction between porcine circovirus type 2 enteritis and porcine proliferative enteropathy caused by *Lawsonia intracellularis. J. Comp. Pathol.* 135:176–182.

22. Kennedy, S., Moffett, D., McNeilly, F., Meehan, B., Ellis, J., Krakowka, S. and Allan, G. M. 2000. Reproduction of lesions of PMWS by infection of conventional pigs with PCV alone or in combination with PPV. *J. Comp. Pathol.* 122:9–24.

23. Kennedy, S., Segales, J., Rovira, A., Scholes, S., Domingo, M., Moffett, D., Mechan, B., O'Neill, R., McNeilly, F. and Allan, G. 2003. Absence of evidence of porcine circovirus infection in pigs with congenital tremors. *J. Vet. Diagn. Invest.* 15:151–156.

24. Kim, J. and Chae, C. 2001. Differentiation of PCV 1 and 2 in formalin-fixed paraffin-wax-embedded tissues from pigs with PMWS by ISH. *Res. Vet. Sci.* 70:265–269.

25. Kim, J. and Chae, C. 2003. Multiplex nested PCR compared with *in situ* hybridization for the differentiation of porcine circoviruses and porcine parvovirus from pigs with PMWS. *Canadian J. Vet. Res.* 67:133–137.

26. Kim, J. and Chae, C. 2004. A comparison of virus isolation, PCR, IHC and ISH for the detection of PCV2 and PPV in experimentally and naturally co-infected pigs. *J. Vet. Diagn. Invest.* 16:45–50.

27. Krakovka, S., Ellis, J. A., Meehan, S., Kennedy, S., McNeilly, F. and Allan, G. 2000. Viral wasting syndrome of swine: Experimental reproduction of postweaning multisystemic wasting syndrome in gnotobiotic swine by co-infection with porcine circovirus2 and porcine parvovirus. *Vet. Pathol.* 37:254–263.

28. Larochelle, R., Antaya, M., Morin, M. and Magar, R. 1999. Typing of PCV in clinical specimens by multiplex PCR. *J. Virol. Meth.* 80:69–75.

29. Larochelle, R., Bielanski, A., Muller, P. and Magar, R. 2000. PCR detection and evidence of shedding of porcine circovirus type 2 in boar semen. *J. Clin. Microbiol.* 38:4629–4632.

30. Madec, F., Albina, E., Cariolet, R., Hamon, L., Mahe, D., Truong, C., Jestin, A., Amenna, N. and Morvan, H. 2000. Postweaning multisystemic wasting syndrome in the pig: A new challenge for veterinary research and practice. *The Pig J.* 45:69–75.

31. Magar, R., Larochelle, R., Thibault, S. and Lamontagne, L. 2000. Experimental transmission of porcine circovirus type 2 (PCV2) in weaned pigs: A sequential study. *J. Comp. Pathol.* 123:258–269.

32. Mankertz., A., Caliskan., R., Hattermann., K., Hillenbrand, B., Kurzendoerfer, P., Mueller, B., Schmitt, C., Steinfeldt, T. and Finsterbusch, T. 2004. Molecular biology of porcine circovirus: Analyses of gene expression and viral replication. *Vet. Microbiol.* 98:81–88.

33. O'Connor, B., Grauvreau, H., West, K., Bogdan, J., Ayroud, M., Clark, E. G., Konoby, C., Allan, G. and Ellis, J. A. 2001. Multiple PCV2-associated abortions and reproductive failure in a multisite swine production unit. *Canadian Vet. J.* 42:551–553.

34. Opriessnig, T., Yu, S., Gallup, J. M., Evans, R. B., Fenaux, M., Pallares, F., Thacker, E. L., Brockus, C. W., Ackermann, M. R., Thomas, P., Meng, X. J. and Halbur, P. G. 2003. Effect of vaccination with selective bacterins on conventional pigs infected with type 2 porcine circovirus. *Vet. Pathol.* 40:521–9.

35. Opriessnig, T., McKeown, N. E., Zhou, E. M., Meng, X. J. and Halbur, P. G. 2006a. Genetic and experimental comparison of porcine circovirus type 2 (PCV2) isolates from cases with and without PCV2-associated lesions provides evidence for differences in virulence. *J. Gen. Virol.* 87:2923–2932.

36. Opriessnig, T., Fenaux, M., Thomas, P., Hoogland, M. J., Rothschild, M. F., Meng, X. J. and Halbur, P. G. 2006b. Evidence of breed-dependant differences in susceptibility to porcine circovirus type-2 associated disease and lesions. *Vet Pathol.* 43:281–293.

37. Pallares, F. J., Halbur, P. G., Opriessnig, T., Sorden, S. D., Villar, D., Janke, B. H., Yaeger, M. J., Larson, D. J., Schwartz, K. J., Yoon, K. J. and Hoffman, L. J. 2002. Porcine circovirus type 2 (PCV2) coinfections in US field cases of postweaning multisystemic wasting syndrome (PMWS). *J. Vet. Diagn. Invest.* 14:515–9.

38. Park, J. S., Kim, J., Ha, Y., Jung, K., Choi, C., Lim, J. K., Kim, S. H. and Chae, C. 2005. Birth abnormalities in pregnant sows infected intranasally with PCV-2. *J. Comp. Pathol.* 132:139–144.

39. Pensaert, M. B., Sanchez, R. E. Jr., Ladekjaer-Mikkelsen, A. S., Allan, G. M. and Nauwynck, H. J. 2004. Viremia and effect of fetal infection with porcine viruses with special reference to porcine circovirus 2 infection. *Vet. Microbiol.* 98:175–83.

40. Quintana, J., Segales, J., Rosell, C., Calsamiglia, M., Rodriguez-Arrioja, G., Chianini, F., Folch, J. M., Maldonado, J., Canal, M., Plana-Duran, J. and Domingo, M. 2001. Clinical and pathological observations on pigs with postweaning multisystemic wasting syndrome. *Vet. Rec.* 149:357–361.

41. Roca, M., Balasch, M., Segales, J., Calsamiglia, M., Viaplana, E., Urniza, A., Hattermann, K., Mankertz, A., Plana-Duran, J. and Domingo, M. 2004. *In vitro* and *in vivo* characterization of an infectious clone of a European strain of PCV2. *J. Gen. Virol.* 85:1259–1266.

42. Rodriguez-Arrioja, G. M., Segales, J., Calsamiglia, M., Resendes, A., Balasch, M., Plana-Duran, J., Casal, J. and Domingo, M. 2002. Dynamics of porcine circovirus type 2 (PCV2) infection in a postweaning multisystemic wasting syndrome (PMWS) affected farm. *Amer. J. Vet. Res.* 63:354–357.

43. Rodriguez-Arrioja, G., M., Segales, J., Rosell, C., Rovira, A. Pujols, J., Plana-Duran, J. and Domingo, M. 2003. Retrospective study on porcine circovirus type 2 infection in pigs from 1985 to 1997 in Spain. *J. Vet. Med.* B 50:99–101.

44. Rosell, C., Segales, J., Plana-Duran, J., Balasch, M., Rodriguez-Arrioja, G. M., Kennedy, S., Allan, G. M., McNeilly, F., Zatimer, K. S. and Domingo, M. 1999. Pathological, immunohistochemical, and *in situ* hybridization studies of natural cases of PMWS in pigs. *J. Comp. Pathol.* 120:59–78.

45. Rosell, C., Segales, J., Folch, J. M., Rodriguez-Arrioja, G., M., Domingo, M., Ramos-Vara, J. A., Duran, C. O., Balasch, M. and Plana-Duran, J. 2000. Identification of PCV in tissues of pigs with porcine dermatitis and nephropathy syndrome. *Vet. Rec.* 146:40–43.

46. Sanchez, R. E., Nauwynck H., J. and Pensaert M. B. 2001. Proc Conference of ssDNA Viruses, Plants, Birds, Pigs and Primates, 122.

47. Sanchez, R. E., Nauwynck, H. J., McNeilly, F., Allan, G. M. and Pensaert, M. B. 2001. Porcine circovirus 2 infection in swine foetuses inoculated at different stages of gestation. *Vet. Microbiol.* 83:169–176.

48. Sanchez, R. E. Jr., Meerts, P., Nanwynck, H. J., Ellis, J. A. and Pensaert M. B. 2004. Characteristics of porcine circovirus 2 replication in lymphoid organs of pigs inoculated in late gestation or postnatally and possible relation to clinical and pathological outcome of infection. *J Vet Diagn. Invest.* 16:175–85.

49. Segales, J., Alonso, F., Rosell, C., Pastor, J., Chianini, F., Campos, E., Lopez-Fuertes, L., Quintana, J., Rodriguez-Arrioja, G., Calsamiglia, M., Pujols, J., Dominguez, J. and Domingo, M. 2001. Changes in peripheral blood leukocyte populations in pigs with natural postweaning multisystemic wasting syndrome (PMWS). *Vet. Immunol. Immunopathol.* 81:37–44.

50. Segales, J., Calsamiglia, M., Olvera, A., Sibila, M. Badiella, L. and Domingo, M. 2005. Quantification of porcine circovirus type 2 (PCV2) DNA in serum and tonsillar, nasal, tracheo-bronchial, urinary and faecal swabs of pigs with and without postweaning multisystemic wasting syndrome (PMWS). *Vet. Microbiol.* 111:223–229.

4. PORCINE CIRCOVIRUS 2–ASSOCIATED DISEASES

51. Segales, J., Calsamiglia, M., Rosell, C., Soler, M., Maldonado, J., Martin, M. and Domingo, M. 2002. Porcine reproductive and respiratory syndrome virus (PRRSV) infection status in pigs naturally affected with post weaning multisystemic wasting syndrome (PMWS) in Spain. *Vet. Microbiol.* 85:23–30.

52. Sharma, R. and Saikumar, G. 2008. Porcine circovirus 2 associated reproductive failure in Indian pigs. *Indian J. Anim. Sci.* 78:1238-40.

53. Stevenson, G. W., Kiupel, M., Mittal, S. K., Choi, J., Latimer, K. S. and Kanitz, L. 2001. Tissue distribution and genetic typing of porcine circoviruses in pigs with naturally occurring congenital tremors. *J. Vet. Diagn. Invest.* 13:57–62.

54. Tischer, I., Rasch, R. and Tochterman, G. 1974. Characterization of papovavrius and picornavirus like particles in permanent pig kidney cell lines. *Zentbl. Bakteriol.* 226:153–167.

55. Tischer, I., Gelderblom, H., Vettermann, W. and Koch, M. A. 1982. A very small porcine virus with circular single-stranded DNA. *Nature* 295:64–66.

56. Todd, D., Niagro, F. D., Ritchie, B. W., Curran, W., Allan, G. M., Lukert, P. D. Latimer, K. S., Steffens, W. L. 3rd and McNutty, M. S. 1991. Comparison of three animal viruses with circular single-stranded DNA genomes. *Arch. Virol.* 117:129–135.

57. Vincent, I. E., Carrasco, C. P., Herrmann, B., Meehan, B. M., Allan, G. M. Summerfield, A. and McCullough, K. C. 2003. Dendritic cells harbour infectious porcine circovirus type 2 in the absence of apparent cell modulation or replication of the virus. *J. Virol.* 77:13288–13300.

5. Porcine Epidemic Diarrhea

Rinku Sharma, and G. Saikumar

Introduction
Porcine epidemic diarrhea (PED) is an infectious and highly contagious viral disease of pigs described for the first time in Great Britain in 1971 and characterized by acute watery diarrhea, depression, and anorexia (Oldham, 1972). Presently, the virus is widely distributed throughout Europe and Asia, but it has not been detected in USA. PED virus (PEDV) is an extremely important pathogen causing an enteric disease in pigs of all ages and clinically resembles transmissible gastroenteritis (TGE). The mortality in piglets may reach up to 90%. Besides the mortality, PEDV infection causes important economic losses due to decrease in the productive indexes.

Etiology
PEDV is a single-stranded, enveloped RNA virus of the family Coronaviridae, order Nidovirales, which also includes transmissible gastroenteritis virus (TGEV), feline infectious peritonitis virus (FIPV), and human respiratory coronavirus 229E (HCV 229E) (Murphy et al., 1999). The sequence of the entire genome of strain CV777 is 28,033 nucleotides in length (excluding the poly A-tail) (Kocherhans et al., 2001). The envelope contains four main viral structural proteins: glycoprotein spike S (180-220 kDa) found in the viral protrusions (corona), nucleocapsid phosphoprotein N (45-57 kDa), membrane M (27-32 kDa), and small membrane sM (7 kDa) (Locker et al., 1992; SangGeon et al., 2003). Four major open reading frames (ORFs) have been identified in the 4 kb nearest to the 3' end of the genome. Three of them encode the distinctive coronavirus structural proteins N, sM, and M. The spike protein gene (S) has a central role in the induction of the immune response, and it also mediates essential biological functions such as recognition of target cells and fusion of viral and cellular membranes. There is only a single serotype of PEDV. Replication of the virus occurs in the host cell cytoplasm. Assembly of virus occurs by budding through intracytoplasmic membranes.

Epizootiology
PEDV is transmitted mainly by feco-oral route from infected animals. Entrance of the virus in a farm occurs by infected animals by way of transport trucks, virus-contaminated boots, or other infected fomites.

The virus is stable between pH 5.0 and 9.0 at 4°C and between pH 6.5 and 7.5 at 37°C. Cell-culture adapted PEDV loses infectivity when heated to 60°C for thirty minutes but is moderately stable at 50°C. PEDV is inactivated by most virucidal disinfectants, including cresol, sodium hydroxide (2.0%), formalin (1.0%), sodium carbonate (4.0% anhydrous or 10.0% crystalline, with 0.1% detergent), ionic and nonionic detergents, and strong iodophors (1.0%) in phosphoric acid and lipid solvents such as chloroform. Enzootic forms of the disease have also been described. After an acute outbreak, the virus can disappear or persist causing an enzootic infection. The disease occurs usually between November and April. However, the enzootic form of PED, which may be a sequel to the epizootic form, is becoming a major problem in persistent preweaning diarrhea and occurs all year-round (Chae et al., 2000). Antibodies against PEDV have been detected in swine sera from Belgium, England, the Federal Republic of Germany, France, the Netherlands, Switzerland, Bulgaria, and Taiwan but not from Sweden, North Ireland, the United States, Australia, and Hungary (De bouck et al., 1982). It has been suggested that PCV-2 may be involved in the pathogenesis of PEDV infection in neonatal piglets (Jung et al., 2005).

OCCURRENCE

In West Germany, blood samples collected from 158 farms with a history of recent outbreaks of diarrhea revealed that 28% had antibodies against PEDV (Prager and Witte, 1983). In Belgium, about 7% of the outbreaks in which diarrhea and death in baby pigs was observed were found to be caused by PEDV (Pensaert, 1992). A serological survey carried out in 1993–1994 in Spain detected antibodies against the virus in 54% of the breeding herds (Carvajal et al., 1995). The PED has been reported in England (Wood, 1977), Belgium (Pensaert and De bouck, 1978), Canada (Turgeon et al., 1980), Hungary (Horvath and Mocsari, 1981), Germany (Pospischil et al., 1981), and Japan (Sueyoshi et al., 1995). Several outbreaks of the disease have been reported in Western Europe and Korea (De bouck et al., 1982; Chae et al., 2000). In Europe, PEDV antibodies were recorded in about 19–28% pigs. Seroprevalence of enteric viruses of pigs in Assam, India, was studied by Barman et al. (2003), and a high percentage of serum samples were positive for rotavirus (51.1%), followed by TGEV (39.4%), and PEDV (21.2%). About 13.6% of the individual pig serum samples were shown to have antibodies against all the three viruses. A comparatively higher percentage of seroreactors were detected in pigs reared under intensive farming system than that of open grazing system.

SYMPTOMATOLOGY

The main clinical sign in suckling piglets is watery diarrhea, possibly preceded by vomiting. Most fattening pigs and weaners recover from the disease, but some may remain unthrifty. In adults, anorexia, lethargy, and diarrhea are seen, but mortality is very low. Outbreaks on breeding farms may show much variation in morbidity and mortality. On some farms, animals of all ages become sick with morbidity approaching 100%. The disease is then very similar to TGE, except for a slower spread and a lower mortality in baby piglets. Piglets up to one week of age may die from dehydration after the diarrhea has lasted three to four days. Older animals recover after about one week. Comparing high morbidity, the mortality is usually low in adult pigs (3%), which can recover within a week. However, when suckling pigs are involved, mortality is normally about 50% and can reach up to 90% in very severe outbreaks. PEDV infection causes acute enteritis in swine of all ages and is often fatal in neonatal piglets. Much less variation is observed during an outbreak on fattening farms. All fattening animals within the herd show diarrhea and recover after one week. A mortality rate of 1–3% is seen in fattening animals. They die acutely, usually in the early stages of diarrhea or even prior to the appearance of diarrhea. The highest mortality rate is found on farms with stress-sensitive animals. In general, PEDV replication starts more easily in the intestine of feeder and fattening pigs than in baby pigs. Consequently, fattening animals are more susceptible to the virus, and 100% morbidity during an outbreak is common (Pensaert, 1992).

PATHOGENESIS

Oral infection results in viral replication in the epithelial cells of the small intestinal villi. Cells on colonic villi also become infected. No other tissue tropism has been shown. The virus infects and replicates in the cytoplasm of differentiated enterocytes in the villi of the small intestine (Song et al., 2006). This leads to villus atrophy and malabsorption, maldigestion, severe diarrhea, and dehydration. Replication may also take place in the crypts and mesenteric lymph nodes, but the infection at these sites always remained scattered and is possibly nonproductive. A reduction of villous height-crypt depth ratio from the normal 7:1 value to 3:1 could be observed in experimentally infected piglets. No cell degeneration is seen in the colonic epithelial cells. The pathogenetic features of PEDV in the small intestine of piglets are very similar to those of TGEV. Since viral replication and progress of the infection in the small intestine with PEDV occurs at a slower rate, a longer incubation period is observed. PEDV replication in piglets has not been detected in cells outside the intestinal tract. The virus is excreted in the feces.

The pathogenesis of PEDV in older swine has not been studied in much detail, but fluorescence is found in the epithelial cells of small intestinal and colonic villi of conventional fattening swine after experimental as well as natural infection.

Pathogenetic explanation cannot be given for sudden death with acute back muscle necrosis often observed in finishing pigs and adult animals (Pensaert, 1992). It is suggested that numerous cytosolic enzymes are released into the membrane early in the course of PEDV infection. Therefore, increased enzymatic activities may result from rapid destruction of PEDV-infected villous enterocytes. After sloughing of infected villous enterocytes in late infection, enzymatic activities are significantly decreased in jejunal villous enterocytes from PEDV-inoculated pigs compared to negative control pigs (Jung et al., 2006a).

PATHOLOGY
GROSS LESIONS
The lesions are confined to the small intestine, which is distended with yellow fluid. The intestine of diarrheic piglets is distended with yellowish watery contents and sometimes may contain flecks of curdled, undigested milk. The intestinal wall becomes thin and transparent, and the mucosa is congested. The stomach may also get distended, and wall becomes thin. The mesenteric vessels are congested, and the mesenteric lymph nodes are occasionally enlarged and edematous (Coussement et al., 1982). Occasionally, a few sows may die acutely and show back muscle necrosis at necropsy.

MICROSCOPICAL LESIONS
Microscopically, vacuolation and exfoliation of enterocytes on the small intestinal villi is observed at the time of onset of diarrhea. This is followed by shortening of the villi. The most consistent and predominant lesion in the diarrheic piglets is moderate to severe multifocal to diffuse villous atrophy in the distal portion of the jejunum and proximal portion of the ileum. Villi are often fused and covered with a degenerated or regenerated flattened epithelium. Rarely, villi are seen that lack an epithelial lining. Vacuolated enterocytes are seen on the tip of the villi or spread over the entire villi in the jejunum. Moderate numbers of exfoliated enterocytes are seen on scattered villi. The lamina propria is infiltrated with small numbers of eosinophils and neutrophils. The crypts of Lieberkuhn appear normal. The cecum and colon show no apparent changes except for vacuolation of the superficial enterocytes. No lesions are seen in other tissues (Kim and Chae, 2000). Both TGEV and PEDV infections can cause severe villous atrophy in the proximal and distal jejunum and also in the ileum. This is in contrast to rotavirus infection, where villous atrophy is found only in the distal jejunum and ileum (Pospischil et al., 1981). Congenital infection with PCV-2 produced a longer clinical course and more severe histopathological lesions in pigs infected postnatally with PEDV (Jung et al., 2006b).

ULTRASTRUCTURAL LESIONS

PED viral particles in infected piglets are observed as numerous pleomorphic coronavirus-like particles, which are generally spherical to oval, enveloped, and centrally depressed. They are surrounded by a single fringe of regularly spaced petal or club-shaped projections attached to the particles by a short, thin stalk. The virions range in size from 80–150 nm. Intracellular viral particles are observed inside intracytoplasmic vesicles or between lamellae of endoplasmic reticulum. Extracellular viral particles range in diameter from 60–90 nm. They consist of an outer unit membrane, separated by a narrow clear zone from an inner dense core. The inner core often shows a central clear halo. Intracellular virus formation is seen by budding through membranes of the endoplasmic reticulum. Ultrastructural changes occur mainly in the cytoplasm of enterocytes (Pospischil et al., 1981) in which cell organelles show decreased electron translucent areas. In the colon, some cellular changes are observed in enterocytes containing virus particles, but no exfoliation is seen (Pensaert, 1992). The cisternae of endoplasmic reticulum often are dilated. Mitochondria become rounded, with distorted cristae. The nuclei are slightly swollen. The Golgi complex often appears with a multilaminated, onionlike structure surrounded by numerous vesicles. The microvilli are short and irregular, and the terminal web is fragmented. The cell loses its columnar shape and has an irregular outline. Sometimes, the tripartite junctions also lose contact, and the cell is released from the epithelium into the gut lumen (Ducatelle et al., 1982). Ultrastructural lesions in the colon may contribute to the severity of the diarrhea.

DIAGNOSIS

A diagnosis of PED cannot be made on a clinical basis alone. Acute PED outbreak in which diarrhea is observed in animals of all ages cannot be clinically differentiated from TGE. Hence, suitable diagnostic methods should be applied for proper diagnosis of PED.

LABORATORY DIAGNOSIS

An etiologic diagnosis can be made in the laboratory by direct demonstration of PEDV and/or its antigens by detection of antibodies. A sensitive and reliable method for diagnosis in older animals as well as in piglets is the ELISA test on fecal material or intestinal contents. Fecal material should be collected from several animals, preferably during the acute phase of diarrhea.

The blocking ELISA is more sensitive than fixed-cell ELISA and highly discriminating between infected and noninfected pigs. The test is recommended for routine diagnostic testing and serologic surveys of PED. Even though serum-neutralization test (SNT) shows high specificity, it is not useful for mass screening of swine sera for diagnosis of PED and is time-consuming and labor-intensive immunoassay. The ELISA has been shown to detect IgG, including maternal antibodies at a very low level, but it detects IgM antibodies to a lesser degree. In contrast, the SNT detects both IgM and IgG antibodies. Keeping in view the advantages and disadvantages of both the assays, the PEDV-ELISA is considered to be more reliable for the detection of PEDV antibody with high sensitivity and specificity for serodiagnosis of PEDV infection, especially on a large scale (Jin sik oh et al., 2005). Indirect ELISA is also helpful to determine the seroprevalence of PEDV (Barman et al., 2003). The use of a Mab-based ELISA for PEDV antigen allows the detection of virus shedding for longer periods (Carvajal et al., 1995).

Immunohistochemical detection of PEDV antigen in formalin-fixed, paraffin-embedded tissues provides a rapid means of confirmation of a histopathological diagnosis of PEDV infection because PEDV is difficult to isolate in cell culture (Hofmann and Wyler, 1988). Specific PEDV antigens can be detected in high concentration in the cytoplasm of enterocytes, mainly in the small intestinal mucosa by the streptavidin-biotin (SAB) technique. The infected enterocytes tend to be less numerous in severe than in moderate villus atrophy. Polyclonal (Sueyoshi et al., 1995) or monoclonal (Kim et al., 1999) antibody-based immunohistochemical detection of PEDV antigen in intestinal tissues can be attempted. Positive enterocytes are distributed over the tip and along the sides of atrophied or fused villi in the jejunum and ileum. A direct fluorescent antibody test (FAT) on cryostat sections has been reported as the most sensitive and reliable method for detection of PEDV (Pensaert, 1992). However, formaldehyde fixation simplifies handling of tissue specimens and allows improvement of quality of the sections.

In situ hybridization (ISH) is a valuable adjunct to standard RNA extraction techniques for evaluating gene expression in tissues and cells. Digoxigenin-labeled (DIG-labeled) DNA probes can be used for generating hybridization signals, which are observed mainly in villus enterocytes of jejunum and ileum of naturally and experimentally infected piglets (Kim and Chae, 2000; Kim and Chae, 2003). In contrast to immunohistochemistry (IHC), ISH is less susceptible to structural alteration caused by fixation. Although antigenic cross-reactivity might not be a problem with ISH, the specificity of nucleic acid hybridization has its own limitations. To avoid nonspecific hybridization of the probe, both reverse transcription and the PCR must be performed under stringent conditions. The greater sensitivity of ISH than IHC has been attributed to higher quantities of PEDV nucleic acid than of proteins. Early in the viral cycle, quantities of viral nucleic acid may predominate over protein (Lai, 1990).

Immune electron microscopy (IEM) and immuno-gold conjugate (IGC) IEM techniques have been used for the detection of PEDV in feces and intestinal contents (Kim et al., 1995). Both IEM and IGC-IEM techniques are rapid and sensitive methods for detection and identification of PEDV. Counterimmunoelectrophoresis (CIE) can be used for diagnosis of PEDV infection in fecal samples. RT-PCR assay can detect virus in the very early stage of infection in natural and experimentally infected pigs (Ishikawa et al., 1997; Kweon et al., 1997; Kim and Chae, 1999). A multiplex RT-PCR for rapid differential detection of PEDV, TGEV, and porcine group A rotavirus has been developed (Song et al., 2006). RT-PCR-based dot blot hybridization can increase the sensitivity by a hundred—to a thousandfold (Jung and Chae, 2005).

Virus isolation is often considered to be the gold standard of viral diagnostic techniques. However, there are inherent difficulties in isolating PEDV in cell culture. The growth of the virus in Vero cell cultures is trypsin dependent. PEDV cannot be cultured in Vero cells without adaptation after several passages. Isolation and propagation of PEDV in cell culture is essential to provide large quantities of virus for detailed characterization of virus and control of the disease. Viral replication leads to characteristic cytopathic effects such as vacuolation, formation of syncytia, and fusion of cells. PEDV is unable to grow in porcine cell cultures (Hofmann and Wyler, 1988; Kim and Chae, 1999). However, propagation of a strain of PEDV, P-5V, which is utilized as a live virus vaccine in Japan, was attempted in swine cell lines KSEK6 and IBRS-2 cells. A clear cytopathic effect (CPE) characterized by cellular destruction was observed in the infected cells on two to three days postinfection (DPI), and affected cells were completely degenerated on 4 days postinfection. The virus was serially passaged in the cells even without addition of trypsin. Small but clear plaques were formed under an agar overlay medium on the cells (Kadoi et al., 2002).

PREVENTION AND CONTROL
Specific therapy for PED is not recommended. Symptomatic treatment of diarrhea should be done, including free access to water to diminish dehydration and withholding of feed, particularly in growing swine. Sanitary

measures should be taken to prevent introduction of PEDV to the farm. Introduction of persistently infected pigs poses the highest risk, and disease can also spread by human personnel movement between affected units. After diagnosis of PED, because of the slow spread of disease, the primary concern should be initiation of preventive measures to temporarily prevent virus entrance into farrowing units. Artificial exposure of pregnant sows to feces from PEDV-infected pigs stimulates lactogenic immunity and helps to postpone infection of these sows' piglets until they are older, resulting in fewer deaths. If persistence of the virus is diagnosed in consecutive litters of weaned piglets after an outbreak has occurred, virus elimination can be attempted by removing pigs immediately after weaning to another site for at least four weeks. Recently, the immunoprophylactic effects of chicken egg yolk immunoglobulin (IgY) against PEDV were investigated in neonatal pigs. Administration of IgY was associated with reduced mortality and increased survival rate in piglets after challenge exposure to PEDV. This suggests that IgY against PEDV might be an alternative prophylactic measure similar to stimulated lactogenic immunity. Live vaccines for PED are used in Korea (KPEDV-9) and Japan (P-5V) due to endemic nature of the disease (Kweon et al., 1999; Kadoi et al., 2002).

REFERENCES

1. Barman, N. N., Barman, B., Sarma, D. K. and Pensaert, M. B. 2003. Prevalence of rotavirus, TEGV and PEDV antibodies in pigs of Assam, *Indian J. Anim. Sci.* 73:576–578.
2. Carvajal, A., Lanza, I., Diego, R., Rubio, P. and Carmenes, P. 1995. Seroprevalence of PEDV infection among different types of breeding swine farms in Spain. *Prev. Vet. Med.* 23:33–40.
3. Chae, C., Kim, O., Choi, C., Min, K., Cho, W. S., Kim, J. and Tai, J. H. 2000. Prevalence of PEDV and TEGV infection in Korean pigs. *Vet. Rec.* 147:606–608.
4. Coussement, W., Ducatelle, R., De bouck, P. and Hoorens, J. 1982. Pathology of experimental CV777 coronavirus enteritis in piglets. I. Histological and histochemical study. *Vet. Pathol.* 19:46–56.
5. De bouck, P., Callebaut, P. and Pensaert, M. 1982. Prevalence of PED virus in the pig population of different countries. *Proc. Int. Pig. Vet. Soc. Congr.* 7:53.
6. Ducatelle, R., Coussement, W., De bouck, P. and Hoorens, J. 1982. Pathology of experimental CV777 Coronavirus enteritis in piglets. II. Electron microscopic study. *Vet. Pathol.* 19:57–66.
7. Hofmann, M. and Wyler, R. 1988. Propagation of the virus of porcine epidemic diarrhea in cell culture. *J. Clin. Microbiol.* 26:2235–2239.
8. Horvath, I. and Mocsari, E. 1981. Ultrastructural changes in the small intestinal epithelium of suckling pigs affected with a TGE-like disease. *Arch. Virol.* 68:103–113.
9. Ishikawa, K., Sekiguchi, H., Ogino, T. and Suzuki, S. 1997. Direct and rapid detection of PEDV by RT-PCR. *J. Virol. Methods.* 69:191–195.
10. Jin sik Oh., Song, D. S., Yang, J. S., Song, J. Y., Moon, H. J., Kim, T. Y. and Park, B. K. 2005. Comparison of an ELISA with serum neutralization test for serodiagnosis of PEDV infection. *J. Vet. Sci.* 6:349–352.
11. Jung, K. and Chae, C. 2005. RT-PCR based dot blot hybridization for the detection and differentiation between PEDV and TEGV in fecal samples using a non-radioactive digoxigenin c-DNA probe. *J. Virol. Methods.* 123:141–146.

12. Jung, K., Kim, J., Ha, Y., Choi, C. and Chae, C. 2006. The effects of transplacental porcine circovirus type-2 infection on porcine epidemic diarrhea virus-induced enteritis in preweaning piglets. *The Vet. J.* 171:445–450.

13. Jung, K., Ahn, K. and Chae, C. 2006a. Decreased activity of brush-border membrane-bound digestive enzymes in small intestines from pigs experimentally infected with PED virus. *Res. Vet. Sci.* 81:310–315.

14. Jung, K., Ha, Y., Ha, S. K., Kim, J., Kim, S. H. and Chae, C. 2006b. Identification of PCV type-2 in retrospective cases of pigs naturally infected with porcine epidemic diarrhea virus. *The Vet. J.* 171: 166–168.

15. Kadoi, K., Sugioka, H., Satoh, T. and Kadoi, B. K. 2002. The propagation of a PEDV in swine cell lines. *Microbiol.* 25:285–290.

16. Kim, O. and Chae, C. 1999. Application of RT-PCR to detect porcine epidemic diarrhea virus in Vero cell culture. *J. Vet. Diagn. Invest.* 11:537–538.

17. Kim, O. and Chae, C. 2000. In-situ hybridization for the detection and localization of PEDV in the intestinal tissues from naturally infected piglets. *Vet. Pathol.* 37:62–67.

18. Kim, O. and Chae, C. 2003. Experimental infection of piglets with a Korean strain of porcine epidemic diarrhea virus. *J. Comp. Pathol.* 129:55–60.

19. Kim, O., Chae, C. and Kweon, C. H. 1999. Monoclonal antibody-based immunohistochemical detection of PEDV antigen in formalin-fixed, paraffin-embedded intestinal tissues. *J. Vet. Diagn. Invest.* 11:458–462.

20. Kim, J. H., Hwang, E. K., Bae, T. C., Son, H. J., Park, J. W. and Yoon, Y. D. 1995. Detection of PEDV by immuno-electron microscopy and immuno-gold conjugate immuno-electron microscopy. *Korean J. Vet. Res.* 35:575–581.

21. Kocherhans, R., Bridgen, A., Ackermann, M. and Tobler, K. 2001. Completion of the porcine epidemic diarrhea coronavirus (PEDV) genome sequence. *Virus Gen.* 23:137–144.

22. Kweon, C. H., Lee, J. G., Han, M. G. and Kang, Y. B. 1997. Rapid diagnosis of PEDV infection by PCR. *J. Vet. Med. Sci.* 59:231–232.

23. Kweon, C. H., Kwon, B. J., Lee, J. G., Kwon, G. O. and Kang, Y. B. 1999. Derivation of attenuated PEDV as vaccine candidate. *Vaccine* 17:2546–2553.

24. Lai, M. M. C. 1990. Coronavirus: Organization, replication and expression of genome. *Ann. Rev. Microbiol.* 44:303–333.

25. Locker, J. K., Rose, J. K., Horzinek, M. C. and Rottier, P. J. M. 1992. Membrane assembly of the triple-spanning coronavirus M protein. Individual transmembrane domains show preferred orientation. *J. Biol. Chem.* 267:21911–21918.

26. Murphy, F. A., Gibbs, E. P. J., Horzinek, M. C. and Studdert, M. J. 1999. Viral taxonomy and nomenclature. In *Veterinary virology*, ed. F. A. Murphy et al., 23–42. San Diego, EE UU: Academic Press.

27. Oldham, J. 1972. *Pig farming*, Oct. Suppl. 72–73.

28. Pensaert, M. B. 1992. Porcine epidemic diarrhea. In *Diseases of swine*, ed. A. D. Leman, B. E. Straw, W. L. Mengeling, S. D. Allaire, and D. J. Taylor, 293–298. London: 7th Wolfe Publishing Ltd.

29. Pensaert, M. B. and De bouck, P. 1978. A new coronavirus-like particle associated with diarrhea in swine. *Arch. Virol.* 58:243–247.

30. Pijipers, A., Niustadt, A. Von, P., Terpstra, S., Verheijden, J. H. M., and Van Nieuwstadt, A. P. 1993. PEDV as a cause of persistent diarrhea in herd of breeding and finishing pigs. *Vet. Rec.* 132:129–131.

31. Pospischil, A., Hess, R. G. and Bachmann, P. A. 1981. Light microscopy and ultrahistology of intestinal changes in pigs infected with epizootic diarrhea virus 32. (EVD): Comparison with transmissible gastroenteritis (TGE) virus and porcine rotavirus infections. *Zentralblatt fur Veterinarmedizin* B 28:564–577.

32. Prager, D. and Witte, K. 1983. Die Haufigkeit von TGE–und Epizootische virusdiarrhoe-(EVD)-Virusinfektionen als Ursachen-Seuchenhafter Durchfaelle in Westfaelischen Schweinenzucht-und-mastbestaenden. *Tieraerztl. Umschau.* 38:155–158.

33. Sang-Geon, Y., Mercedes, H., Peter, J. K. and Eva, N. 2003. Cloning and sequence analysis of spike gene of PEDV Chinju 99. *Virus Genes* 26:239–246.

34. Song, D. S., Kang, B. K., Oh, J. S., Ha, G. W., Yang, J. S., Moon, H. J., Jang, Y. S. and Park, B. K. 2006. Multiplex RT-PCR for rapid differential detection of PEDV, TEGV and porcine group A rotavirus. *J. Vet. Diagn. Invest.* 18:278–281.

35. Sueyoshi, M., Tsuda, T., Yamazaki, K., Yoshida, K., Nakazawa, M., Sato, K., Minami, T., Iwashita, K., Watanabe, M., Suzuki, Y. and Mori, M. 1995. An immunohistochemical investigation of PED. *J. Comp. Path.* 113:59–67.

36. Turgeon, D. C., Morin, M., Jolette, J., Higgins, R., Marsolais, G. and Difranco, E. 1980. Coronavirus-like particles associated with diarrhea in baby pigs in Quebec. *Can. Vet. J.* 21:100–101.

37. Wood, E. N. 1977. An apparently new syndrome of porcine epidemic diarrhea. *Vet. Rec.* 100:243–244.

6. Porcine Parvovirus Disease

Rinku Sharma, and G. Saikumar

Introduction
Porcine parvovirus (PPV) is the major cause of SMEDI (*S*, stillbirth; *M*, mummification; *ED*, embryonic death; *I*, infertility) syndrome. It also leads to neonatal mortality and occasional abortions in sows. It was first associated with reproductive losses in swine by Cartwright and Huck (1967). Porcine parvovirus disease is an important infectious cause of reproductive failure in swine throughout the world, and the outbreaks lead to severe economic losses.

Etiology
PPV is a member of the family Parvoviridae, subfamily Parvovirinae, genus *Parvovirus*, which includes small nonenveloped, single-stranded DNA viruses (Berns, 1996). Although PPV is distinguishable from parvoviruses of all other species, it is antigenically related to some. The virion has a cubic symmetry with a diameter of 20±1 nm. The genome comprises of about 5000 bp, encodes five proteins, two of which are capsid proteins and the other three are the nonstructural (NS) proteins. The genome contains two large open reading frames (ORFs), both located in the same frame of the complementary strand. The left ORF encodes the nonstructural protein NS1, and the right ORF encodes the three-capsid proteins (Ranz et al., 1989, Bergeron et al., 1993). Structural proteins VP1 and VP2 may vary between some strains of PPV (Bergeron et al., 1996).

All isolates of PPV that have been compared to date have been found to be antigenically similar if not identical, and so it appears that there is a single serotype (Mengeling et al., 2000). Differences have been reported with regard to the relative virulence of a few isolates. The virulent strain of PPV, IAF-A54, is associated with dermatitis (Kresse et al., 1985). The NADL-2 strain is nonpathogenic and causes limited viremia and is used currently as an attenuated vaccine, while Kresse is a pathogenic strain, which kills immunocompetent fetus (Choi et al., 1987). Viral replication takes place in the nucleus and requires host cell functions of late S phase or early G2 phase of the cell division cycle. Infection leads to large intranuclear inclusion bodies. PPV agglutinates human, monkey, guinea pig, cat, chicken, rat, and mouse erythrocytes.

Epizootiology
The virus is infective via the oronasal, transplacental, and venereal routes. The oronasal route is believed to be the most important. Virus is shed for

about two weeks after infection, in feces, urine, semen, and nasal secretions. The greatest source of infection is the fluids and fetal membranes of farrowed sows. The virus can persist for four months or more in the environment. Introduction of virus to susceptible herds results in 100% infection rate within three months. Viruses are very stable, resisting 60°C for sixty minutes and pH 3–9.

If a pig becomes infected for the first time when it is not pregnant, there are no clinical signs. However, if the animal is pregnant and exposed for the first time in the first fifty-five days of pregnancy, the virus crosses the placenta killing piglets selectively. If the fetus is infected at less than thirty-five days of age, death and complete resorption may occur, and ultimately a small litter is born. If infection takes place between thirty and fifty-five days of pregnancy, the fetuses die and become mummified. It takes ten to fourteen days from first infection for PPV to reach the piglets inside the uterus. From seventy days of age, the immune system of the piglet develops, and it can therefore respond and protect itself from the virus. Thus, if pregnant sows are infected for the first time after fifty-five days of pregnancy, there will be little evidence of disease. Once inside the uterus, PPV spreads slowly from one fetus to another, and as a result, the size of mummified pigs varies within the litter.

PPV outbreaks usually resolve because of developing herd immunity, but congenitally infected excretors may form a reservoir of infection. In endemically infected herds, 98–100% of adult pigs show serological evidence of active immunity. Active immunity is associated with high persistent levels of hemagglutination-inhibiting (HI) antibody (greater than 256), piglets suckling immune sows acquiring HI titers between 10 000 and 40 000 (Johnson et al., 1976). Boars play a significant role in dissemination of PPV by shedding the virus in semen during acute infection (McAdaragh and Anderson, 1975). Antibodies to PPV have also been detected in wild boars (Roi et al., 2005).

OCCURRENCE
PPV infection has been reported from a large number of countries of the world like Australia, New Zealand, Yugoslavia, Canada, Philippines, Japan, Hungary, Czechoslovakia, Norway, Finland, Sweden, Netherlands, Switzerland, Germany, Panama, and Mozambique. PPV was isolated from U.S. farms with neonatal losses, partially mummified, aborted, stillborn, myoclonic and splayed leg piglets, piglets with atrophy of the intestinal mucosa, and hare-hipped piglets by Johnson and Collings (1971). PPV infection was confirmed in 46/203 litters obtained from slaughtered sows in an U.S. abbatoir

(Mengeling, 1978). PPV infection was detected in 45% of the 602 macerated and mummified fetuses and stillborn piglets obtained from Danish breeding herds with reproductive disorders (Sorensen and Askaa, 1981).

In Korea, PPV was isolated from 27.7% cases of abortion and stillbirths examined in an eight-year period study (Huang et al., 1998). PPV has been isolated not only from herds with a history of stillbirths, neonatal losses, infertility or abortions but also from piglets with myofibrillar hypoplasia, sows with abnormal vaginal discharges, the semen of boars with low fertility and sows with respiratory disorders, loss of condition (Cartwright et al., 1969), dermatitis (Kresse et al., 1985), and enteric diseases (Duhamel et al., 1991). In a recent study conducted in this laboratory, PPV infection was diagnosed in 7.14% litters from an organized farm in Northern India showing reproductive failure characterized by mummified fetuses, small litter size, and neonatal mortality (Sharma, 2007).

Clinical Signs

In case of an acute outbreak of the disease, the reproductive problems are characterized by small litters associated with embryo loss before thirty-five days, mummified pigs of varying size (30–160mm), and increased numbers of stillbirths. These signs are associated with the delay in farrowing, which occurs because of the presence of mummified piglets. Abortions associated with PPV infection are uncommon. There may be an increase in low birth-weight piglets, which may sometimes die within two days of age. Infected sows show no clinical symptoms. The weaners and growers do not exhibit any clinical signs.

Pathogenesis

The susceptible pigs are infected either by oronasal or venereal route. The infection is followed by viremia and sometimes leucopenia. The virus replicates in the epithelium of the alimentary tract with viremia, without causing clinical signs in fattening and breeding stock. PPV replicates in lymph nodes, tonsils, thymus, spleen, lungs, salivary glands, and other organs. It replicates well in peripheral blood lymphocytes and stimulate their proliferation, thereby increasing the viral load. PPV causes persistent infection with chronic shedding.

Transplacental infection can occur with embryonic and fetal death and intrauterine spread of the virus. The virus adheres to the zona pellucida of the embryos. The result of infection in an individual gilt or sow depends on the gestational stage. Fetuses infected before seventy days gestation, i.e., before the estimated stage of immunocompetance for PPV usually die, whereas fetuses infected later in gestation develop antibodies to PPV and usually survive (Bachman et al., 1975; Mengeling and Paul, 1981).

PATHOLOGY
GROSS LESIONS
No gross or microscopic lesions have been reported in nonpregnant pigs (Brown et al., 1980). Gross lesions have not been reported in pregnant dams. In case of embryos, death occurs followed by resorption of fluids and then soft tissues. If the fetuses are infected before they develop immunocompetence, then they show many lesions. These include stunting, loss of condition, an increased prominence of blood vessels over the surface of the fetus due to congestion and leakage of blood into contiguous tissues, congestion, edema, and hemorrhage with accumulation of serosangineous fluid in body cavities, hemorrhagic discoloration becoming progressively darker after death and dehydration (mummified). Many of these changes may also be observed in the placenta. The liver may be enlarged and congested with a mottled appearance. The heart shows paleness, enlargement, rounding due to dilatation, or eccentric hypertrophy of one or both the ventricles (van Leengoed et al., 1983).

MICROSCOPIC LESIONS
Stillborn and aborted fetuses infected with PPV reveal meningoencephalitis characterized by perivascular cuffing with proliferating adventitial cells, histiocytes, and a few plasma cells in the gray and white matter of the cerebrum and in the leptomeninges. Heart shows diffuse infiltration of mononuclear cells with only local perivascular cuffing in the myocardium and occasionally in the endocardium of the ventricles and the atrium (Narita et al., 1975). Microscopic lesions in gilts killed after fetuses are infected by transuterine inoculation of virus include focal accumulation of mononuclear cells adjacent to the endometrium and in deeper layers of the lamina propria (van Leengoed et al., 1983).

The findings in naturally infected mummified and neonatal piglets include presence of serosanaguineous fluid in the body cavities; edematous, noncollapsible, congested lungs with hemorrhages; mild necrotizing interstitial pneumonia; enlarged heart with prominent myocardial congestion and hemorrhages, increased pericardial fluid, myocarditis; severely congested or pale friable liver, hemorrhages, congested sinusoids, disorientation of hepatic cords, degenerated hepatocytes; congested or pale swollen kidneys, multiple areas of diffuse hemorrhages, severe degeneration of epithelial cells of PCTs; meningeal congestion, mild perivascular cuffing, multifocal areas of malacia, and focal gliosis in the subependymal region (Sharma, 2007).

DIAGNOSIS

1. *Clinical and pathological diagnosis.* Based on history of reproductive failure and the gross and histopathological findings, a presumptive diagnosis of PPV infection can be made. Definitive diagnosis requires laboratory tests such as immunostaining on fetal tissues, isolation in cell culture, HA on feces, rising antibody titers in paired serum samples by hemagglutination inhibition, PCR, and in situ hybridization.

2. *Laboratory Diagnosis.* Polymerase chain reaction is very sensitive and can be used to identify a segment of the PPV genome under conditions that preclude virus isolation, e.g., in the presence of neutralizing antibody. PCR can detect the virus in a variety of fetal tissues like lung, liver, kidney, and body fluids. PCR using primers coding for the major structural protein VP2 has been developed (Molitor et al., 1991 and Arnauld et al., 1998). Nested PCR detects the PPV DNA with an approximately three hundred times more sensitivity than the standard PCR assay (Belak et al., 1998; Lelesius et al., 2007). In another study, Soares et al. (1999) developed a PCR and nested-PCR assay using primers directed to the highly conserved nonstructural coding region of the virus. In comparison with HA test, PCR proved to be highly specific and sensitive in detecting PPV (Zhao et al., 2003). PCR revealed fragment of VP1 gene of PPV in lung and tonsil tissues of mummified and day-old piglets from an organized farm experiencing reproductive failure in Northern India (Sharma, 2007).

Immunohistochemistry for detection of viral antigen is carried out by direct fluorescent antibody test using polyclonal antibody or by indirect immunoperoxidase staining, using either polyclonal or monoclonal antibodies. The lung is the organ of choice as it is easily collected even from mummified fetuses and has minimum of autofluorescence. Tissues from mummified fetuses less than 16 cm in length are generally preferred. In experimentally inoculed one-day-old piglets, PPV antigen could be demonstrated in germinal centers of lymph nodes, lamina propria and submucosa of gastrointestinal tract, liver, lung, pancreas, testis, and adrenal gland (Cutlip and Mengeling, 1975). In naturally infected piglets, PPV antigen was demonstrated by direct FAT and indirect IPT in formalin-fixed, paraffin-embedded tissue sections in lungs, heart, and kidney tissues (Sharma, 2007).

In situ hybridization (ISH) is an increasingly popular technique to localize and identify nucleic acid in paraffin-embedded, formalin-fixed tissues.

Since it does not depend on the antigen, the host's antibodies cannot mask the target. Waldvogel et al. (1995) employed ISH using biotinylated probe to detect PPV nucleic acid in formalin-fixed, paraffin-embedded tissue sections of heart and lung of affected fetuses. ISH with a nonradioactive digoxigenin-labeled probe has been used to detect PPV nucleic acid in macrophages of lymph node, spleen, thymus, and tonsil tissue sections of PCV2-infected weaned pigs with naturally occurring PMWS (Choi and Chae, 2000). The PPV genome could be demonstrated in lungs, heart, liver, kidney, and spleen of naturally infected mummified and neonatal piglets by DIG-labeled ISH in formalin-fixed, paraffin-embedded tissue sections (Sharma, 2007).

Virus isolation can be done on wide range of sample types. PPV has a tropism for the actively dividing cells (Bachman, 1972). Early passage cells are generally thought to be more susceptible than established cell lines. Fetal porcine kidney cell cultures, PK15, swine testicle cell lines, and IBRS-2 are commonly used for virus detection and propagation. Viral replication is cytocidal and is characterized by rounding up, pyknosis, and lysis of cells (Mengeling et al., 2000) and can also be detected by immunofluorescence test. PPV was successfully isolated in PK 15 cells, and viral replication was detected by direct FAT, indirect IPT, and DIG-ISH in the infected cover slip preparations (Sharma, 2007). Serological tests like serum neutralization (SN), HI test, ELISA, and immunodiffusion tests are used when mummified fetuses are not available. The SN test has been reported to be more sensitive than HI test (Joo et al., 1975).

Genetic analysis of the VP2 gene of PPV in Brazil revealed the existence of at least two virus lineages among the isolates in spite of high sequence similarity. These results highlight the need for close surveillance on PPV genetic drift, with an assessment of its potential ability to modify the antigenic makeup of the virus (Soares et al., 2003).

PREVENTION AND CONTROL

PPV-free herds must isolate new animals for at least three weeks in case their source herd has recently become infected. Purchase of pregnant sows should be avoided because of the risk of infection by endemic virus. PPV can be controlled by natural challenge. PPV is a resilient virus that persists in the environment. It may be excreted in the feces of weaners at eight to twelve weeks of age. Therefore, if the gilt is exposed to field challenge, particularly once maternal antibodies are declining, natural immunity will occur. This can be measured on an individual or group basis by routine serology. If natural challenge is not achieved, then commercial vaccines can be applied. In an acute outbreak, immediately vaccinate the breeding herd to prevent infection in those animals that are still seronegative. It takes ten days for the first dose of vaccine to take effect. Vaccination and stimulation of immunity by natural infection is sufficient to protect the litter from disease.

PPV vaccines are highly effective at controlling the diseases and are cost effective as well. A number of inactivated and live vaccines are available to prevent PPV infection. One of the latest killed vaccines can be used from five months of age and two initial doses (three to four weeks apart) gives protection for two years. It is important to vaccinate boars as well as sows if control is to be effective. The vaccination of seronegative sows and boars is also recommended. Mainly, the inactivated adjuvant vaccines are being currently used in UK and the live attenuated in USA. Some of the commercially available vaccines in Canada include, Parvo Shield and Parvo Shield L5E. All progeny from an infected litter should be disposed of as congenitally infected animals (which are persistently infected and intermittently shed virus) may survive from an outbreak.

References

1. Arnauld, C., Legeay, O., Laurian, Y., Thiery, R., Denis, M., Blandchard, P. and Jestin, A. 1998. Development of a PCR-based method coupled with a microplate colorimetric assay for the detection of PPV and application to diagnosis in piglet tissues and human plasma. *Mol. Cellul. Probes* 12:407–416.

2. Bachmann, P. A. 1972. PPV infection *in vitro*: A study model of the replication of parvoviruses. I. Replication at different temperatures. *Proc. Soc. Exp. Biol. Med.* 140:1369–1374.

3. Bachmann, P. A., Sheffy, B. E. and Vaughan, J. T. 1975. Experimental *in vitro* infection of fetal pigs with a PPV. *Infect. Immun.* 12:455–460.

4. Belak, S., Rivera, E., Ballagi-Pordany, A., Hanzhong, W., Widen, F. and Soos, T. 1998. Detection of challenge virus in fetal tissues by nested PCR as a test of the potency of a PPV vaccine. *Vet. Res. Commun.* 22:139–146.

5. Bergeron, J., Hebert, B. and Tijssen, P. 1996. Genome organization of the Kresse strain of PPV: Identification of the allotropic determinant and comparison with those of NADL-2 and field isolates. *J. Virol.* 70:2508–2515.

6. Bergeron, J., Menezes, J. and Tijssen, P. 1993. Genome organization of mapping of transcription and translation products of the NADL-2 strain of PPV. *Virology* 197:86–98.

7. Berns, K. I. 1996. Parvoviridae: The virus and their replication. In *Fields virology.* 3rd ed., ed. B. N. Fields, D. M. Knipe, P. M. Homley, R. M. Chanock, J. L. Melnick, T. P. Monath, B. Roizman, and S. E. Straus, 2173–2197. Philadelphia: Lippincott-Raven Publishers.

8. Roi, B., Cajavec, S., Ton, J., Madi, J., Lipej, Z., Jemer, L., Lojki, M., Mihaljevi, Z., Cac, Z., and Sostaric, B. 2005. Prevalence of antibodies to PPV in wild boars *in Croatia. J. Wildlife Dis.* 41:796–799.

9. Brown, T. T., Paul, P. S. and Mengeling, W. L. 1980. Response of conventionally raised weaning pigs to experimental infection with a virulent strained strain of PPV. *Am. J. Vet. Res.* 41:1221–1224.

10. Cartwright, S. F. and Huck, R. A. 1967. Viruses isolated in association with herd infertility, abortions and stillbirths in pigs. *Vet. Rec.* 81:196–197.

11. Cartwright, S. F., Lucas, M. and Huck, R. A. 1969. A small haemagglutinating porcine DNA virus. Isolation and properties. *J. Comp. Pathol.* 79:371–377.

12. Choi, C. and Chae, C. 2000. Distribution of PPV in PCV2 infected pigs with PMWS as shown by *in situ* hybridization. *J. Comp. Pathol.* 123:302–305.

13. Choi, C. S., Molitor, T. W., Joo, H. S. and Gunther, R. 1987. Pathogenicity of a skin isolate of PPV in swine fetuses. *Vet. Microbiol.* 15:19–29.

14. Cutlip, R. C. and Mengeling, W. L. 1975. Experimentally induced infection of neonatal swine with PPV. *Am. J. Vet. Res.* 36:1179–1182.

15. Duhamel, G. E. Bargar, T. W., Schmitt, B. J., Molitor, T. W. and Lu, W. 1991. Identification of PPV-like particles in intestinal crypt epithelial cells of pigs with diarrhea. *J. Vet. Diagn. Invest.* 3:96–98.

16. Huang, E., JaeHoon, K., ByoungHan, K., ChoiKyu, P. and Choi, S. 1998. Infectious agents associated with swine abortions and stillbirths in Korea. *RDA J. Vet. Sci.* 40:48–53.

17. Johnson, R. H. and Collings, D. F. 1971. Transplacental infection of piglets with PPV. *Res. Vet. Sci.* 12:570–572.

18. Johnson, R. H., Donaldson-Wood, C. and Allender, U. 1976 Observations on the epidemiology of PPV. *Aust. Vet. J.* 52:80–84.

19. Joo, H. S., Donaldson-Wood, C. R., Johnson, R. H. and Campbell, R. S. F. 1977. Pathogenesis of PPV infection: Pathology and immunofluorescence in the fetus. *J. Comp. Pathol.* 87:383–391.

20. Joo, H. S., Donaldson-Wood, C. R. and Johnson, R. H. 1975. A microneutralization test for the assay of PPV antibody. *Arch. Virol.* 47:337–341.

21. Kresse, J. I., Talylor, W. D., Stewart, W. W. and Eernisse, K. A. 1985. PPV infection in pigs with necrotic and vesicle-like lesions. *Vet. Microbiol.* 10:525–531.

22. Lelesius, R., Sereika, V. and Stankevicius, A. 2007. Detection of PPV by nested PCR in Lithuania. *Vet. Zoo.* 39:61.

23. McAdaragh, J. P. and Anderson, G. A. 1975. Transmission of viruses through boar semen. Proc. 18th Annu. Meet. Am. Assoc. Vet. Lab. Diagn., 69–76.

24. Mengeling, W. L. 1978. Prevalence of PPV-induced reproduction failure: An abattoir study. *J. Am. Vet. Med. Assoc.* 172:1291–1294.

25. Mengeling, W. L., Lager, K. M. and Vormald, A. C. 2000. The effect of PPV and PRRSV on porcine reproductive performance. *Ani. Reprod. Sci.* 60–61:199–210.

26. Mengeling, W. L. and Paul, P. S. 1981. Reproductive performance of gilts exposed to PPV at 56 or 70 days of gestation. *Am. J. Vet. Res.* 42:2074–2076.

27. Molitor, T. W., Draveerakul, K., Zhang, Q. Q., Choi, C. S. and Ludemann, L. R. 1991. PCR amplificiation for the detection of PPV. *J. Virol. Methods* 32:201–211.

28. Narita, M., Inui, S., Kawakami, Y., Kitamura, K. and Maeda, A. 1975. Histopathological changes of the brain in swine fetuses naturally infected with PPV. *Natl. Inst. Ani. Hlth. Q.* 15:24–28.

29. Ranz, A. I., Manclus, J. J., Diaz Aroca, E. and Casal, J. I. 1989. PPV: DNA sequence and genome organization. *J. Gen. Virol.* 70:254–2553.

30. Soares, R. M., Cortez, A., Heinemann, M. B., Sakamoto, S. M., Martins, V. G., Bacui M. Jr., Fernandes, F. M. C. and Richtzenhain, L. J. 2003. Genetic variability of PPV isolates revealed by analysis of partial sequences of the structural coding gene VP2. *J. Gen. Virol.* 84:1505–1515.

31. Soares, R. M., Durigon, E. L., Bersano, J. G. and Richtzenhain, L. J. 1999. Detection of PPV DNA by the PCR assay using primers to the highly conserved nonstructural protein gene NS-1. *J. Virol. Methods* 78:191–198.

32. Sorensen, K. J. and Askaa, J. 1981. Fetal infection with PPV in herds with reproductive failure. *Acta Vet. Scand.* 22:162–170.

33. Sharma, R. 2007. Studies on pathology and diagnosis of important viral diseases causing reproductive failure and preweaning mortality in swine. PhD thesis, IVRI, Deemed University.

34. van Leengoed, L. A., Vos, J., Gruys, E., Rondhuis, P. and Brand, A. 1983. PPV infection: Review and diagnosis in a sow herd with reproductive failure. *Vet. Q.* 5:131–141.

35. Waldvogel, A. S., Broll, S., Rosskopf, M., Schwyzer, M. and Pospischil, A. 1995. Diagnosis of fetal infection with PPV by *in situ* hybridization. *Vet. Microbiol.* 47:377–365.

36. Zhao, J., Chen, H., Lu, J., Qiu, D. and Zhou, F. 2003. Development of PCR technique for detecting PPV infection. *Chinese J. Vet. Sci.* 23:142–144.

7. Porcine Reproductive and Respiratory Syndrome

H. Kothalawala, and E. Gruys

Introduction

Porcine reproductive and respiratory syndrome (PRRS) is characterized by reproductive loses of sows and respiratory problems of piglets and growing pigs (Benfield et al., 1999). The disease was first documented in 1987 (Keffaber, 1989) in the United States of America (USA), where it is known as mystery swine disease because of the indefinable nature of its causal agent, but later was called swine infertility and respiratory syndrome. During the winter of 1990–1991, the disease emerged in Western Europe, where it spread rapidly and acquired many more names, including Abortus blauw, blue-eared pig disease, and porcine epidemic abortion and respiratory syndrome (Christianson and Joo, 1994). The name "PRRS" was generally accepted by the international veterinary community since 1998 (OIE, 2004). The presence of PRRS has been reported from various countries in Asia and a few countries in South America. Australia, New Zealand, Sweden, and Switzerland are reported to be free from PRRS viral infection (OIE, 2004).

Porcine Reproductive and Respiratory Syndrome Virus (PRRSV)

The virus that causes PRRS was first isolated in the Netherlands in June 1991(Paton et al., 1991; Wensvoort et al., 1991) The causative agent of PRRS is classified as a member of the order Nidovirales, family Arteriviridae, genus *Arterivirus* (Van Regenmortel et al., 2000; Brinton et al., 2000). It has a predilection to grow in porcine alveolar macrophages, both in vivo and in vitro. The virus is an enveloped, positive-standard RNA virus with a diameter of 50–70 nm. The genomic sequence of the virus has been determined (Conzelmann et al., 1993); the viral RNA is approximately 15 kb long and encodes eight open reading frames (ORF). Three major structural proteins have been identified: a nucleocapsid protein (N, ORF 7) of 14–15 kDa, a membrane protein (M, ORF 6) of 18–19 kDa, and an envelope glycol protein (E; ORF 5) of 24–25 kDa (Meulenberg et al., 1993). Three other less abundant structural glycoproteins are encoded by ORFs 4, 3, and 2 (Snijder and Meulenberg 1998; Dea et al; 2000). The European strains of the virus are antigenically closely related to each other, but distinct from American strains of the virus (Benfield et al., 1992; Wensvoort et al., 1992). However, the two PRRSV isolates share only 55–70% nucleotide identity in their genes (Kwang et al., 1994; Mardassi et al., 1994; Meng et al., 1994, 1995a; Morozov et al., 1995; Murtaugh et al; 1995; Ganon and Dea, 1998; Nelson et al., 1999). Among the American isolates, nucleotide homology of the ORF region was found to be 90% or even less (Murtaugh et al., 1995; Andreyev et al., 1997; Meng, 2000; Dee et al., 2001). European PRRS viruses were originally considered to be less heterogenic (Suarez et al., 1996; Indik et al., 2000) until quite recently several studies proved equally large or even larger genetic differences (70–90% homology) between European strains (Forsberg et al., 2002; Stadejek et al., 2002).

Host and Transmission

Since natural infection of birds not been discovered, domesticated pig and wild pig remain the only animals known to experience natural infection with PRRSV (Oslage et al., 1994). The primary transmission route is via close contact between carrier and susceptible pigs. Such contacts are greatly enhanced by intensive animal movements. Infection probably takes place through nose-to-nose contact or direct contact of urine or feces. The virus has been detected in nasal and fecal swabs or in urine from pigs challenged experimentally (Rossow et al., 1994). Arial transmission is another important route of transmission (Rossow et al., 1998; Lager et al., 2000). Airborne spread is generally enhanced during winter. Low-temperature wind speed and ultraviolet irradiation together with high humidity have been creating favorable condition to virus spreading in winter (Komijn et al., 1991). Transmission via insemination with contaminated semen is documented (Yeager et al., 1993; Swenson et al., 1995, Benfield et al., 2000). Several experiments have shown that virus can be present in semen from infected boars up to thirty-five days postinfection (Yeager et al., 1993; Swenson et al., 1995).

Clinical Manifestation and Pathogenesis of PRRSV Infection

Detailed clinical manifestation and lesions resulting from PRRSV infection of pigs of different age groups have been reviewed (Benfield et al., 1999; Done et al., 1996; Rossow et al., 1994). Briefly, PRRSV-infected neonatal pigs show dyspnea but also a variety of other signs such as conjunctivitis, fever, rough hair coat, anorexia, diarrhea, cutaneous erythema, eyelid edema, and mortality, which may be high. In weaned and grower pigs, fever, pneumonia, failure of thrives, and increases in mortality from concurrent bacterial infections were observed. Subclinical infections were more common in finishing pigs, boars, and unbred replacement gilts and sows.

In PRRSV-infected boars and boars that have been vaccinated with live, attenuated vaccine, PRRSV can be shed in semen, and changes in sperm morphology and function have been described. Mortality associated with PRRSV infection of adult swine has been reported.

The reproductive disease was fairly understood. Various research groups have repeatedly shown a causal relationship between PRRSV infection and reproductive failures in breeding herds, and the disease can be reproduced experimentally. Infection in the last third of gestation period seems to cause the most problems, manifested by the birth of dead or weak piglets that die soon after birth (Collins et al., 1992; Wensvoort et al., 1991). It was not clear whether infections earlier in gestation might cause reproductive failures or repeat breeding problems. The clinical and pathological differences between North American and European isolates and within genotypes are dramatic; in piglets, European and some North American PRRSV isolates may induce only mild fever and dyspnea while other American strains induce severe respiratory disease (Halbur et al., 1995, 1996). Reproductive problems in sow are also heavily strain dependent (Mengeling et al., 1996). Both apathogenic isolates (Ohlinger et al., 1992; Van Alstine, 1992) and extremely virulent isolates causing "abortion storms," also called atypical or acute PRRS, are found in the field (Mengeling et al., 1998; Osorio et al., 1998). However, meaningful interpretation of the connection between pathogenicity and nucleotide sequence has not been established.

The importance of the respiratory infection is less well understood. It has been difficult to constantly reproduce significant respiratory disease with the virus alone, and the increase susceptibility to bacterial infection attributed to PRRSV infection has been difficult to reproduce experimentally in pigs. Some studies have reported differences in severity of clinical signs and in gross and microscopic lesions following experimental inoculation of pigs with different PRRSV isolates (Halbur et al., 1994; Halbur et al., 1995).

GROSS AND MICROSCOPIC PATHOLOGY OF PRRSV INFECTION

Gross and microscopic lesions consistent with PRRSV infection are mostly observed in neonatal and nursery pigs. In older pig, lesions may be similar but less marked. Gross lesions associated with PRRSV vary. Lung lesions vary from none to diffuse consolidation and are more commonly complicated by concurrent bacterial infections.

Affected lymph nodes, most commonly in young pigs, can be markedly enlarged. Microscopic lesions, rather nonspecific, most commonly involve lung and lymphoid tissue. Lung lesions are characterized by multifocal interstitial pneumonia showing alveolar septal infiltration by mononuclear cells, type 2 pneumocyte hypertrophy and hyperplasia, and marked accumulation of inflammatory and necrotic alveolar exudate. Lymph nodes demonstrate follicular hyperplasia, foci of follicular necrosis, and debris within follicles; vesicular, heart, and brain lesions have also been described. Inconsistently observed fetal lesions are characterized by vasculitis, myocarditis, and encephalitis. It is important to note that PRRSV infection is but one infectious agent that has been associated with interstitial pneumonia in pigs. Postweaning multisystemic wasting syndrome, associated with porcine circovirus type 2 infection is now commonly related to interstitial pneumonia and lymphadenitis in pigs (Halbur et al., 1995, 1996).

IMMUNE RESPONSE AGAINST THE DISEASE

In general, antibodies seem to have limited protective value. Infected pigs can remain viremic for four to six weeks after infection and can transmit the virus to other pigs. It is not known whether maternal antibodies can protect against early infection, but viremia in pigs born from seropositive females can be detected from week 4 onward (Cristopher-Hennings et al., 1995, 1998, 2001).

However, some levels of protection is seen in piglets with maternal antibody, and a rise in neutralizing antibody titers often corresponds to a decline in virus titers in the blood. In short, the relationship between antibody titers and protection is not very well understood. Cell-mediated immunity has not been widely studied but is thought to play a protective role. PRRSV infection, however, appears to result in weak adaptive cellular immune response. An intriguing aspect of PRRSV infection is the prolonged duration of viremia and subsequent transmission of the virus to contact animals in comparison with other viral infections. Virus is eventually cleared from the circulation but persistent infection is maintained in lymphoid tissues (Cristopher-Hennings et al., 1995, 1998, 2001). However, it is generally agreed that lifelong persistence of infection does not seem to occur (Wills et al., 2003).

PRRS DIAGNOSIS

1. *Agent identification.* Virological diagnosis of PRRS is difficult. This is mainly because the cell of choice for virus isolation is the porcine alveolar macrophage, which needs to be harvested from pigs (preferably specific pathogen free (SPF) under six to eight weeks of age (Wensvoort et al., 1991; Yoon et al., 1992). Not all laboratories have a ready supply of such pigs available, and continuous cell lines cannot fully replace the alveolar

macrophages because these cell lines are generally less susceptible to the virus. In addition, different batches of macrophages are not always equally susceptible to the virus. Certain monkey kidney cell lines (e.g., MA-104) can be a good substitute for macrophages (Bautista et al., 1993; Kim et al., 1993), but such cell lines do not support the growth of all isolates, especially European strains.

Immunohistochemistry and immunoflourescence to detect PRRSV antigen in tissues have been reported. These tests are more rapid than virus isolation and do not necessitate cell culture infrastructure. In addition immunohistochemistry (Halbur et al., 1994; Larochelle and Marger, 1995) performed on formalin-fixed tissue enables the visualization of antigen together with histological lesions and permits retrospective analysis on archival specimens. In situ hybridization capable of detecting and differentiating North American and European PRRSV genotypes in formalin-fixed tissues has been reported (Larochelle and Marger, 1997; Suret al., 1966; Kothalawala et al., 2006). Reverse transcription–polymerase chain reaction (RT-PCR) and nested PCR are highly sensitive tests for detecting viral RNA (Christopher-Hennings et al., 1997; Kono et al., 1966; Larochelle and Marger, 1997; Mardassi et al., 1994) and are now more commonly used on different tissues, including serum. These tests are also useful when virus isolation is challenging, such as when testing semen (Christopher-Hennings et al., 1995) and when testing tissues degraded by autolysis or by heat during transportation of specimens for virus isolation. A multiplex PCR assay has been designed to differentiate North American and European PRRSV isolates (Wesley et al., 1998).

2. *Serological tests.* A variety of tests for the detection of serum antibodies to PRRSV have been described. Serological diagnosis is, in general, easy to perform, with good specificity and sensitivity, especially on a herd basis (Mortensen et al., 2000). Sera of individual pigs sometimes cause difficulties because of nonspecific reactions, but this problem may be solved by re sampling the pig after two to three weeks. Serology is generally performed with a binding assay, such as immunoperoxidase monolayer assay (IPMA), immunofluorescence assay, or the enzyme-linked immunoabsorbant assay (ELISA) of which many varieties are described (Albina et al., 1992; Cho et al., 1997; Denac et al., 1997; Houben et al., 1995; Nodelijk et al., 1996).

CONTROL

Treatment of viral disease is a very difficult task; most viruses have challenged antiviral drug development. Viruses are able to replicate using the replication strategy of their host cell, and obviously the drug that interferes with viral replication nearly always interferes with essential cell functions. Thus, vaccination is the widely practiced method to control and prevention of the PRRSV infection. Several PRRS vaccines are currently available that are producing mixed results regarding the efficacy of these vaccines against the genetically diversified field strains of PRRSV. RespPRRS/Repro (Boehringer Ingelheim), a modified live virus (MLV), is recommended for use in three-to eighteen-week-old pigs and in nonpregnant females. The Prime Pac PRRS vaccine (Schering Plough Animal Health Corporation) is also an MLV, which has been shown to reduce the severity and duration of disease following challenge. However, it did not prevent infection of vaccinated pigs by a virulent heterologous strain. A live vaccine based on a European isolate of PRRSV (Porcilis PRRS) was found to protect fattening pigs against the respiratory manifestations of PRRS. These vaccines confer protection against clinical disease, but not against the infection. However, the great genetic diversity found in American and European strains suggest that the humoral immune response generated by a vaccine that contains only a single PRRSV strain cannot be expected to cover whole antibody spectrum of current field strains. Modified live vaccines would be expected be superior to inactivated vaccines since they induce a more complete cellular immune response. This assumption is supported by several recent clinical trials (Menegeling et al., 2003; Medveczky et al., 2002; Roof et al., 2000). In the future, it may become necessary to develop vaccines that contain more than one strain to cover the whole spectrum of antibodies (Pesh et al., 2005).

CONCLUSION

Porcine reproductive and respiratory syndrome (PRRS) is one of the most economically devastating diseases affecting swine industry worldwide. PRRS virus (PRRSV) is member of Arteriviridae that, like other members of the family, has the ability to infect macrophages and to persist in tissues for at least several months after an acute stage of infection subsides. As a consequence of complex epidemiologic profile of the agent, it creates extreme difficulty in disease control under the usual conditions. The objective of this review is to summarize the current knowledge in PRRS virus (PRRSV) infection in pigs with emphasizing on causative agent, pathogenesis, diseases manifestation, diagnostic techniques, and control.

REFERENCES

1. Albina, E., Leforban, Y., Baron, T., Plana-Duran, J. aqnd Vannir, P. 1992. An enzyme linked immunosorbant assay (ELISA) for detection of antibodies to the porcine reproductive and respiratory syndrome (PRRS) virus. *Ann. Res. Vet.* 23:167–176.

2. Andreyev, V. G., Wesley, R. D., Mengeling, W, L., Vorwald, A. C. and Lager, K. M. 1997. Genetic variation and phylogenic relationships of 22 porcine reproductive and respiratory syndrome virus (PRRSV) field strainsbased on sequence analysis of open reading frame5. *Arch. Virol.* 142:993–1001.

3. Bautista, E. M., Goyal, S. M., Yoon, I. J., Joo, H. S. and Collins, J. E. 1993. Comparison of porcine alveolar macrophages and CL 2621 for the detection of porcine reproductive and respiratory syndrome (PRRS) virus and anti-PRRS antibody. *J. Vet. Diagn. Invest.* 5, 163–165.

4. Benfield, D. A., Collins, J. E., Dee, S. A., Hallbur, P. G., Joo, H. S., Lager, K. M., Menegeling, W. L., Murtaugh, M. P., Rossow, K. D., Stevenson, G. W. and Zimmerman, J. J. 1999. Porcine reproductive and respiratory syndrome. In *Diseases of swine.* 8th ed., ed. B. E. Straw, S. D'Allaire, W. L. Mengeling, and D. J. Taylor, 201–232. Iowa, USA: Iowa State University Press Ames.

5. Benfield, D. A., Nelson, E., Collines, J. E., Harris, L., Goyal, S. M., Robinson, D., Christainson, W. T., Morrison, R. B., Gorcyca, D. and Chladek, D. 1992. Characterization of swine infertility and respiratory syndrome (SIRS) virus (isolate ATCC VR-2332). *J. Vet. Diagn. Invest.* 4, 127–133.

6. Benfield, D. A., Nelson, J. K., Rossow, K. R., Nelson, C., Steffen, M., and Rowland, R. R. 1999. Diagnosis of persistent or prolonged porcine reproductive and respiratory syndrome virus infections. Proceedings of the Third International Symposium on PRRS and Aujeszky's Diseases, Ploufragan, France, 151–152.

7. Benfield, D. A., Nelson, C., Steffen, M. and Rowland, R. R. 2000. Transmission of PRRSV by artificial insemination using extended semen seeded with different concentrations of PRRSV. Proceedings of the 31st Annual Meeting of American Association of Swine Practitioners. Indianapolis, Indiana, 405–408.

8. Brinton, M. A., Godeny, E. K., Horzinek, M. C., Meulenberg, J. J. M., Murtaugh, M. P., Plagemann P. G. W. and Snijder, E. J. 2000. Arteriviridae. In *Virus Taxonomy.* Seventh Report of the International Committee on Taxonomy of Viruses, van Regenmortel USA, 851–857.

9. Cho, H. J., McNab, B., Dubac, C., Jordan, L., Afshar, A., Magar, R., Prince, S. and Eernisse K. 1997. Comparative study of serological methods for detection antibodies to porcine reproductive and respiratory syndrome virus. *Can. J. Vet. Res.* 61:161–166.

10. Collins, J. E., Benefield, D. A., Christianson, W. T., Harris, L., Hennigs J. C., Shaw, D. P., Goyal, S. M., McCullough, S., Morrison, R. B., Joo, H. S., Gorcyca, D. and Chladek D. 1992. Isolation of swine infertility and respiratory syndrome virus (isolate ATCC VR-2332) in North America and experimental reproduction of the disease in gnotobiotic pigs. *J. Vet. Diagn. Invest.* 4:117–126.

11. Conzelmann, K. K., Visser, N., Van Woense, l. P. and Thiel, H. J. 1993. Molecular characterization of porcine reproductive and respiratory syndrome virus, a member of arterivirus group. *Virology* 193:329–339.

12. Cristianson, W. T. and Joo, H. S. 1994. Porcine reproductive and respiratory syndrome. *Swine Health Prod. (AASP)* 2:10–28.

13. Cristopher-Hennings, J., Nelson, E. A., Nelson, J. K. and Benfield, D. A. 1997. Effect of a modified-live virus vaccine against porcine reproductive and respiratory syndrome in boars. *Am. J. Vet. Res.* 61:161–166.

14. Cristopher-Hennigs, J., Nelson, E. A., Nelson, J. K., Hines, R. J., Swenson, S. L., Hill, H. T., Zimmerman, J. J., Katz, J. B., Yaeger, M. J., Chase, C. C. L. and Benefield, D. A. 1995. Detection of porcine reproductive and respiratory syndrome virus in boar semen by PCR. *J. Clin. Microbiol.* 33:1730–1734.

15. Christopher-Hennings, E. A., Nelson, J. K., Nelson, K. D., Rossow, J. L. Shivers, M. J. Yaeger et al. 1998. Identification of porcine reproductive and respiratory syndrome virus in semen and tissues from vasectomized and nonvasectomized boars. *Vet. Pathol.* 35:260–267.

16. Christopher-Hennings, L. D. Holler, D. A., Benfield and E. A. Nelson. 2001. Detection and duration of porcine reproductive and respiratory syndrome virus in semen, serum, peripheral blood mononuclear cells, and tissues from Yorkshire, Hampshire and Landrace boars. *J. Vet. Diagn. Invest.* 13:133–142.

17. Christopher-Hennings, E. A. Nelson, J., Nelson, Hines, R. J., Swenson, S. L., Hill, H. T. et al. 1995. Detection of porcine reproductive and respiratory syndrome virus in boar semen by PCR. *J. Clin. Microbiol.* 33:1730–1734.

18. Dea, S., Ganon, C. A., Mardassi, H., Pirzadeh, B. and Rogan, D. 2000. Current knowledge on the structural proteins of porcine reproductive and respiratory syndrome virus: Comparison of North American and European isolates. *Arch. Virol.* 145:659–688.

19. Dee, S. A., Torremorell, M., Rossow, K., Mahlum, C., Otake, S. and Faaberg, K. 2001. Identification of genetically diverse sequences (ORF) of porcine reproductive and respiratory syndrome virus in swine herd. *Can. J. Vet. Res.* 65:254–260.

20. Denac, H., Moser, C., Tratschin, J. D. and Hofmann, M. A. 1997. An indirect ELISA for detection of antibodies against porcine reproductive and respiratory syndrome virus using recombinant nucleocapsid protein as antigen. *J. Virol. Methods* 65:169–181.

21. Done, S. H., Paton, D. J. and White, M. E. C. 1996. Porcine reproductive and respiratory syndrome (PRRS): A review with emphasis on pathological, virological and diagnostic aspects. *Brit. Vet. J.* 152:153–174.

22. Drew, T. W., Meulenberg, J. J. M., Sands, J. J. and Paton, D. J. 1995. Production, characterization and reactivity of monoclonal antibodies to porcine reproductive and respiratory syndrome virus. *J. Gen Virol.* 76:1361–1369.

23. Forsberg, R., Storgaard, T., Nielsen, H. S., Oleksiewicz, M. B., Corodioli, P., Sala, G., Hein. J. and Botner, A. 2002. The genetic diversity of European type PRRSV is similar to that of North American type but is geogeaphically skewed within Europe. *Virology* 29:38–47

24. Ganon, C. A. and Dea, S. 1998. Differentiation between porcine reproductive and respiratory syndrome virus isolates by restriction fragment length polymorphism of their ORFs 6 and 7 genes. *Can. J. Vet. Res.* 62:110–116.

25. Halbur, P. G., Andrews, J. J., Huffman, E. L., Paul, P. S., Meng, X. L. and Niyo, Y. 1994. Development of a straptavidin-biotin immunoperoxidase procedure for the detection of porcine reproductive and respiratory syndrome virus antigen in porcine lung. *J. Vet Diagn., Invest.* 6:254–257.

26. Halbur, P. G., Paul, P. S., Frey, M. L., Landgraf, J., Eetnisse, K., Meng, X. J., Lum, M. N., Andrew, J. J. and Rathje, J. A. 1995. Comparative pathogencity of nine U.S. porcine reproductive and respiratory syndrome virus (PRRSV) isolates in a five-week-old cesarean-derived colostrums-deprived pig model. *J. Vet. Diagn. Invest.* 8:11–20.

27. Halbur, P. G., Paul, R. S., Frey, M. L., Landgraf, J., Eernisse, K. and Meng, X. J. 1996. Comparison of the antigen distribution of two US porcine reproductive and respiratory syndrome virus isolate with that of the Lelystad virus. *Vet. Pathol.* 33:159–170.

28. Houben, S., Callebaut, P. and Pensaert, M. B. 1995. Comparative study of a blocking enzyme enzyme linked immunosorbant assay and the immunoperoxidase monolayer assay for the detection of antibodies to the porcine reproductive and respiratory syndrome virus in pigs. *J. Virol. Methods* 51:125–128.

29. Indik, S., Valicek, L., Klein, D. and Klanova, J. 2000. Variation in the major envelope glycoprotein GP5 of Czech strains of porcine reproductive and respiratory syndrome virus. *J. Gen. Virol.* 81:2497–2502.

30. Keffaber, K. K. 1989. Reproductive failure of unknown etiology. *American Association Swine Practice News Letter* 1:1–9.

31. Kim, H. S., Kwang, J., Yoon, I. J., Joo, H. S. and Frey, M. L. 1993. Enhanced replication of porcine reproductive and respiratory syndrome virus in a homogenious subpopulation of MA–104 cell line. *Arch. Virol.* 133:477–483.

32. Komijn, R. E., Van Klinik, E. G. M. and Van Der Sande, W. J. H. 1991. The possible effect of weather conditions on the spread of the new pig disease in the Netherlands. Report of a seminar on the new pig disease (PRRS), Brussels (Belgium). 28–31.

33. Kono, Y., Kanno, T., Shimzu, M., Yamad, S., Ohashi, S., Nakamine, M. and Shirai, J. 1996. Nested PCR for the detection and typing of porcine reproductive and respiratory syndrome (PRRS) virus in pigs. *J. Vet. Med. Sci.* 58:540–543.

34. Kothalawala, H., Toussient, M. J. M., van Asten, A. J. A. M., and Gruys, E. 2006. Detection of PRRSV genotypes in tissue sections of piglet with respiratory lesions using cDNA oligonucleotide probes of Lelystad and VR 2332 viruses. *Vet. Pathol.* 43:860–864.

35. Kwang, J., Kim, H. S. and Jo, H. S. 1994. Clonning, expression, and sequence analysis of the ORF gene of the porcine porcine reproductive and respiratory syndrome virus MN–1b. *J. Vet. Diagn. Invest.* 6:293–296.

36. Lager, K. M. and Mengeling, W. L. 2000. Experimental aerosol transmission of pseudorabies virus and porcine reproductive and respiratory syndrome virus. Proceedings of the American Association of Swine Practitioner's Annual Meeting 2000, 409–410.

37. Larochelle, R. and Marger, R. 1995. Comparison of immunogold silver staining (IGSS) with two immunoperoxidase staining systems for the detection of porcine reproductive and respiratory syndrome virus antigens in formaline fixed tissues. *J. Vet. Diagn. Invest.* 7:540–543.

38. Larochelle, R. and Magar, R. 1997. Differentiation of North American and European porcine reproductive and respiratory syndrome virus genotypes by in situ hybridization. *J. Virol. Methods* 68:161–168.

39. Mardassi, H., Wilson, L., Mounir, S. and Dea, S. 1994. Detection of porcine reproductive and respiratory syndrome virus and efficient differentiation between Canadian and European strains by reverse transcription and PCR amplification. *J. Clin. Microbiol.* 32:2197–2203.

40. Meng, X. J., Paul, P. S. and Halbur, P. G. 1994. Molecular cloning and nucleotide sequencing of the 3'-terminal genomic RNA of the porcine reproductive and respiratory syndrome virus. *J. Gen Virol.* 75:1795–1801.

41. Meng, X. J., Paul, P. S., Halbur, P. G. and Morozov, I. 1995a. Phylogenetic analysis of the putative M (ORF 6) and N (ORF 7) genes of porcine reproductive and respiratory syndrome virus (PRRSV): Implication for the existence of genotypes of PRRSV in the USA and Europe. *Arch. Virol.* 140:745–755.

42. Meng, X. J. 2000. Heterogenecity of porcine reproductive and respiratory syndrome virus: Implications for current vaccine efficacy and future vaccine development. *Vet. Microbiology* 74:309–329.

43. Mengeling, W. L., Vorwald, A. C., Lager, K. M. and Brockmeier, S. I. 1996a. Comparison among strains of porcine reproductive and respiratory syndrome virus for their ability to cause reproductive failure. *Am. J. Vet. Res.* 57:834–839.

44. Medveczky, I., Kulscar, G., Makaranski, L., Glavitis, R., Gorcyca, D. and Schutz, B. 2002. Efficacy of a PRRS modified live virus vaccine (US strain) against the heterologous infection by a virulent PRRS virus (EU strain): Reproductive performance. Proceedings of the 17th International Pig Veterinary Society Congress (IPVS), Ames, Iowa, USA, 77.

45. Mengeling, W. L., Lager, K. M., Vorwald, A. C. and Clouser, D. F. 2003. Comparative safety and efficacy of attenuated single strain and multi strain vaccines for porcine reproductive and respiratory syndrome. *Vet. Microbiol.* 93:25–38.

46. Mengelling, W. L., Lager, K. M. and Vorwald, A. C. 1998. Clinical effects of porcine reproductive and respiratory syndrome virus on pigs during early post natal interval. *Am. J. Vet. Res.* 59:52–55.

47. Meulenberg, J. J. M., Hulst, M. M., De Meijer, E. J., Moonen, P. J. L. M., Den Besten, A., De Kluyver, E. P., Wensvoort, G. and Moonmann, R. J. M. 1993. Lelystad virus the causative agent of porcine epidemic abortion and respiratory syndrome (PEARS) is related to LDV and EAV. *Virology* 192:62–72.

48. Morozov, I., Meng, X. J. and Paul P. S. 1995. Sequence analysis of open reading frames (ORFs) 2–4 of a US isolates of porcine reproductive and respiratory virus. *Arch. Virol.* 140:1313–1319.

49. Mortensen, S., Strandbygaard, B. and Botner, A. 2000. Herd-level criteria for European and American PRRSV subtype status based on serology. Proceedings of the 16th Congress of the International Pig Veterinary Society, Australia, 584.

50. Murtaugh, M. P., Elam, M. R. and Kakach, L. T. 1995. Comparison of the structural protein coding sequence of the VR-2332 and Leylystad virus strains of the PRRS virus. *Arch. Virol.* 140:1451–1460.

51. Nelson, C. J., Murtaugh, M. P. and Faaberg, K. S. 1999. Porcine reproductive and respiratory syndrome virus comparison: Divergent evolution on two contienents. *J. Virol.* 73:270–280.

52. Nodelijk, G., Wensvoort, G., Kroese, B., Van Leengoed, L., Colijn, E. and Verheijden, J. 1996. Comparison of a commercial ELISA and an immunoperoxidase monolayer assay to detect antibodies directed against porcine respiratory and reproductive syndrome virus. *Vet. Microbiol.* 49:285–295.

53. Ohlinger, V., Hass, B., Saalmulter, A., Beyer, J., Teufferet, J., Visser, N. and Weiland F. 1992. In vivo in vitro studies on the immunopathology of PRRS. *Proc. of American Association of Swine Practitioners 1st Int. PRRS Symp.* 4: 24.

54. Oslage, V., Dahale, Th., Muller, M., Kramer, M., Beier, D. and Liess, B. 1994. Antibody prevalence of hog cholera, Aujesky's disease and porcine reproductive and respiratory syndrome virus in wild boar in the federal states of Sachsen-anhalt and Bradenburg (Germany). *Dtsch. Tierarztl. Wochenschr.* 101:33–38.

55. Osorio, F. A., Zuckerman, F., Wills, R., Meier, W., Chiristian, S., Galeota, J. and Doste, A. 1998. PRRSV: Comparison of commercial vaccines in their ability to induce protection against current PRSSV strains of high virulence. *Allen D. Leman Swine Conference* 25:176–182.

56. OIE. 2004. *Manual of diagnostic tests and vaccines for terrestrial animals*, 5th ed.

57. Paton, D. J., Brown, I. H., Edwards, S. and Wenswoort, G. 1991. "Blue ear" disease of pigs. *Vet. Rec.* 128, 617.

58. Pesh, S., Meyer, C. and Ohlinger, V. F. 2005. New sights in to the genetic diversity of European porcine reproductive and respiratory syndrome virus (PRRSV) *Vet. Microbiol.* 107:31–48.

59. Roof, M. B., Gorcyca, D. and Wensvoort, D. 2000. Efficacy of a virus vaccine (Ingelvac PRRS MLV) against heterologous virulent Leylstad challenge. In *Proceedings of the 16th International Pig Veterinary Society Congress, Melbourne*, ed. C. Cargill and S. McOrist, 641. Australia.

60. Rossow, K. D. 1998. Porcine reproductive and respiratory syndrome. *Vet. Pathol.* 35:1–20.

61. Rossow, K. D., Bautista, E. M., Goyal, S. M., Molitor, T. W., Murtaugh, M. P., Morrison, R. B., Benfield, D. A., and Collins, J. E. 1994. Experimental porcine reproductive and respiratory virus infection in one-, four-, and 10-week-old pigs. *J. Vet. Diagn. Invest.* 6:3–12.

62. Snijder, E. J. and Meulenberg, J. J. M. 1998. The molecular biology of arteriviruses. *J. Gen. Virol.* 79:961–979.

63. Stadejek, T., Stakevicius, A., Storgaard, T., Oleksiewicz, M. B., Belak, S., Drew, T. W. and Pejsak, Z. 2002. Identification or radically different variants of porcine reproductive and respiratory syndrome virus in Eastern Europe: Towards a common ancestor for European and American viruses. *J. Gen. Virol.* 83:1861–1873.

64. Suarez, P., Zaradoya, R., Martin, M. J., Prieto, C., Dopazo, J., Solana, A. and Castro, J. M. 1996. Phylogenetic relationships of European strains of porcine reproductive syndrome virus inferred from DNA sequences of putative ORF-5 and ORF 7 genes. *Virus Res.* 42:159–165.

65. Sur, J. H., Cooper, V. L., Galeota, J. A., Hesse, R. A., Doster, A. R., and Osorio, F. A. 1996. *In vivo* detection of porcine reproductive and respiratory syndrome virus RNA by in situ hybridization at different time post infection *J. Clin. Microbiol.* 34:2280–2286.

66. Swenson, S., Zimmerman, J. J., Evans, L., Bechtol, D., Hopkins, S., Wills, R., Yoon, K. J., Schwatz, K., Hill, H. and McGinley, M. 1995. Exposure to gilts to PRRS virus by artificial insemination. Proceedings of the Second International Symposium on Porcine Reproductive and Respioratory Syndrome (PRRS), Copenhagen, Denmark, 42.

67. Van Alstine, W. 1992. Isolation of SIRS virus from nursery pigs of two herds without current reproductive failure. Proc. Annu. Meet. *Livest. Conserv. Inst.* 1:253–259.

68. Van Regenmortel, M. H. V., Fauquet, C. M., Bishop, D. H. L., Carstens, E. B., Estes, M. K., Lemon, S. M., Maniloff, J., Mayo, M. A., McGeoch, D. J., Pringle, C. R. and Wickner, R. B. 2000. In *Virus Taxonomy: The classification and nomenclature of viruses*. The seventh report of the International Committee on Taxonomy of Viruses. M. H. V. Virus Taxonomy, VIIth report of the ICTV, 1677. San Diego: Academic Press.

69. Wensvoort, G., Terpstra, C., Po, J. M. A., Ter Laak, E. A., Bloemraad, M., De Kluyver, E. P., Kragten, C., Van Buiten, L., Den Besten, A., Wagenaar, F., Broekhuijsen, J. M., Moonen, P. L. J. M., Zetstra, T., De Boer, E. A., Tibben, H. J., De Jong, M. F., Van't Veld, P., Groenland, G. J. R., Van Gennep, J. A., Voets,

M. Th., Verheijden, J. H. M. and Braamskamp, J. 1991. Mystery swine disease in the Netherlands: The isolation of Lelystad virus. *Vet. Q.* 13:121–130.

70. Wensvoort, G., de Kluyver, E. P., Luitze, E. A., Den Besten, A., Harris, L., Collins, J. E., Christianson, W. T. and Chaadek, D. 1992. Antigenic comparison of Lelystad virus and swine infertility and respiratory syndrome (SIRS) virus. *J. Vet. Diagn. Invest.* 4:134–138.

71. Wesley, R. D., Mengeling, W. L., Lager, K. M., Clouser, D. F., Landgraf, J. G., and Frey, M. L. 1998. Differentiation of a porcine reproductive and respiratory syndrome virus vaccine strain from North American field strains by restriction fragment length polymorphism analysis of ORF 5. *J. Vet. Diagn. Invest.* 10:140–144.

72. Wills, R. W., Doster, A. R., Galeota, J. A., Sur, J. H. and Osario, F. A. 2003. Duration of infection and proportion of pigs persistently infected with porcine reproductive and respiratory syndrome virus. *J. Clin Microbiol.* 41:58–62.

73. Yeager, M. J., Prieve, T., Collins, J. E., Christopher-Hennigs, J., Nelson, E., and Benfield, D. 1993. Evidence for the transmission of porcine reproductive and respiratory syndrome virus in boar semen. *Swine Health Production* 1:7–9.

74. Yoon, I. J., Joo, H. S., Christianson, W. T., Kim, H. S., Collins, J. E., Morrison, R. B. and Dial G. D. 1992. An indirect fluorescent antibody test for the detection of antibody to swine infertility and respiratory syndrome virus in swine sera. *J. Vet. Diagn. Invest.* 4:144–147.

8. Pseudorabies (Aujeszky's Disease)

P. K. Dash, and S. Nandi

Introduction

Pseudorabies, also known as Aujeszky's disease, is one of the most important infectious reportable diseases of swine (Kluge et al., 1999). Apart from swine, it also infects most warm-blooded mammals such as, cattle, sheep, dog, cats, goats, raccoons and opossums, skunks and rodents, horses, and carnivores, including wild felines (Pansaert and Kluge, 1989; Wittmann and Rziha, 1989). Experimentally, rabbits, guinea pigs, mouse, monkey, chickens, nonhuman primates such as rhesus monkeys and marmosets can be infected. However, humans and tailless apes such as chimpanzees are not susceptible to infection.

It is endemic in many parts of the world, causing huge economic losses. Though eradicated from few countries, it is still reported from Belarus, Brazil, Cuba, France, Hungary, Italy, Mexico, Panama, Poland, Portugal, Romania, Russia, Slovakia, Slovenia, Taiwan, and Ukraine.

In the nineteenth century, a disease characterized by heavy itching termed as "mad itch" was first reported among cattle from United States. Later in 1902, a Hungarian veterinarian, Aladar Aujeszky, isolated pseudorabies (PRV) from ox, dog, and cat and reproduced the disease in laboratory animals (Aujeszky, 1902). However, it was only in 1931 that Shope identified mad itch as the same as Aujeszky's disease (Pomeranz et al., 2005). It has since become known as pseudorabies because of some apparent resemblance of clinical syndrome to rabies.

Etiology

Pseudorabies is caused by pseudorabies virus (PRV) (Suid herpesvirus 1), a virus belonging to genus *Varicellovirus,* subfamily Alphaherpesvirinae, and family Herpesviridae (Pomeranz et al., 2005). This virus is also known as Aujeszky's disease virus. Only one serotype of pseudorabies virus is recognized, although strain differences are reported among PRV.

The size of pseudorabies virus (PRV) varies from 200–250 nm. It has a linear double-stranded DNA genome of approximately 143 kbp. The mature virion consists of four morphologically distinct structural components, viz, DNA, capsid, tegument, and envelope. The DNA of the virus is enclosed within an icosahedral capsid to form a nucleocapsid. The capsid is surrounded by tegument. Tegument comprises of at least fourteen viral proteins along with cellular actin. These proteins are organized into two distinct layers, the inner layer interacting closely with capsid and outer layer with the envelope. Tegument proteins play important role in viral entry and morphogenesis (Mettenleiter, 2002). The tegument is surrounded by a lipid bilayer known as envelope. Several membrane proteins are embedded into the envelope. Eleven membrane proteins are glycosylated (designated as gB, gC, gD, gE, gG, gH, gI, gK, gL, gM, and gN), and four transmembrane proteins are not glycosylated (UL20, UL43, US9, and UL24). These proteins play important role in viral entry, fusion, egress, and cell-to-cell spread. These glycoproteins also represent dominant targets for the host's immune defense (Mettenleiter, 1996).

CLINICAL SIGNS

PRV causes clinical infections in both domestic and wild animals. However, it is more pronounced in swine, where the recovered pig remains latently infected following clinical recovery. The disease is manifested by various degrees of nervous disorder accompanied frequently by intense pruritus along with respiratory symptoms of rhinitis and pneumonia. It is almost always fatal. PRV affects both respiratory and nervous system of swine, and viral particles enter sensory nerve endings of the infected nasal and oropharyngeal mucosa (Masic et al., 1965). Morbidity and mortality associated with PRV infection depends on various factors such as age of the pig, health status, viral strain involved, infectious dose and previous exposure. Case fatality rate up to 100% was recorded in piglets up to two weeks of age. It progressively decreases with the increasing age. Mortality in older pigs is rare and only reported with some virulent strains of PRV. In general, younger swine (four to five weeks) are the most susceptible and typically exhibit symptoms of central nervous infection, whereas older swine exhibit symptoms of respiratory disease (Kluge et al., 1999). The mortality is less than 50% among weaned pigs (three to nine weeks of age), though they exhibit symptoms similar to younger pigs. The mortality is even lower in well-nursed pigs. The weaned pigs also develop high temperatures with respiratory signs such as sneezing, nasal discharge, severe cough, and difficulty in breathing. There is also significant decrease in body weight, leading to economic loss for swine producers.

In adult swine, respiratory signs are the hallmark of PRV infection. The morbidity reaches up to 100% with 1–2% mortality. Typically, clinical signs include high fever, listlessness, and anorexia, with mild to severe respiratory signs. The respiratory signs include dyspnea, rhinitis, sneezing, nasal discharge, coughing, and labored breathing, ultimately leading to pneumonia (Baskerville et al., 1971). There is also great loss of body weight leading to financial losses (Kluge et al., 1999). In rare cases, adult swine may exhibit central nervous system abnormalities varying from mild muscle tremors to violent convulsions.

Pregnant sows infected in the first trimester of pregnancy will usually reabsorb the fetuses in utero. If infection occurs within second and third trimester of pregnancy, it results in abortion, stillbirths, and mummified or macerated fetuses. The infertility results from the transplacental transmission of virus (Kluge et al., 1999; Gordon and Luke, 1955).

PATHOGENESIS
The natural route is through nasal infection, though experimentally it can be produced by all routes of inoculation (Lee and Wilson, 1979). During an acute infection, viral particles replicate in the oropharyngeal mucosa. The virus gains entry into the sensory nerve endings innervating the site of infection, following which it enters the central nervous system (CNS) via maxillary branch of the trigeminal nerve, glossopharyngeal nerve, and the olfactory nerve (Mcferran and Dow, 1965). Virus transfer along nerve fibers takes place within the axoplasm and through Schwann cells and fibroblasts of the endoneurium. Other pathways of viral dissemination throughout the body include the lymphatics, and further viral multiplication occurs in lymph nodes and the vascular system. PRV establishes a lifelong infection in a variety of the nervous tissues. The predominant sites of PRV latency are the trigeminal ganglia and the sacral ganglia. Latent PRV genomes can be detected in the other neural tissues such as the olfactory bulb, brain stem, and tonsillar lymph nodes (Tomishima and Enquist, 2002; Wheeler and Osorio, 1991). Reactivation and shedding of virus in latently infected animals frequently occurs after stressful experiences (Azmi et al., 2002). Recovery by swine from pseudorabies confers resistance for at least twelve months. Reexposure may result in reinfection, but it is usually asymptomatic.

PATHOLOGY
No gross lesions characteristic of pseudorabies are consistently found.
The pathology is primarily characterized by meningeal and cerebral vascular congestion, accompanied by edema in the brain (Lee and Wilson, 1979). Some strains also produce inflammatory and necrotic changes in the upper respiratory tract mucosa and lungs. Small grayish white spots of focal necrosis are also observed in the liver, spleen, tonsils, lungs, and various lymph nodes. Microscopically, there is nonsuppurative meningoencephalomyelitis with neuronal degeneration and necrosis, gliosis, and perivascular cuffing by mononuclear cell. Intranuclear inclusions may be found in neurons,

astrocytes, Purkinje cells, pulmonary macrophages, and lymph node macrophages (Dow and Mcferran, 1962).

Diagnosis

The diagnosis of a severe PRV outbreak among swine is relatively easy through appearance of typical symptoms in newborn piglets with heavy mortality. The diagnosis is strengthened further if dogs, cats, cattle, or horses are also found affected. However, diagnosis of milder outbreaks mostly in grower-finisher herds where there are no sucking piglets is difficult. Its clinical resemblance with many other infections of swine, including transmissible gastroenteritis (TGE), porcine reproductive and respiratory syndrome (PRRS), influenza, etc., confounds the diagnosis. However, simultaneous occurrence of reproductive problem in sow and neurological signs in suckling pigs are highly suggestive of pseudorabies. A battery of diagnostic assays is usually followed for confirmatory diagnosis of pseudorabies in a laboratory. These include viral isolation from infected tissues samples, immunofluorescence assays on tissue sections and nasal swabs, and serologic assays. PRV tends to replicate rapidly with cytopathic effects in a matter of hours in many cells. There are accumulations of birefringent cells, followed by complete detachment of the cell monolayer. Syncytia also develop, the appearance and size of which are variable. Presence of acidophilic intranuclear inclusions is regarded as highly significant diagnostically. Though isolation is considered gold standard, however, failure in isolation does not guarantee freedom from infection. Fluorescent antibody tests and peroxidase tests are performed on tissues from affected organs like tonsils, olfactory bulb, pons, nasal mucosa, cervical lymph nodes, and trigeminal nerve. Serum-neutralization test (SNT) with paired sera is the most confirmatory serological assay for PRV. A significant rise in antibodies between the paired serum samples, first taken during early stage of infection and the second three to four weeks later, confirms the infection. Serologic assays also include latex agglutination tests and enzyme-linked immunosorbent assays (ELISA). Of late, ELISA has replaced SNT and widely used for rapid screening of meat juice as well as serum. The gE-specific ELISA are now widely carried out to distinguish vaccinated cases from naturally infected cases (Kluge et al., 1999). Cutaneous allergic test is very useful to detect carrier animals (Smith and Mengeling, 1977). Recent advances in molecular techniques, like polymerase chain reaction (PCR), provide a rapid alternative to the virus isolation technique (Ishikawa et al., 1995). Further, a number of modifications of PCR such as nested PCR, multiplex PCR, and quantitative real-time PCR assays, which provide increased sensitivity and are very useful in diagnosis of latent cases, are reported (Yoon et al., 2005; Thiery et al., 1996).

TREATMENT

There is no treatment or antiviral therapy available specifically against PRV. No other treatment is effective in suckling pigs. However, antibiotics are prescribed to prevent secondary infections particularly of the respiratory system and also reduce bacterial damage. Chlortetracycline and oxytetracycline can be added in the breeding ration for three to four weeks.

PROPHYLAXIS

Successful protection of herds against PRV requires vaccination in conjunction with other measures, including routine testing and selective culling of infected animals. Different types of vaccines containing either modified live or inactivated virus antigens are available for the control of pseudorabies. Recently, modified attenuated live virus vaccines are widely used, which are developed by deletion of PRV UL23, the gene encoding the viral thymidine kinase (TK) and/or glycoprotein E (gE), gG, or gC (Mettenleiter et al., 1989). TK is critical for viral replication in nonmitotic cells like neurons. The glycoprotein gE is an important neurovirulence factor (Kritas et al., 1994). These gene-deleted marker vaccines have the advantage over conventional whole virus vaccines that it is possible to distinguish vaccinated (gE-null vaccine strain-infected) animals from those from virulent field strain-infected animals (Quint et al., 1987). A gE-null, TK-null double knockout vaccine strain (PRV-Begonia) was developed by deleting both gE and TK gene (Visser and Lutticken, 1989). Vaccination with Begonia strain imparts protective immunity against virulent field strain challenge, significantly decreases the excretion of challenge virus, and also guards against the growth retardation. This vaccine is safe in all ages and pregnant sows. This is also safe for cattle, sheep, dogs, and cats (Visser and Lutticken, 1989; Marchioli et al., 1987). Protective immune response is also elicited through use of subunit vaccine consisting of gC or gD (Matsuda et al., 1992), which are important targets for cytotoxic T cells. The DNA vaccines, which provide high degree of biological safety compared to conventional vaccine, are also reported for PRV. Plasmids encoding PRV gC was reported to be very efficient in induction of protective response against wild-type infections in swine (Gerdts et al., 1997). It elicits both humoral and cellular immunity, resulting in full protection of animals against a challenge (Andries et al., 1978). The intradermal inoculation of plasmid DNA also led to higher degree of seroconversion compared to the intramuscular route. This route of immunization facilitates vaccination of large herd of animals in a shorter time period.

EPIZOOTIOLOGY

PRV is a highly stable virus, and under favorable conditions, it can remain viable in hay and wood for up to forty-six days. Drinking water, bedding, and other objects such as clothing and instruments may become contaminated, which make the environment a continuous source of contamination. Aerosolization of the virus and transmission by fomites may also occur. The virus can persist for up to seven hours in air with a relative humidity of ≥55% and can spread on the wind several kilometers leading to potential threat of farm biosecurity. It can also be easily transmitted from infected animals to susceptible animals through injection and inhalation route. However, it is not spread through feces or urine. Transmammary spread of PRV from nonsymptomatic sows to their offspring through milk was also demonstrated. Coital transmission was also earlier documented. Lateral spread of virus between pigs and raccoons, pigs and opossums, and vice versa was also well documented. The carrier state of pigs is also a major source of infection as latent carriers shed virus following stressful conditions such as transportation over long distances, concurrent disease, overcrowding, farrowing, and steroid medication. The coincidence of some outbreaks with environmental extremes is also recorded.

CONTROL OF INFECTION

The introduction of the disease can be minimized by strict restriction on the movement of people, animals, and objects into the farm. All equipments and clothes should be decontaminated with a good disinfectant before introduction. New animal must be purchased from known free herds and be vaccinated before arrival or in isolation. They should undergo quarantine and introduced after being certified pseudorabies free. The infected dead pigs should be disposed by a deep burial or incineration. Isolation and whole-herd depopulation of infected animals is the best way to control the infection. The appearance of an outbreak in nearby area demands immediate vaccination and must be given top priority. Vaccination helps to prevent the establishment of the virus. In enzootic and high-risk areas, routine vaccination is practiced and may be compulsory as part of an eradication scheme. Vaccination also prevents placental transmission of virus to fetus. Piglets that are suckled by vaccinated sows receive passive protection through colostrums to some extent. This gives protection for about six to ten weeks, which is the critical susceptible age for PRV. Special commercially available serological test kits can distinguish antibodies that have been stimulated by the marker vaccine from those that have been stimulated by natural infection with a gene-complete wild virus. Successful eradication of PRV is primarily achieved in many countries, including through selective culling of PRV-positive herds, sustained vaccination programs with marker viruses (gE-null vaccine strains), routine testing, restricted swine import, and improved management practices including isolation of domestic swine from potential wild reservoirs such as wild swine (Pomeranz et al., 2005).

CONCLUSION

Though successfully eradicated from few countries such as Germany and the Netherlands, PRV still remains a potential threat to swine industry across the globe. The latent state of infection in pigs serves as the major hurdle in successful eradication (Maes et al., 1997). However, international attention must be focused for the start of an eradication program through use of marker vaccine and routine surveillance around all the affected regions of the world. Further research on the molecular biology and pathogenesis of the virus will undoubtedly lead to development of better and effective control strategies for the eradication of this scourge of swine.

REFERENCES

1. Andries, K., Pensaert, M. B. and Vandeputte, J. 1978. Effect of experimental infection with pseudorabies (Aujeszky's disease) virus on pigs with maternal immunity from vaccinated sows. *Am. J. Vet. Res.* 39:1282–1285.
2. Aujeszky, A. 1902. Ueber eine neue Infektions-krankheit bei Haustieren. *Zentralbl. Bakterio.* 32:353–357.
3. Azmi, M. L. M., Zeenathul, N. A., Ali, A. W. S., Mohamed, C. A. R. and Kamarudin, A. I. 2002. A restrictive virus tropism, latency and reactivation of pseudorabies virus following irreversible deletion of *Bsr I* restriction site in the thymidine-kinase gene. *J. Microbiol.* 40:1–10.
4. Baskerviile, A., Mccracken, R. M. and Mccracken, J. B. 1971. The histopathology of experimental rhinitis in pigs produced by a strain of Aujeszky's disease virus. *Res. Vet. Sci.* 12:323–326.
5. Dow, C. and Mcferran, J. B. 1962. The neuropathology of Aujeszky's disease in the pig. *Res. Vet. Sci.* 3:436–468.
6. Gerdts, V. A., Makoschey, J. B., Visser, N. and Mettenleiter, T. C. 1997. Protection of pigs against Aujeszky's disease by DNA vaccination. *J. Gen. Virol.* 78:2139–2146.
7. Gordon, W. M. and Luke, D. 1955. An outbreak of Aujeszky's disease in swine with heavy mortality in piglets, illness in sows and death in uterus. *Vet. Rec.* 67:591–597.
8. Ishikawa, K., Jin-yama, M., Saitoh, A., Takagi, M., Muramatsu, M. and Itoh, O. 1995. Differentiation between glycoprotein III gene-deleted vaccine and wild-type strains of pseudorabies virus by polymerase chain reaction (PCR). *J. Virol. Meth.* 51:267–76.
9. Kluge, J. P., Beran, G. W., Hill, H. T. and Platt, K. B. 1999. Pseudorabies (Aujeszky's disease). In *Diseases of swine*, 8th ed., ed. B. E. Straw, S. D'Allaire, W. L. Mengeling, and T. J. Taylor, 233–46. Ames, Iowa: Iowa State University Press.
10. Kritas, S. K., Pensaert, M. B. and Mettenleiter, T. C. 1994. Role of envelope glycoproteins gI, gp63 and gIII in the invasion and spread of Aujeszky's disease virus in the olfactory nervous pathway of the pig. *J. Gen. Virol.* 75:2319–2327.
11. Lee, J. Y. S. and Wilson, M. R. 1979. A review of pseudorabies (Aujeszky's disease) in pigs. *Canadian Vet. J.* 20:65–69.
12. Maes, R. K., Sussman, M. D., Vilnis, A. and Thacker, B. J. 1997. Recent developments in latency and recombination of Aujeszky's disease (pseudorabies) virus. *Vet. Microbiol.* 55:13–27.

13. Marchioli, C. C., Yancey, R. J., Wardley, R. C., Thomsen, D. R. and Post, L. E. 1987. A vaccine strain of pseudorabies virus with deletions in the thymidine kinase and glycoprotein genes. *Am. J. Vet. Res.* 48:1577–1583.

14. Masic, M., Ercegan, M. and Petrovic, M. 1965. The significance of the tonsils in the pathogenesis and diagnosis of Aujeszky's disease in pigs. *Zentralbl. Veterinarmed.* B 12:398–405.

15. Matsuda, T. A., Katayama, S., Okada, N., Okabe, T. and Sasaki, N. 1992. Protection from pseudorabies virus challenge in mice by a combination of purified gII, gIII and gVI antigens. *J. Vet. Med. Sci.* 54:447–452.

16. Mcferran, J. B. and Dow, C. 1965. The distribution of virus of Aujeszky's disease (pseudorabies) in experimentally infected swine. *Am. J. Vet. Res.* 26:631–635.

17. Mettenleiter, T. C. 1996. Immunobiology of pseudorabies (Aujeszky's disease). *Vet. Immunol. Immunopathol.* 54:221–229.

18. Mettenleiter, T. C. 2002. Herpesvirus assembly and egress. *J. Virol.* 76:1537–1547.

19. Mettenleiter, T. C., Lomniczi, B., Zsak, L., Medveczky, I., Ben-Porat, T. and Kaplan, A. S. 1989. Analysis of the factors that affect virulence of pseudorabies virus. In *Vaccination and control of Aujeszky's disease*, ed. J. T. van Oirschot, 3–11. Dordrecht, the Netherlands: Kluwer Academic Publishers.

20. Pensaert, M. B., and Kluge, J. P. 1989. Pseudorabies virus (Aujeszky's disease). In *Virus infections of porcines*, ed. M. B. Pensaert, 39–64. Amsterdam, the Netherlands: Elsevier Science Publishers.

21. Pomeranz, L. E., Reynolds, A. E. and Hengartner, C. J. 2005. Molecular biology of pseudorabies virus: Impact on neurovirology and veterinary medicine. *Microbiol. Molecular Biol. Rev.* 69:462–500.

22. Quint, W., Gielkens, A., Van Oirschot, J., Berns, A. and Cuypers, H. T. 1987. Construction and characterization of deletion mutants of pseudorabies virus: A new generation of "live" vaccines. *J. Gen. Virol.* 68:523–534.

23. Smith, P. C. and Mengeling, W. L. 1977. A skin test for pseudorabies virus infection in swine. *Can. J. Comp. Med.* 41:364–368.

24. Thiery, R., Pannetier, C., Rziha, H. J. and Jestin, A. A. 1996. Fluorescence-based quantitative PCR method for investigation of pseudorabies virus latency. *J Virol. Meth.* 61:79–87.

25. Tomishima, M. and Enquist, L. W. 2002. In vivo egress of an alphaherpesvirus from axons. *J. Virol.* 76:8310–8317.

26. Visser, N. and Lutticken, D. 1989. Experiences with a gI-/TK-modified live pseudorabies virus vaccine: Strain begonia. In *Vaccination and control of Aujeszky's disease*, ed. J. T. van Oirschot, 37–44. Dordrecht, the Netherlands: Kluwer Academic Publishers.

27. Wheeler, J. G. and Osorio, F. A. 1991. Investigation of sites of pseudorabies virus latency using polymerase chain reaction. *Am. J. Vet. Res.* 52:1799–1803.

28. Wittmann, G. and Rziha, H. J. 1989. Aujeszky's disease (pseudorabies) in pigs. In *Herpesvirus diseases of cattle, horses and pigs*, vol. 9, ed. D. M. Knipe and P. M. Howley, 230–325. Boston, Mass.: Kluwer Academic Publishers.

29. Yoon, H. A., Eo, S. K., Aleyas, A. G., Park, S. O., Lee, J. H., Chae, J. S., Cho, J. G. and Song, H. J. 2005. Molecular survey of latent pseudorabies virus infection in nervous tissues of slaughtered pigs by nested and real-time PCR. *J. Microbiol.* 43:430–6.

9. Swine Influenza

Thankam Mathew, K. Dhama, H. Kothalawala, E. Gruys, and M. Mahendran

Introduction

Swine influenza (SI), caused by swine influenza virus (SIV) belonging to Orthomyxoviridae family, is an acute and febrile respiratory disease of swine with high morbidity and relatively low mortality (Easterday and Van Reeth, 1999; Mathew et al., 2006). It is commonly known as swine flu or hog flu and is prevalent throughout the world. Swine influenza was first observed in 1918 in USA, Hungary, and China (Choi et al., 2002c; Karasin et al., 2000, 2002; Vincent et al., 2008). The first SIV from swine has been isolated way back in 1930 (Shope, 1931; Kothalawala et al., 2006). Influenza virus A, the etiological agent of SI, comes under the porcine respiratory disease complex (PRDC) pathogens that consist of porcine respiratory and reproductive syndrome virus (PRRSV), porcine circovirus (PCV), and *Mycoplasma hyopneumoniae* (Woeste and Gross Beilage, 2007; Mellencamp et al., 2008; Nakharuthai et al., 2008). Swine influenza virus is capable of producing flu in humans, animals, and birds also. A viral hemagglutinin protein is responsible for attachment of the virus to the host cell and for fusion of the viral envelope with the host cell membrane, which results in agglutination of red blood cells. A viral neuraminidase protein is responsible for elution of virus from erythrocytes and may also play a role in the release of virus from infected cells. The antigenic characteristics of these two viral surface glycoproteins form the basis for dividing the virus into subtypes. Four main subtypes, which have been isolated in swine, are H1N1, H1N2, H3N2, and H1N7. Other subtypes that have been identified in pigs include H3N1, H4N6, and H9N2 (Kothalawala et al., 2006). The subtypes—namely, H1N1, H1N2, and H3N2 viruses—found in Europe are antigenically and genetically different from those found in the United States of America (Castrucci et al., 1993; Brown et al., 1998). The influenza pandemic in humans, nicknamed Spanish flu, that claimed twenty million lives worldwide in the same year and was initially thought to be having similar etiology with that of influenza affecting pigs coincided with the swine influenza outbreak of 1918. The viruses that caused 1957 and 1968 human influenza pandemics resulted from reassortment events of SIV as per numerous reports available (Webster et al., 1972; Scholtissek et al., 1978; Kawaoka et al., 1989). Taubenberger et al. (1997) analyzed the gene fragments of these viruses, which revealed that they were closely related to swine viruses from that periods and therefore could be transmitted to humans from pigs.

ETIOLOGY

Actually, type A influenza viruses causes swine influenza. The etiological agent is a segmented RNA virus with a lipid envelope and helical nucleocapsid belonging to the family Orthomyxoviridae that are divided into three groups as type A, type B, or type C influenza viruses according to antigenic characteristics of the core proteins, of which only type A viruses will infect pigs (Easterday and Van Reth, 1999; Kothalawala, et al., 2006; Mathew, et al., 2006). Influenza A viruses infects a variety of animal species, including humans, pigs, horses, marine mammals, and birds also (Alexander and Brown, 2000).

The surface of the virus is covered by structural proteins called spikes, which are of two distinct types: hemagglutinin (H) and an enzyme, neuraminidase (N). These surface glycoproteins are the most important antigens for inducing protective immunity in the host (Alexander and Brown, 2000). Generally, antibodies are produced against the hemagglutinin, which helps in preventing reinfection (Kaplan and Webster, 1977; Kothalawala et al., 2006). Based on the H and N glycoprotein, the virus is subtyped into H1N1, H1N2, H3N2, H1N7, etc. As the RNA core is located in eight separate single-stranded segments, genetic reassortment can occur during mixed infections with generation of different influenza A subtypes. This property of the virus is responsible for the appearance of major antigenic and biologic variations. Genetic drift occurs particularly in the genes encoding the external glycoproteins (Alexander and Brown, 2000; Brown, 2000).

EPIDEMIOLOGY

Swine play an important role in the disease ecology of influenza. Having cellular receptors common with birds and humans, swine provide opportunity for mixed infections and potential for genetic reassortment between avian, human, and porcine influenza (Hall et al., 2008). During the period extending from 1978–1984, there has been an expansion of global distribution of swine influenza. SIVs or their antibodies have been reported in swine population from many countries like Czechoslovakia, UK, Poland, Kenya, Russia, Canada, China, Brazil, Italy, Columbia, Taiwan, Japan, and Iran (Shortridge and Webster, 1979; Easterday and Van Reeth, 1999). Epidemiological study held in Germany suggested that SIV infections in wild boar seem to be no serious threat for domestic pigs (Kaden et al., 2008). As per Pasma (2008), in countries like Canada, the herds with outbreaks of swine influenza are located by using a geographic information system (GIS) and analyzed by using spatial analysis software.

Outbreaks with H1N1 and H3N2 viruses have been reported in countries like Belgium, France, USA, Germany, Netherlands, Sweden, Japan, Thailand,

Taiwan, Korea, and Denmark (Brown et al., 1997; Choi et al., 2002a; Jo et al., 2007; Saito et al., 2008; Chutinimitkul et al., 2008; Lee et al., 2008a; Shieh et al., 2008). Influenza virus infections with subtypes H1N1, H3N2, and H1N2 are very common in domestic pigs in Europe (Loeffen et al., 2009). Similarly, swine influenza has been an endemic disease of pigs in USA for more than sixty-five years after it was first observed (Vincent et al., 2008). Till 1997, only H1N1 SIV circulated widely in the swine population of North America. However, it has been observed that since 1997, novel viruses of three different subtypes and five different genotypes have emerged among pigs. This should be considered remarkable as there were no substantial changes in the overall epidemiology for over sixty years prior to this time. Dramatic antigenic shift occurred with the emergence of H3N2 viruses in 1997, particularly the H3N2 viruses with genes derived from human, swine, and avian viruses (Olsen, 2002; CDC, Atlanta, 2005). The triple reassortant H3N2 viruses were isolated for the first time from pigs in 1998 and are known to be endemic in swine and turkey populations in the United States (Vincent et al., 2006; Yassine et al., 2007; Newman et al., 2008). Poljak et al. (2008a) pointed out that the epidemiology of influenza in the North American swine population has changed since the emergence of this triple-reassortant H3N2 influenza virus.

TRANSMISSION

Being a highly contagious viral infection of pigs, swine influenza has significant economic impact on the affected herd (Easterday and Van Reeth, 1999). The young pigs have a major role in maintaining the SIV in farms, and the disease can remain enzootic. Transmission of SI is through contact with aerosols by coughing or sneezing, nasal discharge, and fomites. Nasal secretions are laden with virus during the acute febrile stage, and nasal shedding of the virus can occur within twenty-four hours of infection. The virus is also carried and spread by avian species, particularly waterfowl or by humans. The incubation period is about three days, and the infection is more common during the fall and winter months. Influenza virus can be shed for thirty days postinoculation and has been recovered from clinically normal animals also. Pigs serve as major reservoirs of H1N1 and H3N2 influenza viruses and are often involved in interspecies transmission of influenza viruses. They are known to have receptors in their respiratory tract, which can bind swine, human, and avian influenza viruses. Hence, pigs have been nicknamed as mixing vessels as they pave way for the development of new influenza viruses by the process of recombination (Scholtissek et al., 1983; Alexander and Brown, 2000; Kothalawala et al., 2006). The maintenance of these viruses in pigs and interspecies transmission could be important in the generation of new strains of human influenza viruses that may be capable of rapid transmission, producing devastating pandemics.

Symptoms and Pathogenesis
The infection causes respiratory disease that is characterized by coughing, sneezing, rapid and difficult breathing, nasal discharge, pyrexia, lethargy, depressed appetite, and prostration (Easterday and Van Reeth, 1999; Kothalawala et al., 2006). In some cases, SI may be associated with reproductive disorders, including abortion. If the virus is introduced for the first time into susceptible herds, then acute infections occur and may result in severe outbreaks.

In swine, two forms of the disease can occur: epidemic or endemic. In the epidemic form, the virus quickly moves through the swine population with rapid recovery provided there are not complicating factors like secondary bacterial infections. In the endemic form, clinical signs may be less obvious, and not all pigs may demonstrate the classical signs. Morbidity can reach up to 100% with SIV infections, and mortality rates are usually found to be low (OIE, 2004). However, secondary bacterial infections can exacerbate the clinical manifestations, and after two to six days infected pigs might recover if the condition has not been complicated.

The replication of SIV is generally restricted to the respiratory tract of pigs, the primary area of infection being the respiratory epithelium, which lines the airways. After inhalation, the virus gets deposited on the surface of the lower respiratory tract. In the classic acute form, the virus multiplies in bronchial epithelium within sixteen hours of infection and causes focal necrosis of the bronchial epithelium, focal atelectasis, and gross hyperemia of the lungs (Kothalawala et al., 2006). Bronchial exudates and widespread atelectasis seen grossly as plum-colored lesions affecting individual lobules of apical and intermediate lobes occur after twenty-four hours. After infection, the lesions continue to develop until seventy-two hours, after which the virus becomes more difficult to demonstrate (Easterday and Van Reeth, 1999).

Lesions
There is a demarcation noted between normal and affected lung tissue on the examination of the gross lesions during postmortem examination (Easterday and Van Reeth, 1999; Kothalawala et al., 2006). The involved areas are often purple and firm, and interlobular edema can be appreciated. The airways may be filled with blood-tinged fibrinous exudates, and there is considerable enlargement and edema of bronchial, cervical, mediastinal, and mesenteric lymph nodes. The mucosa of the pharynx and larynx are hyperemic and covered with tenacious mucus (Shope, 1931). Severe cases of swine influenza may result in interstitial pneumonia and fibrinous pleuritis. Microscopic lesions usually consist of widespread congestion of lung parenchyma, thickened alveolar septa, degenerative changes in the epithelium of small

bronchi, necrosis of bronchial epithelium, focal atelectasis, and emphysema (Easterday and Van Reeth, 1999; Kothalawala et al., 2006). Moreover, peribronchial and perivascular cellular infiltrations are noted.

IMMUNE RESPONSES

Defined clinical signs were not seen in most of the SIV infections. The absence of clinical signs in swine suggests that many influenza infections remain subclinical, resulting in immunity for the rest of pig's life span. Or this could be due to protection by maternally derived antibodies during early infection that might have caused absence of clinical signs (Brown and Mc Millen, 1994; Kothalawala et al., 2006), whereas another study did not show protection or level of protection depending on the level of maternally derived antibodies (Renshaw, 1975). Besides the differences in levels of maternally derived antibodies, the age at infection or the influenza strain often influence the immune responses toward the infection (Easterday and Van Reeth, 1999; Kothalawala et al., 2006). Piglets with high levels of maternally derived antibodies developed weaker immunity than pigs without or with low levels of maternally derived antibodies as per the studies of Loeffen et al. (2003). Thus, as per such findings, the advantage of sow herd vaccination to increase piglet's protection against SIV infection is an issue of debate.

Studies on both innate and adaptive immune responses of pigs to influenza virus contribute, therefore, to a better control of these infections. Proinflammatory cytokines–including type I interferon (IFN), tumor necrosis factor-alpha (TNF-alpha), and interleukin-6 (IL-6)–were found in lung secretions of influenza virus infected pigs, and together with this the infection induced long-lived increment of lung CD8+ T cells and local lymphoproliferative responses (Charley et al., 2006). Also, in vivo depletion of alveolar macrophages in pigs resulted in 40% mortality when pigs are infected, giving proof that alveolar macrophages are essential for controlling influenza virus infection in pigs (Kim et al., 2008).

It has been identified that humoral and cellular immune responses equally play a key role in the inflammatory process against the infection in pigs. IgG, IgA, and HI titers obtain peak levels after two to three weeks of primary infection; the predominant virus-specific isotype in serum being IgG (Kothalawala et al., 2006). Besides, pigs responded with IgG and IgA in their upper and lower respiratory tracts, among which IgA was the predominant isotype at both the sites (Schorr et al., 1994).

Further, cross-protection against some SIV subtypes has been documented. It has been reported that postinfection immunity to H1N1 and/or H3N2 viruses provide cross-protection against H1N2 infection (Kothalawala et al., 2006). Also, H1N2 show "double reassortment" with genes of different donor strains. The immune response against the internal proteins, which are relatively conserved in H1N1 and H3N2, may have a role in the cross-protection against H1N2 SIV infections (Van Reeth et al., 2003).

DIAGNOSIS AND TREATMENT

Swine influenza virus infections can be diagnosed based on a combination of clinical signs, typical gross and histopathologic lesions, diagnostic tests to detect live virus, nucleic acid or antigen, and serologic assays (Easterday and Van Reeth, 1999). From the clinical and pathological findings, a presumptive diagnosis can be made. In acute cases, the postmortem investigation shows pneumonic lesions, mainly in the apical and cardiac lobes, and presents edematous mediastinal lymph nodes. Affected areas of lungs become firm and swollen with a purplish color. On microscopical examination, exudative bronchitis and interstitial pneumonia can be seen. For the laboratory confirmation, nasal swabs, lung tissue, and acute and convalescent sera are to be collected. Only pigs with acute disease with high temperatures of 105°F or higher should be swabbed for virus detection. Virus can be isolated from tissues or swabs in cell cultures or embryonated chicken eggs. Virus isolation can be conducted in cell lines susceptible to SIV infection. Madin Darby canine kidney (MDCK) is the preferred cell line, but primary swine kidney, swine testicle, or swine lung epithelial cell lines can also be used (OIE, 2004; Landolt et al., 2005; Kothalawala et al., 2006; Nakharuthai et al., 2008). The SIV can be isolated by inoculation of suspected samples, like nasal swabs, in ten—to eleven-day-old embryonated chicken eggs through the allantoic cavity or amniotic route (Easterday and Van Reeth, 1999; Choi et al., 2002a; Suriya et al., 2008). Hermann et al. (2006) reported that optimized sampling parameters and specific compounds like ethylene glycol can influence the recovery and detection of SIV.

Most important and commonly used serological technique for the diagnosis of SIV infection is hemagglutination inhibition (HI) test (OIE, 2004; Kothalawala et al., 2006; Van Reeth et al., 2006; Poljak et al., 2008b). Hemagglutination inhibition (HI) test, which is the primary serological test for SIV, is sufficiently specific to discriminate between infections with the three subtypes–H1N1, H3N2, and H1N2—in swine populations if properly employed. Commercially available antigen-capture ELISAs can also detect the type A influenza viruses (Poljak et al., 2008b). However, as per Skibbe et al. (2004), a new SIV isolate representing current SIV strains circulating in the field should be used to replace the older isolates used in the HI and ELISA to increase the accuracy for serodiagnosis of SIV. Also, Yoon et al. (2004)

suggested that commercial ELISA may not always identify positive animals at the early stage of infection as effectively as the HI test. ELISA performed with recombinant HA protein, generated using baculovirus system, has been identified as a better tool for swine influenza surveillance (Wan et al., 2008). Leuwerke et al. (2008) recently pointed out the importance of revamping the conventional techniques like ELISA, HI, and SNT to enable subtype-specific detection of antibodies elicited by multiple isolates.

Likewise, detection of SIV from tissues, particularly lung, can be achieved using immunohistochemistry and fluorescent antibody techniques (OIE, 2004; Nakharuthai et al., 2008). The presence of SIV nucleic acid in specimens can be ascertained by polymerase chain reaction (PCR) using suitable primers (Fouchier et al., 2000). HA subtyping of influenza viruses also could be determined by reverse transcription–PCR (RT-PCR) reactions (Horimoto and Kawaoka, 1995; Choi et al., 2002c; Foni et al., 2003; Nakharuthai et al., 2008) each using a set of primers specific to one HA subtype (Lee et al., 2001; Chiapponi et al., 2003). The sensitivity of PCR testing for influenza virus detection in clinical samples appears to exceed virus isolation as per Erickson et al. (2004). Besides, real-time RT-PCR assay is a fast and accurate test for screening numerous nasal-swab specimens for swine influenza virus (Landolt et al., 2005). Likewise, a multiplex RT-PCR (mRT-PCR) assays have been developed that could detect and identify twelve hemagglutinin (H1–H12) and nine neuraminidase (N1–N9) subtypes that are commonly isolated from avian, swine, and human influenza A viruses (Choi et al., 2002b; Chang et al., 2008; Lee et al., 2008b). Meanwhile, Reichmuth et al. (2008) reported that microchip-based portable electrophoretic immunoassays can be used for sensitive and rapid detection of influenza viruses. This technique allows concentration and detection of viruses simultaneously, using a microfluidic chip with an integrated nanoporous membrane.

Because of the zoonotic nature of SIV, different diagnostic methods have been employed for the tissue-based detection of SIV antigen in formalin-fixed, paraffin-embedded forms by monoclonal and/or polyclonal antibody-based immunohistochemical procedures (Haines et al., 1993; Larochelle et al., 1994; Vincent et al., 1997). During such tests, the potentially infectious specimens must be handled carefully to avoid transmission of virus to humans. SIV infections in humans, some of which were fatal, have been documented in USA and Europe (Eason et al., 1980; Dacso et al., 1984; De Jong et al., 1988; Wenworth et al., 1997; Kimura et al., 1998). Another approach for detection of SIV is the application of in situ hybridization (Kothalawala et al., 2006). It is a valuable tool in addition to standard RNA extraction techniques for evaluating gene expression in tissue and cells, the major advantage being the ability to determine tissues or cells in a mixed population expressing the RNA of interest.

Molecular characterization, by gene sequencing, followed by phylogenetic analysis of genes of SIV has been found helpful to characterize the virus. Genome phylogeny of SIV has helped in indicating a sister relationship of the 1918 human flu strain with the classic swine H1N1 lineage (Vana and Westover, 2008). Based on the sequencing of matrix (M), nonstructural (NS), HA and NA genes of subtype H3N2 SIV, it was identified that the virus was a reassortant one, especially of H3N2 human influenza virus and classical H1N1 swine influenza virus (Yao et al., 2007). Phylogenetic analysis also indicated that swine H9N2 viruses formed novel HA and neuraminidase sublineages that were related closely to those of earlier chicken H9 viruses (Cong et al., 2007). Similarly, phylogenetic analysis of the Korean isolates H1N1, H1N2, and H3N2 proved that they are closely related to viruses from North America (Jo et al., 2007; Lee et al., 2008a). Using sequencing studies, Liu et al. (2008a) assessed that majority of SIV HA gene had high homology to the strain of humanlike SIV (99%), while others had high homology to the classical SIV. Likewise, phylogenetic analysis of viral gene segments can also indicate multiple reassortant lineages (Pascua et al., 2008; Shi et al., 2008).

There is no specific treatment for swine influenza. However, drugs approved for the treatment of influenza viruses in general are the influenza M2 channel inhibitors (amantadine and rimantadine) and the influenza neuraminidase inhibitors (oseltamivir and zanamivir) (Leyssen et al., 2008). But treatment for SIV infections is based on supportive therapy and can include steps for reducing stress and body temperatures and ensuring that the affected pigs are maintained in a comfortable environment. Careful nursing and dust-free bedding should be provided to the affected animals. Expectorants are used as herd treatment and can be administered in drinking water. Antibiotics and antimicrobials have been used to control concurrent or secondary bacterial infections. Drugs to prevent ascariasis are recommended to reduce the losses that may incur due to the interaction of migrating ascaris larvae and SIV.

PREVENTION AND CONTROL

The best way to deal with swine influenza is to prevent the occurrence and spread of the disease. Prevention is based on good management practices to reduce the risk of SIV entering the herd and includes good biosecurity measures such as limiting people and vehicle traffic on the premises, properly cleaning and disinfecting animal trucks, and quarantining new pigs before placing them in the farm. Since pigs are vulnerable to infection from both human and avian influenza viruses, it is essential to continue surveillance and monitoring of SIV infection in the swine population to downsize the pandemic threat too (Easterday and Van Reeth, 1999; Gregory et al., 2003; Nakharuthai et al., 2008). Early detection and warning systems and the quick implementation of sanitary measures, including stamping out, remain key issues in the control of highly contagious porcine diseases like influenza (Vannie et al., 2007).

Swine are commonly infected during herd replacements in the farm or during exhibitions (Easterday and Van Reeth, 1999). There are certain important parameters that one should follow to prevent the disease entering a herd like avoiding purchase of new stock and taking animals to exhibitions without proper precautionary measure. During infection, avoid moving animals within the barn to eliminate excess stress that could exacerbate the condition. If any new herd is added to a preexisting herd, be sure to isolate these animals, preferably in a separate building. Screen these animals by employing serological techniques for determining any previous exposure to swine influenza viruses.

Standard sanitary measures can also help prevent and control the spread of SIV. Influenza viruses are inactivated by soap, heat, and formalin. They are very sensitive, and hence, disinfectants such as sodium hypochlorite are effective in disinfecting the farm premises. Vehicles such as trucks, trailers, and any equipment, which may be contaminated, should also be thoroughly disinfected. Along with this, routine use of hand hygiene systems and boot dips will help prevent entry of the virus into the herd.

Vaccination is another mode of controlling swine influenza. However, vaccination of pigs is not commonly practiced. There have been commercial vaccines available throughout Europe, which gave satisfactory protection from SIV infection following vaccination. Large-scale monolayer or suspension cell systems, operated under strict temperature-controlled, aseptic conditions, and defined production methods are used to produce inactivated vaccines as per OIE guidelines (OIE, 2004). Results from various studies show that vaccinated animals exposed to SIV have markedly reduced nasal shedding, virus infection in lung tissue, and lung pathology in comparison to nonvaccinated animals. Thacker and Janke (2008) have recently pointed out that control of swine influenza can be achieved through the vaccination of dam to protect young pigs by generating maternal antibodies. Studies have also shown that maternally derived antibody in vaccinated sows protects five-week-old pigs from clinical disease (Brown and Mc Millen, 1994). But influenza viruses continue to circulate in pigs after the decay of maternal antibodies, providing a continuing source of virus on a herd basis

(Thacker and Janke, 2008). Further, the presence of maternal antibodies at vaccination had a negative impact on vaccine efficacy as fever and clinical signs were prolonged along with SIV-induced pneumonia as per Kitikoon et al. (2006).

Also, at this juncture, SIV vaccine inducing cross-protective immunity between different subtypes and strains is highly desirable (Richt et al., 2006) as SIVs of H1N1, H3N2, and H1N2 subtypes, with antigenically different hemagglutinins, are currently circulating in pigs in many parts of the world (Van Reeth et al., 2006). The efficacy of the present commercial vaccines may also need to be improved to provide sufficient protection against emerging SIV variants (Lee et al., 2007). However, with the increasing number of novel subtypes and genetic variants, the control of swine influenza, using vaccination strategy alone, has become increasingly difficult (Vincent et al., 2008).

Molecular biology and technical advances in DNA recombination have ushered in a new era in vaccinology (Vannie et al., 2007). Regarding the influenza immunoprophylactics, ongoing research is there for the development of novel vaccines such as DNA, live-virus, or vectored vaccines (Thacker and Janke, 2008; Li et al., 2008). Wesley et al. (2004) reported that replication-defective adenovirus recombinants could be developed into potential vaccines against H3N2 influenza viruses in pigs, and they have an additional advantage over commercial vaccines that suckling piglets have no preexisting maternal antibodies to block piglet vaccination. Wesley and Lager (2005) later developed a recombinant human adenovirus-5 vaccine for protecting weaned pigs against swine influenza virus subtype H3N2. Richt et al. (2006) have recently developed an H3N2 SIV containing a deleted NS1 gene expressing a truncated NS1 protein of 126 amino acids for attenuation in swine, indicating its potential use as a DIVA (differentiate infected from vaccinated animals) vaccine. Also, it has the potential for use as a modified live-virus vaccine (MLV) in pigs (Vincent et al., 2007). Studies also indicate that the deletion of amino acids 191 to 195 of the NS1 protein is critical for the attenuation of the SIV in chickens (Zhu et al., 2008). Similarly, the baculovirus insect cell-mediated protein production and viruslike particle (VLP) can be exploited for rapid vaccine production, which is particularly suitable for influenza vaccines (Galarza et al., 2005; Cox, 2008). Regarding human influenza, using baculovirus system, a VLP vaccine bearing the surface glycoproteins HA and NA of the 1918 influenza A virus has been developed into a safe and immunogenic vaccine (Galarza et al., 2005; Matassov et al., 2007). Aside to this, antibody responses to VLP vaccine could be enhanced if the vaccine is formulated with adjuvants like IL-12 (Galarza et al., 2005). Likewise, reassortant technology was recently used to obtain three interspecific reassortant influenza viruses containing H1, H3, and H9 antigens from human, swine, and avian influenza viruses respectively, and the trivalent vaccine made out of it offered multiprotection against different influenza viruses synchronously (Du et al., 2008). In search of a subunit vaccine, Liu et al. (2008b) expressed HA protein in *E. coli* and during antibody response studies; they found that mouse produced antibodies against the target peptide. As per Kitikoon et al. (2008), the influenza matrix 2 (M2) protein is a potential subunit vaccine candidate to induce protective immunity against broader strains of influenza viruses in pigs. Aside to these, the successful rescue of SIV, using reverse genetics technique, can help the scientific world to generate novel SIV as vaccine candidate (Yang et al., 2007; Peng et al., 2008; Masic et al., 2009).

Besides, due to IFN-mediated antiviral and immunomodulatory effects, the use of IFN or IFN inducers may also prove an efficient strategy for a better control of influenza in pigs (Charley et al., 2006). Together with this, novel technologies such as pig gene microarrays, single nucleotide polymorphism (SNP) panels, and advanced bioinformatics should be used to identify new health candidate genes or detection of the infectious agent so that this economically important disease of swine could be effectively checked (Belak, 2005, 2007; Mellencamp et al., 2008). The development of padlock probes and microarrays, as well as ultrarapid PCR and sequencing methods, can further improve the arsenal of nucleic acid–based molecular diagnosis (Belak, 2005, 2007) in order to rejuvenate the field of virus detection systems.

INTERSPECIES TRANSMISSION AND PANDEMIC THREAT

Influenza viruses can infect many species of animals, such as avian, swine, equines, and humans. Avian influenza viruses (AIV) infect not only chickens and ducks but also pigs (Choi et al., 2004). It has been shown that not all but most of the AIV replicate in the upper respiratory tract of pigs (Manzoor et al., 2009). It is clear that the swine influenza outbreak in Hong Kong in 1998 was the result of AIV crossing the species barrier to pigs (Olsen et al., 2002). Gene sequencing was employed to identify the relationship between H9N2 avian and porcine influenza viruses; the study gave ample evidence for avian-to-pig interspecies transmission of H9N2 viruses (Cong et al., 2008). As pigs are susceptible to infection with both avian and human influenza A viruses, they have been proposed to be an intermediate host for the adaptation of avian influenza viruses to humans (Yu et al., 2008b). Also, to mention it more crucially, humans have faced major influenza pandemics in the twentieth century (Perez et al., 2005). The sudden emergence of antigenically different strains in humans, due to antigenic shift, has occurred on four occasions—in 1918 (H1N1), 1957 (H2N2), 1968 (H3N2), and 1977 (H1N1)—each resulting in a severe pandemics (Alexander and Brown, 2000; Kilbourne, 2006). Pandemic influenza occurs at irregular and unpredictable intervals and is the result of a major antigenic change known as antigenic shift, which occurs only in influenza A viruses as per Hampson and Mackenzie (2006). Even though viruses of each of the sixteen influenza A HA subtypes are potential human pathogens, only viruses of the H1, H2, and H3 subtypes are known to have been successfully established in humans (Ma et al., 2007). Even though the transmission of swine influenza to humans appears to be a rare event, swine have been proposed as an intermediate host for the generation of pandemic influenza viruses (Gregory et al., 2003; Komadina et al., 2007).

The probable introduction of classical swine influenza viruses (H1N1) to turkeys from infected pigs has been reported from North America (Hinshaw et al., 1983). Serological studies have revealed antibodies to classical swine H1 influenza virus in both turkeys and pigs. Genetic analyses of H1N1 viruses from turkeys in the United States have revealed a high degree of genetic exchange and reassortment of influenza A viruses from turkeys and pigs (Wright et al., 1992). Also, the isolation of swinelike H3N2 influenza viruses from turkeys raises new concerns for the generation of novel viruses that could affect humans (Webby et al., 2000). These reports suggest the ability of this versatile virus to jump from swine to avian population apart from human beings. Recently, it has been identified that pigs had low susceptibility to infection with the avian H5N1 HPAI viruses (Lipatov et al., 2008).

The SIVs are known for the ability to jump from one species to another as in case of other influenza viruses, and hence the identification of genetic changes responsible for transmission between mammals will be an important task for the near future (de Wit and Fouchier, 2008). Prevalence of antibodies to swine influenza virus in humans has been reported (Ayora-Talavera et al., 2005). Also, cross-species transfer of swine influenza to humans have been noticed on several occasions, but luckily, these viruses lacked the ability to spread from human-to-human (Van Reeth, 2007). However, following interspecies transmission to pigs, some influenza viruses may be genetically unstable, giving rise to variants, but eventually a stable lineage may be derived from the dominant variant and become established in pigs (Brown, 2000).

There is considerable evidence that transmission from pigs to humans does occur. Early theories suggest that the transmission of virus from pigs to humans resulted in the 1918 pandemic (Taubenberger et al., 1997). It was not until 1976 that further evidence for such transmissions became available. Sporadic clinical cases of swine influenza can occur in humans, with a case-fatality rate of 14% (Myers et al., 2007). At Fort Dix, New Jersey, USA, pigs were implicated as the source of infection when an H1N1 virus was isolated from a soldier who had died of influenza. The virus was very much identical to the viruses isolated from pigs in the region. Furthermore, five other servicemen and five hundred personnel at Fort Dix were infected with the same virus (Hodder et al., 1977). Antibodies to swine H1 viruses have been detected in people who had close contact with pigs (Schnurrenberger et al., 1970). Robinson et al. (2007) recently reported that influenza A virus (H3N2) of swine origin was isolated from a seven-month-old child, who recovered uneventfully.

By gene sequencing, the H3N2 viruses from Guangdong Province of China were identified to be descendants of human viruses, and this proved that there occurs interspecies transmission of human influenza viruses to pigs also (Yu et al., 2007). Further, a humanlike H1N1 swine virus was isolated from pigs in Guangdong Province that was directly derived from about two thousand human H1N1 influenza viruses (Yu et al., 2009). As per the analysis of De Jong et al. (2007), the antigenic evolution of swine viruses occurred at a rate approximately six times slower than the rate in human viruses, even though the rates of genetic evolution were similar for human and swine H3N2 viruses.

In swine, genetic reassortment to create novel influenza subtypes by mixing avian, human, and swine influenza viruses is possible as per Richt et al. (2006). It has been identified that occupational exposure to pigs greatly increases workers' risk of SIV infection (Gray and Baker, 2007). Swine industry workers who seldom used gloves or who smoked most frequently had evidence of H1N1 swine virus (Ramirez et al., 2006). Considering such factors, the swine workers should be included in pandemic surveillance and in antiviral and immunization strategies (Myers et al., 2006; Gray et al., 2007a). Further, swine and poultry professionals may expose swine and poultry to human influenza viruses and facilitate the generation of novel influenza viruses to accelerate human influenza epidemics (Gray et al., 2007a). Also to mention, the control of influenza virus infection in poultry and swine is critical to the reduction of potential cross-species adaptation and spread of influenza viruses, which will minimize the risk of animals being the source of the next pandemic (Thacker and Janke, 2008). To conclude, cross-species transmission of influenza viruses alone is insufficient to start a human influenza pandemic, and it requires dramatic but largely unknown genetic changes to become established in the human population (Van Reeth, 2007).

REASSORTMENT OF SWINE INFLUENZA VIRUSES

There were several reports of SIV being isolated from humans with respiratory illness (Dacso et al., 1984) and occasionally with fatal consequences (Rota et al., 1989). All cases examined followed contact with sick pigs and were due to viruses related most closely to classical swine H1N1 influenza virus, which suggests a successful reassortment between the human IV and SIV. Due to the segmented genome of the influenza viruses, genetic reassortment can occur between different subtypes, resulting in antigenic shift, which is an abrupt and major change in the influenza A viruses, resulting in a new hemagglutinin or new hemagglutinin and neuraminidase proteins. This results in a new influenza A subtype. Reassortant viruses with some characteristics of human H1 viruses have been isolated from pigs in England (Brown et al., 1998). H3N2 is one of the main subtypes of influenza virus that circulates in human and swine population throughout the world, indicating the reassortment between H3N2 human and H1N1 swine influenza viruses (Sun et al., 2008). Influenza viruses of subtype H3N2 are endemic in most pig populations worldwide, where they persist for many years after their antigenic counterparts have disappeared from humans. Pigs can be infected with both human and swine influenza viruses, and a new reassortant influenza virus can emerge to which the human population does not have protective antibodies, and this can very well lead to pandemics of devastating potential.

Gene mutation and reassortment of genes have been considered as the key factors responsible for influenza A virus virulence and host tropism change (He et al., 2008). Pigs are capable of harboring the influenza virus of human and avian origin facilitating reassortment of the viruses within their body by acting as a mixing vessel for the generation of pandemic influenza viruses or adaptation to the mammalian host (Easterday and Van Reeth, 1999; Alexander and Brown, 2000; Suriya et al., 2008; Yu et al., 2008a). It has been proven beyond doubt that the genetic reassortment between avian and human influenza viruses, which is an important mechanism for the emergence of new pandemic human strains, frequently occurs in pigs in nature (Van Reeth, 2006; Suriya et al., 2008). The coexistence of humanlike and reassortant viruses provides further evidence that pigs serve as intermediate hosts or mixing vessels (Yu et al., 2008a). This concept is also supported by the detection of human-avian reassortant viruses in

European pigs with some evidence for subsequent transmission to the human population (Brown, 2000). Also, it has been identified that the European H1N2 SIVs arose after multiple reassortment steps involving a porcine influenza virus with avian-influenza-like internal segments and human H1N1 and H3N2 viruses in 1994 (Zell et al., 2008a). Analysis of GenBank sequence data also reveals numerous reassortment events in recent years, demonstrating ongoing evolution of swine influenza viruses (Zell et al., 2008b).

Apart from human influenza viruses, influenza viruses of avian origin can also get into the swine population and get reassorted. In 1979, an H1N1 avian influenza virus crossed the species barrier, establishing a new lineage in European swine population (Stetch et al., 1999). Two H3N3 Ontario swine flu isolates had genes that are most closely related to avian influenza (bird flu) isolates from North America. The H3 is most closely related to avian H3 isolated from mallards and pintails. The N3, however, is most closely related to avian species isolated from Texas as well as British Columbia (www.recombinomics.com, 2005).

The pig is the primary mammalian species that is domesticated, reared in abundance, and susceptible to avian and human influenza viruses and allows productive replication of such viruses (Hinshaw et al., 1983; Zhou et al., 1999; Suriya et al., 2008), whereas other mammalian species such as felines can also become infected and spread avian influenza too (Rimmelzwaan et al., 2006). Swine have receptors to which both avian and mammalian influenza viruses bind, which increases the potential for viruses to exchange genetic sequences and produce new reassortant viruses in swine (Thacker and Janke, 2008). Pigs have both avian (alpha 2–3 linked sialic acid to galactose) and human (alpha 2–6 linked sialic acid) influenza virus receptors, which supports their role as mixing vessels for reassortment between human and avian viruses (Kundin et al., 1970; Schultz et al., 1991; Kida et al., 1994; Van Reeth, 2006; Thacker and Janke, 2008). This can result in modification of the receptor-binding specificities of avian influenza viruses from 2, 3 to 2, 6 linkages (Ito et al., 1998). The latter is the native linkage in the human respiratory tract, thereby providing a potential bridge from birds to humans.

These observations support the potential role of the pig as a mediator for reassortment of influenza viruses originating from different species. The avian influenza viruses are adapted to the avian digestive tract, which carries 2, 3 sialic acid receptors, and do not possess the 2, 6 sialic acid receptors required for virus attachment to human respiratory epithelial cells (Beare and Webster, 1991; Van Reeth, 2006). Hence, pigs are the best candidate for this role because they possess both the receptors and are equally susceptible to infection by both avian and human influenza viruses (Kida et al., 1994; Thacker and Janke, 2008). Furthermore, avian viruses can contribute genes in the generation of reassortants when coinfecting pigs with a swine influenza virus too. Reassortant viruses of H1N2 subtype derived from human and avian viruses or H1N7 subtype derived from human and equine viruses (Brown and Alexander, 1994) supports this fact. Also, phylogenetic analyses of human H3N2 viruses circulating in Italian pigs revealed that genetic reassortment had been occurring between avian and humanlike viruses since 1983 (Castrucci et al., 1993).

STEPS TO REDUCE INTERSPECIES TRANSMISSION

The swine influenza virus vaccines used nowadays may not induce strong immunity nor completely eliminate clinical signs of infection in swine. But vaccination of pigs can reduce the levels of virus shed by infected animals and thus reduce the potential for human exposure and zoonotic infections (Gray and Baker, 2007). Conversely, vaccination of farmworkers with human vaccines will reduce the amounts of viruses they shed if infected during human influenza outbreaks and thereby limit the potential for human influenza virus infection of pigs.

In swine houses, the ventilation systems should be designed to minimize recirculation of air within rooms, which is important to reduce the exposure of pigs to viruses from other pigs, and to reduce their exposure to human influenza viruses and, conversely, to reduce exposure of workers to swine influenza viruses. Basic hygiene practices need to be followed. Workers should change clothes prior to leaving swine barns. In addition, hand-to-face contact should be minimized and hand-washing stations should be available throughout the animal housing areas (Gray et al., 2007b) as the influenza viruses are spread not just by inhalation of aerosolized virus but also by eye and nose contact with droplets of respiratory secretions.

Similarly, steps to reduce interspecies transmission of SIV to birds include bird-proofing, water treatment, separation of pig and bird production, separation of pig and bird production, feed security, and worker biosecurity (Olsen, 2004; Thacker and Janke, 2008). All doorways, windows, and airflow vents in swine housing units should be adequately sealed to prevent entrance of birds. Although small birds such as sparrows, swallows, and finches are not thought to be important in the overall ecology of influenza viruses, they may act as mechanical vectors for the influenza viruses. Untreated surface water should not be used as either drinking water or water for cleaning in swine barns because of fecal contamination with influenza viruses by waterfowl. Keep pig feed in closed containers to prevent contamination with feces from overflying waterfowl. Finally and more importantly, it is unwise to raise pigs and domestic fowl on the same premises.

SWINE FLU: THE CURRENT 2009 SCENARIO

Novel influenza A (H1N1) is a new flu virus of swine origin that was first detected in April 2009. The virus is infecting people and is spreading from person to person and has sparked a growing outbreak of illness in the United States with an increasing number of cases being reported internationally as well. Before April 2009, sporadic human infections with swine influenza have been occasionally reported. Cases of swine flu have most commonly occurred in people with direct exposure to pigs, but some cases of human-to-human transmission have been reported. However, in the current swine flu outbreak, WHO says the virus is being spread from human to human, not from contact with infected pigs.

The current situation regarding the outbreaks of type A (H1N1) swine influenza is evolving rapidly, and countries from different regions of the globe have been affected. Also human-to-human transmission has been demonstrated along with the ability of the virus to cause community-level outbreaks, which together suggest the possibility of sustained human-to-human transmission. In response to an intensifying outbreak in the United States and internationally caused by a new influenza virus of swine origin, the World Health Organization raised the worldwide pandemic alert level to *phase 5*. A phase 5 alert is a "strong signal that a pandemic is imminent and that the time to finalize the organization, communication, and implementation of the planned mitigation measures is short."

The situation continues to evolve rapidly. Till May 13, 2009, thirty-three countries have officially reported 5,728 cases of influenza A (H1N1) infection. Mexico has reported 2,059 laboratory-confirmed human cases of infection, including 56 deaths. The United States has reported 3,352 laboratory-confirmed human cases from forty-five states, including 3 deaths. Canada has reported 358 laboratory-confirmed human cases, including 1 death. Costa Rica has reported 8 laboratory-confirmed human cases, including 1 death.

The following countries have reported laboratory-confirmed cases with no deaths: Argentina (1), Australia (1), Austria (1), Brazil (8), China (2, comprising 1 in China, Hong Kong Special Administrative Region, and 1 in Mainland China), Colombia (3), Denmark (1), El Salvador (4), France (13), Germany (12), Guatemala (1), Ireland (1), Israel (7), Italy (9), Jan (4), Netherlands (3), New Zealand (7), Norway (2), Panama (16), Poland (1), Portugal (1), Republic of Korea (3), Spain (95), Sweden (2), Switzerland (1), and the United Kingdom (55) (*http://www.cdc.gov/h1n1flu/*; *http://www.who.int/csr/don/2009_05_13/en/index.html* Influenza A(H1N1)—update 27).

Pigs most commonly get infected with flu viruses from other pigs (swine flu) but also can get infected with flu viruses from birds (avian flu) and from people (human flu). This cross-species spread of flu viruses can lead to new types of flu viruses. The current swine flu virus originated in pigs and has genes from human, bird, and pig viruses. The new strain is an apparent *reassortment* of four strains of *influenza A virus subtype H1N1*. Analysis by the *CDC* identified the four component strains as one *endemic in humans*, one *endemic in birds*, and two *endemic in pigs (swine)*. However, other scientists have stated that analysis of the 2009 swine flu (A/H1N1) viral genome suggests that all *RNA* segments are of swine origin. Scientists don't know exactly how it jumped to humans. It's thought that novel influenza A (H1N1) flu spreads in the same way that regular seasonal influenza viruses spread, mainly through the coughs and sneezes of people who are sick with the virus.

It is likely that most people, especially those who do not have regular contact with pigs, do not have immunity to swine influenza viruses, that can prevent the virus infection. If a swine virus establishes efficient human-to-human transmission, it can cause an influenza pandemic.

There are no vaccines that contain the current swine influenza virus causing illness in humans. It is not known whether current human seasonal influenza vaccines can provide any protection. Influenza viruses change very quickly. It is important to develop a vaccine against the currently circulating virus strain for it to provide maximum protection to the vaccinated people.

In humans, clinical symptoms are similar to seasonal influenza, but reported clinical presentation ranges broadly from asymptomatic infection to severe pneumonia resulting in death. People infected with flu typically have fever (often high), cough, body aches, headaches, fatigue, and runny or stuffy nose. Vomiting and diarrhea may also occur.

For the ongoing outbreak, the use of oseltamivir or zanamivir is recommended for treatment of the disease. WHO has started distributing its stockpile of two million treatments of the antiviral drug Tamiflu to regional offices. Influenza viruses are not known to be transmissible to people through eating properly handled and prepared pork-processed pork or other food products derived from pigs. The SIV is killed by cooking temperatures of 160°F/70°C or other such products.

The World Health Organization has now suggested using the term "swine flu" to avoid confusion over the danger posed by pigs: "Rather than calling this swine flu the technical scientific name H1N1 influenza A is proposed." Killing pigs "will not help to guard against public or animal health risks" presented by the virus and "is inappropriate" because the current swine flu virus has now gained human-to-human spread.

Conclusion

Swine Influenza is an economically important disease that can lead to significant losses in swine production units. It causes respiratory infection and in some cases reproductive disorders, leading to abortion in sows. A major concern with swine influenza is the economic burden as a result of uneven growth and prolonged finishing time. Adult pigs are the main culprits to maintain the virus and pass it to young susceptible animals. In combination with other viruses and bacteria, the causative agent is capable of producing complex respiratory syndromes too. H1N1 and H3N2 subtype influenza viruses are endemic in pig populations worldwide and are responsible for one of the most prevalent respiratory diseases in pigs. As a result of heterogeneity and reassortments, the vaccination is often not proving out to be successful in case of SIV infections; hence, novel vaccinology tools have to be given due consideration in this regard. Strict biosecurity measures play a major part in controlling the disease, which is essential in preventing infection entering disease-free swine population. The pig has been a contender for the role of intermediate host or mixing vessel for reassortment of influenza viruses of avian and human origin since the pig represents the major mammalian species which is domesticated, reared in abundance, and is susceptible to avian and human influenza viruses and allows productive replication of such viruses. Apart from the disease in swine, the maintenance of SIV and the frequent exchange of virus segments between pigs and other species facilitated directly by improper swine husbandry practices can lead to the emergence of new and much more virulent strains of influenza viruses that has the potential to spread between humans, animals, and birds. To conclude, the research for the future need to target the factors that limit the transmission of influenza viruses from one species to another and should assess the possible reassortment events that could lead to the generation of pandemic influenza viruses.

REFERENCES

1. Alexander, D. J. and Brown, I. H. 2000. Recent zoonoses caused by influenza A viruses. *Rev. Sci. Tech.* 19:197–225.
2. Ayora-Talavera, G., Cadavieco-Burgos, J. M. and Canul-Armas, A. B. 2005. Serologic evidence of human and swine influenza in Mayan persons. *Emerg. Infect. Dis.* 11:158–161.
3. Beare, A. S. and Webster, R. G. 1991, Replication of avian influenza viruses in humans. *Arch Virol.* 119:37–42.
4. Belak, S. 2005. The molecular diagnosis of porcine viral diseases: A review. *Acta Vet. Hung.* 53:113–124.
5. Belak, S. 2007. Molecular diagnosis of viral diseases, present trends and future aspects A view from the OIE Collaborating Centre for the Application of Polymerase Chain Reaction Methods for Diagnosis of Viral Diseases in Veterinary Medicine. *Vaccine* 25:5444–5452.
6. Brown, G. B. and McMillen, J. 1994. Maxivac-Flu: Evaluation of the Safety and Efficacy of a Swine Influenza Vaccine. *Proc. AASP.* 7–39.
7. Brown, I. H. and Alexander, D. J. 1994. Swine influenza virus in Europe. *Proc. AASP.* 246–249.
8. Brown, I. H., Ludwig, S., Olsen, C. W., Hannoun, C., Scholtissek, C. and Hinshaw, V. S. 1997. Antigenic and genetic analyses of H1N1 influenza A viruses from European pigs. *J Gen Virol.* 78:553–562.
9. Brown, I. H., Harris, P. A., McCaulery, J. M. and Alexander, D. J. 1998. Multiple genetic reassortment of avian and human influenza A viruses in European pigs, resulting in the emergence of the H1N2 virus of novel genotype. *J. Gen. Virol.* 79:2947–2955.
10. Brown, I. H. 2000. The epidemiology and evolution of influenza viruses in pigs. *Vet. Microbiol.* 74:29–46.
11. Castrucci, M. R., Donatelli, I., Sidoli, L., Barigazzi, G., Kawaoka, Y. and Webster, R. G. 1993. Genetic reassortment between avian and human influenza A viruses in Italian pigs. *Virology* 193:503–506.
12. Centers for Disease Control and Prevention (CDC) 2005. Transmission of Influenza A viruses between animals and people. Atlanta, USA.
13. Chang, H. K., Park, J. H., Song, M. S., Oh, T. K., Kim, S. Y., Kim, C. J., Kim, H., Sung, M. H., Han, H. S., Hahn, Y. S. and Choi, Y. K. 2008. Development of multiplex rt-PCR assays for rapid detection and subtyping of influenza type A viruses from clinical specimens. *J. Microbiol. Biotechnol.* 18:1164–1169.
14. Charley, B., Riffault, S. and Van Reeth, K. 2006. Porcine innate and adaptive immune responses to influenza and coronavirus infections. *Ann. NY. Acad. Sci.* 1081:130–136.
15. Choi, Y. K., Goyal, S. M. and Joo, H. S. 2002a. Prevalence of swine influenza virus subtypes on swine farms in the United States. *Arch. Virol.* 147:1209–1220.
16. Choi, Y. K., Goyal, S. M., Kang, S. W., Farnham, M. W. and Joo, H. S. 2002b. Detection and subtyping of swine influenza H1N1, H1N2 and H3N2 viruses in clinical samples using two multiplex RT-PCR assays. *J. Virol. Methods* 102:53–59.
17. Choi, Y. K., Goyal, S. M., Farnham, M. W. and Joo, H. S. 2002c. Phylogenetic analysis of H1N2 isolates of influenza A virus from pigs in the United States. *Virus Res.* 87:173–179.

18. Choi, Y. K., Lee, H. J., Erickson, G., Goyal, S. M., Joo, H. S., Webster, R. and Webby, R. J. 2004. H3N2 influenza virus transmission from swine to turkeys, United States of America. *Emerg. Infect. Dis.* 10:2156–2160.

19. Chiapponi, C., Fallacara, F. and Foni, F. 2003. Subtyping of H1N1, H1N2 and H3N2 swine influenza viruses by 2 multiplex RT-PCR. *4th International symposium on emerging and re-emerging pig diseases, Rome, 2003* 1:2–4.

20. Chutinimitkul, S., Thippamom, N., Damrongwatanapokin, S., Payungporn, S., Thanawongnuwech, R., Amonsin, A., Boonsuk, P., Sreta, D., Bunpong, N., Tantilertcharoen, R., Chamnanpood, P., Parchariyanon, S., Theamboonlers, A. and Poovorawan, Y. 2008. Genetic characterization of H1N1, H1N2 and H3N2 swine influenza virus in Thailand. *Arch. Virol.* 153:1049–1056.

21. Cong, Y. L., Pu, J., Liu, Q. F., Wang, S., Zhang, G. Z., Zhang, X. L., Fan, W. X., Brown, E. G. and Liu, J. H. 2007. Antigenic and genetic characterization of H9N2 swine influenza viruses in China. *J. Gen. Virol.* 88:2035–2041.

22. Cong, Y. L., Wang, C. F., Yan, C. M., Peng, J. S., Jiang, Z. L. and Liu, J. H. 2008. Swine infection with H9N2 influenza viruses in China in 2004. *Virus Genes* 36:461–469.

23. Cox, M. M. 2008. Progress on baculovirus-derived influenza vaccines. *Curr. Opin. Mol. Ther.* 10:56–61.

24. Dacso, C. C., Couch, R. B., Six, H. R., Young, J. F., Quarles, J. M. and Kasel, J. A.1984. Sporadic occurrence of zoonotic swine influenza virus infection. *J. Clin. Microbiol.* 20:883–835.

25. De Jong, J. C., Paccaud, M. F., de Ronde-Verloop, F. M., Huffels, N. H., Verwei, C., Weijers, T. F., Bangma, P. J., van Kregten, E., Kerckhaert, J. A. M., Wicky, F. and Wunderli, W. 1988. Isolation of swine like influenza A (H1N1) viruses from man in Switzerland and the Netherlands. *Ann. Inst. Pasteur Virol.* 139:429–437.

26. De Jong, J. C., Smith, D. J., Lapedes, A. S., Donatelli, I., Campitelli, L., Barigazzi, G., Van Reeth, K., Jones, T. C., Rimmelzwaan, G. F., Osterhaus, A. D. and Fouchier, R. A. 2007. Antigenic and genetic evolution of swine influenza A (H3N2) viruses in Europe. *J. Virol.* 81:4315–4322.

27. De Wit, E. and Fouchier, R. A. 2008. Emerging influenza. *J. Clin. Virol.* 41:1–6.

28. Du, N., Li, W., Li, Y., Liu, S., Sui, Y., Qu, Z., Wang, Y., Du, Y. and Xu, B. 2008. Generation and evaluation of the trivalent inactivated reassortant vaccine using human, avian, and swine influenza A viruses. *Vaccine* 26:2912–2918.

29. Easterday, B. C. and Van Reeth, K. 1999. Swine influenza. In *Diseases of swine*, ed. B. E. Straw, S. D'Allaire, W. L. Mengeling, and D. J. Taylor, 277–290. Iowa, USA: Iowa State University Press.

30. Eason, R. J. and Sage, M. D. 1980. Deaths from influenza A, subtype H1N1, during the Auckland epidemic. *NZ Med J.* 91:129–131.

31. Erickson, G., Grammer, M. and Janke, B. 2004. SIV diagnostics: Recent findings at three top laboratories. *Focus* 7:1–7.

32. Foni, F., Chiapponi, C., Fratta, E., Gabriano, C., Barigazzi, G. and Merenda, M. 2003. Detection of swine influenza virus by RT-PCR and Standard methods. *4th International symposium on emerging and re-emerging pig diseases,* Rome, 2003:5–8.

33. Fouchier, R. A., Bestebroer, T. M., Herfst, S., Van Der Kemp, L., Rimmelzwaan, G. F. and Osterhaus, A. D. 2000. Detection of influenza A viruses from different species by PCR amplification of conserved sequences in the matrix gene. *J. Clin. Microbiol.* 38:4096–4101.

34. Galarza, J. M., Latham, T. and Cupo, A. 2005. Virus-like particle vaccine conferred complete protection against a lethal influenza virus challenge. *Viral Immunol.* 18:365–372.

35. Gray, G. C. and Baker, W. S. 2007. The importance of including swine and poultry workers in influenza vaccination programs. *Clin. Pharmacol. Ther.* 82:638–641.

36. Gray, G. C., Trampel, D. W. and Roth, J. A. 2007a. Pandemic influenza planning: Shouldn't swine and poultry workers be included? *Vaccine* 25:4376–4381.

37. Gray, G. C., McCarthy, T., Capuano, A. W., Setterquist, S. F., Olsen, C. W. and Alavanja, M. C. 2007b. Swine workers and swine influenza virus infections. *Emerg. Infect. Dis.* 13:1871–1878.

38. Gregory, V., Bennett, M., Thomas, Y., Kaiser, L., Wunderli, W., Matter, H., Hay, A. and Lin, Y. P. 2003. Human infection by a swine influenza A (H1N1) virus in Switzerland. *Arch. Virol.* 148:793–802.

39. Haines, D. M., Waters, E. H. and Clark, E. G. 1993. Immuno-histochemical detection of swine influenza virus in formalin fixed and paraffin-embedded tissues. *Can. J. Vet. Res.* 57:33–36.

40. Hall, J. S., Minnis, R. B., Campbell, T. A., Barras, S., Deyoung, R. W., Pabilonia, K., Avery, M. L., Sullivan, H., Clark, L. and McLean, R. G. 2008. Influenza exposure in United States feral swine populations. *J. Wildl. Dis.* 44:362–368.

41. Hampson, A. W. and Mackenzie, J. S. 2006. The influenza viruses. *Med. J. Aust.* 185:39–43.

42. He, C. Q., Han, G. Z., Wang, D., Liu, W., Li, G. R., Liu, X. P. and Ding, N. Z. 2008. Homologous recombination evidence in human and swine influenza A viruses. *Virology* 380:12–20.

43. Hermann, J. R., Hoff, S. J., Yoon, K. J., Burkhardt, A. C., Evans, R. B. and Zimmerman, J. J. 2006. Optimization of a sampling system for recovery and detection of airborne porcine reproductive and respiratory syndrome virus and swine influenza virus. *Appl. Environ. Microbiol.* 72:4811–4818.

44. Hinshaw, V. S., Webster, R. G., Bean, W. J., Dowdle, J. and Senne, D. A. 1983. Swine influenza viruses in turkeys—a potential source of virus for humans? *Science* 220:206–208.

45. Hodder, R. A., Graydos, G. C., Allen, R. G., Top, F. H., Nowosiwsky, T. and Russell, P. K. 1977. Swine influenza at Fort Dix, New Jersey (Jan.–Feb. 1976). Extent of spread and duration of the outbreak. *J. Infect. Dis.* 136:369–375.

46. Horimoto, T. and Kawaoka, Y. 1995. Direct reverse transcriptase RT-PCR to determine virulence potential influenza A viruses in birds. *J. Clin. Microbiol.* 33:748–751.

47. Ito, T., Nelson, J., Couceiro, S. S., Kelm, S., Baum, L. G., Krauss, S., Castrucci, M. R., Donatelli, I., Kida, H., Paulson, J. C., Webster, R. G. and Kawaoka, Y. 1998. Molecular basis for the generation in pigs of influenza A viruses with pandemic potential. *J. Virol.* 72:7367–7373.

48. Jo, S. K., Kim, H. S., Cho, S. W. and Seo, S. H. 2007. Genetic and antigenic characterization of swine H1N2 influenza viruses isolated from Korean pigs. *J. Microbiol. Biotechnol.* 17:868–872.

49. Kaden, V., Lange, E., Starick, E., Bruer, W., Krakowski, W. and Klopries, M. 2008. Epidemiological survey of swine influenza A virus in selected wild boar populations in Germany. *Vet. Microbiol.* 131:123–132.

50. Kaplan, M. M. and Webster, R. G. 1977. The epidemiology of influenza. *Sci. Am.* 237:88–105.

51. Karasin, A. I., Olsen, C. W. and Anderson, G. A. 2000. Genetic characterization of an H1N2 influenza virus isolated from a pig in Indiana. *J. Clin. Microbiol.* 38:2453–2456.

52. Karasin, A. I., Landgraf, J., Swenson, S., Erickson, G., Goyal, S., Woodruff, M., Scherba, G., Anderson, G. and Olsen, C. W. 2002. Genetic characterization of H1N2 influenza A viruses isolated from pigs throughout the United States. *J. Clin. Microbiol.* 40:1073–1079.

53. Kawaoka, Y., Krauss, S. and Webster, R. G. 1989. Avian-to human transmission of the PB1 gene of influenza A virus in the 1957 and 1968 pandemics. *J. Virol.* 63:4603–4608.

54. Kida, H., Ito, T., Yasuda, J., Shimizu, Y., Itakura, C., Shortridge, K. F., Kawaoka, Y. and Webster, R. G. 1994. Potential for transmission of avian influenza viruses to pigs. *J. Gen. Virol.* 75:2183–2188.

55. Kilbourne, E. D. 2006. Influenza pandemics of the 20th century. *Emerg. Infect. Dis.* 12:9–14.

56. Kim, H. M., Lee, Y. W., Lee, K. J., Kim, H. S., Cho, S. W., van Rooijen, N., Guan, Y. and Seo, S. H. 2008. Alveolar macrophages are indispensable for controlling influenza viruses in lungs of pigs. *J. Virol.* 82:4265–4274.

57. Kimura, K., Adlakha, A. and Simon, P. M. 1998. Fatal case of swine influenza virus in an immunocompetent host. *Mayo Clinic. Proc.* 73:243–245.

58. Kitikoon, P., Nilubol, D., Erickson, B. J., Janke, B. H., Hoover, T. C., Sornsen, S. A. and Thacker, E. L. 2006. The immune response and maternal antibody interference to a heterologous H1N1 swine influenza virus infection following vaccination. *Vet. Immunol. Immunopathol.* 112:117–128.

59. Kitikoon, P., Strait, E. L. and Thacker, E. L. 2008. The antibody responses to swine influenza virus (SIV) recombinant matrix 1 (rM1), matrix 2 (M2), and hemagglutinin (HA) proteins in pigs with different SIV exposure. *Vet. Microbiol.* 126:51–62.

60. Komadina, N., Roque, V., Thawatsupha, P., Rimando-Magalong, J., Waicharoen, S., Bomasang, E., Sawanpanyalert, P., Rivera, M., Iannello, P., Hurt, A. C. and Barr, I. G. 2007. Genetic analysis of two influenza A (H1) swine viruses isolated from humans in Thailand and the Philippines. *Virus Genes* 35:161–165.

61. Kothalawala, H., Toussaint, M. J. M. and Gruys, E. 2006. An overview of swine influenza. *Vet. Q.* 28:45–53.

62. Kundin, W. D. 1970. Hong Kong A-2 influenza virus infection among swine during a human epidemic in Taiwan. *Nature* 228:857–859.

63. Landolt, G. A., Karasin, A. I., Hofer, C., Mahaney, J., Svaren, J. and Olsen, C. W. 2005. Use of real-time reverse transcriptase polymerase chain reaction assay and cell culture methods for detection of swine influenza A viruses. *Am. J. Vet. Res.* 66:119–124.

64. Larochelle, R., Sauvageau, R. and Mager, R. 1994. Immuno-histochemical detection of swine influenza virus and porcine reproductive and respiratory syndrome virus in porcine proliferative and necrotizing pneumonia cases from Québec. *Can. Vet. J.* 35:513–515.

65. Lee, M. S., Chang, P. C., Shien, J. H., Cheng, M. C. and Shieh, H. K. 2001. Identification and subtyping of avian influenza viruses by reverse transcription-PCR. *J. Virol. Methods* 2:13–22.

66. Lee, J. H., Gramer, M. R. and Joo, H. S. 2007. Efficacy of swine influenza A virus vaccines against an H3N2 virus variant. *Can. J. Vet. Res.* 71:207–212.

67. Lee, C. S., Kang, B. K., Kim, H. K., Park, S. J., Park, B. K., Jung, K. and Song, D. S. 2008a. Phylogenetic analysis of swine influenza viruses recently isolated in Korea. *Virus Genes* 37:168–176.

68. Lee, C. S., Kang, B. K., Lee, D. H., Lyou, S. H., Park, B. K., Ann, S. K., Jung, K. and Song, D. S. 2008b. One-step multiplex RT-PCR for detection and subtyping of swine influenza H1, H3, N1, N2 viruses in clinical samples using a dual priming oligonucleotide (DPO) system. *J. Virol. Methods* 151:30–34.

69. Leuwerke, B., Kitikoon, P., Evans, R. and Thacker, E. 2008. Comparison of three serological assays to determine the cross-reactivity of antibodies from eight genetically diverse U.S. swine influenza viruses. *J. Vet. Diagn. Invest.* 20:426–432.

70. Leyssen, P., De Clercq, E. and Neyts, J. 2008. Molecular strategies to inhibit the replication of RNA viruses. *Antiviral Res.* 78:9–25.

71. Li, G. X., Tian, Z. J., Yu, H., Jin, Y. Y., Hou, S. H., Zhou, Y. J., Liu, T. Q., Hu, S. P. and Tong, G. Z. 2008. Fusion of C3d with hemagglutinin enhances protective immunity against swine influenza virus. *Res. Vet. Sci.* 2008 Nov. issue [Epub ahead of print].

72. Lipatov, A. S., Kwon, Y. K., Sarmento, L. V., Lager, K. M., Spackman, E., Suarez, D. L. and Swayne, D. E. 2008. Domestic pigs have low susceptibility to H5N1 highly pathogenic avian influenza viruses. *PLoS Pathog.* 4:e1000102.

73. Liu, D. F., Liu, M., Liu, C. G., Yang, T. and Liu, D. C. 2008a. Cloning and phylogenetic analysis of the entire gene of an H1N1 subtype swine influenza virus isolated from Guangdong Province. *Bing. Du. Xue. Bao.* 24:358–363.

74. Liu, H., Xing, J., Pan, J., Yang, Q. and Zhao, Y. 2008b. Construction and immunogenicity analysis of antigenic epitopes of swine influenza virus. *Sheng. Wu. Gong. Cheng. Xue. Bao.* 24:690–694.

75. Loeffen, W. L., Heinen, P. P., Bianchi, A. T. J., Hunneman, W. A. and Verheijden, J. H. M. 2003. Effects of maternally derived antibodies on the clinical signs and immune response in pigs after primary and secondary infection with an influenza H1N1 virus. *Vet. Immunol. Immunopathol.* 20:23–35.

76. Loeffen, W. L., Hunneman, W. A., Quak, J., Verheijden, J. H. and Stegeman, J. A. 2009. Population dynamics of swine influenza virus in farrow-to-finish and specialised finishing herds in the Netherlands. *Vet. Microbiol.* 2009 Jan. issue [Epub ahead of print].

77. Ma, W., Vincent, A. L., Gramer, M. R., Brockwell, C. B., Lager, K. M., Janke, B. H., Gauger, P. C., Patnayak, D. P., Webby, R. J. and Richt, J. A. 2007. Identification of H2N3 influenza A viruses from swine in the United States. *Proc. Natl. Acad. Sci. USA.* 104:20949–20954.

78. Manzoor, R., Sakoda, Y., Nomura, N., Tsuda, Y., Ozaki, H., Okamatsu, M. and Kida, H. 2009. PB2 protein of a highly pathogenic avian influenza virus strain A/chicken/Yamaguchi/7/2004 (H5N1) determines its replication potential in pigs. *J. Virol.* 83:1572–1578.

79. Masic, A., Babiuk, L. A. and Zhou, Y. 2009. Reverse genetics-generated elastase-dependent swine influenza viruses are attenuated in pigs. *J. Gen. Virol.* 90:375–385.

80. Matassov, D., Cupo, A. and Galarza, J. M. 2007. A novel intranasal virus-like particle (VLP) vaccine designed to protect against the pandemic 1918 influenza A virus (H1N1). *Viral Immunol.* 20:441–452.

81. Mathew, T., Mahendran, M., Dhama, K., Kataria, J. M., Kothawala, H. and Gruys, E. 2006. Swine influenza. (Chapter VI). In *Advances in medical and veterinary virology, immunology and epidemiology.* Vol. 6 *Influenza and its global public health significance*, ed. T. M. Mathew and T. Mathew, 94–111. West Orange, NJ: Thajema Publishers.

82. Mellencamp, M. A., Galina-Pantoja, L., Gladney, C. D. and Torremorell, M. 2008. Improving pig health through genomics: A view from the industry. *Dev. Biol.* (Basel) 132:35–41.

83. Myers, K. P., Olsen, C. W. and Gray, G. C. 2007. Cases of swine influenza in humans: A review of the literature. *Clin. Infect. Dis.* 44:1084–1088.

84. Myers, K. P., Olsen, C. W., Setterquist, S. F., Capuano, A. W., Donham, K. J., Thacker, E. L., Merchant, J. A. and Gray, G. C. 2006. Are swine workers in the United States at increased risk of infection with zoonotic influenza virus? *Clin. Infect. Dis.* 42:14–20.

85. Nakharuthai, C., Boonsoongnern, A., Poolperm, P., Wajjwalku, W., Urairong, K., Chumsing, W., Lertwitcharasarakul, P. and Lekcharoensuk, P. 2008. Occurrence of swine influenza virus infection in swine with porcine respiratory disease complex. *Southeast Asian J. Trop. Med. Public Health* 39:1045–1053.

86. Newman, A. P., Reisdorf, E., Beinemann, J., Uyeki, T. M., Balish, A., Shu, B., Lindstrom, S., Achenbach, J., Smith, C. and Davis, J. P. 2008. Human case of swine influenza A (H1N1) triple reassortant virus infection, Wisconsin. *Emerg. Infect. Dis.* 14:1470–1472.

87. OIE 2004. *Manual of diagnostic tests and vaccines for terrestrial animals.* Chapter 2.10.11.

88. Olsen, C. W. 2002. The emergence of novel swine influenza viruses in North America. *Virus Res.* 85:199–210.

89. Olsen, C. W., Brammer, L., Easterday, B. C., Arden, N., Belay, E., Baker, I. and Cox, N. J. 2002. Serologic evidence of H1 swine influenza virus infection in swine farm residents and employees. *Emerg. Infect. Dis.* 8:814–819.

90. Olsen, C. W. 2004. Influenza: Pigs, people and public health. Public health fact sheet. *National Pork Board* vol. 2: no. 6.

91. Pascua, P. N., Song, M. S., Lee, J. H., Choi, H. W., Han, J. H., Kim, J. H., Yoo, G. J., Kim, C. J. and Choi, Y. K. 2008. Seroprevalence and genetic evolutions of swine influenza viruses under vaccination pressure in Korean swine herds. *Virus Res.* 138:43–49.

92. Pasma, T. 2008. Spatial epidemiology of an H3N2 swine influenza outbreak. *Can. Vet. J.* 49:167–176.

93. Peng, Y., Zhou, H., Li, C. and Jin, M. 2008. The rescue of H1N1 subtype swine influenza virus. *Sheng. Wu. Gong. Cheng. Xue. Bao.* 24:857–861.

94. Perez, D. R., Sorrell, E. M. and Donis, R. O. 2005. Avian influenza: An omnipresent pandemic threat. *Pediatr. Infect. Dis. J.* 24:208–216.

95. Poljak, Z., Dewey, C. E., Martin, S. W., Christensen, J., Carman, S. and Friendship, R. M. 2008a. Prevalence of and risk factors for influenza in southern Ontario swine herds in 2001 and 2003. *Can. J. Vet. Res.* 72:7–17.

96. Poljak, Z., Friendship, R. M., Carman, S., McNab, W. B. and Dewey, C. E. 2008b. Investigation of exposure to swine influenza viruses in Ontario (Canada) finisher herds in 2004 and 2005. *Prev. Vet. Med.* 83:24–40.

97. Ramirez, A., Capuano, A. W., Wellman, D. A., Lesher, K. A., Setterquist, S. F. and Gray, G. C. 2006. Preventing zoonotic influenza virus infection. *Emerg. Infect. Dis.* 12:996–1000.

98. Reichmuth, D. S., Wang, S. K., Barrett, L. M., Throckmorton, D. J., Einfeld, W. and Singh, A. K. 2008. Rapid microchip-based electrophoretic immunoassays for the detection of swine influenza virus. *Lab Chip.* 8:1319–1324.

99. Renshaw, H. W. 1975. Influence of antibody mediated immune suppression on clinical, viral, and immune responses to swine influenza infection. *Am. J. Vet. Res.* 36:5–13.

100. Richt, J. A., Lekcharoensuk, P., Lager, K. M., Vincent, A. L., Loiacono, C. M., Janke, B. H., Wu, W. H., Yoon, K. J., Webby, R. J., Solorzano, A. and Garcia-Sastre, A. 2006. Vaccination of pigs against swine influenza viruses by using an NS1-truncated modified live-virus vaccine. *J. Virol.* 80:11009–11018.

101. Rimmelzwaan, G. F., Van Riel, D., Baars, M., Besteboer, T., Van Amerongen, G., Fouchier, R. A. M., Osterhaus, A. D. E. and Kuiken, T. 2006. Influenza A virus (H5N1) infection in cats causes systemic disease with potential novel routes of virus spread within and between hosts. *Am. J. Pathol.* 168:176–183.

102. Robinson, J. L., Lee, B. E., Patel, J., Bastien, N., Grimsrud, K., Seal, R. F., King, R., Marshall, F. and Li, Y. 2007. Swine influenza (H3N2) infection in a child and possible community transmission, Canada. *Emerg. Infect. Dis.* 13:1865–1870.

103. Rota, P. A., Rocha, E. P., Harmon, M. W., Hinshaw, V. S., Sheerer, M. G. and Kawaoka, Y. 1989. Laboratory characterization of a swine influenza virus isolated from a fatal case of human influenza. *J. Clin. Microbiol.* 27:1413–1416.

104. Saito, T., Suzuki, H., Maeda, K., Inai, K., Takemae, N., Uchida, Y. and Tsunemitsu, H. 2008. Molecular characterization of an H1N2 swine influenza virus isolated in Miyazaki, Japan, in 2006. *J. Vet. Med. Sci.* 70:423–427.

105. Schorr, E. and Hinshaw, V. S. 1994. Use of polymerase chain reaction to detect swine influenza virus in nasal specimens. *Am. J. Vet. Res.* 55:952–956.

106. Schultz, U., Fitch, W. M., Ludwig, S., Mandler, J. and Scholtissek, C. 1991. Evolution of pig influenza viruses. *J. Virol.* 183:61–73.

107. Schnurrenberger, P. R., Woods, G. T. and Martin, R. J. 1970. Serologic evidence of human infection with swine influenza virus. *Am. Rev. Respir. Dis.* 102:356–361.

108. Scholtissek, C., Rhode, W., Von Hoyningen, V. and Ron, R. 1978. On the origin of the human influenza virus subtype a H2N2 and H3N2. *Virology* 87:13–20.

109. Scholtissek, C., Burger, H., Bachmann, P. A. and Hannoun, C. 1983. Genetic relatedness of hemagglutinins of the H1 subtype of influenza A viruses isolated from swine and birds. *Virology* 129:521–523.

110. Shi, W. F., Gibbs, M. J., Zhang, Y. Z., Zhang, Z., Zhao, X. M., Jin, X., Zhu, C. D., Yang, M. F., Yang, N. N., Cui, Y. J. and Ji, L. 2008. Genetic analysis of four porcine avian influenza viruses isolated from Shandong, China. *Arch. Virol.* 153:211–217.

111. Shieh, H. K., Chang, P. C., Chen, T. H., Li, K. P. and Chan, C. H. 2008. Surveillance of avian and swine influenza in the swine population in Taiwan, 2004. *J. Microbiol. Immunol. Infect.* 41:231–242.

112. Shope, R. E. 1931. Swine influenza. Experimental transmission and pathology. *J. Exp. Med.* 54:349–359.

113. Shortridge, K. F. and Webster, R. G. 1979. Geographical distribution of swine (H1N1) and Hongkong (H3N2) influenza virus variants in pigs in South East Asia. *Intervirol.* 11:9–15.

114. Skibbe, D., Zhou, E. M. and Janke, B. H. 2004. Comparison of a commercial enzyme-linked immunosorbent assay with hemagglutination inhibition assay for serodiagnosis of swine influenza virus (H1N1) infection. *J. Vet. Diagn. Invest.* 16:86–89.

115. Stetch, J., Xiong, X., Scholtissek, C. and Webster, R. G. 1999. Independence of evolutionary and mutational rates after transmission of avian influenza viruses to swine. *J. Virol.* 73:1878–1884.

116. Sun, L., Zhang, G., Shu, Y., Chen, X., Zhu, Y., Yang, L., Ma, G., Kitamura, Y. and Liu, W. 2008. Genetic correlation between H3N2 human and swine influenza viruses. *J. Clin. Virol.* 2008 Dec. issue [Epub ahead of print].

117. Suriya, R., Hassan, L., Omar, A. R., Aini, I., Tan, C. G., Lim, Y. S. and Kamaruddin, M. I. 2008. Seroprevalence and risk factors for influenza A viruses in pigs in Peninsular Malaysia. *Zoon. Pub. Health.* 55:342–351.

118. Taubenberger, J., Reid, A. H. and Krafft, A. E. 1997. Initial genetic characterization of the 1918 "Spanish" influenza virus. *Science* 275:1793–1796.

119. Thacker, E. and Janke, B. 2008. Swine influenza virus: Zoonotic potential and vaccination strategies for the control of avian and swine influenzas. *J. Infect. Dis.* 197:19–24.

120. Vana, G. and Westover, K. M. 2008. Origin of the 1918 Spanish influenza virus: A comparative genomic analysis. *Mol. Phylogenet. Evol.* 47:1100–1110.

121. Vannie, P., Capua, I., Le Potier, M. F., Mackay, D. K., Muylkens, B., Parida, S., Paton, D. J. and Thiry, E. 2007. Marker vaccines and the impact of their use on diagnosis and prophylactic measures. *Rev. Sci. Tech.* 26:351–372.

122. Van Reeth, K., Gregory, V., Hay, A. and Pensaert, M. 2003. Protection against a European H1N2 swine influenza virus in pigs previously infected with H1N1 and or/ H3N2 subtypes. *Vaccine* 21:1375–1381.

123. Van Reeth, K., Labarque, G. and Pensaert, M. 2006. Serological profiles after consecutive experimental infections of pigs with European H1N1, H3N2, and H1N2 swine influenza viruses. *Viral Immunol.* 19:373–382.

124. Van Reeth, K. 2006. Avian influenza in swine: A threat for the human population? *Verh. K Acad. Geneeskd. Belg.* 68:81–101.

125. Van Reeth, K. 2007. Avian and swine influenza viruses: Our current understanding of the zoonotic risk. *Vet. Res.* 38:243–260.

126. Vincent, L. L., Janke, B. H., Paul P. S. and Halbur, P. G. 1997. A monoclonal antibody based immunohistochemical method for the detection of swine influenza virus in formalin fixed paraffin embedded tissues. *J. Vet. Diagn. Invest.* 9:191–197.

127. Vincent, A. L., Lager, K. M., Ma, W., Lekcharoensuk, P., Gramer, M. R., Loiacono, C. and Richt, J. A. 2006. Evaluation of hemagglutinin subtype 1 swine influenza viruses from the United States. *Vet. Microbiol.* 118:212–222.

128. Vincent, A. L., Ma, W., Lager, K. M., Janke, B. H., Webby, R. J., Garcia-Sastre, A. and Richt, J. A. 2007. Efficacy of intranasal administration of a truncated NS1 modified live influenza virus vaccine in swine. *Vaccine* 25:7999–8009.

129. Vincent, A. L., Ma, W., Lager, K. M., Janke, B. H. and Richt, J. A. 2008. Swine influenza viruses a North American perspective. *Adv. Virus Res.* 72:127–154.

130. Wan, C., Liu, M., Liu, C., Zhang, X., Yang, T., Liu, D., Chen, H., Qi, J. and Qiao, C. 2008. Baculovirus expression and establishment of the indirect ELISA for the HA gene of swine influenza virus H1 subtype. *Wei. Sheng. Wu. Xue. Bao.* 48:220–225.

131. Webby, R. J., Swenson, S. L., Krauss, S. L., Gerrish, P. J., Goyal, S. M. and Webster, R. G. 2000. Evolution of swine H3N2 influenza viruses in the United States. *J. Virol.* 74:8243–8251.

132. Webster, R. G. and Lever, W. G. 1972. Studies on the origin of pandemic influenza. Antigenic analysis of A2 influenza viruses isolated before and after the appearance of Hong Kong influenza using antisera to the isolated heamaglutinin subunits. *Virology* 48:433–444.

133. Wentworth, D. E., McGregor, M. W., Macklin, M. D., Neumann, V. and Hinshaw, V. S. 1997. Transmission to swine influenza virus to humans after exposure to experimentally infection pigs. *J. Infect. Dis.* 175:715.

134. Wesley, R. D., Tang, M. and Lager, K. M. 2004. Protection of weaned pigs by vaccination with human adenovirus 5 recombinant viruses expressing the hemagglutinin and the nucleoprotein of H3N2 swine influenza virus. *Vaccine* 22:3427–3434.

135. Wesley, R. D. and Lager, K. M. 2005. Evaluation of a recombinant human adenovirus-5 vaccine administered via needle-free device and intramuscular injection for vaccination of pigs against swine influenza virus. *Am. J. Vet. Res.* 66:1943–1947.

136. Woeste, K. and Grosse Beilage, E. 2007. Transmission of agents of the porcine respiratory disease complex (PRDC) between swine herds: A review. Part 2—Pathogen transmission via semen, air and living/nonliving vectors. *Dtsch. Tierarztl. Wochenschr.* 114:364–366.

137. Wright, S. M., Kawaoka, Y., Sharp, G. B., Senne, D. A. and Webster, R. G. 1992. Interspecies transmission and reassortment of influenza A viruses in pigs and turkeys in the United States. *Am. J. Epidemiol.* 136:488–497.

138. A commentary "Ontario swine flu related to British Columbia bird flu." Jan. 3, 2005. www.recombinomics.com, 2005.

139. Yang, T., Liu, M., Liu, C. G., Zhang, Y., Liu, D. F., Chen, H. and Tong, G. Z. 2007. Generation of cell culture high-yield recombinant H3N2 subtype swine influenza vaccine candidate by reverse genetics. *Bing. Du. Xue. Bao.* 23:471–476.

140. Yao, Y., Zhang, G. H., Liu, W. J., Chen, T. Q. and Sun, L. 2007. Genome sequence analysis of an H3N2 subtype swine influenza virus isolated from Guangdong province in China. *Wei Sheng Wu Xue Bao.* 47:805–809.

141. Yassine, H. M., Al-Natour, M. Q., Lee, C. W. and Saif, Y. M. 2007. Interspecies and intraspecies transmission of triple reassortant H3N2 influenza A viruses. *Virol. J.* 4:129.

142. Yoon, K. J., Janke, B. H., Swalla, R. W. and Erickson, G. 2004. Comparison of a commercial H1N1 enzyme-linked immunosorbent assay and hemagglutination inhibition test in detecting serum antibody against swine influenza viruses. *J. Vet. Diagn. Invest.* 16:197–201.

143. Yu, H., Hua, R. H., Zhang, Q., Liu, T. Q., Liu, H. L., Li, G. X. and Tong, G. Z. 2008a. Genetic evolution of swine influenza A (H3N2) viruses in China from 1970 to 2006. *J. Clin. Microbiol.* 46:1067–1075.

144. Yu, H., Hua, R. H., Wei, T. C., Zhou, Y. J., Tian, Z. J., Li, G. X., Liu, T. Q. and Tong, G. Z. 2008b. Isolation and genetic characterization of avian origin H9N2 influenza viruses from pigs in China. *Vet. Microbiol.* 131:82–92.

145. Yu, H., Zhang, G. H., Hua, R. H., Zhang, Q., Liu, T. Q., Liao, M. and Tong, G. Z. 2007. Isolation and genetic analysis of human origin H1N1 and H3N2 influenza viruses from pigs in China. *Biochem. Biophys. Res. Commun.* 356:91–96.

146. Yu, H., Zhou, Y. J., Li, G. X., Zhang, G. H., Liu, H. L., Yan, L. P., Liao, M. and Tong, G. Z. 2009. Further evidence for infection of pigs with human-like H1N1 influenza viruses in China. *Virus Res.* 2009 Jan. issue [Epub ahead of print].

147. Zell, R., Motzke, S., Krumbholz, A., Wutzler, P., Herwig, V. and Durrwald, R. 2008a. Novel reassortant of swine influenza H1N2 virus in Germany. *J. Gen. Virol.* 89:271–276.

148. Zell, R., Bergmann, S., Krumbholz, A., Wutzler, P. and Durrwald, R. 2008b. Ongoing evolution of swine influenza viruses: A novel reassortant. *Arch. Virol.* 153:2085–2092.

149. Zhou, N. N., Senne, D. A., Landgraf, J. S., Swenson, S. L., Erickson, G. and Rossow, K. 1999. Genetic reassortment of avian, swine, and human influenza A viruses in American pigs. *J. Virol.* 73:8851–8856.

150. Zhu, Q., Yang, H., Chen, W., Cao, W., Zhong, G., Jiao, P., Deng, G., Yu, K., Yang, C., Bu, Z., Kawaoka, Y. and Chen, H. 2008. A naturally occurring deletion in its NS gene contributes to the attenuation of an H5N1 swine influenza virus in chickens. *J. Virol.* 82:220–228.

151. http://www.cdc.gov/h1n1flu/

152. http://www.who.int/csr/don/2009_05_13/en/index.html Influenza A(H1N1) update 27.

10. Swine Pox

D. Nandi, S. Nandi, and Thankam Mathew

Introduction
Swine pox (SP) is a highly contagious acute viral disease of pigs characterized by cutaneous pock lesions. The disease mostly affects younger pigs. It has relatively lower prevalence and mild clinical manifestations. However, the disease is gaining importance particularly in developing countries because of importation of exotic breeds for cross-breeding purposes, which in turn leads to inflow of large number of susceptible population (Olufemi et al., 1981; Garg et al., 1989).

Etiology
The disease is caused by swine pox virus (SPV) of the genus *Suipoxvirus* under Poxviridae family. SPV is an immunologically distinct member of pox group viruses and is host specific (Datt, 1964a; Alfonso et al., 2002). After the eradication of smallpox (vaccinia virus), swine pox is exclusively caused by a host-specific poxvirus.

Causative Virus
Morphologically, swine pox virus resembles vaccinia virus and is prismatic, brick or ovoid in shape with a dimension of around 310×240 nm (Cheville, 1966a). The structural components include a core, lateral bodies, surface protein, and membranes. The 146.0-kbp SPV genome consists of a central coding region bounded by identical 3.7-kbp inverted terminal repeats and contains 150 putative genes. Comparison of SPV with chordopoxviruses reveals 146 conserved genes encoding proteins involved in basic replicative functions, viral virulence, host range, and immune evasion (Alfonso et al., 2002). The core (nucleoid) is composed of deoxyribonucleic acid (DNA) and protein. The nucleoid is biconcave in vertical section, and the DNA is double stranded with a molecular weight of 80×10^6 Da (Kasza, 1986). Due to the large size of the virus, it has been used successfully as recombinant vector for delivery of various antigenic proteins of different viruses, namely, feline luekemia (Winslow et al., 2003), E_2 protein of classical swine fever virus (Hahn-Jung et al., 2001), and Aujeszky's disease (pseudorabies) virus gene insert coding for gp50 and gp63 glycoproteins (Leek et al., 1994; Tripathy, 1999).

Physical Properties of the Virus
The virus s very resistant to environmental influences and can thrive for about two weeks at 37°C. Scabs containing the virion retain infectivity for up to one year at room temperature (Mayr et al., 1984).

HOST RANGE

Unlike vaccinia virus, SPV has a very restricted host range; only pigs are naturally infected by the virus. It does not produce any infection or lesions in horse, calves, pigeon, fowl, sheep, goat, rabbit, rat, guinea pig, chick embryo, or human (McNutt et al., 1929; Datt, 1964a; Garg, 1971; Meyer and Conroy, 1972; Copeland, 1974; Kasza, 1986). Kasza et al. (1960) were not able to grow the SPV on CAM. But vaccinia can also produce pox in swine, and that virus can easily be cultivated on the CAM (Narayana, 1964). However, Mathew (1967 and 1976) failed to grow true swine pox on CAM.

TISSUE CULTURE

Swine kidney tissue cultures have been used successfully for the isolation and cultivation of SPV (Kasza et al., 1960). According to Kasza et al. (1960), they were able to cultivate the virus in the pig embryo testis, lung, and brain tissue culture, and it produced very small plaques. SPV could produce CPE only in the various swine tissue culture. Garg and Meyer (1972) successfully adapted SPV in a continuous cell line of porcine kidney cells (PK-15) and obtained titer comparable with that of diploid swine kidney cell cultures. Maltseva et al. (1966) also suggested the same result. Mathew (1967 and 1977) also reported that she also could not succeed in growing SP virus in four mammalian primary tissue culture systems, namely, monkey kidney, rabbit kidney, hamster kidney, and human amnion. However, attempts to grow the SP virus in rabbit kidney cells (Kasza et al., 1960), HeLa cells (Meyer and Conroy, 1972), or MDMK cell line (Garg and Meyer, 1972) failed. A single report of successful growth of SPV in cells of monkey origin claimed that the virus was able to grow in cells other than swine origin (Nicholas, 1970). Cytopathic effects (CPE) produced in tissue culture are intracytoplasmic inclusions, vacuoles in the nuclei, and margination of chromatin. Cytoplasmic inclusions are variable in size, granular, indistinct in outline, and may not be always evident in all infected cells. The inclusions are usually eosinophilic; however, neutrophilic inclusions are also observed. The cytoplasmic inclusions give positive fluorescent reaction in direct florescent antibody test (FAT) and greenish fluorescence when stained by acridine orange. The virus may produce very large intracytoplasmic crystalline bodies (800 nm in diameter) as a unique feature. In addition to the A and B types of inclusion, the intranuclear vacuoles were produced by the SP virus in the skin tissues (Blackemore and Abdussalam, 1956; Kasza et al., 1960). Destruction of monolayer occurs five to seven days after inoculation of the virus in cell culture (Munz and Dumbell, 2004). Mathew (1967 and 1977) when compared the hemadsoption in the various tissue culture systems with various species erythrocytes with buffalo pox(BP), cowpox (CP), vaccinia, goat pox, SP., and fowl pox viruses, swine pox did not produce any CPE or hemadsorption in the various tissue culture systems, neither in the primary or secondary passages.

SEROLOGICAL PROPERTIES

SPV does not cross-react with vaccinia, cowpox, and fowl pox antisera in precipitation tests, but it reacts with homologous antisera. It is generally agreed that virus of swine pox is antigenically distinct from vaccinia and other animal poxviruses. Mathew (1967 and 1987) also reported that true swine pox do not show any antigenic cross reaction in gel diffusion with other poxviruses like buffalo pox, cowpox, sheep pox, goat pox, and fowl pox. Vaccinia and SP viruses share a common antigen as demonstrated by agar gel precipitation test (Datt and Orlans, 1958) and conglutinin complement absorption test (Datt, 1964b). These two viruses do not reveal cross-protection in pigs and rabbits (Datt, 1964b). Eight separate precipitinogens have been recorded during analysis of soluble antigens of SPV by immunodiffusion and acrylamide gel electrophoresis (Goel et al., 1972). SP viruses do not agglutinate fowl red blood cells, whereas vaccinia viruses do (Datt, 1964c; Garg, 1971). Pigs infected with vaccinia virus remain fully susceptible to SPV and vice versa (Radostits et al., 2007). No hemadsoption was seen with swine pox, goat pox, and fowl pox in a comparative study of hemadsoption with fowl pox, rabbit pox, with human O, and guinea pig RBC (Mathew,1967).

EPIZOOTIOLOGY

HISTORY AND PREVALENCE

The earliest report of swine pox outbreak was documented in European literature by Spinola (1842). Subsequently, the virus has been reported from Morocco (Velu, 1916), North America (McNutt et al., 1929), Japan (Akazawa and Matsumura, 1935), England (Blakemore and Glover, 1937), Kenya (Piercy, 1951), and many other countries in the European Union and the rest of the world. Now the disease is worldwide in distribution, and mostly outbreaks are associated with intensive system of management with definite breach in biosecurity. The outbreak of the disease has been reported from Andra Pradesh, India, during the 1960s (Venkatnarayana, 1962). Later on, similar outbreaks were also reported from other parts of India (Manickam and Mohan, 1987; Verma et al., 1987). Incidences of swine pox have also been reported from pig farms in Ibadan, Nigeria (Olufemi et al., 1981), and Western Australia (Fallon, 1992).

TRANSMISSION

Direct contact is reckoned as the primary route of transmission of the virus from infected to susceptible pigs (Chakrabarti, 2007). Biting lice (*Haematopinus suis*) may mechanically transmit the disease by producing open wound or damaging the skin (Munz and Dumbell, 2004; Radostits et al., 2007). Lice may remain as the source of infection for weeks or months after contracting the virus, but the possibilities for vertical transmission of the virus in lice is ignored. Other biting insects like *Stmoxys* species can also help in the process of disease transmission in a herd. Virus is shed in various excretions and secretions of the ailing pigs like lachrymal fluid, saliva, nasal discharges, etc. Visible unruptured pox lesions and scabs or crusts during the recovery stage from the disease remain highly infective and act as major source of infection in the environment. Congenital infection has been reported in newborn piglets born of an infected sow (Borst et al., 1990). Colostral antibody protects piglets from early infection before the protective titer wanes (Munz and Dumbell, 2004). Recovered pigs achieve a solid and long-lasting immunity. Appearance of antibody in the circulation following a natural spate of infection is a slow process; however, virus-neutralizing and precipitating titers are detectable from twenty days postinfection with peak levels by about six weeks. Cell-mediated immunity also plays significant role in protection from the disease.

PATHOGENESIS
The virus has specific affinity for epithelial cells, and in some rare cases they may invade upper gastrointestinal or respiratory tract. The incubation period of the disease varies from four to fourteen days (McNutt et al., 1929). However, incubation period is only four days when pigs are inoculated intravenously with tissue culture adapted SPV (Kasza and Griessemer, 1962). Scab suspension inoculated intradermally produce lesions by five days in pig (Tewari et al., 1974). The course of the disease is around three to five weeks in absence of any secondary complications.

CLINICAL SIGNS
Affected animals become dull, depressed with high fever (105–107°F). The disease shows only local reactions with fever and lymphadenitis are the only systemic manifestations (Chakrabarti, 2007). Small areas of erythema (4–5 mm diameter) appear on ventral abdominal skin, which increase rapidly in size and pass through papular, vesicular, and pustular stages to ultimately form scabs with central depression by eight to twelve days of infection. The resultant crust soon falls off, and in uncomplicated cases healing occurs with minimal scar formation by two to four weeks. However, the lesions produced due to SPV do not induce itching sensation in animal if not inflicted by secondary bacteria. The morbidity rate is high in young stock, but mortality generally does no exceed 3% in uncomplicated cases. Morbidity has been reported up to 80% without any mortality (McNutt et al., 1929; Murray, 1937). No significant difference exists in mortality or morbidity pattern among male and female pigs, though slightly higher values are observed with males (Olufemi et al., 1981; Manickam and Mohan, 1987). Pock lesions may be located on the skin over maxilla or external ear apart from inner aspects of thigh, ventral abdomen, snout, and eyelids (Venkatnarayana,

1962). In severe cases, vesicles may be seen in buccal cavity, pharynx, esophagus, stomach, trachea, and bronchi (Chatterjee, 1989). Congenital swine pox is characterized by striking pock lesions present on entire body surface in piglets at birth (Borst et al., 1990). Ballooning degeneration of keratinocytes, cytoplasmic inclusions, and intranuclear vacuolization were observed histologically, and poxvirus particles were detected by electron microscopy and further confirmed by restriction endonuclease digestion of genomic DNA in congenitally infected piglets (Borst et al., 1990).

Lesions

Gross Lesions
On gross examination, lesions caused due to SPV progress from a papule through pustule to crusting stage with the passage of time. Papules on skin may attain a size of 0.5–1.0 cm in diameter. By twenty-one days postinfection, most of the crusts desquamated, leaving small spots. The inguinal lymph nodes become swollen and palpable. SPV usually do not produce any characteristic lesions in visceral organs; however, swelling and hyperplasia of regional lymph glands and congestion and petechiae of visceral organs may be observed on postmortem examination (Narayana, 1964; Copeland, 1974; Manickam and Mohan, 1987).

Histopathology
The epidermis is focally thickened up to 1 mm due to hydropic degeneration in stratum spinosum. In histological sections, hyperplasia of the epidermis is seen, and the cytoplasm of the affected cells contains both acidophilic and basophilic inclusions with characteristic vacuoles in nuclei in some occasions (Garg and Meyer, 1973b). Electron and immunoelectron microscopy reveals presence of fibrillar structures within nuclear vacuoles and aggregates of virus particles in cytoplasm (Kim et al., 1977; Verma et al., 1987). Presence of PAS-positive (periodic acid Schiff–positive) cytoplasmic structures are noticed in the infected cells under light microscope (Cheville, 1966b). Basophilic intracytoplasmic inclusions in swine pox may be of two types: one that occurs most frequently with variable sizes and resembles type A poxvirus inclusions and the other which is rare, oval or spherical in shape resembling type B poxvirus inclusions. In advanced papular stage infiltration of the dermis with lymphocytes, neutrophils, eosinophils, and histiocytes along with vascular dilatation is observed.

Diagnosis
Diagnosis should be based on clinically evident pock lesions, differentiation with similar clinical conditions and confirmation of the agent by virus isolation and identification.

DIFFERENTIAL DIAGNOSIS

Swine pox should be differentiated from cutaneous infections caused due to *Staphylococcus* spp. and *Streptococcus* spp. and the lesions produced by mites (like *Demodex phylloides*) and fungi. Mites of the genus *Tryoglyphid* spp. may produce similar lesions, which should be confirmed by skin-scraping examination. Lesions produced by *Sarcoptes scabiei* essentially have itching sensation, which is absent in SPV infection. In ringworm infection, lesions are characteristically round, and presence of fungal spore is obvious under the microscope.

Cutaneous manifestation of other diseases like foot-and-mouth disease, vesicular disease, vesicular stomatitis, vesicular exanthema, hog cholera, erysipelas, pityriasis rosea, vegetative dermatitis, sunburn, parasitic, allergic and nutritional skin diseases should also be considered for differentiation (Kasza, 1986).

CONFIRMATORY DIAGNOSIS

The serological tests for identification of SP virus are neutralization test, agar gel diffusion, and precipitation tests. Swine pox virus antigen in the cytoplasm and nucleus of established cell lines was detected by indirect immunoperoxidase technique using a protein A-horseradish peroxidase (HRPO) conjugate (Mohanty et al., 1989). Monoclonal antibodies against various epitopes of SPV have been used for the detection of swine pox virus antigens (Ouchi et al., 1992). Counterimmunoelectrophoresis and enzyme immunoassay have been used for the rapid detection of antibodies against swine pox virus (Verma and Rai, 1988, 1990). Fluorescent antibody test and conglutinin complement absorption tests are also used for serological diagnosis of swine pox (Datt, 1964b; Garg and Meyer, 1973a).

TREATMENT AND PREVENTION

No specific treatment or control measures are in vogue, although attempts to immunize pigs with cell-culture adapted virus showed promising results (Kubin, 1972; Chakrabarti, 2007). Pigs recovered from swine pox generally develop resistance to subsequent infection by the same virus, and newborn pigs acquire maternal immunity from immune dam. Measures should be adopted to keep the swine population free from lice by routine application of acaricides. Infected sows and their litter must be isolated to prevent further spread of infection, and their pens should be disinfected with 3–4% iodophore solution or any other standard disinfectant (Evans et al., 1972). Segregation of affected animals and isolation of sows until their piglets are above six weeks of age help in containing the spread of the disease (Blakemore and Blover, 1937).

REFERENCES

1. Akazawa, S. and Matsumura, T. 1935. Swine pox in Chosen. *J. Jap. Soc. Vet. Sci.* 14:1–19.
2. Alfonso, C. L., Tulman, E. R., Lu, Z., Zsak, L., Osorio, F. A., Balinsky, C., Kutish, G. F. and Rock, D. L. 2002. The genome of swinepox virus. *J. Virol.* 76:783–790.
3. Blackemore, F. and Abdussalam, M. 1956. Morphology of the elementary bodies and cell inclusions in swine pox. *J. Comp. Path.* 66:373–377.
4. Blakemore, F. and Glover, R. E. 1937. Variola in the pig. *Vet Rec.* 49:750–752.
5. Borst, G. H., Kimman, T. G., Gielkens, A. L., and van der Kamp, J. S. 1990. Four sporadic cases of congenital swinepox. *Vet. Rec.* 127:61–63.
6. Chakrabarti, A. 2007. Swinepox. In *A textbook of preventive veterinary medicine*. Kalyani Publishers, Ludhiana, India, 106–108.
7. Chatterjee, A. 1989. In *Skin infections in domestic animals*. Moitri Publications, Calcutta, India.
8. Cheville, N. F. 1966a. Immunofluorescent and morphological studies on swinepox. *Pathol. Vet.* 3:556–564.
9. Cheville, N. F. 1966b. The cytopathology of swinepox in the skin of swine. *Am. J. Pathol.* 49:339–352.
10. Copeland, J. W. 1974. Swine pox in Papua New Guinea. *Trop. Anim. Hlth. Prod.* 6:153–157.
11. Datt, N. S. 1964a. Comparative studies on pigpox and vaccinia viruses I: Host range pathogenicity. *J. Comp. Pathol.* 74:62–69.
12. Datt, N. S. 1964b. Comparative studies on pigpox and vaccinia viruses II. *J. Comp. Pathol.* 74:70–80.
13. Datt, N. S. 1964c. Haemagglutination reaction with vaccinia virus. Agglutinability of red cells from Turkeys. *Nature* 203:1406–1407.
14. Datt, N. S. and Orlans, E. S. 1958. The immunological relationship of the vaccinia and pig viruses demonstrated by gel diffusion. *Immunology* 1:81–86.
15. Evans, D. H., Stuart, P. and Roberts, D. H. 1972. Disinfection of animal viruses. *British Vet. J.* 133:356–359.
16. Fallon, G. R. 1992. Swinepox in pigs in northern Western Australia. *Aust. Vet. J.* 69:233.
17. Garg, S. K. and Meyer, R. C. 1972. Adaptation of swine pox virus to an established cell line. *Appl. Microbiol.* 23:180–182.
18. Garg, S. K. and Meyer, R. C. 1973a. Studies on swine pox virus: Fluorescence and light microscopy of infected cell cultures. *Res. Vet. Sci.* 14:216–219.
19. Garg, S. K. and Meyer, R. C. 1973b. Plaque formation by swine pox virus adapted to PK-15 cells. *Indian J. Exp. Biol.* 11:344–345.
20. Garg, S. K. 1971. Studies on swine pox virus. *Dissertation Abstracts International* (1972) 32B: 4932–4933.
21. Garg, S. K., Chandra, R. and Rao, V. D. P. 1989. Swinepox. *Vet. Bull.* 59:441–448.
22. Goel, M. C., Singh, I. P. and Sambyal, D. S. 1972. Soluble antigen of pig pox virus. *Ind. J Microbiol.* 12:215–222.
23. Hahn-Jung, H., Park-Se, H., Song-Jae, Y., An-Soo, H. and Ahn-Byung, Y. 2001. Construction of recombinant swinepox viruses and expression of the classical swine fever virus E2 protein. *J. Virol. Methods.* 93:49–56.
24. Kasza, L. 1986. Swinepox. In *Diseases of swine*, 6th ed., ed. A. D. Leman, B. Straw, R. D. Glock, W. L. Mengeling, R. H. C. Penny, and E. Sholl, 315–321. Ames, Iowa: Iowa State University Press.
25. Kasza, L. and Griessemer, R. A. 1962. Experimental swine pox. *Am. J. Vet. Res.* 23:443–451.(Where in the text referred?)
26. Kasza, L., Hoiel, E. H. and Jones, D. O. 1960. Isolation and cultivation of swinepox virus in primary cell culture of swine origin. *Am. J. Vet. Res.* 21:269–273.
27. Kim, U. H., Mukhajonpan, V., Nii, S. and Kato, S. 1977. Ultra structural study of swinepox and orf viruses. *Biken J.* 20:57–67.

28. Kubin, G. 1972. Immunisierung der Schweine gegen Schweinepoocken mit kulturadaptietm virs. *Wiener Tierarztliche Monatsschrift.* 59:317–319.

29. Leek, M. L., Feller, J. A., Sorensen, G., Isaacson, W., Adams, C. L., Borde, D. J., Pfeiffer, N., Tran, T., Moyer, R. W. and Gibbs, E. P. J. 1994. Evaluation of swinepox virus as a vaccine vector in pigs using an Aujeszky's disease (pseudorabies) virus gene insert coding for glycoproteins gp50 and gp63. *Vet. Rec.* 134:13–18.

30. Maltseva, N. N., Shelukhina, A., Yumasheva, M. A. and Marennikova, S. S. 1966. *J. Hyg. Epidemiol. Microbiol. Immunol.* 10:202.

31. Manickam, R. and Mohan, M. 1987. A note on outbreak of swinepox in large white Yorkshire piglets. *Indian J. Vet. Med.* 7:71–72.

32. Mathew, T. 1967. Cultivation and immunological studies on pox group of viruses with special reference to buffalo pox viruses. PhD thesis, University of Madras.

33. Mathew, T. 1976. Comparative studies on the propagation of pox viruses in the chick embryos with special reference to buffalo pox virus. *Kerala J. Vet. Sci.* 7:48–56.

34. Mathew, T. 1977. A comparison of the propagation of buffalo pox with other pox viruses in different cell cultue systems. *Kerala J. Vet. Sci.* 8:189–198.

35. Mathew, T. 1987. In *Advances in medical and veterinary virology, immunology and epidemiology. Cultivation and immunological studies on pox group of viruses with special reference to buffalo pox virus.* Vol. 1:19-122. Thajema publishers, India.

36. Mayr, A., Eissner, G. and Mayr-Bibrack, B. 1984. *Handbuch der Schutzimpfungen in der Tiermedizin.* Berlin, Hamburg: Verlag Paul Parey.

37. McNutt, S. H., Murray, C. and Purwin, P. 1929. Swinepox. *J. Am. Vet. Med. Assoc.* 74:752.

38. Meyer, R. C. and Conroy, J. D. 1972. Experimental swinepox in gnotobiotic piglets. *Res. Vet. Sci.* 13:334–338.

39. Mohanty, P. K., Verma, P. C. and Rai, A. 1989. Detection of swinepox and buffalo pox viruses in cell culture using a protein A-horseradish peroxidase conjugate. *Acta Virol.* 33:290–296.

40. Munz, E. and Dumbell, K. 2004. Swinepox. In *Infectious diseases of livestock*, 2nd ed., vol. 2, J. A. W. Coetzer and R. C. Tustin, 1293–1295. Oxford, UK: Oxford University Press.

41. Murray, C. 1937. Swine pox. *J. Am. Vet. Med. Assoc.* 90:426–331.

42. Narayana, J. V. 1964. Preliminary studies on an outbreak of swinepox in large white Yorkshires in Andra Pradesh. *Indian Vet. J.* 41:71–75.

43. Nicholas, A. H. 1970. A pox virus of primates I. Growth of the virus *in vitro* and comparison with other pox viruses. *J. Natl. Cancer Inst.* 45:897–905.

44. Olufemi, B. E., Ayoade, G. O., Ikede, B. O., Akpavie, S. O. and Nwufoh, K. J. 1981. Swinepox in Nigeria. *Vet. Rec.* 109:278–80.

45. Ouchi, M., Fujiwara, M., Hatano, Y., Yamada, M. and Nii, S. 1992. Analysis of swinepox virus antigens using monoclonal antibodies. *J. Vet. Med. Sci.* 54:731–737.

46. Piercy, S. E. 1951. A pox like condition of swine in Kenya. *Vet. Rec.* 63:574–575.

47. Radostits, O. M., Gay, C. C., Hinchcliff, K. W. and Constable, P. D. 2007. *Veterinary Medicine: A textbook of the diseases of cattle, sheep, pigs, goats and horses*, 10th ed. 1256. Philadelphia: WB Saunders.

48. Spinola, M. 1842. *Krankheiten der Schweine A.* Berlin: Hieschwald. 204.

49. Tewari, S. C., Singh, I. P. and Kaduskar, S. P. 1974. A note on aetiological study of pox in swine. *Ind. J. Anim. Sci.* 44:220–221.

50. Tripathy, D. N. 1999. Swinepox virus as a vaccine vector for swine 3–6 pathogens. *Adv. Vet. Med.* 41:463–480.

51. Velu, T. O. 1916. A contribution to the study of the etiology of pox in pigs. *Recueil de Medecine Veterinaire* 92:24.

52. Venkatnarayana, J. 1962. Annual Technical Report of Disease Investigation Office. Pigs. Andra Pradesh, India.

53. Verma, P. C. and Rai, A. 1988. Enzymeimmunoassay for estimation of antibodies against swinepox virus in pig sera. *Indian J. Virol.* 4:46–49.
54. Verma, P. C. and Rai, A. 1990. Counterimmunoelectrophoresis for the rapid detection of antibodies against swinepox virus. *Indian Vet. Med. J.* 14:81–83.
55. Verma, P. C., Rai, A. and Satish, K. 1987. Electron and immunoelectron microscopy of swinepox virus of Indian origin. *Indian J. Vet. Pathol.* 11:69–71.
56. Winslow, B. J., Cochran, M. D., Holzenburg, A., Sun, J. C., Junker, D. E. and Collisson, E. W. 2003. Replication and expression of a swinepox virus vector delivering feline leukemia virus gag and env to cell lines of swine and feline origin. *Virus Res.* 98:1–15.

11. Swine Rotavirus

K. Dhama, M. Mahendran, and S. Nandi

Introduction
The common causes of infectious enteritis and diarrhea in swine are Escherichia coli, rotavirus, coronavirus, and Clostridium perfringens (Dewey et al., 2003). Among these, neonatal diarrhea due to rotavirus can inflict significant economic loss to intensive pig-rearing units by causing piglet mortality or lack of proper weight gain (Ramos et al., 1998). Rotavirus-associated enteritis and diarrhea are common in one to four-week-old piglets or in recently weaned ones (Bohl et al., 1978; Bergeland and Henry, 1982; Teodoroff et al., 2005). In 1975, viruses that are morphologically similar to reoviruses were first seen in the feces of diarrheic pigs in United Kingdom (Wood and Bridger, 1975). Subsequently, rotaviruses have been identified to have worldwide distribution in swine population. The porcine rotaviruses (PRV) isolated from different parts of the world have been classified in groups A, B, C, and E; among which, group A rotaviruses are most prevalent, OSU and Gottfried being the popular strains (Holland, 1990; Steele et al., 2004; Martella et al., 2007). The OSU strain have antigenic similarity to the equine rotaviruses but were found distinct from other mammalian and avian strains, while the Gottfried strain have antigenic relatedness to human, canine, and simian rotavirus strains (Bohl et al., 1984; Holland, 1990). Among all the etiological agents causing diarrhea, rotaviruses have a significant role and are considered as pathogens with the potential to cause huge economic losses to the livestock industry besides causing death of millions of children in developing countries (Holland, 1990; Dodet et al., 1997; Chauhan et al., 2008).

After group A, group C rotaviruses have been detected in swine (Saif et al., 1980; Bridger and Brown, 1985; Holland, 1990), but they occurred less than half as often as group A rotaviruses. Serological analysis also supports the relatively less frequency of occurrence of group C rotavirus in the swine population. Further, the rotaviruses identified by Bridger (1980) were antigenically distinct from group A rotavirus and genetically distinct from porcine group C viruses and hence were designated as group B virus. However, during the experimental infection in swine, the lesions induced by group B rotavirus have been found to be less severe than the group A rotavirus–mediated infection (Theil et al., 1985; Holland, 1990).

Epidemiology and Etiology

Rotaviruses are ubiquitously present in most of the swine-rearing units having almost 100% seroconversion in adult stock. Antibodies to group A rotavirus can be found in 90–100% swine population (Gaul et al., 1982). Besides, the most important epidemiological aspect is the persistence of the rotaviruses outside the herd, which is particularly due to the extreme environmental resistance exhibited by the virus and due to its resistance to many disinfectants. So the outbreaks of rotavirus infection may be commonplace and can be observed in neonatal piglets of two to four weeks of age (Ramos et al., 1998). The presence of rotavirus infection has been reported from countries like USA (Saif et al., 1980; Winiarczyk et al., 2002), United Kingdom (Bridger, 1980), Brazil (Racz et al., 2000), France (Corthier et al., 1980), Denmark (Svensmark, 1983), Canada (Leece and King, 1980; Dewey et al., 2003), Belgium (Debouck and Pensaert, 1983), Japan (Teodoroff et al., 2005), Italy (Martella et al., 2007), and Argentina (Parra et al., 2008). Besides group A rotavirus infections, viruses of groups B and C may also cause an epizootic infection, especially in seronegative piglets (Smitalova et al., 2006).

The etiological agent porcine rotavirus (PRV), a nonenveloped virus coming under the family Reoviridae, has RNA genome consisting of eleven double-stranded RNA segments protected by a triple-layered wall, out of which two layers are contributed by the icosahedral capsid proteins (Murphy, 1999). The viral genome has the ability to code for structural as well as nonstructural proteins. The protein VP2 forms the first layer of the virion, covering the proteins VP1 and VP3, which functions for virus transcription. VP6 protein is responsible for forming the second layer, and the outermost protein layer is composed of the structural proteins VP7 and spike protein VP4. VP7 (denoted as 'G'-glycoprotein) and VP4 (denoted as 'P'-protease sensitive protein) are capable of generating neutralizing antibodies. VP4 has the ability to undergo proteolytic cleavage, and this phenomenon has been found to drastically enhance the infectivity of rotaviruses (Steele et al., 2004; Desselberger et al., 2005). Among nonstructural proteins (NSP), NSP4, a viral enterotoxin, has a special property to induce diarrhea by acting on intestinal epithelial cells (enterocytes) (Desselberger et al., 2005).

The PRV, based on antigenic specificities, has been classified into groups, subgroups, and serotypes. The group and subgroup specificity conferred by viral protein VP6 differentiate the rotaviruses into seven groups (A to G) and into two subgroups (mainly subgroup I or II) (Steele et al., 2004; Desselberger et al., 2005). Groups A, B, and C rotaviruses are observed in herds, with the group A viruses causing most casualties, approximately 90% of all rotavirus diarrhea in commercial swine production units (Dewey et al., 2003). Regarding the serotypes, G1, G2, G3, G4 and G5, with P serotypes ranging from P (21–26) have been reported (Holland, 1990; Khamrin et al., 2007; Steyer et al., 2007). However, swine may be commonly infected with serotypes 3, 4, and 5 (Dewey et al., 2003). Also, multiple serotypes of group A rotaviruses can affect the same herd, and both group A and nongroup A rotaviruses could be seen in the herd simultaneously (Dewey et al., 2003). In countries like Japan, group A PRVs belonging to G9 serotype have been reported to predominate in young pigs (Teodoroff et al., 2005). Further, the role of PRV in generating reassortants (genetic shift) with other animal and human rotaviruses has been suggested (Ciarlet et al., 2001; Varghese et al., 2006; Mascarenhas et al., 2007; Parra et al., 2008). Other than genetic shift, variations in genome due to rearrangement of RNA segments has also been reported among group A PRVs, and genetic shift and rearrangements are the main reasons for their high antigenic versatility (Mattion et al., 1988; Murphy et al., 1999).

Further, the physicochemical properties of rotaviruses have been analyzed, and it could be stated that these viruses are having the properties to exhibit high stability and resistance. It has been found that rotaviruses having a buoyant density of 1.36 g/cm^3 are stable at pH 3, relatively heat tolerant, and resistant to ether, chloroform, quarternary ammonium compounds, and chlorination procedures, but they are sensitive to phenol and formaldehyde (Murphy et al., 1999; Steele et al., 2004).

TRANSMISSION

The resistance and the extreme stability permit the persistence of the rotavirus in environment, and these seems to be the key factors that favor the transmission of disease to susceptible piglets. Further, it is suggested that porcine rotavirus can retain their infectious nature for eight to nine months in feces, if maintained at a lower temperature. The main route of virus transmission is fecal-oral after the excretion of the virus in feces, and the excretion of the virus can be for long periods of time, favoring the maintenance and persistence of the infection in herds (Ramos et al., 1998).

CLINICAL SIGNS

The clinical form of rotavirus infection is common in piglets of two to four weeks of age, and pigs of all age groups are susceptible to the infection (Smitalova et al., 2006). The disease lasts for about three to four days and results in low weaning weights and poor average daily gain in piglets, with about 60% decrease in body weight by nine days postinfection (Dewey et al., 2003). Usually, the affected piglets show clinical manifestations like anorexia, yellowish white diarrhea, and dehydration. The diarrhea may contain mucus or sometimes blood. If enteropathogenic strains of *E. coli* are simultaneously present, then the severity of the disease could be enhanced, and rate of mortality will be high. Concurrent infection with rotavirus can increase the enteropathogenictiy of *E. coli* also (Lecce et al., 1982).

Age resistance to the clinical disease has been noticed in swine, similar to other animals. The reason could be due to the development of active immunity in adult pigs as a result of natural exposure or due to the increased rate of regeneration of villi, both of these factors acting together to reduce the disease severity and clinical signs (Dewey et al., 2003). In adult pigs or in piglets of above one month of age, the PRV may cause clinical disease; if complicated by secondary pathogens and in mature animals, inappetence and diarrhea lasting for few days can be observed (Smitalova et al., 2006).

PATHOGENESIS

Like all other animal rotaviruses, the PRV also gain entry to the body through ingestion, after which replication commences when it reaches the intestine, especially in mature villus epithelium of the small intestine. Further, the dual capsid protein coat makes the virus very resistant to the pH and the digestive enzymes in the gastrointestinal tract. Regarding the cellular receptors, rotaviruses contain tripeptide amino acid sequences in outer capsid proteins that can act as ligands for integrins 2 1 and 4 1 (Hewish et al., 2000). Also, it has been suggested that a lipid-bound sialic acid moiety in the neonatal intestine may act as receptor for porcine rotavirus (Rolsma et al., 1998). The invasiveness of the virus is enhanced by the proteolytic cleavage of the viral protein VP4. Trypsin has been found capable in digesting VP4 into subunits called VP5 and VP8, thus enabling the penetration of virus into cells (Desselberger et al., 2005; Smitalova et al., 2006). The invasion and replication of the virus in the epithelial cells at the edges of the intestinal villi cause lysis of the host intestinal cells (enterocytes), thereby impairing the nutrient absorption (Dewey et al., 2003; Steele et al., 2004). After cell lysis, the progeny virions are excreted via feces within a period of two to five days postexposure. Diarrhea, a significant manifestation, primarily occurs due to the destruction of mature enterocytes and replacement by immature epithelial cells from the crypts, which lack disaccharidases and have impaired absorptive ability (Murphy et al., 1999; Steele et al., 2004; Desselberger et al., 2005). Intestinal content cannot be digested or absorbed, and severe malabsorption may occur. Loss of sodium and chloride into the intestinal lumen contributes to increased osmotic pressure, drawing more fluid into the intestine. Ultimately, net fluid loss exceeds absorption, and diarrhea results (Dewey et al., 2003). Also, one of the nonstructural proteins called NSP4 has been attributed as a major cause of rotavirus-mediated pathogenesis.

NSP4, an enterotoxin, is capable of causing diarrhea. This viral enterotoxin, released in the lumen of the intestine, interacts with adjacent enterocytes, leading to enhanced chloride secretion and thereby diarrhea (Mori et al., 2002). Also, the mutations taking place in NSP4 could act as a factor for variation of virulence among ARV isolates (Zhang et al., 1998). Besides all these, protein-energy malnutrition (PEM) can also be inferred as a stimulating factor for the rotavirus infection in neonatal pigs, which simulates chronic small intestinal stress in malnourished piglets (Zijlstra et al., 1997).

The replicative mechanism of rotaviruses, by which it affects the host cells, has also been ascertained (Desselberger et al., 2005). The PRV gets entry to the intestinal epithelial cells via endocytosis and is encapsulated in endosomal vesicles. Then, the proteins in the outer layer disrupt the endosomal membrane by altering the calcium ion concentration, after which the breakdown of VP7 into single protein subunits occurs. This creates a double-layered particle (DLP), with VP2 and VP6 proteins covering the viral RNA. After this, the virus produces mRNAs, with the help of RNA-dependent RNA polymerase, to facilitate both translation and replication processes. Later, most of the rotavirus proteins get accumulated in structures known as viroplasms, where replication occurs and DLPs are assembled, which then migrates to the endoplasmic reticulum to obtain the outer layer (VP7 and VP4) to develop into a complete infectious virus particle.

LESIONS
The major pathological lesions of the rotavirus enteritis in swine are intestinal inflammation together with the atrophy of villous cells. The gross lesions are not prominent but may be often seen due to the secondary bacterial infections that occur in the intestinal tract. Histological interpretations reveal vacuolation of enterocytes, separation of enterocytes from lamina propria (desquamation), and infiltration of inflammatory cells in lamina propria. Replacement of columnar cells by cuboidal or squamous cells from the crypts can also be observed. Also, the length of the villi in duodenum and jejunum may be considerably shortened, with a drastic loss of microvilli.

DIAGNOSIS
For isolation of porcine rotaviruses, cell lines like MA104 or PK-15 (Eagle's medium, MEM with 10 µg/ml trypsin), and various diagnostic methods like electron microscopy, viral RNA polyacrylamide gel electrophoresis (PAGE), enzyme-linked immunosorbent assay (ELISA), immunofluorescence test, immunoperoxidase test, and dot blot hybridization can be employed (Herring et al., 1982; Bohl et al., 1984; Terrett et al., 1987; Holland, 1990; Murphy et al., 1999; Malik et al., 2005; Smitalova et al., 2006). Differences between

group A, B, and C of rotaviruses can be determined by electropherotypes of viral RNA (Herring at al., 1982; Smitalova et al., 2006). For antigenic characterization of PRVs, virus-neutralization tests or cross-protection assays could be performed for identifying the emergence of novel serotypes (Bohl et al., 1984, Holland, 1990). Presently, the diagnosis as well as molecular typing is performed using serotype-specific reverse transcription–polymerase chain reaction (RT-PCR), nested/multiplex RT-PCR, and restriction fragment length polymorphism (RFLP) (Murphy et al., 1999; Steele et al., 2004; Smitalova et al., 2006). Gene sequencing (VP6 and VP7) and oligonucleotide microarray hybridization can also be used to identify mixed rotavirus infections (Fischer and Gentsch, 2004). Also, rotaviral diarrhea has to be differentially diagnosed from infectious diarrhea of piglets caused by *E. coli*, *C. perferingens*, calici, corona-, or astroviruses (Holland, 1990; Smitalova et al., 2006), for which employing multiplex RT-PCR can be considered as a suitable option (Song et al., 2006).

PREVENTION AND CONTROL

For an effective control of the disease in piglets, environmental stress factors have to be kept minimal (Holland, 1990). In infected herds, antibiotic therapy has to be initiated to control secondary infections such as *E. coli*. Electrolyte and fluid therapy together with provision of dry, warm, and comfortable lying areas are essential to keep the infection under check. Due attention has to be given for minimizing the chances of temperature fluctuations. Good management practices, like all-in-all-out procedures and cleaning and disinfection of sty, coupled with vaccinating the dam, few weeks before parturition have to be practiced for preventing the PRV infection in swine population. The maternally derived antibodies have a major role in protecting young ones, especially during the initial few weeks of life (Saif and Fernandez, 1996). Protection depends mainly on milk immunoglobulin (Ig) A antibody. Piglets acquire all their maternal antibodies postnatally via colostrum; therefore, the quantity and quality of colostrum received is critical. Colostrum-fed pigs show less severe clinical disease, with circulating maternal antibody being significant in mitigating clinical disease, depending on the antibody titer, for at least the first one or two weeks after birth (Dewey et al., 2003). But due to the lack of an efficient vaccine and the resistance of the virus, the control of the rotavirus infection becomes a difficult task (Ramos et al., 1998). However, modified live rotavirus vaccines are available in some countries. Researchers have tried various options for developing immunization strategies to tackle the problem of rotavirus diarrhea in swine. A single-gene substitution reassortant generated from two porcine rotaviruses, OSU (serotype 5) and Gottfried (serotype 4), after oral administration has been found to induce a high level of neutralizing antibodies to the both common strains (Hoshino et al., 1988).

Later, a recombinant VP6-microsphere-based (MS-based) subunit vaccine has been developed, which provided mucosal immunity by inducing high levels of VP6-specific IgA antibodies similar to live PRV vaccines (Kim et al., 2002). Also, a live rotavirus prime/DNA boost vaccine regimen has been formulated, which exploited the use of plasmid DNA vaccine coding for the VP6 gene of PRV (Yuan et al., 2005).

CONCLUSION

The porcine rotaviruses exhibit a complex epidemiology primarily as a result of cocirculation of different groups and serotypes in a geographical area. Besides, changes can occur in viral genome due to the accumulation of point mutations and gene reassortment (genetic shift), enabling the swine rotaviruses to exhibit significant antigenic variation as seen in case of avian influenza viruses. Both of these phenomena are playing a key role in generating ample diversity among rotaviruses. Further, the high stability of the virus and its environmental resistance are adding to the difficulty of developing a proper eradication program. However, developing vaccines against this infection may help in countering the persistence of the virus in the environment to moderate levels. Also, development of new-generation vaccines using the immunogenic antigens of SRV has to be explored and given due importance. Regarding the diagnosis of this infection, novel detection tools have to be developed and judiciously employed so that a rapid diagnosis is facilitated. Even though the rotaviruses are difficult to completely get eradicated from poultry environment, strict sanitation and hygiene could favor in minimizing its incidence in swine population.

REFERENCES

1. Kohler, E. M., Saif, L. J., Cross, R. F., Agnes, A. G. and Theil, K. W. 1978. Rotavirus as a cause of diarrhea in pigs. *J. Am. Vet. Med. Assoc.* 172:458–463.
2. Bohl, E. H., Theil, K. W. and Saif, L. J. 1984. Isolation and serotyping of porcine rotaviruses and antigenic comparison with other rotaviruses. *J. Clin. Microbiol.* 19:105–111.
3. Bridger, J. C. 1980. Detection by electron microscopy of caliciviruses, astroviruses and rotavirus-like particles in the faeces of piglets with diarrhoea. *Vet. Rec.* 107:532–533.
4. Bridger, J. C. and Brown, J. F. 1985. Prevalence of antibody to typical and atypical rotaviruses in pigs. *Vet. Rec.* 116:50.
5. Chauhan, R. S., Dhama, K. and Mahendran, M. 2008. Pathobiology of rotaviral diarrhea in calves and its diagnosis and control: A review. *J. Immunol. Immunopathol.* 10:1–13.
6. Ciarlet, M., Ia, P., Conner, M. E. and Liprandi, F. 2001. Antigenic and molecular analyses reveal that the equine rotavirus strain H-1 is closely related to porcine, but not equine, rotaviruses: Interspecies transmission from pigs to horses? *Virus Genes* 22:5–20.
7. Corthier, G., Cohen, J. and Scherrer, R. 1980. Isolation of pig rotavirus in France identification and experimental infections. *Ann. Rech. Vet.* 11:45–48.

11. SWINE ROTAVIRUS

8. Debouck, P. and Pensaert, M. 1983. Rotavirus excretion in suckling pigs followed under field circumstances. *Ann. Rech. Vet.* 14:447–448.

9. Desselberger, U., Gray, J. and Estes, M. K. 2005. Rotaviruses. In *Topley and Wilson's microbiology and microbial infection*, ed. B. W. J. Mahy and V. T. Meulen, 946–958. USA: ASM Press.

10. Dewey, C., Carman, S., Pasma, T., Josephson, G. and McEwen, B. 2003. Relationship between group A porcine rotavirus and management practices in swine herds in Ontario. *Can. Vet. J.* 44:649–653.

11. Dodet, B., Heseltine, E., Mary, C. and Saliou, P. 1997. Rotaviruses in human and veterinary medicine. *Sante* 7:195–199.

12. Fischer, T. K. and Gentsch, J. R. 2004. Rotavirus typing methods and algorithms. *Rev. Med. Virol.* 14:71–82.

13. Gaul, S. K., Simpson, T. F., Woode, G. N. and Fulton, R. F. 1982. Antigenic relationships among some animal rotaviruses: Virus neutralization in vitro and cross-protection in piglets. *J. Clin. Microbiol.* 16:495–503.

14. Herring, A. J., Inglis, N. F., Ojeh, C. K., Snodgrass, D. R. and Menzies, J. D. 1982. Rapid diagnosis of rotavirus infection by direct detection of viral nucleic acid in silver-stained polyacrylamide gels. *J. Clin. Microbiol.* 16:473–477.

15. Hewish, M. J., Takada, Y. and Coulson, B. S. 2000. Integrins 2 1 and 4 1 can mediate SA11 rotavirus attachment and entry into cells. *J. Virol.* 74:228–236.

16. Holland, R. E. 1990. Some infectious causes of diarrhoea in young farm animals. *Clin. Microbiol. Rev.* 3:345–375.

17. Hoshino, Y., Saif, L. J., Sereno, M. M., Chanock, R. M. and Kapikian, A. Z. 1988. Infection immunity of piglets to either VP3 or VP7 outer capsid protein confers resistance to challenge with a virulent rotavirus bearing the corresponding antigen. *J. Virol.* 62:744–748.

18. Khamrin, P., Maneekarn, N., Peerakome, S., Chan-it, W., Yagyu, F., Okitsu, S. and Ushijima, H. 2007. Novel porcine rotavirus of genotype P[27] shares new phylogenetic lineage with G2 porcine rotavirus strain. *Virology* 361:243–252.

19. Kim, B., Bowersock, T., Griebel, P., Kidane, A., Babiuk, L. A., Sanchez, M., Attah-Poku, S., Kaushik, R. S. and Mutwiri, G. K. 2002. Mucosal immune responses following oral immunization with rotavirus antigens encapsulated in alginate microspheres. *J. Control. Release* 85:191–202.

20. Lecce, J. G., Balsbaugh, R. K., Clare, D. A. and King, M. W. 1982. Rotavirus and hemolytic enteropathogenic *Escherichia coli* in weanling diarrhea of pigs. *J. Clin. Microbiol.* 16:715–723.

21. Lecce, J. G. and King, M. W. 1980. Persistent rotaviral infection producing multiple episodes of diarrhoea in weanling pigs reared in isolation. Proc. 3rd Intern. Symp. on Neonatal Diarrhoea. Vet. Infect. Dis. Org. Univ. Saskatchewan, Saskatoon, Canada, 21–36.

22. Malik, S. V. S., Barbuddhe, S. B., Rawool, D. B., Vaidya, V. M. and Sahare, A. M. 2005. Data sheet on Rotaviruses (Global status of Rotavirus infections in man and animals). In *Animal Health and Production Compendium, CAB International*, Wallingford, UK.

23. Martella, V., Banyai, K., Lorusso, E., Bellacicco, A. L., Decaro, N., Camero, M., Bozzo, G., Moschidou, P., Arista, S., Pezzotti, G., Lavazza, A. and Buonavoglia, C. 2007. Prevalence of group C rotaviruses in weaning and post-weaning pigs with enteritis. *Vet. Microbiol.* 123:26–33.

24. Mascarenhas, J. D., Leite, J. P., Lima, J. C., Heinemann, M. B., Oliveira, D. S., Araujo, I. T., Soares, L. S., Gusmao, R. H., Gabbay, Y. B. and Linhares, A. C. 2007. Detection of a neonatal human rotavirus strain with VP4 and NSP4 genes of porcine origin. *J. Med. Microbiol.* 56:524–532.

25. Mattion, N., Gonzalez, S. A., Burrone, O., Bellinzoni, R., La Torre, J. L. and Scodeller, E. A. 1988. Rearrangement of genomic segment 11 in two swine rotavirus strains. *J. Gen. Virol.* 69:695–698.

26. Mori, Y., Borgan, M. A., Ito, N., Sugiyama, M. and Minamoto, N. 2002. Diarrhea-inducing activity of avian rotavirus NSP4 glycoproteins, which differ greatly from mammalian rotavirus NSP4 glycoproteins in deduced amino acid sequence, in suckling mice. *J. Virol.* 76:5829–5834.

27. Murphy, F. A., Gibbs, E. P. J., Horzinek, M. C. and Studdert, M. J. 1999. Reoviridae. In *Veterinary Virology*, 391–404. USA: Academic Press.

28. Parra, G. I., Vidales, G., Gomez, J. A., Fernandez, F. M., Parreno, V. and Bok, K. 2008. Phylogenetic analysis of porcine rotavirus in Argentina: Increasing diversity of G4 strains and evidence of interspecies transmission. *Vet. Microbiol.* 126:243–250.

29. Racz, M. L., Kroeff, S. S., Munford, V., Caruzo, T. A., Durigon, E. L., Hayashi, Y., Gouvea, V. and Palombo, E. A. 2000. Molecular characterization of porcine rotaviruses from the southern region of Brazil: Characterization of an atypical genotype G[9] strain. *J. Clin. Microbiol.* 38:2443–2446.

30. Ramos, A. P. D., Stefanelli, C. C., Linhares, R. E. C., Brito, B. G. and Nozawa, C. M. 1998. The infectivity of pig rotavirus in stools. *Braz. J. Vet. Res. Anim. Sci.* 35:84–87.

31. Rolsma, M. D., Kuhlenschmidt, T. B., Gelberg, H. B. and Kuhlenschmidt, M. S. 1998. Structure and function of a ganglioside receptor for porcine rotavirus. *J. Virol.* 72:9079–9091.

32. Saif, L. J. and Fernandez, F. M. 1996. Group A rotavirus veterinary vaccines. *J. Infect. Dis.* 174:98–106.

33. Saif, L. J., Bohl, E. H., Theil, K. W., Cross, R. F. and House, J. A. 1980. Rotavirus-like, calicivirus-like, and 23-nm viruslike particles associated with diarrhea in young pigs. *J. Clin. Microbiol.* 12:105–111.

34. Smitalova, R., Rodak, L., Psikal, I. and Smid, B. 2006. Isolation, immunochemical demonstration of fieldstrains of porcine group A rotaviruses and electrophoretic analysis of RNA segments of group A and C rotaviruses. *Veterinar. Med.* 51:288–295.

35. Song, D. S., Kang, B. K., Oh, J. S., Ha, G. W., Yang, J. S., Moon, H. J., Jang, Y. S. and Park, B. K. 2006. Multiplex reverse transcription-PCR for rapid differential detection of porcine epidemic diarrhea virus, transmissible gastroenteritis virus, and porcine group A rotavirus. *J. Vet. Diagn. Invest.* 18:278–281.

36. Steele, A. D., Geyer, A. and Gerdes, G. H. 2004. Rotavirus infections. In *Infectious diseases of livestock*, ed. J. A. W. Coetzer and R. C. Tustin, 1256–1264. Southern Africa: Oxford University Press.

37. Steyer, A., Poljsak-Prijatelj, M., Barlic-Maganja, D., Jamnikar, U., Mijovski, J. Z. and Marin, J. 2007. Molecular characterization of a new porcine rotavirus P genotype found in an asymptomatic pig in Slovenia. *Virology* 359:275–282.

38. Svensmark, B. 1983. Prevalence rate of porcine rotavirus in Danish swine herds. *Ann. Rech. Vet.* 14:433–436.

39. Teodoroff, T. A., Tsunemitsu, H., Okamoto, K., Katsuda, K., Kohmoto, M., Kawashima, K., Nakagomi, T. and Nakagomi, O. 2005. Predominance of porcine rotavirus G9 in Japanese piglets with diarrhea: Close relationship of their VP7 genes with those of recent human G9 strains. *J. Clin. Microbiol.* 43:1377–1378.

40. Terrett, L. A., Saif, L. J., Theil, K. W. and Kohler, E. M. 1987. Physicochemical characterization of porcine pararotavirus and detection of virus and viral antibodies using cell culture immunofluorescence. *J. Clin. Microbiol.* 25:268–272.

41. Theil, K. W., Saif, L. J., Moorehead, P. D. and Whitmoyer, R. E. 1985. Porcine rotavirus-like virus (group B rotavirus): Characterization and pathogenicity for gnotobiotic pigs. *J. Clin. Microbiol.* 21:340–345.

42. Varghese, V., Ghosh, S., Das, S., Bhattacharya, S. K., Krishnan, T., Karmakar, P., Kobayashi, N. and Naik, T. N. 2006. Characterization of VP1, VP2 and VP3 gene segments of a human rotavirus closely related to porcine strains. *Virus Genes* 32:241–247.

43. Winiarczyk, S., Paul, P. S., Mummidi, S., Panek, R. and Gradzki, Z. 2002. Survey of porcine rotavirus G and P genotype in Poland and the United States using RT-PCR. *J. Vet. Med. B Infect. Dis. Vet. Public Health* 49:373–378.

44. Woode, G. N. and Bridger, J. C. 1975. Viral enteritis of calves. *Vet. Rec.* 96:85–88.

45. Yuan, L., Azevedo, M. S., Gonzalez, A. M., Jeong, K. I., Van Nguyen, T., Lewis, P., Iosef, C., Herrmann, J. E. and Saif, L. J. 2005. Mucosal and systemic antibody responses and protection induced by a prime/boost rotavirus-DNA vaccine in a gnotobiotic pig model. *Vaccine* 23:3925–3936.

46. Zhang, M., Zeng, C. Q., Dong, Y., Ball, J. M., Saif, L. J., Morris, A. P. and Estes, M. K. 1998. Mutations in rotavirus nonstructural glycoprotein NSP4 are associated with altered virus virulence. *J. Virol.* 72:3666–3672.
47. Zijlstra, R. T., Donovan, S. M., Odle, J., Gelberg, H. B., Petschow, B. W. and Gaskins, H. R. 1997. Protein-energy malnutrition delays small-intestinal recovery in neonatal pigs infected with rotavirus. *J. Nutr.* 127:1118–1127.

12. Swine Vesicular Disease

D. Nandi, and S. Nandi

Introduction

Swine vesicular disease (SVD) is a contagious viral disease of swine caused due to enteroviral infection. It is indistinguishable clinically from foot-and-mouth disease (FMD), vesicular stomatitis (VS), and vesicular exanthema (VE) of pigs. The disease is characterized by formation of vesicles on different parts of the body of the pig (Lin and Kitching, 2000).

Etiology

Causative Virus

Swine vesicular disease virus (SVDV) belongs to genus *Enterovirus* and family Picornaviridae. The virus is placed in list A disease by OIE (Office International des-Epizooties, World Organization for Animal Health, Paris, France) due to its similarities in clinical signs and pathology with other members in the list, most notably foot-and-mouth disease (OIE, 2004). Different strains of SVDV vary in virulence, and the disease produced may be subclinical, mild, or severe in manifestation. The virus is thought to be a variant manifestation of human coxsackie B5 virus due to its obvious antigenic similarities with the same (Brown et al., 1973; Zhang et al., 1993; Verdaguer et al., 2003; Jimenez-Clavero et al., 2005). Though the human virus does not infect animals, the swine virus has the propensity to cause human infections. Until now, though only a single serotype of SVDV is found to exist, different isolates collected from various parts have been found to belong to at least four phylogenetically distinct groups on the basis of differences in nucleotide sequence in VP1 or 3BC genes (Bocchi et al., 1997; Zhang et al., 1999). Complete nucleotide sequence data reveals that SVDV has approximately 75–85% homology with coxsackie B5 virus (Knowles and McCauley, 1997), and upon phylogenetic analysis, a common ancestral link has been established with the human coxsackie B5 virus during the period between 1945 and 1965 (Zhang et al., 1999; Ye et al., 2005).

Physical Properties of the Virus

The SVDV is an acid and ether-stable RNA virus of about 30–32 nm diameter, slightly larger than foot-and-mouth virus (FMDV). SVDV is a spherical particle with 150S sedimentation rate and a buoyant density of 1.34 g/ml in cesium chloride compared to 1.43 g/ml for FMDV. The virus is stabilized at 50°C by 1M MgCl₂. SVDV consists of a naked capsid with isometric symmetry, containing a central core of single-stranded RNA. Unlike FMD and other related viruses, SVDV is stable at pH 5.

Host Range

Human and swine are only naturally infected by the virus, and the disease can be produced experimentally in pigs by inoculating the agent in feet epithelium (Dekker, 2000). In human, the symptoms simulate with that observed in case of coxsackie B5 infection. The day-old mice can be readily infected by intracerebral or intraperitoneal inoculation of the virus (Kado, 1983). Among animals, only sheep can be experimentally infected with production of disease signs; however, they do not play any role in the epizootiology of the disease (Burrows et al., 1974).

Tissue Culture

SVD virus can grow and propagate well in primary culture of pig kidney cell origin (Nardelli et al., 1968). Vesicular fluid and extracts of vesicular epithelium from both naturally and experimentally infected swine produce cytopathic effects (CPE) in both primary or secondary pig kidney cell cultures and established cell lines. CPE can be visualized as soon as six hours with complete cell lysis by twenty-four hours. There is characteristic pyknosis, rounding up of cells into small foci or microplaques formation, and ultimately complete disruption of monolayer cell culture leading to cellular detachment from glass surfaces. Unlike FMD virus, SVDV do not produce any CPE in calf kidney, calf thyroid, or the BHK 21 cell lines (Dekker, 2000).

Serological Properties

The virus is serologically and biologically related to human enterovirus coxsackie B5 (Graves, 1973). All strains of SVDV are readily neutralized by antisera prepared in horse against human coxsakie B5, and sera recovered from pigs that suffered an episode of SVD is able to neutralize coxsackie B5 virus in tissue cultures or in mice inoculation. Different strains of SVDV show some differences in complement fixation (CF), neutralization, and in double-diffusion precipitation tests.

Epizootiology

History and Prevalence

The first infection due to SVDV was identified in 1966 from Lombardy, Italy, and subsequently in Hong Kong in the original name of porcine enteroviral infection (Nardelli et al., 1968; Mowat et al., 1972). In Hong Kong, the disease was seen in farms where pigs were vaccinated recently with homologous type O strains of FMD vaccine antigen (Mowat et al., 1972). Subsequently, the viral etiological agent responsible was identified as a new member of the genus *Enterovirus* and the name given as SVD virus in 1972 (Anonymous, 1972). In the 1990s, outbreaks occurred in number of European countries due to long-distance movement of pigs between member states of European Union (EU). Worldwide, the disease is still present in Taiwan Province of China, Hong Kong, and possibly in other Far East countries (Radostits et al., 2007). The occurrence of SVD has also been reported from the British Islands, France, Poland, Austria, Germany, Switzerland, Japan, Malta, Greece, Spain, and Italy (Valpreda and Moda, 1992; Espuna et al., 1993; Wandurski, 1996; Dekker, 2000; Lin and Kitching, 2000; Mackay, 2004). However, extensive serological surveys conducted during 1993 using virus-neutralization tests did not find any serological evidence of the infection in the pigs in UK, Denmark, Portugal, and Greece following adoption of strict control measures (Davies, 1994; Mackay et al., 1995).

TRANSMISSION

A close association is observed between incidence of the disease and importations of pork or pigs from countries where the disease is prevalent. Spread of SVD in England was worked out to be due to transport of pigs by a livestock vehicle that previously transported SVDV-infected swine and remained contaminated even after cleaning. Spread between herds has been primarily by contact of susceptible pigs with infected ones via excretions and secretions. Virus persists in all tissues of a suffering pig, and therefore, feeding of garbage, swill, or pork happens to be the potential route of transmission of the infective agent. Virus can survive well in pork products and by-products even after treatment like smoking or drying (Panina, 1995). Pigs slaughtered during the incubation period of the disease or those fostering subclinical infection possess large number of infective agent in all tissues sufficient to cause new infections in healthy pigs that consume the pork without proper processing (Farez and Morley, 1997). An infected premise or environment is a source of infection to pigs. Abrasions in feet are major avenues for entry of the virus into body from infective source. Incubation period of the disease varies between two to fourteen days; however, virus shedding starts even before appearance of clinical signs. Following a brief period of viremia, virus excretion commences through natural orifices like nasal and oral secretions or via feces. Indirect contact with contaminated feed, water, fomites, or other farm appliances also serves as potential source of infection. However, unlike FMD, the virus does not seem to transmit through air, and thus virus spread is less rapid than FMDV. The dose of virus required to initiate infection across damaged skin is as little as 10 PFU which, is one-thousand-fold less than that required for oral route of infection (Burrows et al., 1974). Resistance of the virus or its persistence in the environment for comparatively long period allows for its spread through various mechanical means. However, vertical transmission of the virus in host has been ruled out (Radostits et al., 2007). Recycling of virus through garbage feeding with subsequent spread to other piggeries has been a major source of new outbreaks of the disease in England. In an epizootiologiocal field study in Great Britain, it has been found that the main source of SVDV infection was movement of pigs (48%) either due to transport of infected pig (16%) or use of contaminated transport vehicle (21%) or because of contact with ailing pig at marketplaces (11%) and the other source (15%) being the feeding of contaminated waste food (Dekker, 1995a, 2000). After an infective episode, virus generally does not persist in host longer than two weeks, but persistence for more than three months has also been reported in natural infection (Gourreau et al., 1975). Recently, persistence of infection was confirmed under experimental situation by detecting viral RNA (vRNA) by reverse transcription-nested–polymerase chain reaction (RT-nPCR) in tissue samples long after exposure to infection providing preliminary evidence of a carrier state in swine vesicular disease (Lin et al., 1998). However, the rate of persistent infection and carrier state development is relatively a rare confrontation (Lin et al., 2001). SVDV is reported to be present in boar semen during viremic stage of the infection, which in turn plays important role in disease transmission through natural mating or artificial insemination (Rijn et al., 2004; Guerin and Pozzi, 2005).

PATHOGEN RISK FACTORS

The virus is extremely resistant to chemical and physical influences and can remain infective in the environment particularly in pig excreta for more than six months. However, the virus is susceptible to extremes of pH, disinfectants like 2.00% sodium hydroxide, 8.00% formaldehyde, and 0.04% sodium hypochlorite in the absence of organic materials. The virus survives processing of pork and pork products but can be destroyed by heating at temperature greater than 68°C (Panina, 1995; Farez and Morley, 1997).

ECONOMIC SIGNIFICANCE

Even though the disease does not pose much economic threats, the cost involved in slaughter to ensure eradication during large-scale outbreak is the major cause of concern. Mortality due the disease is not high, and morbidity, though high, usually runs a brief course. The major importance of the disease is attached to its close proximity in clinical features with FMD or VS and subsequent imposition of ban in trade with other countries. This necessitates a prompt differentiation from related diseases and subsequent confirmation of the exact etiology using sophisticated laboratory techniques, which is an expensive venture. Wooldridge et al. (2006) described a method for estimating economic losses due to SVD in pig.

PATHOGENESIS

Different parts of the body in pig differ in susceptibility to invasion by SVDV with damaged skin being the most vulnerable site. Infection is followed by a brief period of viremia, subsequent to which the virus propagates to several sites of the body, most notably the epithelium of coronary band, tongue, lip, snout, and myocardium. Though lesions may also be seen in brain stem, clinical signs suggestive of neuronal invasion are not evident. Incubation period of SVD is usually two to four days for the appearance of vesicles at the site of virus inoculation and some more days for generalization with visible vesicle formation at secondary sites (Burrows et al., 1973). Lesions develop soon after thirty hours of inoculation through intravenous route and a week following oral ingestion (McKercher and Graves, 1979). Virus has been recovered from the feces of infected animal even after three weeks of infection (Burrows et al., 1974). Recovery from SVD is rapid, and normal health status may be resumed by three to four weeks except hoof deformity and lameness as sequel in some cases. Antibody in serum of SVD-infected pig can be quantified from the seventh day postinfection till the twenty-eight day postinfection, and neutralizing antibody persists in recovered pigs as long as sixty days after infection (Burrows et al., 1974; McKercher and Graves, 1979).

CLINICAL SIGNS

The disease is usually mild in manifestation with morbidity rate ranging between 25–65%. Transient fever (temperature around 105°F), dullness, and inappetance may be followed by lameness and back arching in suffering pigs. Vesicles appear following viremic stage in predilection sites like coronary band, claws, heel, udder, lip, tongue, belly, and legs. They measure nearly 1–3 mm in diameter and often coalesce and rupture, leading to development of ulcer. However, healing is usually rapid in uncomplicated cases, and many pigs experience complete and uneventful recovery. Nervous signs like circling, paralysis, ataxia, head pressing, and convulsions may be seen as a rare consequence.

Lesions

Gross Lesions

On gross examination, vesicles of varying sizes are observed in and around coronary band and interdigital spaces of one or more feet. Cutaneous ulcers may extend to the metacarpus or metatarsus with loosening of sole pad. Vesicles are also seen on teat, buccal mucosa, tongue, and snout; some of them may rupture leaving a raw, denuded bleeding ulcer (Graves, 1986).

Histopathology

Microscopic features of vesicles are same as in gross examination, which consist of areas of coagulative necrosis with intraepithelial vesicle formation. Additional necrotic foci are present in the tonsils, renal pelvis, bladder, salivary glands, pancreas, and myocardium. Lesions in brain consist of diffuse nonpurulent encephalomyelitis, perivascular cuffing with lymphocytes, and formation of neuroglial cell foci (Graves, 1986). Necrotic foci with infiltration of neutrophils are seen in myocardium. Intranuclear inclusion bodies are present in the ganglion amphicytes (Radostits et al., 2007). However, it is difficult to differentiate SVD and FMD in swine on the basis of gross and histological findings.

Diagnosis

Diagnosis of SVD should definitely rest on history of contact with an ailing animal by any means, clinical signs, histopathological findings, differentiation with similar diseases, and subsequent confirmation with the aid of improved laboratory techniques.

Differential Diagnosis

SVD should be differentiated from other vesicular diseases of swine like FMD, VS, and VE. These diseases in pigs cannot be distinguished reliably on clinical grounds alone. Differentiation in the laboratory should be based on antigen detection and serological tests like enzyme-linked immunosorbent assay (ELISA), growth characteristics in cell culture, complement fixation test (CFT), virus-neutralization tests (VNT), counterimmunoelectrophoresis (CIEP), nucleic acid detection by reverse transcriptase–polymerase chain reaction (RT-PCR), and nucleotide sequence analysis. Other nonviral causes of vesicular conditions like photosensitivity and allergy should be considered for differentiation.

CONFIRMATORY DIAGNOSIS

Confirmatory diagnosis of SVD should be based on isolation of virus from samples of epithelium collected from ruptured or intact vesicles. Viral antigen can be detected by ELISA (Ferris and Dawson, 1988) as soon as four hours after the receipt of a sample by the diagnostic laboratory. A 10% suspension of lesion material in phosphate buffered saline may be inoculated on to monolayer of IB-RS-2 porcine cells and observed for cytopathic effects (OIE, 2004). Samples can also be sent to FAO World Reference Laboratory (WRL) for FMD at Institute for Animal Health, Pirbright, Surrey, United Kingdom, for investigation of SVD. Isolates of SVDV are characterized antigenically and genomically for the purpose of molecular epidemiological study of the disease (Brocchi et al., 1997). The VNT, double immunodiffusion test (DID), radial immunodiffusion test (RID), CIEP, and ELISA are recommended by OIE for the detection of antibody against SVD (Golding et al., 1976; Donaldson et al., 1983; Brocchi et al., 1995). Blood and fecal samples may be collected and used for serology and virus isolation. Lots of modifications has been executed over the existing diagnostic techniques to enhance sensitivity and specificity in order to suit rapid diagnosis of SVD. Liquid-phase blocking sandwich ELISA has been developed and correlated with virus-neutralization test for the detection and quantification of antibodies against swine vesicular disease virus (Dekker et al., 1995b; Armstrong and Barnett, 2001). By using ELISA based on monoclonal antibodies directed against particular isolate of SVDV, it has been possible to compare different SVDV isolates and with that of antigenically related coxsackie viruses (Marquardt and Ohlinger, 1995; Brocchi et al., 1995; Chenard et al., 1998; Borrego et al., 2002). Approximately one in around ten thousand pigs react positively for antibody to SVDV, despite never being exposed to the agent. Such singleton reactors cause problems in serological surveys and international trade, which can be minimized by using a combined regime of ELISA and VNT or radioimmunoprecipitation assays (RIPA) and VNT (Moonen et al., 2000) or by combined VNT, monoclonal antibody-based cELISA (MAC—ELISA), and isotype-specific ELISA (De Clercq, 1998). Determination of isotype of antibody in pig sera by MAC or isotype-specific trapping-indirect ELISA helps in detection of singleton reactor as most of the singleton reactors are found to be positive for IgM antibody (Brocchi et al., 1995; De Clercq 1998; Niedbalski, 2002). Automated real-time RT-PCR may be employed for the diagnosis of SVDV from a range of samples like vesicular epithelium, serum, nasal swabs, or feces (Reid et al., 2004b). Single-tube RT-PCR system and digoxigenin (DIG) PCR-ELISA are considered highly sensitive for the detection of the virus (Callens and De Clercq, 1999). A similar type of assay based on fluorogenic probe is found highly sensitive and specific for detection of SAVDV in cerebrospinal fluid (Verstrepen et al., 2002). Multiplexed RT-PCR microsphere array has been exploited for the diagnosis of swine vesicular disease, and FMD in pigs (Hole et al., 2006; Hindson et al., 2008). Fernández et al. (2008) developed and standardized a highly sensitive and specific one-step multiplex RT-PCR assay for simultaneous detection and differential of most important vesicular diseases affecting pigs. Experimental study had shown that the method can diagnose the diseases even before the first vesicular lesions appear. Reid et al. (2004a) reported the usefulness of real-time RT-PCR assays using independent sets of primers and probes as a supplement to the routine procedures of ELISA and virus isolation for the detection of swine vesicular disease virus and its differentiation from closely related diseases. A real-time PCR assay based on primer-probe energy transfer (PriProET) is developed to identify phylogenetically divergent strains of SVDV (Hakhverdyan et al., 2006; Rasmussen et al., 2006). Blomström et al. (2008) developed a rapid, sensitive, and specific one-step reverse transcriptase loop-mediated isothermal amplification (RT-LAMP) assay for the detection of SVDV. A similar method using padlock probes and microarrays is in use for simultaneous detection and differentiation of SVD, FMD, and VS of swine in a single reaction (Banér et al., 2007). Lomakina et al. (2004) described the application of universal primers for identification of SVDV and FMDV by PCR and PCR-ELISA. Thermal—(TaqMan, molecular beacons, primer-probe energy transfer, and light-upon-extension fluorogenic primers) and nonthermal-amplification-based real-time PCR methods have been described for the diagnosis of a wide range of transboundary animal diseases (TADs) of livestock, including SVD (Belak, 2005; Belak, 2007). With the introduction of nucleic acid extraction and pipetting robotics coupled with multichannel real-time PCR machines, the diagnostic procedures have become rapid, robust, and automated to meet national and international standards, thereby contributing immensely toward reduction of losses due to such transboundary viral diseases (Belak et al., 2005; La Rosa et al., 2006). The development of additional methods, like padlock probes and microarrays, are further improving the arsenal of nucleic acid–based novel molecular diagnostic tests for TADs (Belak et al., 2007). Dekker et al. (1995b) recommend that in addition to serological tests, virus isolation from pig tonsils should be carried out to study the epizootiology of SVD in farms where the infection is present. Cell culture, ELISA, PCR, or quantitative RT-PCR are considered most accurate and widely used methods for detection of SVDV directly in batches of semen from suspected herd (Rijn et al., 2004; Guerin and Pozzi, 2005).

TREATMENT AND PREVENTION

Generally, no specific therapy exists for SVD. However, antiseptics like potassium permanganate solution (1%), povidone iodine (2–4%), and copper sulfate (2%) may be applied on the affected body parts repeatedly to ensure quick recovery. Stringent monitoring of trade, quarantine, serodiagnosis, vaccination, and hygiene are the mainstay of prevention of SVD. The control of the disease can be achieved by preventing the introduction of the virus from infected into free zone. Before allowing entry of pigs from an area unknown for SVDV status, serological tests must be carried out in all cases, and the pigs should undergo a quarantine period of sufficient duration before being allowed into the mainstream of the farm. Breeding animal supplying germ plasma or semen intended for use in artificial insemination should be free from the virus. Additionally, the importation of pig products or by-products from unknown or infected zone should be banned. Thorough cooking of swill and cleansing of inanimate objects are essential measures to contain the spread of the virus. Hygiene at all levels of management and pig husbandry should be ensured to prevent entry of the pathogen by any means into a naive farm. Personal hygiene for persons working in a pig farm should be maintained. In the event of confirm introduction of the disease in to a premise, strict quarantine and elimination of infected and contact animals should be carried out.

Sodium hydroxide is the choice of long-term disinfectant where presence of organic material like feces is a problem in virus elimination. Oxidizing agents, iophores, and acids can be used where organic material is not interference. Quaternary ammonium compound with 0.05% or 0.10% NaOH is effective against SVDV (Shirari et al., 1977, 2003). SVDV is more stable to heat disinfection than FMD, and a temperature of above 68°C is necessary for inactivation of the virus. SVD is a notifiable disease; therefore, all suspected outbreaks should be reported to the concerned authority (OIE, 2004). In some countries, stamping-out policy in adopted during the time of an outbreak. All pigs in an infected zone are slaughtered at the earliest, and the carcasses are destroyed in situ by burial or incineration. A thorough cleaning and disinfection of premises is carried out, and the process is repeated in two weeks. Final disinfection of noninflammable surfaces with a flame gun is recommended. In European Union, generally two zones of restrictions are built in the event of a confirmed outbreak. An area of 3-km radius from the original site of infection is perceived as protection zone, and a surveillance zone of 10-km radius is built surrounding it. Movement within the protected zone is strictly prohibited, and pigs in that zone are slaughtered, and serological surveillance is carried out in the zone of surveillance to observe any spread of infection (Mackay, 2004). Once no such spread is detected, embargo on movement is lifted within twenty-one days of cleansing and disinfection operation or completion of sero-surveillance, whichever is earlier. In countries where the disease has become established, eradication is achieved by test and slaughter policy (Mackay, 2004). The serological testing is only of value in detecting residual subclinical pockets of infection. Experimental vaccines have shown varying degree of promise in protecting against SVD, but they are not tested in field conditions. Experimental inactivated vaccines against SVD have been tried (McKercher and Graves, 1979). Attenuated vaccine has also been developed using a temperature-sensitive mutant strain of the virus (Preston and Garland, 1979). In countries where the disease is endemic and existing animal husbandry practices do not allow eradication by stamping-out policy, vaccination may be a realistic option for controlling the disease.

PUBLIC HEALTH ASPECTS
Swine vesicular disease virus has zoonotic potential. Human is susceptible to infection by SVDV if exposed to relatively large quantity of the virus. In human, the virus produce flulike symptoms of mild fever, cold, abdominal pain, muscle cramps, aseptic meningitis, weakness, and weight loss (Lin and Kitching, 2000).

CONCLUSION
The importance of swine vesicular disease is due mostly to its similarities in clinical manifestation with other related disease of pigs. Therefore, efforts should be directed toward confirming an outbreak of SVD by differentiation using approved sophisticated laboratory tools at the earliest to adopt suitable control measures. A good animal husbandry practice with strict imposition of hygiene and biosecurity at all levels of animal rearing and subsequent operations need to be ensured to contain or alleviate the chances of an outbreak.

REFERENCES

1. Anonymous. 1972. Monitor: New disease masquerades as foot-and-mouth disease. *The New Scientist* 56:684.
2. Armstrong, R. M. and Barnett, I. T. 2001. An enzyme-linked immunosorbent assay (ELISA) for the detection and quantification of antibodies against swine vesicular disease virus (SVDV). *J. Gen. Virol.* 82:417–424.
3. Banér, J., Gyarmati, P., Yacoub, A., Hakhverdyan, M., Stenberg, J., Ericsson, O., Nilsson, M., Landegren, U. and Belák, S. 2007. Microarray-based molecular detection of foot-and-mouth disease, vesicular stomatitis and swine vesicular disease viruses, using padlock probes. *J. Virol. Methods* 143:200–206.

4. Belák, S. 2005. The molecular diagnosis of porcine viral diseases: A review. *Acta Vet. Hung.* 53:113–124.

5. Belák, S. 2007. Experiences of an OIE collaborating centre in molecular diagnosis of transboundary animal diseases: A review. *Dev. Biol.* (Basel) 28:103–112.

6. Blomström, A. L., Hakhverdyan, M., Reid, S. M., Dukes, J. P., King, D. P., Belák, S. and Berg, M. 2008. A one-step reverse transcriptase loop-mediated isothermal amplification assay for simple and rapid detection of swine vesicular disease virus. *J. Virol. Methods* 147:188–193.

7. Borrego, B., Garcia-Ranea, J. A., Douglas, A. and Brocchi, E. 2002. Mapping of linear epitopes on the capsid proteins of swine vesicular disease virus using monoclonal antibodies. *J. Gen. Virol.* 83:1387–1395.

8. Brocchi, E., Berlinzani, E., Gamba, D. and Simonede De, F. 1995. Development of two monoclonal antibody based ELISAs for the detection of and the identification of swine isotypes against swine vesicular disease. *J. Virol. Methods* 52:155–167.

9. Brocchi, E., Zhang, G., Knowles, N. J., Wilsden, G., McCauley, J. W., Marquardt, O., Ohlinger, V. F. and De, S. 1997. Molecular epidemiology of recent outbreaks of swine vesicular disease: Two genetically and antigenically different distinct variants in Europe, 1987–1994. *Epidemiol. Infect.* 118:51–61.

10. Brown, F., Talbot, P. and Burrows, R. 1973. Antigenic difference between isolates of swine vesicular disease virus and their relationship to Coxsakie B5 vrus. *Nature* 245:315–316.

11. Burrows, R., Greig, A. and Goodridge, D. 1973. Swine vesicular disease. *Res. Vet. Sci.* 15:141–144.

12. Burrows, R., Mann, J. A., Goodridge, D. and Chapman, W. G. 1974. Swine vesicular disease: Attempts to transmit infection to cattle and sheep. *J. Hygiene* 73:101–107.

13. Callens, M. and De Clercq, K. 1999. Highly sensitive detection of swine vesicular disease virus based on a single tube RT-PCR system and DIG-ELISA detection. *J. Virol. Methods* 77:87–99.

14. Chénard, G., Bloemraad, M., Kramps, J. A., Terpstra, C. and Dekker, A. 1998. Validation of a monoclonal antibody-based ELISA to detect antibodies directed against swine vesicular disease virus. *J. Virol. Methods* 75:105–112.

15. Davies, G. 1994. Eradication of epidemic pig diseases in the European Union. *Vet. Rec.* 135:567–568.

16. De Clercq, K. 1998. Reduction of singleton reactors against swine vesicular disease virus by a combination of virus neutralisation test, monoclonal antibody-based competitive ELISA and isotype specific ELISA. *J. Virol. Methods* 70:7–18.

17. Dekker, A. 2000. Swine vesicular disease, studies on pathogenesis, diagnosis, and epizootiology: A review. *Vet. Quart.* 22:189–192.

18. Dekker, A., Moonen, P., de Boer-Luijtze, E. A. and Terpstra, C. 1995a. Pathogenesis of swine vesicular disease after exposure of pigs to an infected environment. *Vet. Microbiol.* 45:243–250.

19. Dekker, A., Moonen, P. L. J. M. and Terpstra, C. 1995b. Validation of a screening liquid phase blocking ELISA for swine vesicular disease. *J. Virol. Methods* 51:343–348.

20. Donaldson, A. I., Ferris, N. P., Knowles, N. J. and Barett, I. T. R. 1983. Comparative studies of United Kingdom isolates of swine vesicular disease virus. *Res. Vet. Sci.* 35:295–300.

21. Espuna, E., Alemany, R., Riera, P., Artigas, C., Rosell, R., Pujols, J., Sanmartin, J. and San-Gabriel, A. 1993. Isolation of the swine vesicular disease virus in Spain. *Medicina-Veterinaria.* 10:657–662.

22. Farez, S. and Morley, R. S. 1997. Potential animal health hazards of pork and pork products. *Rev. Sci. Tech. Off. Int. Epiz.* 16:65–78.

23. Fernández, J., Agüero, M., Romero, L., Sánchez, C., Belák, S., Arias, M. and Sánchez-Vizcaíno, J. M. 2008. Rapid and differential diagnosis of foot-and-mouth disease, swine vesicular disease, and vesicular stomatitis by a new multiplex RT-PCR assay. *J. Virol. Methods* 147:301–311.

24. Ferris, N. P. and Dawson, M. 1988. Routine application of enzyme linked immunosorbent assay in comparison with complement fixation for the diagnosis of foot-and-mouth and swine vesicular disease. *Vet. Microbiol.* 16:201–209.

25. Golding, S. M., Hedger, R. S., Talbot, P. and Watson, J. 1976. Radial immunidiffusion and serum neutralization techniques for the assay of antibodies to swine vesicular disease. *Res. Vet. Sci.* 20:142–147.

26. Gourreau, J. M., Berthand, N., Mishra, V., Jaco, B. and Vallet, C. 1975. Persistence of swine vesicular disease virus in pig. *Recuil de Medicine Veterinaire* (Afort) 51:283–287.

27. Graves, J. H. 1973. Serological relationship of swine vesicular disease virus and human Coxsakie B5 virus. *Nature* 245:314.

28. Graves, J. H. 1986. Swine vesicular disease. In *Diseases of swine*, 6th ed., ed. A. D. Leman, B. Straw, R. D. Glock, W. L. Mengeling, R. H. C. Penny and E. Sholl, 348–353. Ames, Iowa: Iowa State University Press.

29. Guerin, B. and Pozzi, N. 2005. Viruses in boar semen: Detection and clinical as well as epidemiological consequences regarding disease transmission by artificial insemination. *Theriogenology* 63:556–572.

30. Hakhverdyan, M., Rasmussen, T. B., Thorén, P., Uttenthal, A. and Belák, S. 2006. Development of a real-time PCR assay based on primer-probe energy transfer for the detection of swine vesicular disease virus. *Arch. Virol.* 151:2365–2376.

31. Hindson, B. J., Reid, S. M., Baker, B. R., Ebert, K., Ferris, N. P., Tammero, L. F., Lenhoff, R. J., Naraghi-Arani, P., Vitalis, E. A., Slezak, T. R., Hullinger, P. J. and King, D. P. 2008. Diagnostic evaluation of a multiplexed RT-PCR microsphere array assay for the detection of foot-and-mouth and look-alike disease viruses. *J. Clin. Microbiol.* (In Press).

32. Hole, K., Clavijo, A. and Pineda, L. A. 2006. Detection and serotype-specific differentiation of vesicular stomatitis virus using a multiplex, real-time, reverse transcription-polymerase chain reaction assay. *J. Vet. Diag. Invest.* 18:139–146.

33. Jimenez-Clavero, M. A., Escribano-Romero, E., Ley, V. and Spiller, O. B. 2005. More recent swine vesicular disease virus isolates retain binding to Coxsackie-adenovirus receptor, but have lost the ability to bind human decay-accelerating factor (CD55). *J. Gen. Virol.* 86:1369–1377.

34. Kado, K. 1983. The propagation of a strain of SVDV in one day old mice. *Jap. J. Vet. Sci.* 45:821–823.

35. Knowles, N. J. and McCauley, J. W. 1997. Coxsackievirus B5 and their relationship to swine vesicular disease virus. *Curr. Topics Microbiol. Immunol.* 223:153–167.

36. La Rosa, G., Muscillo, M., Di Grazia, A., Fontana, S., Iaconelli, M. and Tollis, M. 2006. Validation of RT-PCR assays for molecular characterization of porcine teschoviruses and enteroviruses. *J. Vet. Med. B Infect. Dis. Vet. Public Hlth.* 53: 257–265.

37. Lin, F. and Kitching, R. P. 2000. Swine vesicular disease: An overview. *The Vet. J.* 160:192–201.

38. Lin, F., Mackay, D. K. and Knowles, N. J. 1998. Persistence of swine vesicular disease virus in pigs. *Epidemiol. Infect.* 121:459–472.

39. Lin, F., Mackay, D. K., Knowles, N. J. and Kitching, R. P. 2001. Persistent infection is a rare sequel following infection of pigs with swine vesicular disease virus. *Epidemiol. Infect.* 127:135–145.

40. Lomakina, N. F., Fallacara, F., Pacciarini, M., Amadori, M., Lomakin, A. I., Timina, A. M., Shcherbakova, L. O. and Drygin, V. V. 2004. Application of universal primers for identification of foot-and-mouth disease virus and swine vesicular disease virus by PCR and PCR-ELISA. *Arch. Virol.* 149:1155–1170.

41. Mackay, D. K. J. 2004. Swine vesicular disease. In *Infectious diseases of livestock*, 2nd ed., vol. 2, ed. J. A. W. Coetzer and R. C. Tustin, 1313–1318. Oxford, UK: Oxford University Press.

42. Mackay, D. K. J., Armstrong, R. M. and Kilner, C. G. 1995. Serological survey for swine vesicular disease in the UK. *Vet. Rec.* 136(10): 248–249.

43. Marquardt, O. and Ohlinger, V. F. 1995. Differential diagnosis and genetic analysis of the antigenically related swine vesicular disease virus and coxsackie viruses. *J. Virol. Methods* 53:189–199.

44. McKercher, P. D. and Graves, J. H. 1979. In *Enterovirus of animals and their zoonotic aspects. Handbook of zoonosis*. Section B. Viral Zoonosis. CRC Press, Florida, 161–167.

45. Moonen, P., Van Poelwijk, F., Moormann, R. and Dekker, A. 2000. Singleton reactors in the diagnosis of swine vesicular disease: The role of coxsackievirus B5. *Vet. Microbiol.* 76:291–297.

46. Mowat, G. N., Darbyshire, J. H. and Huntley, J. F. 1972. Differentiation of a vesicular disease of pigs in Hong Kong from foot and mouth disease. *Vet. Rec.* 90:618–621.

47. Nardelli, L., Lodetti, E., Gualandi, G. L., Burrows, R., Goodridge, D., Brown, F. and Cartwright, B. 1968. A foot and mouth disease syndrome in pigs caused by an enterovirus. *Nature* 219:1275–1276.

48. Niedbalski, W. 2002. Diagnostic value of the isotype-specific ELISA for the detection of antibodies against swine vesicular disease virus (SVDV). *Bull. Vet. Inst. Puawy* 46:37–44.

49. OIE. 2004. *Manual of diagnostic tests and vaccines for terrestrial animals.* Office-International-des-Epizooties. 5th ed., vol. 1, Paris, France, 136–141.

50. Panina, G. F. 1995. Resistance of swine disease viruses in uncooked and cured meat products. *Atti-del-XXII-Meeting-Annuale-della-Societa-Italiana-di-Patologia-ed-Allevamento-dei-Suini,-Reggio-Emilia-23-34-Marzo* 73–90.

51. Preston, K. J. and Garland, A. J. M. 1979. In vivo and in vitro studies on temperature sensitive mutants of swine vesicular disease virus. *J. Hygiene* 83:319–330.

52. Radostits, O. M., Gay, C. C., Hinchcliff, K. W. and Constable, P. D. 2007. In *Veterinary Medicine: A textbook of the diseases of cattle, sheep, pigs, goats and horses.* 10th ed., WB Saunders, Philadelphia, 1066–1068.

53. Rasmussen, T. B., Uttenthal, A. and Agüero, M. 2006. Detection of three porcine vesicular viruses using multiplex real-time primer-probe energy transfer. *J. Virol. Methods* 134:176–182.

54. Reid, S. M., Ferris, N. P., Hutchings, G. H., King, D. P. and Alexandersen, S. 2004a. Evaluation of real-time reverse transcription polymerase chain reaction assays for the detection of swine vesicular disease virus. *J. Virol. Methods* 116:169–1676.

55. Reid, S. M., Paton, D. J., Wilsden, G., Hutchings, G. H., King, D. P., Ferris, N. P. and Alexandersen, S. 2004b. Use of automated real-time reverse transcription-polymerase chain reaction (RT-PCR) to monitor experimental swine vesicular disease virus infection in pigs. *J. Comp. Pathol.* 131:308–317.

56. Rijn, P. A., Wellenberg, G. J., Hakze-van-der-Honing, R., Jacobs, L., Moonen, P. L. J. M. and Feitsma, H. 2004. Detection of economically important viruses in boar semen by quantitative real-time PCRTM technology. *J. Virol. Methods* 120:151–160.

57. Shirai, J., Kanno, T., Inoue, T., Mitsubayashi, S. and Seki, R. 1997. Effects of quarternary ammonium compounds with 0.1% sodium hydroxide on swine vesicular disease virus. *J. Vet. Med. Sci.* 59:323–328.

58. Shirai, J., Kanno, T., Tsuchiya, Y., Mitsubayashi, S. and Seki, R. 2003. Effects of chlorine, iodine, and quaternary ammonium compound disinfectants on several exotic disease viruses. *J. Virol.* 77:5475–5486.

59. Valpreda, M. and Moda, G. 1992. A current risk for Italian pig farming: Swine vesicular disease. *Praxis Veterinaria Milano* 13:23–24.

60. Verdaguer, N., Jimenez-Clavero, M. A., Fita, I. and Ley, V. 2003. Structure of swine vesicular disease virus: Mapping of changes occurring during adaptation of human coxsackie B5 virus to infect swine. *J. Virol.* 77:9780–9789.

61. Verstrepen, W. A., Kuhn, S., Kockx, M. M., Van de Vyvere, M. E. and Mertens, A. H. 2002. Rapid detection of enterovirus RNA in cerebrospinal fluid specimens with a novel single-tube real-time reverse transcription-PCR assay. *J. Virol. Methods* 103:101–107.

62. Wandurski, A. 1996. Swine vesicular disease outbreak in a large scale unit. *Med. Vet.* 52:113–115.

63. Wooldridge, M., Hartnett, E., Cox, A. and Seaman, M. 2006. Quantitative risk assessment case study: Smuggled meats as disease vectors. *Rev. Sci. Tech. Off. Int. Epiz.* 25:105–117.

64. Ye, G. S., Liu, X. T., Zhang, Y. M., Ma, Y. H., Zhang, M. T., Han, X. Q., Zhang, Y. G. and Xie, Q. G. 2005. Determination and analysis of complete nucleotide sequence of swine vesicular disease virus. *Chinese J. Virol.* 21:69–71.

65. Zhang, G., Haydon, D. T., Knowles, N. J. and McCauley, J. W. 1999. Molecular evolution of swine vesicular disease virus. *J. Gen. Virol.* 80:639–651.
66. Zhang, G., Wilsden, G., Knowles, N. J. and McCauley, J. W. 1993. Complete nucleotide sequence of a Coxsakie B5 virus and its relationship to swine vesicular disease virus. *J. Gen. Virol.* 74:845–853.

13. Transmissible Gastroenteritis in Pigs

S. Nandi, and P. K. Dash

Introduction

Transmissible gastroenteritis (TGE), an important and highly contagious acute infectious disease of piglets less than two weeks of age, is characterized by vomition, diarrhea, and high mortality. Clinical signs of the disease are not observed in cats, dogs, and foxes, though serve as potential carrier. It is classified under OIE list B disease. The TGE virus was first isolated in USA in 1946 from outbreaks of acute diarrhea with high mortality in piglets (Doyle and Hutchings, 1946). Since then, it has been reported in most parts of the world where intensive pig farming is practiced, including Asia (Japan, Korea, Malaysia, and Taiwan), America (North, Central, and South), and Africa (Zaire and Ghana) and major cause of death in piglets in USA, Europe, and elsewhere. It is never reported in Southern Africa and Australia (OIE, 2004).

Since 1984, a distinct respiratory variant of the transmissible gastroenteritis virus (TGEV) known as porcine respiratory coronavirus (PRCV) has spread throughout many parts of the world. This virus is a mutant of TGEV, which resulted from a large deletion in the surface protein S gene (Pensaert et al., 1986; Schwegmann-Wessels and Herrler, 2006). Though PRCV does not appear to be an important primary pathogen, it has greatly complicated the diagnosis of TGE, particularly by serological means. As PRCV is a mutant of TGE virus, a large proportion of pig population has acquired immunity to PRCV and TGEV (Pensaert et al., 1986). The endemicity of PRCV has greatly reduced the clinical symptoms and economic importance of TGE. Two other antigenically distinct coronaviruses are the porcine epidemic diarrhea virus (PEDV) and the hemagglutinating encephalitis virus (HEV) (OIE, 2004).

Etiology

TGE virus (TGEV) is under the genus *Coronavirus* and family Coronaviridae. The prototype of the family avian infectious bronchitis is one of the most infectious of all viruses and causes an acute respiratory disease that can be explosive, affecting all the birds in a flock at about the same time because of respiratory transmission and a very short incubation period. Similarly, TGE virus of swine affects piglets more severely, spread very quickly, and cause major economic losses. The coronaviruses were so named because large club-shaped paplomers projecting from the envelope give the particle the appearance of a solar corona. Virions are enveloped, roughly spherical with a diameter of 60–160 nm, and club-shaped projections 12–25 nm in lengths are present on the surface (Murphy et al., 1999). The genome consists of a single copy of positive-sense ssRNA of 28.5 kb (Laude et al., 1993; Enjuanes et al., 2005). The virions are composed of three structural proteins: the nucleocapsid protein (N), a small membrane glycoprotein (M or E1), and a large glycoprotein constituting the viral projections (S or E2). The S glycoprotein bears the different epitopes responsible for inducing both neutralizing and nonneutralizing antibodies (Delmas et al., 1986).

There is only one serotype of TGE virus, although some antigenic variation exists between field strains of different geographical origins and between virulent and attenuated strains. The TGE virus is closely related to PRCV, canine coronavirus, and feline infectious peritonitis virus (coronavirus) and distantly related to human coronavirus (Pereira, 1989).

The virus is sensitive to lipid solvent and various disinfectants, viz, formaldehyde, sodium hypochloride, iodine, and quarternary ammonium compounds. The virus is inactivated within few hours in sunlight and few days at 37°C. Most of the strains of the TGE virus are moderately sensitive to trypsin but stable at pH 3 (Saif and Bohl, 1986; Bohl, 1989).

The TGE virus can be grown in primary cultures of porcine kidney and thyroid cells. A swine testis cell line (ST) or pig kidney cell line (SK6) can permit the growth of TGE virus. The cytopathic effects are rounding of the affected cells and syncytia formation.

TRANSMISSION

The introduction of infected pigs into a farm usually initiates the outbreaks. Subclinically infected animals can be a source of infection, and recovered pigs often become carriers and can shed the virus for two to three weeks in their feces. Large amounts of virus are excreted in the feces of infected animals. Some of the important mechanisms of transmission includes feco-oral contamination, transfer through milk from infected sows, and contaminated litter. Indirect mechanical transmission is also documented through infected farm machinery and materials such as dirty boots, trucks, and vehicles. The virus may be transported even up to one mile through air current. *Musca domestica* (house fly) can also act as vector since the virus can multiply in it. Infected dogs, cats, foxes, and birds also shed virus in their feces for two to three weeks, contaminating the environment. However, the virus is very susceptible to disinfectants particularly iodine-based ones and quaternary ammonia compounds (Saif and Bohl, 1986).

PATHOGENESIS

After gaining entry into the body, the virus passes unharmed through the stomach and replicates in the enterocytes of villous tips of small intestine causing rapid and massive epithelial cell necrosis, shortening or atrophy of villous, malabsorption, and diarrhea. Dehydration due to vomiting and diarrhea, especially in piglets up to one week of age, is the cause of death. The mortality rate in older pigs is lower because enterocytes are less susceptible to infection and have greater regenerative capacity. There is impairment of transport activity of the intestinal epithelium due to diarrhea. Intestines fail to transport Na+ and Cl-, and there is a defect in the glucose-mediated Na+ ion transport. Mixed infection with TGE virus and other enteric viruses or bacteria, particularly *E. coli*, seldom occur in neonatal piglets. Pigs that recover from enteric infections with TGE virus develop serum antibodies and secretory antibodies. It is the antibodies in the intestinal secretions (IgA) but not in serum that provide protection. The recovered pigs develop immunity for at least six months. Animals reinfected usually show mild or subclinical form of the disease. During enteric infections of sows, lymphocytes stimulated by viral antigens that migrate to the mammary gland become plasma cells and produce IgA antibodies against TGE virus and are excreted through sow's milk throughout lactation. Piglets that ingest milk from an immune mother are protective against TGE as long as they consume milk. The passive protection is afforded only if the sow has undergone intestinal infection as viral antigens inoculated parenterally induce little or no IgA in milk (Haelterman, 1972; Pansaert et al., 1970).

CLINICAL SIGNS

The clinical signs of TGE in pigs in epidemic situation differ from those endemically infected. In epidemic situation, TGE is characterized by sudden onset of acute diarrhea in pigs of all ages, but neonatal animals are severely affected. After an incubation period of twenty-four hours, the pigs show signs of vomition along with watery diarrhea. Young piglets are thirsty and continue to suckle. They die after two to three days due to dehydration. The mortality may reach up to 100% in the piglets infected during first week of life but almost nil in piglets older than two weeks of age. Sows may be subclinically infected and develop diarrhea, agalactia, and anorexia. In growing and finishing pigs, a watery diarrhea last for five to seven days.

In endemic situation, sows are immune and show no signs of illness. Piglets are also protected by antibodies present in milk. Piglets become susceptible to infection two to three weeks after weaning. These animals show diarrhea and transmit the virus to recently weaned piglets. The piglets (three to eight days old) born to nonimmune or partially immune sows or gilts may also develop diarrhea (Saif and Wesley, 1999).

PATHOLOGY

TGEV enters through feco-oral route and multiplies in the enterocytes lining the small intestine. The sialic acid–binding activity of S protein allows TGEV to overcome the mucus barrier in the gut and to get access to the intestinal epithelium for initiation of infection. It destroys the villi by producing villous atrophy (Perlman, 1998). Extraintestinal sites of virus multiplication include the respiratory tract and mammary tissues (Sestak et al., 1999), but the virus is most readily isolated from the intestinal tract and from feces. By contrast, PRCV is most readily isolated from the upper respiratory tract, the tonsils, or the lungs, and little (if any) enteric multiplication of virus occurs.

Gross lesions are confined to the gastrointestinal tract, except for the dehydration. Stomach is distended with curdled milk. It may be congested with a small area of hemorrhage on diaphragmatic surface. Small intestine is distended with foamy yellow fluid containing curdled milk. In some cases, the intestinal wall becomes thin and translucent due to severe atrophy of intestinal villi. There is massive infiltration of inflammatory cellular components with vacuolization of enterocytes. Hematological profile of the diseased animals shows a remarkable lymphopenia and a moderate neutrophilia (Perlman, 1998).

DIAGNOSIS

The diagnosis of TGE is extremely important to control its spread. Though the clinical picture of acute disease along with the rapid spread is almost diagnostic, however, laboratory support is always required for confirmatory diagnosis of TGE.

Laboratory diagnosis of TGE is achieved through isolation of virus, detection of the viral antigen, nucleic acid—and/or virus-specific antibodies (Sirinarumitr et al., 1997). The virus isolation is always considered as gold standard. Isolation is attempted in young piglets or in tissue culture using suspected samples such as feces or small intestinal tissues, particularly loops of affected small intestine. The pig testis cell line (ST) is generally the most sensitive method for virus isolation (McClurkin and Norman, 1966), but pig kidney cell line (SK6) can also be used. However, virus isolation is often difficult and not very reliable because not all field isolates replicate in cell cultures (Voets et al., 1980). The demonstration of viral antigen is achieved through indirect immunofluorescence (IFA), immunoperoxidase, and immunogold silver staining. IFA is a rapid, sensitive, and specific assay for identification of viral antigens in intestine (Pensaert et al., 1981). A peroxidase-antiperoxidase method is also developed for demonstration of TGEV (Shoup et al., 1996). Coronavirus particles can also be detected in negatively stained preparations of feces from piglets with diarrhea by transmission electron microscopy. However, TGE and porcine endemic diarrhea (PED) virus cannot be differentiated unless immune-electron microscopy is used. A double-antibody sandwich ELISA using a capture monoclonal antibody and a polyclonal enzyme-linked detector antibody is preferred in many laboratories for the detection of fecal virus antigens. In situ hybridization (ISH) and RT-PCR methods have been described for the direct detection of TGEV in clinical samples with differentiation from PRCV. The PCR is the most widely used molecular assay for confirmation of TGE. The sensitivity of PCR is further improved by a second round of amplification adopting a nested PCR protocol. A duplex RT-PCR is also reported for the simultaneous detection of TGEV and porcine epidemic diarrhea virus. For immunological methods, paired sera are required for confirmatory diagnosis. The techniques include virus neutralization, indirect ELISA, and competitive ELISA based on TGEV/PRCV group-specific monoclonal antibodies (Nelson and Kehling, 1984). Serological assays are widely used for demonstration of TGE-free status for trade purpose (Brown and Paton, 1991).

In some farm, the disease becomes a low-level endemic problem of postweaning diarrhea, which is more difficult to diagnose. The emergence of PRCV has further complicated the diagnosis of TGE. However, the differentiation between TGEV and PRCV can be accomplished by a discriminatory RT-PCR, TGEV-specific cDNA probes, or by blocking ELISA (Saif and Wesley 1999; Kim et al., 2000). TGE in the weaning and growing pig is clinically indistinguishable from porcine epidemic diarrhea (PED). In comparison to TGE, PED is less acute with lower mortality in suckling pigs. Where TGE has become chronic in pigs, the differentiation from other diarrheal disease is difficult and needs laboratory confirmation. The differential diagnosis should also be considered for hemagglutinating encephalomyelitis, classical swine fever, coli-bacillosis, rotavirus infection, and swine dysentery.

TREATMENT

As for any other viral disease, there is no specific treatment for TGE. Treatment regime is focused on alleviating dehydration and starvation. Antibiotics are generally provided to reduce secondary infections. Water containing electrolyte and antibiotic such as neomycin should be provided to the affected animals. Other supportive care includes provision of extra heat and deep bedding to reduce the weights of infection from the diarrhea.

RISK

The greatest risk of introducing TGE is through the importation of pigs from endemically infected countries. Endemic herds remain infected for months to years and can serve as a source of virus for other outbreaks. The virus can survive for several days in manure and body secretions and for several months in cold or freezing conditions. Therefore, import of fresh or frozen pork from infected countries could represent a potential source. The OIE has recommendations on the trade of semen and embryo although there is no formal evidence that these materials are at risk.

CONTROL

TGE is well controlled in farms where good all-in-all-out procedures are practiced in farrowing houses and grower accommodation. The risk of spread can be reduced through introduction of animals from serologically negative herds. Though vaccination against TGE is carried out in several countries, however, it is not yet successful (Saif, 2004). The main reason for failures was their inability to stimulate high levels of secretory IgA (SIgA) antibodies in milk analogous to the naturally infected lactating sows and inadequate protection to sows themselves. As PRCV shares some epitopes for neutralizing antibodies with TGEV, it acts like a nature-made vaccine against TGEV resulting in a drastic reduction of TGE outbreaks in Europe (Schwegmann-Wessels and Herrler, 2006). However, use of PRCV strains as vaccine candidates for TGE has shown a lack of efficacy or only partial cross-protection (Sestak et al., 1996). New-generation recombinant DNA technology based vaccines, were also developed with limited success.

Subunit vaccines and live recombinant viral or bacterial vectors–based vaccine were developed, which express important immunogenic proteins (Shoup et al., 1997; Sestak et al., 1999). Unfortunately, despite long-term efforts, effective vaccines to prevent TGE infections remain elusive. So far, oral and injectable attenuated live virus vaccines appear to be better at boosting immunity, rather than inducing a primary immune response. However, live modified and killed vaccines are utilized in some countries to maintain immunity in the colostrum.

When an outbreak strikes, good hygiene practices can help reducing the impact of the disease, though it appears to be difficult to eradicate the disease. One approach consists of preventing contamination of newborn piglets by isolation. The other approach aims to minimize the duration of the disease by exposing all the pregnant sows to the disease to develop transplacental immunity of farrows. Immediate transfer of noninfected sows (that are within three weeks of farrowing) from the farm before they become infected could help in escaping the disease. Postinfection, thorough disinfection of pens should be carried out using an iodine based disinfectant.

TGE remains one of the important viral infections of swine. In the absence of an effective vaccine, rapid diagnosis can play an important role in the control of this infection. Strict biosecurity precautions should also be followed throughout the year to prevent the occurrence of infection.

REFERENCES

1. Bohl, E. H. 1989. Transmissible gastroenteritis virus (Classical enteric variant). In *Virus infections of porcines*, ed. M. B. Pensaert. Amsterdam, Oxford, New York, Tokyo: Elsevier Science Publishers.
2. Brown, I. H. and Paton, D. J. 1991. Serological studies of transmissible gastroenteritis in Great Britain, using a competitive ELISA. *Vet. Rec.* 128, 500–503.
3. Delmas, B., Gelfi, J. and Laude, H. 1986. Antigenic structure of transmissible gastroenteritis virus. II. Domains of the peplomer glycoprotein. *J. Gen. Virol.* 67:1405–1418.
4. Doyle, L. P. and Hutching, L. M. 1946. A transmissible gastroenteritis in pigs. *J. Amer. Vet. Med. Assoc.* 108:257–259.
5. Enjuanes, L., Sola, I., Alonso, S., Escors, D. and Zúñiga, S. 2005. Coronavirus reverse genetics and development of vectors for gene expression. *Curr Top Microbiol Immunol.* 287:161–97.
6. Haelterman, E. O. 1972. On the pathogenesis of TGE of swine. *J. Amer. Vet. Med. Assoc.* 160:534–540.
7. Kim, L., Chang, K-OK, Sestak, K., Parwani, A. and Saif, L. J. 2000. Development of a reverse transcription-nested polymerase chain reaction assay for differential diagnosis of transmissible gastroenteritis virus and porcine respiratory coronavirus from feces and nasal swabs of infected pigs. *J. Vet. Diagn. Invest.* 12:385–388.
8. Laude, H., Vanreeth, K. and Pensaert, M. 1993. Porcine respiratory coronavirus: Molecular features and virus-host interactions. *Vet. Res.* 24:125–150.
9. McClurkin, A. W. and Norman, J. O. 1966. Studies on transmissible gastroentetitis in swine. II. Selected characteristics of a cytopathogenic virus common to five isolates from transmissible gastroenteritis. *Canadian J. Com. Med.* 30:190–198.
10. Murphy, F. A., Gibbs, E. P. J., Horzinek, M. and Studdert, M. J. 1999. In *Veterinary virology*, 3rd ed. New York: Academic Press.
11. Nelson, L. D. and Kehling, C. L. 1984. Enzyme-linked immunosorbent assay for detection of transmissible gastroenteritis virus antibody in swine sera. *Am. J. Vet. Res.* 45:1645–1657.

12. OIE. 2004. Transmissible gastroenteritis. In *OIE Manual of diagnostic tests and vaccines for terrestrial animals*. Fifth Edition, 2004, 792–801.

13. Pensaert, M., Callebaut, P. and Vergote, J. 1986. Isolation of a porcine respiratory, non-enteric coronavirus related to transmissible gastroenteritis. *Vet. Q.* 8:257–261.

14. Pensaert, M. B., DeBouck, P. and Reynolds, D. J. 1981. An immunoelectron microscopic and immunofluorescent study on the antigenic relationship between the coronavirus-like agent CV777 and several coronaviruses. *Arch. Virol.* 68:45–52 1981.

15. Pensaert, M. B., Haelterman, E. O. and Burnstein, T. 1970. Transmissible gastroenteritis of swine: Virus intestinal cell interactions: I. Immunofluorescence, histopathology and virus production in the small intestine through the course of infection. *Arch. Ges. Vriusforsch.* 31:321–334.

16. Pereira, H. G. 1989. Coronaviridae. In *Andrew's viruses of vertebrates*, 5th ed., ed. J. S. Porterfield. London, Philadelphia: Bailliere Tindall.

17. Perlman, S. 1998. Pathogenesis of coronavirus-induced infections. Review of pathological and immunological aspects. *Adv. Exp. Med. Biol.* 440:503–13.

18. Saif, L. J. and Bohl, E. H. 1986. Transmissible gastroenteritis. In Diseases of swine, 6th ed., A. D. Leman, B. Straw, R. D. Glock, W. L. Mengeling, R. H. Penny, and E. Scholl. Ames, Iowa: Iowa State University Press.

19. Saif, F. L. J. and Wesley, R. D. 1999. Transmissible gastroenteritis and porcine respiratory coronavirus, In Diseases of swine, 8th ed., 295–325. Ames, Iowa, USA: Iowa State University Press.

20. Saif, L. J. 2004. Animal coronavirus vaccines: Lessons for SARS. *Dev. Biol.* (Basel) 119:129–40.

21. Schwegmann-Wessels, C. and Herrler, G. 2006. Transmissible gastroenteritis virus infection: A vanishing specter. *Dtsch Tierarztl Wochenschr.* 113:157–159.

22. Sestak, K., Lanza, I., Park, S. K., Weilnau, P. and Saif, L. J. 1996. Contribution of passive immunity to porcine respiratory coronavirus to protection against transmissible gastroenteritis virus challenge exposure in suckling pigs. *Am. J. Vet. Res.* 5:664–671.

23. Sestak, K., Meister, R. K., Hayes, J. R., Kim, L., Lewis, P. A., Myers, G. and Saif, L. J. 1999. Active immunity and T-cell populations in pigs intraperitoneally inoculated with baculovirus-expressed transmissible gastroenteritis virus structural proteins. *Vet. Immunol. Immunopathol.* 70:203–221.

24. Shoup, D., Jackwood, D. J. and Saif, L. J. 1997. Active and passive immune responses to transmissible gastroenteritis virus (TGEV) in swine inoculated with recombinant baculovirus-expressed TGEV spike glycoprotein vaccines. *Am. J. Vet. Res.* 58:242–250.

25. Shoup, D. I., Swayne, D. E., Jackwood, D. J. and Saif, L. J. 1996. Immunohistochemistry of transmissible gastroenteritis virus antigens in fixed paraffin-embedded tissues. *J. Vet. Diagn Invest.* 8:161–167.

26. Sirinarumitr, T., Paul, P. S., Halbur, P. G. and Kluge, J. P. 1997. An overview of immunological and genetic methods for detecting swine coronaviruses, transmissible gastroenteritis virus and porcine respiratory coronavirus in tissues. *Adv. Exp. Med. Biol.* 412:37–46.

27. Voets, M. T., Pensaert, M. B. and Rondhuis, P. R. 1980. Vaccination of pregnant sows against transmissible gastroenteritis with two attenuated virus strains and different inoculation routes. *Vet. Q.* 2:211–219.

SECTION D

LIST OF TROPICAL VIRAL DISEASES OF CAMELS
R. S. Chawan, K. Dhama, and M. Mahendran

INTRODUCTION

OTHER VIRAL DISEASES OF CAMEL

Tropical Viral Diseases of Camels

R. S. Chauhan, K. Dhama, and M. Mahendran

Introduction

Camels are known to provide the human population with meat, milk, fiber, and fuel and serve as a transportation vehicle in arid regions of different parts of the world. They are highly adapted to the inclement environments and can function in such environments better than other livestock. Mostly camels are managed on rangelands, community lands, or restricted pasture lands (Saini et al., 2006). Camels also adapt well to contained management with a unique ability to obtain nourishment from harsh forages during the time of free-range grazing (Dorman, 1984; Fowler, 1996; Al-Ani, 2004). Physiologically, this desert dweller has so many features that enable them to survive and work for about fourteen to sixteen hours per day in their respective environment. The body temperature of camels can fluctuate from 35–39°C so as to acclimatize them with the environmental temperature. Generally, it will be lowest in the morning hours and highest in afternoon; and hence, a high temperature in early hours can be an indicative of fever (Tefera, 2004). Also, the stored fat in hump provides metabolic water during scarce periods. Regarding the reproductive performances, the bull camel attains puberty at five years with a reproductive span of ten years, while the female reaches puberty at four years of age. The age at first calving is five years, calving interval is two years, lactation period is one year, and the reproductive span may go up to fifteen years in females. The average milk yield of camel is recorded around 2.5 L per day, and the price of camel's milk is higher than that of cow's milk. Further, the adult camels may weigh about 500 kg with a dressing percentage of 52%.

It has been identified that the economics of camel rearing could be negatively affected by various disease conditions (Brown, 2004). The economic losses due to some diseases are immense as camels play a major role in providing most of the needs of people dwelling in arid regions of the globe (Mochabo et al., 2005). The diseases most commonly encountered are camel pox, contagious pustular dermatitis, trypanosomiasis, dermatomycosis, and mange mite or tick infestation (Tefera and Gebreah, 2001; Mochabo et al., 2006). These diseases incur losses in the form of low production of milk, meat and fat, low-quality hides, and general sale-based depreciation of animals. Also, losses due to infertility and cost of treatment are encountered.

Even though camels have been once considered resistant to most of the pathogens affecting livestock, now it is understood that they might also be susceptible, especially against certain pathogenic agents. In a much recent study conducted in Sudan, it has been shown that generally mange was the most prevalent disease (31.36%), followed by helminthiases (23.24%), wounds and abscesses (8.44%), night blindness (7.53%), dermatomycoses (5.82%), pneumonia and cough (4.39%), mastitis (4.21%), and lameness (2.56%). Also other diseases like calf diarrhea, contagious ecthyma, trypanosomiasis, poxvirus infection, and papillomatosis have been observed (Agab and Abbas, 1999; Agab and Abbas, 2001). This was further confirmed during a cross-sectional study conducted in camels of Morocco and Kenya (Bengoumi et al., 2000; Chemuliti et al., 2003). Recently, Sena et al. (2006) has reported that neonatal care of calves up to three months of age can reduce the incidences of such diseases and thereby can reduce mortality to significant levels.

Regarding the etiological agents, pneumonia, mastitis, and calf diarrhea are the most common infections caused by bacterial pathogens. Likewise, camel pox, contagious echthyma, papillomatosis, and rabies are the most common viral diseases in camels (McGrane and Higgins, 1985; Al-Ani and Chauhan, 2004). However, rinderpest, bluetongue, African horse sickness, and Rift Valley fever has been demonstrated to exist by serological methods (Abbas and Omer, 2005). Serological evidence of exposure to other viral agents, including parainfluenza, bovine respiratory syncytial virus, bovine herpesvirus I, bovine viral diarrhea, and influenza A, have also been identified but without any associated clinical disease (Thedford and Johnson, 1989). Generally, such viral pathogens damage host cells by invading them and replicating using the host cellular machinery (Al-Ani and Chauhan, 2004). The viral proteins present on the surface can bind to host receptors situated at major entry ports like respiratory or digestive systems, and the absence or the presence of such receptors will determine the viral tropism. After entry, the viruses cause harmful effects to the host cells in a number of ways, viz, inhibition of the synthesis of cellular DNA or RNA, damage to the integrity of cellular functions, and by lyses of host cells after replication.

Further, when compared to bacterial diseases, viral diseases are considered more important due to the fact that such agents cannot be kept under control by common therapeutic measures. Only vaccination, with live or inactivated vaccines, is a feasible option. Moreover, some of the viral agents of camels may also get disseminated to the human population in the form of zoonotic infections (Abbas et al., 1987; Murphy et al., 1999). Studies have indicated that some viral diseases like Crimean-Congo hemorrhagic fever (CCHF) and Rift Valley fever (RVF) are circulating in camels, and these diseases can pose potential zoonotic risks (Mariner et al., 1995). Apart from these, the orthopoxviruses that cause camel pox infection can be pathogenic for humans (Mayr, 2003; Panning et al., 2004). Three genera of *Poxviridae* are known to cause human zoonoses: orthopoxviruses, parapoxviruses, and Yata poxvirus (Murphy et al., 1999). But most cases are occupational, sporadic, and have few cutaneous lesions with low morbidity, except the monkey poxvirus (Lewis-Jones, 2004). Further, the camel poxvirus is the closely related to variola virus, the cause of smallpox (Gubser and Smith, 2002). Bioterrorist attacks with poxviruses occupy a special place among the innumerable potential types of unleashing terror. Stocks of camel poxvirus, which is very similar to smallpox virus and was intended for biological warfare, were discovered during the Gulf War in 1991. Besides, the reemergence of camel pox is a real danger among camelids, and contingency planning is needed to define prophylactic and therapeutic strategies to prevent economically devastating epidemics (Georges and Georges-Courbot, 1999).

Considering all these facts, a proper knowledge of individual viral diseases is crucial for the maintenance of a healthy camel herd and human population as well. Also, considerable improvement in disease surveillance and control measures followed by effective management programs has to be implemented by the veterinary health care officials so as to reduce the prevalence as well as the consequences of such diseases, and this could finally pave way for improving the productivity of these desert dwellers in the years to come.

1. Camel Pox

Introduction

Camel pox is an economically important and contagious viral disease of camels. The disease, with low mortality and a high morbidity, caused by orthopoxviruses, is characterized by the presence of pock lesions in skin and the affected animals showing weakness, fever, and anorexia (Chauhan and Kaushik, 1987; Chauhan, 1995; Chauhan and Mahipal, 1995; Chandra et al., 1998; Al-Ani and Chauhan, 2004). The orthopoxviruses belong to the subfamily Chordopoxvirinae and family Poxviridae, and the important viruses in this family are camel poxvirus (*Orthopoxvirus*) and orf (contagious ecthyma) virus (*Parapoxvirus*) (McGrane and Higgins, 1985; Mattson, 1994; Al-Ani and Chauhan, 2004). The etiological agent camel poxvirus (CPV) are ovoid or brick-shaped and measure 260–280 nm, have the ability to remain intact within the dried scabs, and be infectious for long periods (Rosliakov, 1972; Al-Ani and Chauhan, 2004).

Etiology

The camel poxviruses have a genome consisting of a single molecule of linear double-stranded DNA, and it is has the status of a separate species within the Poxiviridae family (Afonso et al., 2002). The 205 kbp genome has 211 putative genes and consists of a central region bound by identical inverted terminal repeats of approximately 7 kb. Also, the viral genome has inverted terminal repeats (ITRs) of 6045 bp and has 206 predicted open reading frames (ORFs). The central region of the genome has genes that are highly conserved. In contrast, genes toward either terminus are more variable and encode proteins involved in host range, virulence, or immunomodulation (Gubser and Smith, 2002). A high degree of similarity in gene order, gene content, and amino acid composition indicates a close structural and functional relationship between CPV and other known orthopoxviruses (OPVs). Notably, CPV contains a unique region of approximately 3 kb, which encodes three orfs that are absent in other OPVs. Among OPVs, CMLV is the most closely related to variola virus (VARV), sharing all genes involved in basic replicative functions and other host-related functions. However, the genome structure and phylogenetic analysis of DNA sequences for all the orfs indicate that CPV is clearly distinct from variola virus and vaccinia viruses and hence demands a separate status (Afonso et al., 2002).

The physicochemical attributes of CPV have been identified, and it has been reported that they are often sensitive to chloroform but resistant to ether and can be easily be destroyed by 0.5–2.5% sodium hydroxide, 0.5–2.5% sulfuric acid, 2.0% calcium hypochlorite, or 5.0% potassium permanganate within a few minutes (Falluji et al., 1979; Al-Ani and Chauhan, 2004). Usually, the CPVs do not agglutinate red blood cells but do for some strains that agglutinate chicken RBCs at low virus titers. Further, the CPVs can be grown in cell lines like HeLa, MA104, HK-21, and Vero cells, with characteristic cytopathic effects, including rounding of cells, syncytia formation, and presence of intracytoplasmic inclusions or in chorioallantoic membrane (CAM) of embryonated chicken eggs (Al-Ani and Chauhan, 2004). Nguyen et al. (1989) reported that the VD47 viral strain of CPV in Niger had the following characteristic properties: heat sensitive, ether resistant, chloroform and induced formation of syncytia, and retracted cell foci with hemadsorption test positive. Later, Renner-Muller et al. (1995) studied CPV isolates from different geographic regions of Africa and Asia in order to identify their biological and genomic attributes. The behavior of the isolates in various cell cultures and the type of pock lesions on the chorioallantoic membrane of embryonated chicken eggs were examined for biologic characterization (Renner-Muller et al., 1995).

EPIDEMIOLOGY

The camel poxvirus is known to spread by either direct contact or by indirect means. The indirect mode of infection is obtained through contaminated feed, pastures, and fomites (Al-Ani and Chauhan, 2004). Also, poxviruses are infamous for affecting novel host species and between populations of the same species (Regnery, 2007). The host range of poxviruses varies from extremely narrow to exceedingly broad, and they have been shown to enter the host by either respiratory or cutaneous route.

The pox infection in camels has been widely reported from different parts of the world especially in countries like India, Pakistan, Afghanistan, Turkmenistan, Russia, Iran, Iraq, Niger, Kenya, Egypt, Somalia, Sudan, Saudi Arabia, UAE, Burkina Faso, and Morocco (Tantawi et al., 1974; Falluji et al., 1979; Kriz, 1982; Davies et al., 1985a; Chauhan et al., 1986; Chauhan and Kaushik, 1987; Pfeffer et al., 1996; Gitao, 1997; Abu Elzein et al., 1999; Agab and Abbas, 2001; Chemuliti et al., 2003). The disease, which is considered notifiable in countries like Iran, Oman, Burkina Faso, and Russia, can infect only camels and not other livestock, and majority of the CPV strains are reported to be highly pathogenic (Al-Ani and Chauhan, 2004). In some cases, human beings may get camel pox infection, especially while consuming milk, and this can give rise to the development of ulcers on the lips and mouth. Also, during one study, it was observed that the camels inoculated with smallpox virus have been found to resist a severe challenge with camel poxvirus, suggesting a close relationship between these two viruses as described earlier (Baxby et al., 1975).

In camels, the pox infection can occur as both benign and malignant forms (Munz, 1992; Khanna et al., 1996). The outbreaks often appear and occur to be related to the stress of weaning in young ones and in adults; it might be due to the stress of long-distance travel (Gitao, 1997). The infection may generally occur in young animals at an age of about three years. However, a devastating outbreak of camel pox has been documented in India that affected a group of camels between twelve to eighteen years of age. But mostly the morbidity and mortality rates of CPV infection are recorded as less than 10 and 1%, respectively (Al-Ani and Chauhan, 2004). However, in another pox outbreak that occurred in Turkmenistan, 30% mortality has been recorded. Also, many outbreaks have been recorded in United Arab Emirates during 1995 and 1996, which resulted in camels showing severe generalized lesions and mortality (Wernery, 1995; Wernery and Kaaden, 1995) Even though the mortality rate is usually low, when compared to morbidity, if the infected animals get exposed to wet conditions, it can lead to abscess and septicemia, and this may ultimately result in the death of the animals.

PATHOGENESIS

The poxviruses have an affinity for the epithelial layer of skin and cause hyperplasia of the stratum spinosum layer of epidermis. Poxvirus tropism at the cellular level seems to be regulated by intracellular events downstream of virus binding and entry rather than at the level of host receptors as in the case seen with many other viruses (McFadden, 2005). The prolific multiplication in the predilection site results in the formation of papules or nodular eruptions on the skin. This is followed by hydropic degeneration of the hyperplastic cells that generate vesicles, which are later converted into pustules (Al-Ani and Chauhan, 2004). These pustules get dried to form scabs and are shed within a period of two weeks from the initiation of infection. As the infection starts, viremia can also occur, manifested as fever in infected camels. Generally, the disease runs a course of one to three weeks, but instances have been presented when it went for up to a period of two months; but this depended on the severity of the infection.

The severity of infection in camels vary dramatically, causing anywhere from a local, self-limiting infection to a devastating disease, like smallpox. Although the immune response to poxvirus infections are very similar to that seen in other viral infections, the poxviruses, unlike most other viruses, have been shown to carry a repertoire of proteins involved in immune evasion and immune modulation. Poxviruses encode proteins involved in blocking many of the strategies employed by the host to combat viral infections; they encode for proteins that block activity of many chemokines, cytokines, serine proteases, and even the complement system (Smith and Kotwal, 2002). Camel poxvirus gene 176R encodes a protein with sequence similarity to murine schlafen (m-slfn) proteins. In vivo, short and long members of the m-slfn family inhibited T-cell development, and thus v-slfn should be considered as a CPV virulence factor that have negative influence on the host immune responses (Gubser et al., 2007).

CLINICAL SIGNS

The incubation period of pox infection in camels is about three to fifteen days. Clinical manifestations like fever, anorexia, restlessness, weakness, nasal discharge, lacrimation, a tendency to drool saliva, and characteristic pock lesions are observed. In lips, there can be diffuse edema and pock lesions; and on the skin surface, there may be present different stages of lesions like papule, vesicle, pustules, and diffuse edema (Chauhan and Mahipal, 1995; Al-Ani and Chauhan, 2004). As a result of itching sensation, the animal may rub their lips against other body parts or against any hard objects, leading to rupture of intact lesions that may lead to secondary bacterial infections. In some cases, there can be enlargement of mandibular lymph nodes or presence of neck edema. Depending on the disease severity, abortions, orchitis, and mortality in young camels may also be observed. During the recovery stages, the animals may be debilitated and lose the strength and work efficiency to a considerable extent.

Clinically, distinct types of infection can be experienced, namely, (1) the severe generalized form, which appears more frequently among young animals; and (2) the milder localized form encountered more often in older camels (Jezek et al., 1983). They also suggested that higher incidence of illness and a twice-higher case fatality rate were observed among male camels. In Kenya (1992), camel pox has been detected in 1,100 camels in two principal camel-rearing regions, and in all the cases, there was 100% morbidity in the affected herds. When young camels were involved, the main lesions were confined to the mouth, nose, and muzzle as distinct pustular lesions. In adults, there was also extensive edema of the head and neck (Gitao, 1997). Highly virulent camel poxvirus strains have been isolated from the lungs of camels in Saudi Arabia and the experimentally infected camels developed severe generalized pox (Wernery and Zachariah, 1999). In another study on the outbreak of camel pox in Syria, the clinical symptoms started with fever, salivation, and general exanthema. The main features were edema of face and legs, pustules on the mucosa of the lips, and a high rate of abortion (Al-Zi'abi et al., 2007).

Also, a slow-spreading and mild form of camel pox has been observed in Saudi Arabia, which caused only a morbidity rate of 10% without any mortality (Alhendi et al., 1994). An eruptive moderate form of camel pox infection has also been reported in camels aged three to four years from Saudi Arabia. The clinical signs were moderate (between mild and severe form), and the morbidity rate was 100% while there was no fatality (Abu Elzein et al., 1999).

GROSS LESIONS AND HISTOPATHOLOGY
The lesions of pox in camels are observed as papular eruptions that later become vesicles, pustules, and crusts. Lesions are commonly observed on lips, nose, oral and nasal cavity, eyelids, flexor surface of legs, scrotum, udder, and vagina (Al-Ani and Chauhan, 2004). Presence of vesicle, which later rupture to form bleeding ulcers, is the early lesion in oral cavity. In nasal cavity, the mucosa may present inflammation and membranous plaques as well. In rare occasions, ocular lesions are also observed, which may lead to opacity of cornea. However, during disease severity, the pock lesions could be seen in trachea, esophagus, and even in the lungs. Mild local exanthemas and generalized poxlike lesions were observed in a dromedary camel herd in Giza, Egypt. Skin lesions including scabs and crusty materials were observed in nose, upper and lower lips, upper and lower parts of the neck, and the external sides of the hind limbs of affected two-to three-year-old camels (Gabry, 2003). Histologically, the lesions include hydropic degeneration of epidermal cells, necrosis of cells of stratum spinosum, together with the infiltration of polymorphonuclear cells and lymphocytes (Alhendi et al., 1994; Al-Ani and Chauhan, 2004). In such cells, intracytoplasmic inclusion bodies can also be seen. Histopathological lesions in the lungs consist of small, sometimes confluent foci of proliferated bronchial epithelium, necrosis and fibrosis, and infiltration of macrophages; the immunohistochemical examination showed numerous poxvirus-antigen-positive cells in the bronchial epithelium (Kinne et al., 1998).

DIAGNOSIS
Camel pox can be diagnosed by observing the clinical signs and lesions present on skin or on mucous membrane. Even though the detection of camel pox is relatively easier when compared to other diseases, differential diagnosis has to be performed accurately because mycotic dermatitis, necrobacillosis, and mange may show similar lesions, and the infection has also to be differentiated from viral diseases like foot-and-mouth disease (FMD) and contagious ecthyma (Al-Ani and Chauhan, 2004). The CPV infection can be confirmed by observing the virus in scabs collected from the infected animal, using electron microscopy (el Harrak et al., 1991; Gitao, 1997). Also, the virus can be isolated using cell lines or by growing it on chorioallantoic membrane (CAM) of embryonated chicken eggs (Ramyar and

Hessami, 1972; Davies et al., 1975; el Harrak et al., 1991; Gitao, 1997; Gabry, 2003; Al-Ani and Chauhan, 2004). While infecting a nine-to eleven-day-old embryo, after few days, there can be seen numerous round and raised white pock lesions on the CAM. The CPV strains often produce pock lesions localized on infected area of CAM, without generalized lesions or death of embryos (Tantawi et al., 1978). The CPV can also be isolated using Vero cell cultures, using the highest positive dilutions (Baky et al., 2006b).

Besides, serological detection methods like agar gel precipitation test (AGPT) and enzyme-linked immunosorbent assay (ELISA) can demonstrate the antigen or antibodies (Munz et al., 1986a; Gabry, 2003; Al-Ani and Chauhan, 2004). An ELISA can be developed for the detection of total and IgG and IgM antibodies to camel poxvirus, with the ability to differentiate between orthopox and parapoxvirus infections in camels. Hence, it is considered that the ELISA technique is justified for serodiagnosis of camel pox (Azwai et al., 1996). Other than for detection, ELISA can also be used for the quantification of camel poxviruses (Pfahler et al., 1986). Likewise, serum samples can also be tested by serum-neutralization test (SNT) for detection of specific neutralizing and precipitating antibodies of CPV (Gabry, 2003). Similarly, CPV in skin scrapings of camels can be detected using indirect fluorescent antibody (IFA) test (Baky et al., 2006b).

During recent years, the detection of pox infection has been performed using molecular detection tools, which identify CPV viral genes. Molecular detection and characterization using polymerase chain reaction (PCR) and other subsequent techniques like gene sequencing provides accurate phylogenetic identification of various CPV isolates (Lewis-Jones, 2004; Al-Zi'abi et al., 2007). Rapid identification and differentiation of orthopoxviruses can be achieved with primers based on gene sequences encoding the hemagglutinin (HA) protein. For this, PCR conditions were developed on the basis of base sequence differences within the HA genes of ten species of orthopoxviruses, which enabled production of a single DNA fragment of different size that indicated the specific species (Ropp et al., 1995). Similarly, orthopoxvirus species can be detected and differentiated by PCR amplification of acidophilic-type inclusion body (ATI) gene; the amplicons ranging in size from 500 to 1,600 base pairs depending on the species (Meyer et al., 1997). Based on these observations, PCR has been considered a powerful tool to detect and differentiate orthopoxviruses, and real-time PCR has further brought in advantages like rapid turn around time, low risk of contamination, capability of strain differentiation, and use of multiplexing (Panning et al., 2004; Scaramozzino et al., 2007). Also, nested PCR has been developed that have a direct bearing on the specificity of the

PCR technique (Sanchez-Seco et al., 2006). Likewise, a differential diagnosis of various orthopoxviruses (OPV) can be made feasible in a one-stage rapid identification method using the properties of multiplex polymerase chain reaction (m-PCR). In m-PCR, different pairs of oligonucleotide primers representing DNA of different species of OPVs are used concurrently for assaying (Shchelkunov et al., 2005).

Aside from detection, characterization of poxviruses have been exhaustively performed using restriction endonuclease (RE) analysis of genomic DNA fragments. Specific endonucleases have the ability to digest DNA to generate electropherograms with different digestion patterns, and this enables differentiation of various orthopoxviruses (Loparev et al., 2001). Esposito and Knight (1985) have reported that the RE *Hind* III can cleave the DNA of various OPVs to generate a meaningful differentiation. They also suggested the use of other enzymes like *Sma* I, *Bgl* I, *Sac* I, *Kpn* I, *Xho* I, and *Sal* I to provide a basis for discerning species, strains, and variants. Similarly, *Rsa* I and *Taq* I are also capable in differentiating various orthopoxviruses. (Ropp et al., 1995). Renner-Muller et al. (1995) has additionally, created maps with REs like *Hind* III and *Xho* I were established. The data obtained from DNA analyses demonstrated minor differences between the five isolates and confirm previous reports suggesting that orthopoxviruses of camels constitute a separate species within the genus *Orthopoxvirus* (Renner-Muller et al., 1995). Further, the RE analysis can characterize various isolates of CPVs (Kinne et al., 1998). Their DNA patterns were virtually identical, displaying only slight variations in the terminal fragments, and such analysis could also differentiate the vaccine strains from the field strains (Pfeffer et al., 1996). Also, comparison of physical maps established for enzymes *Hind* III and *Xho* I revealed deletions accounting for a total of 22 kbp in attenuated strains of CPV (Otterbein et al., 1996). Later, a restriction fragment length polymorphism (RFLP) assay has been developed to identify and differentiate the orthopoxviruses from CPVs. The assay used amplicons of cytokine response modifier B (crmB) gene of forty-three different OPV strains (Loparev et al., 2001). Aside from RE-based characterization, hybridization probe pair with a specific sensor probe that allows reliable differentiation of orthopoxviruses has also been developed (Olson et al., 2004).

Currently, species-specific detection of orthopoxviruses is done using microarrays, which hybridizes a fluorescent-labeled amplified DNA specimen with the oligonucleotide DNA probes immobilized on a microchip. The probes identified species-specific sites within the crmB gene encoding the viral analogue of tumor necrosis factor receptor, and the whole procedure took about six hours (Lapa et al., 2002). Likewise, another oligonucleotide microarray has been developed for the detection and differentiation of OPVs (Riabinin et al., 2006). Genus-specific and orthopoxvirus-species-specific regions of the genes encoding chemokine-binding and alpha/beta-interferon–binding proteins were used as a target, and this microarray allowed the differentiation of variola, monkey pox, cow pox, vaccinia, and camel poxviruses, with a high degree of reliability. Thus, microarray method can perform as a valuable tool for accurate detection and differentiation of camel pox viruses from other orthopoxviruses.

Treatment, Prevention, and Control

During the progress of infection, antibiotic application to the skin surface is desirable in order to prevent secondary bacterial complications and favor a speedy recovery (Al-Ani and Chauhan, 2004). Supportive therapy with vitamins and minerals may help improve healing of lesions in a rapid manner. Fluid therapy is recommended when the infected camels are anorectic or anorexic due to the severity of infection. Therapeutic agents, particularly nucleoside propionate such as cidofovir, have action against poxviruses (Lewis-Jones, 2004). However, cidofovir-resistant forms of camel poxvirus have been observed during prolonged passage of the virus in Vero cells in the presence of drug (Smee et al., 2002). The latest antipoxvirus drugs like kinase inhibitors are known to block or egress (exit) of poxviruses from infected cells (Sliva and Schnierle, 2007).

For control of camel pox, isolation of infected camels and quarantine of contacts are found highly effective (Al-Ani and Chauhan, 2004). Further, cleaning and disinfecting of premises and decontamination of materials can effectively check the spread of disease. For preventive purposes, live or inactivated camel poxvirus vaccine can be employed, and camels aged six months or older should be vaccinated annually. A Saudi isolate of CPV, serially propagated on monolayers of camel kidney cell culture, have been attenuated by the seventy-eighth passage; this live vaccine was tested in two susceptible camels, and the inoculated camels showed no postchallenge clinical symptoms and formed neutralizing antibodies against camel poxvirus. These results indicated the safety and potency of the seventy-eighth passage of the Saudi isolate of CPV can be used for production of live attenuated cell culture camel pox vaccine, using at least 10^3 TCID$_{50}$ as a recommended field dose (Hafez et al., 1992). Similarly, the safety and immunogenicity of the attenuated live CPV strain has been tested in Mauritania, and it has been reported that a dose of $10^{3.7}$ TCID$_{50}$ could be useful in preventing the infection in herds (Nguyen et al., 1996). Also, the efficacies of two commercially available camel pox vaccines (live and inactivated one) produced in South Africa were assessed. Camels vaccinated with both vaccines and later challenged with a virulent CPV showed no clinical signs of disease or pox lesions. Based on serum-neutralization and passive hemagglutination tests, humoral antibody response started on the second week after vaccination for both vaccines; a booster dose increased antibody titers significantly (Khalafalla and El-Dirdiri, 2003). Recently, attention has been shifted to make available laboratory animals like rabbits and guinea pigs in order to replace camels for evaluating the immunogenicity of tissue culture vaccines against camel poxvirus (Baky et al., 2006a).

Further, the camel poxvirus nonessential thymidine kinase (TK) gene can be removed for developing vaccine vector that could insert genes from other camel viruses to generate bivalent vaccines. Binns et al. (1992) has suggested the utility of TK-negative camel poxvirus as a vaccine vector for the expression of genes from other pathogens of camel. Besides, poxviruses have potential in cancer immunotherapy, and their ability to evade host-cell immune responses may provide a basis for new antipoxvirus therapies (Lewis-Jones, 2004).

2. CAMEL CONTAGIOUS PUSTULAR DERMATITIS

INTRODUCTION

Contagious pustular dermatitis (orf) is a viral disease affecting mainly sheep and goats, and it can occasionally affect camelids too. The disease, which is also known as contagious ecthyma, scabby mouth, or sore mouth, is characterized by pustule formation on the lips, gums, and tongue (Hartung, 1980; Al-Ani and Chauhan, 2004).

ETIOLOGY

Orf virus, belonging to the genus *Parapoxvirus* and family Poxviridae, is the etiological agent of contagious pustular dermatitis of camels. It was Dashtseren et al. (1984) who initially observed pustular dermatitis caused among camels in Mongolia. The orf virus can infect llamas and alpacas too. Mortality among camel calves should be considered as a serious problem faced by camel herdsmen, and although there are several reasons for mortality, outbreaks of contagious ecthyma in camels in Kenya gave clear indication of specific involvement of the disease with calf mortality (Gitao, 1994). However, contagious ecthyma may resolve spontaneously, and the mortality rate could be generally low, but fatality rates of 10% have been reported (Al-Ani and Chauhan, 2004). Deaths may be due to the result of complications from secondary infections, and the morbidity rate as high as 80% could be experienced in unvaccinated herds. Also, when dealing with infected animals, it is important to realize that contagious ecthyma can be passed to humans. Orf virus can infect man through direct contact with infected fomites. In man, signs are first seen three to seven days after handling diseased animals. It appears as ulcerative lesions on the fingers, limbs, or face of the affected person. If the lesions are not infected, they will heal in two to four weeks and leave no scars.

EPIDEMIOLOGY

The orf virus, which is found in skin lesions and scabs, is thought to enter the skin through cuts and abrasions. Clinically, normal sheep as well as sick animals can carry the virus. It can be transmitted by direct contact or via fomites. Concurrent outbreaks of contagious pustular dermatitis have also been reported in goat kids housed with camels (Khalafalla et al., 1994). The orf virus remains viable on the wool and hides for approximately one month after the lesions have healed, and the virus is considered to be highly resistant to inactivation in the environment and has been recovered from dried crusts even after twelve years (Al-Ani and Chauhan, 2004).

The disease has been reported in various camel-rearing countries such as Mongolia, Kenya, Somalia, Sudan, and Saudi Arabia (Dashtseren et al., 1984; Gitao, 1994; Moallin and Zessin, 1988). It is highly contagious and affects mainly young camels, producing lesions on the mouth and nostrils (Khalafalla and Mohamed, 1997). However, these lesions may spread to other parts of body also. The recovered animals do not contract the disease again, which indicates lifelong immunity. The orf virus can be transmitted directly through contact with the scab lesions or indirectly by skin wounds. Other fomites—including contaminated tools, cloth, and herd attendants—are also responsible for spread of the virus. In camels, the morbidity rate is about 60–100% while the mortality rate is 5–20%. Calves may die due to the inability to graze or suckle their dam.

PATHOGENESIS

The virus infects the skin of the mouth and replicates in the epidermal epithelium in the wall of the follicles. The infection can then spread laterally throughout the depth of epidermis and form nodular lesions on lips (Al-Ani and Chauhan, 2004). The tissue-level responses could be necrosis that is followed by sloughing of the affected epidermis. Later, pustules are developed, and exudation occurs to form crusts. The mucous membrane of the oral cavity is also affected with hemorrhages and ulcerations.

CLINICAL SIGNS

Within two to three days of contact with the orf virus, the first signs of the disease can be seen. By eleventh day, scabs are evident, which may stay for a couple of weeks. The morbidity in adults ranged from 10–80%, and it reached 100% in young camels of one year or below (Dashtseren et al., 1984). Morbid calves were unable to suckle properly and got debilitated, eventually leading to high calf mortality (Gitao, 1994). The clinical features of the contagious ecthyma in camel calves in the Sudan were investigated. The animals were anorectic, emaciated, and slightly anemic (Ali et al., 1991). Even though the disease is generally mild and self-limiting, in some cases the clinical signs can be severe. Localized lesions at the commissures of the mouth and nostrils are characteristic of the disease; however, generalized lesions have been observed. Further, the acute form of the disease features swelling of the head with proliferative nodular lesions around lips that occasionally extends into the mucosa of the mouth and nostrils (Al-Ani and Chauhan, 2004). The lesions soon convert into pustules and fissured crusts. Papules develop to pustules and become encrusted. In young camels, lesions may be generalized and occur all over the body, in particular on the distal area of the leg, inner thighs, and the vagina. Superficial lymph nodes can also become enlarged in young animals.

LESIONS

In the beginning, pustules developed around the mouth followed by papular elevations and scab formation (Dashtseren et al., 1984). The skin lesions are painful and often occur on the mouth and muzzle. Lesions on the udder may result in the abandonment of offspring, and foot lesions can cause transient lameness. Secondary bacterial infections can occur, and in rare cases, the lesions may extend into the internal organs. Secondary infection of the pustules could be commonly seen in affected calves. In calves, the principal lesions were distinct or largely coalesced pustules on the mouth, nose, and muzzle (Gitao, 1994). Enlargement of superficial parotid, submaxillary, and cervical lymph nodes have been reported due to ecthyma virus. The oral mucosa may become hemorrhagic and ulcerated (Ali et al., 1991). On histopathology, ballooning degeneration of keratinocytes and eosinophilic cytoplasmic inclusions are seen, and there could be vacuolar changes in the epithelial layers (Al-Ani and Chauhan, 2004).

DIAGNOSIS

Clinical signs and lesions present on mouth and nostrils can assist in making a diagnosis in young camels. The typical parapoxvirus particles are diagnosed in scabs, using electron microscopy (EM). EM-based diagnosis of contagious ecthyma virus has been performed by many workers (Munz et al., 1986b; Gitao, 1994). Direct EM of infected scabs or negative contrast EM has proven to be an extremely useful procedure for quick differential diagnosis (Ali et al., 1991; Gitao, 1994). Also, there are reports of isolation of camel ecthyma virus on the chorioallantoic membrane (CAM) of embryonated eggs or on tissue cultures. However, no cytopathic effect has been observed after passages in Vero cell culture (Many et al., 1986). But the virus grows well on the chorioallantoic membrane (CAM) of eleven-day-old chick embryos (Dashtseren et al., 1984).

Serological tests are available for detection of contagious ecthyma (orf) in camels. An enzyme-linked immunosorbent assay (ELISA) is available for the detection of specific IgG and IgM antibodies to the contagious ecthyma virus in camel sera and for identifying the seroreactive viral antigens (Al-Ani and Chauhan, 2004). Two viral antigenic determinants (22 and 40 kDa) were shared by the Western blotting patterns of all the positive camel sera tested, and another viral antigenic component of 28 kDa was shared by the positive sera with high ELISA titers (Azwai et al., 1995).

Molecular detection based on PCR and characterization and phylogenetic analysis based on sequencing of the genes have been performed for contagious ecthyma. Nucleotide sequence of DNA extracted from pustules, saliva, and blood of camels presented with contagious ecthyma in Bahrain and also from a sample of infected tissue from a camel that had presented with contagious ecthyma in 1998 in Saudi Arabia. Sequence and phylogenetic analysis enabled the differentiation of orf viruses from closely related viruses like the pseudocowpox virus (PCPV), which infects sheep, goats, and other animal species (Abubakr et al., 2007). Further, the contagious ecthyma in camels should be differentiated from camel pox, mange, and mycotic infections.

TREATMENT, PREVENTION, AND CONTROL

Application of antiseptic solutions on the affected areas is recommended so that it may help in the control of secondary bacterial infections. For an effective control, isolation of infected animals should be done in order to prevent the disease spread (Al-Ani and Chauhan, 2004). Cleaning and disinfecting all contaminated materials related to the infected animals has to be practiced. The orf virus is considered as a very difficult customer to eradicate once it has entered a flock or herd. So to prevent an entry, fresh stock of animals should be quarantined, and tests should be performed to identify carriers. Also, the practice of rearing sheep and goats together with camels has to be discouraged. Regarding preventive measures, vaccination has been practiced in some regions of the world. Vaccines often contain live virus prepared from dried scabs, or it may be based on viruses propagated in tissue culture systems. The vaccines that are available for sheep and goats can also be used safely for camels. But vaccines should be used only on premises where infection have earlier occurred, and recently vaccinated animals should be isolated from unvaccinated herd. However, even after vaccination, outbreaks have occurred in vaccinated animals, which might be due to the emergence of more virulent strain (Dashtseren et al., 1984). Recently, efforts are being made to develop a bivalent recombinant vaccine with camel poxvirus as a vector to control contagious ecthyma and pox, simultaneously (Al-Ani and Chauhan, 2004).

3. CAMEL PAPILLOMATOSIS

INTRODUCTION

Papillomavirus in the family Papovaviridae is the cause of papilloma (warts) in different animal species (Lancaster and Olson, 1982). Many domestic and wild species of mammals can be infected by one or more species-specific papillomaviruses (Sundberg et al., 2000). They cause a variety of tumors in mucosal and cutaneous epithelium (Nicholls and Stanley, 2000). Infectious papillomatosis are contagious in the animals in which they naturally occur. Moreover, certain papillomavirus types have been found associated with lesions capable of malignant conversion in response to secondary physical or chemical factors (Smith and Campo, 1985). Papillomatosis in camels is characterized by the presence of warts or nodules on the head, neck, shoulder, and udder.

ETIOLOGY

The papillomaviruses represent genus A of the family Papovaviridae, while the polyoma viruses constitute genus B. It is a DNA virus, which is ether resistant, acid and heat stable, and having high host specificity. Papillomaviruses are naked icosahedral capsids of approximately 50 nm in diameter. They have a buoyant density of 1.34 g/ml in CsCl. The papillomavirus genome is a covalently closed circular DNA molecule with molecular weight of 4.5×10^6 Da. Ten polypeptides have been resolved by dodecyl sulfate polyacrylamide gel electrophoresis. The major structural polypeptides have molecular weights in the range of 50–kDa (Lancaster and Olson, 1982).

EPIDEMIOLOGY

Transmission of virus occurs through contact, and the virus enters through the abraded skin of animals. The disease may occur in any-age camel, but the young are more susceptible. Outbreaks of papillomatosis are mainly observed during the rainy season. During the progress of infection, the morbidity rate is more, and mortality rate is low, and high morbidity may be seen in camel calves of less than one year of age. If once recovered, subsequent infection may not occur. The disease has been reported in camels from Somalia, India, UAE, and Jordan (Munz et al., 1990). Till date, there are no reports available on the zoonotic potential of camel papillomaviruses.

PATHOGENESIS

Papillomaviruses (PVs) are highly species-specific and site-specific pathogens. Tumorigenesis due to papillomavirus (PV) infection was first demonstrated in rabbits and cattle (Campo, 2002). The virus targets only the stratified squamous epithelium. Initially, the virus enters through abraded skin, and due to its affinity, it harbors on the stratum spinosum of the epidermis. The virus then multiplies in epithelial cells, and this will lead to hyperplastic lesions visible as nodular eruptions on skin (Al-Ani and Chauhan, 2004). The nodules are persistent, but often remain benign and controlled. But the infected cells show an increase in the size and number of desmosomes and tonofibrils, whereas other epithelial cells show degenerative changes with loss of tonofibrils, detachment of desmosomes, and cytoplasmic vacuolization. Electron microscopic analysis can reveal virions in a crystalline array in nuclei of degenerated cells in the keratinizing layer. In the granular layer, nuclear degeneration is evident, with margination and condensation of chromatin. Typically, the benign warts undergo spontaneous, immune-mediated regression, most likely effected by T-cells, whereas humoral immunity may prevent new infections (Nicholls and Stanley, 2000).

Induction of papillomas and their neoplastic progression has been experimentally demonstrated, and virus-cofactor interactions have been elucidated, much recently. The oncoprotein E5 has been found to play a major role in contributing to the transformation of cells. E5 activate the growth-factor receptors and numerous kinases and down regulates expression of MHC class I molecules. Thus, it helps in the establishment of viral infection by promoting both cell proliferation and immune evasion (Campo, 2002). Very recently, it has been reported that E6 and E7 proteins can function though a number of direct and indirect interactions with cellular proteins, a number of which are well-known cellular tumor suppressors (Wise-Draper and Wells, 2008).

CLINICAL SIGNS

Appearance of papilloma nodules on head, nose, mouth, udder, scrotum, and neck regions is characteristic of the disease. These lesions may create itching sensation, and the affected animal will rub against hard objects, which may lead to hemorrhages and extensive skin excoriation. Such lesions may cause the camel calves to remain away from their dams or show lack of interest in feed consumption or grazing. Further, the presence of papilloma on eyelids can lead to conjunctivitis due to secondary bacterial infection, with marked edema of the head and swelling of the mandibular and cervical lymph nodes (Al-Ani and Chauhan, 2004). In some cases, cauliflower-like lesions may appear on nostrils and lips, and this can persist for long periods of time before eventually dropping off.

LESIONS

From experimental infectivity studies, the first reaction of the skin has been identified as fibroblastic stimulation, which accompanied inflammatory response with congestion, edema, and leukocyte infiltration (Lancaster and Olson, 1982). Later, the inflammatory reaction subsided, and fibroblastic stimulation continued. The epithelium overlying the area of dermal hyperplasia begins to proliferate and shows acanthosis and hyperkeratosis, which later develop to nodular lesions (Lancaster and Olson, 1982). Presence of nodular papilloma (warts) on skin of mouth, nostrils, udder, neck, head, and legs are considered as the important lesions of this disease. Oral papillomas can be multifocal, small, soft, light pink, oval, slightly raised flat sessile lesions on the ventral lingual surfaces (Sundberg et al., 2000). These lesions are regarded as either hyperplasia or benign neoplasms since they do not metastasize and kill the host. There are hemorrhages if the lesions are rubbed against hard objects. Papilloma lesions, appearing in some instances as cauliflower-like growths, are present on lips and nostrils. However, some of these lesions, particularly those affecting mucosal epithelia, may progress to squamous cell carcinomas.

Microscopic examination reveals hyperplasia of epidermal layers, with little mononuclear cell infiltration, hyperkeratinization, and degenerative changes. Histologically, the areas of epidermal hyperplasia are flat (Sundberg *et al.*, 2000). Thickening of the stratum granulosum with formation of prominent pleomorphic amphophilic granules are evident in many lesions. Within the granular layer, individual cells were swollen, having an abundance of clear cytoplasm around nuclei (koilocytes). Further, the productively infected keratinocytes degenerated into koilocytes. These features are characteristic of the general cytopathic effect of PV infections. Sundberg et al. (2000) also observed that the main difference between the histologic features of cutaneous and mucosal papillomas was the prominence of large inclusion bodies in the cytoplasm of mucosal koilocytes.

DIAGNOSIS
Diagnosis is mainly based on the presence of gross and microscopic lesions present on camel skin. Electron microscopic (EM) investigations revealed typical papillomavirions in skin lesions. EM proves to be a useful tool to differentiate papillomatosis from pox and contagious ecthyma. Biopsy of skin papilloma is always helpful in diagnosis as it reveals hyperplasia, degeneration, and hyperkeratinization. Hence, the histopathological sections showed alterations that could be regarded as pathognomonic for warts. Aside from this, PCR technique that amplifies a selective gene of the whole genome of the virus could also support a definitive diagnosis.

Treatment, Prevention, and Control

Although spontaneous recovery may occur, topical treatment with iodine ointment can reduce the duration of the disease. Maintenance of hygienic conditions on farms and segregation of sick animals are always helpful in containing the disease. Wart vaccines can also be used as an aid in the control of viral papillomas. Such vaccines are formalin-inactivated one that contain virus-laden tissue extracts derived from camel papillomas. A dose of 5 ml injected subcutaneously and a repeated in two to three weeks can serve the purpose.

Many experimental vaccines are being developed against papillomaviruses. In principle, two different types of vaccine are being envisaged: one for the prophylactic purposes that would elicit virus-neutralizing antibodies and the other being therapeutic vaccines that would induce regression of established lesions before progression to malignancy (Campo et al., 1993; Campo and Jarrett, 1994). Vaccination can be achieved with live virus, formalin-inactivated virus, synthetic viruslike particles, and by DNA vaccination. There has been much recent progress in the development of such vaccines for papillomavirus infections in animals (Nicholls and Stanley, 2000). Using recombinant DNA technique, such vaccines can be developed against camel papillomaviruses. Viruslike particles can be produced in insect cells containing either the L1 and L2 capsid proteins of papillomavirus together or the L1 protein alone. This could prove to be an extremely effective prophylactic measure against papilloma infection in camels (Kirnbauer et al., 1996). In another study, it was suggested that prophylactic vaccination with the N terminus (aa 11-200) of the minor capsid protein L2 even could prevent papillomavirus infection (Gaukroger et al., 1996).

Recently, the nonenveloped papillomavirus capsid composed of virally encoded major coat protein, L1, and a minor coat protein L2 are coassembled and, when expressed in mammalian cells, was found to encapsidate any plasmid of <8 kb size. This utility could be exploited for developing papillomavirus-based gene transfer vectors. The resulting vectors have utility for in vitro, as well as in vivo gene delivery applications (Buck and Thompson, 2007).

4. CAMEL RABIES

INTRODUCTION

Rhabdoviridae family consists of single-stranded RNA viruses that are considered as important animal pathogens causing diseases like rabies and vesicular stomatitis. Rabies is an infectious viral disease of all warm-blooded animals caused by genus *Lyssavirus*. The disease is transmitted through bite of a rabid dog/wild animal, and characterized by nervous signs, paralysis, and ends with fatal results.

ETIOLOGY

The *Lyssavirus* of the family Rhabdoviridae is bullet shaped, having a length of 180 nm. It is a neurotropic virus and causes lesions only in nervous tissue. However, they are fragile and are highly susceptible to most disinfectants and are destroyed within a few hours in dried saliva. The strains of rabies virus isolated from naturally occurring cases are referred to as street virus and attenuated laboratory strains are referred to as fixed virus.

EPIDEMIOLOGY

Rabies has a significant position among all viral diseases primarily due to the fatality and also due to its zoonotic significance. The disease is widely prevalent in African and Asian continents. In camels, rabies has been reported from many countries including India, Jordan, Iraq, Iran, Afghanistan, Tunisia, and Niger (Bah et al., 1981; Hameid, 1991; Bloch and Diallo, 1995; Al Qudah et al., 1996; Kumar and Jindal, 1997; Al-Rawashdeh et al., 2000). The most frequent animals responsible for the transmission of rabies to camels are stray dogs and wild carnivores (including wolves, foxes, and hyenas) and the mode of transmission is by bite of such infected animals. As the camels are generally reared in areas where it is difficult to completely eliminate wildlife, the danger of rabies always exist. Rabies is considered a fatal disease as the case fatality rate is 100%. In an outbreak of rabies in Mauritania, eighteen animals died of the infection, and twelve other affected camels were exposed to euthanasia. In Jordan, eight cases of rabies were reported, following a fox attack (Al-Ani et al., 1998; Al-Ani and Chauhan, 2004). Similarly, seven camels in a herd in Niger died within a short period after the exposure, but they have shown manifestations including unusual behavior, aggression, pica, ptyalism, and terminal paralysis; and it was postulated that canine rabies could have been transmitted to the camels in the herd (Bloch and Diallo, 1995).

PATHOGENESIS

When the virus-laden saliva comes in contact with an open wound or abraded skin surface, the virus enters the host and replicates initially in myocytes. After multiplication, they travel to the brain tissue by way of the nervous system and enter the nerve cell at motor end plates and bind to the acetylcholine (neurotransmitter) receptors. Then, the virus travels in axon of the neurons to the ventral horn of the spinal cord at a rate of 3–4 mm/hr and replicates in this location. After replication in spinal cord, it spreads to brain tissue, to salivary glands, the brain stem, cerebral cortex, and hippocampus. In salivary gland, the virus rapidly replicates, and the infected saliva serves as a major source of infection. The lesions are mainly produced in the central nervous system, and death occurs due to respiratory paralysis.

CLINICAL SIGNS

The incubation period of rabies can range from one to several months. The furious form of rabies is more commonly observed rather than the dumb form. In furious form, the affected camels show behavioral changes including viciousness, hyperexcitability, and signs of irritation or agitation that may lead to attacking of inanimate objects, exhibiting pica, and self-infliction of bites on forelimbs (Afzal et al., 1993). Signs may also include drooling of saliva, paralysis of throat, difficulty in swallowing, colic symptoms, recumbency in sternal position, paralysis of the hind legs, followed by fatal results within three to seven days after the initial observation of symptoms.

LESIONS

The gross lesions are often not appreciable. But microscopic lesions are seen that consist of necrosis of neurons along with presence of specific intracytoplasmic inclusion bodies in the affected nerve cells. Also, there can be seen perivascular cuffing and neuronophagia in the brain stem and hippocampus. The presence of Babès' nodules is characteristic, which consists of proliferating glial cells encroaching upon the neurons.

DIAGNOSIS

Determining the history of a bite, observing clinical signs, and visualizing characteristic lesions make a tentative diagnosis of rabies infection. For further confirmation, fluorescent antibody testing (FAT) of brain smears and enzyme-linked immunosorbent assay can be employed (Al-Ani et al., 1998). FAT-based detection of rabies virus has been performed in brain tissues of affected camels by Al-Rawashdeh et al. (2000). Further, the presence of eosinophilic intracytoplasmic inclusion bodies called Negri bodies in brain cells is of considerable diagnostic value.

Treatment, Prevention, and Control

There is no treatment for rabid animals. Since rabies is a highly zoonotic disease, all persons handling such animals must be vaccinated according to the guidelines of the World Health Organization (WHO). Vaccination against rabies is the safest, easiest, and surest protection against the incidence of the disease in camels. Moreover, to control rabies, mass vaccination of stray dogs and immediate elimination of any camel suspected of being rabid is essential. Preexposure vaccination of veterinarians and other personnel at risk has become a standard practice in endemic areas. (Refer to "Rabies in Bovines and Ovines" section of this book for more information).

5. CAMEL RIFT VALLEY FEVER

INTRODUCTION

Rift Valley fever (RVF) is a peracute or acute disease of domestic animals characterized by abortion and death among young animals. The infection is considered to be having zoonotic significance as they cause an influenza-like disease in man. People with RVF typically have either no symptoms or a mild illness associated with fever and liver abnormalities. However, in some cases, it can progress to a hemorrhagic condition or encephalitis in man. Presence of the RVF virus has been reported in camels (Mariner et al., 1995).

ETIOLOGY

Rift Valley fever is caused by *Phlebovirus* belonging to the family Bunyaviridae. It is under arbovirus, and arthropod vectors like mosquitoes, ticks, or flies transmit these viruses.

EPIDEMIOLOGY

It is a fact that RVF, initially occurred in Rift Valley (Kenya), have spread to other regions of the African continent to cause serious disease threats to animals as well as humans. It is an arboviral disease and several species of *Aedes* and *Culex* mosquitoes act as vectors of this virus. The virus commonly infects sheep, goat, buffalo, cattle, camels, and man (Abdo-Salem et al., 2006). It is generally found in regions of Eastern and Southern Africa where sheep and cattle are raised, but the virus also exists in most countries of sub-Saharan Africa (Al-Ani and Chauhan, 2004). The epidemics usually coincide with factors like population density, presence and spread of vectors, and the survival of the virus in infected animals. In Mauritania, significant correlation was found between serological evidence of RVF virus infection and the presence of large expanses of stagnant water, which provide a suitable habitat for the vectors of the disease (Saluzz et al., 1987). Epizootics or serological evidence of RVF infection has been reported from Kenya, Mauritania, Senegal, Sudan, Egypt, Congo, Zambia, Mozambique, Madagascar, Saudi Arabia, and Yemen (Hedger et al., 1980; Abd El-Rahim et al., 1999; Al-Ani and Chauhan, 2004). Within the focus of infection, the antibody prevalence rates were 33% in camels, 16% in goats, 14% in sheep, and 13% in cattle.

CLINICAL SIGNS

In camels, the disease may occur as a subclinical one, but there can be significant increase in abortion and mortality, especially during epizootics. However, clinical signs could not be seen following experimental infection of camels (Al-Ani and Chauhan, 2004). In Egypt, serological surveys have indicated that during outbreaks, the incidence rate of RVF could range from 7–27%. Significant lesions are not commonly observed in RVF infection of camelids.

DIAGNOSIS

Serological tests and isolation of the RVF virus can give a confirmatory diagnosis of the infection. In Vero cell lines, the characteristic cytopathic effects can be observed within forty-eight hours of inoculation of suspension of liver and splenic tissues obtained from infected animals. Serological tests like serum-neutralization test (SNT), hemagglutination-inhibition test (HI), and complement fixation test (CFT) are commonly employed for the diagnosis of RVF in animals. Using SNT, Davies et al. (1985b) has reported that serum-neutralizing antibodies were detected in 22% of camels in a herd. Similarly, employing HI test, Olaleye et al. (1996) has reported the presence of hemagglutination-inhibiting antibodies in camels. Aside from these techniques, fluorescent antibody test (FAT) can also detect the presence of RVF virus in infected tissues or cell cultures. Further, researchers have developed and validated sandwich and capture ELISAs for the detection of IgG and IgM antibodies to Rift Valley fever virus (Paweska et al., 2003a). Also, an indirect ELISA for identifying antibodies against RVF virus has been developed (Paweska et al., 2003b). Based on the experiences, it can be concluded that when compared to SNT and HI test, ELISA is a better option due to their sensitivity in detection as well as the ability for identifying earliest immunological responses. Moreover, the technique is robust and highly accurate and can be employed in disease surveillance and control programs in a most suitable and comprehensive manner (Paweska et al., 2005). Apart from ELISA, the PCR detection of RVF viral genome is another useful option for a specific and sensitive detection.

PREVENTION AND CONTROL

Isolation of the infected herds or individuals has to be strictly practiced. Also, it is not advisable to rear camels along with sheep and cattle, especially in endemic areas. As the mosquitoes play a key role in the spread of infection, strong vector control option has to be followed, employing residual insecticides in pens and barns. Killed and live virus vaccines are available for the prevention of RVF in animals, but all the susceptible animals should be vaccinated, more importantly those dwelling in high-risk zones. However, vaccination as to be carefully performed as abortion of pregnant animals may occur following administration of live vaccines. (For more information refer "Rift Valley Fever" of bovine diseases in this book).

6. CAMEL RINDERPEST

INTRODUCTION
Rinderpest is an acute and highly contagious viral infection of bovines, which is characterized by fever, prostration, fetid diarrhea, and presence of erosions and vesicular eruptions on lips, tongue, and dental pad. The etiological agent, the rinderpest virus, is a member of genus *Morbillivirus* within the Paramyxoviridae family (Scott and Macdonald, 1962; Smith, 1970b; Al-Ani and Chauhan, 2004). It is closely related to the viruses causing peste des petits ruminants in small ruminants, canine distemper in dogs, and measles in human beings.

EPIDEMIOLOGY
Water buffalo and cattle are the most susceptible species to the infection, and the disease is still persisting in some African and Asian countries. Airborne infection occurs in the case of rinderpest, which spreads rapidly by direct contact between sick and healthy animals. It has been reported that the virus is highly fragile and even gets easily destroyed in presence of sunlight (Ismail et al., 1992). It has been postulated that camels can become infected when they are in close proximity with infected bovines. The occurrence of rinderpest in camels has been suggested since earlier days (Haji, 1923; El-Shinnawy et al., 1993). There were also some reports of the disease in early 1960s, which elicited signs and lesions similar to rinderpest. But the experimentally administered rinderpest virus could not produce any clinical disease in camels (Smith, 1970a) even though seroconversion has been reported, and the antibodies against rinderpest virus have been detected in camel sera (Al-Ani and Chauhan, 2004).

PATHOGENESIS
Pathogenesis of rinderpest virus is not well established in camels. However, in other animals, the virus multiplies in tonsils and regional lymph nodes, and viremia can occur, and mononuclear cells containing the virus can spread to other parts of body to produce erosions and vesicles in oral and gastrointestinal mucosa, followed by severe diarrhea.

CLINICAL SIGNS
In camels, the earlier reports suggest that rinderpest is clinically characterized by high fever, prostration, fetid diarrhea, and vesicular eruptions on lips, tongue, and dental pad. Aside from these signs, there was the presence of excessive lacrimation. The affected camels were unable to consume feed because of the ulcerated vesicular lesions in oral mucosa. Mortality rate

of 20–40% has been reported in camels. In India, during a ten-year period (1948–1958), data have revealed the occurrence of 17 outbreaks of rinderpest, which affected 128 camels and caused 60 deaths (Dhillon, 1959). However, researchers failed to infect camels experimentally with a virulent rinderpest strain. Experimental infections in camels by Chauhan et al. (1985) could not generate the disease. In another study, Taylor (1968) intravenously injected with a virulent rinderpest strain, which resulted in viremia of short duration, and later, the virus was reisolated between the third and eighth day.

Lesions

Similar to the lesions observed in bovines, camels also exhibit lesions that include erosions and vesicles in oral mucosa, congestion of the intestines, hemorrhagic enteritis, and presence of zebra markings in the large intestine. Enlargement of lymph nodes and congestion of the conjunctival mucous membrane is also observed in infected camels.

Diagnosis

The rinderpest can be diagnosed on the basis of clinical signs and lesions. Laboratory confirmation of rinderpest can be obtained by virus isolation or by detecting the viral antigens using the agar gel immunodiffusion (AGID) test. Detection of antibodies in sera using an ELISA or diagnosis based on the detection of genomic DNA of the rinderpest virus utilizing the molecular techniques like PCR can also be effectively done.

Treatment and Control

Camels rarely develop clinical signs, but treatment may be needed if diarrhea and dehydration are severe, for which fluid an electrolyte therapy is of much significance. In order to prevent the secondary bacterial infections, antibiotic therapy can be initiated. In endemic regions, camels should not be reared along with cattle and buffaloes. Similar to the vaccines used for bovines, studies should be targeted to identify the possibilities of live tissue culture vaccine (Kabete-O strain) for prevention of this disease in camelids, which could well protect these species, especially in endemic areas. (For more information, refer to "Rinderpest" diseases of bovines in this book).

7. OTHER VIRAL DISEASES OF CAMEL

A. FOOT-AND-MOUTH DISEASES (FMD)

Aphthovirus belonging to family Picornaviridae is the etiological agent of FMD, which is considered as an economically important disease of cloven-footed animals (Wernery and Kaaden, 2004). FMD affects mainly cattle, buffalo, and swine. Sheep and goats are also affected, and outbreaks have been experienced in wild ruminants, particularly deer and Arabian oryx. The disease is highly contagious and is characterized by vesicular and ulcerative lesions in mouth and foot. Seven FMD virus (FMDV) types—viz, O, A, C, SAT1, SAT2, SAT3, and Asia 1—are responsible for FMD in animals dwelling in different parts of the world. In affected animals, the vesicles appear principally on the mucous membranes of the mouth, muzzle, interdigital space, teats, and occasionally on the surface of the udder (Al-Ani and Chauhan, 2004). Presence of FMD in camels has been reported by many workers (Paling et al., 1979; Wernery et al., 2006). Nasser et al. (1980) reported that FMDV strain O was detected in the feces of camels three to six days postinfection. Also, Moussa et al. (1987) suggested that dromedary are susceptible to natural infection when they observed ruptured vesicles and ulcers on the upper lips, and FMDV, strain O was identified as the causative agent. However, many other studies prove that camel sera could be positive for FMDV strains C and SAT2 (Al-Ani and Chauhan, 2004). Even though the FMD virus may affect camels, most of the time, infected camel could remain asymptomatic. This has been observed during an outbreak of FMD (2001–2002) in cattle and sheep in different Arab countries; the camels kept in close contact with naturally infected cattle and sheep did not develop clinical signs. Similarly, the llama and alpaca can be infected with FMDV, but they are not very susceptible and do not pose a risk in transmitting FMD to susceptible animal species. However, the Office International des Epizooties (OIE) includes camelids as being susceptible species to FMD and suggests their potential involvement in the epidemiology of FMD (Wernery and Kaaden, 2004). In such a scenario, further studies are required to clarify the role of camels in spreading FMDV, especially in Mediterranean and African regions. Serological investigations have to be heightened in connection with susceptible contact animals as well as by observing the epidemiological niche of the FMDV (Wernery and Kaaden, 2004). (Refer "Foot-and-Mouth Diseases of Bovines" in this book).

B. INFLUENZA

The family Orthomyxoviridae comprises the genera *Influenzavirus* and among the types A, B, and C. Influenza A viruses are known to be causing majority of infections in domestic animals and poultry. Antibodies against the influenza viruses have been detected in camel sera (Yamnikova et al., 1993; Anchlan et al., 1996). In 1979, a severe influenza epizootic has occurred among camels in Mongolia (Yamnikova et al., 1993). The infection presented signs like fever, dry cough, bronchitis, and pneumonia, followed by discharge from nose and eyes. Occasional deaths have been reported in camels, and the pregnant camels may get abortions. In another study on the incidence of influenza in camels (Nigeria), serological surveys have indicated 6% antibodies against influenza A and 12% for influenza B; the human strain, H1N1 influenza A virus has also been isolated from camels (Al-Ani and Chauhan, 2004). The isolated H1N1 viruses were virtually indistinguishable from the human A/USSR/90/77 strain. A genetic sequence analysis revealed that among the eight gene segments, the PBI, HA, and NA genes, were almost identical with the similar genes of the USSR/77 strain, and the PB2, PA, NP, M, and NS genes were almost identical with those of the A/PR/8/34 strain. (For more information, refer to *Influenza and Its Global Public Health Significance* book by Tripthi M. Mathew and Thankam Mathew, Thajema Publishers, 2006.)

C. PARAINFLUENZA

Parainflueza is a common infectious viral disease of cattle characterized by watery yellow-colored discharges from the eyes and nose, coughs, respiratory distress, and fever. The infection is often relatively mild and may not lead to death of the animals. The disease can also affect camelids like camels and llamas. The etiological agent is parainfluenza virus 3 (PI-3), belonging to family Paramyxoviridae. Parainfluenza has been reported in camels (Afzal and Sakkir, 1994; Al-Ani and Chauhan, 2004), and the infection has been observed to be uncomplicated and asymptomatic. Serological surveys indicate that camels in Somalia, Sudan, and Tunisia have the antibodies against PI-3 virus. In a study in Nigeria—which was meant for identifying major respiratory viruses of camel—when compared to adenovirus, influenza virus, and respiratory syncytial virus, parainfluenza viral antibodies have predominated in camel sera (Paling et al., 1979; Olaleye et al., 1989). Another important factor that to be noted is that the PI-3 virus infection may predispose to secondary bacterial infections of respiratory tract, and transportation and other stressful situations may flare it up. Treatment by antibiotic may become necessary during secondary infections. For prevention, a wide variety of killed and attenuated live vaccines are available for cattle, but there are no reports of such vaccines being used in camels (Scholtissek, 1995).

D.   Vesicular Stomatitis (VS)

It is a disease that commonly affects domestic animals and free-living antelopes. The etiology of is vesicular stomatitis virus (VSV), a member of the genus *Vesiculovirus* in the family Rhabdoviridae. Equines, bovines, swine, camelids, and humans can be affected by VSV. Morbidity rate may reach up to 90% in a herd, but mortality rate is considerably low. Insect vectors, particularly sand flies and blackflies, could transmit VSV. Transovarial transmission has been demonstrated in such vectors. VSV has been isolated from mosquitoes and grasshoppers too. As a disease, the incubation period is two to eight days, and vesicles, characteristic of the disease, may develop within twenty-four hours. The animals show excessive salivation in initial stages, which is followed by presence of vesicles on the lips, mouth, nostrils, hooves, and teats. Based on manifestations, the vesicular stomatitis closely resembles foot-and-mouth disease (FMD), swine vesicular disease, and vesicular exanthema of swine. One natural infection, vesicular stomatitis has been reported in camelids (Gomez, 1964). Also, experimental infection of llama and alpacas by intradermal inoculation into the dorsum of the tongue produced localized vesicles with signs like elevated body temperature and anorexia (Al-Ani and Chauhan, 2004). (For more information, refer "Bovine and Ovine Tropical Viral Diseases" of this book).

E.   Herpesvirus Infection

Herpesvirus infections have been reported in camels and llamas. They are bovine rhinotracheitis caused by bovine herpesvirus 1 and equine herpesvirus 1. Both the viruses have a single linear molecule of a double-stranded DNA (Rebhun et al., 1988; Rosadio et al., 1993; Bildfell et al., 1996). In an epidemiological study conducted in Tunisia, about 6% of camels had antibody titers to bovine herpesvirus-1. Another serological survey stated that 16.7% of llamas and 16.2% of alpacas that grazed on the same pasture with cattle developed antibody titer to infectious bovine rhinotracheitis (IBR). This points to the fact that cattle may be the source of infection to camels when they are grazing together. Also, a herpesvirus indistinguishable from equine herpesvirus 1 was isolated from llamas and alpacas that had suffered from blindness and central nervous system disorders consisting of nystagmus, torticollis, and paralysis. Nonsuppurative meningoencephalitis with vasculitis, necrosis, and edema in a Bactrian camel has been caused by equine herpesvirus 1 (Al-Ani and Chauhan, 2004). Also, intranuclear inclusions typical of EHV-1 can be detected in neurons and glial cells. Besides, EHV-1 antigens can be located in neurons and lymphocytes.

F.   Bluetongue

Bluetongue (BT) is an infectious viral disease of small ruminants caused by *Orbivirus* belonging to Reoviridae family. The vector mosquito, belonging to *Culicoides* sp., transmits the disease. The viral RNA genome is characteristically double stranded (ds) having segments of different sizes. The disease is of noncontagious nature and occurs in both wild and domestic ruminants, including camelids. Characteristic signs include transient fever, edema of the face, lips, muzzle, and ears; excessive salivation; and hyperemic oral mucosa. Swelling of the lips and tongue gives the tongue a bluish tinge, and hence, the disease has its name. BT virus antibodies have been detected in serum samples of camels from Botswana (81.0%), Saudi Arabia (67.0%), Sudan (14.6%), Egypt (14.3%), Yemen (13.0%), and Iran (5.9%) (Simpson, 1979; Al-Ani and Chauhan, 2004). Using the agar gel immunodiffusion (AGID) test, rapid detection of bluetongue virus antigen has been done in infected camels (Abu Elzein, 1984). However, in camels, the characteristics signs are not appreciated, and hence it is concluded that BT infection may cause clinical disease in sheep, while it is probably subclinical or inapparent in camels (Eisa et al., 1979). Other than AGID, competitive enzyme-linked immunosorbent assay (cELISA) can also be developed for the detection of serum antibodies against bluetongue virus (BTV) in camels (Chandel et al., 2003; Al-Ani and Chauhan, 2004). In India, one study reports that out of 176 sera tested, 12.5% and 19.3% were positive for group-specific bluetongue antibodies when tested by AGID and cELISA, respectively (Chandel et al., 2003). (For more information, refer to "Bluetongue" on the bovine diseases section of this book).

G.   African Horse Sickness

African horse sickness (AHS) is an infectious, arthropod-borne disease of animals belonging to the family Equidae (Binepal et al., 1992; Baba et al., 1992). The etiological agent is *Orbivirus* belonging to the family Reoviridae. Nine antigenically distinct virus types have been identified. The disease, usually transmitted by mosquitoes, results in high mortality in horses, often up to 90%. AHS virus has not been isolated from camels, but AHS virus type 9 was isolated from *Hyalomma dromedarii* ticks that fed on camels (Al-Ani and Chauhan, 2004). Serological surveys indicate the AHS incidence in camels as 23% in Sudan, 10% in Nigeria, and 5% in Egypt (Salama et al., 1986). In another observation, 10% of the sera samples from camels were tested as positive while using the hemagglutination inhibition test (HI) (Baba et al., 1993). In another survey in Egypt, imported camels showed the presence of AHS virus antibodies as 12% by agar gel precipitation and 10% by complement fixation and hemagglutination-inhibition test (Al-Ani and Chauhan, 2004). To conclude, the prevalence of antibody to AHS virus detected in camels suggests that they might act as reservoirs of the virus and could have an influence upon the epidemiology of the disease in Africa (Baba et al., 1993).

H.   RESPIRATORY SYNCYTIAL VIRUS (RSV)

A virus belonging to the genus *Pneumovirus*, subfamily Pneumovirinae, and family Paramyxoviridae causes respiratory syncytial virus (RSV) infection. The disease has been recognized in cattle worldwide as being associated with bovine respiratory disease. The agent causes disease of respiratory tract and produces syncytial lesions in lungs. RSV is a negative-sense, enveloped RNA virus. RSV also reduces the resistance of the respiratory tract and makes the animal susceptible to secondary infections like bronchiolitis and pneumonia. RSV-infected animals are considered the principal reservoirs of the disease. As the disease is manifested as a respiratory one, transmission from one animal to another is thought to be via aerosol route. However, the virus is unstable in the environment and can get readily inactivated with soap and other disinfectants. Respiratory syncytial (RS) viruses have been a problem for human beings, cattle, goats, and sheep. Even though many reports are not available in camels, antibody to RSV has been detected in Nigeria but with an incidence of only 0.6% (Al-Ani and Chauhan, 2004).

I.   PESTE DES PETITS RUMINANTS (PPR)

PPR is a highly contagious, systemic disease of goats and sheep very similar to rinderpest. The disease is caused by a closely related *Morbillivirus* that belongs to the Paramyxoviridae family (Scott and Macdonald, 1962; Smith, 1970). The etiological agent causes a severe disease in sheep and goats with a mortality rate 50–80%. The disease is spread by direct contact between infected and susceptible population. Infection with PPRV results in an acute, highly contagious disease characterized by fever, anorexia, necrotic stomatitis, diarrhea, purulent ocular and nasal discharges, and respiratory distress. The PPRV is found to be closely related to rinderpest virus (RPV), canine distemper virus, and human measles virus. In camels, the serological surveys have indicated the presence of antibodies to PPR. The PPRV-specific antibody prevalence in camels has been reported by many workers (Haroun et al., 2002; Abraham et al., 2005).

J.   ROTAVIRUS DIARRHEA

Rotavirus belonging to family Reoviridae is the cause of diarrhea in newborn animals including calf herds in many camel herds. The etiological agent is having a double-stranded RNA genome. Other than camels, a wide range of mammalian species can be infected with rotaviruses. In recent years, the importance of rotaviruses in the etiology of diarrhea in young animals has been well established. Rotavirus has been isolated from cases of diarrhea in newborn camel calves in Sudan (Mohin et al., 1983). Rotavirus induces diarrhea primarily due to malabsorption based on the destruction of mature enterocytes, activation of enteric nervous system, and also due to secretion of a viral enterotoxin known as nonstructural protein 4 (NSP4) (Chauhan et al., 2008).

K.   CORONAVIRAL INFECTIONS

The *Coronavirus* that comes under the family Coronaviridae causes enteritis and diarrheic conditions in camels and other animals. Numerous viral particles, approximately 140 nm in diameter, with clublike projections can be detected in the diarrheic feces of affected camels by electron microscopy (Al-Ani and Chauhan, 2004). During another observation, Wunschmann et al. (2002) reported a case of enteric coronavirus infection in a six-week-aged dromedary calf. The diarrhea persisted for five days, and the calf died in spite of the providing symptomatic treatment. These characteristics were consistent with coronavirus infections. Immunohistochemical reactivity with coronavirus-specific antibodies confirmed the presence of viral antigen in colonic epithelial cells (Wunschmann et al., 2002).

L.   ENCEPHALOMYOCARDITIS

The disease is caused by *Cardiovirus* that belongs to the family Picornaviridae. The natural hosts of encephalomyocarditis virus (EMCV) are rodents, and the virus gets transmitted from rodents to humans and other animals (Bildfell et al., 1996). EMCV, which has caused death of many species of animals in zoological parks, is a slow, progressive, inflammatory disease of the central nervous system and myocardium. It has been suggested that the disease could be present in both dromedary and bactrian camels. The serum-neutralization test (SNT) is the best serodiagnostic technique for the identification of EMCV infection. Vaccination with a genetically engineered, live attenuated *Mengovirus*, which is serologically indistinguishable from the field strain of EMCV, has been occasionally used to control the disease. However, the vaccine response might be variable, with high virus-neutralizing antibody titer responses shown in some primate species and mixed to poor responses for other species (Backues et al., 1999).

M.   WESSELSBORN DISEASE

Flavivirus, in the family Flaviviridae, is the causative agent of Wesselsborn disease (WSL). An arthropod vector transmits the disease, and it has been shown that *Aedes* sp. has a major role in the disease transmission. Infection is common, but clinical disease is infrequent. Infection in adults is usually subclinical, but disease may be severe in the presence of preexisting liver pathology. Occasional abortion, together with congenital malformation of the

CNS with arthrogryposis and hydrops amnii, also seen. After an incubation period of one to three days in newborn lambs, nonspecific signs of illness, including fever, anorexia, listlessness, weakness, and increased respiration, become evident. Antibodies against WSL virus have been encountered in human and animal population in many African countries. The presence of WSL virus infections in camels has been reported (Baba et al., 1995). Also, an epidemiological survey in Nigeria using hemagglutination test indicated antibody prevalence against WSL virus to be 60.2% (Al-Ani and Chauhan, 2004). The disease, with an incubation period of 24 to 120 hours, shows a febrile condition that lasts for about 48 hours. No other symptoms are observed, but there can be abortion in pregnant animals, and congenital anomalies may also be observed in newborn animals (Al-Ani and Chauhan, 2004). To conclude, high antibody titer to flaviviruses in camels suggests a potential danger to meat handlers, camel-rearing farmers, and veterinarians.

N. BOVINE VIRAL DIARRHEA (BVD/MD)

BVD/MD virus is a *Pestivirus* that infects cattle in many countries of the world. The disease is characterized by fever, yellowish discharge from the nose and eyes, erosions of the muzzle and mouth, and diarrhea with the presence of mucus and blood. The virus has the capability to readily cross into other species of animals. Serological surveys have been conducted in different countries, and they reveal the presence of antibodies to BVD/MD in camel sera in Sudan (15.5%), United Arab Emirates (9.2%), Oman (6.7%), Tunisia (3.9%), and Somalia (3.4%) (Zaghawa, 1998). Also, neutralizing antibodies have been demonstrated in the serum of white-tailed deer, sheep, and goats (Al-Ani and Chauhan, 2004). Wernery and Wernery (1990) have reported that when compared to the breeder herds, racing camels have more prevalence of BVD infection. In another study, Zhagawa (1998) has reported the prevalence of neutralizing antibodies to BVD virus to 52.0% in camels (Zaghawa, 1998). However, during all such incidences, it has been identified that BVD/MD virus may cause only an inapparent infection in camels. (For more information, refer to "Bovine Viral Diarrhea—Mucosal Disease Complex" of bovine viral diseases section of this book).

O. ADENOVIRAL INFECTIONS

Adenoviruses that comes under the family Adenoviridae causes upper or lower respiratory tract diseases in many animal species. Adenovirus-mediated respiratory infections have also been observed in camelids. Serological examination of camelids has revealed the presence of adenovirus antibodies in camels, and there are reports from Nigeria indicating that camels intended for slaughter showed presence of serum antibodies to adenovirus (Al-Ani and

Chauhan, 2004). In another serologic analysis, involving llamas, prevalence of antibodies to the adenoviruses was 93% (Mattson, 1994). However, most adenovirus infections could be asymptomatic or may be presented as mild infection. The diagnosis of adenovirus infections is often performed by virus isolation, serological tests, detection of viral antigen in tissues by immunofluorescence, or by the detection of virions by electron microscopy.

P.   CRIMEAN-CONGO HEMORRHAGIC FEVER

It is a severe hemorrhagic viral disease of humans that is acquired from infected ticks, tissues of infected animals, and from contact with people who are infected. The disease was first described in Crimea (1944) and was given the name Crimean hemorrhagic fever. In 1969, the pathogen caused similar disease in Congo, and hence the disease got its name as Crimean-Congo hemorrhagic fever (CCHF). The causative agent, *Nairovirus* belonging to family Bunyaviridae, is transmitted by ixodid ticks, especially those of the genus Hyalomma, serving as reservoir and vector for the CCHF virus. Numerous wild and domestic animals, such as cattle, goats, sheep, and hares, serve as amplifying hosts for the virus. CCHF has been reported in humans in Iraq, UAE, Russia, Pakistan, and Nigeria. There has been reports of the isolation of CCHF virus from the *Hyalomma anatolicum* that commonly infest camels (Al-Ani and Chauhan, 2004). A seroepidemiological survey to determine the prevalence of CCHF virus and its circulation among camels in Iraq has been carried out during 1980s, and it was identified that 23% camel sera were found positive (Tantawi et al., 1981). During another study, conducted during 1986–87, CCHF infection among camels imported into Egypt from Sudan and Kenya has been tested for CCHF antibodies by the agar gel immunodiffusion (AGID) and indirect fluorescent antibody (IFA) techniques, and virus-specific antibodies have been demonstrated in 14% of the camels (Al-Ani and Chauhan, 2004). Similarly, the prevalence of CCHF viral antibodies among camels has been reported by many other workers (Morril et al., 1990; Mariner et al., 1995).

Q.   WEST NILE VIRUS INFECTION

The disease is caused by West Nile virus (WNV), which belongs to genus *Flavivirus* within the family Flaviviridae. It mainly infects birds but may infect humans, horses, and other animals. The infection may be asymptomatic, febrile, or neuroinvasive. The virus is transmitted through mosquito vectors (*Culex* sp.), which bite and infect birds. The birds are amplifying hosts, developing sufficient viral levels to transmit the infection to other biting mosquitoes, which go on to infect other birds and also humans. The West Nile virus may not show symptoms, but if present, they include fever, body aches and headaches, skin rashes, and swollen lymph glands. When the virus spreads to brain, it can be fatal as it causes encephalitis or meningitis. Regarding the infection in camels, during a survey, Olaleye et al. (1990) reported a seroprevalence of WNV antibodies as 26%. In another study, Vasilev et al. (2005) suggested that based on the serological detection, hemagglutination test detected the prevalence of WNV infection as 5% while the neutralization test has detected it to be 42% (For more information, refer to "West Nile Virus Infection of Horses" of this book).

R.   AKABANE DISEASE

Akabane disease is caused by *Bunyavirus* that belongs to family Bunyaviridae. The virus is a mosquito-borne (*Culicoides* sp.) agent that primarily infects cattle, sheep, and goats to cause abortion or congenital anomalies, which are the hallmarks of this disease. The anomalies include arthrogryposis, hydranencephaly, and microencephaly of the newborn animal (Al-Ani and Chauhan, 2004). Muscle atrophy, exophthalmos, excessive lacrimation, torticolis, scoliosis, kyphosis, and abnormal vocalization may also been seen. These abnormalities are usually the first to be seen during an outbreak. The mortality rate could be very high in affected newborn animals. This disease has been serologically identified in camels from African as well as Mediterranean regions. Serum-neutralizing antibodies have been detected against the virus in camels from Kenya and Oman, with a prevalence of 70 and 50%, respectively (Davies and Jessett, 1985; Al-Bushidy et al., 1988). The disease is endemic in animals in Middle East countries, Turkey, Australia, Japan, and Kenya (Al-Ani and Chauhan, 2004).

S.   YELLOW FEVER

The disease is caused by yellow fever virus (YFV), which belongs to genus *Flavivirus* within the family Flaviviridae. Yellow fever has caused large epidemics among human population in Africa and the American continents. Thirty-three countries, with a cumulative population of 500 million, are at risk in Africa, while in American continent, countries like Bolivia, Brazil, Colombia, Ecuador, and Peru are considered to be having higher risk. Humans and monkeys are the principal host of the virus, and they are transmitted horizontally from one animal by biting mosquitoes, especially the *Aedes* sp. Serological evidences of the YFV has been reported in camels (Adu et al., 1990). Serum samples from camels have been tested positive for yellow fever virus antibodies when counterimmunoelectrophoresis was performed. This test was confirmed by both single radial hemolysis and serum-neutralization tests.

T. RETROVIRUS INFECTIONS

Retrovirus in the family Retroviridae is known to cause enzootic leukemia in camels. Wernery and Kaaden (1995) have reported the occurrence of lymphatic leukemia in camels in United Arab Emirates. All affected camels were over eight years old and had lymphocytic leukocytosis. During necropsy, tumor masses were present in the lungs, spleen, and lymph nodes. However, the detection of retrovirus by serological examination or viral isolation has been found to yield negative results.

CONCLUSION

Aside from the above-mentioned viral diseases of camel, various other viral infections have been reported in camels, even though their pathogenic potential is not fully understood. Serological tests have revealed the presence of antibodies against *Chittor virus* in camels, a virus that is associated with human illness, and this suggests that camels could act as a carrier for this virus. Similarly, *Thogotovirus* and *Dhorivirus* have also been isolated from camel tick *Hyalomma dromedarii*. Also, there are serological evidences for the presence of *Chikungunyavirus* in camels. Some workers have even reported the presence of *Quaranfilvirus* in camel tick, *H. dromedarii* especially in countries like Kuwait, Iraq, and Yemen (Converse and Moussa, 1982). Further, antibodies against *Orungovirus* and *Ifevirus* have been detected in camels (Ezeifeka et al., 1984, 1989). Very recently, *Torque teno virus* (TTV), isolated from camel specimens from the United Arab Emirates (UAE), has been studied for its relation with the human TTV (Al-Moslih et al., 2007). Phylogenetic analysis revealed that the similarity between isolates from camels and humans is between 92–97%, prompting to conclude that camels and humans share a common source of TTV infection. Taking all this into consideration, the presence of many viruses in camels warrants more rapid detection, characterization, and preventive tools, for which the conventional techniques have to be replaced with new-generation diagnostics and prophylactic agents.

As per the current scenario, the rapid developments in molecular biology have led to the introduction of highly sensitive and speedy diagnostic approaches as well as effective prophylactic measures for tackling important viral diseases of camels. For diagnosis, techniques like isolation by cell culture and detection of virus-specific antibodies using serological techniques such as agar gel immunodiffusion, enzyme-linked immunosorbent assay, fluoresent antibody test and neutralization tests have been initially performed. However, in recent years, novel technologies for the detection of viruses in clinical specimens are being employed. Molecular detection techniques started with evolution of nucleic acid hybridization, which is the combination of labeled, single-stranded

DNA or RNA molecules (probes) binding specifically with target viral nucleic acid in the specimen (Sall et al., 2002). Further, the polymerase chain reaction (PCR) and allied techniques like real-time and multiplex-PCR along with gene sequencing has become popular for detection and characterization of viral pathogens. Such techniques are widely used because of being highly sensitive and can be performed rapidly in a cost-effective manner. Several other techniques like nucleic acid sequence–based amplification (NASBA), biosensor-based detection, and microarray analysis have become popular during recent years. Even though conventional assays are still used routinely, the molecular techniques have broadened the scope of viral diagnostics and have assisted in the comprehensive analysis of viral pathogens. Also, the advancements in high-throughput technologies arising from knowledge of viral genomics is enabling the analysis of the genome and proteome as well in order to gain a better understanding of the molecular pathways of various pathogens and host-pathogen interactions.

Besides, the precise knowledge of the molecular conformation and structural details of viral pathogens and the assessment of the immunological parameters of the host have ushered a new era in vaccine development. Various novel techniques have been applied to develop vaccines that are safer and at the meantime could ably elicit specific immune responses that are desirable for a complete protection. The drawbacks of the conventional vaccines, in the long run, have forced researchers to evolve newer alternatives, among which nucleic acid–based or recombinant protein-based vaccines holds a prominent position. Utilizing a prokaryotic or eukaryotic system, immunogenic proteins of viral pathogens are expressed for developing subunit vaccines. The recombinant DNA technology has also enabled the researchers to develop DNA vaccines (Dhama et al., 2008) and virus vector vaccines as well that are capable of eliciting sufficient immune response in host, with long duration of immunity and without any adverse implications, thus generating a ray of hope for creating reliable and efficacious vaccines to combat viral diseases of camels in the coming decades.

REFERENCES

1. Abbas, B., el Zubeir, A. E. and Yassin, T. T. 1987. Survey for certain zoonotic diseases in camels in Sudan. *Rev. Elev. Med. Vet. Pays. Trop.* 40:231–233.
2. Abbas, B. and Omer, O. H. 2005. Review of infectious diseases of the camel. *Vet. Bulletin* 75:1–16.
3. Abd EI-Rahim, I., Abd EI-Hakim, U. and Hussein, M. 1999. An epizootic of Rift Valley fever in Egypt in 1997. *Rev. Sci. Tech. Off. Int. Epiz.* 18:741–748.
4. Abdo-Salem, S., Gerbier, G., Bonnet, P., Al-Qadasi, M., Tran, A., Thiry, E., Al-Eryni, G. and Roger, F. 2006. Descriptive and spatial epidemiology of Rift Valley fever outbreak in Yemen 2000–2001. *Ann. NY. Acad. Sci.* 1081:240–242.

7. OTHER VIRAL DISEASES OF CAMEL

5. Abraham, G., Sintayehu, A., Libeau, G., Albina, E., Roger, F., Laekemariam, Y., Abayneh, D. and Awoke, K. M. 2005. Antibody seroprevalences against peste des petits ruminants (PPR) virus in camels, cattle, goats and sheep in Ethiopia. *Prev. Vet. Med.* 70:51–57.

6. Abu Elzein, E. M. 1984. Rapid detection of bluetongue virus antigen in the sera and plasma of camels, sheep and cattle in the Sudan, using the gel immunodiffusion test. Brief report. *Arch. Virol.* 79:131–134.

7. Abu Elzein, E. M., Gameel, A. A., Ramadan, R. O. and Housawi, F. M. 1999. An eruptive moderate form of camelpox infection in dromedary camels (Camelus dromedarius) in Saudi Arabia. *Rev. Sci. Tech.* 18:749–752.

8. Abubakr, M. I., Abu-Elzein, E. M., Housawi, F. M., Abdelrahman, A. O., Fadlallah, M. E., Nayel, M. N., Adam, A. S., Moss, S., Forrester, N. L., Coloyan, E., Gameel, A., Al-Afaleq, A. I. and Gould, E. A. 2007. Pseudocowpox virus: The etiological agent of contagious ecthyma (Auzdyk) in camels (Camelus dromedarius) in the Arabian peninsula. *Vect. Borne Zoon. Dis.* 7:257–260.

9. Adu, F., Esan, J. and Baba, S. S. 1990. Seroepidemiological survey for yellow fever antibodies in domestic animals. *Rev. Roum. Virol.* 41:147–150.

10. Afonso, C. L., Tulman, E. R., Lu, Z., Zsak, L., Sandybaev, N. T., Kerembekova, U. Z., Zaitsev, V. L., Kutish, G. F. and Rock, D. L. 2002. The genome of camelpox virus. *Virology* 295:1–9.

11. Afzal, M. and Sakkir, M. 1994. Survey of antibodies against various infectious disease agents in racing camels in Abu Dhabi, United Arab Emirates. *Rev. Sci. Tech.* 13:787–792.

12. Afzal, M., Khan, I. A. and Salman, R. 1993. Symptoms and clinical pathology of rabies in the camel. *Vet. Rec.* 133:220.

13. Agab, H. and Abbas, B. 2001. Epidemiological studies on camel diseases in eastern Sudan: Diseases encountered among pastoralist camels during 1991–1992. *Camel-Newsletter* 18:31–43.

14. Agab, H. and Abbas, B. 1999. Epidemiological studies on camel diseases in the eastern Sudan. *World Anim. Rev.* 92:42–51.

15. Al-Ani, F. K., Sharrif, L. A., Al-Rawashdeh, O., Al-Qudah, K. and Al-Hammi, Y. 1998. Camel diseases in Jordan. Proceeding of the 3rd Ann. Meeting Anim. Prod. Arid Conditions. United Arab Emirates, 77–92.

16. Al-Ani, F. K. 2004. Camel management and husbandry. In *Camel: Management and diseases*, ed. F. K. Al-Ani, 69–90. Baghdad, Iraq.

17. Al-Ani, F. K. and Chauhan, R. S. 2004. Viral diseases. In *Camel: Management and diseases*, ed. F. K. Al-Ani, 367–384. Baghdad, Iraq.

18. Al-Bushidy, S. M., Mellor, P. S. and Tayler, W. 1988. Prevalence of neutralizing antibodies to Akabane virus in the Arabian Peninsula. *Vet. Microbiol.* 17:141–149.

19. Alhendi, A. B., Abuelzein, E. M., Gameel, A. A., Hassanein, M. M. 1994. A slow-spreading mild form of camel pox infection. *Zentr. Veter. B.* 41:71–73.

20. Ali, O. A., Kheir, S. A., Abu Damir, H. and Barri, M. E. 1991. Camel (Camelus dromedarius) contagious ecthyma in the Sudan. A case report. *Rev. Elev. Med. Vet. Pays Trop.* 44:143.

21. Al-Moslih, M. I., Perkins, H. and Hu, Y. W. 2007. Genetic relationship of Torque Teno virus (TTV) between humans and camels in United Arab Emirates (UAE). *J. Med. Virol.* 79:188–191.

22. Al-Rawashdeh, O. F., Al-Ani, F. K., Sharrif, L. A., Al-Qudah, K. M., Al-Hami, Y. and Frank, N. 2000. A survey of camel (Camelus dromedarius) diseases in Jordan. *J. Zoo Wildl. Med.* 31:335–338.

23. Al-Qudah, K., Al-Rawashdeh, O., Abdul-Majeed, M. and Al-Ani, F. K. 1996. An epidemiological investigation of rabies in Jordan. *Acat. Vet. Beograd* 47:12.

24. Al-Zi'abi, O., Nishikawa, H. and Meyer, H. 2007. The first outbreak of camelpox in Syria. *J. Vet. Med. Sci.* 69:541–543.

25. Anchlan, D., Ludwig, S. and Nymadawa, P. 1996. Previous H1N1 influenza A virus circulating in the Mongolian population. *Arch. Virol.* 141:1553–1569.

26. Azwai, S. M., Carter, S. D. and Woldehiwet, Z. 1995. Immune responses of the camel (Camelus dromedarius) to contagious ecthyma (Orf) virus infection. *Vet. Microbiol.* 47:119–131.

27. Azwai, S. M., Carter, S. D., Woldehiwet, Z. and Wernery, U. 1996. Serology of orthopoxvirus cameli infection in dromedary camels: Analysis by ELISA and western blotting. *Comp. Immunol. Microbiol. Infect. Dis.* 19:65–78.

28. Baba, S. S., Akinyele, H. A. and Olaleye, O. D. 1992. Prevalence of complement-fixing antibody to the African horse sickness virus in domestic animals in Nigeria. *Beitr. Trop. Landwir. Veterinar.* 30:471–477.

29. Baba, S. S., Olaleye, O. D. and Ayanbadejo, O. A. 1993. Haemagglutination-inhibiting antibodies against African horse sickness virus in domestic animals in Nigeria. *Vet. Res.* 24:483–487.

30. Baba, S. S., Fagbami, A. H., Ojeh, C. K., Olaleye, O. D. and Omilabu, S. A. 1995. Wesselsbron virus antibody in domestic animals in Nigeria: Retrospective and prospective studies. *New Microbiol.* 18:151–162.

31. Backues, K. A., Hill, M., Palmenberg, A. C., Miller, C., Soike, K. F. and Aguilar, R. 1999. Genetically engineered Mengo virus vaccination of multiple captive wildlife species. *J. Wildl. Dis.* 35:384–387.

32. Bah, S. O., Chamoiseau, G., Biha, M. L. O. and Fall, S. M. 1981. A focus of camel rabies in Mauritania. *Rev. Elev. Med. Vet. Pays Trop.* 34:263–265.

33. Baky, M. H. A., Al-Sukayran, A., Mazloum, K. S., Al-Bokmy, A. M. and Al-Mujalli, D. M. 2006a. Immunogenicity of camel pox virus, Jouf-78 vaccine-strain in Boskat rabbits and guineapigs. *Assiut Vet. Med. J.* 52:194–202.

34. Baky, M. H. A., Al-Sukayran, A. M., Mazloum, K. S., Al-Bokmy, A. M. and Al-Mujalli, D. M. 2006b. Isolation and standardization of camel pox virus from naturally infected cases in the central region of Saudi Arabia 2004. *Assiut Vet. Med. J.* 52:183–193.

35. Baxby, D., Hessami, M., Ghaboosi, B. and Ramyar, H. 1975. Response of camels to intradermal inoculation with smallpox and camelpox viruses. *Infect. Immun.* 11:617–621.

36. Bengoumi, M., Gandega, E. B., El-Abrak, A., Berrada, J. and Faye, B. 2000. Study of camel calf mortality in South Morocco: Retrospective survey. *Rev. Elev. Med. Vet. Pays. Trop.* 53:132–135.

37. Bildfell, R., Yason, C., Haines, D. and McGowan, M. 1996. Herpes virus encephalitis in a camel (*Camelus bacterianus*). *J. Zoo Wildl. Med.* 27:409.

38. Binepal, V. S., Wariru, B. N., Davies, F. G., Soi, R. and Olubayo, R. 1992. An attempt to define the host range for African horse sickness virus (Orbivirus, Reoviridae) in east Africa, by a serological survey in some equidae, camelidae, loxodontidae and carnivore. *Vet. Microbiol.* 31:19–23.

39. Binns, M., Mumford, J. and Wernery, U. 1992. Analysis of the camelpox virus thymidine kinase gene. *Brit. Vet. J.* 148:541–546.

40. Bloch, N. and Diallo, I. 1995. A probable outbreak of rabies in a group of camels in Niger. *Vet. Microbiol.* 46:281–284.

41. Brown, A. 2004. A review of camel diseases in Central Australia. Technical Bulletin: Dept. of Business, Industry and Resource Development, Northern Territory Government. 314:1–16.

42. Buck, C. B. and Thompson, C. D. 2007. Production of papillomavirus-based gene transfer vectors. Chapter 26. In *Current Protocols in Cellular Biology.* Unit 26.1.

43. Campo, M. S. 2002. Animal models of papillomavirus pathogenesis. *Virus Res.* 89:249–261.

44. Campo, M. S. and Jarrett, W. F. 1994. Vaccination against cutaneous and mucosal papillomavirus in cattle. *Ciba Found. Symp.* 187:61–73.

45. Campo, M. S., Grindlay, G. J., O'Neil, B. W., Chandrachud, L. M., McGarvie, G. M. and Jarrett, W. F. 1993. Prophylactic and therapeutic vaccination against a mucosal papillomavirus. *J. Gen. Virol* 74:945–953.

46. Chandel, B. S., Chauhan, H. C. and Kher, H. N. 2003. Comparison of the standard AGID test and competitive ELISA for detecting bluetongue virus antibodies in camels in Gujarat, India. *Trop. Anim. Health Prod.* 35:99–104.

7. OTHER VIRAL DISEASES OF CAMEL

47. Chandra, R., Chauhan, R. S. and Garg, S. K. 1998. Camel pox—a review. *Camel-News Letter* 14:34–45.

48. Chauhan, R. S. 1995. Health, production and management of camels in Haryana State, India. In *Livestock production and diseases in the tropics livestock production and human welfare*, ed. K. H. Zessin, 255. Association of Institution of Tropical Veterinary Medicine.

49. Chauhan, R. S. and Kaushik, R. K. 1987. Isolation of camel pox virus in India. *Brit. Vet. J.* 143:581–582.

50. Chauhan, R. S. and Mahipal, S. K. 1995. Infectious diseases of camels in India: A review. In *Advances in animal health and production*, ed. R. S. Chauhan, P. C. Sharma, R. Rakesh Kumar, R. Sharma, and S. K. Mahipal, 163–172.

51. Chauhan, R. S., Kulshrestha, R. C. and Kaushik, R. K. 1985. Epidemiological studies of viral diseases of livestock in Haryana state. *Indian J. Virol.* 1:10–16.

52. Chauhan, R. S., Kaushik, R. K., Gupta, S. C., Satija, K. C. and Kulshreshtha, R. C. 1986. Prevalence of different diseases in camels (*Camelus dromedaries*) in India. *Camel-News Letter* 3:10–14.

53. Chauhan, R. S., Dhama, K. and Mahendran, M. 2008. Pathobiology of rotaviral diarrhea in calves and its diagnosis and control: A review. *J. Immunol. Immunopathol.* 10:1–13.

54. Chemuliti, J. K., Njiru, Z. K. and Bukachi, S. 2003. Disease conditions of camels in non-traditional camel keeping areas of Kajiado District in Kenya: A case study. *J. Camel Pract. Res.* 10:207–210.

55. Converse, J. D. and Moussa, M. I. 1982. Quaranfil virus from *Hyalmma dromedarii* (Acari: *Ixodidae*) collected in Kuwait, Iraq and Yemen. *J. Med. Entomol.* 19:209–210.

56. Dashtseren, T., Solovyev, B. V., Varejka, F. and Khokhoo, A. 1984. Camel contagious ecthyma (pustular dermatitis). *Acta Virol.* 28:122–127.

57. Davies, F. G. and Jessett, D. M. 1985. A study of the host range and distribution of antibody to Akabane virus (genus bunyavirus, family Bunyaviridae) in Kenya. *J. Hyg.* (Lond) 95:191–196.

58. Davies, F. G., Mbugua, H., Atema, C. and Wilson, A. 1985a. The prevalence of antibody to camel pox virus in six different herds in Kenya. *J. Comp. Pathol.* 95:633–635.

59. Davies, F. G., Koros, J. and Mbugua, H. 1985b. Rift Valley fever in Kenya: The presence of antibody to the virus in camels (Camelus dromedarius). *J. Hyg.* (Lond) 94:241–244.

60. Davies, F. G., Mungai, J. N. and Shaw, T. 1975. Characteristics of a Kenyan camelpox virus. *J. Hyg.* (Lond) 75:381–385.

61. Dhama K., Mahendran M., Gupta, P. K. and Rai A. 2008. DNA vaccines and their applications in veterinary practice: Current perspectives. *Vet. Res. Commun.* (2008) (In Press).

62. Dhillon, S. S. 1959. Incidence of rinderpest in camels in Hissar district. *Indian Vet. J.* 36:603–607.

63. Dorman, A. E. 1984. The camel in health and disease. 2. Aspects of the husbandry and management of the genus Camelus. *Brit. Vet. J.* 140:616–633.

64. Eisa, M., Karrar, A. E. and Abd Elrahim, A. H. 1979. Incidence of bluetongue virus precipitating antibodies in sera of some domestic animals in the Sudan. *J. Hyg.* (Lond) 83:539–545.

65. El-Shinnawy, M. M., Abd Ed-Hady, O. A., Mouaz, M. A., Zaghawa, A. A., Khodeir, M. and Khadr, A. M. 1993. Some serological studies on rinderpest in Egypt. Proceedings of the Second Scientific Congress, Egyptian Society for Cattle Diseases, 1993. *Assiut. Egypt* 257–265.

66. El-Harrak, M., Loutfi, C. and Bertin, F. 1991. Isolation and identification of camel pox virus in Morocco. *Ann. Rech. Vet.* 22:95–98.

67. Esposito, J. J. and Knight, J. C. 1985. Orthopoxvirus DNA: A comparison of restriction profiles and maps. *Virology* 143:230–251.

68. Ezeifeka, G. O., Umoh, J. U., Belino, E. D. and Ezeokoli, C. D. 1984. Complement fixing antibodies to Orungo virus in food animals of Northern Nigeria. *Int. J. Zoonoses* 11:149–154.

69. Ezeifeka, G. O., Umoh, J. U., Ezeokoli, C. D. and Gomwalk, N. E. 1989. Serological evidence of Ife virus infection in Nigerian indigenous domestic ruminants. *Trop. Anim. Health Prod.* 21:55–57.

70. Falluji, M. M., Tantawi, H. H. and Shony, M. O. 1979. Isolation, identification and characterization of camelpox virus in Iraq. *J. Hyg.* (Lond) 83:267–272.

71. Fowler, M. E. 1996. Husbandry and diseases of camelids. *Rev. Sci. Tech.* 15:155–169.

72. Gabry, G. H. 2003. Some biological properties of camel pox virus. *Vet. Med. J. Giza* 51:5–17.

73. Gaukroger, J. M., Chandrachud, L. M., O'Neil, B. W., Grindlay, G. J., Knowles, G. and Campo, M. S. 1996. Vaccination of cattle with bovine papillomavirus type 4 L2 elicits the production of virus-neutralizing antibodies. *J. Gen. Virol.* 77:1577–1583.

74. Georges, A. J. and Georges-Courbot, M. C. 1999. Biohazards due to orthopoxvirus: Should we re-vaccinate against smallpox? *Med. Trop.* 59:483–487.

75. Gitao, C. G. 1994. Outbreaks of contagious ecthyma in camels (Camelus dromedarius) in the Turkana district of Kenya. *Rev. Sci. Tech.* 13:939–945.

76. Gitao, C. G. 1997. An investigation of camelpox outbreaks in two principal camel (Camelus dromedarius) rearing areas of Kenya. *Rev. Sci. Tech.* 16:841–847.

77. Gomez, U. D. 1964. Test on the sensitivity of South American camelids to vesicular stomatitis. *An. Segun. Congr. Vet. Zootec.* 403–406.

78. Gubser, C., Goodbody, R., Ecker, A., Brady, G., O'Neill, L. A., Jacobs, N. and Smith, G. L. 2007. Camelpox virus encodes a schlafen-like protein that affects orthopoxvirus virulence. *J. Gen. Virol.* 88:1667–1676.

79. Gubser, C. and Smith, G. L. 2002. The sequence of camelpox virus shows it is most closely related to Variola virus, the cause of smallpox. *J. Gen. Virol.* 83:855–872.

80. Hafez, S. M., al-Sukayran, A., dela Cruz, D., Mazloum, K. S., al-Bokmy, A. M., al-Mukayel, A. and Amjad, A. M. 1992. Development of a live cell culture camelpox vaccine. *Vaccine* 10:533–539.

81. Haji, C. S. G. 1923. Rinderpest in camels. *Indian Vet. J.* 9:13–14.

82. Hameid, O. A. 1991. Rabies in Sudan: An epidemiological review. *Vet. Rec.* 128:61–62.

83. Haroun, M., Hajer, I., Mukhtar, M. and Ali, B. E. 2002. Detection of antibodies against peste des petits ruminants virus in sera of cattle, camels, sheep and goats in Sudan. *Vet. Res. Commun.* 26:537–541.

84. Hartung, J. 1980. Contagious ecthyma of sheep, cases in man, dog, alpaca and camel. *Tierarztl. Prax.* 8:435–438.

85. Hedger, R. S., Barnett, I. T. R. and Gray, D. F. 1980. Some virus diseases of domestic animals in the Sultanate of Oman. *Trop. Anim. Health Prod.* 12:107–114.

86. Ismail, T. M., Hassan, H. B., Youssef, N. M. A., Rakha, G. M., El-Halim, M. M. A., Fatehia, M. M. and Abd El-Halim, M. M. 1992. Studies on prevalence of rinderpest and peste-des-petits ruminants antibodies in camel sera in Egypt. *Vet. Med. J. Giza* 40:49–53.

87. Jezek, Z., Kriz, B. and Rothbauer, V. 1983. Camelpox and its risk to the human population. *J. Hyg. Epidemiol. Microbiol. Immunol.* 27:29–42.

88. Khalafalla, A. I. and El-Dirdiri, G. A. 2003. Laboratory and field investigations of a live attenuated and an inactivated camel pox vaccine. *J. Camel Pract. Res.* 10:191–200.

89. Khalafalla, A. I. and Mohamed, M. E. 1997. Epizootiology of camel contagious ecthyma in eastern Sudan. *Rev. Elev. Med. Veter. Pays Trop.* 5:99–103.

90. Khalafalla, A. I., Agab, H. and Abbas, B. 1994. An outbreak of contagious ecthyma in camels (*Camelus dromedaries*) in eastern Sudan. *Trop. Anim. Health Prod.* 26:253–254.

91. Khanna, N. D., Uppal, P. K., Sharma, N. and Tripathi, B. N. 1996. Occurrence of pox infections in camels. *Indian Vet. J.* 73:813–817.

92. Kinne, J., Cooper, J. E. and Wernery, U. 1998. Pathological studies on camelpox lesions of the respiratory system in the United Arab Emirates (UAE). *J. Comp. Pathol.* 118:257–266.

93. Kirnbauer, R., Chandrachud, L. M., O'Neil, B. W., Wagner, E. R., Grindlay, G. J., Armstrong, A., McGarvie, G. M., Schiller, J. T., Lowy, D. R. and Campo, M. S. 1996. Virus-like particles of bovine papillomavirus type 4 in prophylactic and therapeutic immunization. *Virology* 219:37–44.

94. Kriz, B. 1982. A study of camelpox in Somalia. *J. Comp. Pathol.* 92:1–8.

95. Kumar, A. and Jindal, N. 1997. Rabies in a camel—a case report. *Trop. Anim. Health Prod.* 29:34.

96. Lancaster, W. D. and Olson, C. 1982. Animal papillomaviruses. *Microbiol. Rev.* 46:191–207.

97. Lapa, S., Mikheev, M., Shchelkunov, S., Mikhailovich, V., Sobolev, A., Blinov, V., Babkin, I., Guskov, A., Sokunova, E., Zasedatelev, A., Sandakhchiev, L. and Mirzabekov, A. 2002. Species level identification of orthopoxviruses with an oligonucleotide microchip. *J. Clin. Microbiol.* 40:753–757.

98. Lewis-Jones, S. 2004. Zoonotic poxvirus infections in humans. *Curr. Opin. Infect. Dis.* 17:81–89.

99. Loparev, V. N., Massung, R. F., Esposito, J. J. and Meyer, H. 2001. Detection and differentiation of old world orthopoxviruses: Restriction fragment length polymorphism of the crmB gene region. *J. Clin. Microbiol.* 39:94–100.

100. Many, E., Schillinger, D., Reimann, M. and Mahnel, H. 1986. Electron-microscopical diagnosis of ecthyma contagious in camels (*Camelus dromedaries*). First report of the disease in Kenya. *Zentr. Vet. Med. J.* 33:73–77.

101. Mariner, J. C., Morrill, J. and Ksiazek, T. G. 1995. Antibodies to hemorrhagic fever viruses in domestic livestock in Niger: Rift Valley fever and Crimean-Congo hemorrhagic fever. *Am. J. Trop. Med. Hyg.* 53:217–221.

102. Mathew, T. M. and Mathew, T. 2006. *Advances in medical and veterinary virology immunology and epidemiology*. Vol. 6 *Influenza and its global public health significance*. USA: Thajema Publishers. 1–201.

103. Mattson, D. E. 1994. Viral diseases. *Vet. Clinic North Am. Food Anim. Pract.* 10:345–351.

104. Mayr, A. 2003. Smallpox vaccination and bioterrorism with pox viruses. *Comp. Immunol. Microbiol. Infect. Dis.* 26:423–430.

105. McFadden, G. 2005. Poxvirus tropism. *Nat. Rev. Microbiol.* 3:201–213.

106. McGrane, U. and Higgins, A. J. 1985. Infectious diseases of the camel viruses, bacteria and fungi. *Br. Vet. J.* 141:529–547.

107. Meyer, H., Ropp, S. L. and Esposito, J. J. 1997. Gene for A-type inclusion body protein is useful for a polymerase chain reaction assay to differentiate orthopoxviruses. *J. Virol. Methods* 64:217–221.

108. Moallin, A. S. M. and Zessin, K. H. 1988. Outbreak of camel contagious ecthyma in central Somalia. *Trop. Anim. Health Prod.* 20:185–186.

109. Mochabo, K. O., Kitala, P. M., Gathura, P. B., Ogara, W. O., Catley, A., Eregae, E. M. and Kaitho, T. D. 2005. Community perceptions of important camel diseases in Lapur Division of Turkana District, Kenya. *Trop. Anim. Health Prod.* 37:187–204.

110. Mochabo, M. O., Kitala, P. M., Gathura, P. B., Ogara, W. O., Eregae, E. M., Kaitho, T. D. and Catley, A. 2006. The socio-economic impact of important camel diseases as perceived by a pastoralist community in Kenya. *Onder. J. Vet. Res.* 73:269–274.

111. Mohin, L., Schwers, A., Chadli, M., Maenhoudt, M. and Pastoret, P. P. 1983. Susceptibility of the dromedary (*Camelus dromedarius*) to rotavirus infection. *Rev. Elev. Med. Vet. Pays Trop.* 36:251–252.

112. Morrill, J. C., Soliman, A. K., Imam, I. Z., Botros, B. A., Moussa, M. I. and Watts, D. M. 1990. Serological evidence of Crimean-Congo haemorrhagic fever viral infection among camels imported into Egypt. *J. Trop. Med. Hyg.* 93:201–204.

113. Moussa, A., Daoud, A. and Omar, N. 1987. Isolation of foot and mouth disease virus from camels with ulcerative disease syndromes. *J. Egypt. Vet. Med. Ass.* 47:219–229.

114. Munz, E. 1992. Pox and pox-like diseases in camels. Proc. 1st Int. Camel Conf. United Arab Emirates, 43–46.

115. Munz, E., Kropp, E. M. and Reimann, M. 1986a. Detection of antibodies to orthopoxvirus cameli in the sera of East African dromedaries with ELISA. *Zentr. Veterinar.* B 33:221–230.

116. Munz, E., Schillinger, D., Reimann, M. and Mahnel, H. 1986b. Electron microscopical diagnosis of Ecthyma contagiosum in camels (Camelus dromedarius). First report of the disease in Kenya. *Zentr. Veterinar.* B 33:73–77.

117. Munz, E., Moallin, A. S., Mahnel, H. and Reimann, M. 1990. Camel papillomatosis in Somalia. *Zentr. Veterinar.* B 37:191–196.

118. Murphy, F. A., Gibbs, E., Horzinek, M. and Studdert, M. 1999. In *Veterinary virology*, 3rd ed. Academic Press, San Diego, USA.

119. Nasser, M., Moussa, M. and Abdeir, M. 1980. Secretion and persistence of foot and mouth disease virus in feces of experimentally infected camels and ram. *J. Egypt. Vet. Med. Assoc.* 40:5–13.

120. Nguyen, B. V., Richard, D. and Gillet, J. P. 1989. Properties of an orthopoxvirus strain isolated from camels in Niger. *Rev. Elev. Med. Vet. Pays Trop.* 42:19–25.

121. Nguyen, B. V., Guerre, L. and Saint-Martin, G. 1996. Preliminary study of the safety and immunogenicity of the attenuated VD47/25 strain of camelpoxvirus. *Rev. Elev. Med. Vet. Pays Trop.* 49:189–194.

122. Nicholls, P. K. and Stanley, M. A. 2000. The immunology of animal papillomaviruses. *Vet. Immunol. Immunopathol.* 73:101–127.

123. Olaleye, O. D., Omilabu, S. A., Ilomechina, E. N. and Fagbami, A. H. 1990. A survey for haemagglutination-inhibiting antibody to West Nile virus in human and animal sera in Nigeria. *Comp. Immunol. Microbiol. Infect. Dis.* 13:35–39.

124. Olaleye, O. D., Tomori, O. and Schmitz, H. 1996. Rift Valley fever in Nigeria: Infections in domestic animals. *Rev. Sci. Tech.* 15:937–946.

125. Olaleye, O. D., Baba, S. S. and Omolabu 1989. Preliminary survey of antibodies against respiratory viruses among slaughter camels (*Camelus dromedarius*) in northeastern Nigeria. *Rev. Sci. Tech.* 8:779–783.

126. Olson, V. A., Laue, T., Laker, M. T., Babkin, I. V., Drosten, C., Shchelkunov, S. N., Niedrig, M., Damon, I. K. and Meyer, H. 2004. Real-time PCR system for detection of orthopoxviruses and simultaneous identification of smallpox virus. *J. Clin. Microbiol.* 42:1940–1946.

127. Otterbein, C. K., Meyer, H., Renner-Muller, I. C. and Munz, E. 1996. *In vivo* and *in vitro* characterization of two camelpoxvirus isolates with decreased virulence. *Rev. Elev. Med. Vet. Pays Trop.* 49:114–120.

128. Paling, R. W., Jessett, D. M. and Health, B. R. 1979. The occurrence of infectious diseases in mixed farming of domesticated, wild herbivores and domestic herbivores including camels in Kenya 1. Viral diseases serological survey with special reference to foot and mouth disease. *J. Wildl. Dis.* 15:351–358.

129. Panning, M., Asper, M., Kramme, S., Schmitz, H. and Drosten, C. 2004. Rapid detection and differentiation of human pathogenic orthopox viruses by a fluorescence resonance energy transfer real-time PCR assay. *Clin. Chem.* 50:702–708.

130. Paweska, J. T., Burt, F. J., Anthony, F., Smith, S. J., Grobbelaar, A. A., Croft, J. E., Ksiazek, T. G. and Swanepoel, R. 2003a. IgG-sandwich and IgM-capture enzyme-linked immunosorbent assay for the detection of antibody to Rift Valley fever virus in domestic ruminants. *J. Virol. Methods* 113:103–112.

131. Paweska, J. T., Smith, S. J., Wright, I. M., Williams, R., Cohen, A. S., Van Dijk, A. A., Grobbelaar, A. A., Croft, J. E., Swanepoel, R. and Gerdes, G. H. 2003b. Indirect enzyme-linked immunosorbent assay for the detection of antibody against Rift Valley fever virus in domestic and wild ruminant sera. *Onder. J. Vet. Res.* 70:49–64.

132. Paweska, J. T., Mortimer, E., Leman, P. A. and Swanepoel, R. 2005. An inhibition enzyme-linked immunosorbent assay for the detection of antibody to Rift Valley fever virus in humans, domestic and wild ruminants. *J. Virol. Methods* 127:10–18.

133. Pfahler, W. H., Reimann, M. and Munz, E. 1986. A biotin-avidin amplified enzyme immunoassay for detection and quantitation of orthopox virus camel antibodies in dromedaries. *Zentr. Veterinar.* B 33:477–484.

134. Pfeffer, M., Meyer, H., Wernery, U. and Kaaden, O. R. 1996. Comparison of camelpox viruses isolated in Dubai. *Vet. Microbiol.* 49:135–146.

135. Ramyar, H. and Hessami, M. 1972. Isolation, cultivation and characterization of camel poxvirus. *Zentr. Veterinar.* B 19:182–189.

136. Rebhun, W. C., Jenkins, R. C. and Riis, R. 1988. An epizootic of blindness and encephalitis associated with a herpes virus indistinguishable from equine herpes virus-l in a herd of alpacas and llama. *J. Am. Vet. Med. Assoc.* 192:953–956.

137. Regnery, R. L. 2007. Poxviruses and the passive quest for novel hosts. *Curr. Top. Microbiol. Immunol.* 315:345–361.

138. Renner-Muller, I. C., Meyer, H. and Munz, E. 1995. Characterization of camelpoxvirus isolates from Africa and Asia. *Vet. Microbiol.* 45:371–381.

139. Riabinin, V. A., Shundrin, L. A., Kostina, E. V., Laassri, M., Chizhikov, V. E., Maksakova, G. A., Baturina, O. A., Pozdniakova, L. D., Feshchenko, M. V., Shchelkunov, S. N., Chumakov, K. M. and Siniakov, A. N. 2006. An oligonucleotide microarray for detection and discrimination of orthopoxviruses based on oligonucleotide sequences of two viral genes. *Mol. Gen. Mikrobiol. Virusol.* 4:23–30.

140. Ropp, S. L., Jin, Q., Knight, J. C., Massung, R. F. and Esposito, J. J. 1995. PCR strategy for identification and differentiation of small pox and other orthopoxviruses. *J. Clin. Microbiol.* 33:2069–2076.

141. Rosadio, R., Rivera, H. and Manchego, A. 1993. Prevalence of neutralizing antibodies to bovine herpesvirus-I in Peruvian livestock. *Vet. Rec.* 132:611–612.

142. Rosliakov, A. A. 1972. Comparative ultrastructure of viruses of camel pox, pox-like disease of camels ("auzdyk") and contagious ecthyma of sheep. *Vopr. Virusol.* 17:26–30.

143. Saini, N., Ram Kumar., Kiradoo, B. D., Singh, N., Bhardwaj, A. and Sahani, M. S. 2006. Camel rearing practices—a survey study in arid western agro-ecosystem of Rajasthan. *J. Camel Pract. Res.* 13:179–184.

144. Salama, S. A., Abdallah, S. K., El-Bakry, M. and Hassanun, M. M. 1986. Serological studies on African horse sickness virus in camels. *Assiut. Vet. Med. J.* 16:379–390.

145. Sall, A. A. and Macondo, E. 2002. Use of reverse transcriptase PCR in early diagnosis of Rift Valley fever. *Clin. Diag. Lab. Immunol.* 9:713–715.

146. Saluzz, J. F., Digoutte, J. P. and Chartier, C. 1987. Focus of Rift Valley fever virus transmission in Southern Mauritania. *Lancet* 8531:504.

147. Sanchez-Seco, M. P., Hernandez, L., Eiros, J. M., Negredo, A., Fedele, G. and Tenorio, A. 2006. Detection and identification of orthopoxviruses using a generic nested PCR followed by sequencing. *Brit. J. Biomed. Sci.* 63:79–85.

148. Scaramozzino, N., Ferrier-Rembert, A., Favier, A. L., Rothlisberger, C., Richard, S., Crance, J. M., Meyer, H. and Garin, D. 2007. Real-time PCR to identify variola virus or other human pathogenic orthopox viruses. *Clin. Chem.* 53:606–613.

149. Scholtissek, C. 1995. Potential hazards associated with influenza virus vaccines. *Dev. Biol. Stand.* 84:55–58.

150. Scott, G. R. and Macdonald, J. 1962. Kenya camels and Rinderpest. *Bull. Epiozoot. Dis. Africa* 10:490.

151. Sena, D. S., Gorakh-Mal., Sharma, N. and Sahani, M. S. 2006. Calf mortality in camels: A report. *J. Camel Pract. Res.* 13:171–172.

152. Shchelkunov, S. N., Gavrilova, E. V. and Babkin, I. V. 2005. Multiplex PCR detection and species differentiation of orthopoxviruses pathogenic to humans. *Mol. Cell Probes* 19:1–8.

153. Simpson, V. R. 1979. Bluetongue antibody in Botswana's domestic and game animals. *Trop. Anim. Health Prod.* 11:43–49.

154. Sliva, K. and Schnierle, B. 2007. From actually toxic to highly specific-novel drugs against poxviruses. *Virol. J.* 4:8.

155. Smee, D. F., Sidwell, R. W., Kefauver, D., Bray, M. and Huggins J. W. 2002. Characterization of wild-type and cidofovir-resistant strains of camelpox, cowpox, monkeypox, and vaccinia viruses. *Antimicrob. Agents Chemother.* 46:1329–1335.

156. Smith, V. M. 1970a. Experimental rinderpest in camels. A preliminary report. *Bull. Epiozoot. Dis. Africa* 15:19–23.

157. Smith, V. M. 1970b. Rinderpest. *J. Agr. West. Aust.* 11:147–148.

158. Smith, K. T. and Campo, M. S. 1985. Papillomaviruses and their involvement in oncogenesis. *Biomed. Pharmacother.* 39:405–414.

159. Smith, S. A. and Kotwal, G. J. 2002. Immune response to poxvirus infections in various animals. *Crit. Rev. Microbiol.* 28:149–185.

160. Sundberg, J. P., Van Ranst, M., Montali, R., Homer, B. L., Miller, W. H., Rowland, P. H., Scott, D. W., England, J. J., Dunstan, R. W., Mikaelian, I. and Jenson, A. B. 2000. Feline papillomas and papillomaviruses. *Vet. Pathol.* 37:1–10.

161. Tantawi, H. H., El-Dahaby, H. and Fahmy, L. S. 1978. Comparative studies on poxvirus strains isolated from camels. *Acta Virol.* 22:451–457.

162. Tantawi, H. H., Saban, M. S., Reda, I. M. and Dahaby, H. E. 1974. Camel poxvirus in Egypt. I-isolation and characterization. *Bull. Epizoot. Dis. Africa* 22:315–319.

163. Tantawi, H. H., Shony, M. O. and Al-Tikriti, S. K. 1981. Antibodies to Crimean-Congo haemorrhagic fever virus in domestic animals in Iraq: A sero-epidemiological survey. *Int. J. Zoonoses.* 8:115–120.

164. Taylor, W. P. 1968. The susceptibility of the one humped camel (*Camelus dromedarus*) to infection with rinderpest virus. *Bull. Epizoot. Dis. Africa* 16:405–410.

165. Tefera, M. and Gebreah, F. 2001. A study on the productivity and diseases of camels in eastern Ethiopia. *Trop. Anim. Health. Prod.* 33:265–274.

166. Tefera, M. 2004. Observations on the clinical examination of the camel (Camelus dromedarius) in the field. *Trop. Anim. Health prod.* 36:435–449.

167. Thedford, T. R. and Johnson, L. W. 1989. Infectious diseases of New-World camelids (NWC). *Vet. Clin. North Am. Food Anim. Pract.* 5:145–157.

168. Vasilev, A. V., Shchelkanov, M., Dzharkenov, A. F., Aristova, V. A., Galkina, I. V., L'vov, D. N., Morozova, T. N., Kovtunov, A. I., Grenkova, E. P., Zhernovoi, A. V., Shatilova, V. P., Slavskiǐ, A. A., Petrenko, M. S., Chirkizov, P. F., Dybal, V. D., Leont'ev, E. A., Gabbasov, F. B., Odolevskiǐ, E. A., Ibragimov, R. M., Idrisova, R. Z., Sokolova, N. N., Artiukh, N. P., Andreeva, N. I., Bondarev, A. D., Deriabin, P. G., Gromashevskiǐ, V. L., Nepoklonov, E. A., Aliper, T. I. and L'vov, D. K. 2005. West Nile virus infection of agricultural animals in the Astrakhan region, as evidenced by the 2001–2004 serological surveys. *Vopr. Virusol.* 50:36–41.

169. Wernery, U. 1995. Viral infections in camels—a review. *J. Camel Pract. Res.* 2:1–12.

170. Wernery, U. and Wernery, R. 1990. Seroepidemiologic studies of the detection of antibodies to Brucella, Chlamydia, Leptospira, BVD/MD virus, IBR/IPV virus and enzootic bovine leukosis virus (EBL) in dromedary mares (Camelus dromedarius)]. *Dtsch. Tierar. Wochen.* 97:134–135.

171. Wernery, U. and Kaaden, O. 1995. In *Infectious diseases of camelids*. 1st ed. Blackwell Wissenschafts-Verlag. Berlin.

172. Wernery, U. and Zachariah, R. 1999. Experimental camel pox infection in vaccinated and unvaccinated dromedaries. *Zentr. Veterinar.* B 46:131–135.

173. Wernery, U. and Kaaden, O. R. 2004. Foot-and-mouth disease in camelids: A review. *Vet. J.* 168:134–142.

174. Wernery, U., Nagy, P., Amaral-Doel, C. M., Zhang, Z. and Alexandersen, S. 2006. Lack of susceptibility of the dromedary camel (Camelus dromedarius) to foot-and-mouth disease virus serotype O. *Vet. Rec.* 158:201–203.

175. Wise-Draper, T. M. and Wells, S. I. 2008. Papillomavirus E6 and E7 proteins and their cellular targets. *Front. Biosci.* 13:1003–1017.

176. Wunschmann, A., Frank, R., Pomeroy, K. and Kapil, S. 2002. Enteric coronavirus infection in a juvenile dromedary (*Camelus dromedarius*). *J. Vet. Diagn. Invest.* 14:441–444.

7. OTHER VIRAL DISEASES OF CAMEL

177. Yamnikova, S. S., Mandler, J., Bekh-Ochir, Z. H., Dachtzeren, P., Ludwig, S., Lvov, D. K. and Scholtissek C. 1993. A reassortant H1N1 influenza A virus caused fatal epizootics among camels in Mongolia. *Virology* 197:558–563.
178. Zaghawa, A. 1998. Prevalence of antibodies to bovine viral diarrhoea virus and/or border disease virus in domestic ruminants. *Zentr. Veterinar.* B 45:345–351.

INDEX

A

acanthosis, 178, 728
  papillary. *See* papillomatosis, equine: aural
    plaques, 178
acidosis, 248, 360, 407, 409, 447
Actnobacillus equuli, 66
acyclovir, 84, 87
ADCC (antibody-dependent cell-mediated
    cytotoxicity), 382
Adenoviridae, 63, 72
adenovirus, equine
  clinical signs, 68–69
  diagnosis, 69–70
  epidemiology, 65–67
  etiology, 63–65
  pathogenesis and pathology, 67–68
  prevention and control, 70
Aedes, 264
  Aedes aegypti, 17, 374
  Aedes albopictus, 374
  Aedes vexans, 93, 523
Aeromonas hydrophila, 356
African green monkey, 268, 333, 336, 362
African horse sickness
  equine, 12, 31, 35
    clinical findings, 20–21
    diagnosis, 23–26
    epidemiology, 15–16
    microscopic lesions, 22–23
    necropsy findings, 21–22
    pathogenesis, 19
    prevention and control, 26–30
    public health considerations, 30
    therapy, 26
    transmission and spread, 16–18
  virus, 11–20, 23–26, 29–38
AGID (agar gel immunodiffusion) test, 24,
    159–62, 166, 170, 249, 424, 504, 736,
    740, 744
AGPT (agar gel precipitation test), 70, 120,
    154, 159, 538, 541, 561–62, 670, 718
Agrimi, P., 356, 370
AHSV (African horse sickness virus). *See*
    African horse sickness, virus
AHV-2 (asinine herpesvirus 2), 119–20, 126
AIDS virus, 25, 152, 166, 302

AINV (Aino virus), 344
AIV (avian influenza virus), 133, 651, 655
Alfuy virus, 323, 373
Aljofan, M., 301, 304
Alloherpesviridae, 111
Alphaherpesvirinae, 77, 85, 111, 633
Alphavirus, 90–91, 107, 279, 287, 289, 291
alphaviruses, 90–92, 95–96, 102, 104–6,
    108–9, 118, 124, 280, 282, 289–90
ALV (attenuated live vaccine), 29, 42, 738
amantadine, 54–55, 60, 146, 648
amantadine sulphate, 52
amphoterin, 46, 57
Andrews, C., 310
Anopheles, Anopheles stephensi, 17
Anthomyiidae, 264
anthrax, 12, 26, 301
antibody-dependent cell-mediated
    cytotoxicity, 382
Aphthovirus, 224–25, 235, 239
Arboviruses, 322
Archambault, D., 248
arctigenin, 334, 343
arginine, 207, 324
Arteriviridae, 241, 255, 627–28
Arterivirus, 241
arteriviruses, 242, 255, 631
ASF (African swine fever). *See* swine fever,
    African
ASFV (African swine fever virus). *See* swine
    fever, African: virus
asinine herpesvirus 2, 119–20, 126
ASP (acid-stable picornaviruses), 225–26
ataxia, 44, 53, 98, 100, 156, 158, 169, 207–8,
    246, 292, 295, 297, 329, 348, 376, 378
atelectasis, 68, 644
Aujeszky's disease. *See* pseudorabies
Australian bat virus, 204
avidin-biotin-peroxidase techniques, 250
avipox virus, 310
Ayerst, 216

B

babesiosis, 26, 415, 423, 482
Bacillus, 66
  Bacillus thuringensis, 28, 35

Webb, P. A., 269
WEE (Western equine encephalomylelitis)
    virus, 90, 92, 99
WEEV. *See* WEE (Western equine
    encephalomylelitis), virus
Wekesa, S. N., 280
Wen, J. S., 280
Wesselsborn disease, 742
Westcott, D., 251
Wilson, A., 18
Witte, J., 39, 196
WNV (West Nile virus), 258, 309, 323, 333,
    336, 340, 342, 344, 372, 374, 378, 381,
    384–92
    clinical signs, 377–78
    diagnosis, 379–81
    epidemiology, 376–77
    etiology, 373–74
    pathogenesis and pathology, 378–79
    prevention and control, 382, 384
    role of birds and mosquitoes in
        transmission, 374–75
    therapy, 382
    tissue culture susceptibility, 374
Wohlsein, P., 19
WTBE (Western European tickborne
    encephalitis), 346

X

xanthochromia, 121
Xiao, C., 300
Xu, K., 303

Y

Yaounde virus, 373
Yatapox, 313
YF (yellow fever), 383, 745

Z

Zhou, E. M., 269
Zientara, S., 381
Zwick, W., 39, 61
Zwick vaccine, 52

www.ingramcontent.com/pod-product-compliance
Lightning Source LLC
Chambersburg PA
CBHW031808170526
45157CB00001B/2